Robbins and Cotran Review of Pathology

ROBBINS AND COTRAN REVIEW OF PATHOLOGY

Second Edition

EDWARD C. KLATT, MD

Professor and Academic Administrator
Department of Biomedical Sciences
Florida State University College of Medicine
Tallahassee, Florida

VINAY KUMAR, MBBS, MD, FRCPath

Alice Hogge and Arthur A. Baer Professor
Chairman, Department of Pathology
The University of Chicago
Pritzker School of Medicine
Chicago, Illinois

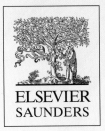

ELSEVIER
SAUNDERS

ELSEVIER
SAUNDERS

An Imprint of Elsevier

The Curtis Center
170 S Independence Mall W 300E
Philadelphia, Pennsylvania 19106

NOTICE

Medicine is an ever-changing field. Standard safety precautions must be followed, but as new research and clinical experience broaden our knowledge, changes in treatment and drug therapy may become necessary or appropriate. Readers are advised to check the most current product information provided by the manufacturer of each drug to be administered to verify the recommended dose, the method and duration of administration, and contraindications. It is the responsibility of the treating physician, relying on experience and knowledge of the patient, to determine dosages and the best treatment for each individual patient. Neither the publisher nor the authors assume any liability for any injury and/or damage to persons or property arising from this publication.

Previous edition copyrighted 2000

Publishing Director: William Schmitt
Managing Editor: Rebecca Gruliow
Developmental Editor: Susan Kelly
Design Manager: Ellen Zanolle

Printed in China

Last digit is the print number: 9 8 7 6 5 4 3 2 1

To our students, for constant
challenge and stimulation

Preface

This book is designed to provide a comprehensive review of pathology through multiple-choice questions and explanations of the answers. The source materials are the seventh editions of Kumar, Abbas, Fausto *Robbins and Cotran Pathologic Basis of Disease* (PBD7) and Kumar, Cotran, Robbins *Robbins Basic Pathology* (BP7). It is intended to be a useful resource for students at a variety of levels in the health sciences.

In keeping with the style used by the USMLE, we have included single best answer questions, most with a clinical vignette, followed by a series of homogenous choices. This approach emphasizes an understanding of pathophysiologic mechanisms and manifestations of disease in a clinical context. We have incorporated relevant laboratory, radiologic, and physical diagnostic findings in the questions to emphasize clinicopathologic correlations. For each question, the correct answer is provided with a brief explanation of why this answer is "correct" and why the other choices are "incorrect." Each answer is referenced by page numbers to *Robbins and Cotran Pathologic Basis of Disease* and to *Robbins Basic Pathology* (both the current, 7th, and the previous, 6th, editions) to facilitate and encourage a more complete reading of the topic. Pathology is a visually oriented discipline; hence, we have used full-color images in many of the questions. The illustrations are taken mainly from the *Robbins* textbooks, so students can reinforce their study of the illustrations in the texts with questions that utilize the same images.

Many questions in this second edition are new, some reflecting new topics and others new understanding of disease processes. Some of the older questions have been rewritten to improve clarity and offer increased numbers of choices. The questions are intentionally fairly difficult, with the purpose of "pushing the envelope" of student understanding of pathology. We are pushing it further by addition of a new, final "super review" chapter, which draws on information from the entire book. Many of the questions require a "two-step" process: first, interpreting the information presented to arrive at a diagnosis, and then solving a problem based on that diagnosis. We must hasten to add that no review book is a substitute for textbooks and other course materials provided by individual instructors. This book should be used after a thorough study of *Robbins and Cotran Pathologic Basis of Disease* and/or *Robbins Basic Pathology* and course materials. Finally, we hope that students and instructors will find this review book to be a useful adjunct to the learning of pathology.

Edward C. Klatt, MD

Vinay Kumar, MD

To Our Students

Although medical knowledge has increased exponentially over the past 100 years, the desire to learn and apply this knowledge to the service of others has not changed. The study and practice of healing arts require persistence more than brilliance. By continuing as a lifelong student, it is possible to become a better health practitioner with the passage of time. Use this book to find where you are on the path to excellence and be inspired to continue down that path.

Common mistakes made by students in answering questions include (1) inappropriate use of a single finding as an exclusionary criterion, and (2) ignoring important diagnostic information. Remember that medicine is mostly analogue, not digital. The information you obtain occurs along a continuum of probability. Four key elements are involved in arriving at a correct answer: (1) read the question thoroughly, (2) define the terms (use your vocabulary), (3) rank order possible answers from common to uncommon, and (4) recognize key diagnostic information that differentiates the answers.

There are no magic formulas for academic achievement. The most important thing you can do is to spend some time each day in a learning process. The brain is subject to the second law of thermodynamics, which states that entropy in a system always increases. Learning requires modification of synaptic interfaces at the dendritic level, and for learning to occur, there are a finite number of synaptic modifications that can be established per unit time, above which entropy increases and total comprehension is reduced. Increasing the rate or length of information delivery diminishes the efficiency of learning. Lack of break periods and "all nighters" presage onset of entropy, particularly when least desirable—during an examination. There is also decay of learning over time, with inevitable random loss of data elements. The key branch points in learning where review with reinforcement can reduce data loss occur at 20 to 40 minutes (transfer to intermediate memory) and at 24 to 48 hours (transfer to long-term memory) following initial learning.

We hope, therefore, that this review will be useful not only in preparing for examinations but also for courses you take and for your career. It is our sincere hope that this review book will make you a better health practitioner in your chosen career.

Edward C. Klatt, MD

Vinay Kumar, MD

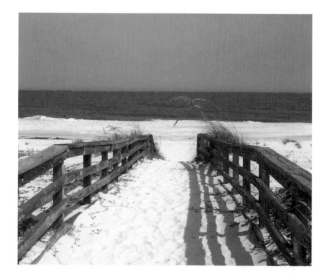

Acknowledgments

We are very grateful to Susan Kelly, our Developmental Editor, and William Schmitt, Publishing Director, Medical Textbooks, Elsevier Science, for their support of this project. We are grateful to our families and colleagues for graciously accepting this additional demand on our time.

Edward C. Klatt, MD

Vinay Kumar, MD

Acknowledgments

Contents

UNIT III ◉ Final Examination

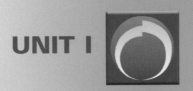

General Pathology

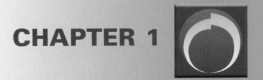

Cellular Pathology

1 A 17-year-old boy infected with hepatitis A experiences mild nausea for about 1 week and develops very mild scleral icterus. On physical examination, he has minimal right upper quadrant tenderness. Laboratory findings include a serum AST of 68 U/L, ALT 75 U/L, and total bilirubin 5.1 mg/dL. The increase in this patient's serum enzyme levels most likely results from which of the following changes in the hepatocytes?

- ❏ (A) Dispersion of ribosomes
- ❏ (B) Autophagy by lysosomes
- ❏ (C) Swelling of the mitochondria
- ❏ (D) Clumping of nuclear chromatin
- ❏ (E) Defects in the cell membrane

2 A 16-year-old boy sustained blunt trauma to the abdomen when the vehicle he was driving struck a bridge abutment at high speed. Peritoneal lavage shows a hemoperitoneum, and at laparotomy, a small portion of the left lobe of the liver is removed because of the injury. Several weeks later, a CT scan of the abdomen shows that the liver has nearly regained its size prior to the injury. Which of the following processes best explains this CT scan finding?

- ❏ (A) Apoptosis
- ❏ (B) Dysplasia
- ❏ (C) Fatty change
- ❏ (D) Hydropic change
- ❏ (E) Hyperplasia
- ❏ (F) Hypertrophy
- ❏ (G) Metaplasia

3 On a routine visit to the physician, an otherwise healthy 51-year-old man has a blood pressure of 150/95 mm Hg. If the patient's hypertension remains untreated for years, which of the following cellular alterations will most likely be seen in the myocardium?

- ❏ (A) Atrophy
- ❏ (B) Hyperplasia
- ❏ (C) Metaplasia
- ❏ (D) Hemosiderosis
- ❏ (E) Hypertrophy

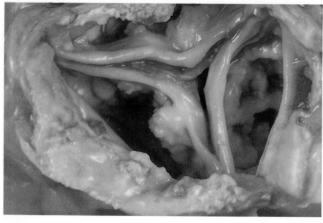

4 A 72-year-old man died suddenly and unexpectedly from congestive heart failure. At autopsy, the heart weighed 580 g and showed marked left ventricular hypertrophy and minimal coronary arterial atherosclerosis. A serum chemistry panel ordered prior to death showed no abnormalities. Which of the following pathologic processes best accounts for the appearance of the aortic valve seen in the figure?

❏ (A) Amyloidosis
❏ (B) Dystrophic calcification
❏ (C) Lipofuscin deposition
❏ (D) Hemosiderosis
❏ (E) Fatty change

5 A 69-year-old woman has had transient ischemic attacks for the past 3 months. On physical examination, she has an audible bruit on auscultation of the neck. A right carotid endarterectomy is performed. The curetted atheromatous plaque has a grossly yellow-tan, firm appearance. Microscopically, which of the following materials can be found in abundance in the form of crystals that produce long, cleft-like spaces?

❏ (A) Glycogen
❏ (B) Lipofuscin
❏ (C) Hemosiderin
❏ (D) Immunoglobulin
❏ (E) Cholesterol

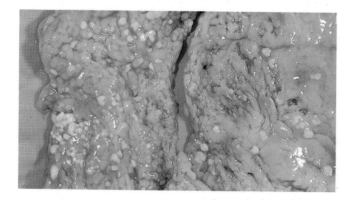

6 A 38-year-old woman experienced severe abdominal pain with hypotension and shock that led to her death within 36 hours after the onset of the pain. From the gross appearance of the mesentery, seen in the figure, which of the following events has most likely occurred?

❏ (A) Hepatitis B virus infection
❏ (B) Small intestinal infarction
❏ (C) Tuberculous lymphadenitis
❏ (D) Gangrenous cholecystitis
❏ (E) Acute pancreatitis

7 In an experiment, cells are subjected to radiant energy in the form of x-rays. This results in cell injury caused by hydrolysis of water. Which of the following cellular enzymes protects the cells from this type of injury?

❏ (A) Phospholipase
❏ (B) Glutathione peroxidase
❏ (C) Endonuclease
❏ (D) Lactate dehydrogenase
❏ (E) Protease

8 A 47-year-old woman has had worsening dyspnea for the past 5 years. A chest CT scan shows panlobular emphysema. Laboratory studies show the PiZZ genotype of α_1-antitrypsin deficiency. A liver biopsy specimen examined microscopically shows abundant PAS-positive globules within periportal hepatocytes. Which of the following molecular mechanisms is most likely responsible for this finding in the hepatocytes?

❏ (A) Excessive hepatic synthesis of α_1-antitrypsin
❏ (B) Retention in the endoplasmic reticulum because of poorly folded α_1-antitrypsin
❏ (C) Decreased catabolism of α_1-antitrypsin in lysosomes
❏ (D) Inability to metabolize α_1-antitrypsin
❏ (E) Impaired dissociation of α_1-antitrypsin from chaperones

9 A 68-year-old woman suddenly lost consciousness and, on awakening 1 hour later, she could not speak or move her right arm and leg. Two months later, a head CT scan showed a large cystic area in the left parietal lobe. Which of the following pathologic processes has most likely occurred in the brain?

❏ (A) Fat necrosis
❏ (B) Coagulative necrosis
❏ (C) Apoptosis
❏ (D) Liquefactive necrosis
❏ (E) Karyolysis

10 A 30-year-old man sustains a left femoral fracture in a skiing accident, and his leg is placed in a plaster cast. After the leg has been immobilized for several weeks, the diameter of the left calf has decreased. This change is most likely to result from which of the following alterations in the calf muscles?

❏ (A) Aplasia
❏ (B) Hypoplasia
❏ (C) Atrophy
❏ (D) Dystrophy
❏ (E) Hyalinosis

11 An experiment analyzes cells for enzyme activity associated with sustained cellular proliferation. Which of the following cells is most likely to have the highest telomerase activity?

❏ (A) Endothelial cells
❏ (B) Germ cells
❏ (C) Neurons
❏ (D) Neutrophils
❏ (E) Erythrocytes

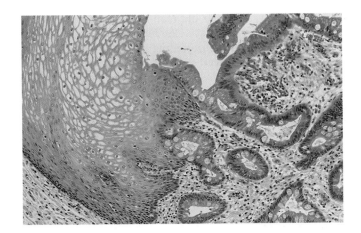

12 A 32-year-old man experiences "heartburn" and gastric reflux after eating a large meal. After many months of symptoms, he undergoes upper gastrointestinal endoscopy, and a biopsy specimen of the esophageal epithelium is obtained. Which of the following pathologic changes, seen in the figure, has most likely occurred?

☐ (A) Squamous metaplasia
☐ (B) Mucosal hypertrophy
☐ (C) Columnar epithelial metaplasia
☐ (D) Atrophy of lamina propria
☐ (E) Goblet cell hyperplasia

13 On day 28 of her menstrual cycle, a 23-year-old woman experiences onset of menstrual bleeding that lasts for 6 days. She has had regular cycles for many years. Which of the following processes is most likely occurring in the endometrium just before the onset of bleeding?

☐ (A) Apoptosis
☐ (B) Caseous necrosis
☐ (C) Heterophagocytosis
☐ (D) Atrophy
☐ (E) Liquefactive necrosis

14 In a clinical trial, a chemotherapeutic agent is given to patients with breast cancer metastases. Samples of the cancer cells are obtained and assessed for the presence of death of tumor cells by apoptosis. Mutational inactivation of which of the following products is most likely to render tumor cells resistant to the effects of such an agent?

☐ (A) BCL-2
☐ (B) p53
☐ (C) NF-κB
☐ (D) Cytochrome P-450
☐ (E) Granzyme B

15 After the birth of her first child, a 19-year-old woman breast-fed the infant for about 1 year. Which of the following processes that occurred in the breast during pregnancy allowed her to breast-feed the infant?

☐ (A) Stromal hypertrophy
☐ (B) Lobular hyperplasia
☐ (C) Epithelial dysplasia
☐ (D) Intracellular accumulation of fat
☐ (E) Ductal epithelial metaplasia

16 A 22-year-old woman has a congenital anemia that has required multiple transfusions of RBCs for many years. On physical examination, she now has no significant findings; however, liver function tests show reduced serum albumin. Which of the following findings would most likely appear in a liver biopsy specimen?

☐ (A) Steatosis in hepatocytes
☐ (B) Bilirubin in canaliculi
☐ (C) Glycogen in hepatocytes
☐ (D) Amyloid in portal triads
☐ (E) Hemosiderin in hepatocytes

17 A 50-year-old man experienced an episode of chest pain 6 hours before his death. A histologic section of left ventricular myocardium taken at autopsy showed a deeply eosinophilic-staining area with loss of nuclei and cross-striations in myocardial fibers. There was no hemorrhage or inflammation. Which of the following conditions most likely produced these myocardial changes?

☐ (A) Viral infection
☐ (B) Coronary artery thrombosis
☐ (C) Blunt chest trauma
☐ (D) Antibodies directed against myocardium
☐ (E) Protein-deficient diet

18 A 69-year-old man has had difficulty with urination, including hesitancy and frequency, for the past 5 years. A digital rectal examination reveals that the prostate gland is palpably enlarged to about twice normal size. A transurethral resection of the prostate is performed, and the microscopic appearance of the prostate "chips" obtained is that of nodules of glands with intervening stroma. Which of the following pathologic processes has most likely occurred in the prostate?

☐ (A) Apoptosis
☐ (B) Dysplasia
☐ (C) Fatty change
☐ (D) Hyperplasia
☐ (E) Hypertrophy
☐ (F) Metaplasia

19 A 54-year-old man experienced onset of severe substernal chest pain over a period of 3 hours. An ECG showed changes consistent with an acute myocardial infarction. After thrombolytic therapy with tissue plasminogen activator (t-PA), his serum creatine kinase (CK) level increased. Which of the following events most likely occurred following t-PA therapy?

☐ (A) Reperfusion injury
☐ (B) Cellular regeneration
☐ (C) Chemical injury
☐ (D) Increased synthesis of CK
☐ (E) Myofiber atrophy

20 A 33-year-old woman has had increasing lethargy and decreased urine output for the past week. Laboratory studies show serum creatinine level of 4.3 mg/dL and urea nitrogen level of 40 mg/dL. A renal biopsy is performed, and the specimen is examined using electron microscopy. Which of the following morphologic changes most likely suggests a diagnosis of acute tubular necrosis?

☐ (A) Mitochondrial swelling
☐ (B) Plasma membrane blebs
☐ (C) Chromatin clumping
☐ (D) Nuclear fragmentation
☐ (E) Ribosomal disaggregation

21 A 40-year-old man had undifferentiated carcinoma of the lung. Despite chemotherapy, the man died of widespread metastases. At autopsy, tumors were found in many organs. Histologic examination showed many foci in which individual tumor cells appeared shrunken and deeply eosinophilic. Their nuclei exhibited condensed aggregates of chromatin under the nuclear membrane. The process affecting these shrunken tumor cells was most likely triggered by the release of which of the following substances into the cytosol?

- ❏ (A) Lipofuscin
- ❏ (B) Cytochrome *c*
- ❏ (C) Catalase
- ❏ (D) Phospholipase
- ❏ (E) *BCL-2*

22 A 70-year-old man died suddenly and unexpectedly. At autopsy, multiple tissue sites were sampled for microscopic analysis. Examination of the tissues showed noncrystalline amorphous deposits of calcium salts in gastric mucosa, renal interstitium, and alveolar walls of lungs. Which of the following conditions is most likely to explain these findings?

- ❏ (A) Chronic hepatitis
- ❏ (B) Chronic glomerulonephritis
- ❏ (C) Disseminated tuberculosis
- ❏ (D) Generalized atherosclerosis
- ❏ (E) Normal aging process
- ❏ (F) Pulmonary emphysema

23 A 63-year-old man has a 2-year history of worsening congestive heart failure. An echocardiogram shows mitral stenosis with left atrial dilation. A thrombus is present in the left atrium. One month later, he experiences left flank pain and notes hematuria. Laboratory testing shows elevated serum AST. Which of the following patterns of tissue injury is most likely to be present?

- ❏ (A) Liquefactive necrosis
- ❏ (B) Caseous necrosis
- ❏ (C) Coagulative necrosis
- ❏ (D) Fat necrosis
- ❏ (E) Gangrenous necrosis

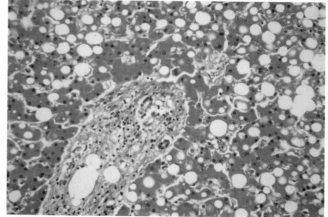

Courtesy of Dr. James Crawford, Department of Pathology, Brigham and Women's Hospital, Boston, MA.

24 At autopsy, a 40-year-old man has an enlarged (2200 g) liver with a yellow cut surface. The microscopic appearance of this liver is shown in the preceding figure. Before death, the man's total serum cholesterol and triglyceride levels were normal, but he had a decreased serum albumin concentration and increased prothrombin time. Which of the following activities most likely led to these findings?

- ❏ (A) Injecting heroin
- ❏ (B) Playing basketball
- ❏ (C) Drinking beer
- ❏ (D) Smoking cigarettes
- ❏ (E) Ingesting aspirin

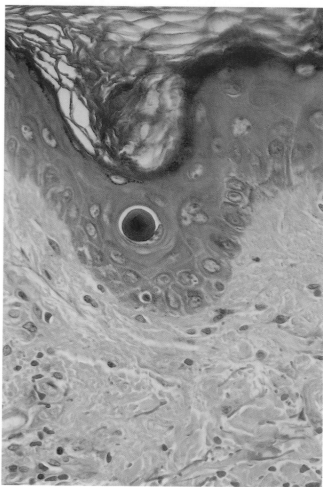

Courtesy of Dr. Scott Granter, Department of Pathology, Brigham and Women's Hospital, Boston, MA.

25 A 22-year-old woman with leukemia undergoes bone marrow transplantation and receives partially mismatched donor marrow. One month later, she has a scaling skin rash. Examination of a skin biopsy specimen reveals the cellular change shown in the figure. This change most likely results from which of the following biochemical reactions?

- ❏ (A) Activation of caspases
- ❏ (B) Reduction of ATP synthesis
- ❏ (C) Increase in glycolysis
- ❏ (D) Activation of lipases
- ❏ (E) Lipid peroxidation

26 At autopsy, the heart of a 63-year-old man weighs only 250 g and has small right and left ventricles. The myocardium is firm, with a dark chocolate-brown color throughout. The coronary arteries show minimal atherosclerotic changes. An excessive amount of which of the following substances will most likely be found in the myocardial fibers of this heart?

- ❏ (A) Melanin
- ❏ (B) Hemosiderin
- ❏ (C) Glycogen
- ❏ (D) Lipofuscin
- ❏ (E) Bilirubin

27 A 69-year-old woman has had a chronic cough for the past year. A chest radiograph shows a 6-cm mass in the left lung, and a needle biopsy specimen of the mass shows carcinoma. A pneumonectomy is performed, and examination of the hilar lymph nodes reveals a uniform, dark-black cut surface. Which of the following factors is most likely to account for the appearance of the lymph nodes?

- ❏ (A) Smoking
- ❏ (B) Bleeding disorder
- ❏ (C) Liver failure
- ❏ (D) Aging
- ❏ (E) Metastases

28 A 38-year-old man has had headaches and nausea for the past 2 months. Laboratory findings show hypercalcemia and hypophosphatemia and normal serum albumin. Urine microscopic analysis shows deposition of calcium salts in the renal tubular epithelium. Which of the following processes has most likely produced this change in the kidney?

- ❏ (A) Dystrophic calcification
- ❏ (B) Renal tubular atrophy
- ❏ (C) Autophagocytosis
- ❏ (D) Metastatic calcification
- ❏ (E) Cellular aging

29 An experiment introduces a "knockout" gene mutation into a cell line. The frequency of shrunken cells with chromatin clumping and cytoplasmic blebbing is increased, compared with a cell line without the mutation. Overall survival of the mutant cell line is reduced. Which of the following genes is most likely to be affected by this mutation?

- ❏ (A) *BAX*
- ❏ (B) *BCL-2*
- ❏ (C) *C-MYC*
- ❏ (D) *FAS*
- ❏ (E) *p53*

30 A 53-year-old man has had marked chest pain for the past 3 hours. Laboratory findings include elevated serum creatine kinase-MB (CK-MB). He receives thrombolytic therapy with tissue plasminogen activator. After the therapy, the CK-MB further increases. Which of the following is the most likely biochemical basis for this observed rise in CK-MB?

- ❏ (A) Reduced protein synthesis
- ❏ (B) Increased generation of oxygen-derived free radicals
- ❏ (C) Increased activity of catalase
- ❏ (D) Reduced oxidative phosphorylation
- ❏ (E) Release of calcium from endoplasmic reticulum

31 A chest radiograph of an asymptomatic 37-year-old man showed a 3-cm nodule in the middle lobe of the right lung. The nodule was excised with a pulmonary wedge resection, and sectioning showed the nodule to be sharply circumscribed with a soft, white center. Culture of tissue from the nodule grew *Mycobacterium tuberculosis.* Which of the following pathologic processes has most likely occurred in this nodule?

- ❏ (A) Apoptosis
- ❏ (B) Caseous necrosis
- ❏ (C) Coagulative necrosis
- ❏ (D) Fat necrosis
- ❏ (E) Fatty change
- ❏ (F) Gangrenous necrosis
- ❏ (G) Liquefactive necrosis

32 The nonpregnant uterus of a 20-year-old woman measures $7 \times 4 \times 3$ cm. The woman becomes pregnant and just before delivery of a term infant, the uterus measures $34 \times 18 \times 12$ cm. Which of the following cellular processes has contributed most to the increase in uterine size?

- ❏ (A) Endometrial glandular hyperplasia
- ❏ (B) Myometrial fibroblast proliferation
- ❏ (C) Endometrial stromal hypertrophy
- ❏ (D) Myometrial smooth muscle hypertrophy
- ❏ (E) Vascular endothelial hyperplasia

33 A 40-year-old woman has had chronic congestive heart failure for the past 3 years. In the past 2 months, she developed a cough productive of rust-colored sputum. A sputum cytology specimen shows numerous hemosiderin-laden macrophages. Which of the following subcellular structures in macrophages is most important for the accumulation of this pigment?

- ❏ (A) Lysosome
- ❏ (B) Endoplasmic reticulum
- ❏ (C) Ribosome
- ❏ (D) Golgi apparatus
- ❏ (E) Chromosome

34 In an experiment, a large amount of a drug is administered to subjects and is converted by cytochrome P-450 to a toxic metabolite. The accumulation of this metabolite leads to increased lipid peroxidation within cells, causing damage to cell membranes and cell swelling. Depletion of which of the following substances by this mechanism within the cytosol exacerbates the cellular injury?

- ❏ (A) ADP
- ❏ (B) Calcium
- ❏ (C) Glutathione
- ❏ (D) NADPH oxidase
- ❏ (E) Nitric oxide synthase
- ❏ (F) mRNA
- ❏ (G) Sodium

35 An experiment is conducted in which cells in tissue culture are subjected to high levels of ultraviolet radiant energy. Electron microscopy shows cellular damage in the form of increased cytosolic aggregates of denatured proteins. In situ hybridization reveals that protein components in these aggregates are also found in proteasomes. Which of the following substances is most likely to bind to the denatured proteins, targeting them for catabolism by cytosolic proteasomes?

☐ (A) Adenosine monophosphate
☐ (B) Calcium
☐ (C) Caspase
☐ (D) Granzyme B
☐ (E) Hydrogen peroxide
☐ (F) Ubiquitin

ANSWERS

1 (E) Irreversible cell injury is associated with loss of membrane integrity. This allows intracellular enzymes to leak into the serum. All other morphologic changes listed are associated with reversible cell injury, in which the cell membrane remains intact.

BP7 22-24   BP6 6-8   PBD7 11-12   PBD6 7-9

2 (E) The liver is one of the few organs in the human body that can partially regenerate. This is a form of compensatory hyperplasia. The stimuli to hepatocyte mitotic activity cease when the liver has attained its normal size. Apoptosis is single cell death and frequently occurs with viral hepatitis. Dysplasia is disordered epithelial cell growth that can be premalignant. Fatty change can lead to hepatomegaly; this is not a regenerative process, but is the result of toxic hepatocyte injury. Hydropic change, or cell swelling, does not produce regeneration. Hepatocytes can reenter the cell cycle and proliferate to regenerate liver; they do not just increase in size.

BP7 13   BP6 22   PBD7 6-7   PBD6 32-33

3 (E) The pressure load on the left ventricle results in an increase in myofilaments in the existing myofibers. The result of continued stress from hypertension is eventual heart failure with decreased contractility, but the cells do not decrease in size. Metaplasia of muscle does not occur, although loss of muscle occurs with aging as myofibers are replaced by fibrous tissue and adipose tissue. Hemosiderin deposition in the heart is a pathologic process resulting from increased iron stores in the body.

BP7 12-13   BP6 22   PBD7 7-9   PBD6 33-35

4 (B) The valve is stenotic because of nodular deposits of calcium. The process is "dystrophic" because calcium deposition occurs in damaged tissues. The damage in this patient is a result of the wear and tear of aging. Amyloid deposition in the heart typically occurs within the myocardium and the vessels. The amount of lipofuscin increases within myocardial

fibers (not valves) with aging. Hereditary hemochromatosis is a genetic defect in iron absorption that results in extensive myocardial iron deposition (hemosiderosis). Fatty change is uncommonly seen in myocardium, but infiltration of fat cells between myofibers can occur.

BP7 21   BP6 20   PBD7 41   PBD6 43-44

5 (E) Cholesterol is a form of lipid commonly deposited within atheromas in arterial walls, imparting a yellow color to these plaques. Glycogen is a storage form of carbohydrate seen mainly in liver and muscle. Lipofuscin is a brown pigment that increases with aging in cell cytoplasm, mainly in cardiac myocytes and in hepatocytes. Hemosiderin is a storage form of iron that appears in tissues of the mononuclear phagocyte system (e.g., marrow, liver, spleen) but can be widely deposited with hereditary hemochromatosis. Immunoglobulin occasionally may be seen as rounded globules in plasma cells (i.e., Russell bodies).

BP7 18   BP6 18   PBD7 37   PBD6 40

6 (E) The focal, chalky-white deposits are areas of fat necrosis resulting from the release of pancreatic lipases in a patient with acute pancreatitis. Viral hepatitis does not cause necrosis in other organs, and hepatocyte necrosis from viral infections occurs mainly by means of apoptosis. Intestinal infarction is a form of coagulative necrosis. Tuberculosis produces caseous necrosis. Gangrenous necrosis is mainly coagulative necrosis but occurs over an extensive area.

BP7 25-26   BP6 12-13   PBD7 22   PBD6 16-17

7 (B) Intracellular mechanisms exist that deal with free-radical generation, as can occur with radiant injury from irradiation. Glutathione peroxidase reduces such injury by catalyzing the breakdown of hydrogen peroxide. Phospholipases decrease cellular phospholipids and promote cell membrane injury. Proteases can damage cell membranes and cytoskeletal proteins. Endonucleases damage nuclear chromatin. Lactate dehydrogenase is present in a variety of cells, and its elevation in the serum is an indicator of cell death.

BP7 10   BP6 9-11   PBD7 16-18   PBD6 12-14

8 (B) Mutations in the α_1-antitrypsin gene give rise to α_1-antitrypsin molecules that cannot fold properly. In the PiZZ genotype, both alleles have the mutation. The partially folded molecules accumulate in the endoplasmic reticulum and cannot be secreted. Impaired dissociation of the CFTR protein from chaperones causes many cases of cystic fibrosis. There is no abnormality in the synthesis, catabolism, or metabolism of α_1-antitrypsin in patients with α_1-antitrypsin deficiency.

PBD7 38   PBD6 41

9 (D) The high lipid content of central nervous system tissues results in liquefactive necrosis as a consequence of ischemic injury, as in this case of a "stroke." Fat necrosis is seen in breast and pancreatic tissues. Coagulative necrosis is the typical result of ischemia in most solid organs. Apoptosis affects single cells and typically is not grossly visible. Karyolysis refers to fading away of cell nuclei in dead cells.

BP7 25-26   BP6 12-13   PBD7 22   PBD6 16-17

10 (C) Reduced workload causes shrinkage of cell size because of loss of cell substance, a process called atrophy. Aplasia refers to lack of embryonic development; hypoplasia describes poor or subnormal development. Dystrophy of muscles refers to inherited disorders of skeletal muscles that lead to muscle weakness and wasting. Hyaline change (hyalinosis) refers to a nonspecific, pink, glassy eosinophilic appearance of cells.

BP7 11-12   BP6 21-22   PBD7 9-10   PBD6 35-36

11 (B) Germ cells have the highest telomerase activity, and the telomere length therefore can be stabilized in these cells. This allows testicular germ cells to retain the ability to divide throughout life. Normal somatic cells have no telomerase activity, and telomeres progressively shorten with each cell division until growth arrest occurs.

BP7 29-30   PBD7 43   PBD6 47

12 (C) Inflammation from reflux of gastric acid has resulted in replacement of normal esophageal squamous epithelium by intestinal-type columnar epithelium with goblet cells. Such conversion of one adult cell type to another cell type is called metaplasia. The cells are not significantly increased in size (hypertrophic). The lamina propria has some inflammatory cells but is not atrophic. Goblet cells are not normal constituents of the esophageal mucosa.

BP7 14   BP6 22-23   PBD7 10-11   PBD6 36-37

13 (A) The onset of menstruation is an example of orderly, programmed cell death (apoptosis) through hormonal stimuli. The endometrium breaks down, sloughs off, and then regenerates. Caseous necrosis is typical of granulomatous inflammation, resulting most commonly from mycobacterial infection. Heterophagocytosis is typified by the clearing of an area of necrosis through macrophage ingestion of the necrotic cells. With cellular atrophy, there is often no visible necrosis, but the tissues shrink, something that occurs in the endometrium after menopause. Liquefactive necrosis can occur in any tissue after acute bacterial infection or in the brain after ischemia.

BP7 26-28   BP6 13-14   PBD7 26-27   PBD6 18-19

14 (B) When DNA damage is induced by chemotherapeutic drugs (or other agents), normal *p53* genes trigger the cells to undergo apoptosis. When *p53* is inactivated, this pathway of cell death can be blocked, rendering the chemotherapy less effective. *BCL-2* and NF-κB activity favor cell survival. Cytochrome P-450 does not affect apoptosis. Granzyme B can trigger apoptosis, but it is found in cytotoxic T cells and not in tumor cells.

BP7 187-188   BP6 155-156   PBD7 31-32   PBD6 25

15 (B) Lobules increase under hormonal influence (mainly progesterone) to provide for normal lactation. The breast stroma plays no role in lactation and may increase with pathologic processes. Epithelial dysplasia denotes disordered growth and maturation of epithelial cells that may progress to cancer. Accumulation of fat within cells is a common manifestation of sublethal cell injury or, uncommonly, of inborn errors in fat metabolism. Epithelial metaplasia in the breast is a pathologic process.

BP7 13-14   BP6 22   PBD7 6-7   PBD6 32-33

16 (E) Each unit of blood contains about 250 mg of iron. The body has no mechanism for getting rid of excess iron. About 10 to 20 mg of iron per day is lost with normal desquamation of epithelia; menstruating women lose slightly more. Any excess iron becomes storage iron, or hemosiderin. Over time, hemosiderosis involves more and more tissues of the body, particularly the liver. Initially, hemosiderin deposits are found in Kupffer cells and other mononuclear phagocytes in the bone marrow, spleen, and lymph nodes. With great excess of iron, liver cells also accumulate iron. Steatosis usually occurs with ingestion of hepatotoxins, such as alcohol. Bilirubin, a breakdown product of blood, can be excreted in the bile so that a person does not become jaundiced. Glycogen storage diseases are inherited and present in childhood. Amyloid is an abnormal protein derived from a variety of precursors, such as immunoglobulin light chains.

BP7 20   BP6 19   PBD7 39-40   PBD6 42-43

17 (B) The deep eosinophilic staining, loss of nuclei, and loss of cell structure suggest an early ischemic injury, resulting in coagulative necrosis. This finding is typically caused by loss of blood flow. Viral infection could cause necrosis of the myocardium, but this is usually accompanied by an inflammatory infiltrate consisting of lymphocytes and macrophages. Blunt trauma produces hemorrhage. An immunologic injury may produce focal cell injury but not widespread ischemic injury. Lack of protein leads to a catabolic state with gradual decrease in cell size, but it does not cause ischemic changes.

BP7 25-26   BP6 6-7   PBD7 21-22   PBD6 7

18 (D) Nodular prostatic hyperplasia (also known as benign prostatic hyperplasia, or BPH) is a common condition in older men that results from proliferation of both prostatic glands and stroma. The prostate becomes more sensitive to androgenic stimulation with age. This is an example of pathologic hyperplasia. Apoptosis results in a loss, not an increase, in cells. Dysplasia refers to disordered epithelial cell growth and maturation. Fatty change in hepatocytes may produce hepatomegaly. Although BPH is often called "benign prostatic hypertrophy," this term is technically incorrect; it is the number of glands and stromal cells that is increased rather than the size of existing cells. A change in the glandular epithelium to squamous epithelium would be an example of metaplasia.

BP7 13-14   BP6 22   PBD7 6-7   PBD6 32-33

19 (A) If the existing cell damage is not great after myocardial infarction, the restoration of blood flow can help prevent further damage. However, the reperfusion of damaged cells results in generation of oxygen-derived free radicals, causing a reperfusion injury. The elevation in the creatine kinase level is indicative of myocardial cell necrosis, because this intracellular enzyme does not leak in large quantities from intact cells. Myocardial fibers do not regenerate to a significant degree, and atrophic fibers would have less enzyme to release. Tissue plasminogen activator does not produce a chemical injury; it induces thrombolysis to restore blood flow in blocked coronary arteries.

BP7 9-10   BP6 9-10   PBD7 24   PBD6 12-13

20 (D) Loss of the nucleus results in cell death. All other cellular morphologic changes listed represent reversible cellular injury. The plasma membrane and intracellular organelles remain functional unless severe damage causes loss of membrane integrity.

BP7 22-23   BP6 11-12   PBD7 12, 19   PBD6 8-10

21 **(B)** This histologic picture is typical of apoptosis produced by chemotherapeutic agents. The release of cytochrome from the mitochondria is a key step in many forms of apoptosis, and it leads to the activation of caspases. *BCL-2* is an antiapoptotic protein that prevents cytochrome *c* release and prevents caspase activation. Lipofuscin is a pigmented residue representing undigested cellular organelles in autophagic vacuoles. Catalase is a scavenger of hydrogen peroxide. Phospholipases are activated during necrosis and cause cell membrane damage.

BP727-29   BP6 13-15   PBD7 29-31   PBD6 22-24

22 **(B)** The microscopic findings suggest metastatic calcification, with deposition of calcium salts in tissues that have physiologic mechanisms for losing acid, creating an internal alkaline environment that favors calcium precipitation. Hypercalcemia can have a variety of causes, including hyperparathyroidism, bone destruction due to metastases, paraneoplastic syndromes, and, less commonly, vitamin D toxicity or sarcoidosis. Chronic renal disease reduces phosphate excretion by the kidney, resulting in an increase in serum phosphate. Because the solubility product of calcium and phosphorus must be maintained, the serum calcium is depressed, triggering increased parathyroid hormone output to increase the calcium level, which promotes calcium deposition. Chronic hepatitis leads to hyperbilirubinemia and jaundice. The granulomas of tuberculosis have caseous necrosis with dystrophic calcification. Another form of dystrophic calcification occurs when atherosclerotic lesions calcify. Dystrophic calcification is seen more often in the elderly, but it is the result of a lifetime of pathologic changes, not aging itself. Pulmonary emphysema can lead to respiratory acidosis that is compensated by metabolic alkalosis, with the result that the serum calcium level remains relatively unchanged.

BP7 22   BP6 20   PBD7 41-42   PBD6 45

23 **(C)** Embolization of the thrombus led to blockage of a renal arterial branch, causing an acute renal infarction in this patient. An ischemic injury to most internal organs produces a pattern of cell death called coagulative necrosis. Liquefactive necrosis occurs following ischemic injury to the brain and is also the pattern seen with abscess formation. Caseous necrosis can be seen in various forms of granulomatous inflammation, typified by tuberculosis. Fat necrosis is usually seen in pancreatic and breast tissue. Gangrenous necrosis is a form of coagulative necrosis that usually results from ischemia and affects limbs.

BP7 25-26   BP6 12-13   PBD7 21-22   PBD6 16-18

24 **(C)** The appearance of lipid vacuoles in many of the hepatocytes is characteristic of fatty change (steatosis) of the liver. Abnormalities in lipoprotein metabolism can lead to steatosis. Alcohol is a hepatotoxin that produces hepatic steatosis. Decreased serum albumin levels and increased prothrombin time suggest alcohol-induced hepatocyte damage. Substance abuse with heroin produces surprisingly few organ-specific pathologic findings. Exercise has little direct effect on

hepatic function. Smoking directly damages lung tissue but has no direct effect on the liver. Aspirin has a significant effect on platelet function but not on hepatocytes.

BP7 16-17   BP6 17-18   PBD7 35-36   PBD6 39-40

25 **(A)** This cell is shrunken and has been converted into a dense eosinophilic mass. The surrounding cells are normal, and there is no inflammatory reaction. This pattern is typical of apoptosis. Caspase activation is a universal feature of apoptosis, regardless of the initiating cause. Apoptosis induced in recipient cells from donor lymphocytes occurs with graft-versus-host disease. Reduced ATP synthesis and increased glycolysis occur when a cell is subjected to anoxia. These changes are reversible. Lipases are activated in enzymatic fat necrosis. Lipid peroxidation occurs when the cell is injured by free radicals.

BP7 26-28   BP6 13-14   PBD7 29-31   PBD6 18-20

26 **(D)** Lipofuscin is a "wear-and-tear" pigment that increases with aging, particularly in liver and myocardium. The pigment has minimal effect on cellular function in most cases. Rarely, there is marked lipofuscin deposition in a small heart, a so-called brown atrophy. Melanin pigment is responsible for skin tone: the more melanin, the darker the skin. Hemosiderin is the breakdown product of hemoglobin that contains the iron. Hearts with excessive iron deposition tend to be large. Glycogen is increased in some inherited enzyme disorders, and when the heart is involved, heart size increases. Bilirubin, another breakdown product of hemoglobin, imparts a yellow appearance (icterus) to tissues.

BP7 20   BP6 19   PBD7 39-40   PBD6 42

27 **(A)** Anthracotic pigmentation is common in lung and hilar lymph nodes and occurs when carbon pigment is inhaled from polluted air. The tar in cigarette smoke is a major source of such carbonaceous pigment. Resolution of hemorrhage can produce hemosiderin pigmentation, which imparts a brown color to tissues. Hepatic failure may result in jaundice, characterized by a yellow color. Older persons generally have more anthracotic pigment, but this is not inevitable with aging—persons living in rural areas with good environmental air quality will have less pigment. Metastases impart a tan to white appearance to tissues.

BP7 19   BP6 19   PBD7 39   PBD6 42

28 **(D)** Deposition of calcium in normal healthy tissues as a result of prolonged hypercalcemia is called metastatic calcification. This process may occur in hyperparathyroidism. Dystrophic calcification refers to calcium deposition in injured tissues, with normal serum calcium levels. Atrophy decreases cell size but is not accompanied by calcium deposition. Autophagocytosis yields more golden-brown lipofuscin pigment in the cytoplasm, particularly in hepatocytes and myocardial fibers, a process that becomes more apparent with aging.

BP7 22   BP6 20   PBD7 41-42   PBD6 45

29 **(B)** These histologic findings are typical of apoptosis. The *BCL-2* gene product inhibits cellular apoptosis by binding to Apaf-1. The *BAX* gene product promotes apoptosis. The *C-MYC* gene is involved with oncogenesis. The *FAS* gene encodes for a cellular receptor for *FAS* ligand, which signals apoptosis.

p53 gene activity normally stimulates apoptosis, but mutation favors cell survival.

BP7 27-28   BP6 19   PBD7 29-30   PBD6 26, 36

30 **(B)** Reperfusion injury is clinically important in myocardial infarction and stroke. Paradoxically, the oxygen that flows in with blood can be converted to free radicals by parenchymal and endothelial cells and infiltrating leukocytes. Catalase is a scavenger of free radicals. All other changes listed occur in sublethal cell injury.

BP7 9   BP6 11   PBD7 24   PBD6 14-15

31 **(B)** The cheese-like appearance gives this form of necrosis its name—caseous necrosis. In the lung, tuberculosis and fungal infections are most likely to produce this pattern of tissue injury. Apoptosis involves individual cells, without extensive or localized areas of tissue necrosis. Coagulative necrosis is more typical of ischemic tissue injury. Fat necrosis most often occurs in the breast and pancreas. Fatty change is most often a feature of hepatocyte injury, and the cell integrity is maintained. Gangrene characterizes extensive necrosis of multiple cell types in a body region or organ. Liquefactive necrosis is seen in abscesses or ischemic cerebral injury.

BP7 25-26   BP6 13   PBD7 22   PBD6 17

32 **(D)** The increase in uterine size is primarily the result of an increase in myometrial smooth muscle cell size. The endometrium also increases in size, but it remains as a lining to the muscular wall and does not contribute as much to the change in size. There is little stroma in myometrium and a greater proportion in endometrium, but this contributes a smaller percentage to the gain in size than does muscle. The vessels are a minor but essential component in this process.

BP7 12-13   BP6 22   PBD7 7-9   PBD6 33-35

33 **(A)** Heterophagocytosis by macrophages requires that endocytosed vacuoles fuse with lysosomes to degrade the engulfed material. With congestive failure, extravasation of RBCs into alveoli occurs, and pulmonary macrophages must phagocytose the RBCs, breaking down the hemoglobin and recycling the iron by hemosiderin formation.

BP7 9, 20   BP6 15-16   PBD7 32-33   PBD6 25-26

34 **(C)** Glutathione in the cytosol helps to reduce cellular injury from many toxic metabolites and free radicals. ADP is converted to ATP by oxidative and glycolytic cellular pathways to provide energy that drives cellular functions, and a reduction in ATP leaves the cell vulnerable to injury. Calcium influx into a cell promotes injury. NADPH oxidase generates superoxide, which is used by neutrophils in killing bacteria. Nitric oxide synthase in macrophages produces nitric oxide, which aids in destroying organisms undergoing phagocytosis. Protein synthesis in cells depends on mRNA for longer survival and to recover from damage from free radicals. Failure of the sodium pump leads to increased cytosolic sodium and cell swelling with injury.

BP7 10   BP6 10   PBD7 17-18   PBD6 13-14

35 **(F)** Heat shock proteins provide for a variety of cellular "housekeeping" activities, including recycling and restoration of damaged proteins, as well as removal of denatured proteins. Ubiquitin targets denatured proteins and facilitates their binding to proteasomes, which then break down the proteins to peptides. ADP increases when ATP is depleted, helping to drive anaerobic glycolysis. Cytosolic calcium levels may increase with cell injury that depletes ATP; the calcium activates phospholipases, endonucleases, and proteases, which damage the cell membranes, structural proteins, and mitochondria. Caspases are enzymes that facilitate apoptosis. Granzyme B is released from cytotoxic T lymphocytes and triggers apoptosis. Hydrogen peroxide is one of the activated oxygen species generated under conditions of cellular ischemia, producing nonspecific damage to cellular structures, particularly membranes.

BP7 16-17   PBD7 37-38

CHAPTER 2

Acute and Chronic Inflammation

PBD7 Chapter 2: Acute and Chronic Inflammation

PBD6 Chapter 3: Acute and Chronic Inflammation

BP7 and BP6 Chapter 2: Acute and Chronic Inflammation

1 In a 6-month randomized trial of a pharmacologic agent, one group of patients receives a cyclooxygenase-2 (COX-2) inhibitor and a control group does not. Laboratory measurements during the trial show no significant differences between the groups in WBC count, platelet count, hemoglobin, and creatinine. However, the group receiving the drug reports subjective findings different from those of the control group. Which of the following findings was most likely reported by the group receiving the drug?

- ❏ (A) Ankle swelling
- ❏ (B) Increased bouts of asthma
- ❏ (C) Easy bruisability
- ❏ (D) Reduced urticaria
- ❏ (E) Increased febrile episodes
- ❏ (F) Reduced arthritis pain

2 An experiment introduces bacteria into a perfused tissue preparation. Leukocytes then leave the vasculature and migrate to the site of bacterial inoculation. The movement of these leukocytes is most likely to be mediated by which of the following substances?

- ❏ (A) Bradykinin
- ❏ (B) Chemokines
- ❏ (C) Histamine
- ❏ (D) Prostaglandins
- ❏ (E) Complement C3a

3 A 53-year-old woman has had a high fever and cough productive of yellowish sputum for the past 2 days. Her vital signs include temperature of 37.8°C, pulse 83/min, respirations 17/min, and blood pressure 100/60 mm Hg. On auscultation of the chest, crackles are audible in both lung bases. A chest radiograph shows bilateral patchy pulmonary infiltrates. Which of the following inflammatory cell types is most likely to be seen in greatly increased numbers in a sputum specimen?

- ❏ (A) Macrophages
- ❏ (B) Neutrophils
- ❏ (C) Mast cells
- ❏ (D) Small lymphocytes
- ❏ (E) Langhans giant cells

4 A 63-year-old man develops worsening congestive heart failure 2 weeks after an acute myocardial infarction. An echocardiogram shows a markedly decreased ejection fraction. He dies 1 day later. At autopsy, a section of the infarct shows that the necrotic myocardium has largely been replaced by capillaries, fibroblasts, and collagen. Various inflammatory cells are present. Which of the following inflammatory cell types in this lesion plays the most important role in the healing process?

- (A) Macrophages
- (B) Plasma cells
- (C) Neutrophils
- (D) Eosinophils
- (E) Epithelioid cells

5 A 10-year-old child developed a sore throat and fever over a period of 24 hours. Physical examination shows pharyngeal erythema and swelling. Laboratory findings include leukocytosis. The child is given acetylsalicylic acid (aspirin). Which of the following features of the inflammatory response is most affected by this drug?

- (A) Vasodilation
- (B) Chemotaxis
- (C) Phagocytosis
- (D) Emigration of leukocytes
- (E) Release of leukocytes from bone marrow

6 A woman who is allergic to cats visits a neighbor who has several cats. During the visit, she inhales cat dander and within minutes, she develops nasal congestion with abundant nasal secretions. Which of the following substances is most likely to produce these findings?

- (A) Bradykinin
- (B) Complement C5a
- (C) Histamine
- (D) Interleukin-1
- (E) Phospholipase C
- (F) Platelet-activating factor
- (G) Tumor necrosis factor

7 A 32-year-old woman has had a chronic cough with fever for the past month. On physical examination, she has a temperature of 37.5°C, and on auscultation of the chest, crackles are heard in all lung fields. A chest radiograph shows many small, ill-defined nodular opacities in all lung fields. A transbronchial biopsy specimen shows interstitial infiltrates with lymphocytes, plasma cells, and epithelioid macrophages. Which of the following infectious agents is the most likely cause of this appearance?

- (A) *Staphylococcus aureus*
- (B) *Plasmodium falciparum*
- (C) *Candida albicans*
- (D) *Mycobacterium tuberculosis*
- (E) *Klebsiella pneumoniae*
- (F) Cytomegalovirus

8 A 36-year-old man has had midepigastric abdominal pain for the past 3 months. An upper gastrointestinal endoscopy shows a 2-cm, sharply demarcated, shallow ulceration of the gastric antrum. A biopsy specimen of the ulcer base shows angiogenesis, fibrosis, and mononuclear cell infiltrates with lymphocytes, macrophages, and plasma cells. Which of the following terms best describes this pathologic process?

- (A) Acute inflammation
- (B) Serous inflammation
- (C) Granulomatous inflammation
- (D) Fibrinous inflammation
- (E) Chronic inflammation

9 A 5-year-old child reaches up to the stove and touches a pot of boiling soup. Within several hours, there is marked erythema of the skin of the fingers on the child's right hand, and small blisters appear on the finger pads. Which of the following terms best describes this process?

- (A) Fibrinous inflammation
- (B) Purulent inflammation
- (C) Serous inflammation
- (D) Ulceration
- (E) Granulomatous inflammation

10 For the past 2 days, a 41-year-old man has had a severe headache, and he now has a temperature of 39.2°C. A lumbar puncture is performed, and the cerebrospinal fluid obtained has a WBC count of 910/mm^3 with 94% neutrophils and 6% lymphocytes. Which of the following substances is the most likely mediator for the fever observed in this patient?

- (A) Bradykinin
- (B) Leukotriene B$_4$
- (C) Histamine
- (D) Myeloperoxidase
- (E) Nitric oxide
- (F) Phospholipase C
- (G) Tumor necrosis factor

11 A 6-year-old child has a history of recurrent infections with pyogenic bacteria, including *Staphylococcus aureus* and *Streptococcus pneumoniae*. The infections are accompanied by a neutrophilic leukocytosis. Microscopic examination of a biopsy specimen obtained from an area of soft tissue necrosis shows microbial organisms but very few neutrophils. An analysis of neutrophil function shows a defect in rolling. This child's increased susceptibility to infection is most likely caused by a defect in which of the following molecules?

- (A) Selectins
- (B) Integrins
- (C) Leukotriene B$_4$
- (D) Complement C3b
- (E) NADPH oxidase

12 One month after an appendectomy, a 25-year-old woman palpates a small nodule beneath the skin at the site of the healed right lower quadrant incision. The nodule is excised, and microscopic examination shows macrophages, collagen, a few small lymphocytes, and multinucleated giant cells. Polarizable, refractile material is seen in the nodule. Which of the following complications of the surgery best accounts for these findings?

- (A) Chronic inflammation
- (B) Abscess formation
- (C) Suture granuloma
- (D) Ulceration
- (E) Edema

13 A 3-year-old boy and other male relatives have a history of multiple recurrent infections, including *Aspergillus, Staphylococcus, Serratia, Nocardia,* and *Pseudomonas* species. Physical examination shows generalized tender lymphadenopathy. Laboratory findings show normal numbers of morphologically normal circulating WBCs. This child's increased susceptibility to infection is most likely caused by a defect in which of the following steps of the inflammatory response?

❑ (A) Activation of macrophages by interferon-γ
❑ (B) Oxygen-dependent killing of bacteria by neutrophils
❑ (C) Firm adhesion between leukocytes and endothelial cells
❑ (D) Synthesis of lysozyme in neutrophil granules
❑ (E) Opsonization of bacteria by immunoglobulins

14 In an experiment, neutrophils collected from peripheral blood are analyzed for a "burst" of oxygen consumption. This respiratory burst is an essential step for which of the following events in an acute inflammatory response?

❑ (A) Increased production in bone marrow
❑ (B) Attachment to endothelial cells
❑ (C) Opsonization of bacteria
❑ (D) Phagocytosis of bacteria
❑ (E) Generation of microbicidal activity

15 A 20-year-old sexually active woman experiences lower abdominal pain of 24 hours' duration. She has no previous history of this type of pain. Her temperature is 37.9°C, and on palpation, the left lower abdomen is markedly tender. Laboratory findings include a total WBC count of 29,000/mm^3 with 75% segmented neutrophils, 6% bands, 14% lymphocytes, and 5% monocytes. Laparotomy reveals a distended, fluid-filled, reddened left fallopian tube that is about to rupture. A left salpingectomy is performed. Which of the following is most likely to be seen on microscopic examination of the excised fallopian tube?

❑ (A) Fibroblastic proliferation
❑ (B) Langhans giant cells
❑ (C) Liquefactive necrosis
❑ (D) Mononuclear infiltrates
❑ (E) Squamous metaplasia

16 A 9-year-old boy has had a chronic cough and fever for the past month. A chest radiograph shows enlargement of hilar lymph nodes and bilateral pulmonary nodular interstitial infiltrates. A sputum sample contains acid-fast bacilli. A transbronchial biopsy specimen shows granulomatous inflammation within the lung, marked by the presence of Langhans giant cells. Which of the following mediators is most likely to contribute to giant cell formation?

❑ (A) Tumor necrosis factor
❑ (B) Complement C3b
❑ (C) Leukotriene B$_4$
❑ (D) Interferon-γ
❑ (E) Interleukin-1

17 A 5-year-old child has a history of recurrent bacterial infections, including pneumonia and otitis media. Analysis of leukocytes collected from the peripheral blood shows a deficiency in myeloperoxidase. Which of the following is the most likely cause of this child's increased susceptibility to infections?

❑ (A) Defective neutrophil degranulation
❑ (B) Defective production of prostaglandins
❑ (C) Failure to produce hydroxy-halide radicals (HOCl$^-$)
❑ (D) Decreased oxygen consumption after phagocytosis
❑ (E) Failure to produce hydrogen peroxide

18 A 78-year-old woman suffers a sudden loss of consciousness, with loss of movement on the right side of the body. Cerebral angiography shows an occlusion of the left middle cerebral artery. To prevent further ischemic injury to the cerebral cortex, which of the following mediators would be most beneficial?

❑ (A) Thromboxane A$_2$
❑ (B) Bradykinin
❑ (C) Nitric oxide
❑ (D) Platelet-activating factor
❑ (E) Leukotriene E$_4$

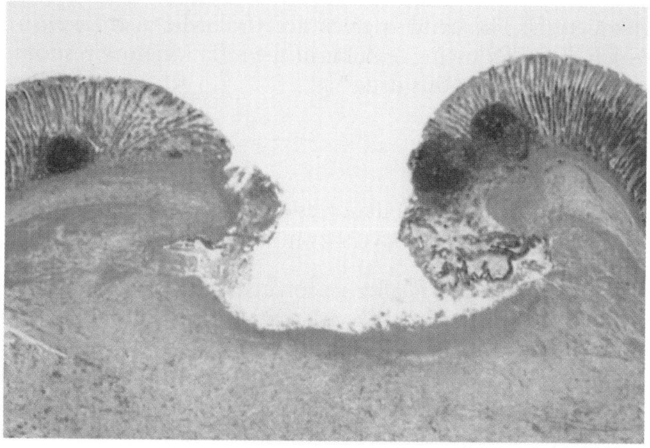

19 A 50-year-old man has experienced midabdominal pain for several weeks. He is afebrile. There is mild upper abdominal tenderness on palpation, and bowel sounds are present. Stool is positive for occult blood. An upper gastrointestinal endoscopy is performed and biopsies taken. Microscopic examination of a biopsy specimen of a duodenal lesion is shown. Which of the following terms best describes this lesion?

❑ (A) Abscess
❑ (B) Caseating granuloma
❑ (C) Chronic inflammation
❑ (D) Purulent exudate
❑ (E) Serous effusion
❑ (F) Ulceration

20 A 72-year-old man with severe emphysema has had worsening right ventricular failure for the past 5 years. He has had fever and increasing dyspnea for the past 4 days. A chest radiograph shows an accumulation of fluid in the pleural spaces. Fluid obtained by thoracentesis has a specific gravity of 1.030 and contains degenerating neutrophils. The most likely cause of this fluid accumulation is an increase in which of the following mechanisms?

❑ (A) Colloid osmotic pressure
❑ (B) Lymphatic pressure
❑ (C) Vascular permeability
❑ (D) Renal retention of sodium and water
❑ (E) Leukocytic diapedesis

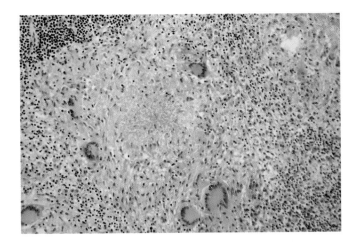

21 A 43-year-old man has had a cough and fever for the past 2 months. A chest radiograph shows bilateral nodular densities, some with calcification, located mainly in the upper lobes of the lungs. A transbronchial lung biopsy is performed, yielding a specimen with the microscopic appearance shown. Which of the following chemical mediators is most important in the pathogenesis of this lesion?

❑ (A) Complement C5a
❑ (B) Interferon-γ
❑ (C) Bradykinin
❑ (D) Nitric oxide
❑ (E) Prostaglandin

22 A 59-year-old man has had a cough and fever for the past week. On physical examination, his temperature is 38.5°C. On auscultation, he has decreased breath sounds and dullness to percussion over the right lung. A chest radiograph shows fluid in the right pleural cavity. Thoracentesis yields 500 mL of cloudy yellow fluid. Which of the following cell types is most likely to be abundant in this fluid?

❑ (A) Macrophages
❑ (B) Neutrophils
❑ (C) CD4 lymphocytes
❑ (D) Plasma cells
❑ (E) Eosinophils

23 In an experiment, peripheral blood T lymphocytes are collected and placed in a medium that preserves their function. The lymphocytes are activated by contact with antigen and incubated for several hours. The supernatant fluid is collected and is found to contain a substance that is a major stimulator of monocytes and macrophages. Which of the following substances is most likely to stimulate these cells?

❑ (A) Leukotriene B$_4$
❑ (B) Histamine
❑ (C) Interferon-γ
❑ (D) Interleukin-1
❑ (E) Nitric oxide
❑ (F) Phospholipase C
❑ (G) Tumor necrosis factor

24 A 90-year-old woman is diagnosed with *Staphylococcus aureus* pneumonia and receives a course of antibiotic therapy. Two weeks later, she no longer has a productive cough, but she still has a temperature of 38.1°C. A chest radiograph shows a 3-cm rounded density in the right lower lobe of the lung whose liquefied contents form a central air-fluid level. There are no surrounding infiltrates. Which of the following terms best describes the outcome of the patient's pneumonia?

❑ (A) Complete resolution
❑ (B) Regeneration
❑ (C) Fibrosis
❑ (D) Abscess formation
❑ (E) Progression to chronic inflammation

25 A 30-year-old woman with a history of a congenital ventricular septal defect has had a persistent temperature of 38.6°C and headache for the past 3 weeks. A head CT scan shows an enhancing 3-cm ring-like lesion in the right parietal lobe. Which of the following actions by inflammatory cells is most likely to produce this CT finding?

❑ (A) Formation of nitric oxide by macrophages
❑ (B) Production of interferon-γ by lymphocytes
❑ (C) Formation of transforming growth factor-β by macrophages
❑ (D) Generation of prostaglandin by endothelium
❑ (E) Release of lysosomal enzymes from neutrophils

26 A 35-year-old man has had increasing dyspnea for the past 24 hours. A chest radiograph shows large, bilateral pleural effusions. Thoracentesis yields 500 mL of slightly cloudy yellow fluid from the right pleural cavity. Cytologic examination of the fluid shows many neutrophils but no lymphocytes or RBCs. Which of the following mechanisms contributes most to the accumulation of the fluid in the pleural space?

❑ (A) Arteriolar vasoconstriction
❑ (B) Neutrophil release of lysosomes
❑ (C) Endothelial contraction
❑ (D) Inhibition of platelet adherence
❑ (E) Lymphatic obstruction

27 A 12-month-old boy with a 6-month history of repeated infections has had a fever and cough for the past 3 days. A Gram stain of sputum shows many gram-positive cocci in chains. CBC shows neutrophilia. Laboratory studies demonstrate that the patient's neutrophils phagocytose and kill organisms normally in the presence of normal human serum but not in his own serum. The neutrophils migrate normally in a chemotaxis assay. Which of the following is the most likely cause of the child's increased susceptibility to infection?

❑ (A) Deficiency of integrins
❑ (B) Neutrophil microtubular protein defect
❑ (C) Immunoglobulin deficiency
❑ (D) Defective neutrophil generation of hydrogen peroxide
❑ (E) Deficiency of selectins

28 A 35-year-old woman takes acetylsalicylic acid (aspirin) for arthritis. Although her joint pain is reduced with this therapy, the inflammatory process continues. The aspirin therapy alleviates her pain mainly through reduction in the synthesis of which of the following mediators?

❑ (A) Complement C1q
❑ (B) Prostaglandins
❑ (C) Leukotriene E$_4$
❑ (D) Histamine
❑ (E) Nitric oxide

29 A 70-year-old woman has had worsening shortness of breath for the past week. On physical examination, her temperature is 38.3°C. On percussion, there is dullness over the left lung fields. Thoracentesis yields 800 mL of cloudy yellow fluid from the left pleural cavity. Analysis of the fluid reveals a WBC count of 2500/mm^3 with 98% neutrophils and 2% lymphocytes. A Gram stain of the fluid shows gram-positive cocci in clusters. Which of the following terms best describes the process occurring in the left pleural cavity?

- ❑ (A) Abscess
- ❑ (B) Chronic inflammation
- ❑ (C) Edema
- ❑ (D) Fibrinous inflammation
- ❑ (E) Purulent exudate
- ❑ (F) Serous effusion

30 A 5-year-old boy has a history of recurrent infections with gram-positive bacteria, including *Staphylococcus aureus*. Genetic testing shows a defect leading to a lack of β_2-integrin production. Which of the following abnormalities of neutrophil function is most likely responsible for these clinical symptoms?

- ❑ (A) Normal neutrophil rolling but inadequate sticking on cytokine-activated endothelial cells
- ❑ (B) Failure of neutrophils to migrate to the site of infection after leaving the vasculature
- ❑ (C) Reduced respiratory burst in neutrophils after phagocytosis of bacteria
- ❑ (D) Diminished phagocytosis of bacteria opsonized with immunoglobulin G
- ❑ (E) Failure to generate hydroxy-halide radicals (HOCl$^-$)

31 An experiment isolates peripheral blood cells into a culture medium that preserves their metabolic activity. After interferon-gamma is added to this culture the cells are incubated. Next, a cell-free supernatant from this culture is added to a second culture medium containing *Escherichia coli* organisms. Which of the following cell types is the most likely source for observed bactericidal activity against *E. coli*?

- ❑ (A) Basophil
- ❑ (B) B lymphocyte
- ❑ (C) CD4 lymphocyte
- ❑ (D) CD8 lymphocyte
- ❑ (E) Macrophage
- ❑ (F) Neutrophil
- ❑ (G) Natural killer cell

ANSWERS

1 **(F)** The cyclooxygenase-2 (COX-2) enzyme is inducible with acute inflammatory reactions, particularly in neutrophils, in synovium, and in the central nervous system. The cyclooxygenase pathway of arachidonic acid metabolism generates prostaglandins, which mediate pain, fever, and vasodilation. Ankle swelling is most likely to be the result of peripheral edema due to congestive heart failure. Asthma results from bronchoconstriction mediated by leukotrienes that are generated by the lipoxygenase pathway of arachidonic acid metabolism. Easy bruisability results from prolonged glucocorticoid administration, which also causes leukopenia. Inhibition of histamine released from mast cells helps reduce urticaria. Fever can be mediated by prostaglandin release, not inhibition.
BP7 47-48   BP6 35-36   PBD7 68-70   PBD6 67-69

2 **(B)** Chemokines include a number of molecules that are chemotactic for neutrophils, eosinophils, lymphocytes, monocytes, and basophils. Bradykinin causes pain and increased vascular permeability. Histamine causes vascular leakage, and prostaglandins have multiple actions, but they do not cause chemotaxis. Complement C3a causes increased vascular permeability by releasing histamine from mast cells.
BP7 40   BP6 31   PBD7 71-72   PBD6 61

3 **(B)** The patient's signs and symptoms suggest acute bacterial pneumonia. Such infections induce an acute inflammation dominated by neutrophils, which gives the sputum its yellowish, purulent appearance. Macrophages become more numerous after acute events, cleaning up tissue and bacterial debris through phagocytosis. Mast cells are better known as participants in allergic and anaphylactic responses. Lymphocytes are a feature of chronic inflammation. Langhans giant cells are seen with granulomatous inflammatory responses.
BP7 40, 57-58   BP6 26   PBD7 77-78   PBD6 51

4 **(A)** Macrophages, present in such lesions, play a prominent role in the healing process. Activated macrophages can secrete various cytokines that promote angiogenesis and fibrosis, including platelet-derived growth factor, fibroblast growth factor, interleukin-1, and tumor necrosis factor. Plasma cells can secrete immunoglobulins and are not instrumental to healing of an area of tissue injury. Neutrophils are most numerous within the initial 48 hours after infarction but are not numerous after the first week. Eosinophils are most prominent in allergic inflammations and in parasitic infections. Epithelioid cells, which are aggregations of activated macrophages, are typically seen with granulomatous inflammation. The healing of acute inflammatory processes does not involve granulomatous inflammation.
BP7 54-55   BP6 41-42   PBD7 79-81   PBD6 79-81

5 **(A)** Aspirin (acetylsalicylic acid) blocks the cyclooxygenase pathway of arachidonic acid metabolism, which leads to reduced prostaglandin generation. Prostaglandins promote vasodilation at sites of inflammation. Chemotaxis is a function of various chemokines, and complement C3b may promote phagocytosis, but neither is affected by aspirin. Leukocyte emigration is aided by various adhesion molecules. Leukocyte release from the marrow can be driven by the cytokines interleukin-1 and tumor necrosis factor.
BP7 47   BP6 37   PBD7 69-70   PBD6 71-72

6 **(C)** Histamine is found in abundance in mast cells, which are normally present in connective tissues next to blood vessels beneath mucosal surfaces in airways. Binding of an antigen (allergen) to IgE antibodies that have previously attached to the mast cells by the Fc receptor triggers mast cell degranulation, with release of histamine. This response causes increased vascular permeability and mucous secretions.

Bradykinin, generated from the kinin system upon surface contact of Hageman factor with collagen and basement membrane from vascular injury, promotes vascular permeability, smooth muscle contraction, and pain. Complement C5a is a potent chemotactic factor for neutrophils. Interleukin-1 and tumor necrosis factor, both produced by activated macrophages, mediate many systemic effects, including fever, metabolic wasting, and hypotension. Phospholipase C, which catalyzes the release of arachidonic acid, is generated from platelet activation.   Platelet-activating factor (PAF) can be released by neutrophils, mast cells, monocytes, macrophages, and endothelial cells, as well as platelets. PAF promotes vascular permeability as well as neutrophil aggregation and platelet activation.

BP7 44   BP6 34   PBD7 63-64   PBD6 66

7 **(D)** These findings suggest a granulomatous inflammation, and tuberculosis is a common cause. Bacteria such as *Staphylococcus* and *Klebsiella* are more likely to produce acute inflammation. *Plasmodium* produces malaria, a parasitic infection without a significant degree of lung involvement. *Candida* is often a commensal organism in the oropharyngeal region and rarely causes pneumonia in healthy (nonimmunosuppressed) individuals. Viral infections tend to produce a mononuclear interstitial inflammatory cell response.

BP7 56-57   BP6 42-43   PBD7 82-83   PBD6 82-83

8 **(E)** One outcome of acute inflammation with ulceration is chronic inflammation. This is particularly true when the inflammatory process continues for weeks to months. Chronic inflammation is characterized by tissue destruction, mononuclear cell infiltration, and repair. In acute inflammation, the healing process of fibrosis and angiogenesis has not begun. Serous inflammation is an inflammatory process involving a mesothelial surface (e.g., lining of the pericardial cavity), with an outpouring of fluid having little protein or cellular content. Granulomatous inflammation is a form of chronic inflammation in which epithelioid macrophages form aggregates. In fibrinous inflammation, typically involving a mesothelial surface, there is an outpouring of protein-rich fluid that results in precipitation of fibrin.

BP7 52   BP6 41   PBD7 78-79   PBD6 79

9 **(C)** Serous inflammation represents the mildest form of acute inflammation. A blister is a good example of serous inflammation. It is associated primarily with exudation of fluid into the subcorneal or subepidermal space. Because the injury is mild, the fluid is relatively protein poor. A protein-rich exudate results in fibrin accumulation. Acute inflammatory cells, mainly neutrophils, exuded into a body cavity or space form a purulent (suppurative) exudate, typically associated with liquefactive necrosis. Loss of the epithelium leads to ulceration. Granulomatous inflammation is characterized by collections of transformed macrophages called epithelioid cells.

BP7 57   BP6 44   PBD7 76   PBD6 84

10 **(G)** Fever is produced by various inflammatory mediators, but the major cytokines that produce fever are interleukin-1 (IL-1) and tumor necrosis factor (TNF), which are produced by macrophages and other cell types. IL-1 and TNF can have autocrine, paracrine, and endocrine effects. They mediate the acute phase responses, such as fever, nausea, and neutrophil release from marrow. Bradykinin, generated from the kinin system upon surface contact of Hageman factor with collagen and basement membrane from vascular injury, promotes vascular permeability, smooth muscle contraction, and pain. Leukotriene B$_4$, generated in the lipoxygenase pathway of arachidonic acid metabolism, is a potent neutrophil chemotactic factor. Histamine released from mast cells is a potent vasodilator, increasing vascular permeability. Myeloperoxidase is contained within the azurophilic granules of neutrophils, and in the presence of halide converts hydrogen peroxide to HOCl$^-$, which destroys phagocytized organisms by halogenation. Nitric oxide generated by macrophages aids in destruction of microorganisms; nitric oxide released from endothelium mediates vasodilation and inhibits platelet activation. Phospholipase C, which catalyzes the release of arachidonic acid, is generated from platelet activation.

BP7 49-50   BP6 40   PBD7 71   PBD6 78

11 **(A)** The patient has a defect in leukocyte rolling, the first step in transmigration of neutrophils from the vasculature to the tissues. Rolling depends on interaction between selectins (P- and E-selectins on endothelial cells, and L-selectin on neutrophils) and their sialylated ligand molecules (e.g., sialylated Lewis X). Integrins are involved in the next step of transmigration, during which there is firm adhesion between neutrophils and endothelial cells. Leukotriene B$_4$ is a chemotactic agent, complement C3b facilitates phagocytosis, and NADPH oxidase is involved in microbicidal activity.

BP7 38-39   BP6 28-29   PBD7 54-55   PBD6 58-63

12 **(C)** The polarizable material is the suture, and a multinucleated giant cell reaction, typically with foreign body giant cells, is characteristic of a granulomatous reaction to foreign material. Chronic inflammation alone is not likely to produce a localized nodule with giant cells. An abscess, typically from a wound infection, would have liquefactive necrosis and numerous neutrophils. An ulceration involves loss of epidermis or other epithelial layer. Edema refers to accumulation of fluid in the interstitial space. It does not produce a cellular nodule.

BP7 56   BP6 42-43   PBD7 82-83   PBD6 83

13 **(B)** Chronic granulomatous disease is characterized by reduced killing of ingested microbes because of inherited defects in the NADPH oxidase system. Two thirds of cases are X-linked, and one third are autosomal recessive. This system generates superoxide anions (O$_2^-$), essential for the subsequent production of microbicidal products such as H$_2$O$_2$, OH, and HOCl$^-$. Macrophage activation by interferon-γ is a key feature of granulomatous inflammation, which is typical of mycobacterial infections. Firm adhesions between leukocytes and endothelium are impaired in leukocyte adhesion deficiency type 1, in which there is a mutation in the β chain of integrins. Lysozyme contained in neutrophil granules is responsible for oxygen-independent killing of bacteria. Impaired opsonization can lead to infections in states of immunoglobulin deficiency.

BP7 43   BP6 32-33   PBD7 60-62   PBD6 62-65

14 (E) The respiratory, or oxidative, burst generates reactive oxygen species (i.e., superoxide anion) that are important in destruction of engulfed bacteria. Myelopoiesis does not depend on generation of superoxide. Endothelial attachment of neutrophils is aided by adhesion molecules on the endothelium and the neutrophil surface. These molecules include selectins and integrins. Bacteria are opsonized by complement C3b and IgG, allowing the bacteria to be more readily phagocytosed.

BP7 42-43 BP6 32-33 PBD7 60-62 PBD6 62-64

15 (C) This patient is experiencing an acute inflammatory response, with edema, erythema, and pain of short duration. Neutrophils form an exudate and release various proteases, which can produce liquefactive necrosis, starting at the mucosa and extending through the wall of the tube. This mechanism results in perforation. Fibroblasts are more likely participants in chronic inflammatory responses and in healing responses, generally appearing more than 1 week after the initial event. Langhans giant cells are a feature of granulomatous inflammation. Mononuclear infiltrates are more typical of chronic inflammation of the fallopian tube, in which rupture is less likely. Epithelial metaplasia is most likely to occur in the setting of chronic irritation with inflammation.

BP7 57-58 BP6 40-41 PBD7 77-78 PBD6 78-79

16 (D) Interferon-γ is secreted by activated T cells and is an important mediator of granulomatous inflammation. It causes activation of macrophages and their transformation into epithelioid cells and then giant cells. Tumor necrosis factor can be secreted by activated macrophages and induces activation of lymphocytes and proliferation of fibroblasts, which are other elements of a granuloma. Complement C3b acts as an opsonin in acute inflammatory reactions. Leukotriene B$_4$ induces chemotaxis in acute inflammatory processes. Interleukin-1 can be secreted by macrophages to produce a variety of effects, including fever, leukocyte adherence, fibroblast proliferation, and cytokine secretion.

BP7 54-55 BP6 42 PBD7 82-83 PBD6 82-83

17 (C) Myeloperoxidase is present in the azurophilic granules of neutrophils. It converts H_2O_2 into $HOCl^-$, a powerful oxidant and antimicrobial agent. Degranulation occurs when phagolysosomes are formed with engulfed bacteria in phagocytic vacuoles within the neutrophil cytoplasm. In contrast, prostaglandin production depends on a functioning cyclooxygenase pathway of arachidonic acid metabolism. Oxygen consumption with an oxidative or respiratory burst after phagocytosis is aided by glucose oxidation and activation of neutrophil NADPH oxidase, resulting in generation of superoxide that is converted by spontaneous dismutation to H_2O_2.

BP7 42-43 BP6 32-33 PBD7 60-62 PBD6 62-64

18 (C) Endothelial cells can release nitric oxide to produce vasodilation. Nitric oxide can also be administered to patients to promote vasodilation in areas of ischemic injury. Thromboxane A$_2$, platelet-activating factor, and leukotriene E$_4$ have vasoconstrictive properties. Bradykinin mainly increases vascular permeability and produces pain.

BP7 50-51 BP6 38-39 PBD7 72-73 PBD6 75

19 (F) Inflammation involving an epithelial surface may cause such extensive necrosis that the surface becomes eroded, forming an ulcer. If the inflammation continues, the ulcer can continue to penetrate downward into submucosa and muscularis. Alternatively, the ulcer may heal or may remain chronically inflamed. An abscess is a localized collection of neutrophils in tissues. A caseating granuloma is a granulomatous inflammation with central necrosis; the necrosis has elements of both liquefaction and coagulative necrosis. Chronic inflammation occurs when there is a preponderance of mononuclear cells, such as lymphocytes, macrophages, and plasma cells, in a process that has gone on for more than a few days—more likely weeks or months—or that accompanies repeated bouts of acute inflammation. Pus, or a purulent exudate, appears semiliquid and yellowish because of the large numbers of granulocytes present. A serous effusion is a watery-appearing transudate that resembles an ultrafiltrate of blood plasma, with a low cell and protein content.

BP7 58 BP6 45 PBD7 77 PBD6 85

20 (C) The formation of an exudate containing a significant amount of protein and cells depends on the "leakiness" of blood vessels, principally venules. The extravascular colloid osmotic pressure increases when exudation has occurred and the protein content of the extravascular space increases, causing extracellular fluid accumulation. The lymphatics scavenge exuded fluid with protein and reduce the amount of extravascular and extracellular fluid. Sodium and water retention helps drive transudation of fluid. Leukocytosis alone is not sufficient for exudation, because the leukocytes must be driven to emigrate from the vessels by chemotactic factors.

BP7 35-36 BP6 26-28 PBD7 50-52 PBD6 52-54

21 (B) The figure shows a granuloma with many epithelioid cells and prominent large Langhans giant cells. Macrophage stimulation and transformation to epithelioid cells and giant cells are characteristic of granuloma formation. Interferon-γ promotes the formation of epithelioid cells and giant cells. Complement C5a is chemotactic for neutrophils. Although occasional neutrophils are seen in granulomas, neutrophils do not form a major component of granulomatous inflammation. Bradykinin, released in acute inflammatory responses, results in pain. Macrophages can release nitric oxide to destroy other cells, but nitric oxide does not stimulate macrophages to form a granulomatous response. Prostaglandins are mainly involved in the causation of vasodilation and pain in acute inflammatory responses.

BP7 56-57 BP6 42-43 PBD7 82-83 PBD6 83-84

22 (B) These findings suggest an acute inflammatory process dominated by the presence of neutrophils. As this process resolves, the number of macrophages will increase. There may be few chronic inflammatory cells, including lymphocytes and plasma cells, but they are not necessarily absent from acute inflammatory processes. Eosinophils form the minority of acute inflammatory infiltrates unless allergic or parasitic stimuli are present.

BP7 57-58 BP6 45 PBD7 76-78 PBD6 84-85

23 (C) Interferon-γ secreted from lymphocytes stimulates monocytes and macrophages, which then secrete their own cytokines that further activate lymphocytes. Interferon-γ is also important in transforming macrophages into epithelioid cells in a granulomatous inflammatory response. Leukotriene B$_4$, generated in the lipoxygenase pathway of arachidonic acid metabolism, is a potent neutrophil chemotactic factor. Histamine released from mast cells is a potent vasodilator, increasing vascular permeability. Interleukin-1 and tumor necrosis factor, both produced by activated macrophages, mediate many systemic effects, including fever, metabolic wasting, and hypotension. Nitric oxide generated by macrophages aids in destruction of microorganisms; nitric oxide released from endothelium mediates vasodilation and inhibits platelet activation. Binding of agonists such as epinephrine, collagen, or thrombin to platelet surface receptors activates phospholipase C, which catalyzes the release of arachidonic acid from two of the major membrane phospholipids, phosphatidylinositol and phosphatidylcholine.

BP7 49, 55   BP6 42-43   PBD7 82-83   PBD6 82-83

24 **(D)** The formation of a fluid-filled cavity after an infection with *Staphylococcus aureus* suggests that liquefactive necrosis has occurred. The cavity is filled with tissue debris and viable and dead neutrophils (pus). Localized, pus-filled cavities are called abscesses. Some bacterial organisms, such as *S. aureus,* are more likely to be pyogenic, or pus-forming. With complete resolution, the structure of the lung remains almost unaltered. Lung tissue, unlike liver, is not capable of regeneration. Scarring or fibrosis may follow acute inflammation as the damaged tissue is replaced by fibrous connective tissue. Most bacterial pneumonias resolve, and progression to continued chronic inflammation is uncommon.

BP7 57-58   BP6 40-41   PBD7 77-78   PBD6 78-79, 85

25 **(E)** This patient has infective endocarditis with septic embolization, producing a cerebral abscess. The tissue destruction that accompanies abscess formation as part of acute inflammatory processes occurs from lysosomal enzymatic destruction, aided by release of reactive oxygen species. Nitric oxide generated by macrophages aids in destruction of infectious agents. Interferon-γ released from lymphocytes plays a major role in chronic and granulomatous inflammatory responses. Transforming growth factor-β formed by macrophages promotes fibrosis. Prostaglandins produced by endothelium promote vasodilation.

BP7 50-51   BP6 33   PBD7 77-78   PBD6 64-65

26 **(C)** Exudation of fluid from venules and capillaries is a key component of the acute inflammatory process. Several mechanisms of increased vascular permeability have been proposed, including formation of interendothelial gaps by contraction of endothelium. This is caused by mediators, such as histamine and leukotrienes. The vessels then become more "leaky," and the fluid leaves the intravascular space to accumulate extravascularly, forming effusions in body cavities or edema in tissues. Arteriolar vasoconstriction is a transient response to injury that diminishes blood loss. After neutrophils reach the site of tissue injury outside of the vascular space, they release lysosomal enzymes. Platelets adhere to damaged endothelium and promote hemostasis. Lymphatic obstruction results in the accumulation of protein-rich lymph and lymphocytes, producing a chylous effusion.

BP7 35-36   BP6 27-28   PBD7 50-52   PBD6 53-54

27 **(C)** The patient has immunoglobulin deficiency, which prevents opsonization and phagocytosis of microbes. Deficiency of integrins and selectins, or a defect in microtubules, would prevent adhesion and locomotion of neutrophils. H$_2$O$_2$ production is part of the oxygen-dependent killing mechanism. This mechanism is intact in this patient, because the neutrophils are able to kill bacteria when immunoglobulins in normal serum allow phagocytosis.

BP7 42   BP6 32   PBD7 58-59   PBD6 62-64

28 **(B)** Prostaglandins are produced through the cyclooxygenase pathway of arachidonic acid metabolism. Aspirin and other nonsteroidal anti-inflammatory drugs block the synthesis of prostaglandins, which can produce pain. Complement C1q is generated in the initial stage of complement activation, which can eventually result in cell lysis. Leukotrienes are generated by the lipoxygenase pathway, which is not blocked by aspirin. Histamine is mainly a vasodilator. Nitric oxide released from endothelium is a vasodilator.

BP7 47-48   BP6 37   PBD7 68-70   PBD6 70-71

29 **(E)** Bacterial infections often evoke an acute inflammatory response dominated by neutrophils. The extravasated neutrophils attempt to phagocytose and kill the bacteria. In the process, some neutrophils die, and the release of their lysosomal enzymes can cause liquefactive necrosis of the tissue. This liquefied tissue debris and the live and dead neutrophils comprise pus, or purulent exudate. Such an exudate is typical of bacterial infections that involve body cavities. Another term for purulent exudate in the pleural space is empyema. An abscess is a localized collection of neutrophils within tissues. Chronic inflammation occurs when there is a preponderance of mononuclear cells, such as lymphocytes, macrophages, and plasma cells, in a process that has gone on for more than a few days—more likely weeks or months—or that accompanies repeated bouts of acute inflammation. Edema refers to increased fluid collection within tissues, leading to tissue swelling. In fibrinous inflammation, exudation of blood proteins (including fibrinogen, which polymerizes to fibrin) gives a grossly shaggy appearance to surfaces overlying the inflammation. A serous effusion is a watery-appearing transudate that resembles an ultrafiltrate of blood plasma, with a low cell and protein content.

BP7 57-58   BP6 45   PBD7 77-78   PBD6 84-85

30 **(A)** During acute inflammation, neutrophils extravasate from the blood vessels. This process depends on adhesion molecules expressed on the neutrophils and endothelial cells. In the first stage of extravasation, the neutrophils "roll over" the endothelium. At this stage, the adhesion between the neutrophils and endothelial cells is not very strong. Rolling is mediated by binding of selectins to sialylated oligosaccharides. The next step, firm adhesion, is mediated by binding of integrins on the leukocytes to their receptors, intracellular adhesion molecule-1 or vascular cell adhesion molecule-1 (VCAM-1), on endothelial cells. Integrins have two chains, α and β. A genetic lack of β chains prevents firm adhesion of leukocytes to endothelial cells. Neutrophil migration to a site of infection depends on the presence of chemotactic factors that bind to the neutrophil and activate phospholipase C to begin a series of events that culminate in the influx of calcium, which triggers contractile proteins. The respiratory burst to kill phagocytized organisms is dependent on NADPH oxidase, and a deficiency of this enzyme leads to chronic granulomatous disease. Phagocytosis of opsonized organisms is dependent on engulfment, which requires contractile proteins in the neutrophil cytoplasm. Formation of $HOCL^-$ requires myeloperoxidase released from neutrophil granules.

BP7 38-39   BP6 28-29   PBD7 53-55   PBD6 57-59

31 (E) Macrophages contain cytokine-inducible nitric oxide synthase (iNOS), which generates nitric oxide. Nitric oxide, by itself and upon interaction with other reactive oxygen species, has antimicrobial activity. CD4 or CD8 lymphocytes can be the source for interferon-gamma (IFN-γ), which stimulates macrophage production of NOS. Endothelial cells contain a form of NOS (eNOS) that acts to promote vasodilation. B lymphocytes produce immunoglobulins that can opsonize bacteria. Basophils release histamine and arachidonic acid metabolites, which participate in the acute inflammatory process. Neutrophils can phagocytize microbes, but use NAPDH oxidase and enzymes other than NOS to kill the microbes. Natural killer cells have Fc receptors and can lyse IgG-coated target cells; they also generate IFN-γ.

BP7 50-51   BP6 38-39   PBD7 72-73   PBD6 75-76

Tissue Renewal and Repair: Regeneration, Healing, and Fibrosis

---

PBD7 Chapter 3: Tissue Renewal and Repair: Regeneration, Healing, and Fibrosis

PBD6 Chapter 4: Tissue Repair: Cellular Growth, Fibrosis, and Wound Healing

BP7 Chapter 3: Tissue Repair: Cell Regeneration and Fibrosis

BP6 Chapter 3: Repair: Cell Regeneration, Fibrosis, and Wound Healing

---

1 In an experiment, surgical incisions are made in a study group of laboratory rats. Observations about the wounds are recorded over a 2-week period using a variety of chemical mediators. Which of the following steps in the inflammatory-repair response is most likely affected by neutralization of transforming growth factor-β?

- ❑ (A) Leukocyte extravasation
- ❑ (B) Increase in vascular permeability
- ❑ (C) Production of collagen
- ❑ (D) Chemotaxis of lymphocytes
- ❑ (E) Migration of epithelial cells

2 A 60-year-old woman developed chest pain that persisted for 4 hours. A radiographic imaging procedure showed an apparent myocardial infarction involving a 3 × 4 cm area of the posterior left ventricular free wall. Laboratory findings showed serum creatine kinase of 600 U/L. The patient received both anti-arrhythmic and pressor agents to treat the decreased cardiac output while in the hospital. Which of the following pathologic findings would most likely be seen in the left ventricle 1 month later?

- ❑ (A) Abscess
- ❑ (B) Complete resolution
- ❑ (C) Coagulative necrosis
- ❑ (D) Nodular regeneration
- ❑ (E) Fibrous scar

3 An experiment infects one group of test animals with viral hepatitis. Two months later, complete recovery of the normal liver architecture is observed when the livers from these animals are examined microscopically. A second test group is infected with bacterial organisms, and after the same period of time, fibrous scars from resolving abscesses are seen microscopically in the livers. Which of the following factors best explains the different outcomes for the two test groups?

- ❑ (A) Nature of the etiologic agent
- ❑ (B) Extent of liver cell injury
- ❑ (C) Injury to the connective tissue framework
- ❑ (D) Location of the lesion
- ❑ (E) Extent of damage to the bile ducts

4 A 23-year-old woman receiving corticosteroid therapy for an autoimmune disease has an abscess on her upper outer right arm. She undergoes minor surgery to incise and drain the abscess, but the wound heals poorly over the next month. Which of the following aspects of wound healing is most likely to be deficient in this patient?

- ❑ (A) Re-epithelization
- ❑ (B) Fibroblast growth factor elaboration
- ❑ (C) Collagen deposition
- ❑ (D) Serine proteinase production
- ❑ (E) Neutrophil infiltration

5 A cesarean section is performed on a 20-year-old woman to deliver a term infant, and the lower abdominal incision is sutured. The sutures are removed 1 week later. Which of the following statements best describes the wound site at the time of suture removal?

- ❑ (A) Granulation tissue is still present
- ❑ (B) Collagen degradation exceeds synthesis
- ❑ (C) Wound strength is 80% of normal tissue
- ❑ (D) Type IV collagen predominates
- ❑ (E) No more wound strength will be gained

6 A 40-year-old man underwent laparotomy for a perforated sigmoid colon diverticulum. A wound infection complicated the postoperative course, and surgical wound dehiscence occurred. Primary closure was no longer possible, and the wound "granulated in." Six weeks later, the wound is only 10% of its original size. Which of the following processes best accounts for the observed decrease in wound size over the past 6 weeks?

- ❑ (A) Increase in synthesis of collagen
- ❑ (B) Myofibroblast contraction
- ❑ (C) Inhibition of metalloproteinases
- ❑ (D) Resolution of subcutaneous edema
- ❑ (E) Elaboration of adhesive glycoproteins

7 In an experiment involving observations on wound healing, researchers noted that intracytoplasmic cytoskeletal elements, including actin, interact with the extracellular matrix to promote cell attachment and migration in wound healing. Which of the following substances is most likely responsible for such interaction between the cytoskeleton and the extracellular matrix?

- ❑ (A) Epidermal growth factor
- ❑ (B) Fibronectin
- ❑ (C) Integrin
- ❑ (D) Platelet-derived growth factor
- ❑ (E) Type IV collagen
- ❑ (F) Vascular endothelial growth factor

8 In an experiment, release of epidermal growth factor into an area of denuded skin causes mitogenic stimulation of the skin epithelial cells. Which of the following proteins is most likely to be involved in transducing the mitogenic signal from the epidermal cell membrane to the nucleus?

- ❑ (A) G proteins
- ❑ (B) *RAS* proteins
- ❑ (C) Cyclin D
- ❑ (D) Cyclic AMP
- ❑ (E) Cyclin-dependent kinase

9 An experiment analyzes factors involved in the cell cycle during growth factor–induced cellular regeneration in a tissue culture. Cyclin B synthesis is induced; the cyclin B then binds and activates cyclin-dependent kinase 1 (CDK1). The active kinase produced by this process is most likely to control progression in which of the following phases of the cell cycle?

- ❑ (A) G_0 to G_1
- ❑ (B) G_1 to S
- ❑ (C) S to G_2
- ❑ (D) G_2 to M
- ❑ (E) M to G_1

10 An experiment is conducted involving cellular aspects of wound healing. Components of the extracellular matrix are analyzed to determine their sites of production and their binding patterns to other tissue components. Which of the following molecules synthesized by fibroblasts can best bind to cellular integrins and extracellular collagen and attach epidermal basal cells to basement membrane?

- ❑ (A) Heparin
- ❑ (B) Dermatan sulfate
- ❑ (C) Procollagen
- ❑ (D) Fibronectin
- ❑ (E) Hyaluronic acid

11 An 18-year-old man lacerated his left hand and required sutures. The sutures were removed 1 week later. Wound healing continued, but the site became disfigured by a prominent raised, nodular scar that developed over the next 2 months. Which of the following terms best describes the process that occurred during this 2-month period?

- ❑ (A) Organization
- ❑ (B) Dehiscence
- ❑ (C) Resolution
- ❑ (D) Keloid formation
- ❑ (E) Secondary union

12 An experiment involves factors controlling wound healing. Skin ulcerations are observed, and the factors involved in the healing process are analyzed. Which of the following factors is most likely to be effective in promoting angiogenesis?

- ❑ (A) Platelet-derived growth factor
- ❑ (B) Epidermal growth factor
- ❑ (C) Basic fibroblast growth factor
- ❑ (D) Endostatin
- ❑ (E) Interleukin-1

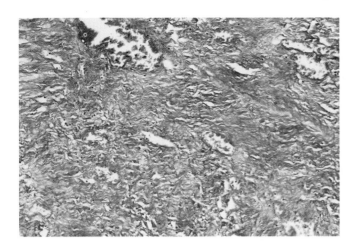

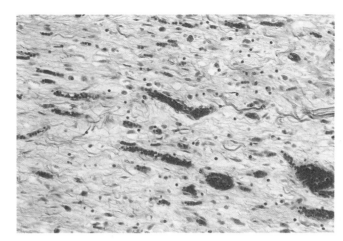

13 A 24-year-old man with acute appendicitis undergoes surgical removal of the inflamed appendix. The incision site is sutured. A trichrome-stained section of the site is shown in the figure above. How long after the surgery would this appearance most likely be seen?

❑ (A) 1 day
❑ (B) 2 to 3 days
❑ (C) 4 to 5 days
❑ (D) 2 weeks
❑ (E) 1 month

14 A 50-year-old woman tests positive for hepatitis A antibody. The serum AST level is 275 U/L, and ALT is 310 U/L. One month later, these enzyme levels have returned to normal. Which phase of the cell cycle best describes the hepatocytes 1 month after infection?

❑ (A) G_0
❑ (B) G_1
❑ (C) S
❑ (D) G_2
❑ (E) M

15 In an experiment, the role of low density lipoprotein (LDL) receptors in uptake of lipids in the liver is studied. A mouse model is created in which the LDL receptor gene is not expressed in the liver. For creating such a "knock out" mouse, which of the following cells will be most useful?

❑ (A) Adult bone marrow mesenchymal progenitor cells
❑ (B) Embryonic stem cells in culture
❑ (C) Hepatic oval cells
❑ (D) Hematopoietic stem cells
❑ (E) Regenerating hepatocytes

16 In an experiment, glass beads are embolized into the coronary arteries of rats, resulting in myocardial injury. After 7 days, sections of the myocardium are studied using light microscopy. The microscopic appearance of one of these sections is shown in the figure above. Which of the following mediators is most likely being expressed to produce this appearance?

❑ (A) Epidermal growth factor
❑ (B) Interleukin-2
❑ (C) Leukotriene-B_4
❑ (D) Thromboxane A_2
❑ (E) Vascular endothelial growth factor
❑ (F) Tumor necrosis factor

17 An experiment is conducted in which the time sequence of events in wound healing is analyzed. Histologic sections are produced from samples of the tissue at the site of a small superficial skin incision in laboratory animals. During the first week, the number of macrophages that are activated to phagocytize tissue debris increases. Which of the following signaling molecules is most likely to play a significant role in producing this finding?

❑ (A) Acetylcholine
❑ (B) Cyclic AMP
❑ (C) Heparan sulfate
❑ (D) Interferon-γ
❑ (E) Transforming growth factor-β

18 In an experiment, various soluble mediators are added to a cell culture containing epidermal cells to determine which of the mediators might be useful for promoting epidermal cell growth. When epidermal growth factor (EGF) is added, it binds to epidermal cell surface receptors, inducing *RAS* protein activation, with subsequent transcription factor translocation and DNA transcription activation. This effect in the epidermal cells is most likely to be mediated through which of the following intracellular pathways?

❑ (A) Calcium ion channel
❑ (B) Cyclic AMP
❑ (C) Cycline-dependent kinase
❑ (D) JAK/STAT system
❑ (E) Mitogen-activated protein kinase

ANSWERS

1 **(C)** Transforming growth factor-β (TGF-β) stimulates many steps in fibrogenesis, including fibroblast chemotaxis and production of collagen by fibroblasts, while inhibiting degradation of collagen. All of the other steps listed are unaffected by TGF-β.

BP7 73-74   BP6 51   PBD7 96-97   PBD6 98

2 **(E)** The elevated creatine kinase level indicates that myocardial necrosis has occurred. The destruction of myocardial fibers precludes complete resolution. The area of myocardial necrosis is gradually replaced by a fibrous scar. Liquefactive necrosis with abscess formation is not a feature of ischemic myocardial injury. Coagulative necrosis is typical of myocardial infarction, but after 1 month, a scar would be present. Nodular regeneration is typical of hepatocyte injury, because hepatocytes are stable cells.

BP7 72   BP6 58   PBD7 110-111   PBD6 111

3 **(C)** Hepatocytes are stable cells with an extensive ability to regenerate. However, the ability to restore normal architecture of an organ such as the liver depends on the viability of the supporting connective tissue framework. If the connective tissue cells are not injured, hepatocyte regeneration can restore normal liver architecture. This regeneration occurs in many cases of viral hepatitis. A liver abscess is associated with liquefactive necrosis of hepatocytes and the supporting connective tissue. It heals by scarring. The other options listed may explain the amount of liver injury but not the nature of the response.

BP7 63-64   BP6 48-49   PBD7 90-91   PBD6 91

4 **(C)** Glucocorticoids inhibit wound healing by impairing collagen synthesis. This is a desirable side effect if the amount of scarring is to be reduced, but it results in the delayed healing of surgical wounds. Re-epithelization, in part driven by epidermal growth factor, is not affected by corticosteroid therapy. Angiogenesis driven by fibroblast growth factor is not significantly affected by corticosteroids. Serine proteinases are important in wound remodeling. Neutrophil infiltration is not prevented by glucocorticoids.

BP7 76   BP6 57-58   PBD7 114   PBD6 110

5 **(A)** At 1 week, wound healing is incomplete, and granulation tissue is still present. More collagen will be synthesized in the following weeks. Wound strength will peak at about 80% by 3 months. Type IV collagen is found in basement membranes.

BP7 75-76   BP6 56-57   PBD7 111-112   PBD6 108-109

6 **(B)** Wound contraction is a characteristic feature of healing by second intention that occurs in larger wounds. Collagen synthesis helps fill the defect but does not contract it. The inhibition of metalloproteinases leads to decreased degradation of collagen and impaired connective tissue remodeling in wound repair. Edema diminishes over time, but this does not result in much contraction. Adhesive glycoproteins such as fibronectin help to maintain a cellular scaffolding for growth and repair, but they do not contract.

BP7 75-76   BP6 56   PBD7 113   PBD6 108-109

7 **(C)** Integrins interact with the extracellular matrix proteins (e.g., fibronectin). Engagement of integrins by extracellular matrix proteins leads to the formation of focal adhesions at which integrins link to intracellular cytoskeletal elements such as actin. These interactions lead to intracellular signals that modulate cell growth, differentiation, and migration during wound healing. Epidermal growth factor stimulates epithelial cell and fibroblast proliferation. Platelet-derived growth factor (PDGF) can be produced by endothelium, macrophages, and smooth muscle cells, as well as by platelets; PDGF mediates migration and proliferation of fibroblasts and smooth muscle cells, as well as migration of monocytes. Type IV collagen is found in basement membranes on which cells are anchored. Vascular endothelial growth factor promotes angiogenesis (capillary proliferation) through endothelial cell proliferation and migration in a healing response.

BP7 67-69   BP6 52   PBD7 104-106   PBD6 100-101

8 **(B)** *RAS* proteins transduce signals from growth factor receptors, such as epidermal growth factor, that have intrinsic tyrosine kinase activity. G proteins perform a similar function for G-protein–linked, seven-spanning receptors. Cyclic AMP is an effector in the G-protein signaling pathway. Cyclins and cyclin-dependent kinases regulate the cell cycle in the nucleus.

BP7 65-66   BP6 51   PBD7 98-99   PBD6 93-94

9 **(D)** Cyclin-dependent kinase 1 (CDK1) controls an extremely important transition point, the G_2 to M transition during the cell cycle, which can be regulated by CDK inhibitors. The other checkpoints are regulated by a distinct set of proteins.

BP7 62-63   BP6 50   PBD7 100-101   PBD6 96

10 **(D)** Fibronectin is a key component of the extracellular matrix and has a structure that looks like a paper clip. Fibronectin can be synthesized by monocytes, fibroblasts, and endothelium. Heparin that is infused has an anticoagulant function. Dermatan sulfate, a glycosaminoglycan, acts to form a gel that provides resilience and lubrication. Procollagen produced by fibroblasts is formed into ropelike strands of collagen that provide tensile strength. Hyaluronic acid binds water to form a gelatinous extracellular matrix.

BP7 69   BP6 52-53   PBD7 103-104   PBD6 100-103

11 **(D)** The healing process sometimes results in an exuberant production of collagen, giving rise to a keloid. This tendency may run in families. Organization occurs as granulation tissue is replaced by fibrous tissue. Dehiscence occurs when a wound pulls apart. If normal tissue architecture is restored, then resolution of inflammation has occurred. Secondary union describes the process by which large wounds fill in and contract.

BP7 76   BP6 58   PBD7 115   PBD6 110

12 **(C)** Basic fibroblast growth factor is a potent inducer of angiogenesis. It can participate in all steps of angiogenesis. Epidermal growth factor and interleukin-1 have no angiogenic activity. Platelet-derived growth factor plays a role in vascular remodeling. Endostatin is an inhibitor of angiogenesis.

BP7 72   BP6 51   PBD7 95-96   PBD6 104-105

13 **(E)** The figure shows dense collagen with some remaining dilated blood vessels, typical of the final phase of wound healing, which is extensive by the end of the first month. On day 1, the wound is filled only with fibrin and inflammatory cells. Macrophages and granulation tissue are seen 2 to 3 days postoperatively. Neovascularization is most prominent by days 4 and 5. Collagen is prominent, and fewer vessels and inflammatory cells are seen by week 2.

BP7 75   BP6 56   PBD7 112-113   PBD6 104, 108

14 **(A)** Hepatocytes are quiescent (stable) cells that can reenter the cell cycle and proliferate in response to hepatic injury, enabling the liver to partially regenerate. Acute hepatitis results in hepatocyte necrosis, marked by elevations in AST and AST. After the acute process has ended, cells return to the G_0 phase, and the liver becomes quiescent again.

BP7 64   BP6 48-49   PBD7 101-103   PBD6 90-91

15 **(B)** Embryonic stem (ES) cells are multipotent and can give rise to all cells, including hepatocytes. Gene targeting to produce "knock out" mice is done in cultures of ES cells that are then injected into mouse blastocysts and then implanted into the uterus of a surrogate mother. Mesenchymal stem cells are also multipotential but not useful for gene targeting. Hematopoietic stem cells can give rise to all hematopoietic cells, but not other types of cells. Hepatocytes and oval cells within the liver can only give rise to liver cells.

PBD7 91

16 **(E)** The figure shows a subacute infarction with granulation tissue formation containing numerous capillaries stimulated by vascular endothelial growth factor, representing a healing response. Epidermal growth factor aids in re-epithelialization of a surface wound. Interleukin-2 mediates lymphocyte activation. Leukotriene B_4 mediates vasoconstriction and bronchoconstriction. Thromboxane A_2 aids vasoconstriction and platelet aggregation. Tumor necrosis factor induces endothelial activation as well as many responses that occur secondary to inflammation, including fever, loss of appetite, sleep disturbances, hypotension, and increased corticosteroid production.

BP7 71-72   BP6 54   PBD7 96, 107-108   PBD6 104-105

17 **(D)** Interferon-γ is a cytokine secreted by lymphocytes at the site of inflammation; it has a paracrine effect that causes transformation of monocytes to activated macrophages. Acetylcholine is a neurotransmitter that does not act on inflammatory cells. Cyclic AMP acts as a "second messenger" within a cell. Heparan sulfate is a component of the extracellular matrix that does not have a signaling function. Transforming growth factor-β has an inhibitory function on growth.

BP7 65-66   PBD7 97

18 **(E)** The mitogen-activated (MAP)–kinase cascade is involved in signaling from activation via cell surface receptors for growth factors. This pathway is particularly important for signaling of epidermal growth factor and fibroblast growth factor. Ligand binding, such as occurs with acetylcholine at a nerve-muscle junction, alters the conformation of ion channel receptors to allow flow of specific ions such as calcium into the cell, changing the electric potential across the cell membrane. Cyclic AMP is a "second messenger" that is typically activated via ligand binding to receptors with seven transmembrane segments that associate with GTP-hydrolyzing proteins; chemokine receptors function in this fashion. Cyclin-dependent kinases act within the nucleus. JAK/STAT pathways are typically recruited by cytokine receptors.

BP7 65-66   BP6 49-50   PBD7 98-99   PBD6 93-94

Hemodynamic Disorders, Thromboebolic Disease, and Shock

PBD7 Chapter 4: Hemodynamic Disorders, Thromboembolic Disease, and Shock

PBD6 Chapter 5: Hemodynamic Disorders, Thrombosis, and Shock

BP7 and BP6 Chapter 4: Hemodynamic Disorders, Thrombosis, and Shock

1 While shaving one morning, a 23-year-old man nicks his lip with a razor. Seconds after the injury, the bleeding stops. Which of the following mechanisms is most likely to reduce blood loss from a small dermal arteriole?

❑ (A) Protein C activation
❑ (B) Vasoconstriction
❑ (C) Platelet aggregation
❑ (D) Neutrophil chemotaxis
❑ (E) Fibrin polymerization

2 A 73-year-old man was diagnosed 1 year ago with pancreatic adenocarcinoma. He now sees his physician because of a transient ischemic attack. On auscultation of the chest, a heart murmur is heard. Echocardiography shows a 1-cm nodular lesion on the superior aspect of the anterior mitral valve leaflet. The valve leaflet appears to be intact. The blood culture is negative. Which of the following terms best describes this mitral valve lesion?

❑ (A) Adenocarcinoma
❑ (B) Atheroma
❑ (C) Chronic passive congestion
❑ (D) Mural thrombus
❑ (E) Petechial hemorrhage
❑ (F) Phlebothrombosis
❑ (G) Vegetation

3 A 21-year-old woman sustains multiple injuries, including fractures of the right femur and tibia and the left humerus, in a motor vehicle collision. She is admitted to the hospital, and the fractures are stabilized surgically. Soon after admission to the hospital, she is in stable condition. However, 2 days later, she suddenly ·becomes severely dyspneic. Which of the following complications is the most likely cause of this sudden respiratory difficulty?

❑ (A) Right hemothorax
❑ (B) Pulmonary edema
❑ (C) Fat embolism
❑ (D) Cardiac tamponade
❑ (E) Pulmonary infarction

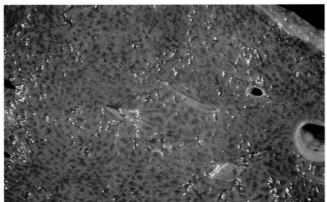

Courtesy of Dr. James Crawford, Department of Pathology, Brigham and Women's Hospital, Boston, MA.

4 For the past week, a 61-year-old man has had increasing levels of serum AST and ALT. On physical examination, he has lower leg swelling with grade 2+ pitting edema to the knees and prominent jugular venous distention to the level of the mandible. Based on the gross appearance of the liver, seen in the figure, which of the following underlying conditions is most likely to be present?

- ❏ (A) Thrombocytopenia
- ❏ (B) Portal vein thrombosis
- ❏ (C) Chronic renal failure
- ❏ (D) Common bile duct obstruction
- ❏ (E) Congestive heart failure

5 A 55-year-old woman has had discomfort and swelling of the left leg for the past week. On physical examination, the leg is slightly difficult to move, but on palpation, there is no pain. A venogram shows thrombosis of deep left leg veins. Which of the following mechanisms is most likely to cause this condition?

- ❏ (A) Turbulent blood flow
- ❏ (B) Nitric oxide release
- ❏ (C) Ingestion of aspirin
- ❏ (D) Hypercalcemia
- ❏ (E) Immobilization

6 A 25-year-old woman who has had altered consciousness and slurred speech for the past 24 hours is brought to the emergency department. A head CT scan shows a right temporal hemorrhagic infarction. Cerebral angiography shows a distal right middle cerebral arterial occlusion. Within the past 3 years, she has had an episode of pulmonary embolism. A pregnancy 18 months ago ended in miscarriage. Laboratory studies show a false-positive serologic test for syphilis, normal prothrombin time, elevated partial thromboplastin time, and normal platelet count. Which of the following is the most likely cause of these findings?

- ❏ (A) Disseminated intravascular coagulation
- ❏ (B) Factor V mutation
- ❏ (C) Hypercholesterolemia
- ❏ (D) Lupus anticoagulant
- ❏ (E) Von Willebrand disease

7 A 66-year-old woman comes to the emergency department 3 hours after the onset of chest pain that radiates to her neck and left arm. She is diaphoretic and hypotensive; the serum troponin I level is elevated. Thrombolytic therapy is begun. Which of the following drugs is most likely to be administered?

- ❏ (A) Tissue plasminogen activator
- ❏ (B) Aspirin
- ❏ (C) Heparin
- ❏ (D) Nitric oxide
- ❏ (E) Vitamin K

8 A 49-year-old man is in stable condition after an infarction of the anterior left ventricular wall. He receives therapy with antiarrhythmic and pressor agents. Three days later, he develops severe breathlessness, and an echocardiogram shows a markedly decreased ejection fraction. He dies 2 hours later. At autopsy, which of the following microscopic changes is most likely to be present in the lungs?

- ❏ (A) Congestion of alveolar capillaries with fibrin and neutrophils in alveoli
- ❏ (B) Congestion of alveolar capillaries with transudate in alveoli
- ❏ (C) Fibrosis of alveolar walls with hemosiderin-laden macrophages in alveoli
- ❏ (D) Multiple areas of subpleural hemorrhagic necrosis
- ❏ (E) Purulent exudate in the pleural space
- ❏ (F) Purulent exudate in the mainstem bronchi

9 A 27-year-old man is on a scuba diving trip to the Caribbean and descends to a depth of 50 m in the Blue Hole off the coast of Belize. After 30 minutes, he has a malfunction in his equipment and quickly returns to the boat on the surface. He soon experiences difficulty breathing, with dyspnea and substernal chest pain, followed by a severe headache and vertigo. About 1 hour later, he develops severe, painful myalgias and arthralgias. These symptoms abate within 24 hours. Which of the following mechanisms is the most likely cause of these symptoms?

- ❏ (A) Disseminated intravascular coagulation
- ❏ (B) Systemic vasodilation
- ❏ (C) Venous thrombosis
- ❏ (D) Tissue nitrogen emboli
- ❏ (E) Fat globules in arterioles

10 A 39-year-old woman comes to the physician because she has noticed a lump in her breast. Over the past 2 months, the left breast has become slightly enlarged compared with the right breast. On physical examination, the skin overlying the left breast is thickened, reddish-orange, and pitted. Mammography shows a 3-cm underlying density, and a fine-needle aspirate of the density indicates carcinoma. Which of the following mechanisms best explains the gross appearance of the left breast?

- ❏ (A) Venous thrombosis
- ❏ (B) Lymphatic obstruction
- ❏ (C) Ischemia
- ❏ (D) Chronic passive congestion
- ❏ (E) Chronic inflammation

11 A 29-year-old woman has a history of frequent nose-bleeds and increased menstrual flow. On physical examination, petechiae and purpura are present on the skin of her extremities. Laboratory studies show normal partial thromboplastin time, prothrombin time, and platelet count, and decreased von Willebrand factor activity. This patient most likely has a derangement in which of the following steps in hemostasis?

❑ (A) Vasoconstriction
❑ (B) Platelet adhesion
❑ (C) Platelet aggregation
❑ (D) Prothrombin generation
❑ (E) Prothrombin inhibition
❑ (F) Fibrin polymerization

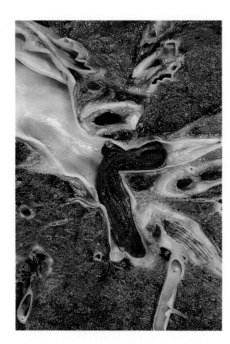

12 A 70-year-old man who was hospitalized 3 weeks ago for a cerebral infarction is ambulating for the first time. Within minutes of returning to his hospital room, he has sudden onset of dyspnea with diaphoresis. He cannot be resuscitated. The gross appearance of the hilum of the left lung at autopsy is shown in the figure. Which of the following risk factors most likely contributed to this finding?

❑ (A) Venous stasis
❑ (B) Pulmonary arterial atherosclerosis
❑ (C) Lupus anticoagulant
❑ (D) Bronchopneumonia
❑ (E) Factor V mutation

13 A 25-year-old woman has had multiple episodes of deep venous thrombosis during the past 10 years and one episode of pulmonary thromboembolism during the past year. Prothrombin time, partial thromboplastin time, platelet count, and platelet function studies are all normal. Which of the following risk factors has most likely contributed to the patient's condition?

❑ (A) Factor V mutation
❑ (B) Antithrombin III deficiency
❑ (C) Mutation in protein C
❑ (D) Hyperhomocysteinemia
❑ (E) Smoking cigarettes

14 A 76-year-old woman is hospitalized after falling and fracturing her left femoral trochanter. Two weeks later, the left leg is swollen, particularly below the knee. She experiences pain on movement of the leg; on palpation, there is tenderness. Which of the following complications is most likely to occur after these events?

❑ (A) Gangrenous necrosis of the foot
❑ (B) Hematoma of the thigh
❑ (C) Disseminated intravascular coagulation
❑ (D) Pulmonary thromboembolism
❑ (E) Fat embolism

15 A 12-year-old boy has a history of multiple soft tissue hemorrhages and acute upper airway obstruction from hematoma formation in the neck. On physical examination, he has decreased range of motion of the large joints, particularly the knees and ankles. He has no petechiae or purpura of the skin. Laboratory studies show normal prothrombin time, elevated partial thromboplastin time, and normal platelet count, but markedly decreased factor VIII activity. Which of the following mechanisms best describes the development of this disease?

❑ (A) Decrease in a reaction accelerator (cofactor) in the coagulation cascade
❑ (B) Decrease in phospholipid necessary for assembly of coagulation factors, cofactors, and calcium
❑ (C) Failure of platelet aggregation
❑ (D) Failure of fibrin polymerization
❑ (E) Inability to neutralize antithrombin III
❑ (F) Inability of platelets to release thromboxane A_2

16 Within 1 hour after a gunshot wound to the abdomen, a 19-year-old man exhibits tachycardia. His skin is cool and clammy to the touch, and blood pressure is 80/30 mm Hg. Which of the following organ-specific changes is most likely to occur within 2 days after this injury?

❑ (A) Acute hepatic infarction
❑ (B) Cerebral basal ganglia hemorrhage
❑ (C) Renal passive congestion
❑ (D) Pulmonary diffuse alveolar damage
❑ (E) Gangrenous necrosis of the lower legs

17 A 56-year-old man with a history of diabetes mellitus goes to the emergency department because he has had left-sided chest pain that radiates to the arm for the past 5 hours. Serial measurements of serum creatine kinase-MB levels show an elevated level 24 hours after the onset of pain. Partial thromboplastin time and prothrombin time are normal. Coronary angiography shows occlusion of the left anterior descending artery. Which of the following mechanisms is the most likely cause of thrombosis in this patient?

❑ (A) Stasis of blood flow
❑ (B) Damage to endothelium
❑ (C) Decreased production of tissue plasminogen activator by intact endothelial cells
❑ (D) Decreased antithrombin III level
❑ (E) Mutation in factor V gene
❑ (F) Circulating antibody acting as an inhibitor to coagulation

18 An experiment is conducted in which platelet function is analyzed. A substance is obtained from the dense bodies (delta granules) of normal pooled platelets from healthy blood donors. When this substance is added to platelets obtained from patients with a bleeding disorder, no platelet aggregation occurs. Adding the substance to platelets from a normal control group induces platelet aggregation. Which of the following substances is most likely to produce this effect?

❑ (A) Adenosine diphosphate
❑ (B) Antithrombin III
❑ (C) Fibronectin
❑ (D) Fibrinogen
❑ (E) Plasminogen
❑ (F) Thromboxane A_2
❑ (G) Von Willebrand factor

19 In an experiment, thrombus formation is studied in areas of vascular damage. After a thrombus forms in an area of vascular injury, the propagation of the thrombus to normal arteries is prevented. Researchers identify a substance that diminishes thrombus propagation by binding to thrombin, converting it to a procoagulant that activates protein C. Which of the following substances is most likely to produce this effect?

❑ (A) Calcium
❑ (B) Fibrin
❑ (C) Platelet factor 4
❑ (D) Prothrombin
❑ (E) Thrombomodulin
❑ (F) Tumor necrosis factor

20 A 44-year-old man has an acute myocardial infarction. Four days later, his ejection fraction is 25%, and cardiac output is reduced. The patient becomes increasingly dyspneic, and a chest radiograph shows bilateral pulmonary edema. These pulmonary findings are most likely caused by which of the following mechanisms?

❑ (A) Lymphatic obstruction
❑ (B) Decreased plasma osmotic pressure
❑ (C) Decreased central venous pressure
❑ (D) Increased hydrostatic pressure
❑ (E) Acute inflammation

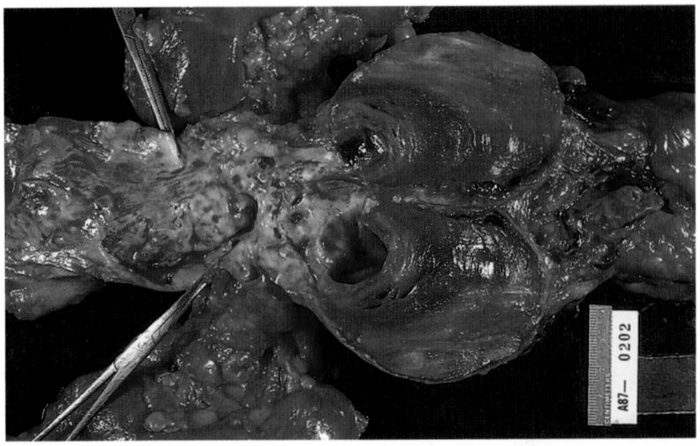

21 A 70-year-old man with a history of diabetes mellitus died of an acute myocardial infarction. The appearance at autopsy of the aorta, opened longitudinally, is seen in the figure above. Which of the following complications associated with aortic disease would most likely have been present during his life?

❑ (A) Renal infarction
❑ (B) Pulmonary thromboembolism
❑ (C) Edema of the left leg
❑ (D) Thrombocytopenia
❑ (E) Popliteal arterial occlusion

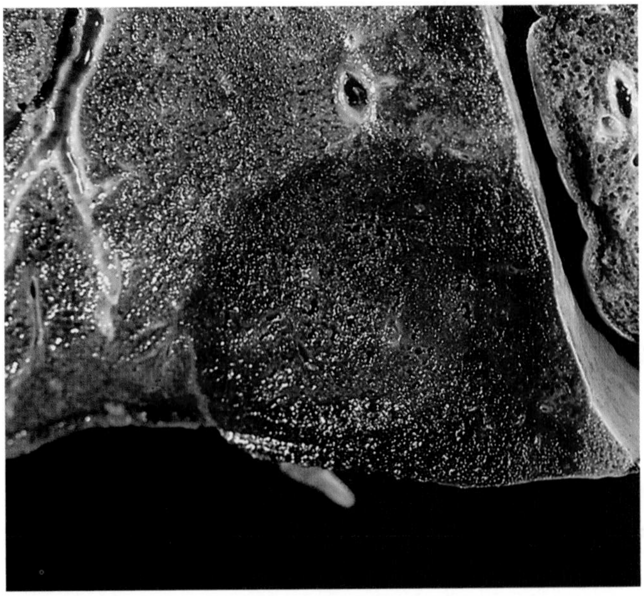

22 A 49-year-old man with congestive heart failure develops *Streptococcus pneumoniae* after a bout of influenza. After recuperating for 2 weeks, he develops pleuritic chest pain. The pain is caused by the development of the lesion shown in the figure above. Which of the following events has most likely occurred?

❑ (A) Pulmonary infarction
❑ (B) Chronic pulmonary congestion
❑ (C) Pulmonary edema
❑ (D) Acute pulmonary congestion
❑ (E) Pulmonary venous thrombosis

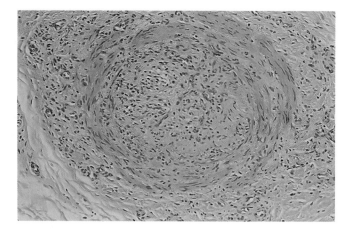

23 A 58-year-old man with hyperlipidemia and severe atherosclerosis has had anginal pain for the past 24 hours. Laboratory findings show no increase in serum troponin I or creatine kinase-MB. Two weeks later, he is in stable condition and has no chest pain, but a small artery in the epicardium has undergone the changes seen in the figure. Which of the following terms best describes this finding in the epicardial artery?

❏ (A) Air embolus
❏ (B) Cholesterol embolus
❏ (C) Chronic passive congestion
❏ (D) Fat embolus
❏ (E) Mural thrombus
❏ (F) Organization with recanalization
❏ (G) Phlebothrombosis

24 A 78-year-old woman falls in the bathtub and strikes the back of her head. Over the next 24 hours, she becomes increasingly somnolent. A head CT scan shows an accumulation of fluid beneath the dura, compressing the left cerebral hemisphere. Which of the following terms best describes this collection of fluid?

❏ (A) Hematoma
❏ (B) Purpura
❏ (C) Congestion
❏ (D) Petechia
❏ (E) Ecchymosis

25 A 28-year-old woman with a 15 year history of recurrent thromobosis from a prothrombin gene mutation develops septicemia following a urinary tract infection with *Pseudomonas aeruginosa*. Despite aggressive therapy, she dies of multiple organ failure. At autopsy, which of the following organs is most likely to be spared from the effects of ischemic injury?

❏ (A) Brain
❏ (B) Liver
❏ (C) Kidney
❏ (D) Heart
❏ (E) Spleen

26 A 58-year-old woman diagnosed with breast cancer in the left breast underwent a mastectomy with axillary lymph node dissection. Postoperatively, she developed marked swelling of the left arm that has persisted for several months.

On physical examination, her temperature is 36.9°C. The left arm is not tender or erythematous, and it is it not painful to movement or touch. Which of the following best describes the mechanism for these findings?

❏ (A) Cellulitis
❏ (B) Congestive heart failure
❏ (C) Decreased plasma oncotic pressure
❏ (D) Lymphedema
❏ (E) Sodium and water retention
❏ (F) Phlebothrombosis

27 A 61-year-old woman has had a fever and felt faint for the past 2 days. On physical examination, her temperature is 38.4°C, pulse 101/min, respirations 17/min, and blood pressure 85/40 mm Hg. She has marked peripheral vasodilation. The serum lactic acid level is 6.8 mg/dL. Which of the following laboratory findings is most likely to be related to the cause of this clinical condition?

❏ (A) Elevated serum creatine kinase
❏ (B) Decreased PO_2 on blood gas measurement
❏ (C) Blood culture positive for *Escherichia coli*
❏ (D) Increased blood urea nitrogen
❏ (E) Decreased hematocrit

28 A 71-year-old man died of pneumonia following a cerebral hemorrhage that left him bedridden for 3 months. At autopsy, a section through a branch of the right main pulmonary artery shows a band of fibrous connective tissue that extends across the lumen. Which of the following events best explains the presence of this finding?

❏ (A) Inflammation with exudation
❏ (B) Hemorrhage
❏ (C) Passive congestion
❏ (D) Ischemia
❏ (E) Hypertension
❏ (F) Thromboembolism

29 A 59-year-old obese woman with a history of diabetes mellitus had a myocardial infarction 3 months ago. She is now taking a low dose of aspirin to reduce the risk of arterial thrombosis. On which of the following steps in hemostasis does aspirin have its greatest effect?

❏ (A) Adhesion of platelets to collagen
❏ (B) Aggregation of platelets
❏ (C) Production of tissue factor
❏ (D) Synthesis of von Willebrand factor
❏ (E) Synthesis of antithrombin III

30 A 60-year-old woman fractured the right femur, pelvis, and left humerus in a motor vehicle collision. The fractures were stabilized, and the patient's recovery was uneventful. During a physical examination 3 weeks later, the physician observes swelling and warmth in the left leg, and there is local pain and tenderness in the left thigh. Which of the following processes is most likely occurring in the femoral vein?

❏ (A) Anasarca
❏ (B) Chronic passive congestion
❏ (C) Fat embolus formation
❏ (D) Mural thrombosis
❏ (E) Organization with recanalization
❏ (F) Phlebothrombosis
❏ (G) Vegetation

31 A 45-year-old woman who works as a bank teller notices at the end of her 8-hour shift that her lower legs and feet are swollen, although there was no swelling at the beginning of the day. There is no pain or erythema associated with this swelling. The woman is otherwise healthy and takes no medications; laboratory testing reveals normal liver and renal function. Which of the following mechanisms best explains this phenomenon?

❑ (A) Increased hydrostatic pressure
❑ (B) Lymphatic obstruction
❑ (C) Secondary aldosteronism
❑ (D) Hypoalbuminemia
❑ (E) Excessive water intake

32 A 23-year-old woman with an uncomplicated pregnancy develops sudden dyspnea with cyanosis and hypotension during routine vaginal delivery of a term infant. She has a generalized seizure and becomes comatose. Her condition does not improve over the next 2 days. Which of the following findings is most likely to be present in the peripheral pulmonary arteries?

❑ (A) Aggregates of red blood cells
❑ (B) Amniotic fluid
❑ (C) Fat globules
❑ (D) Gas bubbles
❑ (E) Thromboemboli

ANSWERS

1 **(B)** The initial response to injury is arteriolar vasoconstriction, but this is transient and the coagulation mechanism must be initiated to maintain hemostasis. Protein C is involved in anticoagulation to counteract clotting. Platelet aggregation occurs with release of factors such as ADP, but this takes several minutes. Neutrophils are not essential to hemostasis. Fibrin polymerization is part of secondary hemostasis after the vascular injury is initially closed.

BP7 84-85   BP6 65-66   PBD7 124-125   PBD6 119

2 **(G)** A thrombotic mass that forms on a cardiac valve (or less commonly, on the cardiac mural endocardium) is known as a vegetation. Such vegetations may produce thromboemboli. Vegetations on the right-sided heart valves may embolize to the lungs; those on the left embolize systemically to organs such as the brain, spleen, and kidney. A so-called paradoxical embolus occurs when a right-sided cardiac thrombus crosses a patent foramen ovale and enters the systemic arterial circulation. Patients with cancer may have a hypercoagulable state (such as Trousseau syndrome, with malignant neoplasms) that favors the development of arterial and venous thromboses. An adenocarcinoma is a malignant neoplasm that arises from glandular epithelium, forming a mass lesion; endocardial metastases are quite rare. Atheromas form in arteries and do not typically involve the cardiac valves. Chronic passive congestion refers to capillary, sinusoidal, or venous stasis of blood within an organ such as the lungs or liver. Mural thrombi are thrombi that form on the surfaces of the heart or large arteries. The term is typically reserved for large thrombi in a cardiac chamber or dilated aorta or large aortic branch; it is not used to describe thrombotic lesions on cardiac valves. A petechial hemorrhage is a grossly pinpoint hemorrhage. Phlebothrombosis occurs when stasis in large veins promotes thrombosis formation.

BP7 92   BP6 71, 326   PBD7 133   PBD6 127

3 **(C)** The mechanism for fat embolism is unknown, in particular, why onset of symptoms is delayed from 1 to 3 days after the initial injury (or even 1 week for cerebral symptoms). The cumulative effect of many small fat globules filling peripheral pulmonary arteries is the same as one large pulmonary thromboembolus. Hemothorax and cardiac tamponade would be immediate complications after traumatic injury, not delayed events. Pulmonary edema severe enough to cause dyspnea would be unlikely to occur in hospitalized patients because fluid status is closely monitored. Pulmonary infarction may cause dyspnea, but pulmonary thromboembolus from deep venous thrombosis is typically a complication of a longer hospitalization.

BP7 96   BP6 74   PBD7 136-137   PBD6 130-131

4 **(E)** The figure shows a so-called nutmeg liver caused by chronic passive congestion. The elevated enzyme levels suggest that the process is so severe that hepatic centrilobular necrosis has also occurred. The physical findings suggest right-sided heart failure. The regular pattern of red lobular discoloration seen in the figure is unlikely to occur in hemorrhage from thrombocytopenia, characterized by petechiae and ecchymoses. A portal vein thrombus would diminish blood flow to the liver, but it would not be likely to cause necrosis because of that organ's dual blood. Hepatic congestion is not directly related to renal failure, and hepatorenal syndrome has no characteristic gross appearance. Biliary tract obstruction would produce bile stasis (cholestasis) with icterus.

BP7 82-83   BP6 63-64   PBD7 122-123   PBD6 116-117

5 **(E)** The most important and the most common cause of venous thrombosis is vascular stasis, which often occurs with immobilization. Turbulent blood flow may promote thrombosis, but this risk factor is more common in fast-flowing arterial circulation. Nitric oxide is a vasodilator and an inhibitor of platelet aggregation. Aspirin inhibits platelet function and limits thrombosis. Calcium is a cofactor in the coagulation pathway, but an increase in calcium has minimal effect on the coagulation process.

BP7 92-94   BP6 69   PBD7 130-131   PBD6 124-125

6 **(D)** These findings are characteristic of a hypercoagulable state. The patient has antibodies that react with cardiolipin, a phospholipid antigen used for the serologic diagnosis of syphilis. These so-called antiphospholipid antibodies are directed against phospholipid-protein complexes and are sometimes called lupus anticoagulant, because they are present in some patients with systemic lupus erythematosus (SLE). However, lupus anticoagulant may occur in persons with no evidence of SLE. Patients with lupus anticoagulant have recurrent arterial and venous thrombosis and repeated miscarriages. In vitro, these antibodies inhibit coagulation by interfering with the assembly of phospholipid complexes. In vivo, the antibodies induce a hypercoagulable state by unknown mechanisms. Disseminated intravascular coagulation is an acute consumptive coagulopathy characterized by elevated prothrombin time and partial thromboplastin time (PTT) and decreased platelet count. The prothrombin time and PTT are normal in patients with factor V (Leiden) mutation. Hypercholesterolemia promotes atherosclerosis over many years, and the risk of arterial thrombosis increases. Von Willebrand disease affects platelet adhesion and leads to a bleeding tendency, not to thrombosis.

BP7 91   BP6 70   PBD7 132   BPD6 126

7 (A) Tissue plasminogen activator is a thrombolytic agent that causes the generation of plasmin, which cleaves fibrin to dissolve clots. Aspirin prevents formation of new thrombi by inhibiting platelet aggregation. Heparin prevents thrombosis by activating antithrombin III. Nitric oxide is a vasodilator. Vitamin K is required for synthesis of certain clotting factors.

BP7 89-90   BP6 65-66   PBD7 129-130   PBD6 118-120

8 (B) Acute left ventricular failure after a myocardial infarction causes venous congestion in the pulmonary capillary bed and increased hydrostatic pressure, which leads to pulmonary edema by transudation in the alveolar space. Neutrophils and fibrin would be found in cases of acute inflammation of the lung (i.e., pneumonia). Fibrosis and hemosiderin-filled macrophages (heart failure cells) would be found in long-standing, not acute, left ventricular failure. Subpleural hemorrhagic necrosis occurs if there are pulmonary thromboemboli. These thromboemboli can cause right-sided heart failure. Purulent exudate in the pleural space (empyema) or draining from bronchi results from bacterial infection, not heart failure.

BP7 80-82   BP6 61-64   PBD7 120-121   PBD6 113-116

9 (D) These findings are characteristic of decompression sickness (the "bends"). At high pressures, such as occur during a deep scuba dive, nitrogen is dissolved in blood and tissues in large amounts. Ascending too quickly does not allow for slow release of the gas, and formation of small gas bubbles causes symptoms from occlusion of small arteries and arterioles. Hemorrhage or thrombosis from disseminated intravascular coagulation is more likely to occur in underlying diseases such as sepsis, and symptoms do not abate so quickly. Systemic vasodilation is a feature of some forms of shock. Venous thrombosis is more typically a complication of stasis, which does not occur in a physically active person. Fat globules in pulmonary arteries are a feature of fat embolism, which usually follows trauma.

BP7 96   BP6 74   PBD7 137   PBD6 131

10 (B) Spread of the cancer to the dermal lymphatics produces a peau d'orange appearance of the breast. Because the breast has an extensive venous drainage, cancer or other focal mass lesions are unlikely to cause significant congestion and edema of the breast. Ischemia is rare in the breast because of the abundant arterial supply. Passive congestion does not involve the breast. Chronic inflammation is rare in breast tissue and is not associated with cancer.

BP7 81   BP6 62   PBD7 121-122   PBD6 115

11 (B) Von Willebrand factor acts as a "glue" between platelets and the exposed extracellular matrix of the vessel wall after vascular injury. None of the other steps listed depends on von Willebrand factor. Because the patient's prothrombin time is normal, a lack of prothrombin or the presence of an inhibitor is unlikely.

BP7 86-87   BP6 65-67   PBD7 126-127   PBD6 118-120

12 (A) The figure shows a large pulmonary thromboembolus. The most common risk factor is immobilization leading to venous stasis. These thrombi form in the large deep leg or pelvic veins, not in the pulmonary arteries. Coagulopathies from acquired or inherited disorders, such as those from lupus anticoagulant (antiphospholipid antibodies) or factor V (Leiden) mutation, are possible causes of thrombosis, but they usually manifest at a younger age. These causes also are far less common risks for pulmonary thromboembolism than is venous stasis. Local inflammation from pneumonia may result in thrombosis of small vessels in affected areas.

BP7 95   BP6 73-74   PBD7 136   PBD6 130

13 (A) Recurrent thrombotic episodes at such a young age strongly suggest an inherited coagulopathy. The factor V (Leiden) mutation affects 2% to 15% of the population, and more than one half of all persons with a history of recurrent deep venous thrombosis have such a defect. Inherited deficiencies of the anticoagulant proteins antithrombin III and protein C can cause hypercoagulable states, but these are much less common than factor V mutation. Although some cancers elaborate factors that promote thrombosis, this patient is unlikely to have cancer at such a young age; a 10-year history of thrombosis is unlikely to occur in a patient with cancer. Hyperhomocysteinemia is a less common cause of inherited risk of thrombosis than is factor V mutation. It is also a risk factor for atherosclerosis that predisposes to arterial thrombosis. Smoking promotes atherosclerosis with arterial thrombosis.

BP790-91   BP6 69-70   PBD7 131   PBD6 125-126

14 (D) The patient has deep and superficial venous thrombosis as a consequence of venous stasis from immobilization. The large, deep thrombi can embolize to the lungs, leading to death. Gangrene occurs from arterial, not venous, occlusion in the leg. Vessels with thrombi typically stay intact; if a hematoma had developed as a consequence of the trauma from the fall, it would be organizing and decreasing in size after 2 weeks. Disseminated intravascular coagulation is not a common complication in patients with thrombosis of the extremities or in those recuperating from an injury. Fat embolism can occur with fractures, but pulmonary problems typically appear 1 to 3 days after the traumatic event.

BP7 93-94   BP6 71-72   PBD7 134-135   PBD6 127-129

15 (A) Factor VIII, tissue factor (thromboplastin), and factor V act as cofactors or reaction accelerators in the clotting cascade. Factor VIII acts as a reaction accelerator for the conversion of factor X and Xa. The platelet surface provides phospholipid for assembly of coagulation factors. Platelet aggregation is promoted by thromboxane A_2 and ADP. Thromboxane A_2 is released when platelets are activated during the process of platelet adhesion. Fibrin polymerization is promoted by factor XIII. Antithrombin III inhibits thrombin to prolong the prothrombin time.

BP7 88   BP6 68   PBD7 127-129; 654-656   PBD6 121

16 (D) The patient is quickly going into shock after trauma. So-called shock lung, with diffuse alveolar damage, is a common occurrence in this situation. Infarction of the liver is uncommon because of this organ's dual blood supply. Basal ganglia hemorrhages are more typical of hypertension, not hypotension with shock. Passive congestion is less likely because of the diminished blood volumes and tissue perfusion that occur in shock. Gangrene requires much longer to develop and is not a common complication of shock.

BP7 101-102   BP6 78-79   PBD7 138-139   PBD6 136-137

17 (B) Atherosclerotic damage to vascular endothelium is the most common cause of arterial thrombosis. Stasis of blood flow is important in the low-pressure venous circulation. Decreased production of tissue plasminogen activator from intact endothelial cells may occur in anoxia of the endothelial cells in veins with sluggish circulation. Decreased levels of antithrombin III and mutation in the factor V gene are inherited causes of hypercoagulability; they are far less common than atherosclerosis of coronary vessels. Inhibitors to coagulation, such as antiphospholipid antibodies, typically prolong the partial thromboplastin time, the prothrombin time, or both.

BP7 90   BP6 69   PBD7 135   PBD6 124-125

18 (A) ADP is released from the platelet dense bodies and is a potent stimulator of platelet aggregation. ADP also stimulates further release of ADP from other platelets. Many other substances involved in hemostasis, such as fibrinogen, von Willebrand factor (vWF), and factor V, are stored in the α granules of platelets. Thromboxane A_2, another powerful aggregator of platelets, is synthesized by the cyclooxygenase pathway; it is not stored in dense bodies. Fibronectin forms part of the extracellular matrix between cells that "glues" them together. Plasminogen is activated to inhibit coagulation. Platelet aggregation requires active platelet metabolism, platelet stimulation by agonists such as ADP, thrombin, collagen, or epinephrine; the presence of calcium or magnesium ions and specific plasma proteins such as fibrinogen or vWF; and a platelet receptor, the glycoprotein IIb-IIIa (GPIIb-IIIa) complex. Thus, platelet stimulation results in the generation of intracellular second messengers that transmit the stimulus back to the platelet surface, exposing protein-binding sites on GPIIb-IIIa. Fibrinogen or vWF then binds to GPIIb-IIIa and crosslinks adjacent platelets to produce platelet aggregates. The patients in this experiment could have Glanzmann's thrombasthenia, in which platelets are deficient or defective in the GPIIb-IIIa complex, do not bind fibrinogen, and cannot form aggregates, although the platelets can be stimulated by ADP, undergo shape change, and are of normal size.

BP7 87   BP6 67   PBD7 126-127   PBD6 120-121

19 (E) Thrombomodulin is present on intact endothelium and binds thrombin, which inhibits coagulation by activating protein C. Calcium is a cofactor that assists clotting in the coagulation cascade (ethylenediaminetetraacetic acid [EDTA] in some blood collection tubes binds calcium to prevent clotting). Fibrin protein forms a meshwork that is essential to thrombus formation. Platelet factor 4 is released from the α granules of platelets and promotes platelet aggregation during the coagulation process. Prothrombin is converted to throm-bin in the coagulation cascade. Tumor necrosis factor is not significantly involved in coagulation.

BP7 86   BP6 66-67   PBD7 125-126   PBD6 119-120

20 (D) Hydrostatic pressure in the pulmonary capillary bed is increased because of the patient's left-sided heart failure. Pulmonary lymphatics are not affected by heart failure. Plasma oncotic pressure is mainly diminished by decreased synthesis of protein in the liver or by loss of protein through the kidney (proteinuria). With right-sided heart failure, central venous pressure is increased, not decreased. Acute inflammation of the lung (pneumonia) can give rise to alveolar exudate. This occurs only if infection supervenes. It is not caused by a myocardial failure.

BP7 80-81   BP6 62-64   PBD7 120-123   PBD6 114-117

21 (E) The figure shows a mural thrombus filling an atherosclerotic aortic aneurysm below the renal arteries. Diabetes mellitus accelerates and worsens atherosclerosis. One of the complications of mural thrombosis is embolization, which occurs when a small piece of the clot breaks off. The embolus is carried distally and may occlude the popliteal artery. Because the thrombus is in the arterial circulation, an embolus will not travel to the lungs. A venous thrombus produces leg swelling from edema. Although platelets contribute to the formation of thrombi, the platelet count does not drop appreciably with formation of a localized thrombus, and a generalized process such as disseminated intravascular coagulation is needed to consume enough platelets to cause thrombocytopenia.

BP7 92-93   BP6 71-72   PBD7 133, 135   PBD6 127-129

22 (A) The figure shows a hemorrhagic infarct on the pleura, a typical finding when a medium-sized thromboembolus lodges in a pulmonary artery branch. The infarct is hemorrhagic, because the bronchial arterial circulation in the lung (derived from the systemic arterial circulation and separate from the pulmonary arterial circulation) continues to supply a small amount of blood to the affected area of infarction. Passive congestion, whether acute or chronic, is a diffuse process, as is edema, which does not impart a red color. Pulmonary venous thrombosis is rare.

BP7 97   BP6 75   PBD7 138-139   PBD6 132-133

23 (F) The figure shows an organizing thrombus in a small artery, with several small recanalized channels. Such a peripheral arterial occlusion was not sufficient to produce infarction, as evidenced by the lack of enzyme elevation. Thrombi become organized over time if they are not dissolved by fibrinolytic activity. Air emboli are uncommon and usually the result of trauma. Those on the arterial side can cause ischemia through occlusion even when very small, whereas on the venous side, more than 100 mL of air trapped in the heart may reduce cardiac output. Air emboli from decompression form when gases that became dissolved in tissues at high pressure bubble out at lower pressure in blood and tissues. Cholesterol emboli can break off from atheromas in arteries and proceed distally to occlude small arteries; however, because these emboli are usually quite small, they are seldom clinically significant. Chronic passive congestion refers to capillary, sinusoidal, or venous stasis of blood within an organ such as the lungs or liver. Fat emboli are globules of lipid that are most likely to form following traumatic injury, typically to long bones. Mural thrombi are thrombi that form on the surfaces of the heart or large arteries. After a thrombus has formed, it may become organized with ingrowth of capillaries, fibroblast proliferation, and macrophage infiltration that eventually clears part or most of the clot, forming one or more new lumens (recanalization).

BP7 92-93 BP6 71-73 PBD7 133-135 PBD6 127-129

24 **(A)** The patient has a subdural hematoma. A hematoma is a collection of blood in a potential space or within tissue. Purpura denotes blotchy hemorrhage on skin, serosal, or mucous membrane surfaces; areas larger than 1 to 2 cm are often called ecchymoses. Congestion occurs when there is vascular dilation with pooling of blood within an organ. Petechiae are pinpoint areas of hemorrhage.

BP7 83 BP6 64 PBD7 123-124 PBD6 117-118

25 **(B)** The liver has a dual blood supply, with a hepatic arterial circulation and a portal venous circulation. Therefore, infarction of the liver caused by occlusion of hepatic artery is uncommon. Cerebral infarction typically produces liquefactive necrosis. Infarcts of most solid parenchymal organs such as the kidney, heart, and spleen demonstrate coagulative necrosis, and emboli from the left heart often go to these organs.

BP7 98 BP6 76 PBD7 137-139 PBD6 133

26 **(D)** The surgery disrupted lymphatic return, resulting in functional lymphatic obstruction and lymphedema of the arm. The lymphatic channels are important in scavenging fluid and protein that have leaked into the tissues from the intravascular space. Although the amount of fluid that is drained through the lymphatics is not great, it can build up gradually. Cellulitis is caused by an infection of the skin and subcutaneous tissue and displays erythema, warmth, and tenderness. Congestive heart failure can lead to peripheral edema, which is most marked in dependent areas such as the lower extremities and over the sacrum (in bedridden patients). Decreased plasma oncotic pressure from hypoalbuminemia, or sodium and water retention with heart or renal failure, leads to more generalized edema. Phlebothrombosis leads to swelling with pain and tenderness, but it is uncommon in the upper extremities.

BP7 81 BP6 62 PBD7 121-122 PBD6 115

27 **(C)** The patient has septic shock with poor tissue perfusion, evidenced by the high lactate level. Vasodilation is a feature of septic shock, typically as a result of gram-negative endotoxemia. Elevated creatine kinase suggests an acute myocardial infarction, which produces cardiogenic shock. Decreased P_{O_2} suggests a problem with lung ventilation or perfusion. Increased blood urea nitrogen concentration is a feature of renal failure, not the cause of renal failure. Decreased hematocrit suggests hypovolemic shock from blood loss.

BP7 100 BP6 77 PBD7 139-141 PBD6 134

28 **(F)** The patient's prolonged immobilized condition placed him at risk for pulmonary thromboembolism; not all such embolic events are symptomatic. Organization with recanalization occurs in a vessel after thrombosis or thromboembolism. A small fibrous band may be all that remains of the clot. An exudate is unlikely to form such a band, and pneumonia is more likely to involve the bronchial tree than vascular lumens. Hemorrhage alone cannot cause fibrosis. Passive congestion of surrounding lung tissue has a negligible effect on arteries. Ischemia could result from the same thromboembolus but would produce a hemorrhagic infarct of the lung. Pulmonary hypertension could occur from the decreased vascular bed resulting from recurrent, widespread thromboembolism to small peripheral pulmonary arteries but not from a single thromboembolic event.

BP7 95 BP6 71 PBD7 133-135 PBD6 127-128

29 **(B)** Aspirin blocks the cyclooxygenase pathway of arachidonic acid metabolism and generation of eicosanoids, including thromboxane A_2, which causes vasoconstriction and promotes platelet aggregation. Platelet adhesion to extracellular matrix is mediated by interactions with von Willebrand factor. Tissue factor (thromboplastin) is released with tissue injury and is not platelet dependent. Endothelial cells produce von Willebrand factor independent of platelet action. Antithrombin III has anticoagulant properties because it inactivates several coagulation factors, but its function is not affected by aspirin.

BP7 87 BP6 37, 66-67 PBD7 126-127
PBD6 71,120-122

30 **(F)** Venous stasis favors the development of phlebothrombosis (venous thrombosis), particularly in the leg and pelvic veins. This is a common complication among hospitalized patients who are bedridden. The obstruction may produce local pain and swelling, or it may be asymptomatic. Such deep thrombi in large veins create a risk for pulmonary thromboembolism. Anasarca refers to marked generalized edema. Chronic passive congestion refers to capillary, sinusoidal, or venous stasis of blood within an organ such as the lungs or liver. Fat emboli are globules of lipid that are most likely to form following traumatic injury, typically to long bones. Mural thrombi are thrombi that form on the surfaces of the heart or large arteries. After a thrombus has formed, it may become organized with ingrowth of capillaries, fibroblast proliferation, and macrophage infiltration that eventually clears part or most of the clot, forming one or more new lumens (recanalization). Phlebothrombosis occurs when stasis in large veins promotes thrombosis formation, typically in leg and pelvic veins; because there is often clinically apparent swelling, warmth, and pain, the term "thrombophlebitis" is often employed regardless of whether true vascular inflammation is present. A vegetation is a localized thrombus formation on cardiac endothelium, typically a valve.

BP7 93-94 BP6 72-73 PBD7 130-131 PBD6 129

31 **(A)** The hydrostatic pressure exerted from standing leads to edema in dependent parts of the body. Lymphatic obstruction from infection or tumor can lead to lymphedema, but this is a chronic process. Secondary aldosteronism results from congestive heart failure and renal hypoperfusion, but this is a generalized process. Hypoalbuminemia leads to more generalized edema, although the effect is more pronounced in dependent areas. In a healthy patient, normal renal function would be sufficient to clear free water ingested orally.

BP7 80-81 BP6 61-62 PBD7 120-121 PBD6 114-115

32 (**B**) Amniotic fluid embolism rarely occurs in pregnancy but has a high mortality rate. The fluid reaches torn uterine veins through ruptured fetal membranes. Aggregates of RBCs are seen in passive congestion. Fat globules are seen in fat embolism, usually after severe trauma. Gas bubbles in vessels from air embolism can be a rare event in some obstetric procedures, but it is unlikely in natural deliveries. Peripheral pulmonary thromboemboli are most likely to produce chronic pulmonary hypertension and develop over weeks to months.

BP7 96   BP6 74-75   PBD7 137   PBD6 131-132

CHAPTER 5

Genetic Disorders

PBD7 Chapter 5: Genetic Disorders

PBD6 Chapter 6: Genetic Disorders

BP7 and BP6 Chapter 7: Genetic and Pediatric Diseases

1 A 22-year-old man who had a myocardial infarction 1 year ago now has chest pain when exercising. His underlying disease is due to an absence of LDL receptors on liver cells, inherited as an autosomal dominant condition. Which of the following laboratory findings is most likely to be present in this patient?

- ❑ (A) Abetalipoproteinemia
- ❑ (B) Hypertriglyceridemia
- ❑ (C) Ketonuria
- ❑ (D) Hypoglycemia
- ❑ (E) Hypercholesterolemia

2 A 27-year-old man comes to the physician for an infertility workup. He and his wife have been trying to conceive a child for 6 years. Physical examination shows bilateral gynecomastia, reduced testicular size, reduced body hair, and increased length between the soles of his feet and the pubic bone. A semen analysis indicates oligospermia. Laboratory studies show increased follicle-stimulating hormone level and slightly decreased testosterone level. Which of the following karyotypes is most likely to be present in this man?

- ❑ (A) 46,X,i(Xq)
- ❑ (B) 47,XYY
- ❑ (C) 47,XXY
- ❑ (D) 46XX/47XX,+21
- ❑ (E) 46,XY,del(22q11)

3 The parents of a male infant come to the physician because of their concern that male children over several generations in the mother's family have been affected by a progressive disorder involving multiple organ systems. These children have had coarse facial features, corneal clouding, joint stiffness, hepatosplenomegaly, and mental retardation, and many died in childhood. At autopsy, some of the children had subendothelial coronary arterial deposits that caused myocardial infarction. Laboratory testing of the infant shows increased urinary excretion of mucopolysaccharides. Bone marrow biopsy is performed, and the accumulated mucopolysaccharides are found in macrophages ("balloon cells" filled with minute vacuoles). Which of the following enzyme deficiencies is most likely to be seen in this infant?

- ❑ (A) Adenosine deaminase
- ❑ (B) α-L-iduronidase
- ❑ (C) Glucocerebrosidase
- ❑ (D) Glucose-6-phosphatase
- ❑ (E) Hexosaminidase A
- ❑ (F) Lysosomal glucosidase
- ❑ (G) Sphingomyelinase

4 A 25-year-old woman stops going to her aerobic exercise class because of severe muscle cramps that have occurred during every session for the past 2 months. Several hours after each session, she notices that her urine is a brown color. On physical examination, she has normal muscle development and strength. An inherited defect in which of the following substances is most likely to explain these findings?

- ❏ (A) Dystrophin
- ❏ (B) Fibrillin
- ❏ (C) Glucose-6-phosphatase
- ❏ (D) Hexosaminidase
- ❏ (E) Lysosomal glucosidase
- ❏ (F) Muscle phosphorylase
- ❏ (G) Spectrin

5 A 25-year-old professional male hockey player who has never won the Lady Byng trophy goes to the physician for a routine physical examination. He is 195 cm (6 ft 5 in) tall and has prominent facial acne scars and four missing teeth. He is married and has two children who show normal development for their ages. Which of the following karyotypes is most likely to be present in this patient?

- ❏ (A) 45,X/46,XY
- ❏ (B) 46,X(fra)Y
- ❏ (C) 47,XXY
- ❏ (D) 47,XYY
- ❏ (E) 47,XX,+21
- ❏ (F) 69,XYY

6 A 19-year-old woman, G 3, P 2, gives birth after an uncomplicated pregnancy to a term male infant. On physical examination soon after birth, the infant is recorded at the 60th percentile for height and weight. The only abnormal finding is a cleft lip. There is no family history of birth defects, and the mother's other two children are healthy with no apparent abnormalities. Which of the following factors is most likely to influence the appearance of this infant?

- ❏ (A) Chromosomal anomaly
- ❏ (B) Early amnion disruption
- ❏ (C) Maternal malnutrition
- ❏ (D) Multifactorial inheritance
- ❏ (E) Single gene defect
- ❏ (F) Teratogenicity

7 A 25-year-old woman with amenorrhea has never had menarche. On physical examination, she is 145 cm (4 ft 9 in) tall. She has a webbed neck, a broad chest, and widely spaced nipples. Strong pulses are palpable in the upper extremities, but there are only weak pulses in the lower extremities. On abdominal MR imaging, the ovaries are small, elongated, and tubular. Which of the following karyotypes is most likely to be present in this patient?

- ❏ (A) 45,X/46,XX
- ❏ (B) 46,X,X(fra)
- ❏ (C) 47,XXY
- ❏ (D) 47,XXX
- ❏ (E) 47,XX,+16

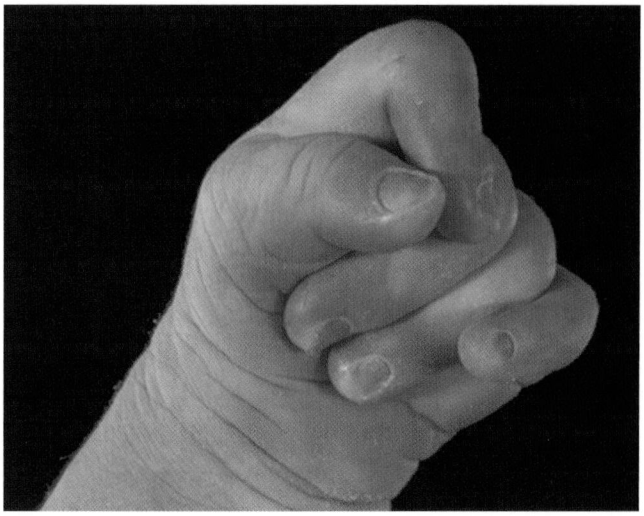

8 A 37-year-old woman gives birth at 35 weeks' gestation to a female infant. Physical examination of the infant soon after delivery shows rocker bottom feet, a small face and mouth, and low-set ears. On auscultation of the chest, a heart murmur is detected. The appearance of the infant's hands is shown in the figure above. The infant dies at 4 months of age. Which of the following karyotypes is most likely to be present in this infant?

- ❏ (A) 45,X
- ❏ (B) 46,XX
- ❏ (C) 47,XX,+18
- ❏ (D) 47,XX,+21
- ❏ (E) 48,XXX

9 A 10-year-old boy who is mentally retarded is able to carry out activities of daily living, including feeding and dressing himself. On physical examination, he has brachycephaly and oblique palpebral fissures with prominent epicanthal folds. A transverse crease is seen on the palm of each hand. On auscultation of the chest, there is a grade III/VI systolic murmur. Which of the following diseases is he most likely to develop by age 20?

- ❏ (A) Acute leukemia
- ❏ (B) Hepatic cirrhosis
- ❏ (C) Chronic renal failure
- ❏ (D) Acute myocardial infarction
- ❏ (E) Aortic dissection

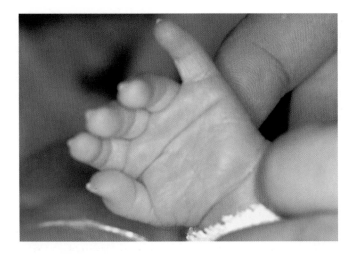

10 The left hand of an infant born at 38 weeks' gestation to a 25-year-old woman, G 2, P 1, has the appearance shown in the figure above. The infant is small for gestational age. Which of the following chromosomal abnormalities is most likely to be present?

- ❏ (A) 45,X
- ❏ (B) 47,XX,+21
- ❏ (C) 47,XY,+18
- ❏ (D) 69,XXY
- ❏ (E) 47,XXY

11 A 19-year-old man is referred to a neurologist because of failing eyesight and progressive muscle weakness. The neurologist takes a history and finds that several of the patient's male and female relatives have similar symptoms. His mother, her brother and sister, and two of the aunt's children are affected, but the uncle's children are not. Which of the following types of genetic disorders is most likely to be present in this patient?

- ❏ (A) Trinucleotide repeat expansion
- ❏ (B) Genetic imprinting
- ❏ (C) X-linked inheritance pattern
- ❏ (D) Mitochondrial mutation
- ❏ (E) Uniparental disomy

12 A healthy 20-year-old woman, G 3, P 2, Ab 1, comes to the physician for a prenatal visit. She has previously given birth to a liveborn infant and a stillborn infant, both with the same karyotypic abnormality. On physical examination, she is at the 50th percentile for height and weight. She has no physical abnormalities noted. Which of the following karyotypic abnormalities is most likely to be present in this patient?

- ❏ (A) Robertsonian translocation
- ❏ (B) Ring chromosome
- ❏ (C) Isochromosome
- ❏ (D) Paracentric inversion
- ❏ (E) Deletion of q arm

13 A 36-year-old woman gives birth at 34 weeks' gestation to a male infant who lives for only 1 hour after delivery. On physical examination, the infant is at the 30th percentile for height and weight. Anomalies include microcephaly, a cleft lip and palate, and postaxial polydactyly, with six fingers on each hand and foot. Which of the following karyotypes is most likely to be present in this infant?

- ❏ (A) 45,X
- ❏ (B) 46,XY
- ❏ (C) 47,XXY
- ❏ (D) 47,XY,+13
- ❏ (E) 47,XY,+18
- ❏ (F) 69,XXY

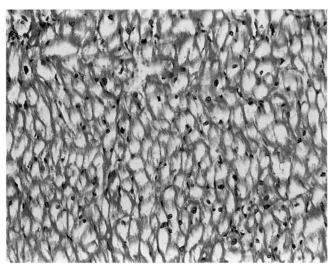

Courtesy of Dr. Trace Worrell, Department of Pathology, University of Texas Southwestern Medical Center, Dallas, TX.

14 A 6-month-old male infant is brought to the physician because of failure to thrive and abdominal enlargement. His parents are concerned that he has shown minimal movement since birth. On physical examination, the infant has marked muscle weakness and hepatosplenomegaly. A chest radiograph shows marked cardiomegaly. He dies of congestive heart failure at the age of 19 months. The microscopic appearance of myocardial fibers at autopsy is shown in the figure above. A deficiency of which of the following enzymes is most likely to be present in this infant?

- ❏ (A) Glucocerebrosidase
- ❏ (B) Glucose-6-phosphatase
- ❏ (C) Hexosaminidase A
- ❏ (D) Homogentisic oxidase
- ❏ (E) Lysosomal glucosidase
- ❏ (F) Myophosphorylase
- ❏ (G) Sphingomyelinase

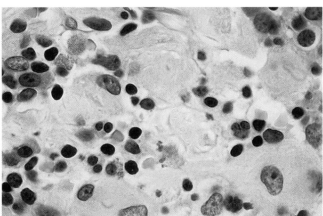

Courtesy of Dr. Matthew Fries, Department of Pathology, University of Texas Southwestern Medical Center, Dallas, TX.

15 A 10-year-old child has had recurrent otitis media for the past 8 years. On physical examination, there is hepatosplenomegaly. No external anomalies are present. Laboratory findings include anemia and leukopenia. A bone marrow biopsy is performed, and high magnification of the sample shows the findings depicted in the figure. An inherited deficiency of which of the following enzymes is most likely to produce these findings?

- (A) Glucocerebrosidase
- (B) Acid maltase
- (C) Glucose-6-phosphatase
- (D) Sphingomyelinase
- (E) Hexosaminidase A

16 Mental retardation has affected several generations of a family, and most of the affected persons have been males. The severity of mental retardation has increased with each passing generation. Genetic testing is performed, and about 20% of the males who have the genetic abnormality are unaffected. Which of the following mechanisms is most likely to produce this genetic condition?

- (A) Trinucleotide repeat mutation
- (B) Frameshift mutation
- (C) Missense mutation
- (D) Point mutation
- (E) Mitochondrial DNA mutation

17 A 15-year-old girl is brought to the physician by her parents, who are concerned because she has developed multiple nodules on her skin. On physical examination, there are 20 scattered, 0.3- to 1-cm, firm nodules on the patient's trunk and extremities. There are 12 light-brown macules averaging 2 to 5 cm in diameter on the skin of the trunk. Slit-lamp examination shows pigmented nodules in the iris. These findings are most likely to be associated with which of the following types of neoplasm?

- (A) Dermatofibroma
- (B) Leiomyoma
- (C) Neurofibroma
- (D) Lipoma
- (E) Hemangioma

18 A 39-year-old woman gives birth to a term infant with a right transverse palmar crease, low-set ears, oblique palpebral fissures, and a heart murmur. The infant survives to childhood and exhibits only mild mental retardation. Which of the following chromosomal abnormalities is most likely to be present in the somatic cells of this child?

- (A) Haploidy
- (B) Monosomy
- (C) Mosaicism
- (D) Tetraploidy
- (E) Triploidy

19 A 23-year-old woman gives birth to a term infant after an uncomplicated pregnancy. On physical examination, the infant has ambiguous external genitalia. The parents want to know the infant's sex, but the physician is hesitant to assign a sex without further information. A chromosomal analysis indicates a karyotype of 46,XX. An abdominal CT scan shows bilaterally enlarged adrenal glands, and the internal genitalia appear to consist of uterus, fallopian tubes, and ovaries. This infant is most likely to have which of the following abnormalities?

- (A) Female pseudohermaphroditism
- (B) Testicular feminization
- (C) Nondisjunctional event with loss of Y chromosome
- (D) Excessive trinucleotide repeats
- (E) Mitochondrial DNA mutation

20 A 1-year-old infant girl is brought to the physician because of failure to thrive, poor neurologic development, and poor motor function. Physical examination shows a "cherry red" spot on the macula of the retina. The infant's muscle tone is poor. Both parents and a brother and sister are healthy, with no apparent abnormalities. However, one brother with a similar condition died at the age of 18 months. This genetic disorder most likely resulted from which of the following underlying abnormalities?

- (A) Mutation in a mitochondrial gene
- (B) Mutation in a gene encoding a lysosomal enzyme
- (C) Mutation in a gene encoding a receptor protein
- (D) Mutation in a gene encoding a structural protein
- (E) Genomic imprinting

21 A 10-year-old boy is brought to the physician because of a cough and earache. The child has a history of recurrent infections, including otitis media, diarrhea, and pneumonia. Physical examination shows an erythematous right tympanic membrane, a cleft palate, and murmur suggestive of congenital heart disease. A thoracic CT scan shows a small thymus. Results of laboratory studies suggest mild hypoparathyroidism. Which of the following diagnostic studies is most likely to be helpful in diagnosing this patient's condition?

- (A) HIV type 1 RNA level
- (B) FISH analysis with a probe for chromosome 22q11.2
- (C) PCR analysis for trinucleotide repeats affecting the X chromosome
- (D) Assay for the enzyme adenosine deaminase in lymphocytes
- (E) Lymph node biopsy

22 A 2-year-old child is brought to the physician after having convulsions. The child has a history of failure to thrive. Physical examination shows hepatomegaly and ecchymoses of the skin. Laboratory studies show a blood glucose level of 31 mg/dL. A liver biopsy specimen shows cells filled with clear vacuoles that stain positive for glycogen. Which of the following conditions is most likely to produce these findings?

- ❑ (A) McArdle syndrome
- ❑ (B) Von Gierke disease
- ❑ (C) Tay-Sachs disease
- ❑ (D) Hurler syndrome
- ❑ (E) Pompe disease

23 An 8-year-old girl is brought to the physician after sustaining a traumatic laceration to the forearm. The wound is 4 cm long and gaping open. On physical examination, the girl's skin is extremely stretchable and fragile. She can bend her thumb back to touch her forearm and can pull the skin of her abdomen out about 8 cm. An inherited disorder involving which of the following is most likely to explain these findings?

- ❑ (A) α_1-Antitrypsin
- ❑ (B) Retinoblastoma (Rb) protein
- ❑ (C) LDL receptor
- ❑ (D) Collagen
- ❑ (E) Factor VIII

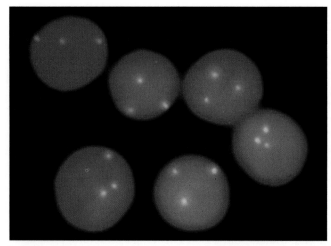

Courtesy of Dr. Vijay Tonk, Department of Pathology, University of Texas Southwestern Medical Center, Dallas, TX.

24 An ultrasound examination of a 29-year-old primigravida performed at 18 weeks' gestation shows a male fetus that is mildly growth retarded. Multiple congenital anomalies are present, including ventricular and atrial septal defects, horseshoe kidney, and omphalocele. Amniocentesis is performed, and the fetal cells obtained are examined using FISH analysis. Based on the findings shown in the figure, which of the following karyotypic abnormalities is most likely to be present in this fetus?

- ❑ (A) 46,XY,der(14;21)(q10.0),+21
- ❑ (B) 47,XY,+18
- ❑ (C) 47,XXY
- ❑ (D) 46,XY,del(22q11)
- ❑ (E) 45,X/46,XX

25 A 22-year-old woman delivers an apparently healthy female infant following an uncomplicated pregnancy. At 4

years of age, the girl is brought to the physician because her parents have observed progressive, severe neurologic deterioration. Physical examination now shows marked hepatosplenomegaly. A bone marrow biopsy specimen shows numerous foamy vacuolated macrophages. Analysis of which of the following factors is most likely to aid in the diagnosis of this condition?

- ❑ (A) Number of LDL receptors on hepatocytes
- ❑ (B) Level of sphingomyelinase in splenic macrophages
- ❑ (C) Rate of synthesis of collagen
- ❑ (D) Level of glucose-6-phosphatase in liver cells
- ❑ (E) Level of α_1-antitrypsin in the liver

26 A 22-year-old primigravida notes absent fetal movement for 2 days. The fetus is delivered stillborn at 19 weeks' gestation. The macerated fetus shows marked hydrops fetalis and a large posterior cystic hygroma of the neck. At autopsy, internal anomalies are seen, including aortic coarctation and a horseshoe kidney. Which of the following karyotypes is most likely to be present in cells obtained from the fetus?

- ❑ (A) 47,XX,+18
- ❑ (B) 48,XXXY
- ❑ (C) 47,XX,+21
- ❑ (D) 47,XYY
- ❑ (E) 45,X
- ❑ (F) 69,XXX

27 A 13-year-old boy has been drinking large quantities of fluids and has an insatiable appetite. He is losing weight and has become more tired and listless for the past month. Laboratory findings include normal CBC and fasting serum glucose of 175 mg/dL. Which of the following is the probable inheritance pattern of this disease?

- ❑ (A) Autosomal dominant
- ❑ (B) Multifactorial
- ❑ (C) X-linked recessive
- ❑ (D) Mitochondrial DNA
- ❑ (E) Autosomal recessive

28 A pregnant woman with a family history of fragile X syndrome undergoes prenatal testing of her fetus. PCR analysis to amplify the appropriate region of the *FMR1* gene is attempted using DNA from amniotic fluid cells, but no amplified products are obtained. Which of the following is the most appropriate next step?

- ❑ (A) Routine karyotyping of the amniotic fluid cells
- ❑ (B) Routine karyotyping of the unaffected father
- ❑ (C) Southern blot analysis of DNA from the amniotic fluid cells
- ❑ (D) PCR analysis of the mother's *FMR1* gene
- ❑ (E) No further testing

29 A 3-year-old boy is brought to the physician because of progressive developmental delay, ataxia, seizures, and inappropriate laughter. The child has a normal karyotype of 46,XY, but DNA analysis shows that he has inherited both of his number 15 chromosomes from his father. These findings are most likely to be present with which of the following?

- ❑ (A) X-linked inheritance pattern
- ❑ (B) Maternal inheritance pattern
- ❑ (C) Mutation of mitochondrial DNA
- ❑ (D) Genomic imprinting
- ❑ (E) Trinucleotide repeat expansion

30 A 22-year-old man has a sudden loss of vision in the right eye. On physical examination, there is a subluxation of the crystalline lens of the right eye. On auscultation of the chest, a midsystolic click is audible. An echocardiogram shows a floppy mitral valve and dilated aortic arch. The patient's brother and his cousin are similarly affected. A genetic defect involving which of the following substances is most likely to be present in this patient?

- (A) Dystrophin
- (B) Collagen
- (C) Fibrillin-1
- (D) NF1 protein
- (E) Spectrin

31 A 24-year-old woman comes to the physician because she has been unable to bear children during her 3 years of marriage. She has never had a menstrual period. On physical examination, she has normal breast development and scanty axillary and pubic hair. Pelvic examination shows a short, blind-ending vagina with no palpable uterus or adnexa. Chromosomal analysis indicates a 46,XY karyotype. Which of the following findings is most likely to be present?

- (A) Abnormal androgen receptor
- (B) Fragile X syndrome
- (C) Gonadal mosaicism
- (D) Hypopituitarism
- (E) Testicular agenesis

32 A 21-year-old primigravida gives birth to a term infant following an uncomplicated pregnancy. The infant is of normal height and weight, and no anomalies are noted. However, the infant fails to pass meconium. Laboratory studies show an elevated sweat chloride level. Genetic testing indicates that a critical protein coded by a gene is missing one phenylalanine amino acid in the protein sequence. Which of the following types of gene mutations is most likely to produce these findings?

- (A) Frameshift
- (B) Nonsense (stop codon)
- (C) Point
- (D) Three–base pair deletion
- (E) Trinucleotide repeat

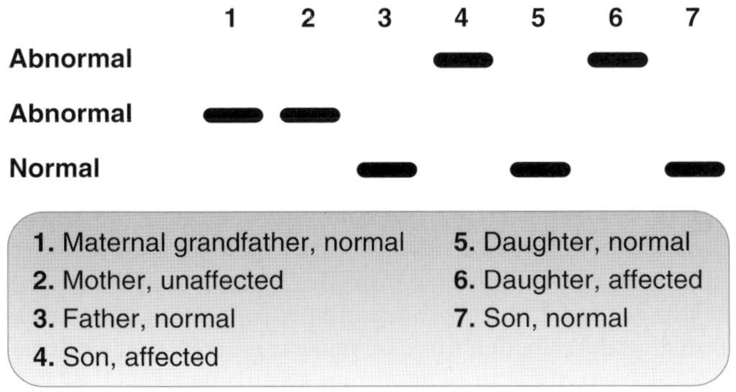

33 Genetic testing of a family is performed using Southern blot with a DNA probe spanning the region of a suspected mutation. The results are shown in the figure above. Based on these findings, which of the following types of gene mutations is most likely to be present in this family?

- (A) Frameshift
- (B) Nonsense (stop codon)
- (C) Point
- (D) Three–base pair deletion
- (E) Trinucleotide repeat

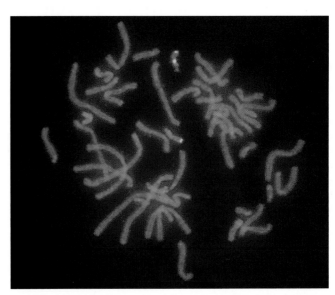

Courtesy of Dr. Nancy R. Schneider and Jeff Doolittle, Cytogenetics Laboratory, University of Texas Southwestern Medical Center, Dallas, TX.

34 A 9-month-old infant has had numerous viral and fungal infections since birth. On physical examination, no congenital anomalies are noted. Laboratory studies show hypocalcemia. FISH analysis of the infant's cells is performed. A metaphase spread is shown in the figure above, with probes to two different regions on chromosome 22. Which of the following cytogenetic abnormalities is most likely to be present?

- (A) Aneuploidy
- (B) Deletion
- (C) Inversion
- (D) Monosomy
- (E) Translocation

ANSWERS

1 (E) Familial hypercholesterolemia results from mutations in the LDL receptor gene, causing LDL cholesterol to be increased in the blood because it is not catabolized or taken up by the liver. Abetalipoproteinemia is rare. Triglycerides are not primarily affected. Ketonuria can occur in starvation or insulin deficiency. The LDL receptors do not play a direct role in gluconeogenesis.

BP7 218-220   BP6 182-183   PBD7 156-158
PBD6 150-153

2 (C) These findings are characteristic of Klinefelter syndrome, one of the more common chromosomal abnormalities, which occurs in about 1 of 850 liveborn males. The

Genetic testing family table (question 33):

	1	2	3	4	5	6	7
Abnormal				▬		▬	
Abnormal	▬	▬					
Normal			▬		▬		▬

1. Maternal grandfather, normal
2. Mother, unaffected
3. Father, normal
4. Son, affected
5. Daughter, normal
6. Daughter, affected
7. Son, normal

findings can be subtle. The 46,X,i(Xq) karyotype is a variant of Turner syndrome (seen only in females), caused by a defective second X chromosome. The 47,XYY karyotype occurs in about 1 in 1000 liveborn males and is associated with taller-than-average stature. A person with a mosaic such as 46,XX/47,XX,+21 has milder features of Down syndrome than a person with the more typical 47,XX,+21 karyotype. The 22q11 deletion syndrome is associated with congenital defects affecting the palate, face, and heart and, in some cases, with T-cell immunodeficiency.

BP7 233   BP6 196   PBD7 179   PBD6 174

3   **(B)** The findings listed are consistent with Hunter syndrome, one of the mucopolysaccharidoses (MPSs) that results from deficiencies of lysosomal enzymes, such as α-L-iduronidase. The glycosaminoglycans that accumulate in MPSs include dermatan sulfate, heparan sulfate, keratan sulfate, and chondroitin sulfate. All of the MPS variants are autosomal recessive, except for Hunter syndrome, which is X-linked recessive. Adenosine deaminase deficiency is a cause of severe combined immunodeficiency (SCID), an immunodeficiency state in which multiple recurrent infections occur following birth. Glucocerebrosidase deficiency is seen in Gaucher disease; in the most common form of the disease, there is no neurologic impairment, and patients have splenomegaly and skeletal disease as a consequence of increased lysosomal glucocerebrosides in cells of the mononuclear phagocyte system. Glucose-6-phosphatase deficiency leads to von Gierke disease, characterized by hepatomegaly, renomegaly, and impaired gluconeogenesis leading to hypoglycemia and hyperlipidemia. Hexosaminidase A deficiency occurs in Tay-Sachs disease; affected persons manifest severe neurologic impairment, poor motor development, and blindness beginning in infancy. Lysosomal glucosidase deficiency, seen in Pompe disease, is associated with marked cardiomegaly and heart failure beginning in infancy. Sphingomyelinase deficiency occurs in Niemann-Pick disease type A, characterized by hepatosplenomegaly, lymphadenopathy, and severe motor and mental impairment.

BP7 224-225   BP6 187-188   PBD7 165   PBD6 159-160

4   **(F)** This woman has McArdle syndrome, a form of glycogen storage disease with onset in young adulthood. In this disorder, a deficiency of muscle phosphorylase enzyme causes glycogen to accumulate in skeletal muscle. Because strenuous exercise requires glycogenolysis and use of anaerobic metabolism, muscle cramps ensue and the blood lactate level does not rise. Myoglobinuria is seen in about one half of cases. A lack of the muscle membrane protein dystrophin characterizes Duchenne muscular dystrophy. A fibrillin gene mutation can lead to Marfan syndrome. Glucose-6-phosphatase deficiency leads to von Gierke disease, characterized by hepatomegaly, renomegaly, and impaired gluconeogenesis leading to hypoglycemia and hyperlipidemia. Hexosaminidase A deficiency occurs in Tay-Sachs disease, causing severe neurologic impairment, poor motor development, and blindness beginning in infancy. Lysosomal glucosidase deficiency is seen in Pompe disease, characterized by marked cardiomegaly and heart failure beginning in infancy. Abnormal spectrin, an RBC membrane cytoskeletal protein, leads to a condition known as hereditary spherocytosis.

BP7 225   BP6 188-189   PBD7 166-167   PBD6 160, 163

5   **(D)** An extra Y chromosome is present in about 1 in 1000 liveborn males. There is a tendency for these males to be tall and prone to severe acne. The missing teeth in this patient are a result of playing hockey and are not related to the extra Y chromosome. There is a controversy about whether such persons exhibit more aggressive behavior than other males. Generally, the behavior of virtually all 47,XYY males is indistinguishable from that of other males. The 45,X/46,XY mosaic is extremely rare. The 46,X(fra)Y karyotype is second only to trisomy 21 as a cause of mental retardation in males. The 47,XXY karyotype occurs in Klinefelter syndrome; affected persons are often infertile. Down syndrome (47,XX,+21) is characterized by mental retardation. In triploidy with 69 chromosomes, survival in utero is unlikely.

BP7 233   BP6 196   PBD7 178   PBD6 174

6   **(D)** Most congenital malformations, including cleft lip, are not determined by a single gene and may be conditioned by environmental influences. This type of multifactorial inheritance accounts for 20% to 25% of all anomalies noted. Of the remaining options, all are more likely to produce multiple defects and reduce fetal growth. Most chromosomal anomalies are not compatible with survival; the few fetuses (e.g., with sex chromosome aneuploidies and autosomal triploidies such as 13, 18, and 21) that do survive to term and beyond manifest multiple anomalies. Early amnion disruption may result in clefts, but more severe defects are present (e.g., gastroschisis and missing digits or limbs), and stillbirth is the usual consequence. Maternal malnutrition typically results in an infant who is small for gestational age. Single gene defects account for less than 10% of anomalies noted at birth. Teratogens account for no more than 1% of congenital anomalies.

BP7 240-241   BP6 190   PBD7 169-170   PBD6 165

7   **(A)** The features described are those of classic Turner syndrome. Persons who reach adulthood may have mosaic cell lines, with some 45,X cells and some 46,XX. A female carrier of the fragile X syndrome, X(fra), is less likely to manifest the disease than a male, but the number of triple repeat sequences (CGG) increases in her male offspring. The 47,XXY karyotype occurs in Klinefelter syndrome; affected persons appear as phenotypic males. The "superfemale" karyotype (XXX) leads to mild mental retardation. Trisomy 16 is a cause of fetal loss early in pregnancy.

BP7 233-234   BP6 196-197   PBD7 179-180
PBD6 174-176

8   **(C)** This spectrum of findings correlates best with trisomy 18 (Edwards syndrome), in which survival is shortened significantly. Turner syndrome (45,X) is associated with the presence of cystic hygroma and hydrops fetalis. The severe anomalies described in this case make it unlikely that a normal 46,XX karyotype is present. Down syndrome (47,XX,+21) is associated with longer survival than is described in this case, and the external features can be quite subtle at birth. The "superfemale" karyotype (XXX) leads to mild mental retardation. Generally, abnormal numbers of sex chromosomes are better tolerated than abnormalities of autosomes.

BP7 231   BP6 182-183   PBD7 177   PBD6 151-152

9 (A) This boy has Down syndrome (trisomy 21), one of the trisomies that can result in a liveborn infant. Although children with Down syndrome can function fairly well, they often have many associated congenital anomalies. Among the more common is congenital heart disease, including ventricular septal defect. There is also a 10- to 20-fold increased risk of acute leukemia. Virtually all persons with Down syndrome who live to the age of 40 will have evidence of Alzheimer disease. Hepatic cirrhosis is a feature of galactosemia. Chronic renal failure may be seen in genetic disorders that produce polycystic kidneys. Myocardial infarction at a young age suggests familial hypercholesterolemia. Aortic dissection is seen in persons with Marfan syndrome.

BP7 230-232   BP6 193-195   PBD7 175-176
PBD6 170-172

10 (B) The figure shows a single palmar flexion crease and a single flexion crease on the fifth digit, both features of trisomy 21. Although there is an increased risk of Down syndrome with increasing maternal age, most infants with Down syndrome are born to younger women because there are far more pregnancies at younger maternal ages. Monosomy X may be marked by a short fourth metacarpal. With trisomy 18, the fingers are often clenched, with digits 2 and 5 overlapping 3 and 4. Triploidy may be marked by syndactyly of digits 3 and 4. There are no characteristic hand features in males with Klinefelter syndrome.

BP7 230-232   BP6 193-194   PBD7 175-176
PBD6 170-172

11 (D) This is a classic pattern of maternal inheritance resulting from a mutation in mitochondrial DNA. Males and females are affected, but affected males cannot transmit the disease to their offspring. Because mitochondrial DNA encodes many enzymes involved in oxidative phosphorylation, mutations in mitochondrial genes exert their most deleterious effects on organs most dependent on oxidative phosphorylation, including the central nervous system and muscles. The other listed options do not exhibit strict maternal inheritance.

BP7 235-236   BP6 178   PBD7 185   PBD6 179-180

12 (A) Almost all of the normal genetic material is present in the case of a robertsonian translocation, because only a small amount of the p arm from each chromosome is lost. Statistically, one of six fetuses in a mother who carries a robertsonian translocation will also be a carrier. In balanced reciprocal translocation, the same possibility of inheriting the defect exists. However, the other listed structural abnormalities are likely to result in loss of significant genetic material, reducing survivability, or to interfere with meiosis.

BP7 230, 232   BP6 192-193   PBD7 174-175
PBD6 168-170

13 (D) Cleft lip and palate, along with microcephaly and polydactyly, are features of trisomy 13 (Patau syndrome). These infants also commonly have severe heart defects. For monosomy X (45,X) to be considered, the infant must be female. The severe anomalies described in this case may occur with a normal karyotype (46,XY), but the spectrum of findings, particularly the polydactyly, suggests trisomy 13. Klinefelter syndrome (47,XXY) results in phenotypic males who are

hard to distinguish from males with a 46,XY karyotype. Infants with trisomy 18 lack polydactyly and are more likely to have micrognathia than are infants with trisomy 13. Triploidy with 69 chromosomes leads to stillbirth in virtually all cases.

BP7 231   BP6 194   PBD7 177   PBD6 172

14 (E) This infant has Pompe disease, a form of glycogen storage disease that results from a deficiency in lysosomal glucosidase (acid maltase). The glycogen stored in the myocardium results in massive cardiomegaly and heart failure within 2 years. Glucocerebrosidase deficiency occurs in Gaucher disease. In the most common form of the disease, there is no neurologic impairment, and patients have splenomegaly and skeletal disease as a consequence of increased lysosomal glucocerebrosides in cells of the mononuclear phagocyte system. Glucose-6-phosphatase deficiency leads to von Gierke disease, characterized by hepatomegaly, renomegaly, and impaired gluconeogenesis leading to hypoglycemia and hyperlipidemia. Hexosaminidase A deficiency occurs in Tay-Sachs disease and is associated with severe neurologic impairment, poor motor development, and blindness beginning in infancy. Homogentisic oxidase deficiency leads to alkaptonuria with ochronosis or to deposition of a blueblack pigment in joints, resulting in arthropathy. Myophosphorylase deficiency leads to McArdle disease, characterized by muscle cramping after strenuous exercise. Sphingomyelinase deficiency occurs in Niemann-Pick disease; affected persons with type A have hepatosplenomegaly, lymphadenopathy, and severe motor and mental impairment.

BP7 225   BP6 188-189   PBD7 166-167   PBD6 160, 163

15 (A) This child has one of the three forms of Gaucher disease. Type 1, seen in this child, accounts for 99% of cases and does not involve the central nervous system (CNS). It is caused by a deficiency of glucocerebrosidase, and infusion with this enzyme reduces severity and progression. Type 2 involves the CNS and is lethal in infancy. Type 3 also involves the CNS, although not as severely as type 2. A deficiency of acid maltase is a feature of Pompe disease. Von Gierke disease results from deficiency of glucose-6-phosphatase. Sphingomyelinase deficiency leads to Niemann-Pick disease types A and B. Type A, the more common form, is associated with severe neurologic deterioration. Type B, the less common form, may resemble the findings in this case, but the appearance of macrophages is different: they contain many small vacuoles. Tay-Sachs disease involves a deficiency of hexosaminidase A and is also associated with severe mental retardation and death before 10 years of age.

BP7 223-224   BP6 187   PBD7 163-165   PBD6 158-159

16 (A) These findings are characteristic of fragile X syndrome, a condition in which there are 250 to 4000 tandem repeats of the trinucleotide sequence CGG. Generally, as the number of trinucleotide repeats increases, the manifestations of the associated conditions worsen or have an earlier onset. The trinucleotide mutations are dynamic; because their number increases during oogenesis, subsequent male offspring have more severe disease compared with, for example, their grandfathers. With a frameshift mutation, one, two, or three nucleotide base pairs are inserted or deleted. As a result, the protein transcribed is abnormal. A missense mutation results from a single nucleotide base substitution, and it leads to elaboration of an abnormal protein. Abnormalities of mitochondrial DNA, typically involving genes associated with oxidative phosphorylation, are transmitted on the maternal side.

BP7 234-235 BP6 176-178 PBD7 181-183
PBD6 143, 177-178

17 **(C)** The patient has neurofibromatosis type 1 (NF-1), characterized by the development of multiple neurofibromas and pigmented skin lesions. Neurofibromas are most numerous in the dermis but also may occur in visceral organs. Patients with NF-1 may also develop a type of sarcomatous neoplasm known as a malignant peripheral nerve sheath tumor (MPNST). Dermatofibromas are subcutaneous masses that typically are small and solitary. Leiomyomas occur most frequently in the uterus. Lipomas can occur almost anywhere in the body, but do so sporadically. Hemangiomas may occur sporadically on the skin; they typically are red-blue masses.

BP7 226-227, 848-849 BP6 189-190 PBD7 168-169
PBD6 162-164

18 **(C)** These features are characteristic of trisomy 21, but the child is not severely affected, which suggests mosaicism. In mosaic persons, greater numbers of potentially normal cells having the proper chromosomal complement are present, which may allow infants with abnormalities of chromosome number to survive to term and beyond. Haploidy is present in gametes. Loss of an autosomal chromosome is devastating; the only monosomy associated with possible survival to term is Turner syndrome (monosomy X). Most aneuploid conditions (trisomies and monosomies) lead to fetal demise; fetuses with trisomy 21 are the most likely to survive to term. Triploid fetuses rarely survive beyond the second trimester and are virtually never liveborn. Likewise, tetraploidy accounts for many first-trimester fetal losses and is not survivable.

BP7 228 BP6 191 PBD7 175-177 PBD6 168

19 **(A)** Physicians must be cautious in assigning sex to an infant with ambiguous genitalia; changing one's opinion is about as popular as an umpire changing the call. True hermaphroditism, with ovarian and testicular tissue present, is rare. This infant has female pseudohermaphroditism, resulting from exposure of the fetus to excessive androgenic stimulation, which in this case is due to congenital adrenal hyperplasia. Both the gonadal and the karyotypic sex are female. Male pseudohermaphroditism has a variety of forms, but the most common is testicular feminization, resulting from androgen insensitivity. Those affected are phenotypically females but have testes and a 46,XY karyotype. Nondisjunctional events lead to monosomies or trisomies. Trinucleotide repeats are seen in males with fragile X syndrome. Abnormalities of mitochondrial DNA have a maternal transmission pattern and do not involve sex chromosomes or sexual characteristics.

PBD7 181 PBD6 176

20 **(B)** The findings listed suggest a severe inherited neurologic disease, and the pattern of inheritance (e.g., normal parents, an affected sibling) is consistent with an autosomal recessive disorder. This inheritance pattern and the cherry red

spot in the retina are characteristic of Tay-Sachs disease, caused by mutations in the gene that encodes a lysosomal enzyme hexosaminidase A. Mitochondrial genes have a maternal pattern of transmission. Mutations in genes affecting receptor proteins and structural proteins typically give rise to an autosomal dominant pattern of inheritance. Genomic imprinting is characterized by a parent-of-origin effect.

BP7 222-223 BP6 186 PBD7 160-162
PBD6 148, 155-156, 179-180

21 **(B)** This child has an immunodeficiency characterized by infection, a small thymus, congenital malformations, and hypoparathyroidism. This cluster is characteristic of the 22q11.2 deletion syndrome, readily diagnosed by FISH. HIV infection can lead to AIDS, but no congenital anomalies are associated with this condition. Trinucleotide repeats of the X chromosome are seen in fragile X syndrome, which manifests with mental retardation in males. Adenosine deaminase deficiency can cause immunodeficiency, but it is not associated with congenital malformations. A lymph node biopsy may show a reduction in T or B cells associated with various forms of immunodeficiency, but this is not a specific test that can aid in confirming a specific diagnosis.

BP7 232 PBD7 176, 178 PBD6 173

22 **(B)** This child has von Gierke disease. Because of the deficiency of glucose-6-phosphatase, glycogen is not metabolized readily to glucose. Affected persons have severe hypoglycemia, which leads to convulsions. Intracytoplasmic accumulations of glycogen occur mainly in the liver and kidney. Another form of glycogen storage disease, McArdle syndrome, results from a deficiency of muscle phosphorylase and leads to muscle cramping. Tay-Sachs disease is characterized by a deficiency in hexosaminidase A and results in severe neurologic deterioration. In Hurler syndrome, the enzyme α-L-iduronidase is deficient. Affected children have skeletal deformities and a buildup of mucopolysaccharides in endocardium and coronary arteries, leading to heart failure. Cardiomegaly and heart failure mark Pompe disease, another form of glycogen storage disease.

BP7 225 BP6 188-189 PBD7 166-167 PBD6 160-163

23 **(D)** This girl has Ehlers-Danlos syndrome, which results from a collagen defect that causes connective tissues to be weak and fragile. A deficiency of α_1-antitrypsin leads to liver and lung disease. A mutated retinoblastoma (Rb) protein is associated with development of neoplasms, including retinoblastoma and osteosarcoma. Inherited defects in the number of LDL receptors result in hypercholesterolemia, leading to early and advanced atherosclerosis. A deficiency of factor VIII occurs in hemophilia A.

BP7 218 BP6 182 PBD7 155-156 PBD6 149-150

24 **(B)** The infant has findings associated with trisomy 18. In the FISH analysis shown, the chromosomes in each cell have been painted with a marker for chromosome 18. In this case, there are three markers per cell, consistent with a trisomy. In reality, many cells would have to be counted to allow for artifacts in preparation. In most cases, trisomy 18 results from nondisjunctional events. Most infants with trisomy 18 are stillborn, and survival beyond 4 months is rare. The other listed options do not account for this FISH analysis or for this spectrum of anomalies.

BP7 231   BP6 194   PBD7 177   PBD6 172

25 **(B)** The clinical features of this child—neurologic involvement, hepatosplenomegaly, and accumulation of foamy macrophages—suggest a lysosomal storage disorder. One such disorder, with which the clinical history is quite compatible, is Niemann-Pick disease type A. It is characterized by lysosomal accumulation of sphingomyelin due to a severe deficiency of sphingomyelinase. In familial hypercholesterolemia, there are fewer numbers of LDL receptors on hepatocytes, leading to early and accelerated atherosclerosis by young adulthood. Collagen synthesis is impaired in persons with Ehlers-Danlos syndrome. The glycogen storage disease known as von Gierke disease results from glucose-6-phosphatase deficiency. Globules of α_1-antitrypsin are seen in the liver cells of persons with inherited deficiency of α_1-antitrypsin.

BP7 223   BP6 186-187   PBD7 163   PBD6 156-158

26 **(E)** The findings listed are characteristic of Turner syndrome (monosomy X), which accounts for a considerable portion of first-trimester fetal losses. The hygroma is quite suggestive of this disorder. Fetuses with this finding are rarely liveborn. Trisomy 18 can be marked by multiple anomalies, but overlapping fingers and a short neck are more typical features. The presence of additional X chromosomes may not cause serious fetal anomalies, because all but one X chromosome is inactive. Down syndrome (47,XX,+21) may be accompanied by a hygroma and hydrops, but ventricular septal defect is more frequent than coarctation, and horseshoe kidney is uncommon. The 47,XXY karyotype (Klinefelter syndrome) does not result in stillbirth, and these males have no major congenital defects. Triploidy with 69 chromosomes typically leads to fetal loss, but hydrops and hygroma are not features of this condition.

BP7 233-234   BP6 196-197   PBD7 179-180
PBD6 174-176

27 **(B)** Type 1 diabetes mellitus has an increased frequency in some families, but the exact mechanism of inheritance is unknown. The risk is about 6% for offspring when first-order relatives are affected. HLA-linked genes and other genetic loci, as well as environmental factors, are considered important. This pattern of inheritance is multifactorial. The other listed inheritance patterns are not seen with diabetes mellitus.

BP7 227, 643-644   BP6 190, 564-565   PBD7 169-170
PBD6 165, 915-916

28 **(C)** Failure to find amplified product by PCR analysis in such a case could mean that the fetus is not affected or that there is a full mutation that is too large to be detected by PCR. The next logical step is a Southern blot analysis of genomic DNA from fetal cells. Routine karyotyping of the amniotic fluid cells is much less sensitive than a Southern blot analysis. Karyotyping of the unaffected father cannot provide information about the status of the *FMR1* gene in the fetus, because amplification of the trinucleotide occurs during oogenesis. For the same reason, PCR analysis of the mother's *FMR1* gene is of no value.

BP7 234-235   PBD7 188-189   PBD6 183-184

29 **(D)** This child has features of Angelman syndrome, and the DNA analysis shows uniparental disomy. The Angelman gene encoded on chromosome 15 is subject to genomic imprinting. It is silenced on the paternal chromosome 15 but is active on the maternal chromosome 15. If the child lacks maternal chromosome 15, there is no active Angelman gene in the somatic cells. This gives rise to the abnormalities typical of this disorder. The same effect occurs when there is a deletion of the Angelman gene from the maternal chromosome 15. The other listed options do not occur in uniparental disomy.

BP7 236-237   BP6 199   PBD7 186-187   PBD6 180-181

30 **(C)** This man has Marfan syndrome, an autosomal dominant condition that is caused by quantitative and qualitative defects in fibrillin from mutations in the fibrillin gene. Genetic mutations in the dystrophin gene are involved in Duchenne and Becker muscular dystrophies. An abnormal collagen gene can cause osteogenesis imperfecta and Ehlers-Danlos syndrome. The NF1 protein is abnormal in neurofibromatosis type 1. Disordered spectrin causes hereditary spherocytosis.

BP7 217-218   BP6 181   PBD7 154-155   PBD6 148-149

31 **(A)** This woman has androgen insensitivity ("testicular feminization") syndrome, which results from X-linked inheritance of a defect in the androgen receptor. The cells of affected persons do not respond to dihydrotestosterone, but they do respond to estradiol, producing a phenotypic female. Testes are present but typically are cryptorchid, and there is an increased risk of testicular neoplasms. Manifestations of fragile X syndrome are more likely to be seen in males. The disorder stems from an abnormality in a triple repeat sequence in the *FMR1* gene, and the most significant consequence is mental retardation. Gonadal mosaicism refers to the presence of a genetic mutation acquired during embryogenesis and present only in germ cells; the person with the mutation does not manifest the disease, but multiple offspring do. Hypopituitarism can lead to hypogonadism and diminished secondary sex characteristics, but a person with a karyotype of 46,XY would be a phenotypic male. Agenesis of the testes does not occur in persons with the androgen insensitivity syndrome, but lack of normal descent may make it difficult to observe the testes in these persons.

PBD7 181

32 **(D)** The infant has cystic fibrosis. The elevated sweat chloride level is related to a defect in the transport of chloride ions across epithelia. The most common genetic defect is a deletion of three base pairs at the ΔF508 position coding for phenylalanine in the CFTR gene. A frameshift mutation involves one or two base pairs, not three, and changes the remaining sequence of amino acids in a protein. A point mutation may change the codon to the sequence of a "stop" codon that truncates the protein being synthesized, typically leading to degradation of the protein. A point mutation typically is a missense mutation that leads to replacement of one amino acid for another in the protein chain; this can lead to abnormal conformation and function of the protein. A trinucleotide repeat sequence mutation leads to amplification of repeats of three nucleotides, so-called tandem repeats, which prevent normal gene expression.

BP7 213-214, 250-251   PBD7 147-149, 151   PBD6 143

33 (E) This is the inheritance pattern for fragile X syndrome, which is caused by triple repeat expansions in the *FMR1* gene. In normal persons, the number of CGG repeats is about 29 and thus the normal band is small. In persons with premutations, there are typically 52 to 200 repeats, and about 80% of males and 50% of females with premutations are affected. Premutations produce larger DNA fragments and hence they migrate more slowly than normal bands on the gel. Carrier males transmit the gene without further expansion of repeats, but carrier females expand the repeats during oogenesis, so that affected persons have the full mutation of 230 to 4000 repeats, and these produce the largest DNA fragments that migrate very slowly and appear at the top of the gel. The other options do not involve a genetic premutation. A frameshift mutation involves one or two base pairs and changes the remaining sequence of amino acids in a protein. A point mutation may change the codon to the sequence of a "stop" codon that truncates the protein being synthesized, typically leading to degradation of the protein. A point mutation typically is a missense mutation that leads to replacement of one amino acid for another in the protein chain; this can lead to abnormal conformation and function of the protein. A deletion of three base pairs leads to loss of a single amino acid in a protein.

BP7 234-235, 261   PBD7 181-183   PBD6 177-179

34 (B) The infant has DiGeorge syndrome, resulting from a chromosome 22q11.2 microdeletion. This is indicated in the metaphase spread by the presence of only three dots, because this region is deleted on one chromosome 22, but both number 22 chromosomes are present. With aneuploidy, there is an abnormal number of chromosomes (trisomy, monosomy), and loss or gain of autosomes tends to produce fetal loss, except for some cases of trisomies 13, 18, and 21 and monosomy X. A chromosome inversion would shift the marked region to a different part of the same chromosome. In monosomy, only one of a pair of chromosomes is present. A translocation is the swapping of genetic material between two chromosomes.

BP7 228-230, 257-258   PBD7 176, 178   PBD6 173, 235

CHAPTER 6

Diseases of Immunity

PBD7 Chapter 6: Diseases of Immunity

PBD6 Chapter 7: Diseases of Immunity

BP7 Chapter 5: Diseases of Immunity

BP6 Chapter 5: Disorders of the Immune System

1 A 25-year-old woman has had increasing malaise, a slight fever, and arthralgias and myalgias for the past month. On physical examination, her temperature is 37.7°C. On auscultation, a friction rub is audible over the chest. There is no joint deformity or swelling. Laboratory findings include hemoglobin 10.8 g/dL, hematocrit 32.5%, platelet count 106,700/mm^3, and WBC count 3420/mm^3. Urinalysis shows 2+ proteinuria. A serologic test for syphilis yields a false-positive result. A chest radiograph shows bilateral pleural effusions. Which of the following problems is most likely to occur as a result of the patient's underlying disease?

- ❑ (A) Photosensitivity
- ❑ (B) Urethritis
- ❑ (C) Esophageal dysmotility
- ❑ (D) Xerostomia
- ❑ (E) Congenital heart disease

2 A 30-year-old woman has had fever and arthralgia for the past 2 weeks. On physical examination, she has a temperature of 37.6°C and an erythematous malar rash. Initial laboratory studies are positive for ANAs at 1:1600 and anti–double-stranded DNA antibodies at 1:3200. Serum creatinine is markedly elevated, and serum complement levels are decreased. A VDRL test for syphilis is positive, and in vitro tests of coagulation (prothrombin time and partial thromboplastin time) are prolonged. Which of the following clinical features of her illness is most likely caused by antibodies that interfere with the coagulation test?

- ❑ (A) Arthritis
- ❑ (B) Recurrent thrombosis
- ❑ (C) Rash
- ❑ (D) Renal failure
- ❑ (E) Fever

3 In epidemiologic studies of HIV infection and AIDS, investigators noticed that certain individuals failed to develop HIV infection despite known exposure to the virus under conditions that caused HIV disease in all other individuals similarly exposed. When CD4+ lymphocytes from resistant individuals are incubated with HIV-1, they fail to become infected. Such resistance to infection by HIV is most likely caused by a mutation affecting genes for which of the following cellular components?

- ❑ (A) T cell receptor
- ❑ (B) Chemokine receptor
- ❑ (C) Interleukin-2 receptor
- ❑ (D) CD28 receptor
- ❑ (E) Fc receptor
- ❑ (F) p24 antigen

4 A 12-year-old boy has had multiple recurrent infections for the past 10 years, including *Pneumocystis carinii* pneumonia, *Streptococcus pneumoniae* otitis media, and *Pseudomonas aeruginosa* urinary tract infection. On physical examination, he has a temperature of 38.5°C and pharyngeal erythema with exudate. Laboratory studies show hemoglobin of 9.1 g/dL, hematocrit 27.6%, platelet count 130,900/mm³, and WBC count 3,440/mm³ with 47% segmented neutrophils, 3% bands, 40% lymphocytes, and 10% monocytes. Serum immunoglobulin levels are IgG 88 mg/dL, IgM 721 mg/dL, and IgA undetectable. A peripheral blood smear shows nucleated RBCs. Which of the following immunologic defects is most likely to produce this disease?

- ❑ (A) Absence of adenosine deaminase
- ❑ (B) Abnormal CD40-CD40L interaction
- ❑ (C) Deletion of chromosome 22q11
- ❑ (D) HIV infection
- ❑ (E) Lack of IgA production by B lymphocytes
- ❑ (F) Mutation in the *BTK* gene

5 Within minutes after a bee sting, a 15-year-old girl suddenly has difficulty breathing. There is marked urticaria and marked edema of the hand that was stung. Which of the following is the best pharmacologic agent to treat these signs and symptoms?

- ❑ (A) Cyclosporine
- ❑ (B) Epinephrine
- ❑ (C) Penicillin
- ❑ (D) Glucocorticoids
- ❑ (E) Methotrexate

6 A 31-year-old woman notices that when she is outside in the sun for more than 1 hour, she develops a rash on her face. Laboratory studies show hemoglobin of 10.9 g/dL, hematocrit 32.9%, platelet count 156,800/mm³, and WBC count 4211/mm³. Urinalysis shows no blood or glucose; there is 3+ proteinuria. The ANA test result is positive with a titer of 1:2048 and a diffuse homogeneous immunofluorescent staining pattern. Which of the following complications is most characteristic of her illness?

- ❑ (A) Bronchoconstriction
- ❑ (B) Cerebral lymphoma
- ❑ (C) Hemolytic anemia
- ❑ (D) Keratoconjunctivitis
- ❑ (E) Sacroiliitis
- ❑ (F) Sclerodactyly

7 A 43-year-old woman has been bothered by a chronic, dry cough for the past 5 years. She has had increasing difficulty with blurred vision for the past year. On physical examination, she has a perforated nasal septum, bilateral mild corneal scarring, and oral cavity fissuring of the tongue and corners of her mouth. Laboratory studies show antibodies to SS-A and SS-B. The serum creatinine is 2.5, and the urea nitrogen is 25 mg/dL. A renal biopsy specimen examined microscopically shows tubulointerstitial nephritis. Which of the following is the most serious condition likely to complicate the course of her disease?

- ❑ (A) Chronic renal failure
- ❑ (B) Endocarditis
- ❑ (C) Non-Hodgkin lymphoma
- ❑ (D) Photosensitivity
- ❑ (E) Sclerodactyly
- ❑ (F) Subcutaneous nodules
- ❑ (G) Urethritis

8 A 48-year-old man has been relatively healthy all of his life, bothered only by an occasional mild diarrheal illness. On physical examination, his temperature is 37.1°C and blood pressure is 125/85 mm Hg. Laboratory studies show a total WBC count of 6900/mm³ with 72% segmented neutrophils, 3% bands, 18% lymphocytes, and 7% monocytes. Serum immunoglobulin levels are IgG 1.9 g/dL, IgM 0.3 g/dL, and IgA 0.01 g/dL. The ANA test result is negative. The skin test result for mumps and *Candida* antigens is positive. This patient is at greatest risk of infection from which of the following agents?

- ❑ (A) *Pneumocystis carinii*
- ❑ (B) *Streptococcus pneumoniae*
- ❑ (C) Hepatitis B virus
- ❑ (D) *Aspergillus flavus*
- ❑ (E) Herpes simplex virus

9 A 37-year-old man who is HIV positive has noticed multiple 0.5- to 1.2-cm plaque-like, reddish-purple, skin lesions on his face, trunk, and extremities. Some of the larger lesions appear to be nodular. These lesions have appeared over the past 6 months and have slowly enlarged. Molecular analysis of the spindle cells found in these skin lesions is likely to reveal the genome of which of the following viruses?

- ❑ (A) Cytomegalovirus
- ❑ (B) Epstein-Barr virus
- ❑ (C) Adenovirus
- ❑ (D) Human herpesvirus-8
- ❑ (E) HIV-1

10 In an experiment, antigen is used to induce an immediate (type I) hypersensitivity response. Cytokines are secreted that are observed to stimulate IgE production by B cells, promote mast cell growth, and recruit and activate eosinophils in this response. Which of the following cells is most likely to be the source of these cytokines?

- ❑ (A) CD4+ lymphocytes
- ❑ (B) Natural killer cells
- ❑ (C) Macrophages
- ❑ (D) Dendritic cells
- ❑ (E) Neutrophils

11 For the past 6 weeks, a 52-year-old woman has had bilateral diffuse pain in her thighs and shoulders. She has difficulty rising from a chair and climbing steps. She has a rash with a violaceous color around the orbits and on the skin of her knuckles. On physical examination, she is afebrile. Muscle strength is 4/5 in all extremities. Laboratory studies show serum creatine kinase of 753 U/L, and the ANA test result is positive with a titer of 1:160. Which of the following tests is most specific for the diagnosis of this patient's underlying condition?

❏ (A) Anti–double-stranded DNA antibodies
❏ (B) Rheumatoid factor
❏ (C) Anti–U1-ribonucleoprotein antibodies
❏ (D) Antihistone antibodies
❏ (E) Anti–Jo-1 antibodies

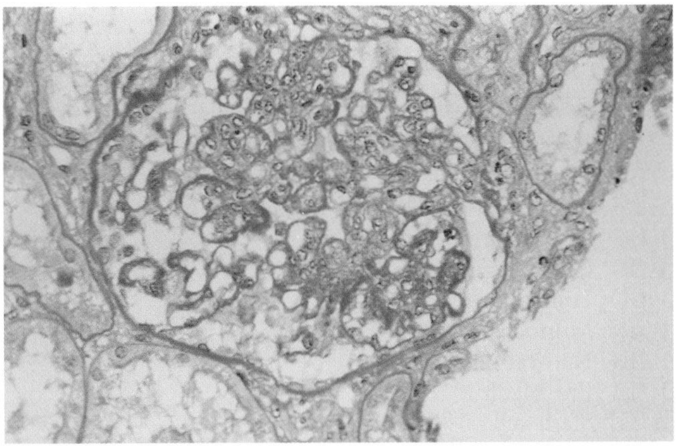

Courtesy of Dr. Helmut Rennke, Department of Pathology, Brigham and Women's Hospital, Boston, MA.

12 A 31-year-old woman has had increasing edema, chest pain, and an erythematous rash for the past 6 months. Laboratory studies show increasing serum creatinine, and urinalysis shows proteinuria with RBC casts. A renal biopsy is performed, and the light microscopic appearance of the PAS-stained specimen is seen in the figure. If present, which of the following antibodies is most helpful in diagnosing this patient's condition?

❏ (A) Scl-70
❏ (B) Anti-Sm
❏ (C) Jo-1
❏ (D) Anti–HLA-B27
❏ (E) Anticentromere

13 A 23-year-old man has had myalgias and a fever for the past week. On physical examination, his temperature is 38.6°C. He has diffuse muscle tenderness but no rashes or joint pain on movement. Laboratory studies show elevated serum creatine kinase and peripheral blood eosinophilia. Larvae of *Trichinella spiralis* are present within the skeletal muscle fibers of a gastrocnemius biopsy specimen. Two years later, a chest radiograph shows only a few small calcifications in the diaphragm. Which of the following immunologic mechanisms most likely contributed to the destruction of the larvae?

❏ (A) Antibody-dependent cellular cytotoxicity
❏ (B) Complement-mediated cell lysis
❏ (C) Formation of Langhans giant cells
❏ (D) Abscess formation with neutrophils
❏ (E) Synthesis of leukotriene C4 in mast cells

14 A 45-year-old man with chronic renal failure received a kidney transplant from his brother 36 months ago. For the next 30 months, he had only minor episodes of rejection that were controlled with immunosuppressive therapy. However, in the past 6 months, he has had increasing serum creatinine and urea nitrogen levels. On physical examination, he is afebrile. Microscopic examination of a urinalysis specimen shows no WBCs. CT scan of the pelvis shows that the allograft is reduced in size. Which of the following immunologic processes most likely accounts for these findings?

❏ (A) Macrophage-mediated cell lysis
❏ (B) Vascular intimal fibrosis
❏ (C) Granulomatous vasculitis
❏ (D) Release of leukotriene C4 from mast cells
❏ (E) Complement-mediated cell lysis

15 A 20-year-old man steps into an elevator full of people who are coughing and sneezing, all of whom appear to have colds or the flu. The influenza viral particles that he inhales attach to respiratory epithelium, and viral transformation reduces the MHC class I molecules on these epithelial cells. Which of the following cells is most likely to respond to destroy the infected cells?

❏ (A) Natural killer cell
❏ (B) Neutrophil
❏ (C) Macrophage
❏ (D) CD4 cell
❏ (E) Dendritic cell

16 A 35-year-old man has a history of mild infections of the upper respiratory tract. He also has had diarrhea for most of his life, although it was not severe enough to cause malabsorption and weight loss. After an episode of trauma with blood loss, he receives a blood transfusion and has an anaphylactic reaction. Which of the following underlying conditions best explains these findings?

❏ (A) Severe combined immunodeficiency
❏ (B) HIV infection
❏ (C) DiGeorge syndrome
❏ (D) Wiskott-Aldrich syndrome
❏ (E) Selective IgA deficiency

17 A laboratory worker who is "allergic" to fungal spores is accidentally exposed to a culture of the incriminating fungus on a Friday afternoon. Within 1 hour, he develops bouts of sneezing, watery eyes, and nasal discharge. The symptoms seem to subside within a few hours of returning home but reappear the next morning, although the laboratory fungus is not present in his home environment. The symptoms persist through the weekend, and on Monday morning, he sees the physician. Which of the following cells is most likely to be seen on microscopic examination of the patient's nasal discharge?

❏ (A) Mast cells and neutrophils
❏ (B) Lymphocytes and macrophages
❏ (C) Neutrophils, eosinophils, and CD4+ lymphocytes
❏ (D) Neutrophils and CD8+ lymphocytes
❏ (E) Mast cells, lymphocytes, and macrophages

18 A 30-year-old man infected with HIV begins to have difficulty with activities of daily living. He has memory problems and decreased ability to perform functions that require fine motor control, such as writing and painting. His CD4 lymphocyte count currently is 150/μL. Which of the following cell types is most important for the dissemination of the infection into the central nervous system?

❑ (A) Natural killer cell
❑ (B) Macrophage
❑ (C) Neutrophil
❑ (D) CD8 lymphocyte
❑ (E) Langerhans cell

19 A 29-year-old man has developed marked abdominal pain over the past week. On physical examination, there is diffuse abdominal tenderness with decreased bowel sounds, but no masses are noted. The stool is negative for occult blood. Laboratory studies show a serum creatinine level of 4.4 mg/dL and urea nitrogen level of 42 mg/dL. Microscopic examination of a renal biopsy specimen shows focal fibrinoid necrosis of the small arterial and arteriolar vascular media as well as intravascular microthrombi. Scattered neutrophils are seen in these areas of necrosis. Which of the following laboratory findings would most likely be present in this patient?

❑ (A) Increased IgE
❑ (B) Neutropenia
❑ (C) Decreased complement C3
❑ (D) Tuberculin skin test positivity
❑ (E) CD4 lymphocytosis

20 A 63-year-old man has had chronic arthritis for the past 15 years. Physical examination shows ulnar deviation with bony ankylosis producing swan-neck deformities of the fingers of his hands. Laboratory studies show 4.2 g of protein in a 24-hour urine collection, serum creatinine of 3.1 g/dL, and urea nitrogen of 3 g/dL. A rectal biopsy is performed, which demonstrates deposition of amorphous pink material in the mucosa. The material stains positive with Congo red. Which of the following best describes this material in the mucosa?

❑ (A) It is within the cytoplasm
❑ (B) It contains >50% P component
❑ (C) It is derived from an acute-phase reactant
❑ (D) It does not show birefringence after Congo red staining
❑ (E) It is derived from λ light chains

21 A 60-year-old woman who undergoes a routine health screening examination has a blood pressure of 155/95 mm Hg. She receives antihypertensive therapy that includes hydralazine. Four months later, she develops arthralgias, myalgias, and a malar erythematous rash. Laboratory findings include an ANA titer of 1:2560 in a diffuse pattern. Anti–double-stranded DNA antibodies are not present. Which of the following autoantibodies has the greatest specificity for her condition?

❑ (A) Anti-Sm
❑ (B) Antihistone
❑ (C) Anti–Jo-1
❑ (D) Anti–U1-riboneucleoprotein
❑ (E) Anticentromere
❑ (F) Anti–SS-A

22 A 4-year-old child has a history of recurrent sinopulmonary infections with *Staphylococcus aureus* and *Streptococcus pneumoniae* since the age of 17 months. He also developed an arthritis that cleared with immunoglobulin therapy. On physical examination, he is at the 30th percentile for height and weight. His temperature is 37.9°C. There is no lymphadenopathy, and lymph nodes are difficult to palpate. There is no hepatosplenomegaly. Laboratory studies show total serum protein of 5.1 g/dL and albumin 4.6 g/dL. A lymph node biopsy specimen shows lymph nodes with rudimentary germinal centers. Over the next 10 years, the child develops arthralgias and erythematous skin rashes and has a positive ANA test result. Which of the following types of cells has most likely failed to differentiate to produce this patient's disease?

❑ (A) CD4+ lymphocyte
❑ (B) CD8+ lymphocyte
❑ (C) Follicular dendritic cell
❑ (D) Monocyte
❑ (E) Natural killer cell
❑ (F) Pre-B cell
❑ (G) Stem cell

23 A 3-month-old boy has had recurrent infections of the respiratory, gastrointestinal, and urinary tracts since birth. The infectious agents have included *Candida albicans*, *Pneumocystis carinii*, *Pseudomonas aeruginosa*, and cytomegalovirus. Despite intensive treatment with antibiotics and antifungal drugs, he dies at the age of 5 months. At autopsy, lymph nodes are small with very few lymphocytes and no germinal centers. The thymus, Peyer patches, and tonsils are hypoplastic. There is a family history of other males with similar findings. Which of the following immunologic alterations best describes the abnormality that caused this patient's illness?

❑ (A) Maternal HIV infection
❑ (B) Loss of chromosome 22q11
❑ (C) Mutation in the common γ chain of cytokine receptors
❑ (D) Mutation in the *BTK* gene
❑ (E) Mutation in CD40 ligand

24 A 34-year-old woman has experienced increasing muscular weakness over the past 5 months. This weakness is most pronounced in muscles that are used extensively, such as the levator palpebrae of the eyelids, causing her to have difficulty with vision by the end of the day. After a night's sleep, her symptoms have lessened. On physical examination, she is afebrile. No skin rashes are noted. Muscle strength is 5/5 initially, but diminishes with repetitive movement. Which of the following is the most likely mechanism for muscle weakness in this patient?

❑ (A) Secretion of cytokines by activated macrophages
❑ (B) Lysis of muscle cells by CD8+ T cells
❑ (C) Antibody-mediated dysfunction of neuromuscular junction
❑ (D) Deposition of immune complexes in the muscle capillaries
❑ (E) Delayed hypersensitivity reaction against muscle antigens

25 A 45-year-old woman has experienced difficulty in swallowing that has increased in severity over the past year. She has also experienced malabsorption, demonstrated by a 5-kg weight loss in the past 6 months. She reports increasing dyspnea during this time. On physical examination, her temperature is 36.9°C, pulse 66/min, respirations 18/min, and blood pressure 145/90 mm Hg. Echocardiography shows a large pericardial effusion. The ANA test result is positive at 1:512 with a nucleolar pattern. Which of the following serious complications of the patient's underlying autoimmune disease is most likely to occur?

❑ (A) Meningitis
❑ (B) Glomerulonephritis
❑ (C) Perforated duodenal ulcer
❑ (D) Adrenal failure
❑ (E) Malignant hypertension

26 A 30-year old woman gives birth at term to a normal-appearing infant girl. One hour after birth, the neonate exhibits tetany. On physical examination, she is at the 55th percentile for height and weight. Laboratory studies show serum calcium of 6.3 mg/dL and phosphorus of 3.5 mg/dL. Over the next year, the infant has bouts of pneumonia caused by *Pneumocystis carinii* and *Aspergillus fumigatus* and upper respiratory infections with parainfluenza virus and herpes simplex virus. Which of the following mechanisms is most likely to be responsible for the development of the clinical features seen in this infant?

❑ (A) Malformation of third and fourth pharyngeal pouches
❑ (B) Failure of maturation of B cells into plasma cells
❑ (C) Lack of adenosine deaminase
❑ (D) Acquisition of maternal HIV infection at delivery
❑ (E) Failure of differentiation of pre-B cells into B cells

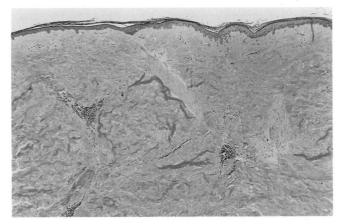

Courtesy of Dr. Trace Worrell, Department of Pathology, University of Texas Southwestern Medical School, Dallas, TX.

27 A 39-year-old woman has fingers that are tapered and clawlike, with decreased motion at the small joints. The microscopic appearance of the skin is shown in the figure. The patient also has diffuse interstitial fibrosis of the lungs, with pulmonary hypertension and cor pulmonale. Which of the following dermal inflammatory cells is the most likely initiator of the process that results in her skin disease?

❑ (A) CD4 lymphocyte
❑ (B) Macrophage
❑ (C) Mast cell
❑ (D) Neutrophil
❑ (E) Natural killer cell

28 A 19-year-old previously healthy woman had an acute illness with fever, myalgia, sore throat, and mild erythematous rash over the abdomen and thighs. The symptoms abated after 1 month, and she remained healthy for 8 years. Now, decreased visual acuity and pain in the right eye lead to a finding of cytomegalovirus retinitis on funduscopy. Assuming that the patient's initial illness and the ocular problem are a part of the same disease process, which of the following laboratory findings would most likely be present after her ocular problems began to appear?

❑ (A) ANA titer 1:1024
❑ (B) Total serum globulin level 650 mg/dL
❑ (C) Positive HLA-B27 antigen
❑ (D) Anticentromere antibody titer 1:512
❑ (E) CD4 lymphocyte count 102/μL

29 A 32-year-old woman with a 10-year history of intravenous drug use has developed a chronic watery diarrhea that has persisted for the past week. On physical examination, she is afebrile and has mild muscle wasting. Her BMI is 18. Laboratory studies of the stool show cysts of *Cryptosporidium parvum*. One month later, she develops cryptococcal meningitis, which is treated successfully. Oral candidiasis is diagnosed 1 month later. This patient is at greatest risk of developing which of the following neoplasms?

❑ (A) Intestinal non-Hodgkin lymphoma
❑ (B) Adenocarcinoma of the lung
❑ (C) Leiomyosarcoma of retroperitoneum
❑ (D) Cervical squamous carcinoma
❑ (E) Cerebral astrocytoma

30 An epidemiologic study is conducted to determine risk factors for HIV infection. The study documents that persons with coexisting sexually transmitted diseases such as chancroid are more likely to become HIV positive. It is postulated that an inflamed mucosal surface is an ideal location for the transmission of HIV during sexual intercourse. Which of the following cells in these mucosal surfaces is most instrumental in transmitting HIV to CD4+ T lymphocytes?

❑ (A) CD8+ cells
❑ (B) Natural killer cells
❑ (C) Dendritic cells
❑ (D) Neutrophils
❑ (E) Plasma cells

31 A 35-year-old woman who has been in the hospital receiving treatment for leukemia has developed an extensive, scaling rash over the past week. A skin biopsy specimen shows keratinocyte apoptosis along the dermal-epidermal junction, with upper dermal lymphocytic infiltrates. She also has jaundice. This patient has most likely recently undergone which of the following procedures?

❑ (A) Tuberculin skin testing
❑ (B) Chemotherapy for malignant lymphoma
❑ (C) Allogeneic bone marrow transplantation
❑ (D) Penicillin therapy for pneumonia
❑ (E) Patch testing for allergen detection

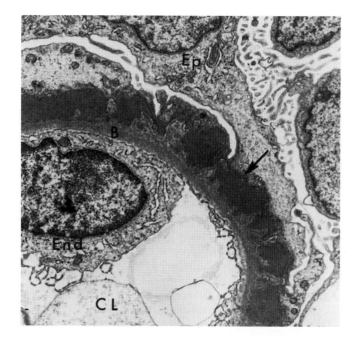

32 A 20-year-old woman has had increasing malaise, oliguria, and peripheral edema for the past week. On physical examination, she has 2+ pitting edema to the knees and puffiness around the eyes. Laboratory studies show serum creatinine of 4.6 mg/dL and urea nitrogen of 42 mg/dL. A renal biopsy specimen shows positive immunofluorescent staining for Ig and complement C3 within the glomeruli. The electron microscopic appearance of the specimen is shown in the figure above. Which of the following immunologic mechanisms has most likely produced the renal damage seen in this patient?

❑ (A) Antibody-dependent cell-mediated cytotoxicity
❑ (B) Immune complex-mediated hypersensitivity
❑ (C) Localized anaphylaxis
❑ (D) Granulomatous inflammation
❑ (E) T-cell–mediated cytotoxicity

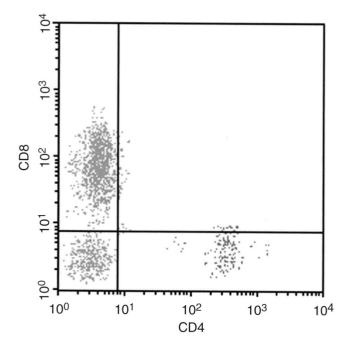

33 In a study of immunodeficient patients, samples of patient blood are collected and analyzed by flow cytometry. The results for one group of patients are shown in the preceding figure. These patients are statistically more likely to develop non-Hodgkin lymphomas. Which diagnosis is most applicable to this group of patients?

❑ (A) Bruton agammaglobulinemia
❑ (B) Common variable immunodeficiency
❑ (C) DiGeorge anomaly
❑ (D) HIV infection
❑ (E) Hyper-IgM syndrome
❑ (F) Postchemotherapy state
❑ (G) Severe combined immunodeficiency

34 A 29-year-old woman has had increasing weakness over the past year and now has difficulty climbing even a single flight of stairs. Her muscles are sore most of the time. However, she has little difficulty writing or typing. During the past 3 months, she has had increasing difficulty swallowing. She has experienced chest pain for the past week. On physical examination, she is afebrile. Her blood pressure is 115/75 mm Hg. Muscle strength is 4/5 in all extremities. No rashes are present. She has 2+ pitting edema to the knees. Rales are auscultated over lower lung fields. Laboratory studies show serum creatine kinase level of 458 U/L and Jo-1 antibodies. Which of the following conditions is she most likely to have?

❑ (A) Bony ankylosis
❑ (B) Myocarditis
❑ (C) Pericarditis
❑ (D) Raynaud phenomenon
❑ (E) Sclerodactyly
❑ (F) Urethritis
❑ (G) Xerophthalmia

35 A 28-year-old woman has a 5-year history of severe psoriasis involving the skin of the face, trunk, and extremities, as well as uveitis. She sees her physician because she has had increasing pain in her hands and left hip for the past 6 months. On physical examination, there is decreased range of motion of the left hip and the distal interphalangeal joints. Her fingers have a sausage-like appearance. Laboratory studies show that she is positive for HLA-B27, but her ANA and rheumatoid factor test results are negative. Which of the following complications is most characteristic of this patient's illness?

❑ (A) Angioedema of skin
❑ (B) Cerebral lymphoma
❑ (C) Hemolytic anemia
❑ (D) Keratoconjunctivitis
❑ (E) Sacroiliitis
❑ (F) Sclerodactyly

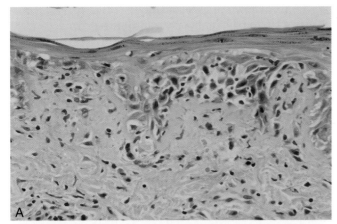

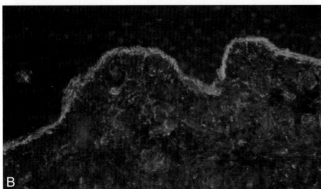

Courtesy of Dr. Richard Sontheimer, Department of Dermatology, University of Texas Southwestern Medical School, Dallas, TX.

36 A 26-year-old woman has had bouts of joint pain for the past 2 years. She also has a rash on the cheeks and bridge of the nose. On physical examination, there is no joint swelling or deformity, although generalized lymphadenopathy is present. Laboratory studies indicate anemia, leukopenia, a polyclonal gammopathy, and proteinuria. The serum ANA test result is positive at a titer of 1:1024 with a rim pattern identified by immunofluorescence. The light microscopic and immunofluorescent (with antibody to IgG) appearances of a skin biopsy are shown. Which of the following is the best information to give this patient about her disease?

- ❏ (A) Blindness is likely to occur within 5 years
- ❏ (B) Avoid exposure to cold environments
- ❏ (C) Joint deformities will eventually occur
- ❏ (D) Chronic renal failure is likely to occur
- ❏ (E) Cardiac valve replacement will eventually be required

37 In a study that examines granuloma formation in the lung in response to infection with *Mycobacterium tuberculosis,* it is observed that cells within the granuloma express MHC class II antigens. These cells elaborate cytokines that promote fibroblastic production of collagen within the granuloma. These class II antigen-bearing cells are most likely derived from which of the following peripheral blood leukocytes?

- ❏ (A) Neutrophil
- ❏ (B) Monocyte
- ❏ (C) B cell
- ❏ (D) Natural killer cell
- ❏ (E) Basophil

38 A 38-year-old man has been infected with HIV for the past 8 years. He has been receiving highly active antiretroviral therapy (HAART) for the past 18 months with a regimen that includes zidovudine, stavudine, and ritonavir. His HIV-1 RNA level initially decreased below 50 copies/μL after initiation of therapy; the current level is 5120 copies/μL. A mutation in the gene for which of the following substances is most likely to have occurred?

- ❏ (A) CD40 ligand
- ❏ (B) Chemokine receptor
- ❏ (C) Cytokine receptor γ chain
- ❏ (D) p24 antigen
- ❏ (E) Protein tyrosine kinase
- ❏ (F) Reverse transcriptase

39 Laboratory tests are ordered for two hospitalized patients. During the phlebotomy procedure, the Vacutainer tubes drawn from these patients are mislabeled. One of the patients receives a blood transfusion later that day. Within 1 hour after the transfusion of RBCs begins, the patient becomes tachycardic and hypotensive and passes pink-colored urine. Which of the following statements best describes how this reaction is mediated?

- ❏ (A) Release of tumor necrosis factor-α into the circulation
- ❏ (B) Antibody-dependent cellular cytotoxicity by natural killer cells
- ❏ (C) Antigen-antibody complex deposition in glomeruli
- ❏ (D) Complement-mediated lysis of RBCs
- ❏ (E) Mast cell degranulation

40 A 45-year-old man has had a fever, cough, and worsening dyspnea for the past few days. On physical examination, his temperature is 39.2°C. Auscultation of the chest shows decreased breath sounds over all lung fields. A bronchoalveolar lavage is performed, and the fluid obtained yields cysts of *Pneumocystis carinii.* Laboratory studies show a CD4 lymphocyte count of 135/μL, total serum globulin concentration 2.5 g/dL, and WBC count 7800/mm³ with 75% segmented neutrophils, 8% bands, 6% lymphocytes, 10% monocytes, and 1% eosinophils. Which of the following serologic laboratory findings is most likely to be positive in this patient?

- ❏ (A) Antineutrophil cytoplasmic autoantibody
- ❏ (B) Rheumatoid factor
- ❏ (C) Antibodies to HIV
- ❏ (D) Antistreptolysin O
- ❏ (E) Anti–double-stranded DNA antibody

41 A 14-month-old child has had multiple infections since birth, including pneumonia with *Pseudomonas aeruginosa*, adenovirus, and *Aspergillus fumigatus;* diarrhea with *Isospora belli;* otitis media with *Haemophilus influenzae;* and urinary tract infection with *Candida albicans*. Laboratory studies show hemoglobin of 13.2 g/dL, hematocrit 39.7%, platelet count 239,100/mm³, and WBC count 3450/mm³ with 85% segmented neutrophils, 6% bands, 2% lymphocytes, and 7% monocytes. Serum immunoglobulin levels are IgG 118 mg/dL, IgM 14 mg/dL, and IgA 23 mg/dL. The child dies of pneumonia. At autopsy, a hypoplastic thymus, small lymph nodes that lack germinal centers, and scant gut-associated lymphoid tissue are seen. Which of the following is the most likely cause of this disease?

❑ (A) Abnormal CD40 ligand
❑ (B) Adenosine deaminase deficiency
❑ (C) *BTK* gene mutation C2
❑ (D) Complement component deficiency
❑ (E) Chromosome 22q11 deletion
❑ (F) HIV infection

42 A 9-year-old girl has experienced pain and swelling of the elbows and knees and a fever for 1 month. On physical examination, her temperature is 38°C. There is decreased range of motion at the elbows and knees, with joint swelling and warmth. Laboratory studies show hemoglobin of 13.4 g/dL, hematocrit 40.3%, platelet count 288,200/mm³, and WBC count 12,560/mm³. The ANA test result is positive, but results for rheumatoid factor, Scl-70, and SS-A serologies are negative. The girl's symptoms abate after 4 years and never recur. Which of the following is the most likely diagnosis?

❑ (A) Systemic sclerosis
❑ (B) Juvenile rheumatoid arthritis
❑ (C) Psoriatic arthropathy
❑ (D) Ankylosing spondylitis
❑ (E) Reiter syndrome

43 A 9-month-old child has a history of recurrent infections with multiple agents, including cytomegalovirus, *Candida* albicans, *Staphylococcus aureus,* and *Staphylococcus epidermidis*. A careful family history and pedigree analysis show this to be a genetic disorder that is inherited in an autosomal recessive pattern. Which of the following laboratory studies is likely to be most useful in establishing the underlying mechanism of immunodeficiency in this infant?

❑ (A) Quantitative serum immunoglobulin levels
❑ (B) Enumeration of B cells in blood
❑ (C) Enumeration of CD3+ cells in blood
❑ (D) Tests of neutrophil function
❑ (E) Adenosine deaminase levels in leukocytes

44 A 12-year-old girl has complained of a sore throat for the past 3 days. On physical examination, she has a temperature of 38.4°C and pharyngeal erythema with minimal exudate. A throat culture grows group A β-hemolytic streptococcus. The pharyngitis resolves, but 3 weeks later, the girl develops fever and chest pain. Her anti–streptolysin O titer is 1:512. Which of the following immunologic mechanisms has most likely produced the chest pain?

❑ (A) Breakdown of T-cell anergy
❑ (B) Polyclonal lymphocyte activation
❑ (C) Release of sequestered antigens
❑ (D) Molecular mimicry
❑ (E) Failure of T-cell–mediated suppression

45 Over the past week, a 32-year-old man has experienced nausea and vomiting and has become mildly icteric. On physical examination, his temperature is 37.4°C. Laboratory studies show serum AST of 208 U/L and ALT of 274 U/L. Serologic findings for HBsAg and HBcAb are positive. A liver biopsy specimen examined microscopically shows focal death of hepatocytes with a portal infiltrate composed mainly of lymphocytes. Which of the following is the most likely mechanism by which the liver cell injury occurs under these conditions?

❑ (A) Recognition of HBsAg by the CD8 molecule of T cells
❑ (B) Recognition of an antigenic peptide presented by MHC class I molecules to natural killer cells
❑ (C) Recognition of an antigenic peptide presented by MHC class I molecule to CD8+ cells
❑ (D) Destruction of HBsAg-expressing cells by anti-HBs IgG antibody
❑ (E) Apoptosis of the liver cells by cytokines released by activated macrophages

46 A 41-year-old man has been bothered by a feeling of dryness in his mouth for the past 3 years. During this time, erythematous rashes have appeared on the skin of his face and upper neck. In the past 6 months, he has developed arthralgias. On physical examination, he is afebrile. There are no joint deformities. Laboratory findings include a positive ANA test result, with a speckled pattern, and high titers of antibodies to U1-ribonucleoprotein. The serum creatinine is 1.1 mg/dL, and the urea nitrogen is 17 mg/dL. Which of the following diseases is most likely to produce these findings?

❑ (A) Dermatomyositis
❑ (B) Discoid lupus erythematosus
❑ (C) Limited scleroderma
❑ (D) Mixed connective tissue disease
❑ (E) Reiter syndrome
❑ (F) Sjögren syndrome
❑ (G) Systemic lupus erythematosus

47 A 28-year-old man has had hemoptysis and hematuria for the past 2 days. On physical examination, his temperature is 36.8°C, pulse 87/min, respirations 19/min, and blood pressure 150/90 mm Hg. Laboratory studies show creatinine of 3.8 mg/dL and urea nitrogen of 35 mg/dL. Urinalysis shows 4+ hematuria, 2+ proteinuria, and no glucose. A renal biopsy specimen examined microscopically shows glomerular damage and linear immunofluorescence with labeled anti-complement and anti-IgG antibody. Which of the following autoantibodies has the greatest specificity for this patient's condition?

❏ (A) Anti–double-stranded DNA
❏ (B) Antihistone
❏ (C) Anti–Jo-1
❏ (D) Anti–U1-riboneucleoprotein
❏ (E) Anti–SS-A
❏ (F) Anti–basement membrane
❏ (G) Anti-phospholipid

48 A 40-year-old man has been infected with HIV for the past 10 years. During this time, he has had several bouts of oral candidiasis but no major illnesses. He is now diagnosed with Kaposi sarcoma involving the skin. He has experienced a 7-kg weight loss in the past 6 months. Laboratory studies show the HIV-1 RNA viral load is currently 60,000 copies/mL. Which of the following types of cells is most depleted in his lymph nodes?

❏ (A) CD4+ lymphocyte
❏ (B) CD8+ lymphocyte
❏ (C) Eosinophil
❏ (D) Follicular dendritic cell
❏ (E) Macrophage
❏ (F) Natural killer cell
❏ (G) Plasma cell

49 For the past 2 years, a 42-year-old woman has had tightening of the skin of her fingers, making them difficult to bend. She has had increasing difficulty swallowing for the past 8 months. During the past winter, her fingers became cyanotic and painful on exposure to cold. On physical examination, the skin on her face, neck, hands, and forearms appears firm and shiny. Her blood pressure is 150/95 mm Hg. A chest radiograph shows prominent interstitial markings, and lung function tests indicate moderately severe restrictive pulmonary disease. The result of the DNA topoisomerase I antibody test is positive. Which of the following conditions is most likely to produce these findings?

❏ (A) Ankylosing spondylitis
❏ (B) Diffuse systemic sclerosis
❏ (C) Discoid lupus erythematosus
❏ (D) Limited scleroderma
❏ (E) Reiter syndrome
❏ (F) Rheumatoid arthritis
❏ (G) Systemic lupus erythematosus

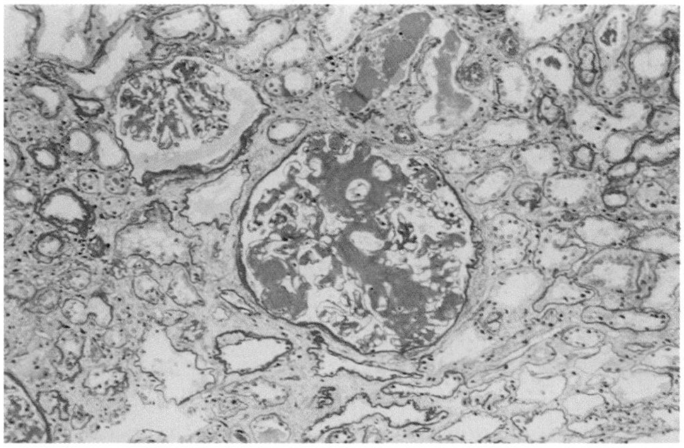

50 A 61-year-old man has had increasing malaise for the past 4 months. On physical examination, he is afebrile and has mild muscle wasting. Laboratory studies show serum creatinine of 4.5 mg/dL and urea nitrogen of 44 mg/dL. Urine dipstick analysis shows no blood, protein, or glucose, but a specific test for Bence Jones proteins yields a positive result. A renal biopsy specimen has the microscopic appearance shown in the figure. Which of the following underlying conditions is most likely to be present in this patient?

❏ (A) Rheumatic fever
❏ (B) Multiple myeloma
❏ (C) Ankylosing spondylitis
❏ (D) Systemic sclerosis
❏ (E) Common variable immunodeficiency

51 A 40-year-old laboratory technician accidentally injects a chemical into his skin. The next day, he notes that an area of erythematous, indurated skin is forming around the site of injection. Two days later, the induration measures 10 mm in diameter. A microscopic section from this area, with immunostaining using antibody to CD4, shows many positive lymphocytes. Which of the following immunologic reactions is most consistent with this appearance?

❏ (A) Systemic anaphylaxis
❏ (B) Arthus reaction
❏ (C) Graft-versus-host disease
❏ (D) Delayed-type hypersensitivity
❏ (E) Serum sickness

52 A 19-year-old woman with chronic renal failure received a cadaveric renal transplantation. One month later, she experienced rising serum creatinine and urea nitrogen levels, and a renal biopsy was performed. She was then treated with corticosteroids, and her renal function improved. Which of the following changes was most likely seen in the biopsy specimen before corticosteroid therapy was initiated?

❏ (A) Interstitial infiltration by CD3+ lymphocytes and tubular epithelial damage
❏ (B) Extensive fibrosis of the interstitium and glomeruli with markedly thickened blood vessels
❏ (C) Fibrinoid necrosis of renal arterioles with thrombotic occlusion
❏ (D) Interstitial infiltration by eosinophils with tubular epithelial damage
❏ (E) Glomerular deposition of serum amyloid–associated protein

53 A 35-year-old woman has had bouts of severe pain and swelling of the small joints of both hands and feet for the past 10 years, although she has had remissions during each of her three pregnancies. She has been bedridden for the past 2 months. On physical examination, there is warmth, swelling, and tenderness of the hands and feet, deformity of the hands, and ulnar deviation and decreased range of motion of metacarpophalangeal and interphalangeal joints. She has no muscle pain or skin rash. A painless 1.5-cm subcutaneous nodule is present behind the elbow joint over the olecranon process. A joint aspirate shows turbid fluid with many neutrophils containing phagocytized immune complexes. Which of the following long-term outcomes of this patient's disease is most likely to occur?

❏ (A) Chronic renal failure
❏ (B) Aortic dissection
❏ (C) Vertebral kyphosis
❏ (D) Adenocarcinoma of the colon
❏ (E) Joint deformities

54 A 45-year-old woman has had a burning sensation with increasing blurring of vision for the past 5 years. On physical examination, she has keratoconjunctivitis. Atrophy of the oral mucosa, with buccal mucosal ulcerations, is also present. A biopsy specimen of the lip shows marked lymphocytic and plasma cell infiltrates in minor salivary glands. Which of the following antibodies is most likely to be identified on laboratory testing?

❏ (A) Anti–double-stranded DNA
❏ (B) Anticentromere
❏ (C) SS-B
❏ (D) Scl-70
❏ (E) Jo-1

55 A 22-year-old man has had a urethral discharge for the past week. A culture of the exudate from the urethra grows *Neisseria gonorrhoeae*. He is treated with penicillin G, but within minutes after injection, he develops itching and erythema of the skin. This is quickly followed by severe respiratory difficulty with wheezing and stridor. Which of the following immunoglobulins has most likely become attached to the penicillin G and mast cells to produce these symptoms?

❏ (A) IgA
❏ (B) IgG
❏ (C) IgM
❏ (D) IgD
❏ (E) IgE

56 A 4-year-old boy has had recurrent respiratory infections with multiple bacterial and viral pathogens for the past 3 years. On physical examination, he has eczema involving the trunk and extremities. Laboratory findings include a platelet count of 71,000/mm³ and WBC count of 3800/mm³ with 88% segmented neutrophils, 6% bands, 3% lymphocytes, and 3% monocytes. Serum immunoglobulin levels are IgG 1422 mg/dL, IgM 11 mg/dL, and IgA 672 mg/dL. This patient is at an increased risk of developing which of the following conditions?

❏ (A) Hypocalcemia
❏ (B) Rheumatoid arthritis
❏ (C) Glomerulonephritis
❏ (D) Malignant lymphoma
❏ (E) Dementia

57 A 17-year-old boy has been sexually active for the past 3 years. Serologic testing shows that he is HIV positive. He is currently healthy and is not an intravenous drug user. Which of the following is the best information to give this patient about his disease?

❏ (A) You should not have unprotected sex with other persons
❏ (B) You will probably develop AIDS within 1 year
❏ (C) Your HIV test may become negative within 1 year
❏ (D) As long as you are clinically well, you can donate blood
❏ (E) The course of your infection is best followed by titers of anti-HIV antibodies

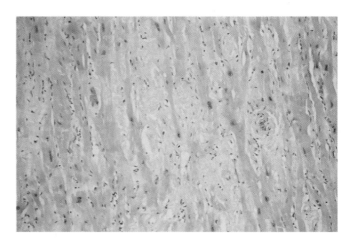

58 A 79-year-old man has experienced worsening congestive heart failure and pulmonary and peripheral edema for the past 4 years. On physical examination, his temperature is 36.9°C, pulse 70/min, respirations 16/min, and blood pressure 120/75 mm Hg. Echocardiography shows cardiomegaly with four-chamber dilation. All laboratory studies, including serum protein electrophoresis and examination of bone marrow smear, are normal. An endomyocardial biopsy specimen has the histologic appearance shown in the figure. Which of the following proteins is most likely to be found in this lesion?

❏ (A) α-Fetoprotein
❏ (B) β₂-Microglobulin
❏ (C) Transthyretin
❏ (D) Calcitonin
❏ (E) IgE

59 A 2-year-old boy has had almost continuous infections since he was 6 months old. These infections have included otitis media, pneumonia, and impetigo. Organisms cultured have included *Haemophilus influenzae*, *Streptococcus pneumoniae*, and *Staphylococcus aureus*. He has also had diarrhea, with *Giardia lamblia* cysts identified in stool specimens. The family history indicates that an older brother with a similar condition died because of overwhelming infections. The boy's two sisters and both parents are normal. Which of the following laboratory findings would most likely be seen in this boy?

❏ (A) Absence of IgA
❏ (B) Decreased complement C3
❏ (C) High titer of HIV-1 RNA
❏ (D) Markedly decreased immunoglobulins
❏ (E) Positive ANA test result

60 A 39-year-old woman sees her physician because of acute onset of severe dyspnea. On physical examination, she is afebrile and has marked laryngeal stridor and severe airway obstruction. The medical history indicates that she has had similar episodes since childhood, as well as episodes of colicky gastrointestinal pain. Her mother and her brother are similarly affected. There is no history of severe or recurrent infections. She does not have urticaria. Laboratory studies show normal WBC count, hematocrit, and platelet count. A deficiency in which of the following plasma components is most likely to produce these findings?

- ❑ (A) ß₂-Microglobulin
- ❑ (B) C1 inhibitor
- ❑ (C) C3
- ❑ (D) 5-Hydroxytryptamine
- ❑ (E) IgA
- ❑ (F) IgE

61 In an experiment, a cell line derived from a human malignant neoplasm is grown in culture. A human IgG antibody is added to the culture, and the tumor cells are observed to be coated by the antibody, but they do not undergo lysis. Next, human cells are added that are negative for CD3, CD19, surface Ig, and T-cell receptor markers, but are positive for CD16 and CD56. The tumor cells are then observed to undergo lysis. Which of the following human cell types added to the tumor cell culture is most likely to produce these findings?

- ❑ (A) B cell
- ❑ (B) CD4 cell
- ❑ (C) CD8 cell
- ❑ (D) Dendritic cell
- ❑ (E) Macrophage
- ❑ (F) Natural killer cell
- ❑ (G) Stem cell

62 During heterosexual intercourse, seminal fluid containing HIV contacts vaginal squamous mucosa. The virions are captured by cells, which then transport the virus via lymphatics to the regional lymph nodes. Within the germinal centers of these lymph nodes, the virions infect CD4 lymphocytes and proliferate, causing CD4 lysis with release of more virions, which are then taken up on the surface of cells having Fc receptors, allowing continued infection by HIV of more CD4 cells passing through the nodes. Which of the following types of cells is most likely to capture HIV onto its surface via Fc receptors?

- ❑ (A) B cell
- ❑ (B) CD8 cell
- ❑ (C) Follicular dendritic cell
- ❑ (D) Langhans giant cell
- ❑ (E) Macrophage
- ❑ (F) Mast cell
- ❑ (G) Natural killer cell

ANSWERS

1 **(A)** This patient has features of systemic lupus erythematosus (SLE). Patients with SLE often have a skin rash on sun-exposed areas. Urethritis is more characteristic of Reiter syndrome, one of the spondyloarthropathies. Difficulty in swallowing is a feature of scleroderma. Xerostomia suggests Sjögren syndrome. Although SLE has genetic associations with complement deficiencies or HLA-DQ, malformations are not a feature of SLE. Congenital heart disease may be seen in DiGeorge syndrome.

BP7 132-136   BP6 103   PBD7 231-233   PBD6 217

2 **(B)** This patient has clinical and serologic features of systemic lupus erythematosus (SLE). She also has a false-positive test result for syphilis, indicating the presence of anticardiolipin antibodies. These antibodies against phospholipid-protein complexes (antiphospholipid antibodies) are also called lupus anticoagulants, because they interfere with in vitro clotting tests. However, in vivo, they are thrombogenic. Hence, these patients can have recurrent thrombosis. Lupus anticoagulants can also occur in the absence of lupus. The other listed options can occur in SLE, but they are not mediated by antiphospholipid antibodies.

BP7 131   BP6 103   PBD7 228-230   PBD6 218

3 **(B)** Entry of HIV into cells requires binding to the CD4 molecule and coreceptor molecules such as CCR5 and CXCR4. These HIV coreceptors are receptors for chemokines on the surface of T cells and macrophages. Mutations in genes encoding these coreceptor molecules cause individuals to be resistant to the effects of HIV infection, because HIV cannot enter lymphocytes and macrophages. The other cell surface receptors are not relevant for HIV entry into cells. The p24 antigen is contained within the HIV virion and is not part of cell entry mechanisms, although its presence aids in detection of HIV infection.

BP7 150-151   BP6 119-120   PBD7 248-249   PBD6 242

4 **(B)** These are features of the hyper-IgM syndrome, which results from lack of isotype switching from IgM to other immunoglobulins. Patients are particularly susceptible to *Pneumocystis* as well as to bacterial infections. The abnormal IgM antibodies in excess can attach to circulating cells and lead to cytopenias. An absence of adenosine deaminase characterizes a form of severe combined immunodeficiency. The deletion of chromosome 22q11 is a feature of the DiGeorge anomaly, which affects T-cell differentiation and maturation. HIV infection can be accompanied by opportunistic infections, particularly *Pneumocystis*, but abnormal immunoglobulin production generally is not seen. A lack of IgA production alone is seen with selective IgA deficiency. Mutations in the *BTK* gene account for Bruton agammaglobulinemia, in which levels of all immunoglobulins are reduced.

BP7 146   BP6 102-104   PBD7 242-243   PBD6 216-218

5 **(B)** This girl has experienced a systemic anaphylactic reaction from a type I hypersensitivity reaction. Epinephrine is the fastest acting agent to treat this life-threatening condition. Cyclosporine is used to minimize transplant rejection. Penicillin is an antibiotic that often induces a type I hypersensitivity reaction. Glucocorticoids can reduce immune reactions, although this occurs over days to weeks, not minutes. Methotrexate is useful in the treatment of graft-versus-host disease.

BP7 112-114   BP6 87-89   PBD7 206-209   PBD6 197-199

6 **(C)** This woman has systemic lupus erythematosus (SLE). Patients with SLE can develop anti–red cell antibodies that can cause hemolytic anemia. Cytopenias, including leukopenia, thrombocytopenia, and anemia, are also common. Bronchoconstriction is a feature of bronchial asthma and can occur in allergies as a predominantly type I hypersensitivity reaction. Cerebral lymphomas are rare but may occur in immunodeficient patients, particularly those with AIDS. Keratoconjunctivitis can be seen in Sjögren syndrome as a result of decreased tear production from lacrimal gland inflammation. Sacroiliitis is a feature of many of the spondyloarthropathies, such as ankylosing spondylitis. Sclerodactyly is seen in scleroderma. When extensive, it is usually part of the spectrum of findings associated with diffuse scleroderma; when it involves only a few areas of the skin (e.g., just the hands), it is more likely to indicate limited scleroderma (CREST syndrome).

BP7 131   BP6 103   PBD7 231-234   PBD6 217

7 **(C)** This woman has Sjögren syndrome, which is characterized by immunologically mediated destruction of salivary and lacrimal glands, as well as other exocrine glands, lining the respiratory and gastrointestinal tracts. Dryness and crusting of the nose can lead to perforation of the nasal septum. In 25% of cases, extraglandular tissues such as lung, skin, kidney, and muscles may be involved. Renal failure is more likely to occur with systemic lupus erythematosus from glomerulonephritis. Libman-Sacks endocarditis is most often a feature of systemic lupus erythematosus (SLE). Photosensitivity is a feature of SLE, with formation of an erythematous rash in sun-exposed areas; it can also be a drug reaction. Sclerodactyly is a feature of scleroderma. When not extensive, it typically indicates limited scleroderma (CREST syndrome); when extensive, diffuse scleroderma, which has a poorer prognosis. Subcutaneous nodules can occur in rheumatic fever as part of the immunologic reaction following some group A beta-hemolytic streptococcal infections. Nongonococcal urethritis is seen in Reiter syndrome, along with conjunctivitis and arthritis.

BP7 139-140   BP6 111-112   PBD7 235-236
PBD6 225-226

8 **(B)** This man has a selective (isolated) IgA deficiency. Such persons are bothered by minor recurrent sinopulmonary infections and by diarrhea. *Pneumocystis* infections are seen in patients with more severe acquired or inherited immunodeficiency disorders, particularly those with AIDS, which affect cell-mediated immunity. Hepatitis infections are not directly related to immunodeficiency states, although AIDS patients with a history of injection drug use are often infected with hepatitis B or C. Resistance against fungal and viral infection is mediated by T cells.

BP7 146   BP6 116   PBD7 242   PBD6 234

9 **(D)** This patient has AIDS, with Kaposi sarcoma of the skin. Kaposi sarcoma is associated with a herpesvirus agent that is sexually transmitted: human herpesvirus 8 (HHV-8), also called the Kaposi sarcoma herpesvirus. Other herpesviruses are not involved in the pathogenesis of Kaposi sarcoma, although infection with these viruses can occur frequently in persons with AIDS. HIV, although present in the lymphocytes and monocytes, is not detected in the spindle cells that proliferate in Kaposi sarcoma. With the exception of the varicella-zoster virus, which is associated with dermatomally distributed skin vesicles known as shingles, skin lesions are not common manifestations of herpesviruses,

which include cytomegalovirus, Epstein-Barr virus, or adenovirus infections.

BP7 156-157   BP6 125   PBD7 256-257   PBD6 248

10 **(A)** CD4 cells of the T_H2 type are essential to the induction of type I hypersensitivity because they can secrete cytokines, such as interleukin (IL)-4, IL-5, IL-3, and granulocyte-macrophage colony-stimulating factor, which are required for the growth, recruitment, and activation of mast cells and eosinophils. Natural killer cells can lyse other cells, such as virus-infected cells, without prior sensitization. Macrophages can secrete a variety of cytokines, but they are not essential to type I hypersensitivity. Dendritic cells trap antigen and aid in antigen presentation. Neutrophils are recruited by cytokines to participate in acute inflammatory reactions.

BP7 112-113   BP6 87   PBD7 206-208   PBD6 196

11 **(E)** This woman has dermatomyositis, a form of inflammatory myopathy in which capillaries are the primary target for antibody and complement-mediated injury. Anti-Jo-1 antibodies, although not present in most cases, are quite specific for inflammatory myopathies. The perivascular and perimysial inflammatory infiltrates result in peripheral muscle fascicular myocyte necrosis. The process is mediated by CD4+ cells and B cells. The heliotrope rash is a characteristic feature of dermatomyositis. Anti–double-stranded DNA is specific for systemic lupus erythematosus (SLE), in which there can be myositis without significant inflammation or necrosis. Rheumatoid factor is present in most patients with rheumatoid arthritis, which is accompanied by inflammatory destruction of joints, not muscle, although muscle may atrophy secondary to diminished movement. The anti–U1-ribonucleoprotein antibodies suggest a diagnosis of mixed connective tissue disease, a condition that can overlap with polymyositis. Antihistone antibodies are associated with drug-induced SLE.

BP7 143-144   BP6 114-115   PBD7 1342-1343
PBD6 230-232

12 **(B)** The figure shows the so-called wire loop glomerular capillary lesions of lupus nephritis. Anti-Sm and anti–double-stranded DNA are specific for systemic lupus erythematosus. However, anti-Sm is present in only 25% of cases. Scl-70 is a marker for diffuse systemic sclerosis. Jo-1 is most specific for polymyositis. HLA-B27 is seen in ankylosing spondylitis. Anticentromere antibody is seen most often with limited scleroderma.

BP7 134-136   BP6 104, 108   PBD7 231-233
PBD6 218, 222

13 **(A)** This is an example of antibody-dependent cell-mediated cytotoxicity directed at a parasitic infection. IgG and IgE antibodies bearing Fc receptors coat the parasite. Macrophages, natural killer cells, and neutrophils can recognize the Fc receptor and lyse the antibody-coated target cells. Complement-mediated lysis is most typical of immune destruction of RBCs with hemolysis. Langhans giant cells are seen in granulomatous inflammation, a form of type IV hypersensitivity. Acute inflammatory reactions with abscess formation have little effect against tissue parasites. Leukotriene C4 is a potent agent that promotes vascular permeability and bronchial smooth muscle contraction in type I hypersensitivity reactions.

BP7 115   BP6 90-91   PBD7 210   PBD6 200-201

14 (**B**) These findings represent chronic rejection. The progressive renal failure results from ischemic changes with vascular narrowing. Cell lysis with macrophages is typical of antibody-dependent cell-mediated cytotoxicity, which does not play a key role in chronic rejection. Granulomatous inflammation is not typical of transplant rejection. Release of leukotriene C4 from mast cells is a feature of type I hypersensitivity. Complement-mediated cell lysis can occur when antidonor antibodies are preformed in the host, as occurs in hyperacute rejection.

BP7 124   BP6 98   PBD7 220-221   PBD6 210

15 (**A**) Natural killer (NK) cells have the ability to respond without prior sensitization. They carry receptors for MHC class I molecules that inhibit their lytic function. When expression of class I MHC molecules is reduced on the cell surface, the inhibitory receptors on NK cells do not receive a negative signal, and the cell is killed. NK cells are often the first line of defense against viral infection. Neutrophils provide a nonspecific immune response, primarily to bacterial infections and not to intracellular viral infections. Macrophages can process antigen and can phagocytize necrotic cells. CD4 cells are helper T cells that assist other cells, such as NK cells, macrophages, and B cells, in the immune response. Dendritic cells aid in antigen presentation.

BP7 107   BP6 83   PBD7 201-202   PBD6 191

16 (**E**) These findings indicate a failure of terminal differentiation of B cells into IgA-secreting plasma cells. Lack of IgA in mucosal secretions increases the risk of respiratory and gastrointestinal infections. IgA antibodies present in serum can lead to a transfusion reaction with IgA in donor serum. Persons with severe combined immunodeficiency would not live as long as this patient with such mild infections. HIV infection is marked by failure of cell-mediated immunity. DiGeorge syndrome manifests in infancy with failure of cell-mediated immunity from lack of functional T cells. Wiskott-Aldrich syndrome is associated with eczema and thrombocytopenia.

BP7 146   BP6 116   PBD7 242   PBD6 234

17 (**C**) This history is typical of the late-phase reaction in type I hypersensitivity. The initial rapid response is largely caused by degranulation of mast cells. The late-phase reaction follows without additional exposure to antigen and is characterized by more intense infiltration by inflammatory cells such as neutrophils, eosinophils, basophils, monocytes, and CD4+ lymphocytes. There is more tissue destruction in this late phase.

BP7 113-114   BP6 88-89   PBD7 206-209   PBD 196-198

18 (**B**) Macrophages can become infected with HIV and are not destroyed like CD4 cells. Instead, macrophages survive to carry the infection to tissues throughout the body, particularly the brain. HIV infection of the brain can result in encephalitis and dementia. Natural killer cells and neutrophils play no significant role in HIV infection. CD8 lymphocytes cannot be infected with HIV. Langerhans

cells in mucosal surfaces may aid in initial HIV infection of CD4 lymphocytes.

BP7 151-153   BP6 120-121   PBD7 252-253
PBD6 241-243

19 (**C**) This patient has a localized immune-complex reaction (Arthus reaction), which activates and depletes complement C3 and C4. IgE concentration is increased in persons with atopy and the potential for type I hypersensitivity. Although neutrophils are being recruited locally to the inflammatory reaction in this case, they are not depleted systemically, and they may be increased in the circulation. Skin tests are measures of type IV hypersensitivity when antigens such as tuberculin are used. CD4 lymphocytes assist in a variety of antibody- and cell-mediated immune reactions, but their numbers in peripheral blood do not change appreciably.

BP7 119   BP6 93-94   PBD7 215   PBD6 204

20 (**C**) In chronic inflammatory conditions such as rheumatoid arthritis, the serum amyloid–associated (SAA) precursor protein forms the major amyloid fibril protein AA. Amyloid is deposited in interstitial locations, not intracellularly. The P component is a minor component of the amyloid. All amyloid demonstrates characteristic "apple-green" birefringence under polarized light microscopy after Congo red staining—anything else would not be amyloid. Amyloid derived from light chains in association with multiple myeloma has AL fibrils.

BP7 159-160   BP6 126-128   PBD7 260, 262
PBD6 251-253

21 (**B**) This patient has a drug-induced systemic lupus erythematosus (SLE)-like condition. Drugs such as procainamide, hydralazine, and isoniazid can cause this condition. Test results for ANA are often positive, but those for anti–double-stranded DNA are negative. Antihistone antibodies are present in many cases. Characteristic signs and symptoms of SLE are often lacking, and renal involvement is uncommon. Remission occurs when the patient stops taking the drug. Anti-Sm antibody shows specificity for SLE. Anti-Jo-1 antibody has specificity for polymyositis/dermatomyositis. Anti-U1-ribonucleotide protein has specificity for mixed connective tissue disease. Anticentromeric antibody is most likely to be present with limited scleroderma (CREST syndrome). Anti-SS-A antibody is most characteristic of Sjögren syndrome.

BP7 131   PBD7 235   PBD6 218, 224-225

22 (**F**) This child has features of X-linked agammaglobulinemia of Bruton. In this condition, B-cell maturation stops after the rearrangement of heavy-chain genes, and light chains are not produced. Complete immunoglobulin molecules with heavy and light chains are not assembled and transported to the cell membrane. The lack of immunoglobulins predisposes the child to recurrent bacterial infections. Because T-cell function remains intact, viral, fungal, and protozoal infections are uncommon. CD4 and CD8 lymphocytes differentiate from precursors in the thymus, which is not affected by the *BTK* gene mutation that gives rise to Bruton agammaglobulinemia. Follicular dendritic cells are a form of antigen-presenting cell that is not affected by B-cell and T-cell disorders. Monocytes may leave the circulation to become tissue macrophages, a process not dependent on B-cell maturation. Natural killer (NK) cells are part of the innate immune system and respond to antibody coating abnormal cells—a process diminished by reduced antibody production—but the NK cells themselves are not directly affected by lack of immunoglobulin. Lack of stem cell differentiation is incompatible with life.

BP7 144-146   BP6 115-116   PBD7 240-242
PBD6 232-233

23 **(C)** This patient has severe combined immunodeficiency (SCID). Because the T-cell and B-cell arms of the immune system are deficient, there are severe and recurrent infections with bacteria, viruses, and fungi. With the family history of males being affected, the patient most likely has X-linked SCID. This form results from mutations in the common γ chain that is a part of many cytokine receptors, such as interleukin (IL)-2, IL-4, IL-7, and IL-15. These cytokines are needed for normal B-cell and T-cell development. The marked lymphoid hypoplasia is not typical of HIV infection. Loss of chromosome 22q11 is seen in DiGeorge syndrome. *BTK* gene mutations give rise to Bruton agammaglobulinemia. Mutation in the CD40 ligand is responsible for hyper-IgM syndrome.

BP7 146-147   BP6 117   PBD7 243-244   PBD6 234-236

24 **(C)** This patient has features of myasthenia gravis, a form of type II hypersensitivity reaction in which antibody is directed against cell surface receptors. Antibodies to acetylcholine receptors impair the function of skeletal muscle motor end plates. Antibodies are produced by B cells, and macrophages are not a significant part of this hypersensitivity reaction; there is little or no inflammation of the muscle in myasthenia gravis. Muscle lysis by CD8+ T cells occurs in polymyositis. Immune complex–mediated injury is a feature of dermatomyositis. Delayed hypersensitivity reactions are more likely in parasitic infestations of muscles.

BP7 115-116   BP6 90   PBD7 210-211   PBD6 201

25 **(E)** This patient has diffuse systemic sclerosis (scleroderma). The small arteries of the kidney are damaged by a hyperplastic arteriolosclerosis that can be complicated by very high blood pressure and renal failure. Meningitis and adrenal failure are not typical features of autoimmune diseases. Glomerulonephritis is a more typical complication of systemic lupus erythematosus. With scleroderma, the gastrointestinal tract undergoes fibrosis, without any tendency to perforation or ulceration.

BP7 142-143   BP6 112-114   PBD7 237-239
PBD6 226-229

26 **(A)** This infant has DiGeorge syndrome, which can involve the thymus, parathyroids, aorta, and heart. T-cell function is deficient, resulting in recurrent and multiple fungal, viral, and protozoal infections. Failure of B-cell maturation to plasma cells is a mode of development of common variable immunodeficiency. Some cases of severe combined immunodeficiency are caused by lack of adenosine deaminase. HIV infection does not explain the hypocalcemia at birth.

Failure of pre-B cell maturation results in Bruton agammaglobulinemia.

BP7 146   BP6 116-117   PBD7 243   PBD6 235

27 **(A)** The CD4 lymphocytes are thought to respond to some unknown antigenic stimulation, releasing cytokines that further activate macrophages and mast cells. The result is extensive dermal fibrosis that produces the clinical appearance of sclerodactyly in scleroderma. Neutrophils and natural killer cells do not participate in this process. Despite scleroderma being an autoimmune disease, inflammation is minimal. The major finding is progressive fibrosis of skin, lung, and gastrointestinal tract.

BP7 141-142   BP6 113-114   PBD7 237-239
PBD6 228-229

28 **(E)** This woman's original symptoms, although nonspecific, are seen in more than one half of adults with acute HIV infection. The average time to development of AIDS is 8 to 10 years; onset of opportunistic infections occurs as the CD4 cell count falls below 200/μL. Spondyloarthropathies and autoimmune diseases such as systemic lupus erythematosus or scleroderma are unlikely to have such a long interval between illnesses and are not as likely to manifest opportunistic infections without immunosuppressive therapy. The ANA is typical of autoimmune diseases. HLA-B27 antigen is associated with spondyloarthropathies. Anticentromere antibody is seen in limited scleroderma. Persons with AIDS may have a polyclonal gammopathy but not marked hypogammaglobulinemia.

BP7 154-155   BP6 122-124   PBD7 253-254
PBD6 245-246

29 **(A)** Opportunistic infections in an intravenous drug abuser suggest a diagnosis of AIDS. The most common neoplasms seen in association with AIDS are B-cell non-Hodgkin lymphoma and Kaposi sarcoma. A rare tumor associated with AIDS in children is leiomyosarcoma. Cervical dysplasias and carcinomas are increased in women with HIV infection, but such lesions are less frequent than lymphoma. Lung cancers at this woman's age are uncommon in any circumstance. Opportunistic infections of the brain and central nervous system lymphomas are common in patients with AIDS, but glial neoplasms are not.

BP7 156-157   BP6 124-126   PBD7 256-258
PBD6 247-250

30 **(C)** Three types of cells can carry HIV: dendritic cells, monocytes, and CD4+ T cells. Mucosal dendritic cells (i.e., Langerhans cells) can bind to the virus and transport it to CD4+ cells in the lymph nodes. Whether the virus is internalized by mucosal dendritic cells is not clear. Monocytes and CD4+ T cells express CD4 and the coreceptors (CCR5 and CXCR4); therefore, HIV can enter these cells. Follicular dendritic cells are distinct from mucosal or epithelial dendritic cells; they trap antibody-coated HIV virions by means of their Fc receptors. The other listed cells cannot be infected by HIV.

BP7 151-153   BP6 83   PBD7 248-250   PBD6 191

31 **(C)** This patient has graft-versus-host disease. The engrafted marrow contains immunocompetent cells that can proliferate and attack host tissues, usually skin, liver, and gastrointestinal epithelium. Tuberculin skin testing is a form of delayed-type hypersensitivity. Some chemotherapy agents can produce a drug reaction with more acute inflammation than was described in this case. Urticaria with type I hypersensitivity is a typical reaction to penicillin therapy. Patch testing is done to determine the type of allergens to which atopic persons may react.

BP7 125   BP6 99   PBD7 222-223   PBD6 210-211

32 (B) These findings are characteristic of immune complex–mediated glomerulonephritis. The immune complexes activate complement and result in acute inflammation. Antibody-dependent cell-mediated cytotoxicity is initiated when IgG or IgE coats a target to attract cells that affect lysis; immune complexes do not form. Localized anaphylaxis is a type I hypersensitivity reaction that is mediated by IgE antibody. Granulomatous inflammation and T-cell cytotoxicity are features of type IV hypersensitivity.

BP7 118-119   BP6 92-93   PBD7 231-233   PBD6 201-203

33 (D) In these patients, the CD4 count is decreased, compared with the CD8 count. HIV selectively infects CD4 cells, eventually leading to a reduced CD4 count that presages AIDS. In agammaglobulinemia, there is a failure of B-cell precursors to differentiate into B cells secreting immunoglobulins, and B cells mark with CD19 and CD20. In common variable immunodeficiency, there are normal numbers of B and T lymphocytes, but they do not interact properly. In DiGeorge anomaly, there is an overall reduction in T cells, not subsets. In hyper-IgM syndrome, there is defective T-cell signaling to induce isotype switching in B cells, but the numbers of lymphocytes are not reduced. Chemotherapy tends to produce a reduction in all lymphocytes, particularly T lymphocytes, but this is not selective for lymphocyte subsets. In severe combined immunodeficiency, there is a reduction in both B and T lymphocytes, with a greater reduction in the latter, which is not selective for subsets.

BP7 150-152   BP6 119-124   PBD7 250-252
PBD6 242-244

34 (B) This patient has polymyositis. Muscle weakness in polymyositis tends to be symmetric, and proximal muscles are involved first. This condition differs from dermatomyositis in that there is no skin involvement, and polymyositis typically affects adults. On biopsy, the skeletal muscle shows infiltration by lymphocytes along with degeneration and regeneration of muscle fibers. The lymphocytes are cytotoxic CD8+ cells. Some patients may have myocarditis, vasculitis, or pneumonitis, but unlike dermatomyositis, the risk of cancer is equivocal. Bony ankylosis is a feature of progressive or recurrent joint inflammation with rheumatoid arthritis. Myocarditis or pericarditis are most likely to be a feature of systemic lupus erythematosus or diffuse systemic sclerosis. Raynaud phenomenon is seen in many autoimmune phenomena, but it is most often a feature of scleroderma. Sclerodactyly is a feature of scleroderma. When not extensive, it typically indicates limited scleroderma (CREST syndrome); when extensive, diffuse scleroderma, which has a poorer prognosis. Nongonococcal urethritis, conjunctivitis, and arthritis are seen in Reiter syndrome. Xerophthalmia (usually with accompanying xerostomia) is seen in Sjögren syndrome.

BP7 143   BP6 115   PBD7 1342-1343   PBD6 229-231

35 (E) This patient has psoriatic arthropathy. The arthritis in this condition may resemble rheumatoid arthritis both clinically and pathologically. Like other spondyloarthropathies, sacroiliitis occurs in patients with psoriatic arthropathy. Hereditary angioedema is associated with a deficiency of complement C1 inhibitor. Cerebral lymphomas are rare, but they can occur in immunodeficiency states, particularly in patients with AIDS. Hemolytic anemia can accompany a wide variety of autoimmune phenomena and can be related to formation of specific RBC antibodies or coating of RBCs with antibody. Keratoconjunctivitis can be seen in Sjögren syndrome as a result of decreased tear production from lacrimal gland inflammation. Sclerodactyly is seen in scleroderma. When extensive, it is usually part of the spectrum of findings in diffuse scleroderma; when it involves only a few areas of the skin (e.g., just the hands), it is more likely a feature of limited scleroderma (CREST syndrome).

BP7 140   BP6 112   PBD7 1256, 1310   PBD6 1252

36 (D) This patient has systemic lupus erythematosus (SLE). Many persons with SLE have glomerulonephritis and eventually develop renal failure. Blindness is uncommon in SLE. Raynaud phenomenon is associated with many autoimmune diseases, but it is most troublesome in scleroderma. Although synovial inflammation is common in SLE, joint deformity is rare. The Libman-Sacks endocarditis associated with SLE tends to be nondeforming and limited, and there is minimal valve damage. It is now uncommon, because of the use of corticosteroid therapy in the treatment of SLE.

BP7 134-135   BP6 106-108   PBD7 227-231
PBD6 220-222

37 (B) Blood monocytes express MHC class II antigens and can migrate into tissues to become macrophages. In tuberculosis, these macrophages transform into epithelioid cells, thus forming a granuloma. Macrophages play an important role in delayed hypersensitivity reactions associated with cell-mediated immunity. Neutrophils are important mainly in acute inflammatory responses, although some may be present in a granulomatous reaction. B cells form plasma cells that secrete immunoglobulin on stimulation and are essential to humoral immunity. Natural killer cells can function without prior sensitization. Basophils may play a role in IgE-mediated responses.

BP7 107,121   BP6 83   PBD7 204, 216-217
PBD6 190-191

38 (F) The reverse transcriptase gene of HIV undergoes mutation on average once per 2000 replications, a very high rate, which can account for the appearance of drug resistance. The absence of CD40 ligand interaction with CD40 explains the hyper-IgM syndrome. Chemokine receptors are important in facilitating initial HIV entry into cells, and mutations in these receptors may help explain variable susceptibility to and progression of HIV infection. The cytokine receptor γ chain is abnormal in severe combined immunodeficiency. The p24 antigen is a component of the HIV virion and is used to detect infection, but it is not a target of drug therapy. Protein tyrosine kinases are involved in signal transduction. They can be abnormal in conditions such as Bruton agammaglobulinemia but not in patients receiving HIV drug therapy; ritonavir is an HIV protease inhibitor.

BP7 149-150   BP6 105-106   PBD7 246-247
PBD6 222-223

39 **(D)** This patient is experiencing a major transfusion reaction resulting from a type II hypersensitivity reaction. The patient's serum contains naturally occurring antibodies to the incompatible donor RBCs. They attach to the donor RBCs and induce complement activation that results in generation of the C5–9 membrane attack complex. Major transfusion reactions are rare, and most result from clerical errors. Tumor necrosis factor-α is not part of hypersensitivity reactions. Natural killer cell lysis is seen with antibody-dependent cell-mediated cytotoxicity. Antigen-antibody complex formation is typical of a type III hypersensitivity reaction. Mast cells degranulate with antigen attachment to IgE in type I hypersensitivity reactions.

BP7 115   BP6 90   PBD7 210   PBD6 199-200

40 **(C)** *Pneumocystis carinii* pneumonia is a common finding in persons with AIDS. This patient's low CD4 count is characteristic of AIDS. Antineutrophil cytoplasmic autoantibody (C-ANCA or P-ANCA) can be seen in patients with vasculitis. Rheumatoid factor is present in most persons with rheumatoid arthritis; however, significant immunosuppression is not seen unless they are treated with highly potent immunosuppressive drugs such as cyclosporine. The anti–streptolysin O titer is elevated in patients with rheumatic fever, but there is no serious immunosuppression. The ANA test result is positive in a variety of autoimmune diseases, but a decrease in CD4 count is not typical of such conditions.

BP7 156   BP6 124-125   PBD7 255   PBD6 247-248

41 **(B)** This child had severe combined immunodeficiency (SCID), which is now treated with allogeneic bone marrow transplantation. The transplanted stem cells in the bone marrow give rise to normal T and B cells. Half of SCID cases are caused by an X-linked mutation in the common γ chain for cytokine receptors, and the rest are due to autosomal recessive mutations in the gene encoding for adenosine deaminase, which leads to accumulation of metabolites toxic to lymphocytes. An abnormal CD40 ligand interaction with CD40 leads to lack of isotype switching in patients with hyper-IgM syndrome. The *BTK* gene product is required for differentiation of pro- and pre-B cells, and a mutation leads to agammaglobulinemia. Persons lacking C2 have some increase in infections but mainly develop a disease resembling systemic lupus erythematosus. The 22q11 deletion is seen in infants with DiGeorge anomaly and results in lack of T-cell development. HIV infection leads to many opportunistic infections, which sometimes occur in infancy and early childhood, but it is mainly CD4 lymphocytes that are diminished.

BP7 146-147   BP6 117   PBD7 243-244   PBD6 235-236

42 **(B)** This child has had juvenile rheumatoid arthritis. About 70% to 90% of cases resolve without joint deformity. Unlike rheumatoid arthritis, juvenile rheumatoid arthritis tends to involve lower and larger joints, and rheumatoid factor is often absent. Systemic sclerosis is a disease of adults that may have features resembling early rheumatoid arthritis, but joint destruction is rare. Psoriatic arthropathy is a disease of adults with features similar to rheumatoid arthritis, but joint involvement is more irregular. Ankylosing spondylitis occurs in older adults and principally affects the vertebral column. Reiter syndrome occurs in young to middle-aged adults; its major features are urethritis, arthritis, and conjunctivitis.

BP7 139   BP6 115   PBD7 1309   PBD6 1251-1252

43 **(E)** This patient is susceptible to bacterial, fungal, and viral infections and most likely has severe combined immunodeficiency (SCID). The autosomal recessive pattern of inheritance implicates adenosine deaminase (ADA) deficiency rather than mutations in the γ chain of cytokine receptors. Low ADA levels in the leukocytes are diagnostic. The other listed options are relevant to the workup of primary immunodeficiencies, but they are not specific to SCID.

BP7 146-147   BP6 117   PBD7 243-244   PBD6 235

44 **(D)** Streptococcal M proteins cross-react with cardiac glycoproteins, resulting in rheumatic heart disease, a form of autoimmunity. Breakdown of T-cell anergy usually occurs when localized tissue damage and inflammation cause upregulation of costimulatory molecules on the target tissues. This is a possible mechanism of autoimmunity in the brain and in pancreatic β cells. Polyclonal lymphocyte activation may be caused by microbial products such as endotoxin or bacterial superantigens. Release of sequestered antigens can cause autoimmunity; this mechanism is likely in autoimmune uveitis. Failure of T-cell–mediated suppression has not yet been shown to cause any autoimmune disease; it remains a potential mechanism. The other listed options are not major immune responses to streptococcal infection.

BP7 128-129   BP6 100-102   PBD7 226-227
PBD6 214-215

45 **(C)** Virus-infected cells are recognized and killed by cytotoxic CD8+ T cells. The T-cell receptor on the CD8 T cells binds to the complex of viral peptide and MHC class I molecules on the surface of the infected cell. Natural killer (NK) cells also recognize MHC class I molecules with self-peptides. This recognition inhibits NK cell killing. The other listed options are not the major immune response to hepatitis infection.

BP7 105,109   BP6 96   PBD7 203-204   PBD6 206

46 **(D)** Mixed connective tissue disease can have features of systemic lupus erythematosus (SLE), polymyositis, rheumatoid arthritis, and Sjögren syndrome. Unlike SLE or diffuse scleroderma, serious renal disease is unlikely. Dermatomyositis causes muscle pain, and the rash is typically a subtle heliotrope rash with a violaceous appearance to the eyelids; Jo-1 antibody is a more typical finding. Discoid lupus erythematosus (DLE) is characterized by a rash similar to SLE, but with immune complex deposition only in sun-exposed areas of the skin, a positive ANA test result in a minority of cases, absence of anti-Sm or anti–double-stranded DNA antibodies, and absence of serious renal disease. Some cases of DLE can progress to SLE. In limited scleroderma (CREST syndrome), anticentromeric antibody is often present. In Reiter syndrome (with conjunctivitis, arthritis, and nongonococcal urethritis), there is often a positive serology for HLA-B27. In Sjögren syndrome, antibodies to SS-A and SS-B are often present. The anti-Sm or anti–double-stranded DNA antibodies are more specific for SLE.

BP7 143   BP6 115   PBD7 239   PBD6 231

47 (F) This patient has Goodpasture syndrome, in which an antibody is directed against type IV collagen in basement membranes of the glomeruli and in the lung. This is a form of type II hypersensitivity reaction. The antibodies attach to the basement membrane and fix complement, thus damaging the glomeruli. Anti–double-stranded DNA antibodies have specificity for systemic lupus erythematosus (SLE), whereas antihistone antibodies are characteristic of drug-induced SLE. Anti-Jo-1 antibody is found in dermatomyositis and polymyositis. The anti-U1-ribonucleoprotein antibody is seen in mixed connective tissue diseases. Anti–SS-A antibody is seen in Sjögren syndrome. Antiphospholipid antibodies are sometimes called "lupus anticoagulant," because they may appear in SLE; such patients have coagulopathies with thrombosis or bleeding, or both.

BP7 473-474   BP6 90   PBD7 210, 212   PBD6 201

48 (A) As HIV infection progresses, there is continuing, gradual loss of CD4 cells. The stage of clinical AIDS is reached when the peripheral CD4 count drops below 200/μL, which usually occurs over a period of 8 to 10 years. At this point, the risk of development of opportunistic infections and neoplasms typical of AIDS increases greatly. The extent of viremia also is an indication of the progression of HIV infection; an increase in HIV-1 RNA levels is seen as immunologic containment of HIV fails. In HIV infection, the numbers of CD8 lymphocytes tend to be maintained. Cells of the granulocytic series, including eosinophils, are relatively unaffected, although patients with AIDS may have cytopenias. Follicular dendritic cells (FDCs) can be infected by HIV and pass the virions to CD4 cells and macrophages, but the FDCs and the macrophages are not destroyed by the virus and become a reservoir for infection. The natural killer cells and plasma cells are not directly affected by HIV.

BP7 155-156   BP6 122-124   PBD7 253-254
PBD6 245-247

49 (B) This patient has cutaneous and visceral manifestations of diffuse systemic sclerosis (diffuse scleroderma). Raynaud phenomenon, skin changes, and esophageal dysmotility can also occur in limited scleroderma (CREST syndrome), but lung and renal involvement typically do not. In diffuse systemic sclerosis, the anti-DNA topoisomerase I antibody is often present, and patients can develop interstitial lung disease and renal disease with hyperplastic arteriolosclerosis. A feature of discoid lupus erythematosus is skin rashes, but usually there is no internal organ involvement. Ankylosing spondylitis is one of the spondyloarthropathies; it is characterized by low back pain from sacroiliitis and positive serology for HLA-B27. Reiter syndrome is characterized by conjunctivitis, arthritis, and nongonococcal urethritis, with a positive serology for HLA-B27. In rheumatoid arthritis, there is often progressive joint deformity; the serologic tests likely to be positive include rheumatoid factor and antibodies to cyclic citrullinated peptide (anti-CCP). The anti-Sm or anti–double-stranded DNA antibodies are more specific for

systemic lupus erythematosus, and renal disease in these patients is most likely due to glomerulonephritis.

BP7 141-143   BP6 114   PBD7 237-239   PBD6 227-228

50 (B) Amyloidosis is most often caused by excessive light chain production with plasma cell dyscrasias such as multiple myeloma (AL amyloid). Chronic inflammatory conditions, such as rheumatic fever, ankylosing spondylitis, and systemic sclerosis, may also result in amyloidosis (AA amyloid), but not in secretion of light chains in urine (i.e., Bence Jones proteinuria). Immunoglobulin levels are generally reduced in patients with common variable immunodeficiency.

BP7 159-160   BP6 127, 130   PBD7 260-261
PBD6 252-255

51 (D) Perivascular accumulation of T cells, particularly CD4+ cells, is typical of delayed hypersensitivity skin reactions, driven by a T_H1 response mediated largely by release of the cytokine interleukin-2. Systemic anaphylaxis typically occurs within minutes after an encounter with the antigen. Systemic and localized immune complex diseases (serum sickness and Arthus reactions) are type III hypersensitivity reactions; they often demonstrate vasculitis. Graft-versus-host disease is characterized by epidermal apoptosis and rash.

BP7 119-120   BP6 94-95   PBD7 216-217   PBD6 204-205

52 (A) Acute rejection of kidney transplants occurs weeks, months, or even years after transplantation. It is characterized by infiltration with CD3+ T cells that include the CD4+ and CD8+ subsets. These cells damage tubular epithelium by direct cytotoxicity and by release of cytokines, such as interferon-γ, that activate macrophages. The reaction is called acute cellular rejection, and it can be readily treated with corticosteroids. Interstitial and glomerular fibrosis, as well as blood vessel thickening, occur in chronic rejection. Fibrinoid necrosis and thrombosis are more typical of hyperacute rejection, which occurs within minutes of placement of the transplant into the recipient. Eosinophils accumulate in acute interstitial nephritis due to drug reactions. Amyloid derived from serum amyloid–associated protein can occur in chronic infections and inflammation.

BP7 122-123   BP6 96-98   PBD7 218-220   PBD6 207-209

53 (E) This patient has rheumatoid arthritis. The pannus of rheumatoid arthritis leads to joint destruction and ankylosis with marked deformity. There are few other organ-specific lesions, although rheumatoid nodules can be found under the skin over bony prominences and in organs such as the lung and heart. Renal failure is more likely in systemic lupus erythematosus. Aortic dissection is more likely in Reiter syndrome. Ankylosing spondylitis is marked by kyphosis. The risk of malignancies is increased in patients with autoimmune diseases, although malignancies are still uncommon.

BP7 136-138   BP6 109-111   PBD7 1305-1309
PBD6 1248-1251

54 (C) This patient has Sjögren syndrome, which primarily involves salivary and lacrimal glands. Antibodies to SS-B are found in 60% to 90% of patients. Anti–double-stranded DNA is a specific autoantibody for systemic lupus erythematosus. Anticentromere antibody is seen in systemic sclerosis. Scl-70 is a marker for diffuse systemic sclerosis. Jo-1 is a marker for polymyositis.

BP7 139-140   BP6 111-112   PBD7 235-237
PBD6 225-226

55 **(E)** This patient is experiencing a systemic anaphylactic reaction, a form of type I hypersensitivity. IgE is bound to mast cells, after previous sensitization, so that a repeat encounter with the antigen results in mast cell degranulation and the release of mediators, such as histamine, that lead to anaphylaxis. IgE is also important in mediating more localized inflammatory reactions such as allergic rhinitis (hay fever). Other immunoglobulins do not bind so readily to mast cells.

BP7 112-114   BP6 87-88   PBD7 209   PBD6 196-198

56 **(D)** These findings point to the X-linked disorder known as Wiskott-Aldrich syndrome, which is characterized by thrombocytopenia, eczema, and decreased IgM. IgA may be increased. As in many immunodeficiency disorders, there is an increased risk of non-Hodgkin lymphoma. Hypocalcemia is seen in neonates with DiGeorge syndrome. Rheumatoid arthritis can complicate isolated IgA deficiency and common variable immunodeficiency, conditions with survival to adulthood. A deficiency of complement component C3 may be complicated by immune-complex glomerulonephritis. Dementia can be seen in patients with AIDS.

BP7 147   PBD7 244   PBD6 236

57 **(A)** Persons infected with HIV are infected for life. They can transmit the virus to others via sexual intercourse even if they appear to be well. The average time for the development of AIDS after HIV infection is 8 to 10 years. Seroreversion in HIV infection does not occur. Screening questionnaires and serologic testing can prevent this person from being a blood donor. HIV infection affects mainly CD4 lymphocytes, with declining CD4 counts presaging the development of clinically apparent AIDS. Antibody titers do not predict clinical illness or complications. Progression of HIV disease is monitored by levels of HIV-1 mRNA in the blood and by CD4+ cell counts.

BP7 155-156   BP6 122-125   PBD7 245-246
PBD6 245-248

58 **(C)** These findings are characteristic of cardiac amyloidosis. Because of the patient's age, a senile cardiac amyloidosis, resulting from deposition of transthyretin, is most likely. α-Fetoprotein is present during fetal life, but it is best known in adults as a serum tumor marker. β_2-Microglobulin contributes to the development of amyloidosis associated with long-term hemodialysis. Calcitonin forms the precursor for amyloid deposited in thyroid medullary carcinomas. Amyloidosis associated with plasma cell dyscrasias results from light-chain production. Although the heart is commonly involved in light-chain amyloidosis, the normal laboratory values and absence of plasma cell collections in the marrow argue against a plasma cell dyscrasia. IgE is not a component of amyloid.

BP7 160-161   BP6 127-130   PBD7 263
PBD6 252-253, 256

59 **(D)** This boy most likely has Bruton agammaglobulinemia, an X-linked primary immunodeficiency marked by recurrent bacterial infections that begin after maternal antibody levels diminish. Selective IgA deficiency is marked by a more benign course, with sinopulmonary infections and diarrhea that are not severe. Deficiency of complement C3 is rare; it leads to greater numbers of infections in children and young adults, but *Giardia* infections are not a feature of this disease. Lack of cell-mediated immunity is more likely to be seen in HIV infection in children. Although some patients with Bruton agammaglobulinemia can develop features of systemic lupus erythematosus, they generally do not have a positive test result for ANA.

BP7 144-145   BP6 115   PBD7 240-242   PBD6 232-233

60 **(B)** This woman has hereditary angioedema, a rare autosomal recessive disorder in which there is a deficiency of antigenic or functional C1 inhibitor, resulting in recurrent episodes of edema. Of the remaining choices, only C3 and IgA have a deficiency state. C3 deficiency is accompanied by recurrent infections with pyogenic bacteria. IgA deficiency leads to mild recurrent gastrointestinal and respiratory tract infections and predisposes to anaphylactic transfusion reaction. β_2-Microglobulin is a component of MHC class I; it can be increased with HIV infection and can be a substrate for amyloid fibrils in patients receiving long-term hemodialysis. 5-Hydroxytryptamine (serotonin) has an effect similar to histamine, which drives vasodilation and edema. IgE participates in localized or systemic anaphylaxis with edema.

BP7 147   BP6 117   PBD7 244-245   PBD6 69

61 **(F)** Natural killer (NK) cells have CD16, an Fc receptor that allows them to bind to opsonized cells and lyse them. This is a form of antibody-dependent cell-mediated cytotoxicity. NK cells comprise 10% to 15% of circulating lymphocytes. NK cells may also lyse human cells that have lost MHC class I expression as a result of viral infection or neoplastic transformation. B cells have surface immunoglobulin, are CD19 positive, and participate in humoral immunity. CD4 cells are T lymphocytes that are "helper" cells; they have T-cell receptors and are CD3 positive. Likewise CD8 cells have T-cell receptors and mark with CD3, but they act as cytotoxic T lymphocytes. Dendritic cells are a form of antigen-presenting cell that expresses large amounts of MHC class II molecules. Macrophages express MHC II and also act as antigen-presenting cells to CD4 cells; they can phagocytize opsonized cells. Stem cells are CD34 positive and can give rise to the whole range of cells in the immune system, as well as blood-forming cells.

BP7 107, 115   BP6 83-84   PBD7 210   PBD6 191

62 **(C)** Dendritic cells are a form of antigen-presenting cell (APC). Dendritic cells in epithelia are known as Langerhans cells, and those within germinal centers are called follicular dendritic cells (FDCs). The FDCs may become infected, but not killed by HIV. They have cell surface Fc receptors that capture antibody-coated HIV virions through the Fc portion of the antibody. These virions attached to the FDCs can infect passing CD4+ lymphocytes. B cells are a component of humoral immunity, and antibody to HIV does not serve a protective function, but allows serologic detection of infection. CD8 cells are cytotoxic lymphocytes that lack the receptor necessary for infection by HIV. Because they survive selectively, the CD4:CD8 ratio is reversed; it is typically <1 with advanced HIV infection. Langhans giant cells are "committees" of activated macrophages that are part of a granulomatous response. Macrophages are a type of antigen presenting cell that can become infected by HIV without destruction. Mast cells have surface-bound IgE, which can be cross-linked by antigens (allergens) to cause degranulation and release of vasoactive amines, such as histamine, as part of anaphylaxis with type I hypersensitivity. Natural killer cells have Fc receptors, but they are not antigen presenting cells.

BP7 107, 153   BP6 83   PBD7 199-200   PBD6 191

Neoplasia

PBD7 Chapter 7: Neoplasia

PBD6 Chapter 8: Neoplasia

BP7 and BP6 Chapter 6: Neoplasia

1 A 40-year-old man has a history of intravenous drug use. Physical examination shows needle tracks in his left antecubital fossa. He has mild scleral icterus. Serologic studies for HBsAg and anti-HCV are positive. He develops hepatocellular carcinoma 15 years later. Which of the following best explains why this patient developed hepatocellular carcinoma?

☐ (A) The consistent integration of these viruses in the vicinity of protooncogenes

☐ (B) The ability of these viruses to capture protooncogenes from the host DNA

☐ (C) Virus-induced injury to liver cells followed by extensive regeneration

☐ (D) The ability of viral genes to inactivate *RB* and *p53* expression

☐ (E) The ability of these viruses to cause immunosuppression of the host

2 A 48-year-old woman notices a lump in her left breast. On physical examination, the physician palpates a firm, nonmovable, 2-cm mass in the upper outer quadrant of the left breast. There are enlarged, firm, nontender lymph nodes in the left axilla. A fine-needle aspiration biopsy is performed, and the cells present are consistent with carcinoma. A mastectomy with axillary lymph node dissection is performed, and carcinoma is present in two of eight axillary nodes. Which

of the following factors is most likely responsible for the lymph node metastases?

☐ (A) Increased laminin receptors on tumor cells

☐ (B) Presence of keratin in tumor cells

☐ (C) Diminished apoptosis of tumor cells

☐ (D) Tumor cell monoclonality

☐ (E) Lymphadenitis

3 A 30-year-old woman who has had multiple sexual partners sees her physician because she has had vaginal bleeding and discharge for the past 5 days. On physical examination, she is afebrile. Pelvic examination shows an ulcerated lesion arising from the squamocolumnar junction of the uterine cervix. A cervical biopsy is performed. Microscopic examination reveals an invasive tumor containing areas of squamous epithelium, with pearls of keratin. In situ hybridization shows the presence of human papillomavirus type 16 (HPV-16) DNA within the tumor cells. Which of the following molecular abnormalities in this tumor is most likely related to infection with HPV-16?

☐ (A) Trapping of the *RAS* protein in a GTP-bound state

☐ (B) Increased expression of laminin receptor genes

☐ (C) Inability to repair DNA damage

☐ (D) Functional inactivation of the *RB1* protein

☐ (E) Increased expression of epidermal growth factor receptor

4 A 47-year-old man has felt increasingly tired and weak for the past 6 months. On physical examination, he appears pale. Laboratory studies show hemoglobin of 10.7 g/dL, hematocrit 32.1%, platelet count 155,000/mm³, and WBC count 167,500/mm³. The peripheral blood smear shows a predominance of mature and immature neutrophilic cells. Cytogenetic analysis of cells obtained through bone marrow aspiration shows a t(9;22) translocation, which has resulted in formation of a hybrid gene, causing potent tyrosine kinase activity. Which of the following genes was translocated from chromosome 9?

- ❏ (A) *p53*
- ❏ (B) *RB*
- ❏ (C) *NF1*
- ❏ (D) *K-RAS*
- ❏ (E) *C-ABL*

5 A 44-year-old woman sees her physician because she feels lumps in the right axilla. The physician notes right axillary lymphadenopathy on physical examination. The nodes are painless but firm. Which of the following is the most likely diagnosis?

- ❏ (A) Ductal carcinoma of the breast
- ❏ (B) Acute mastitis with breast abscess
- ❏ (C) Leiomyosarcoma of the uterus
- ❏ (D) Cerebral glioblastoma multiforme
- ❏ (E) Squamous dysplasia of the larynx

6 A 20-year-old man has a raised, irregular, pigmented lesion on his forearm that has increased in size and become more irregular in color over the past 4 months. Physical examination shows a 0.5 × 1.2 cm black to brown-colored lesion with irregular borders. An excisional biopsy specimen shows a malignant melanoma that extends into the reticular dermis. Family history indicates that the patient's paternal uncle died of metastatic melanoma that spread to the liver after excision of a primary lesion on the foot. His grandfather required enucleation of the left eye because of a "dark brown" mass in the eyeball. Which of the following genes is most likely to have undergone mutation to produce these findings?

- ❏ (A) *BCL2* (antiapoptosis gene)
- ❏ (B) *C-MYC* (transcription factor gene)
- ❏ (C) *IL2* (growth factor gene)
- ❏ (D) *Lyn* (tyrosine kinase gene)
- ❏ (E) *PDGF* (growth factor overexpression)
- ❏ (F) *p53* (DNA damage response gene)
- ❏ (G) *sis* (growth factor overexpression)

7 A 32-year-old woman has experienced dull pelvic pain for the past 2 months. Physical examination shows a right adnexal mass. An abdominal ultrasound scan shows a 7.5-cm cystic ovarian mass. The mass is surgically excised. The surface of the mass is smooth, and it is nonadherent to surrounding pelvic structures. On gross examination, the mass is cystic and filled with hair. Microscopically, there is squamous epithelium, tall columnar glandular epithelium, cartilage, and fibrous connective tissue present. Which of the following is the most likely diagnosis?

- ❏ (A) Adenocarcinoma
- ❏ (B) Fibroadenoma
- ❏ (C) Glioma
- ❏ (D) Hamartoma
- ❏ (E) Mesothelioma
- ❏ (F) Rhabdomyosarcoma
- ❏ (G) Teratoma

8 A 30-year-old man has a 15-year history of increasing numbers of multiple benign skin nodules. On physical examination, the firm nodules average 0.5 to 1 cm and appear to be subcutaneous. Further examination shows numerous oval 1- to 5-cm pigmented skin lesions. Ophthalmoscopic examination shows hamartomatous nodules on the iris. A biopsy specimen of one skin nodule shows a neoplasm that is attached to a peripheral nerve. Which of the following mechanisms of transformation is most likely related to the mutation that this patient has inherited?

- ❏ (A) Persistent activation of the *RAS* gene
- ❏ (B) Increased production of epidermal growth factor
- ❏ (C) Decreased susceptibility to apoptosis
- ❏ (D) Impaired functioning of mismatch repair genes
- ❏ (E) Inactivation of the *RB* gene

9 A study of chemical carcinogenesis shows that repeated application of croton oil containing tetra-decanoylphorbol-acetate (TPA, a phorbol ester), after one application of a mutagenic agent on the skin, promotes carcinogenesis. Which of the following is the most likely mechanism for this phenomenon?

- ❏ (A) Induction of chromosome breaks
- ❏ (B) Inhibition of DNA repair
- ❏ (C) Activation of protein kinase C
- ❏ (D) Activation of endogenous viruses
- ❏ (E) Blockage of TGF-β pathways

10 A 50-year-old woman undergoes screening colonoscopy as part of a routine health maintenance workup. An isolated 1-cm pedunculated polyp is found in the sigmoid colon. The excised polyp histologically shows well-differentiated glands with no invasion of the stalk. Which of the following investigational research procedures can most clearly distinguish whether the polyp represents hyperplasia of the colonic mucosa or a tubular adenoma?

- ❏ (A) Histochemical staining for mucin
- ❏ (B) Flow cytometry to determine the frequency of cells in the S phase
- ❏ (C) Determination of clonality by pattern of X chromosome inactivation
- ❏ (D) Immunoperoxidase staining for keratin
- ❏ (E) Immunoperoxidase staining for factor VIII

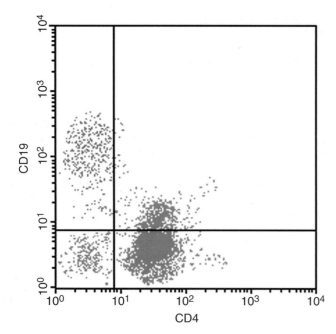

11 A 66-year-old woman has worked all of her life on a small family farm on the Kanto plain near Tokyo. She has had no previous major illnesses, but has been feeling increasingly tired and weak for the past year. On physical examination, she is afebrile but appears pale. Laboratory studies show hemoglobin of 11.3 g/dL, hematocrit 33.8%, platelet count 205,200/mm³, and WBC count 64,000/mm³. Immunophenotyping yields the findings shown in the figure. Assuming that the dominant cell population is clonal, which of the following viral agents is most likely involved in this patient's disease process?

☐ (A) Human papillomavirus
☐ (B) HIV-1
☐ (C) Epstein-Barr virus
☐ (D) Human T-cell lymphotropic virus type 1
☐ (E) Hepatitis B virus

12 A 50-year-old woman saw her physician after noticing a mass in the right breast. Physical examination showed a 2-cm mass fixed to the underlying tissues beneath the areola and three firm, nontender, lymph nodes palpable in the right axilla. There was no family history of cancer. An excisional breast biopsy was performed, and microscopic examination showed a well-differentiated ductal carcinoma. Over the next 6 months, additional lymph nodes became enlarged, and CT scans showed nodules in the lung, liver, and brain. The patient died 9 months after diagnosis. Which of the following molecular abnormalities is most likely to be found in this setting?

☐ (A) Inactivation of one copy of the *BRCA1* gene in fibroblasts cultured from the normal skin
☐ (B) Deletion of one copy of the *p53* gene in all cells of the patient
☐ (C) Amplification of the *ERBB2* (*HER2*) gene in breast cancer cells
☐ (D) Deletion of the *RB* locus in the normal somatic cells of the patient
☐ (E) Fusion of *BCR* and *C-ABL* genes in the cancer cells

13 In a family of five children, a 12-year-old girl and a 14-year-old boy have been affected by skin nodules that have developed over the past 5 years. On physical examination, both children are of appropriate height and weight. The skin lesions are 1- to 3-cm maculopapular nodules that are erythematous to brown-colored and have areas of ulceration. Biopsy specimens of the skin lesions show squamous cell carcinoma. The children have no history of recurrent infections, and their parents and other relatives are not affected. Which of the following mechanisms is most likely to produce neoplasia in these children?

☐ (A) Infection with human papillomavirus
☐ (B) Failure of nucleotide excision repair of DNA
☐ (C) Ingestion of food contaminated with *Aspergillus flavus*
☐ (D) Inactivation of *p53*
☐ (E) Chromosomal translocation

14 A 55-year-old man visits the physician because of hemoptysis and worsening cough. On physical examination, wheezes are auscultated over the right lung posteriorly. A chest radiograph shows a 6-cm perihilar mass on the right. A fine-needle aspiration biopsy yields cells consistent with non–small cell bronchogenic carcinoma. Molecular analysis of the neoplastic cells shows a *p53* gene mutation. Which of the following mechanisms has most likely produced the neoplastic transformation?

☐ (A) Inability to hydrolyze GTP
☐ (B) Microsatellite instability
☐ (C) Lack of necrosis
☐ (D) Loss of cell cycle arrest
☐ (E) Transcriptional activation

15 A 5-year-old child has difficulty with vision in the right eye. On physical examination, there is leukokoria of the right eye, consistent with a mass in the posterior chamber. MR imaging shows a mass that nearly fills the globe. The child undergoes enucleation of the right eye. Molecular analysis of the neoplastic cells indicates absence of both copies of a tumor suppressor gene that controls the transition from the G1 to the S phase of the cell cycle. Which of the following genes is most likely to have the mechanism of action that produced this neoplasm?

☐ (A) *BCR-ABL*
☐ (B) *BCL2*
☐ (C) *hMSH2*
☐ (D) *K-RAS*
☐ (E) *NF1*
☐ (F) *p53*
☐ (G) *RB*

16 A 60-year-old male comes to his physician because he has noted a mass in his neck that has increased rapidly in size over the past 2 months. On physical examination a firm, non-tender 10 cm mass in the left lateral posterior neck is palpated that appears to be fused cervical lymph nodes. Hepatosplenomegaly is noted. A head CT scan reveals a mass in the Waldeyer ring near the pharynx. A biopsy of the neck mass is performed and on microscopic examination shows abnormal lymphoid cells with many mitotic figures and many apoptotic nuclei. He is treated with a cocktail of cell cycle acting chemotherapeutic agents. The cervical and oral masses shrink dramatically over the next month. Based upon his history and response to treatment, the tumor cells are most likely to have which of the following features?

- ❑ (A) Limited capacity to metastasize
- ❑ (B) Polyclonality
- ❑ (C) Poor vascularity
- ❑ (D) High growth fraction
- ❑ (E) Strong expression of tumor antigens

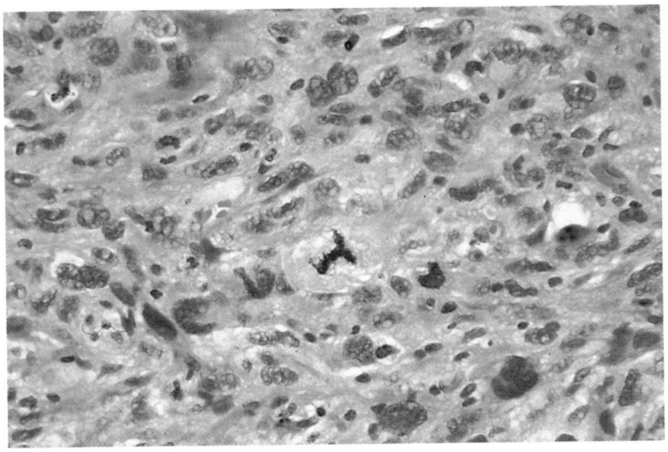

17 A 58-year-old woman has experienced an increasing feeling of fullness in the neck for the past 3 months, and she has noted a 3-kg weight loss during that time. On physical examination, there is a firm, fixed mass in a 3 × 5 cm area in the right side of the neck. CT scan shows a solid mass in the region of the right lobe of the thyroid gland. A biopsy of the mass is performed, and the microscopic appearance of the specimen is shown. All areas of the tumor have similar morphology. Which of the following terms best describes this neoplasm?

- ❑ (A) Adenoma
- ❑ (B) Well-differentiated adenocarcinoma
- ❑ (C) Squamous cell carcinoma
- ❑ (D) Leiomyoma
- ❑ (E) Anaplastic carcinoma

18 A 59-year-old man has recently noticed blood in his urine. Cystoscopy shows a 4-cm exophytic mass involving the right bladder mucosa near the trigone. Biopsy specimens are obtained, and the patient undergoes a radical cystectomy. Examination of the excised specimen shows that a grade IV urothelial cell carcinoma has infiltrated the bladder wall. Which of the following statements regarding these findings is most appropriate?

- ❑ (A) The neoplasm is a metastasis
- ❑ (B) The patient has a poorly differentiated neoplasm
- ❑ (C) A paraneoplastic syndrome is likely
- ❑ (D) The stage of the neoplasm is low
- ❑ (E) The patient is probably cured of the cancer

19 An epidemiologic study analyzes health-care benefits of cancer screening techniques applied to a population. Which of the following diagnostic screening techniques used in health care is most likely to have had the greatest impact on reduction in cancer deaths in developed nations?

- ❑ (A) Chest radiograph
- ❑ (B) Stool guaiac
- ❑ (C) Pap smear
- ❑ (D) Serum carcinoembryonic antigen assay
- ❑ (E) Urinalysis

20 During a routine health maintenance examination, a 46-year-old man is found to have an enlarged, nontender supraclavicular lymph node that is palpable on physical examination. The 2-cm node is excised. Histologically, the nodal architecture is effaced by a monomorphous population of small lymphocytes. Which of the following procedures would best confirm that the patient has a malignancy?

- ❑ (A) Peripheral WBC count and differential cell count
- ❑ (B) Flow cytometry of nodal tissue for DNA content
- ❑ (C) Electron microscopy to determine cellular ultrastructure
- ❑ (D) Southern blot analysis to demonstrate monoclonality
- ❑ (E) Determination of the serum lactate dehydrogenase level

21 An epidemiologic study investigates the potential cellular molecular alterations that may contribute to the development of cancers in a population. Data analyzed from resected colonic lesions show that changes are occurring that demonstrate the evolution of a sporadic colonic adenoma into an invasive carcinoma. Which of the following best describes the mechanism producing these changes?

- ❑ (A) Protooncogenes can be activated by chromosomal translocation
- ❑ (B) Malignant transformation involves accumulation of mutations in protooncogenes and tumor suppressor genes in a step-wise fashion
- ❑ (C) Extensive regeneration of tissues increases the risk of cancer-causing mutations
- ❑ (D) Inherited defects in DNA repair increase the susceptibility to develop cancer
- ❑ (E) Overexpression of growth factor receptor genes is associated with poor prognosis.

22 A 49-year old man has a lump near his right shoulder that has been increasing in size for the past 8 months. On physical examination, the physician palpates a 4-cm firm, nontender mass in the right supraclavicular region. The mass is excised, and microscopically, it is diagnosed as follicular lymphoma. Karyotypic analysis of the cells shows a chromosomal translocation, t(14;18), involving the immunoglobulin heavy-chain gene. Which of the following genes is most likely to have undergone mutation to produce these findings?

- ❑ (A) *APC* (tumor suppressor gene)
- ❑ (B) *BCL1* (cyclin gene)
- ❑ (C) *BCL2* (antiapoptosis gene)
- ❑ (D) *BRCA1* (DNA repair gene)
- ❑ (E) *C-MYC* (transcription factor gene)
- ❑ (F) *ERBB2* (growth factor receptor gene)
- ❑ (G) *IL2* (growth factor gene)
- ❑ (H) *K-RAS* (GTP-binding protein gene)
- ❑ (I) *p53* (DNA damage response gene)

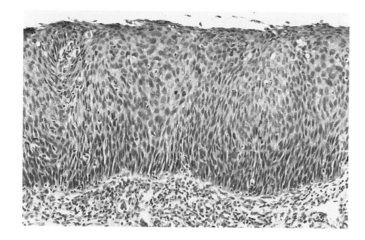

23 A Pap smear obtained from a 29-year-old woman during a routine health maintenance examination is abnormal. She is currently asymptomatic, but has a history of multiple sexual partners. Cervical biopsy specimens are obtained. The representative microscopic appearance of a specimen is shown above. Which of the following is the most likely diagnosis?

❑ (A) Adenocarcinoma
❑ (B) Carcinoma in situ
❑ (C) Hamartoma
❑ (D) Leiomyoma
❑ (E) Melanoma
❑ (F) Mesothelioma
❑ (G) Nevus
❑ (H) Small cell anaplastic carcinoma

24 An epidemiologic study of cancer deaths recorded in the last half of the 20th century is conducted. The number of deaths for one particular type of cancer has been decreasing in developed nations, despite the absence of widespread screening programs. Which of the following neoplasms was most likely to be identified by this study?

❑ (A) Angiosarcoma of the liver
❑ (B) Gastric adenocarcinoma
❑ (C) Glioma of the brain
❑ (D) Leukemia
❑ (E) Lymphoma of the lymph nodes
❑ (F) Pancreatic adenocarcinoma

25 A 26-year-old woman has a lump in the left breast. On physical examination by the physician, there is an irregular, firm, 2-cm mass in the upper inner quadrant of the breast. No axillary adenopathy is noted. A fine-needle aspirate of the mass shows carcinoma. The patient's 30-year-old sister was recently diagnosed with ovarian cancer, and 3 years ago her maternal aunt was diagnosed with ductal carcinoma of the breast and had a mastectomy. Which of the following genes is most likely to have undergone mutation to produce these findings?

❑ (A) *BCL2* (antiapoptosis gene)
❑ (B) *BRCA1* (DNA repair gene)
❑ (C) *EGF* (epidermal growth factor gene)
❑ (D) *ERBB2* (growth factor receptor gene)
❑ (E) *HST1* (fibroblast growth factor gene)
❑ (F) *IL2* (growth factor gene)
❑ (G) *K-RAS* (GTP-binding protein gene)
❑ (H) *Lyn* (tyrosine kinase gene)

26 A 51-year-old man who works in a factory that produces plastic pipe has experienced weight loss, nausea, and vomiting over the past 4 months. On physical examination, he has tenderness to palpation in the right upper quadrant of the abdomen, and the liver span is increased. Laboratory findings include serum alkaline phosphatase of 405 U/L AST, 45 U/L, ALT 30 U/L, and total bilirubin 0.9 mg/dL. An abdominal CT scan shows a 12-cm mass in the right lobe of the liver. A liver biopsy is performed, and microscopic examination shows an angiosarcoma. The patient has most likely been exposed to which of the following agents?

❑ (A) Arsenic
❑ (B) Asbestos
❑ (C) Benzene
❑ (D) Beryllium
❑ (E) Nickel
❑ (F) Vinyl chloride
❑ (G) Naphthalene

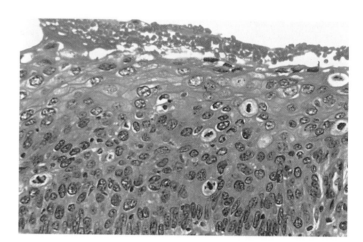

27 A 39-year-old woman underwent a routine health maintenance examination for the first time in many years. A Pap smear was obtained, and the result reported was abnormal. On pelvic examination, a red, slightly raised, 1-cm lesion on the anterior ectocervix at the 2-o'clock position was excised and biopsied. The microscopic appearance on medium-power magnification is shown above. Which of the following statements best characterizes the patient's condition?

❑ (A) A primary site should be sought
❑ (B) This is a high-grade lesion
❑ (C) The cell of origin is a fibroblast
❑ (D) A chest radiograph will show nodules
❑ (E) Local excision will be curative

28 A 61-year-old woman has felt a lump in her breast for the past 2 months. On physical examination, there is a firm 2-cm mass in the right breast. An excisional biopsy specimen of the mass shows carcinoma. Immunoperoxidase stains for protease cathepsin D and matrix metalloproteinase-9 are performed on the microscopic tissue section and show pronounced cytoplasmic staining in the tumor cells. Which of the following characteristics is most likely to be predicted by this marker?

- ❑ (A) Angiogenesis
- ❑ (B) Invasiveness
- ❑ (C) Differentiation
- ❑ (D) Heterogeneity
- ❑ (E) Aneuploidy

29 A 22-year-old woman, who works as a secretary for an accounting firm, has noted a palpable nodule on the side of her neck for the past 3 months. On physical examination, there is a 2-cm firm, nontender nodule involving the right lobe of the thyroid gland. A fine-needle aspiration biopsy specimen of the nodule shows cells consistent with carcinoma of the thyroid. No other family members are affected by this disorder. Which of the following would be considered most relevant in the woman's past medical history?

- ❑ (A) Chronic alcoholism
- ❑ (B) Ataxia telangiectasia
- ❑ (C) Radiation therapy in childhood
- ❑ (D) Blunt trauma from a fall
- ❑ (E) Exposure to arsenic compounds

30 An epidemiologic study is performed to assess risks for cervical carcinoma. The cells from cervical lesions in a population of women are analyzed. Binding of certain viral proteins to *pRB* is found in patients in whom dysplastic cells are present. Viral proteins from which of the following are most likely to bind *pRB*, increasing the risk for dysplasia?

- ❑ (A) Cytomegalovirus
- ❑ (B) Epstein-Barr virus
- ❑ (C) Herpes simplex virus
- ❑ (D) Hepatitis B virus
- ❑ (E) HIV
- ❑ (F) Human papillomavirus
- ❑ (G) JC papovavirus

31 A 62-year-old man with a history of chronic alcoholism has noted a 6-kg weight loss over the past 5 months. Physical examination shows no masses or palpable lymphadenopathy. Laboratory studies include an elevated serum α-fetoprotein level. A stool guaiac test result is negative. Which of the following is the most likely diagnosis?

- ❑ (A) Prostatic adenocarcinoma
- ❑ (B) Pulmonary squamous cell carcinoma
- ❑ (C) Multiple myeloma
- ❑ (D) Pancreatic adenocarcinoma
- ❑ (E) Hepatocellular carcinoma

32 A 49-year-old man experiences an episode of hemoptysis. On physical examination, he has puffiness of the face, pedal edema, and systolic hypertension. A chest radiograph shows a 5-cm mass of the right upper lobe of the lung. A fine-needle aspiration biopsy of this mass yields cells consistent with small cell anaplastic carcinoma. A bone scan shows no metastases. Immunohistochemical staining of the tumor cells is most likely to be positive for which of the following?

- ❑ (A) Parathyroid hormone–related peptide
- ❑ (B) Erythropoietin
- ❑ (C) Corticotropin
- ❑ (D) Insulin
- ❑ (E) Gastrin

33 During a routine health maintenance examination of a 40-year-old man, a stool guaiac test result was positive. A follow-up sigmoidoscopy showed a 1.5-cm circumscribed, pedunculated mass on a short stalk, located in the upper rectum. Which of the following terms best describes this lesion?

- ❑ (A) Adenoma
- ❑ (B) Hamartoma
- ❑ (C) Sarcoma
- ❑ (D) Choristoma
- ❑ (E) Nevus

34 A 40-year-old man notices an increasing number of lumps in the groin and armpit. On physical examination, he has generalized nontender lymph node enlargement and hepatosplenomegaly. An inguinal lymph node biopsy specimen shows a malignant tumor of lymphoid cells. Immunoperoxidase staining of the tumor cells with antibody to *BCL2* is positive in the lymphocytic cell nuclei. Which of the following mechanisms has most likely produced the lymphoma?

- ❑ (A) Increased tyrosine kinase activity
- ❑ (B) Lack of apoptosis
- ❑ (C) Gene amplifications
- ❑ (D) Reduced DNA repair
- ❑ (E) Loss of cell cycle inhibition

35 A 70-year-old woman reported a 4-month history of a 4-kg weight loss and increasing generalized icterus. On physical examination, she is afebrile, and her blood pressure is 130/80 mm Hg. An abdominal CT scan shows a 5-cm mass in the head of the pancreas. Fine-needle aspiration of the mass is performed. On molecular analysis, the neoplastic cells from the mass show continued activation of cytoplasmic kinases. Which of the following oncogenes is most likely to be involved in this process?

- ❑ (A) *MYC*
- ❑ (B) *APC*
- ❑ (C) *RAS*
- ❑ (D) *ERBB2*
- ❑ (E) *sis*

36 A 23-year-old woman has noted a nodule on the skin of her upper chest. She reports that the nodule has been present for many years and has not changed in size. On physical examination, there is a 0.5-cm dark-red, nontender, raised nodule with a smooth surface. Which of the following is the most likely diagnosis?

- ❑ (A) Adenoma
- ❑ (B) Fibroadenoma
- ❑ (C) Hamartoma
- ❑ (D) Hemangioma
- ❑ (E) Leiomyoma
- ❑ (F) Lipoma
- ❑ (G) Melanoma
- ❑ (H) Nevus

37 A 63-year-old man sees the physician because of cough and hemoptysis. He has a 65 pack-year history of smoking. A chest CT scan shows a 5-cm right hilar mass. Bronchoscopy is performed, and lung biopsy specimens show small cell anaplastic lung carcinoma. His family history shows three first-degree maternal relatives who developed leukemia, sarcoma, and carcinoma before the age of 40 years. Which of the following genes is most likely to have undergone mutation to produce these findings?

❏ (A) *APC* (tumor suppressor gene)
❏ (B) *BCL2* (antiapoptosis gene)
❏ (C) *ERBB2* (growth factor receptor gene)
❏ (D) *K-RAS* (GTP-binding protein gene)
❏ (E) *NF1* (GTPase-activating protein)
❏ (F) *p53* (DNA damage response gene)

38 A 70-year-old man has sprayed his orchard with insecticide each spring for 20 years. He recently noticed a rough, erythematous area of skin on the right shoulder. The patch becomes ulcerated and does not heal. He develops weight loss, nausea, and vomiting. The excised lesion is a squamous cell carcinoma. Which of the following was most likely a component of the insecticide that was used by this man?

❏ (A) Arsenic
❏ (B) Benzene
❏ (C) Cadmium
❏ (D) Chromium
❏ (E) Chlorinated biphenyl
❏ (F) Ethylene oxide
❏ (G) Naphthalene

39 In a clinical trial, patients diagnosed with malignant melanoma are treated by infusion of autologous CD8+ T cells that are known to kill melanoma cells but not normal cells. The target antigen recognized by these CD8+ T cells is most likely to be composed of which of the following?

❏ (A) Class I MHC molecules plus a peptide produced by normal melanocytes and melanoma cells
❏ (B) Class I MHC molecules plus a peptide derived from carcinoembryonic antigen
❏ (C) Class II MHC molecules plus a peptide derived from melanoma cells
❏ (D) Class I MHC molecules plus a peptide produced by melanoma cells
❏ (E) A peptide secreted by melanoma cells and presented by laminin receptors on melanoma cells

40 A 62-year-old man has had several episodes of hematuria in the past week. On physical examination, there are no abnormal findings. A urinalysis shows 4+ hematuria, and cytologic examination of the urine shows that atypical cells are present. The urologist performs a cystoscopy and observes a 4-cm sessile mass with a nodular, ulcerated surface in the dome of the bladder. Which of the following terms best describes this lesion?

❏ (A) Papilloma
❏ (B) Carcinoma
❏ (C) Adenoma
❏ (D) Sarcoma
❏ (E) Fibroma

41 A 66-year-old man with chronic cough has an episode of hemoptysis. On physical examination, there are no abnormal findings. A chest radiograph shows a 6-cm mass in the right lung. A sputum cytologic analysis shows cells consistent with squamous cell carcinoma. Metastases from this neoplasm are most likely to be found at which of the following sites?

❏ (A) Chest wall muscle
❏ (B) Splenic red pulp
❏ (C) Hilar lymph nodes
❏ (D) Vertebral bone marrow
❏ (E) Cerebrum

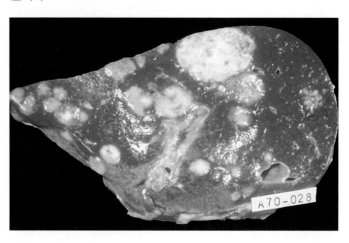

42 A 69-year-old woman has experienced increasing malaise and a 10-kg weight loss over the past year. She dies of massive pulmonary thromboembolism. The gross appearance of the liver at autopsy is shown. Which of the following statements best characterizes the process that led to the patient's death?

❏ (A) A liver biopsy would have shown a dysplasia
❏ (B) This is a multifocal hepatic adenoma
❏ (C) A hepatocellular carcinoma has invaded locally
❏ (D) Colonic adenocarcinoma with metastases was present
❏ (E) The lesions should have been resected

43 A 75-year-old woman has reported a change in the caliber of her stools during the past month. On physical examination, there are no abnormal findings, but a stool sample is positive for occult blood. A colonoscopy shows a constricting mass involving the lower sigmoid colon, and the patient undergoes a partial colectomy. Which of the following techniques used during surgery can best aid the surgeon in determining whether the resection is adequate to reduce the probability of a recurrence?

❏ (A) Fine-needle aspiration
❏ (B) Serum carcinoembryonic antigen assay
❏ (C) Frozen section
❏ (D) Electron microscopy
❏ (E) Flow cytometry

44 A 60-year-old woman has noted a feeling of pelvic heaviness for the past 6 months. On physical examination, there is a nontender lower abdominal mass. An abdominal ultrasound scan shows a 12-cm solid mass in the uterine wall. A total abdominal hysterectomy is performed, and on removal, the mass has the microscopic appearance of a well-differentiated leiomyosarcoma. One year later, a chest radiograph shows a 4-cm nodule on the right lower lung. A biopsy specimen of the nodule shows a poorly differentiated sarcoma. The patient's past medical history indicates that she has smoked cigarettes most of her adult life. Which of the following best explains these findings?

❑ (A) Development of a second primary neoplasm
❑ (B) Inheritance of a defective *RB* gene
❑ (C) Continued cigarette smoking by the patient
❑ (D) Loss of an oncogene
❑ (E) Metastasis from an aggressive subclone of the primary tumor

45 In an experiment, cells from human malignant neoplasms explanted into tissue culture medium continue to replicate. This allows development of "immortal" tumor cell lines that are extremely useful for study of tumor biology and responses to therapeutic modalities. Which of the following molecular alterations that endows these tumor cells with limitless replicative ability both *in vivo* and *in vitro* is most likely to be observed?

❑ (A) Activation of telomerase
❑ (B) Activation of cyclin genes
❑ (C) Inhibition of cyclin activators
❑ (D) Activation of vascular endothelial growth factor (VEGF)
❑ (E) Activation of *BCL2* gene
❑ (F) Inability to repair errors in DNA replication

46 An investigational study reviews cells from patients who had hereditary nonpolyposis colon cancer. The patients typically developed multiple lesions of the colon during middle age. Molecular analysis of the cells from the lesions shows changes in *hPMS1*, *hPMS2*, and *hMLH1* genes. Which of the following principles of carcinogenesis is best illustrated by this study?

❑ (A) Tumor initiators are mutagenic
❑ (B) Tumor promoters induce proliferation
❑ (C) Many oncogenes are activated by translocations
❑ (D) Inability to repair DNA is carcinogenic
❑ (E) Carcinogenesis is a multistep process

47 A 38-year-old woman has abdominal distention that has been worsening for the past 6 weeks. An abdominal CT scan shows bowel obstruction caused by a 6-cm mass in the jejunum. At laparotomy, a portion of the small bowel is resected. Microscopic examination shows that the mass is a Burkitt lymphoma. Flow cytometry analysis of a portion of the tumor shows a high S phase. Mutational activation of which of the following nuclear oncogenes is most likely to be present in this tumor?

❑ (A) *ERBB2*
❑ (B) *p53*
❑ (C) *RAS*
❑ (D) *MYC*
❑ (E) *APC*

48 A 55-year-old female has felt an enlarging lump in her left breast for the past year. A hard, irregular 5 cm mass fixed to the underlying chest wall is palpable in her left breast. Left axillary nontender lymphadenopathy is noted. There is no hepatosplenomegaly. A chest CT scan reveals multiple bilateral pulmonary "cannon ball" nodules. A left breast biopsy is performed and on microscopic examination shows high grade infiltrating ductal carcinoma. The appearance of the nodules in her lungs is most likely related to which of the following?

❑ (A) Proximity of the breast carcinoma to the lungs
❑ (B) Lymphatic connections between the breast and the pleura
❑ (C) Internal mammary artery invasion by carcinoma cells
❑ (D) Pulmonary chemokines that bind carcinoma cell chemokine receptors
❑ (E) Overexpression of laminin receptors on carcinoma cell surfaces
❑ (F) Overexpression of estrogen receptors within the carcinoma cell nuclei

49 A 33-year-old woman undergoes a routine physical examination as part of her health maintenance screening. There are no abnormal findings. A Pap smear is obtained as part of the pelvic examination. Cytologically, the cells obtained on the smear from the cervix show severe epithelial dysplasia. Which of the following statements best explains the significance of these findings?

❑ (A) The lesion could progress to invasive cervical carcinoma
❑ (B) An ovarian teratoma is present
❑ (C) There has been regression of a cervical carcinoma
❑ (D) Antibiotic therapy will cure the lesion
❑ (E) Female relatives are at risk of acquiring the same condition

50 A 53-year-old woman sees her physician because she has noticed a change in her bowel habits. On physical examination, there are no abnormal findings, but the test result for stool guaiac is positive. A colonoscopy is performed, and a 3-cm sessile mass is found in the cecum. A biopsy specimen of the mass shows a moderately differentiated adenocarcinoma confined to the mucosa. An abdominal CT scan shows no lymphadenopathy. Given this information, which of the following is the best course of action?

❑ (A) Perform a limited excision to "shell out" the lesion from its surrounding capsule
❑ (B) Assume that this represents a metastasis and search for a primary tumor elsewhere
❑ (C) Resect the tumor and some of the normal surrounding tissue
❑ (D) Remove the entire colon to prevent a recurrence
❑ (E) Observe the lesion for further increase in size

51 A 50-year-old woman has had easy fatigability and noted a dragging sensation in her abdomen for the past 5 months. Physical examination reveals that she is afebrile. She has marked splenomegaly but no lymphadenopathy. Laboratory studies show her total WBC count is 250,000/mm³ with WBC differential count showing 68% segmented neutrophils, 11% band neutrophils, 6% metamyelocytes, 5% myelocytes, 5% myeloblasts, 3% lymphocytes, and 2% monocytes. A bone marrow biopsy is performed, and karyotypic analysis of the cells reveals a t(9;22) translocation. Medical treatment with a drug having which of the following modes of action is most likely to produce a complete remission in this patient?

❑ (A) Antibody binding to ERB-2 receptor
❑ (B) Inhibiting tyrosine-kinase activity
❑ (C) Selective killing of cells in S-phase
❑ (D) Activating caspases
❑ (E) Preventing translocation of B-catenin to the nucleus
❑ (F) Delivering normal p53 into cells with viral vectors

52 A 35-year-old man with a family history of colon carcinoma undergoes a surveillance colonoscopy. It reveals hundreds of polyps in the colon, and two focal 0.5 cm ulcerated areas. A biopsy from an ulcer reveals irregularly shaped glands that have penetrated into the muscular layer. Which of the following molecular events is believed to occur very early in the evolution of his colonic disease process?

- ❏ (A) Mutations in mismatch repair genes.
- ❏ (B) Inability to hydrolyze GTP-bound *RAS*
- ❏ (C) Activation of the *WNT* signaling pathway
- ❏ (D) Loss of heterozygosity affecting the *p53* gene.
- ❏ (E) Translocation of *BCL2* from mitochondria to cytoplasm.

53 A 56-year-old woman has had vaginal bleeding for 1 week. Her last menstrual period was 10 years ago. On physical examination, a lower abdominal mass is palpated. An abdominal CT scan shows a 6-cm mass in the left ovary. A total abdominal hysterectomy is performed. Microscopically, the ovarian mass is a granulosa-theca cell tumor. The patient also is found to have an endometrial carcinoma, which resulted from increased estrogen production by the ovarian mass. Which of the following best describes the relationship between these two neoplasms?

- ❏ (A) Promotion of carcinogenesis
- ❏ (B) Tumor heterogeneity
- ❏ (C) Paraneoplastic syndrome
- ❏ (D) Genetic susceptibility to tumorigenesis
- ❏ (E) Mutation of a tumor suppressor gene

54 A 67-year-old man has noted a chronic cough for the past 3 months. On physical examination, there is mild stridor on inspiration over the right lung. A chest radiograph shows a 5-cm right hilar lung mass, and a fine-needle aspiration biopsy specimen of the mass shows cells consistent with squamous cell carcinoma. If staging of this neoplasm is denoted as T2N1M1, which of the following statements is most accurate?

- ❏ (A) A CT scan of the head shows a 2-cm right parietal mass
- ❏ (B) Serum chemistry shows an elevated corticotropin level
- ❏ (C) The mass had infiltrated the chest wall
- ❏ (D) The cancer is poorly differentiated
- ❏ (E) The tumor is obstructing the left mainstem bronchus

55 A 33-year-old man has experienced occasional headaches for the past 3 months. He suddenly has a generalized seizure. CT scan of the head shows a periventricular 3-cm mass in the region of the right thalamus. A stereotactic biopsy of the mass yields cells diagnostic of a large B-cell malignant lymphoma. Which of the following underlying diseases is most likely to be found in this patient?

- ❏ (A) Diabetes mellitus
- ❏ (B) AIDS
- ❏ (C) Hypertension
- ❏ (D) Multiple sclerosis
- ❏ (E) Tuberculosis

56 A 76-year-old man has experienced lower back pain for the past year. On physical examination, the physician palpates a firm nodule in the prostate. Laboratory studies show an alkaline phosphatase level of 290 U/L and a serum prostate-specific antigen level of 17 ng/mL. A prostate needle biopsy specimen shows a moderately differentiated adenocarcinoma. Which of the following mechanisms best accounts for these findings?

- ❏ (A) Tumor extension to rectum
- ❏ (B) Paraneoplastic syndrome
- ❏ (C) High tumor grade
- ❏ (D) Metastases to vertebrae
- ❏ (E) Tumor angiogenesis

57 An epidemiologic study of cancer deaths recorded in the last half of the 20th century is conducted. The number of deaths for one particular cancer increased markedly in developed nations. In 1998, more than 30% of cancer deaths in men and more than 24% of cancer deaths in women were caused by this neoplasm. Which of the following neoplasms was most likely identified by this study?

- ❏ (A) Breast carcinoma
- ❏ (B) Bronchogenic carcinoma
- ❏ (C) Cervical squamous cell carcinoma
- ❏ (D) Adenocarcinoma of the colon
- ❏ (E) Melanoma of the skin
- ❏ (F) Prostatic adenocarcinoma

58 The mother of a 5-year-old boy notices that his abdomen is enlarged. On physical examination, the physician palpates an ill-defined abdominal mass. An abdominal CT scan shows a 9-cm mass in the region of the right adrenal gland. The mass is removed and microscopically appears to be a neuroblastoma. Cytogenetic analysis of tumor cells shows many double minutes and homogeneously staining regions. Which of the following genes is most likely to have undergone alterations to produce these findings?

- ❏ (A) *BCL1* (cyclin gene)
- ❏ (B) *BCL2* (antiapoptosis gene)
- ❏ (C) *IL2* (growth factor gene)
- ❏ (D) *Lyn* (tyrosine kinase gene)
- ❏ (E) *K-RAS* (GTP-binding protein gene)
- ❏ (F) *N-MYC* (transcription factor gene)
- ❏ (G) *p53* (DNA damage response gene)

59 A 42-year-old man is concerned about a darkly pigmented "mole" on the back of his hand. The lesion has enlarged and bled during the past month. On physical examination, there is a slightly raised, darkly pigmented, 1.2-cm lesion on the dorsum of the right hand. The lesion is completely excised. Microscopically, a malignant melanoma is present. Which of the following factors presents the greatest risk for the development of this neoplasm?

- ❏ (A) Smoking tobacco
- ❏ (B) Ultraviolet radiation
- ❏ (C) Chemotherapy
- ❏ (D) Asbestos exposure
- ❏ (E) Allergy to latex

60 A clinical study involves patients diagnosed with carcinoma and whose tumor stage is T4N1M1. The patients' survival rate 5 years from the time of diagnosis is less than 50%, regardless of therapy. Which of the following clinical findings is most likely to be characteristic of this group of patients?

- ❑ (A) Cachexia
- ❑ (B) Cardiac murmur
- ❑ (C) Icterus
- ❑ (D) Loss of sensation
- ❑ (E) Splenomegaly
- ❑ (F) Tympany

ANSWERS

1 **(C)** Although the hepatitis B virus (HBV) and hepatitis C virus (HCV) genomes do not encode for any transforming proteins, the regenerating hepatocytes are more likely to develop mutations, such as inactivation of *p53*. HBV does not have a consistent site of integration in the liver cell nuclei, nor does it contain viral oncogenes. Many DNA viruses, such as human papillomavirus, inactivate tumor suppressor genes, but there is no convincing evidence that HBV or HCV can bind to *p53* or *RB* proteins. Also, the HBV-encoded regulatory element, called *HBx*, disrupts normal growth of infected hepatocytes.

BP7 201   BP6 167   PBD7 327   PBD6 313-314

2 **(A)** Several pathologic mechanisms play a role in the development of tumor metastases. The tumor cells must first become discohesive and detach from the primary site and then attach elsewhere to become metastases. Tumor cells tend to have many more laminin receptors than do normal cells, allowing them to attach more readily to basement membranes at distant sites. Keratin is a marker of epithelial differentiation, not metastatic ability.

A reduction in apoptosis allows greater proliferation but not necessarily metastases. Monoclonality is a feature of neoplasia, but further tumor heterogeneity helps to increase the chance for metastases to occur. Inflammation probably does not play a major role in metastasis.

BP7 191-192   BP6 161-162   PBD7 309-313
PBD6 302-304

3 **(D)** The oncogenic potential of human papillomavirus (HPV), a sexually transmissible agent, is related to products of two early viral genes—E6 and E7. E7 binds to *RB* protein to cause displacement of normally sequestered transcription factors, which nullifies tumor suppressor activity of the *RB* protein. E6 binds to and inactivates the *p53* gene product. Trapping of GTP-bound *RAS* protein can occur in many tumors but is not related to HPV infection. Laminin receptor expression correlates with metastatic potential of a malignant neoplasm. Inability to repair DNA damage plays a role in some colon and skin cancers. Increased epidermal growth factor receptor expression is a feature seen in many pulmonary squamous cell carcinomas, and the related *ERBB2* (*HER2*) receptor is seen in some breast carcinomas.

BP7 200   BP6 167   PBD7 324-325   PBD6 311

4 **(E)** This patient has chronic myelogenous leukemia. The t(9;22) causes c-*ABL* on chromosome 9 (the Philadelphia chromosome) to fuse with *BCR* on chromosome 22. Both *p53* and *RB* are tumor suppressor genes, and loss of both alleles is needed to promote cell proliferation. The *NF1* gene is a signal transducer seen in schwannomas. The *RAS* oncogenes are involved with GTP binding and become activated from point mutations.

BP7 195, 197   BP6 150-151   PBD7 297-298
PBD6 285-286

5 **(A)** Lymphatic spread, especially to regional lymph nodes draining from the primary site, is typical of a carcinoma. Infection from a breast abscess can spread to the lymph nodes, but the resulting nodal enlargement is typically associated with pain—a cardinal sign of acute inflammation. Sarcomas uncommonly metastasize to lymph nodes. Central nervous system (CNS) malignancies rarely metastasize outside of the CNS. Dysplasias do not metastasize, because they are not malignancies.

BP7 173   BP6 139-142   PBD7 279-280   PBD6 269-272

6 **(E)** This patient has a family history of malignant melanoma. Familial tumors are often associated with inheritance of a defective copy of one of several tumor suppressor genes. In the case of melanomas, the implicated gene is called *p16*, or *INK4a*. The product of the *p16* gene is an inhibitor of cyclin-dependent kinases. With loss of control over cyclin-dependent kinases, the cell cycle cannot be regulated, favoring neoplastic transformation. *BCL-2* is present in some lymphoid neoplasms. The *C-MYC* gene is mutated in a variety of carcinomas but is not known to be specifically associated with melanomas. The *IL2* mutation is associated with some T cell neoplasms. The *Lyn* mutation is seen in some immunodeficiency states. *p53* mutations occur in many cancers but not specifically in familial melanomas. PDGF can be overexpressed in some central nervous system gliomas and some osteosarcomas.

PBD7 286-287   PBD6 920

7 **(G)** A teratoma is a neoplasm derived from totipotential germ cells that differentiate into tissues that represent all three germ layers: ectoderm, endoderm, and mesoderm. When the elements are all well differentiated, the neoplasm is "mature" (benign). Adenocarcinomas have malignant-appearing glandular elements. Fibroadenomas have both a benign glandular and stromal component; they are common in the breast. Gliomas are found in the central nervous system. Hamartomas contain a mixture of cell types common to a tissue site; the lung is one site for this uncommon lesion. A mesothelioma arises from the lining of thoracic and abdominal body cavities. A rhabdomyosarcoma comprises cells that poorly resemble striated muscle; most arise in soft tissues.

BP7 167-168   BP6 135   PBD7 271-273   PBD6 263-264

8 **(A)** This patient has clinical features of neurofibromatosis type 1. The *NF1* gene encodes a GTPase-activating protein that facilitates the conversion of active (GTP-bound) RAS to inactive (GDP-bound) RAS. Loss of *NF1* prevents such conversion and traps RAS in the active signal-transmitting stage. All other listed mechanisms are also involved in carcinogenesis, although in different tumors.

BP7 181   BP6 153   PBD7 294, 296, 305   PBD6 293

9 (C) Phorbol esters cause tumor promotion by activating protein kinase C. This enzyme phosphorylates several substrates in signal transduction pathways, including those activated by growth factors, and the cells divide. Forced cell division predisposes the accumulation of mutations in cells previously damaged by exposure to a mutagenic agent (initiator). The other listed mechanisms are not operative in this example.

BP7 198   BP6 165   PBD7 321-322   PBD6 309

10 (C) A true neoplasm is a monoclonal proliferation of cells, whereas a reactive proliferation of cells is not monoclonal. Reactive and neoplastic cellular proliferations may have similar histochemical and immunohistochemical staining patterns based on the type of cells that are present. Flow cytometry is effective at indicating the DNA content, aneuploidy, and growth fraction, but does not indicate clonality.

BP7 179, 194   BP6 145-146   PBD7 277, 288, 337
PBD6 277

11 (D) The largest cell population, determined to be clonal, is marking for CD4. This patient has a T-cell leukemia, which develops in approximately 1% of persons infected with human lymphotropic virus type 1. Human papillomavirus is best known for causing squamous epithelial dysplasias and carcinomas. HIV-1 infection causes AIDS. Infection with Epstein-Barr virus is associated with a variety of cancers, including Burkitt lymphoma and nasopharyngeal carcinoma. Infection with hepatitis B virus may result in hepatic cirrhosis, in which hepatocellular carcinoma may arise.

BP7 199-200   BP6 166   PBD7 327-328   PBD6 314

12 (C) Increased expression of *ERBB2* (*HER2*) can be detected immunohistochemically in the biopsy specimen. As many as one third of breast cancers may show this change. Such amplification is associated with a poorer prognosis. Detection of a specific gene product in the tissue has value for determination of prognosis. *BRCA1* and *p53* mutations, if inherited in the germ line, can predispose the patient to breast cancer and other tumors. However, with *BRCA1*, there is family history of breast cancer, and *p53* mutation predisposes to many types of cancers. An inherited deletion of *RB* gene predisposes to retinoblastoma. The *BCR-ABL* fusion product, seen in chronic myeloid leukemia, results from t(9;22).

BP7 180   BP6 151   PBD7 315, 337   PBD6 286

13 (B) The children described in the question have an autosomal recessive condition known as xeroderma pigmentosum (XP). Affected persons have extreme photosensitivity, with a 2000-fold increase in the risk of skin cancers. The DNA damage is initiated by exposure to ultraviolet light; however, nucleotide excision repair cannot occur normally in XP. Human papillomavirus is a sexually transmitted disease that is associated with the development of genital squamous cell carcinomas. *Aspergillus flavus,* found on moldy peanuts and other foods, produces the potent hepatic carcinogen aflatoxin B1. Inactivation of the *p53* tumor suppressor gene is found in many sporadic human cancers and in some familial cancers, but these cancers are not limited to the skin. Chromosomal translocations are often involved in the development of hema-

tologic malignancies, although they are not often seen in skin cancers.

BP7 177, 193   BP6 165   PBD7 307, 323   PBD6 310

14 (D) The *p53* mutation involving both alleles is one of the most common genetic mutations in human cancers, including the most common: lung, colon, and breast cancers. The loss of this tumor suppressor indicates that the cell cycle is not properly arrested in the late G1 phase; thus, when DNA damage occurs, DNA repair cannot be completed before the cell proliferates. Inability to hydrolyze GTP is a result of *RAS* oncogene activation. Microsatellite instability occurs with mutation in genes, such as *hMSH2*, that repair DNA damage. *BCL2* mutation is one of the best known mechanisms for apoptotic arrest in neoplasms. Transcriptional activation is a feature of the *MYC* protooncogene.

BP7 187-188   BP6 153-154   PBD7 302-303
PBD6 290-292

15 (G) The *RB* gene is a classic example of the two-hit mechanism for loss of tumor suppression. About 60% of these tumors are sporadic. Others are familial, and there is inheritance of a mutated copy of the *RB* gene. Loss of the second copy in retinoblasts leads to the occurrence of retinoblastoma in childhood. Researchers do not know why patients who inherit a mutant *RB* gene through the germ line develop retinoblastoma rather than other types of tumors. The *RB* gene controls the G1 to S transition of the cell cycle; with loss of both copies, this important checkpoint in the cell cycle is lost. The *BCR-ABL* fusion gene in chronic myelogenous leukemia is an example of overexpression of a gene product producing neoplasia. The *BCL2* gene is an inhibitor of apoptosis. The *hMSH2* gene is present in most cases of hereditary nonpolyposis colon cancer and functions in DNA repair. Many cancers have the *K-RAS* gene, which acts as an oncogene. The *NF1* gene product acts as a tumor suppressor; this is a component of neurofibromatosis (which usually does not involve the eye), and the neoplasms typically appear at a later age. Many cancers have the *p53* tumor suppressor gene mutation, but this is not typical of childhood ocular neoplasms.

BP7 183-185   BP6 151-154   PBD7 299-302
PBD6 289-290

16 (D) Some neoplasms, including certain lymphomas, have a high proportion of cells in the replicative pool (i.e., have high growth fraction). They grow rapidly and also respond rapidly to drugs that kill dividing cells. Monoclonality rather than polyclonality is typical of malignant tumors. Similarly, poor vascularity would not favor rapid growth. Tumors that are highly antigenic are likely to be controlled by the immune system and hence not be rapidly growing.

PBD7 276

17 (E) The cells shown in the figure demonstrate marked pleomorphism and hyperchromatism (anaplasia). A bizarre tripolar mitotic figure is present. This degree of anaplasia is consistent with a malignancy. An adenoma is a benign tumor of glandular origin. Adenocarcinomas and squamous cell carcinomas show differentiation into glandular or squamous tissues. Leiomyomas are benign mesenchymal tumors of smooth muscle origin.

BP7 169-170   BP6 135-137   PBD7 272-276
PBD6 264-266

18 (B) Cancer grading systems are typically denoted by I to III or I to IV, and increase with worse differentiation (more anaplasia). A transitional cell carcinoma would be expected at this site. Bladder cancers are not commonly associated with paraneoplastic syndromes. Infiltration through the wall indicates a high stage. The cure rate for this high-grade, high-stage cancer is poor. Determination of the presence of metastases is part of staging, not grading.

BP7 206-207   BP6 171   PBD7 335   PBD6 321-322

19 (C) Because Pap smear screening can detect dysplasias and in situ carcinomas that can be treated before progression to invasive lesions, deaths from cervical carcinoma have steadily decreased since this screening method became widely available in the last half of the 20th century. A chest radiograph is an insensitive technique for detecting early lung cancers. Use of stool guaiac has had a minimal effect on rates of death from colorectal carcinomas, but physicians are cautioned not to indicate "rectal deferred" on the physical examination report, and hence contribute to the problem. Serum tumor markers have not proved useful as general screening techniques, although they are useful in selected circumstances. Urine cytology is better than urinalysis for detection of urothelial malignancies, but it does not have a high sensitivity.

BP7 175, 207-208   BP6 142   PBD7 282, 336   PBD6 272

20 (D) Monoclonality is the hallmark of a malignancy. In the diagnosis of a leukemia, the WBC count is helpful but not definitive. The DNA content analysis alone cannot define a malignancy; Southern blot analysis for T- or B-cell receptor gene rearrangements can define monoclonality. Electron microscopy is an adjunct to diagnosis of the type of tumor. Lactate dehydrogenase levels are often increased with lymphoid proliferations but are not diagnostic of the type of proliferation.

BP7 179, 194   BP6 171-174   PBD7 288, 336-338
PBD6 322-325

21 (B) Development of colonic adenocarcinoma typically takes years, during which time a number of mutations occur within the mucosa, including mutations involving such genes as *APC* (adenomatous polyposis coli), *K-RAS*, and *p53*. The accumulation of mutations, rather than their occurrence in a specific order, is most important in the development of a carcinoma. Activation of protooncogenes, extensive regeneration, faulty DNA repair genes, and amplification of growth factor receptor genes all contribute to the development of malignancies, but they are not sufficient by themselves to produce a carcinoma from an adenoma of the colon.

BP7 186-187, 193   BP6 157, 509   PBD7 284, 304, 318
PBD6 296-297, 832

22 (C) This is an example of chromosomal translocation that brings *BCL2*, an anti apoptosis gene, close to another gene (immunoglobulin heavy chain gene). The *BCL2* gene becomes subject to continuous stimulation by the adjacent enhancer element of the immunoglobulin gene, leading to overexpres-

sion. The *APC* gene is mutated in both sporadic colon cancers and those seen in familial polyposis coli. The *BCL1* gene is mutated in mantle zone lymphoma, with t(11;14) that brings the cyclin gene on chromosome 11 to the immunoglobulin enhancer gene on chromosome 14. The *BRCA1* and *ERBB2* gene mutations are seen in some breast cancers. The *IL2* mutation may be present in some T-cell neoplasms. *K-RAS* and *p53* mutations are present in many cancers, but not typically lymphoid malignancies.

BP7 182   BP6 150   PBD7 298   PBD6 285

23 (B) Notice on the figure that the disorderly, atypical epithelial cells involve the entire thickness of the epithelium, but that the underlying basement membrane is intact, with no invasion. Carcinoma in situ is confined to the epithelium; if the basement membrane is breached, the lesion is no longer in situ but rather invasive. An adenocarcinoma is a malignant neoplasm arising from glandular epithelium, such as the endocervix or endometrium, not the ectocervix. A hamartoma contains a mixture of cell types common to a tissue site. Leiomyomas arise from smooth muscle and are most common in the uterus; they are white. Melanomas are malignant and tend to enlarge quickly; many are darkly pigmented. The benign counterpart to the melanoma is the nevus, which is quite common; nevi are usually light brown. A mesothelioma arises from the lining of thoracic and abdominal body cavities. Small cell anaplastic carcinomas of the lung are aggressive neoplasms that are unlikely to be diagnosed in situ.

BP7 169-170   BP6 137   PBD7 275   PBD6 267

24 (B) The decrease in the number of gastric cancers may be related to reduced numbers of dietary carcinogens or a decrease in the prevalence of *Helicobacter pylori* infection; however, the exact reason is obscure. Angiosarcomas of the liver are quite rare; they are epidemiologically linked to vinyl chloride exposure. Cerebral gliomas are not as common as carcinomas; an urban legend links them to cell phone use, but legitimate epidemiologic studies have not made this link. Leukemias and lymphomas are not as common as carcinomas. Pancreatic adenocarcinoma is the sixth most common cause of cancer deaths in men and women, and the death rate is typically double the incidence, because the prognosis for pancreatic cancer is so poor.

BP7 175, 201   BP6 142   PBD7 283, 327-328   PBD6 272

25 (B) Approximately 5% to 10% of breast cancers are familial, and 80% of these cases result from mutations in the *BRCA1* and *BRCA2* genes. Onset of these familial cancers occurs earlier in life than the sporadic cancers. The protein products of these genes are involved in DNA repair. *BCL2* is overexpressed in some lymphoid neoplasms. *ERBB2* overexpression is present in some sporadic breast cancers; other EGF alterations can be seen in lung, bladder, gastrointestinal, ovarian, and brain neoplasms. The *HST1* mutation is seen in some gastric cancers. *IL2* overexpression is associated with some T-cell neoplasms. *K-RAS* overexpression is seen in many cancers, including some breast cancers, but the early age of onset and family history in this case strongly suggest *BRCA* mutations. The *Lyn* mutation is seen in some immunodeficiency states.

BP7 193   BP6 153, 156, 630   PBD7 307-308
PBD6 292, 1106

26 **(F)** Vinyl chloride is a rare cause of liver cancer. However, this causal relationship was easy to demonstrate, because hepatic angiosarcoma is a rare neoplasm. Arsenic is a risk factor for skin cancer. Asbestos exposure is linked to pleural malignant mesothelioma and to bronchogenic carcinomas in smokers. Benzene exposure is linked to leukemias. Beryllium exposure can produce interstitial lung disease and lung cancer. Nickel exposure increases the risk of respiratory tract cancers. Exposure to naphthalene compounds is a risk factor for cancer of the urinary tract.

BP7 197   BP6 144   PBD7 285, 321   PBD6 279, 304

27 **(E)** The figure shows an in situ carcinoma of the squamous cervical epithelium with neoplastic growth above the basement membrane. Such cancers, limited to the epithelium, are noninvasive, and local excision has a 100% cure rate. In situ lesions do not give rise to metastases. Lesions limited to the epithelium are low grade. Because it originated in the epithelium, this neoplasm is not derived from fibroblasts.

BP7 207   BP6 136-138   PBP7 275   BP6 265-268

28 **(B)** The elaboration of a variety of enzymes by tumor cells aids in degradation of extracellular matrix and invasiveness. Cathepsin D is a cysteine proteinase that cleaves a variety of substrates such as fibronectin and laminin. High levels of this enzyme in tumor cells are associated with greater invasiveness. Angiogenesis is mediated mainly by basic fibroblast growth factor and vascular endothelial cell growth factor. Differentiation, heterogeneity, and aneuploidy are regulated by protooncogenes and tumor suppressor genes.

BP7 192   BP6 162   PBD7 310-312   PBD6 303-304

29 **(C)** Radiation is oncogenic. Cancers of thyroid and bone often develop following radiation exposure; leukemias can also occur. Hepatocellular carcinomas can arise in cirrhosis caused by chronic alcoholism. Ataxia telangiectasia is an inherited syndrome that carries an increased risk of development of leukemias and lymphomas. Trauma is not a risk factor for development of cancer, although traumatic episodes often are recalled and irrationally associated with subsequent health problems. Arsenic exposure, which is uncommon, leads to lung and skin cancers.

BP7 199   BP6 165   PBD7 323-324   PBD6 310

30 **(F)** Human papillomavirus (HPV) types 16, 18, and 31 encode proteins that bind $p53$ with high affinity, resulting in loss of tumor suppressor activity. Seventy-five to nearly 100% of squamous epithelial dysplasias and carcinomas of the cervix are associated with HPV infection. Cytomegalovirus and herpes simplex virus do not participate directly in carcinogenesis. Epstein-Barr virus is associated with some malignant lymphomas and nasopharyngeal carcinomas. Hepatitis B virus is associated with hepatocellular carcinomas arising in the setting of regeneration in chronic liver injury. HIV does not affect pRB, but the loss of immune regulation promotes development of lymphomas and Kaposi sarcoma. The JC papovavirus is associated with development of progressive multifocal leukoencephalopathy.

BP7 200   BP6 167   PBD7 324-325   PBD6 311

31 **(E)** α-Fetoprotein is a tumor marker for hepatocellular carcinomas and some testicular carcinomas. The serum prostate-specific antigen is a helpful marker for prostatic adenocarcinoma. Squamous cell carcinomas of any site do not have useful specific tumor markers. A serum immunoglobulin level with protein electrophoresis aids in the diagnosis of myeloma. Gastrointestinal tract adenocarcinomas, including those arising in the pancreas, may be accompanied by elevations in the serum carcinoembryonic antigen level.

BP7 208   BP6 173-174   PBD7 330, 338   PBD6 325

32 **(C)** This patient has Cushing syndrome due to ectopic corticotropin production by the tumor, a form of paraneoplastic syndrome common to small cell carcinomas of the lung. Hypercalcemia from a parathormone-related peptide (PrP) is more typically associated with pulmonary squamous cell carcinomas. Erythropoietin production with polycythemia is more likely to be associated with a renal cell carcinoma. Insulin and gastrin production are most often seen in islet cell tumors of the pancreas.

BP7 205-206   BP6 171   PBD7 333-334   PBD6 320-321

33 **(A)** A discrete small mass such as that described is probably benign. Adenomas arise from epithelial surfaces. A hamartoma is a rare benign mass composed of tissues usually found at the site of origin. A sarcoma is a malignant neoplasm arising in mesenchymal tissues. A choristoma is a benign mass composed of tissues not found at the site of origin. A nevus arises in the skin.

BP7 166-167   BP6 133-134   PBD7 270-272
PBD6 261-262

34 **(B)** Overexpression of the $BCL2$ gene prevents apoptosis, allowing accumulation of cells in lymphoid tissues. Increased tyrosine kinase activity results from mutations affecting the ABL oncogene. Gene amplifications typically affect the $ERBB2$ ($HER2$) and MYC oncogenes. Reduced DNA repair occurs in the inherited disorder xeroderma pigmentosa. Loss of cell cycle inhibition results from loss of tumor suppressor genes such as $p53$.

BP7 188-189   BP6 154-155   PBD7 306   PBD6 294-295

35 **(C)** The RAS oncogene is the most common oncogene involved in the development of human cancers. Mutations of the RAS oncogene reduce GTPase activity, and RAS is trapped in an activated GTP-bound state. RAS then signals the nucleus through cytoplasmic kinases. The MYC oncogene is a transcriptional activator that is overexpressed in many tumors. The APC gene can cause activation of the WNT signaling pathway. The $ERBB2$ oncogene encodes growth factor receptors that are amplified in certain tumors. The sis oncogene encodes platelet-derived growth factor receptor-β, which is overexpressed in certain astrocytomas.

BP7 180-181   BP6 147-148   PBD7 296-297
PBD6 279-281

36 **(D)** The small, discrete nature of this mass and its relatively unchanged size suggest a benign neoplasm. The red color suggests vascularity. A hemangioma is a common benign lesion of the skin. Adenomas arise in glandular epithelium, such as the colon. Fibroadenomas arise in the breast. A hamartoma contains a mixture of cell types common to a tissue site. Leiomyomas, which are white, arise from smooth muscle and are most common in the uterus. Lipomas are yellow fatty tumors. Melanomas are malignant and tend to increase in size quickly; many are darkly pigmented. The benign counterpart to the melanoma is the nevus, which is quite common; nevi are usually light brown.

BP7 166-168   BP6 135   PBD7 270-273   PBD6 263

37 (G) *p53* is the most common target for genetic alterations in human neoplasms. Most are sporadic mutations, although some are inherited. The inheritance of one faulty *p53* suppressor gene predisposes to a "second hit" that eliminates the remaining *p53* gene. Homozygous loss of the *p53* genes dysregulates the repair of damaged DNA, predisposing persons to multiple tumors, as in this case. The *APC* gene is mutated in sporadic colon cancers and in familial polyposis coli. The *BCL2* gene is mutated in some non-Hodgkin lymphomas. The *ERBB2* gene is one of the EGF receptor family members amplified in some breast cancers. The EGF mutation is most often seen in squamous cell carcinomas of the lung. *K-RAS* mutations are present in many cancers but not typically lymphoid malignancies. The *NF1* gene mutation is seen in neurofibromatosis type 1.

BP7 187-188   BP6 153-154   PBD7 302-303
PBD6 290-292

38 (A) Arsenic can cause skin cancer. However, lead arsenate has not been in widespread use for years, and occupational safety measures have reduced risks to workers from the use of chemicals in agriculture and industry. Benzene is linked to leukemias. Cadmium exposure is linked to prostate cancer (dispose of old batteries properly!). Some lung cancers are linked to chromium exposure. Chlorinated biphenyls, contained in many insect sprays, have not been linked directly to cancer. Ethylene oxide exposure carries an increased risk of leukemia. Ethylene oxide has been employed as a ripening agent for some agricultural products, and it is also used as a disinfectant gas for surgical equipment in hospitals. Exposure to naphthalene compounds is a risk factor for urinary tract cancer.

BP7 197   BP6 144   PBD7 285, 323   PBD6 274, 309

39 (D) CD8+ T cells recognize peptides presented by MHC class I antigens. In many tumors, especially melanomas, the tumor cells produce peptides that can be presented by MHC class I molecules. If such peptides are not produced by other cells, the CD8+ T cells specific for such peptides lyse melanoma cells but not normal melanocytes or other normal cells.

BP7 202-204   BP6 168   PBD7 329, 332   PBD6 315-317

40 (B) A large, irregular, ulcerated mass such as that described is most likely malignant, and the epithelium of the bladder gives rise to carcinomas. A papilloma is a benign, localized mass that has an exophytic growth pattern. An adenoma is a benign epithelial neoplasm of glandular tissues. A sarcoma is derived from cells of mesenchymal origin; sarcomas are much less common than carcinomas. A fibroma is a benign mesenchymal neoplasm.

BP7 167-168   BP6 133-134   PBD7 271-273
PBD6 261-262

41 (C) Carcinomas metastasize through lymphatics most often, usually to regional nodes first. However, hematogenous metastases are possible. About half of all cerebral metastases arise from the lung. Soft tissue metastases are rare, as are splenic metastases.

BP7 172-174   BP6 140, 162   PBD7 279-280
PBD6 269-270, 305

42 (D) The figure shows the appearance of metastatic lesions from a malignant neoplasm with multiple tumor masses present. Dysplastic lesions do not produce large masses. Although some benign tumors, such as leiomyomas of the uterus, can be multiple, this is not the rule in the liver, and hepatic adenomas are rare. Although hepatocellular carcinomas can have "satellite" nodules, widespread nodules such as those seen here are more characteristic of metastases. Resection of multiple metastases is usually fruitless.

BP7 172-174   BP6 139-140   PBD7 279-281   PBD6 268

43 (C) The rapid frozen section of resection margins helps to determine whether enough of the colon has been resected. Fine-needle aspiration is used for preoperative diagnosis. Serum tumor markers may aid in preoperative diagnosis or postoperative follow-up of neoplasms. Electron microscopy requires at least 1 day to perform and helps to determine the cell type. Flow cytometry can be performed in several hours, but it is useful mainly for prognostic information and is not a "stat" procedure.

BP7 207-208   BP6 171-173   PBD7 336   PBD6 322-325

44 (E) Although neoplasms begin their careers as monoclonal proliferations, additional mutations occur over time, leading to subclones of neoplastic cells with various properties. This may allow metastases, greater invasiveness, resistance to chemotherapy, and morphologic differences to occur. Because sarcomas of the lung are rare, the lung mass is statistically a metastasis. Inheritance of a mutant *RB* gene is most likely to lead to childhood retinoblastomas. Pulmonary sarcomas are not related to smoking tobacco. Loss of tumor suppressor genes, not oncogenes, is related to tumor development.

BP7 194   BP6 160   PBD7 276-277, 290   PBD6 320

45 (A) Chromosomal telomere shortening in normal human cells limits their replicative potential and gives rise to replicative senescence. This occurs because most somatic cells lack the enzyme telomerase. By contrast, 90% or more human tumor cells show activation of telomerase, explaining continued tumor growth in the body as well as "immortalized" cell lines. All other pathways listed cannot affect telomerase shortening, which is the rate limiting step in indefinite replication of cells.

PBD7 289, 309

46 (D) Patients with hereditary nonpolyposis colon carcinoma (HNPCC) inherit one defective copy of mismatch repair genes. Any of several human mismatch repair genes are involved in the development of HNPCC. Mutations in mismatch repair genes can be detected by the presence of microsatellite instability. The other listed options are not characteristic of HNPCC.

BP7 192-193   BP6 508   PBD7 285, 306-307
PBD6 295-296, 831-833

47 **(D)** The *MYC* oncogene is commonly activated in Burkitt lymphoma because of a t(8;14) translocation. The *MYC* gene binds DNA to cause transcriptional activation of growth-related genes such as that for cyclin D1, resulting in activation of the cell cycle. *ERBB2* (also known as *HER2*) encodes growth factor receptor located on the cell surface. *p53* and *APC* are tumor suppressor genes that are inactivated in many cancers, including colon cancer (*APC*). *RAS* oncogene encodes a GTP-binding protein that is located under the cell membrane.

BP7 182   BP6 149   PBD7 298   PBD6 282

48 **(D)** There is increasing evidence that localization of cancer metastases is influenced by the expression of chemokine receptors by cancer cells and elaboration of their ligands (chemokines) by certain tissues. In the case of breast cancer, the carcinoma cells express CXCR4 chemokines. Vascular, lymphatic, or basement membrane invasion is required for metastases but these characteristics do not dictate accurately the location of metastases.

PBD7 313

49 **(A)** Epithelial dysplasias, especially those that are severe, can be precursors of carcinomas. This is a key reason for Pap smear screening; the incidence of cervical carcinoma decreases when routine Pap smears are performed. Teratomas show well-differentiated elements derived from all the germ cell layers, and they do not manifest as epithelial dysplasias. Severe dysplasias are not amenable to antibiotic therapy. Cervical dysplasias are not hereditary. Regression of a malignancy is a rare event.

BP7 207-208   BP6 137   PBD7 275-276, 282-283
PBD6 266

50 **(C)** A malignant neoplasm has a tendency to invade locally. A benign neoplasm is often well circumscribed, although a true capsule is uncommon, and compressed normal surrounding tissue appears to form a discrete border. Such a solitary mucosal lesion is unlikely to represent a metastasis, and the localized lesion can be easily resected. If there is no family history, a familial cancer with high risk of recurrence from multiple polyps is unlikely; local excision is therefore adequate. The biopsy specimen shows a malignant lesion; therefore, it must be removed before it increases in size and invades locally or metastasizes.

BP7 171-172   BP6 138-139   PBD7 272-274
PBD6 267-268

51 **(B)** This patient has a classic history and t(9;22) translocation with chronic myelogenous leukemia (CML). The translocation causes uncontrolled tyrosine kinase activity of the *Bcr-Abl* fusion gene. Hence, these patients undergo remission with drugs that inhibit tyrosine kinases. Antibodies to *ERB-2* receptors are beneficial in certain breast tumors with amplification of this gene. Agents that activate caspases may theoretically help in many cases especially when apoptosis is blocked as in tumors with *BCL-2* overexpression. Transloca-

tion of β-catenin to the nucleus occurs in colon cancers when there is mutational loss of *APC* genes. Delivery of *p53* into cells by viral vectors has not yet been proven to be of value in cancer treatment and there is no usage in CML.

PBD7 297

52 **(C)** The patient has a classical history of familial adenomatous polyposis (FAP) with numerous adenomatous polyps and malignant transformation. The earliest event in the *APC* → adenocarcinoma sequence is loss of *APC* gene function. This prevents the destruction of β-catenin in the cytoplasm, which then translocates to the nucleus and co-activates transcription of several genes. The *APC* → β-catenin are components of the *WNT* signaling pathway. Mutations in mismatch repair genes give rise to hereditary non-polyposis colon cancer syndrome (HNPCC) from loss of ability to repair DNA damage. Loss of cell cycle G1 arrest occurs with *p53* loss late in the sequence. The *BCL2* gene is not involved in the transition from adenoma to carcinoma. *RAS* activation occurs after the sequence is initiated by the *APC* (gate keeper) gene.

PBD7 304-305

53 **(A)** Estrogen, like many other hormones and drugs, by itself is not carcinogenic, but it is responsible for stimulation of endometrial growth (hyperplasia), which has a promoting effect when mutations occur to produce carcinoma. Tumor heterogeneity does not refer to two separate kinds of neoplasms; it refers to heterogeneity with a given tumor or metastasis. A paraneoplastic syndrome results from ectopic secretion of a hormone by tumor (e.g., lung cancer cells producing corticotropin). Inherited susceptibility can never be completely excluded when a person has two tumors; for example, this can occur in patients with inherited mutations in the *p53* gene. In this case, however, there is a clear hormonal basis for the second tumor. Faulty tumor suppressor genes are not involved in hormonal promotion of a neoplasm.

BP7 198   BP6 164-165   PBD7 323   PBD6 308

54 **(A)** The M1 designation indicates that distant metastases are present. Elevated corticotropin levels indicate secretion of an ectopic hormone that may produce a paraneoplastic syndrome. A T2 designation indicates that the overall size of the tumor is not large. The TNM system is used for staging, not grading.

BP7 207   BP6 171   PBD7 335   PBD6 321-322

55 **(B)** Primary or secondary immunodeficiency diseases carry an increased risk of neoplasia, particularly lymphomas. B-cell lymphomas of the brain are 1000-fold more common in patients with AIDS than in the general population. Patients with diabetes mellitus can experience various complications, although not neoplasia. Hypertension can lead to central nervous system hemorrhages. Multiple sclerosis is a demyelinating disease and carries no significant risk of neoplasia. Tuberculosis as a chronic infection may lead to amyloidosis, not neoplasia.

BP7 157, 199   BP6 169   PBD7 257-258   PBD6 315

56 **(D)** The high alkaline phosphatase concentration in a patient with prostate cancer suggests that there are metastases to bone. Tumor extension to soft tissues and major organs does not produce an elevated alkaline phosphatase level, except in the liver. Prostate cancer is not known for paraneoplastic effects. The grade of the tumor is not a major factor in this process, although higher-grade lesions are more likely to be metastatic. Angiogenesis does not affect alkaline phosphatase.

BP7 207-208   BP6 171-172   PBD7 279-281, 1303
PBD6 320-321

57 (B) Incidence of lung cancers increased dramatically in the 20th century because of the popularity of cigarette smoking. As the number of persons in a population who smoke increases, so do the number of cases of lung cancers. Some cancers of the urinary tract, oral cavity, esophagus, and pancreas are also causally related to smoking. Breast, prostate, and colon cancers remain common in developed nations, but the number of cases has not increased sharply. Pap smear screening markedly decreases numbers of cases of cervical cancers. There has been a marked increase in melanomas, but there are still far fewer cases of melanomas than of lung cancers.

BP7 174-176   BP6 142   PBD7 282-283   PBD6 272

58 (F) Double minutes and homogeneously staining regions seen on a karyotype represent gene amplifications. Amplification of the *N-MYC* gene occurs in 30% to 40% of neuroblastomas, and this change is associated with a poor prognosis. The *BCL1* and *BCL2* genes are mutated in some non-Hodgkin lymphomas. The *IL2* mutation may be present in some T-cell neoplasms. The *Lyn* mutation is seen in some immunodeficiency states. *K-RAS* and *p53* mutations are present in many cancers but not typically childhood neoplasms.

BP7 182   BP6 151   PBD7 299, 315   PBD6 286

59 (B) Worldwide, increasing numbers of skin cancers occur because of sun exposure. The ultraviolet light damages the skin and damages cellular DNA, leading to mutations that escape cellular repair mechanisms. Smoking tobacco is related to many cancers, but skin cancers are not typically associated with this risk factor. Chemotherapeutic agents have carcinogenic potential, particularly the alkylating agents such as cyclophosphamide, but leukemias and lymphomas are the usual result. Asbestos exposure increases lung carcinoma risk in smokers and can lead to rare mesotheliomas of pleura. Allergic reactions do not promote cancer.

BP7 199   BP6 165   PBD7 323   PBD6 310

60 (A) Cachexia is a common finding in advanced cancers, and weight loss without dieting in an adult is a "red flag" for malignancy. The exact cause for this is not known, but increases in circulating factors such as tumor necrosis factor may play a role. Cardiac murmurs may occur in the development of nonbacterial thrombotic endocarditis, a feature of a hypercoagulable state that may occur with advanced malignancies. Icterus is most likely to occur when there is obstruction of the biliary tract by a mass (e.g., as in pancreatic cancer), but metastases are unlikely to cause such an obstruction. Neurologic abnormalities may occur in local tumor growth impinging on nerves, but dull constant pain is the most likely abnormality in malignant neoplasms that invade nerves. Metastases to the spleen are not common. Tympany is not common in cancer, because obstruction by a mass tends to be incomplete and develop over a long time. (Hint: an empty beer keg is tympanitic when percussed.)

BP7 205   BP6 170-171   PBD7 333   PBD6 319-320

Infectious Diseases

PBD7 Chapter 8: Infectious Diseases

PBD6 Chapter 9: Infectious Diseases

BP7 and BP6 Chapter 9: General Pathology of Infectious Diseases

1 A 35-year-old man who received a kidney transplantation was being treated with cyclosporine, azathioprine, and high doses of corticosteroids. While on this regimen, the patient began to experience headaches and became lethargic. A clinical diagnosis of meningoencephalitis was made. He died 7 days later. Autopsy showed a gelatinous meningeal exudate, and on sectioning of the brain, multiple small cyst-like areas were seen. Microscopic examination showed areas containing rounded structures with a prominent capsule that stained brightly with mucicarmine. Which of the following tests would have been most useful for diagnosis of this condition during life?

☐ (A) Examination of CSF with an India ink preparation
☐ (B) Determination of glucose and protein content of CSF
☐ (C) Brain biopsy specimen stained for viral inclusions
☐ (D) Culture of CSF for *Streptococcus pneumoniae*
☐ (E) PCR assay to detect Epstein-Barr virus genome in lymphocytes isolated from CSF

2 Six weeks after a trip to Central America, a 33-year-old woman develops fever with right upper abdominal pain. During the last week of her trip, she had blood-tinged watery diarrhea, but it subsided shortly after her return home. On physical examination, her temperature is 37.6°C. There is moderate tenderness on palpation of the right upper quadrant, and the liver span is increased. Laboratory studies show a total bilirubin level of 5.4 mg/dL, a direct bilirubin concentration of 4.9 mg/dL, and alkaline phosphatase level of 175 U/L. An abdominal CT scan shows a 7-cm right hepatic mass with central necrosis and discrete borders. Which of the following organisms is most likely to produce these findings?

☐ (A) *Giardia lamblia*
☐ (B) *Salmonella typhi*
☐ (C) *Entamoeba histolytica*
☐ (D) *Campylobacter jejuni*
☐ (E) *Yersinia enterocolitica*
☐ (F) *Staphylococcus aureus*

3 A 20-year-old man who has multiple sexual partners and does not use barrier precautions comes to the physician complaining of a nontender ulcer on the penis that has been present for 1 week. On physical examination, the 0.6-cm lesion has a firm, erythematous base and sharply demarcated borders. The lesion is scraped, and darkfield examination is positive for spirochetes consistent with *Treponema pallidum*. Which of the following is most likely to be seen microscopically in the biopsy specimen?

☐ (A) Granulomatous inflammation with suppuration
☐ (B) Granulomatous inflammation with caseation
☐ (C) Acute inflammation with abscess formation
☐ (D) Perivascular inflammation with plasma cells
☐ (E) Gummatous inflammation

4 A 24-year-old man has a fever and a runny nose, sneezing, and coughing that have worsened over the past 4 days. The symptoms abate, and he has sequelae. This infection is most likely to be promoted by binding of which of the following organisms to intercellular adhesion molecule-1 (ICAM-1)?

❑ (A) *Mycoplasma pneumoniae*
❑ (B) *Haemophilus influenzae*
❑ (C) Rhinovirus
❑ (D) Epstein-Barr virus
❑ (E) *Neisseria meningitidis*

5 About 10 months after returning to the US from a vacation to the Costa del Sol near Barcelona, a 45-year-old man experiences malaise and fatigue, which slowly become more noticeable over a 2-month period. He develops occasional diarrhea and a low-grade fever, with abdominal discomfort that worsens over the next month. On physical examination, his vital signs include temperature of 38.3°C, pulse 81/min, respirations 17/min, and blood pressure 130/85 mm Hg. He has pronounced splenomegaly, an increased liver span, and generalized lymphadenopathy. Laboratory studies show hemoglobin of 11.8 g/dL, hematocrit 34.9%, platelet count 89,000/mm³, and WBC count 3350/mm³ with 29% segmented neutrophils, 5% bands, 48% lymphocytes, and 18% monocytes. His total serum protein is 7.6 g/dL, albumin 3.2 g/dL, AST 67 U/L, ALT 51 U/L, alkaline phosphatase 190 U/L, and total bilirubin 1.3 mg/dL. A stool sample is negative for occult blood. Which of the following is the most likely diagnosis?

❑ (A) Borreliosis
❑ (B) Echinococcosis
❑ (C) Leishmaniasis
❑ (D) Lyme disease
❑ (E) Schistosomiasis
❑ (F) Tuberculosis
❑ (G) Typhus

6 A 19-year-old woman develops bloody diarrhea and abdominal pain 3 weeks after returning from a trip to Central America. On physical examination, her temperature is 37.5°C. There is lower abdominal tenderness, but no masses are palpable. On colonoscopy, marked mucosal erythema with focal ulceration is seen from the rectum to the ascending colon. A biopsy is performed, and the microscopic appearance of a specimen is shown in the preceding figure. Which of the following infectious agents is most likely to produce these findings?

❑ (A) Adenovirus
❑ (B) *Campylobacter jejuni*
❑ (C) *Candida albicans*
❑ (D) *Entamoeba histolytica*
❑ (E) *Giardia lamblia*
❑ (F) *Helicobacter pylori*
❑ (G) *Salmonella typhi*
❑ (H) *Vibrio cholerae*

7 A 25-year-old soldier stationed in the Middle East has experienced abdominal enlargement and a 7-kg weight loss over the past 7 weeks. On physical examination, there is hyperpigmentation of skin, hepatosplenomegaly, and generalized lymphadenopathy. Laboratory studies show hemoglobin of 10.0 g/dL, hematocrit 29.9%, platelet count 78,200/mm³, and WBC count 3210/mm³. One month later, he develops a high fever, and *Streptococcus pneumoniae* is cultured from his blood. Which of the following infectious organisms is most likely to produce these findings?

❑ (A) *Borrelia recurrentis*
❑ (B) *Brugia malayi*
❑ (C) *Leishmania donovani*
❑ (D) *Listeria monocytogenes*
❑ (E) *Mycobacterium leprae*
❑ (F) *Plasmodium falciparum*
❑ (G) *Trypanosoma gambiense*

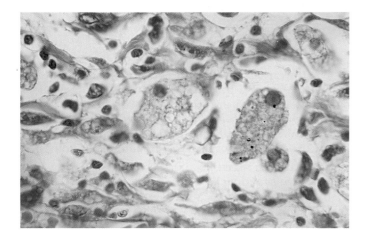

8 A 50-year-old woman comes to the health center because she has observed a small vesicle on her right labium majus. She is sexually active. On physical examination, tender inguinal lymph nodes are palpable. She was diagnosed with lymphoma 10 years ago. A biopsy of one of the lymph nodes is performed to exclude malignancy. Histologically, the biopsy specimen shows multiple abscesses in which central necrosis is surrounded by palisading histiocytes. This morphology, combined with the clinical picture, is most likely to be a complication of which of the following conditions?

❑ (A) *Chlamydia trachomatis* cervicitis
❑ (B) Herpes simplex virus infection of the perineum
❑ (C) Recurrent non-Hodgkin lymphoma
❑ (D) *Candida albicans* vaginitis
❑ (E) *Gardnerella vaginalis* vaginosis

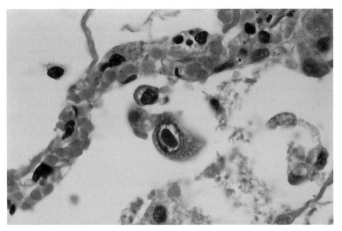

Courtesy of Dr. Arlene Sharpe.

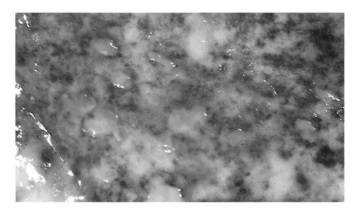

9 A 31-year-old man has had increasing respiratory difficulty for the past 2 days. On physical examination, crackles are auscultated over all lung fields. A chest radiograph shows bilateral interstitial infiltrates. Laboratory studies show that the patient is HIV positive and has a plasma titer of 26,800 copies of HIV-1 RNA/mL. A transbronchial biopsy is performed, and the microscopic appearance of the specimen is shown above. On the basis of the clinical and histologic findings, which of the following is the most likely causative organism of this acute illness?

❑ (A) Epstein-Barr virus
❑ (B) Cytomegalovirus
❑ (C) Respiratory syncytial virus
❑ (D) Herpes zoster virus
❑ (E) Adenovirus

10 A 60-year-old man has had persistent bloody diarrhea, abdominal cramps, and fever for the past week. On physical examination, his temperature is 38.1°C. He has mild diffuse abdominal pain. A stool sample is positive for occult blood. Sigmoidoscopic examination shows mucosal ulceration in the cecum and ascending colon. Microscopic examination of a colonic biopsy specimen shows flask-shaped mucosal ulcers with extensive necrosis and a modest, nonspecific, inflammatory response. The ulcers do not penetrate the muscularis propria. Which of the following infectious organisms is most likely to produce these findings?

❑ (A) *Giardia lamblia*
❑ (B) *Entamoeba histolytica*
❑ (C) *Shigella flexneri*
❑ (D) *Salmonella enteritidis*
❑ (E) *Vibrio cholerae*
❑ (F) *Bacillus cereus*

11 A 24-year-old woman has had bloody diarrhea for the past 4 days. On physical examination, she has a temperature of 38.3°C. The appearance of the rectum and descending colon on colonoscopy is shown above. The patient is treated with antibiotics but develops a chronic arthritis after the diarrhea has resolved. HLA typing is done, and she is found to be HLA-B27 positive. Which of the following organisms is most likely to be identified in her diarrheal stool?

❑ (A) *Vibrio cholerae*
❑ (B) *Shigella flexneri*
❑ (C) *Entamoeba histolytica*
❑ (D) *Salmonella typhi*
❑ (E) *Helicobacter pylori*

12 A 23-year-old woman has had increasing delirium for 2 days and is admitted to the hospital. On physical examination, she has acute pharyngitis with an overlying dirty-white, tough mucosal membrane. Paresthesias with decreased vibratory sensation are present in the extremities. On auscultation, there is an irregular cardiac rhythm. A chest radiograph shows cardiomegaly. A Gram stain of the pharyngeal membrane shows numerous small, gram-positive rods in a fibrinopurulent exudate. Which of the following is the most likely mechanism for development of cardiac disease in this patient?

❑ (A) Microabscess formation
❑ (B) Endotoxin-mediated hypotension and shock
❑ (C) Vasculitis with thrombosis and infarction
❑ (D) Granulomatous inflammation
❑ (E) Elaboration of exotoxin

13 A 15-year-old boy has a small eschar on his left forearm around the site of a tick bite. A hemorrhagic rash develops over the next few days involving the trunk and extremities and even the palms and soles. Small, 0.2- to 0.4-cm foci of skin necrosis develop on the fingers and toes. Which of the following organisms is most likely to produce these findings?

❑ (A) *Rickettsia rickettsii*
❑ (B) *Mycobacterium leprae*
❑ (C) *Yersinia pestis*
❑ (D) *Borrelia burgdorferi*
❑ (E) *Leishmania braziliensis*

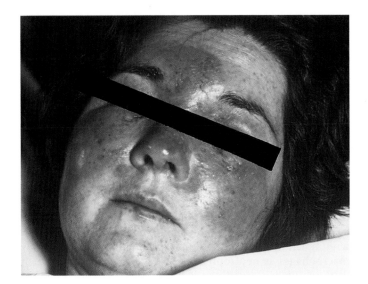

14 A 40-year-old woman has had a high fever and swelling, warmth, and tenderness of the right arm for the past 3 days. On physical examination, she has a temperature of 39.4°C and the appearance shown in the figure. She receives antibiotic therapy and recovers. Which of the following organisms is most likely to produce these findings?

❑ (A) *Clostridium botulinum*
❑ (B) *Escherichia coli*
❑ (C) *Neisseria gonorrhoeae*
❑ (D) *Staphylococcus epidermidis*
❑ (E) *Streptococcus pyogenes*

15 In an epidemiologic study of persons who died in a worldwide pandemic after World War I, many persons were shown to have contracted an influenza pneumonia. Decades later, molecular analysis of samples of tissue showed changes in the virus responsible for this pandemic of influenza. Which of the following changes most likely occurred in this virus?

❑ (A) Mutations in DNA encoding envelope proteins
❑ (B) Increased ability to bind to intercellular adhesion molecule-1 (ICAM-1) receptor
❑ (C) Ability to elaborate exotoxins
❑ (D) Recombination with RNA segments from pig viruses
❑ (E) Acquisition of antibiotic resistance genes

16 A 52-year-old man has a fever and a cough that worsens over several days. On physical examination, his temperature is 38.2°C. On auscultation of the chest, diffuse crackles are heard at the right lung base. Laboratory studies show hemoglobin of 13.3 g/dL, hematocrit 40%, platelet count 291,800/mm³, and WBC count 13,240/mm³ with 71% segmented neutrophils, 7% bands, 16% lymphocytes, and 6% monocytes. *Klebsiella pneumoniae* is cultured from the patient's sputum. His condition improves after a course of antibiotic therapy with gentamicin. Which of the following complications of this infection is the patient most likely to develop?

❑ (A) Gas gangrene
❑ (B) Cavitary granulomas
❑ (C) Abscess formation
❑ (D) Bullous emphysema
❑ (E) Adenocarcinoma

17 For the past 3 days, a 68-year-old woman has had a fever and a cough productive of yellow sputum. On physical examination, there is dullness to percussion at the left lung base. A chest radiograph shows areas of consolidation in the left lower lobe. Despite antibiotic therapy, the course of the disease is complicated by abscess formation, and she dies. At autopsy, there is a bronchopleural fistula surrounded by a pronounced fibroblastic reaction. Small, yellow, 1- to 2-mm "sulfur granules" are grossly visible within the area of abscess formation. Which of the following organisms is most likely to produce these autopsy findings?

❑ (A) *Actinomyces israelii*
❑ (B) *Blastomyces dermatitidis*
❑ (C) *Chlamydia pneumoniae*
❑ (D) *Klebsiella pneumoniae*
❑ (E) *Mycobacterium kansasii*

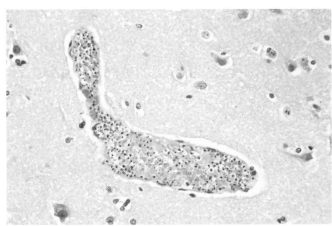

18 An 11-year-old boy had episodic fevers for 1 week and then developed a severe headache. He became progressively more somnolent and died 1 week later. At autopsy, there was marked diffuse cerebral edema with areas of cerebral softening. The microscopic appearance of a cerebral vein is shown. Which of the following organs is most likely to serve as the reservoir for proliferation of the infectious agent producing this disease?

❑ (A) Heart
❑ (B) Liver
❑ (C) Brain
❑ (D) Lymph nodes
❑ (E) Spleen

19 A 29-year-old man has had hematuria for the past month. On physical examination, he is afebrile. There is diffuse lower abdominal tenderness but no palpable masses. An abdominal radiograph shows a small bladder outlined by a rim of calcification. Cystoscopy is performed, and the entire bladder mucosa is erythematous and granular. Biopsy samples are taken. Which of the following histologic findings is most likely to be seen in these samples?

❑ (A) Eggs of *Schistosoma hematobium*
❑ (B) Larvae of *Trichinella spiralis*
❑ (C) *Taenia solium* cysts
❑ (D) Acid-fast bacilli
❑ (E) Migrating *Ascaris lumbricoides*

20 A 24-year-old college student comes to the health service because he has had a cough, fever, and shortness of breath for the past 3 weeks when walking. The results of cardiac examination are normal, but crackles are heard in both lungs. A chest radiograph shows patchy infiltrates in the lungs. Laboratory studies show an elevated cold agglutinin titer. A presumptive clinical diagnosis of *Mycoplasma pneumoniae* is made, and the patient responds to erythromycin therapy. Which of the following histologic changes is most likely responsible for the pulmonary symptoms in this patient?

- (A) Neutrophils within bronchioles, extending into alveoli
- (B) Granulomas with Langhans giant cells
- (C) Pulmonary infarcts with vascular occlusion by microorganisms
- (D) Mononuclear interstitial infiltrate
- (E) Collection of neutrophils and fibrin in the pleural space

21 The "fun ship" leaves port from Miami on a cruise to the Caribbean. On the third day out of port, 10 adult passengers experience sudden onset of nausea and abdominal cramps, followed by periods of watery diarrhea. Some of the affected passengers also experience vomiting, and most have headaches, myalgias, or abdominal pain. On physical examination, five patients have a temperature of 38°C, but there are no other abnormal findings. Stool smears show no RBCs, leukocytes, ova, or cysts. The affected passengers recover without therapy over the next 3 days. Which of the following is the most likely causative agent?

- (A) *Giardia lamblia*
- (B) Norwalk-like virus
- (C) Rotavirus
- (D) *Shigella dysenteriae*
- (E) *Yersinia pseudotuberculosis*
- (F) *Vibrio parahaemolyticus*

22 A 44-year-old woman notices an erythematous papule on her left lower leg that becomes a ringlike rash and then subsides over several weeks. Over the next 5 months, she has migratory joint and muscle pain, substernal chest pain, and an irregular heart rhythm. The problems subside, but 2 years after the initial rash appeared, she develops a chronic arthritis involving the hips, knees, and shoulders. Which of the following is the most likely diagnosis?

- (A) Chagas disease
- (B) Dengue fever
- (C) Leishmaniasis
- (D) Leprosy
- (E) Lyme disease
- (F) Malaria
- (G) Syphilis

23 While repairing a fence on his farm, a 40-year-old man cuts the skin over his shin. The wound heals without any complications. Four days later, he develops muscle spasms of the face and extremities. These spasms worsen to the point of severe contractions. Which of the following actions by a toxin is responsible for the clinical features in this case?

- (A) Degradation of muscle cell membranes by phospholipase C
- (B) Inhibition of acetylcholine release at neuromuscular junctions
- (C) Stimulation of adenylate cyclase production
- (D) Cleavage of synaptobrevin in synaptic vesicles of neurons
- (E) Release of cytokine by T lymphocytes

24 At a convention of veterans, several of the participants begin to develop respiratory difficulty and fever. The affected men are between 58 and 73 years of age, they are all smokers, and many have chronic obstructive lung disease. On physical examination, the men have temperatures ranging from 37.3° to 38.4°C. On auscultation, crackles are heard in the lung bases. Chest radiographs show extensive pulmonary infiltrates with small abscesses. Sputum specimens show as many macrophages as neutrophils on the cytologic smears. Which of the following organisms is most likely to be identified in the sputum samples of these patients?

- (A) Cytomegalovirus
- (B) *Pneumocystis carinii*
- (C) *Legionella pneumophila*
- (D) *Burkholderia cepacia*
- (E) *Listeria monocytogenes*

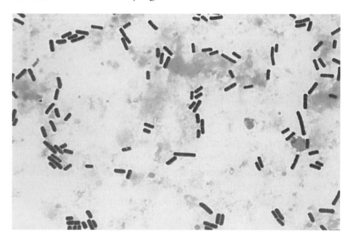

25 A 25-year-old man is involved in a rollover accident in which he is ejected from the vehicle. He sustains a compound fracture of the right humerus and undergoes open reduction with internal fixation of the humeral fracture. Several days later, he has marked swelling of the right arm and crepitus. A Gram stain of exudate from the wound site has the appearance as shown in the figure. Which of the following organisms is the most likely causative agent for this patient's infection?

- (A) *Candida albicans*
- (B) *Listeria monocytogenes*
- (C) *Haemophilus influenzae*
- (D) *Clostridium perfringens*
- (E) *Bacteroides fragilis*

26 For the past 3 weeks, a 52-year-old man has had a chronic cough with a low-grade fever. On physical examination, his temperature is 37.4°C. A chest radiograph shows bilateral, scattered, 0.3- to 2-cm nodules in the upper lobes and hilar adenopathy. A fine-needle aspirate of one of the nodules shows inflammation with mononuclear cells, including macrophages that, with PAS stain, show intracellular, 2- to

5-μm, rounded, yeastlike organisms. Which of the following infectious diseases is most likely to produce these findings?

- ❏ (A) Coccidioidomycosis
- ❏ (B) Candidiasis
- ❏ (C) Cryptococcosis
- ❏ (D) Histoplasmosis
- ❏ (E) Blastomycosis

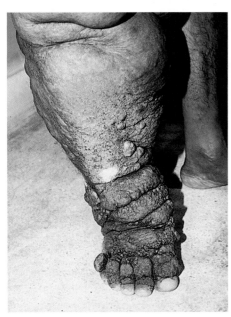

Courtesy of Dr. Willy Pressens, Harvard School of Public Health, Boston, MA.

27 A 40-year-old man has had progressive enlargement of his left leg for the past 6 years, leading to the appearance shown above. On physical examination, he is afebrile. He has inguinal lymphadenopathy and scrotal edema. Infection with which of the following organisms is most likely to be present?

- ❏ (A) *Schistosoma mansoni*
- ❏ (B) *Echinococcus granulosis*
- ❏ (C) *Trichinella spiralis*
- ❏ (D) *Leishmania tropica*
- ❏ (E) *Wuchereria bancrofti*

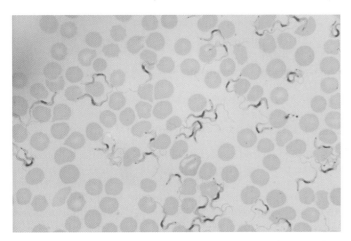

28 A 22-year-old man develops a rubbery, red, 1-cm chancre on his right forearm. Three months later, he develops splenomegaly and lymphadenopathy. Two months later, he succumbs to progressive wasting with cachexia and decreased mentation. At the time of his death, a peripheral blood smear had the appearance shown in the preceding figure. Where is this disease most likely to have been acquired?

- ❏ (A) West Africa
- ❏ (B) Central America
- ❏ (C) Southeast Asia
- ❏ (D) Southern Europe
- ❏ (E) Polynesia

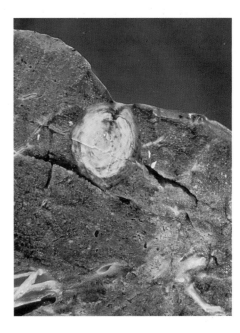

29 A 36-year-old man is singing the blues on Beale Street in Memphis, Tennessee, after a chest radiograph shows a peripheral, 2.5-cm mass in the right lower lobe during a routine health screening examination. He is currently asymptomatic, but he remembers that he had a month-long febrile illness 1 year ago. The gross appearance shown in the figure is representative of the pathologic process in the man's lung. Which of the following mechanisms best explains how this infection was contracted?

- ❏ (A) Mosquito bite on a trip to Africa
- ❏ (B) Transfusion of packed RBCs
- ❏ (C) Injection drug use with shared needles
- ❏ (D) Ingestion of contaminated dairy products
- ❏ (E) Birds roosting on his air conditioner

30 A study of transfusion-related infectious diseases determines that some blood donors appear to have acquired an infection via vertical transmission from mother to child. Laboratory testing strategies are devised to detect the most common of these infections and exclude such persons as blood donors. As a consequence, which of the following infectious agents is most likely to be a significant cause for rejection as a blood donor later in life?

- ❏ (A) *Escherichia coli*
- ❏ (B) Hepatitis B virus
- ❏ (C) *Plasmodium vivax*
- ❏ (D) *Candida albicans*
- ❏ (E) *Pneumocystis carinii*

31 In October 1347, a Genoese trading ship returning from the Black Sea docked at Messina, Sicily. The ship's crew had been decimated by an illness marked by a short time course of days from onset of inguinal lymph node enlargement with overlying skin ulceration to prostration and death. A small, ulcerated pustule ringed by a rosy rash was seen on the lower extremities of some of the crew. Within days, more than one half of the population of the port city had died. Which of the following vectors was most likely responsible for the rapid spread of this disease?

❑ (A) Mosquitoes
❑ (B) Rats
❑ (C) Sand flies
❑ (D) Cats
❑ (E) Ticks

32 A 25-year-old woman has had pelvic pain, fever, and vaginal discharge for 3 weeks. On physical examination, she has lower abdominal adnexal tenderness and a painful, swollen left knee. Laboratory studies show WBC count of 11,875/mm³ with 68% segmented neutrophils, 8% bands, 18% lymphocytes, and 6% monocytes. The patient receives antibiotic therapy and recovers. However, 5 years later she undergoes a workup for infertility. Which of the following infectious agents is most likely to produce these findings?

❑ (A) *Bacteroides fragilis*
❑ (B) *Campylobacter jejuni*
❑ (C) *Candida albicans*
❑ (D) *Entamoeba histolytica*
❑ (E) *Herpes simplex* virus
❑ (F) *Neisseria gonorrhoeae*
❑ (G) *Pseudomonas aeruginosa*
❑ (H) *Toxoplasma gondii*

33 A 9-year-old girl has developed a mild febrile illness with a sore throat over the past 2 days. On physical examination, her temperature is 38.4°C, and she has a mild pharyngitis. The girl's symptoms subside in 1 week without therapy. However, over the next 2 months, she has increasing right-sided facial drooping with inability to close the right eye. Which of the following infectious organisms is most likely to produce these findings?

❑ (A) *Cryptococcus neoformans*
❑ (B) Cytomegalovirus
❑ (C) *Listeria monocytogenes*
❑ (D) Poliovirus
❑ (E) *Toxoplasma gondii*

34 An 18-year-old woman gives birth at 33 weeks' gestation to a stillborn boy. Autopsy shows extensive periventricular cerebral necrosis with calcification and vascular thrombosis in the circle of Willis. Small areas of necrosis also appear in the heart and lung. Which of the following is most likely part of the life cycle of the infection in this stillborn fetus?

❑ (A) Cat
❑ (B) Flea
❑ (C) Pig
❑ (D) Sand fly
❑ (E) Tick
❑ (F) Triatomid bug

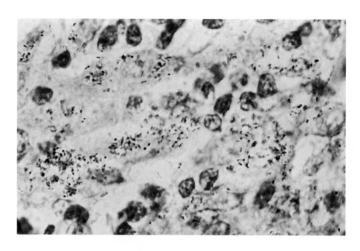

35 A 32-year-old man has maculopapular and nodular skin lesions, mainly involving his face, elbows, wrists, and knees. The nodular lesions have slowly enlarged over the past 10 years and are now beginning to cause deformity. The lesions are not painful, but the patient has decreased to absent sensation in these areas. An acid-fast stain of a biopsy specimen of a nodular lesion is shown. Which of the following is the most likely diagnosis?

❑ (A) Anthrax
❑ (B) Chagas disease
❑ (C) Leishmaniasis
❑ (D) Leprosy
❑ (E) Lyme disease
❑ (F) Onchocerciasis
❑ (G) Syphilis

36 A 9-year-old child who is living in a mud hut in northeastern Brazil has a sore on her face. She is taken to the physician, and physical examination shows an indurated area of erythema and swelling just lateral to the left eye, accompanied by posterior cervical lymphadenopathy. She has unilateral painless edema of the palpebrae and periocular tissues. Two days later, she has malaise, fever, anorexia, and edema of the face and lower extremities. On physical examination 1 week later, there is hepatosplenomegaly and generalized lymphadenopathy. Which of the following pathologic findings is most likely to develop in this patient?

❑ (A) Cerebral abscesses
❑ (B) Chronic arthritis
❑ (C) Dilated cardiomyopathy
❑ (D) Meningitis
❑ (E) Mucocutaneous ulcers
❑ (F) Myositis
❑ (G) Paranasal bony destruction

37 A 50-year-old resident of Phoenix, Arizona, has a cough that has persisted for 1 month. On physical examination, his temperature is 38.1°C. A chest radiograph shows a 3.5-cm opacity with central cavitation in the right apical region. An open lung biopsy is performed to exclude cancer. Microscopic examination of the biopsy specimen shows caseating granulomatous inflammation containing 60-μm spherules filled with smaller, rounded structures. Which of the following infectious organisms is most likely to produce these findings?

- ❑ (A) *Aspergillus fumigatus*
- ❑ (B) *Coccidioides immitis*
- ❑ (C) *Histoplasma capsulatum*
- ❑ (D) *Mycobacterium tuberculosis*
- ❑ (E) *Pseudomonas aeruginosa*
- ❑ (F) *Pneumocystis carinii*
- ❑ (G) *Staphylococcus aureus*
- ❑ (H) *Toxoplasma gondii*

38 A 6-month-old infant has abrupt onset of vomiting followed by profuse, watery diarrhea. On physical examination, the infant has a temperature of 38.3°C. Development is normal for age, and the only abnormal finding is poor skin turgor. Laboratory studies show serum Na$^+$ of 153 mmol/L, K$^+$ 4.4 mmol/L, Cl$^-$ 111 mmol/L, CO$_2$ 27 mmol/L, and glucose 70 mg/dL. Examination of a stool specimen shows mucus but no RBCs or WBCs. Which of the following mechanisms accounts for this diarrhea?

- ❑ (A) Decreased absorption of sodium and water
- ❑ (B) Increased secretion of potassium and water by epithelial cells
- ❑ (C) Presence of Yop virulence plasmid
- ❑ (D) Lysis of colonic epithelial cells
- ❑ (E) Decreased breakdown of lactose to glucose and galactose

39 A 5-year-old girl has a blotchy, reddish-brown rash on her face, trunk, and proximal extremities that developed over the course of 3 days. On physical examination, she has 0.2- to 0.5-cm ulcerated lesions on the oral cavity mucosa and generalized lymphadenopathy. A cough with minimal sputum production becomes progressively worse over the next 3 days. Which of the following viruses is most likely to produce these findings?

- ❑ (A) Mumps
- ❑ (B) Varicella zoster
- ❑ (C) Rubella
- ❑ (D) Epstein-Barr
- ❑ (E) Rubeola

40 A 42-year-old man who is HIV positive has had a fever and cough for the past month. On physical examination, his temperature is 37.5°C. On auscultation of the chest, decreased breath sounds are heard over the right posterior lung. A chest radiograph shows a large area of consolidation with a central air-fluid level involving the right middle lobe. A transbronchial biopsy specimen contains gram-positive filamentous organisms that are weakly acid fast. The patient's course is further complicated by empyema and acute onset of a headache. A head CT scan shows a 4-cm discrete lesion of the right hemisphere with ring enhancement. Which of the following infectious agents is most likely to produce these findings?

- ❑ (A) *Aspergillus fumigatus*
- ❑ (B) *Nocardia asteroides*
- ❑ (C) *Mycobacterium avium-intracellulare*
- ❑ (D) *Staphylococcus aureus*
- ❑ (E) *Mucor circinelloides*

41 A 33-year-old woman who is an injection drug user develops a severe headache and neck stiffness. On physical examination, her temperature is 38.2°C. She has no papilledema. A lumbar puncture is performed, and a Gram stain of the CSF obtained shows many short, gram-positive rods. The patient most likely acquired this illness through which of the following mechanisms?

- ❑ (A) Sharing infected needles
- ❑ (B) Inhalation of droplet nuclei
- ❑ (C) Inoculation through a cut on the skin
- ❑ (D) Ingestion of contaminated dairy products
- ❑ (E) Using a friend's toothbrush

42 A 6-year-old boy developed a rash over his chest that began as 0.5-cm, reddish macules. Within 2 days, the macules became vesicles. A few days later, the vesicles ruptured and crusted over. Over the next 2 weeks, crops of the lesions spread to the face and extremities. Which of the following clinical manifestations of this infection is most likely to appear decades later?

- ❑ (A) Shingles
- ❑ (B) Infertility
- ❑ (C) Paralysis
- ❑ (D) Congestive heart failure
- ❑ (E) Chronic arthritis

43 A 6-year-old boy has had diarrhea for 7 days and is brought to the physician. He has averaged about six stools per day, which appear mucoid and sometimes blood-tinged. On physical examination, his temperature is 37.4°C. He has mild lower abdominal tenderness but no masses. A stool culture is positive for *Shigella sonnei*. Which of the following would most likely be seen in an endoscopic biopsy specimen from this child's colon?

- ❑ (A) Epithelial disruption with overlying exudate of polymorphonuclear leukocytes (neutrophils)
- ❑ (B) Multiple granulomas throughout the colon wall
- ❑ (C) Slight increase in numbers of lymphocytes and plasma cells in lamina propria
- ❑ (D) Intranuclear inclusions in enterocytes
- ❑ (E) Extensive scarring of lamina propria with stricture formation

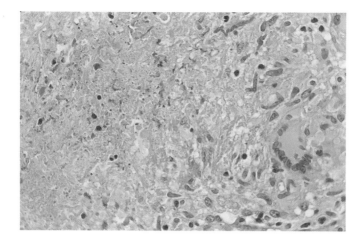

44 A 32-year-old man has had a low-grade fever and a 4-kg weight loss over the course of 3 months. On physical examination, his temperature is 37.5°C. Laboratory studies show elevated AST and ALT, but the serum bilirubin level is not elevated. A liver biopsy is performed, and the sample has the microscopic appearance shown in the figure above. An acid-fast stain of this tissue is positive. This infectious agent is most likely being destroyed by which of the following mechanisms?

- ❏ (A) Phagocytosis by eosinophils
- ❏ (B) Elaboration of nitric oxide by macrophages
- ❏ (C) Generation of NADPH-dependent oxygen-free radicals
- ❏ (D) Complement-mediated lysis
- ❏ (E) Superoxide formation within phagolysosomes

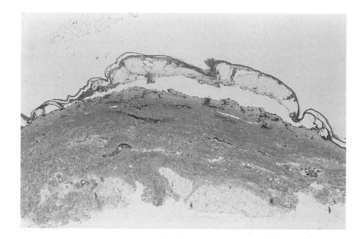

45 A 23-year-old woman has had recurrent vesicular lesions on her labia majora and perineum for several years. On physical examination, she is afebrile. Clusters of clear, 0.2- to 0.5-cm vesicles are present on the labia, with some surrounding erythema. The representative microscopic appearance of one of the lesions under low power is shown above. Which of the following is most likely to be seen under higher magnification of this lesion?

- ❏ (A) Dysplastic epithelial cells that contain human papillomavirus sequences
- ❏ (B) Neutrophils containing ingested gram-negative diplococci
- ❏ (C) Multinucleated (syncytial) cells that contain pink-to-purple intranuclear inclusions
- ❏ (D) Perivascular lymphoplasmacytic infiltrate surrounding arterioles, with endothelial proliferation
- ❏ (E) Mononuclear infiltrate with *Trichomonas vaginalis* organisms

46 In a study of persons living in a subtropical region in which an irrigation project has been completed, it is noted that rice farmers have experienced an increased rate of an infectious illness since the project began. Investigators determine that the infection is acquired through cercaria that penetrate the skin. The cercaria are released from snails living in the irrigation canals. Infected persons develop progressive ascites. Which of the following pathologic findings is most likely to be present in these infected persons as a consequence of the infection?

- ❏ (A) Dilated cardiomyopathy
- ❏ (B) Elephantiasis
- ❏ (C) Hepatic fibrosis
- ❏ (D) Mucocutaneous ulcers
- ❏ (E) Skin anesthesia
- ❏ (F) Squamous cell carcinoma
- ❏ (G) Voluminous watery diarrhea

47 A 66-year-old man incurs extensive thermal burns to his skin and undergoes skin grafting procedures in the surgical intensive care unit. Two weeks later, he has increasing respiratory distress. Laboratory studies show hemoglobin of 13.1 g/dL, hematocrit 39.2%, platelet count 222,200/mm³, and WBC count 4520/mm³ with 15% segmented neutrophils, 3% bands, 67% lymphocytes, and 15% monocytes. A chest radiograph shows extensive bilateral infiltrates with patchy areas of consolidation. Bronchoscopy is performed, and microscopic examination of a transbronchial biopsy specimen shows pulmonary vasculitis and surrounding areas of necrosis with sparse inflammatory exudate. Which of the following infectious agents is most likely to produce these findings?

- ❏ (A) Adenovirus
- ❏ (B) *Coccidioides immitis*
- ❏ (C) *Histoplasma capsulatum*
- ❏ (D) *Mycobacterium tuberculosis*
- ❏ (E) *Pseudomonas aeruginosa*
- ❏ (F) *Pneumocystis carinii*
- ❏ (G) *Streptococcus pneumoniae*
- ❏ (H) *Toxoplasma gondii*

48 A 25-year-old woman has sudden onset of severe, profuse, watery diarrhea. Over the next 3 days, she becomes severely dehydrated. On physical examination, she is afebrile but has poor skin turgor. Laboratory studies of the diarrheal fluid show microscopic flecks of mucus but no blood and few WBCs. A blood culture is negative. The woman is hospitalized and receives intravenous fluid therapy for 1 week. Which of the following is the most likely diagnosis?

- ❑ (A) African trypanosomiasis
- ❑ (B) Amebiasis
- ❑ (C) Aspergillosis
- ❑ (D) Cholera
- ❑ (E) Filariasis
- ❑ (F) Hydatid disease
- ❑ (G) Typhoid fever

49 A previously healthy 21-year-old man has a new-onset seizure disorder. On physical examination, he is afebrile, and there are no localizing neurologic signs. MR imaging of the brain shows multiple, 0.5- to 1.5-cm, cystic periventricular and meningeal lesions. Which of the following infectious organisms is most likely to produce these findings?

- ❑ (A) *Aspergillus fumigatus*
- ❑ (B) *Cryptococcus neoformans*
- ❑ (C) *Plasmodium falciparum*
- ❑ (D) Poliovirus
- ❑ (E) *Taenia solium*
- ❑ (F) *Toxoplasma gondii*
- ❑ (G) *Trypanosoma gambiense*

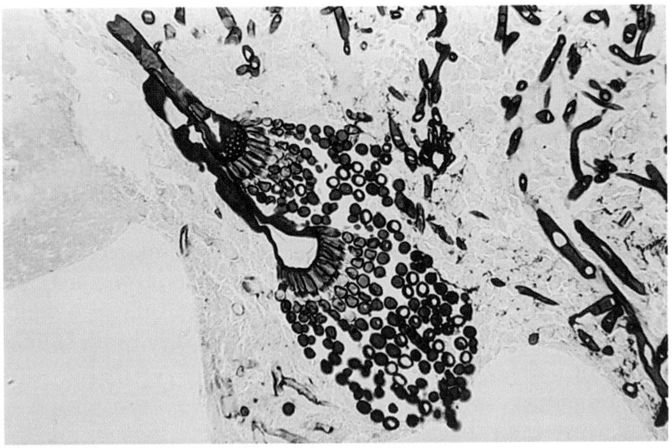

50 A 10-year-old girl with leukemia undergoes allogeneic bone marrow transplantation. She has poor engraftment and 1 month later develops fever and dyspnea. On physical examination, her temperature is 39.0°C. On auscultation of the chest, wheezes and crackles are heard in both lungs. A chest radiograph suggests pulmonary infarcts. Laboratory studies show hemoglobin of 8.8 g/dL, hematocrit 26.5%, platelet count 91,540/mm³, and WBC count 1910/mm³ with 10% segmented neutrophils, 2% bands neutrophils, 74% lymphocytes, and 14% monocytes. The girl's condition worsens, and she dies. At autopsy, pulmonary vessels are occluded by abundant growth of microorganisms, as shown in the figure. Which of the following infectious agents is most likely to produce these findings?

- ❑ (A) *Aspergillus fumigatus*
- ❑ (B) *Coccidioides immitis*
- ❑ (C) *Corynebacterium diphtheriae*
- ❑ (D) *Histoplasma capsulatum*
- ❑ (E) *Mycobacterium tuberculosis*
- ❑ (F) *Pneumocystis carinii*
- ❑ (G) *Streptococcus pneumoniae*

51 A 6-year-old girl who lives in the Yucatan peninsula has developed a high fever over the past 3 days. On physical exam-

ination, she has a temperature of 39.6°C and marked tenderness in all muscles. Laboratory studies shows WBC count of 2950/mm³ with 12% segmented neutrophils, 4% bands, 66% lymphocytes, and 18% monocytes. Over a period of 1 week, she becomes more lethargic, with a decreased level of consciousness, and petechiae and purpura develop over the skin. Further laboratory studies show thrombocytopenia with markedly prolonged prothrombin and partial thromboplastin times. CT scan of the brain shows a hemorrhage in the right parietal lobe. Which of the following is most likely part of the life cycle of the agent causing infection in this patient?

- ❑ (A) Cow
- ❑ (B) Louse
- ❑ (C) Mosquito
- ❑ (D) Pig
- ❑ (E) Snail
- ❑ (F) Tick
- ❑ (G) Tsetse fly

52 An infant born at term to a 33-year-old woman is severely hydropic. On physical examination, there is a diffuse rash with sloughing skin on the palms and soles. Within 2 days, the infant dies of respiratory distress. At autopsy, there is marked hepatosplenomegaly. Microscopic examination of the femur and vertebrae shows periosteitis and osteochondritis. The lungs are pale and poorly aerated, with microscopic interstitial mononuclear infiltrates. A serologic test result for which of the following agents is most likely to be positive in the infant's mother?

- ❑ (A) HIV
- ❑ (B) Herpes simplex type 2
- ❑ (C) *Toxoplasma gondii*
- ❑ (D) Syphilis
- ❑ (E) Cytomegalovirus

53 When Pharaoh did not heed Moses to let the Hebrews go, a series of plagues fell upon the land of Egypt. In the fifth plague, large domesticated mammals including cattle, horses, and sheep died. This was followed by a plague in which the Egyptians developed cutaneous boils that probably appeared as 1- to 5-cm areas of erythema with central necrosis forming an eschar. Some Egyptians may also have developed a mild, nonproductive cough associated with fatigue, myalgia, and low-grade fever over 72 hours, followed by a rapid onset of severe dyspnea with diaphoresis and cyanosis. Vital signs might have included temperature of 39.5°C, pulse 105/min, respirations 25/min, and blood pressure 85/45 mm Hg. On auscultation of the chest, crackles would be heard at the lung bases. A chest radiograph would show a widened mediastinum and small pleural effusions. "Legacy" laboratory findings would include a CBC with WBC count of 13,130/mm³, hemoglobin 13.7 g/dL, hematocrit 41.2%, MCV 91 μm³, and platelet count 244,000/mm³. Despite antibiotic therapy with both ciprofloxacin and doxycycline, many of those affected would die. Which of the following organisms is most likely to produce these findings?

- ❑ (A) *Bacillus anthracis*
- ❑ (B) Herpes simplex virus
- ❑ (C) *Mycobacterium leprae*
- ❑ (D) *Staphylococcus aureus*
- ❑ (E) *Variola major*
- ❑ (F) *Yersinia pestis*

54 A clinical study is conducted involving hospitalized patients with positive blood cultures. A subset of these patients is found to have fever, hypotension, disseminated intravascular coagulopathy, and pulmonary diffuse alveolar damage with respiratory distress. Analysis of the microbiology laboratory findings shows that the organisms cultured from this subset of patients are gram-negative bacilli. Which of the following substances elaborated by these organisms is most likely to cause this complex of clinical findings?

- ❑ (A) Endotoxin
- ❑ (B) Exotoxin
- ❑ (C) Mycolic acid
- ❑ (D) RNA polymerase
- ❑ (E) Superantigen
- ❑ (F) Tumor necrosis factor

55 In the same day, the emergency department is visited by 20 persons, all of whom work in the same building. Over the past day, they all experienced the sudden onset of high fever, headache, backache, and malaise. On examination they are febrile. They do not have lymphadenopathy or hepatosplenomegaly. Over the next 2 days they develop a maculopapular rash on the face, forearms, and mucous membranes of the oropharynx. Despite supportive care, a third of these patients die. Which of the following organisms is the most likely causative agent?

- ❑ (A) Chlamydia psittaci
- ❑ (B) Francisella tularensis
- ❑ (C) Hantavirus
- ❑ (D) Mycobacterium kansasii
- ❑ (E) Rickettsia typhi
- ❑ (F) Variola major

ANSWERS

1 **(A)** The patient developed cryptococcal meningoencephalitis, a complication of his immunocompromised state. *Cryptococcus neoformans* typically has a thick capsule, making it easily visible with the India ink preparation, a procedure that can be performed within a few minutes. The glucose and protein levels of CSF can aid in determining whether an infection is present and what general type of organism is present, but they do not yield a specific cause. A cryptococcal antigen test also would be useful for this patient. Brain biopsies are not commonly performed, and other less invasive methods should be pursued first. Bacterial meningitis is possible, and pneumococcus would be a common bacterial cause, but this description is consistent with cryptococcosis. PCR probes for Epstein-Barr virus are not useful in this case, because acute viral meningitis usually does not cause a visible exudate, the onset of disease is more insidious, and it is not typically associated with immunocompromised states.

BP7 311, 494   BP6 727   PBD7 399   PBD6 379-380

2 **(C)** Amebic liver abscess is an uncommon complication of amebiasis. The colonic lesions typically have disappeared by the time the liver lesions appear. *Entamoeba histolytica* organisms can invade the colonic submucosa, gaining access to venules draining to the portal system. Giardiasis is caused

by an intestinal parasite and produces watery diarrhea. Typhoid fever is a systemic disease that produces splenomegaly more so than hepatomegaly, and abscesses are uncommon. *Campylobacter* and *Yersinia* can produce various presentations of diarrhea, but abscesses would not be expected. Staphylococcal enterotoxin typically produces abdominal pain and diarrhea within hours of ingestion.

BP7 314, 569   BP6 269, 496   PBD7 351, 839-840
PBD6 358-359

3 **(D)** Syphilitic chancres occur in the primary stage of syphilis and are characterized by lymphoplasmacytic infiltrates, as well as by an obliterative endarteritis. Similar lesions may also appear with secondary syphilitic mucocutaneous lesions. Suppurative granulomas are typical of cat scratch disease. Caseating granulomatous inflammation is more characteristic of tuberculosis or fungal infections. Acute inflammation with abscess formation is characteristic of bacterial infections such as gonorrhea. Gummatous inflammation can be seen with tertiary syphilis in adults or in congenital syphilis.

BP7 670-673   BP6 589-592   PBD7 388-390
PBD6 346, 362-364

4 **(C)** Rhinovirus binds to intercellular adhesion molecule-1 (ICAM-1) and accounts for 60% of common colds. *Mycoplasma pneumoniae* also accounts for some colds, but this agent does not bind to ICAM-1 receptors on host cells. *Haemophilus influenzae* can produce sinusitis, otitis media, and bronchopneumonia. Infection with Epstein-Barr virus can produce pharyngitis with infectious mononucleosis, but the course tends to extend over weeks. *Neisseria meningitidis* infections, which produce meningitis, may begin as a mild pharyngitis, but these infections can have a very rapid course over 1 or 2 days.

PBD7 356-357   PBD6 347-348

5 **(C)** Visceral leishmaniasis (kala-azar) is caused by protozoa in the *Leishmania donovani* complex. Of these, only *L. donovani infantum* is endemic to southern Europe and the Mediterranean area. It is transmitted to humans by the sandfly (*Phlebotomus*). The pancytopenia implies bone marrow involvement, possibly enhanced by the enlarged spleen, and the liver function abnormalities suggest liver involvement. Borreliosis causes relapsing fever and is transmitted via body lice. Echinococcal disease is caused by ingestion of tapeworm eggs and can lead to cyst formation in visceral organs. *Borrelia burgdorferi* infection is transmitted via ticks and can cause Lyme disease, characterized by erythema chronicum migrans, meningoencephalitis, and chronic arthritis. Schistosomiasis, which is transmitted via snails, can produce hepatic cirrhosis (*Schistosoma mansoni* or *S. japonicum*) or bladder disease (*S. hematobium*). It would be unusual for a case of tuberculosis not to start with pulmonary signs or symptoms before becoming disseminated. Typhus is a louse-borne rickettsial disease with skin rash that may proceed to skin necrosis.

PBD7 403-405   PBD6 380-381

6 **(D)** This patient's travel history suggests amebiasis as the most likely cause of her dysentery. The amebae can invade the mucosa and sometimes penetrate into submucosal veins. They are then carried to the liver, where they form abscesses.

Adenovirus may produce mild, watery diarrhea. *Campylobacter jejuni* can produce disease very similar to amebiasis, but there is more likely to be involvement of the small intestine. Overgrowth of *Candida* after broad-spectrum antibiotic therapy that alters intestinal flora may lead to pseudomembranous colitis. Giardiasis typically produces self-limited, watery diarrhea. *Helicobacter pylori* lives in the gastric mucus and is associated with gastritis and peptic ulcer disease. Typhoid fever produces ulcerations of Peyer's patches and systemic disease. Cholera is marked by severe, watery diarrhea.

BP7 314, 569   BP6 428   PBD7 839-840   PBD6 380-381

7 (C) This patient has visceral leishmaniasis, or kala-azar. Leishmaniasis is endemic in the Middle East, South Asia, Africa, and Latin America. The organisms proliferate within macrophages in the mononuclear phagocyte system and cause hepatosplenomegaly and lymphadenopathy. Often, there is hyperpigmentation of the skin. Bone marrow involvement and splenic enlargement contribute to reduced production and accelerated destruction of hematopoietic cells, giving rise to pancytopenia. Borreliosis causes relapsing fever and is transmitted via body lice. *Brugia malayi* is a nematode transmitted by mosquitoes that leads to filariasis involving lymphatics to produce elephantiasis. *Leishmania donovani* is transmitted by sand flies and leads to infection of macrophages, which produces hepatosplenomegaly, lymphadenopathy, and bone marrow involvement with pancytopenia. Listeriosis is most often acquired via contaminated food or water. In most adults, it produces mild diarrheal illness, but in some adults and children, and in fetuses, it may produce meningitis or dissemination with microabscess (microgranuloma) formation. *Mycobacterium leprae* causes Hansen disease, with infection of peripheral nerves and skin. In persons with a strong immune response, the tuberculoid form of this disease results in granuloma formation; in those with a weak immune response, the lepromatous form occurs, characterized by large numbers of macrophages filled with short, thin, acid-fast bacilli. Malaria, caused by *Plasmodium falciparum*, produces hemolytic anemia, splenomegaly, and cerebral thrombosis. *African trypanosomiasis* produces sleeping sickness.

PBD7 403-405   PBD6 391-392

8 (A) Infection with *Chlamydia trachomatis* is one of the more common sexually transmitted diseases. Most cases produce only urethritis and cervicitis; however, some strains of *C. trachomatis* can produce lymphogranuloma venereum, a chronic, ulcerative disease that is more endemic in Asia, Africa, and the Caribbean. In this disease, there is a mixed granulomatous and neutrophilic inflammatory reaction, as seen in this patient. In contrast, herpes simplex virus produces clear mucocutaneous vesicles with no exudates and is unlikely to involve lymph nodes. Recurrent lymphoma is characterized by sheets or nodules of pleomorphic lymphocytes without significant inflammation. Candidiasis can produce superficial inflammation with an exudate, but it is rarely invasive or disseminated in nonimmunosuppressed persons. Bacterial vaginosis due to *Gardnerella* produces a whitish discharge that has a "fishy" odor.

BP7 310-311, 675   BP6 595   PBD7 394-395
PBD6 361-362

9 (B) This patient has high HIV-1 RNA levels that are consistent with the diagnosis of AIDS. Although patients with AIDS are susceptible to many microbes, infections with cytomegalovirus (CMV) are particularly common. The biopsy specimen shows an enlarged cell containing a distinct intranuclear inclusion and ill-defined cytoplasmic inclusions, which are typical of CMV infection. Epstein-Barr virus infection frequently is seen in patients with HIV infection, but there are no distinct pulmonary lesions associated with it. Respiratory syncytial virus infections are seen in children but rarely in adults. Herpes zoster infections are most likely to affect the peripheral nervous system, rarely can become disseminated to affect the lungs in immunosuppressed patients, and produce a different appearance than that shown. Adenovirus is a common viral pathogen in adults that may produce a clinically significant pneumonia, and intranuclear inclusions may be present, but the cells are not large, and cytoplasmic inclusions are absent.

BP7 310, 496-497   BP6 429-430   PBD7 366-368
PBD6 726

10 (B) Amebiasis is a common cause of dysentery in developing nations. The *Entamoeba histolytica* trophozoites can attach to colonic epithelium, invade, and lyse the epithelial cells. In some cases, there can be extensive mucosal involvement with characteristic flask-shaped (like an Erlenmeyer flask) ulcerations similar to those seen in other severe inflammatory bowel diseases. Giardiasis tends to involve the small intestine and produces variable inflammation but not ulceration. Shigellosis can produce bloody dysentery with irregular superficial colonic mucosal ulceration, but the organisms typically do not invade beyond the lamina propria. Salmonellosis more typically involves the small intestine and in most cases produces self-limited enteritis, although more severe disease with dissemination to other organs can occur with *Salmonella typhi* infection. Cholera is characterized by massive, secretory diarrhea without intestinal mucosal invasion or necrosis. *Bacillus cereus* is a cause of food poisoning (most often as a contaminant in reheated fried rice) and has a short incubation time.

BP7 314, 569   BP6 496   PBD7 839-840   PBD6 358-359

11 (B) The *Shigella* organisms elaborate a shiga toxin that damages colonic epithelial cells. The colonic mucosa is intensely inflamed, with ulcerations and pseudomembrane formation (pale, white patches). *S. flexneri* infections in persons positive for HLA-B27 can lead to Reiter syndrome, with chronic arthritis. *Vibrio* organisms elaborate an exotoxin and do not invade and destroy intestinal epithelium. *Entamoeba histolytica* can produce bloody diarrhea but not Reiter syndrome. Typhoid fever causes many systemic problems but not arthritis. The presence of *Helicobacter pylori* in gastric mucus drives the processes of chronic gastritis and ulceration of gastric and duodenal mucosal surfaces.

BP7 314, 568-569   BP6 495   PBD7 834-835   PBD6 355

12 (E) This woman has diphtheria. The *Corynebacterium diphtheriae* organisms proliferate in the inflammatory membrane that covers the pharynx and tonsils. These organisms elaborate an exotoxin that produces myocarditis and neuropathy. The organisms do not disseminate to cause inflammation or abscesses or vasculitis elsewhere in the body.

Endotoxins tend to be elaborated by gram-negative bacterial organisms. Granulomatous inflammation is more typical of mycobacterial and fungal infections.

BP7 318-319   BP6 274   PBD7 374-375
PBD6 343, 759, 1276

13 (A) This patient has Rocky Mountain spotted fever, which occurs sporadically in the US in areas other than the Rocky Mountains. Rickettsial diseases produce signs and symptoms from damage to vascular endothelium and smooth muscle similar to a vasculitis. Thrombosis of the affected blood vessels is responsible for foci of skin necrosis. Hansen disease, produced by *Mycobacterium leprae*, results in skin anesthesia that predisposes to recurrent injury. Plague, caused by *Yersinia pestis*, can produce focal skin necrosis at the site of a flea bite. Lyme disease, caused by *Borrelia burgdorferi*, can produce an erythema chronicum migrans of skin at the site of a tick bite. Mucocutaneous leishmaniasis mainly involves the nasal and oral regions.

PBD7 395-397   PBD6 384

14 (E) This rash and edema are manifestations of streptococcal erysipelas. Erysipelas is usually caused by group A or C streptococci. Streptolysins elaborated by these organisms aid in the spread of the infection. *Clostridium botulinum* elaborates an exotoxin that, when ingested, results in paralysis. *Escherichia coli* produces a variety of infections, but skin infections are not common. *Neisseria gonorrhoeae* is best known as a sexually transmitted disease, and a rash is possible, although usually there is no pronounced swelling. *Staphylococcus epidermidis* is usually considered a contaminant in cultures.

PBF7 373-374   PBD6 367-368

15 (D) The influenza pandemic in 1918 resulted from an antigenic shift in the influenza A type. This occurs when there is recombination with RNA sequences of influenza viruses found in animals such as pigs (e.g., "swine flu"). A swine flu virus has been identified as a cause of the 1918 pandemic. Mutations in the envelope genes are responsible for epidemics. These mutations allow evasion from host antibodies. Influenza viruses do not bind to intercellular adhesion molecule-1 (ICAM-1) receptors; rhinoviruses do. Viruses do not make exotoxins and do not acquire antibiotic resistance.

PBD7 751-752   PBD6 348

16 (C) Bacterial infections are marked by suppurative inflammation, and a virulent organism such as *Klebsiella* can lead to tissue destruction with abscess formation. Gas-forming bacteria, such as *Clostridium* organisms, are unusual as a cause of respiratory infections. Granulomatous inflammation is characteristic of mycobacterial or fungal infections. Infections of the lung do not result in emphysema. Carcinomas are not sequelae of bacterial infections.

BP7 319-321   BP6 428-429   PBD7 361-362   PBD6 345

17 (A) Actinomycetes that can produce chronic abscessing pneumonia, particularly in immunocompromised patients, include *Actinomyces israelii* and *Nocardia asteroides*. Sulfur granules, formed from masses of the branching, filamentous organisms, are more likely to be seen in *Actinomyces*. *Blastomyces dermatitidis* infections tend to produce a granuloma-

tous inflammatory process. Chlamydial infections produce an interstitial pattern like that of most viruses. *Klebsiella* infections, like other bacterial infections, can result in abscess formation, although without distinct sulfur granules. *Mycobacterium kansasii* infections are similar to *M. tuberculosis* infections in that granulomatous inflammation is prominent.

BP6 420   PBD7 376, 747   PBD6 335, 722

18 (B) This boy had malaria. After the infective mosquito bite, *Plasmodium falciparum* sporozoites invade liver cells and reproduce asexually. When the hepatocytes rupture, they release thousands of merozoites that infect RBCs. The infected RBCs circulate and can bind to endothelium in the brain. Small cerebral vessels become plugged with the RBCs, resulting in ischemia. The other listed options could also be secondarily involved by vascular thromboses.

BP7 408-409   BP6 352-353   PBD7 401-403
PBD6 389-391

19 (A) *Schistosoma hematobium* is seen in Africa, particularly the Nile Valley, in areas where irrigation has expanded the range of the host snails. It infects the wall of the urinary bladder, causing severe granulomatous inflammation, fibrosis, and calcification. *Trichinella spiralis* infects striated muscle. Cysticercosis can have a wide tissue distribution, but the brain is most often affected. Mycobacterial infections of the urinary tract are uncommon and do not cause bladder fibrosis. Ascariasis involves the lower gastrointestinal tract, and the worms reside in the lumen.

BP7 312   PBD7 408-409   PBD6 396-397

20 (D) *Mycoplasma* infections lead to a primary atypical pneumonia in which there are no alveolar infiltrates, but there is prominent interstitial inflammation with lymphocytes, histiocytes, and plasma cells. Alveolar and bronchiolar neutrophilic exudates suggest a bacterial agent causing pneumonia. Granulomas with Langhans-type giant cells are typical of tuberculosis. Proliferation of microorganisms with vascular occlusion and infarction is most typical of *Aspergillus* fungal infections. An empyema with neutrophils suggests a bacterial cause for pneumonia with spread to pleura.

BP7 310-311, 482-483   BP6 419-420   PBD7 751
PBD6 335, 721-722

21 (B) Norwalk-like viruses (NLVs) are members of the Calciviridae family of viruses (also known as the enteric caliciviruses) and are transmitted by hands contaminated through the fecal-oral route, directly from person to person, through contaminated food or water, or by contact with contaminated surfaces (known as fomites). They are the leading cause of outbreaks of gastroenteritis. Infections occur year-round, with a clear peak in the winter. More than 80% of adults in both developed and developing countries have antibodies to NLVs. Giardiasis usually produces self-limited, watery diarrhea and is acquired from untreated water supplies. Rotavirus is more common in children. Shigellosis typically leads to a more severe, sometimes bloody, diarrhea. *Yersinia pseudotuberculosis* and *Y. enterocolitica* can produce a syndrome of mesenteric adenitis and terminal ileitis with abdominal pain that may mimic acute appendicitis. *Vibrio parahaemolyticus* causes an acute gastroenteritis with explosive watery diarrhea, vomiting, nausea, abdominal cramps, and headaches.

PBD7 832-833   PBD6 354, 807

22 (E) The acute stage of Lyme disease is marked by the appearance of erythema chronicum migrans of the skin. As the *Borrelia burgdorferi* organisms proliferate and disseminate, systemic manifestations of carditis, meningitis, and migratory arthralgias and myalgias appear. These are followed 2 to 3 years after initial infection by arthritis involving the large joints. Chagas disease may be associated with acute and chronic myocarditis leading to heart failure; some patients have esophageal involvement, but arthritis and rash are not features of the disease. Hemorrhagic fever, or Dengue fever, caused by an arbovirus, can produce myositis and bone marrow suppression. Mucocutaneous ulcers may be seen with *Leishmania braziliensis*. Leprosy, or Hansen disease, is associated with skin anesthesia and granuloma formation with nodular deformities of the skin. Malaria is not typically associated with skin lesions. In primary syphilis, a hard chancre may be present at the site of inoculation (usually the external genitalia); in secondary syphilis, a maculopapular rash may be present.

BP7 777   BP6 686-687   PBD7 392-393   PBD6 388-389

23 (D) This man has tetanus. The contamination of a wound with *Clostridium tetani* can result in the elaboration of a potent neurotoxin. This toxin is a protease that cleaves synaptobrevin, a major transmembrane protein of the synaptic vesicles of the inhibitory neurons. *Clostridium perfringens* elaborates a variety of toxins, one of which (tetanospasmin) is a phospholipase. Inhibition of acetylcholine release is not a feature of infection. Cholera is produced when the toxin elaborated by *Vibrio cholerae* stimulates epithelial cell adenylate cyclase. The toxin of *Staphylococcus aureus* is an enterotoxin that acts as a superantigen and stimulates T-cell cytokine release.

PBD7 393   PBD6 368-369

24 (C) The original outbreak for which this disease was named occurred at an American Legion convention in Philadelphia. *Legionella pneumophila* is a facultative parasite of macrophages. A high ratio of macrophages to neutrophils is characteristic of the infection. Persons with immunosuppression are at risk for cytomegalovirus and *Pneumocystis* pneumonia. *Burkholderia cepacia* is most often seen in patients with cystic fibrosis who have extensive bronchiectasis. *Listeria monocytogenes* can produce disseminated disease with meningitis in immunocompromised adults.

BP7 482   BP6 418   PBD7 749-750   PBD6 377-378

25 (D) The large, gram-positive rods seen in the figure are characteristic of *Clostridium perfringens*, which can contaminate open wounds and produce gas gangrene. Candidal infections are typically superficial, and a Gram stain shows gram-positive budding cells with pseudohyphae. Listeriosis can be a congenital or food-borne infection, and the organisms are short, gram-positive rods. *Haemophilus influenzae* is a gram-negative rod best known for causing respiratory and central nervous system infections. *Bacteroides fragilis* can contaminate surgical wounds of the abdomen.

PBD7 393-394   PBD6 369

26 (D) The small yeasts of *Histoplasma capsulatum* are often intracellular. Infections can be disseminated, involving tissues of the mononuclear phagocyte system. In the lung, histoplasmosis can mimic primary or secondary tuberculosis. The spherules of *Coccidioides* are larger and are not intracellular. *Candida albicans* produces budding cells with pseudohyphae. *Cryptococcus neoformans* organisms have narrow-based budding and are two to three times larger than organisms of *H. capsulatum*. Organisms of *Blastomyces dermatitidis* exhibit broad-based budding and are slightly larger than *C. neoformans* organisms.

BP7 493-495   BP6 425-426   PBD7 754-755
PBD6 352-353

27 (E) This patient has elephantiasis, which results from lymphatic obstruction in the presence of an inflammatory reaction to the adult filarial worms *Wuchereria bancrofti*. Schistosomiasis may affect the liver or bladder most severely. *Echinococcus* produces hydatid disease of the liver, lungs, or bone. *Trichinella* encysts in striated muscle. *Leishmania* can involve the skin, causing ulceration, and can enlarge parenchymal organs.

BP7 81   PBD7 409-410   PBD6 397-398

28 (A) The findings are consistent with African trypanosomiasis, or sleeping sickness. The eradication of the tsetse fly vector has been a priority for decades. Filarial worms endemic in parts of Central America, Southeast Asia, and Polynesia can also appear in blood, but are smaller in size and do not lead to chronic wasting. Filariasis is not endemic in Europe.

PBD7 405   PBD6 337, 393

29 (E) The figure shows a small, so-called coin lesion of the lung produced by a granulomatous inflammatory process. On chest radiographs, the lesion appears sharply demarcated and rounded like a Canadian or US dollar coin. A cause for this process is infection with *Histoplasma capsulatum*. Bird droppings, especially from pigeons, are a rich source of dusts contaminated with *H. capsulatum*. Mosquitoes generally are not known as vectors for diseases that cause granulomatous inflammation. Fungal and mycobacterial infections are not acquired by transfusion or other parenteral routes, such as sharing intravenous needles. Contaminated milk is a source of *Mycobacterium bovis*, but this is a rare pulmonary infection.

BP7 493-495   BP6 425-427   PBD7 754-755
PBD6 352-353

30 (B) Testing for hepatitis B and C is part of routine screening of blood donors. This form of transmission for hepatitis B is most common in developing nations. *Escherichia coli* can be a congenital infection, but it leaves no major significant lasting sequelae in infants who survive. Malaria, candidal infection, and pneumocystosis are not congenital infections.

BP7 601-603   BP6 526   PBD7 369   PBD6 339

31 (B) This incident marks the first appearance of the Black Death in Europe, a disease that persisted during the 14th and 15th centuries. The plague spread through Italy and across the European continent. By the following spring, it had reached as far north as England, and within 5 years, it had killed 25 million people, one third of the European population. Rodents form the reservoir of infection. Flea bites and aerosols transmit the infection very efficiently. The causative organism, *Yersinia pestis*, secretes a plasminogen activator that promotes its spread. Plague was endemic in East Asia at the beginning of the 20th century and was carried to San Francisco. Seeking to avoid a panic that could be bad for business and tourism, California's governor at the time did not enforce a quarantine. As a consequence, plague is endemic in wild rodents in the western US, but fortunately it accounts for only occasional sporadic human infections. Mosquitoes are best known as vectors of malaria, sand flies of leishmaniasis, cats of toxoplasmosis, and ticks of Lyme disease.

PBD7 379-380   PBD6 387-388

32   (F) This patient has pelvic inflammatory disease (PID), which may occur as a result of infection with *Neisseria gonorrhoeae* or *Chlamydia trachomatis*. Both organisms cause sexually transmitted diseases, and chronic inflammation may lead to PID. Complications of PID include peritonitis, adhesions with bowel obstruction, sepsis with endocarditis, meningitis, arthritis, and infertility. Of the remaining organisms listed, *Candida* can produce vaginitis with a curdlike discharge, but it does not typically produce PID. Herpes simplex virus can produce painful vesicles, usually on the external genitalia, and is often recurrent. The other listed organisms often are not present in the female genital tract.

BP7 310-311, 675   BP6 593, 613   PBD7 394-395
PBD6 362

33   (D) Poliomyelitis is an enterovirus spread through fecal-oral contamination. The virus infects the oropharynx first. It then spreads to spinal cord anterior horn cells and bulbar nuclei to produce the paralysis typical of polio. In places where vaccination in routinely available, this disease is rare. Cryptococcosis most often involves the lungs and meninges. Cytomegalovirus infection can be congenital; in immunocompromised adults, it can involve many organs, principally the gastrointestinal tract, brain, and lungs. Listeriosis is most often acquired via contaminated food or water; in most adults, it produces mild diarrheal illness, but in some adults and children, and in fetuses, it can produce meningitis or dissemination with microabscess (microgranuloma) formation. Toxoplasmosis can be a congenital infection. In immunocompromised adults, it can produce inflammation in multiple tissues, but most often, it causes chronic abscessing inflammation in brain.

PBD7 364   PBD6 373

34   (A) Toxoplasmosis is the "T" in the TORCH mnemonic for congenital infections (*t*oxoplasmosis, *o*ther infections, *r*ubella, *c*ytomegalovirus infection, and *h*erpes simplex). The *Toxoplasma gondii* organisms can cross the placenta to affect the fetus. The mother is typically asymptomatic. The cat is the natural host for *T. gondii*. Fleas can be vectors for infections, such as those caused by some *Rickettsiae*, and for the Black Death, caused by *Yersinia pestis*. The pig can be involved in the life cycle of *Taenia solium* and of *Trichinella spiralis*. The sand fly is a vector for *Leishmania* infections. Ticks can transmit typhus and Lyme disease. Triatomid bugs harbor *Trypanosoma cruzi* organisms, which cause Chagas disease.

BP7 242   PBD7 477, 480   PBD6 382-383

35   (D) Leprosy, also known as Hansen disease, is caused by the small, acid-fast organism *Mycobacterium leprae*, which chronically infects peripheral nerves and skin. This organism cannot be cultured in artificial media. Diagnosis is made by biopsy of a skin lesion. There are two polar forms of leprosy: tuberculoid and lepromatous. In the tuberculoid form, a delayed hypersensitivity reaction gives rise to granulomatous lesions that resemble tuberculosis. Acid-fast bacilli are rare in such lesions. In contrast, in the lepromatous form, shown in the figure, T-cell immunity is markedly impaired and, therefore, granulomas are not formed. Instead, there are large aggregates of lipid-filled macrophages that are stuffed with acid-fast bacilli. Leprosy is poorly transmissible through aerosols (not from direct contact), probably requires some genetic susceptibility, and, like most diseases throughout human history, is linked to poverty. Cutaneous anthrax, caused by *Bacillus anthracis*, produces a necrotic skin lesion with eschar at the site of inoculation. The reduviid bug carries *Trypanosoma cruzi*, which causes Chagas disease. Its bite may cause a localized area of skin erythema and swelling. Mucocutaneous ulcers may be seen with *Leishmania braziliensis* infection, which is transmitted via sand flies. The area of the tick bite that introduces *Borrelia burgdorferi* spirochetes, the cause of Lyme disease, may manifest erythema chronicum migrans. Onchocerciasis occurs as a result of infection with the filarial nematode *Onchocerca volvulus* and leads to formation of a subcutaneous nodule.

BP7 321   BP6 276   PBD7 387-388   PBD6 385-387

36   (C) This child is infected with *Trypanosoma cruzi*, resulting in Chagas disease. The vector is the reduviid (triatomid) bug. The organisms can damage the heart by direct infection or by inducing an autoimmune response that affects the heart because of the existence of cross-reactive antigen. Acute myocarditis rarely occurs, but most deaths in acute Chagas disease are due to heart failure. In 20% of infected persons, cardiac failure can occur 5 to 15 years after the initial infection. The affected heart is enlarged, and all four chambers are dilated. A cerebral abscess or acute meningitis is typically a complication of a bacterial infection with septicemia. Chronic arthritis can be seen in Lyme disease, which is transmitted by deer ticks. Mucocutaneous ulcers may be seen in *Leishmania braziliensis* infection, which is transmitted via sand flies. Myositis can be the result of infection with *Trichinella spiralis*, which is acquired from poorly cooked pork. Paranasal sinus infection may be caused by *Mucor circinelloides*.

BP7 383-384   PBD7 405-406   PBD6 393-394

37   (B) Inhaling the arthrospores of *Coccidioides immitis* can lead to coccidioidomycosis. This disease is endemic to the southwestern US. The infection typically results in granuloma formation, but most persons have subclinical infections. About 10% may be symptomatic with respiratory symptoms, including cough and pleuritic chest pain. Dissemination to extrapulmonary sites occurs in only 1% of cases. *Aspergillus* organisms have branching septate hyphae. *Histoplasma capsulatum* organisms are about 2 to 4 μ (roughly the size of the endospores of *C. immitis*) and are often found within macrophages. *Mycobacterium tuberculosis* organisms are identified with acid-fast stains to highlight the rodlike bacterial shape. *Pseudomonas aeruginosa* is a gram-negative rodlike bacterium. *Pneumocystis carinii* produces 7-μ cysts that are seen with Gomori methenamine silver stain. *Staphylococcus aureus* grows as clusters of gram-positive cocci. *Toxoplasma gondii* produces pseudocysts filled with tachyzoites, but the pseudocyst does not have a thick wall. *T. gondii* is a rare pulmonary infection that produces small, focal, mixed inflammatory exudates.

BP7 493-495   BP6 427   PBD7 755   PBD6 353

38 (A) Rotavirus, an encapsulated RNA virus, is a major cause of diarrhea in infancy. The villous destruction with atrophy leads to decreased absorption of sodium and water. The development of antibodies from secretory immunity in the bowel to rotavirus surface antigens causes older children and adults to be relatively resistant to rotavirus infection. Such antibodies are present in maternal milk and confer some degree of resistance to infants who breast feed. Rotavirus infection occurs worldwide. By the age of 3 years, virtually every individual has been infected by rotaviruses at least once. Most rotavirus infections are subclinical or cause mild gastrointestinal illnesses that do not require hospitalization. The first infection is the most likely to be symptomatic; subsequent infections are often mild or asymptomatic. Many enteroviruses also produce diarrhea by inhibiting the intestinal absorption of intraluminal sodium and water. Most older children and adults have immunity. Cholera is the result of secretion of an exotoxin by the *Vibrio cholerae* organism, which potentiates the epithelial cell production of adenylate cyclase and causes secretory diarrhea with sodium chloride and water loss. The Yop plasmid confers infectivity to *Yersinia* organisms. Amebae can lyse epithelium, and the diarrhea can be bloody. Decreased breakdown of lactose occurs in disaccharidase deficiency and gives rise to an osmotic diarrhea.

BP6 493-494   PBD7 832-833   PBD6 354, 815

39 (E) The rash and the Koplik spots on the buccal mucosa are characteristic findings in measles, a childhood infection. It occurs only sporadically when immunizations have been administered to a large part of the population. The severity of the illness varies, and a measles pneumonia may complicate the course of the disease, which in some cases can be life threatening. Mumps produces parotitis and orchitis. Varicella-zoster virus infections in children manifest as chickenpox. Rubella, also called German measles, is a much milder infection than rubeola. Mononucleosis, which results from Epstein-Barr virus infection, is more likely to occur in adolescence.

PBD7 363-364   PBD6 370

40 (B) Although nocardial infections typically begin in the lungs, they often become disseminated, particularly to the central nervous system. These infections are most often seen in immunocompromised patients. Aspergillosis can also affect immunocompromised persons, but the fungal hyphae are easily distinguishable on hematoxylin and eosin stains. *Mycobacterium avium-intracellulare* infections are seen in persons with AIDS, but these are short, acid-fast rods that produce poorly formed granulomas. Bacterial pneumonias should also be considered in immunocompromised patients, and septicemia can complicate them, but *Staphylococcus aureus* organisms form clusters of cocci on Gram stain. *Mucor*

organisms have broad, nonseptate hyphae and are seen most often in patients with diabetes or burn injuries.

BP6 420   PBD7 376-377   PBD6 334, 722

41 (D) The result of the Gram stain is diagnostic for *Listeria monocytogenes*, an organism that is more likely to produce disseminated disease in persons who are immunocompromised. Such persons include injection drug users, who are at a high risk of HIV infection. Listeriosis is not known to be acquired parenterally or by the other listed routes, although it can be a congenital infection.

BP7 825   BP6 726   PBD7 375   PBD6 378

42 (A) The skin lesions are typical of chickenpox, a common childhood infection caused by varicella-zoster virus infection. The infection can remain dormant for years in dorsal root ganglia, only to reactivate when immune status is diminished. Infertility is a complication of mumps orchitis. Paralysis can complicate poliovirus infection. Rheumatic heart disease can appear after group A β-hemolytic streptococcal infection. A chronic arthritis can be seen with Lyme disease after *Borrelia burgdorferi* infection.

PBD7 368   PBD6 373-374

43 (A) Shigellosis results in bloody dysentery because the *Shigella* organisms can invade and destroy the mucosa. There is typically a mononuclear infiltrate extending to the lamina propria, with a neutrophilic exudate overlying the ulcerated areas. Granulomatous inflammation may be seen with granulomatous colitis (Crohn disease) and intestinal tuberculosis (rare). An increase in mononuclear inflammatory cells may be seen with milder forms of enterocolitis caused by viruses, *Giardia*, and *Salmonella* spp. Intranuclear inclusions in enterocytes point to infection with DNA viruses, such as herpesviruses. Stricture formation may follow intestinal tuberculosis.

BP7 314, 568-569   BP6 495   PBD7 834-835   PBD6 355

44 (B) The figure shows a granuloma. Activated macrophages are the key cellular component within granulomas. CD4 cells secrete interferon-γ, which activates macrophages to kill organisms with reactive nitrogen intermediates. Eosinophils are not a major component of most granulomas, and they cannot destroy mycobacteria. NADPH-dependent reactive oxygen species are important in the lysis of bacteria by neutrophils. Complement-mediated lysis is not involved in the destruction of intracellular bacteria such as *Mycobacterium tuberculosis*. However, complement activation on the surface of *M. tuberculosis* can opsonize the bacteria for uptake by macrophages. *M. tuberculosis* organisms reside in phagosomes, which are not acidified into phagolysosomes. Inhibition of acidification is caused by the urease secreted by mycobacteria.

BP7 321   BP6 421-423   PBD7 381-386   PBD6 349-351

45 (C) The figure shows a vesicle that has resulted from herpes simplex virus (HSV) infection. Most genital infections are caused by HSV-1; HSV-2 is responsible for most cases of herpetic gingivostomatitis. The viral cytopathic effect results in formation of intranuclear inclusions, multinucleated cells, and cell lysis with vesicle formation in the epithelium. Cervical dysplasias do not produce vesicular lesions and are the result of another sexually transmitted disease—human papillomavirus infection. Gram-negative diplococci are characteristic of *Neisseria gonorrhoeae* infection, also a sexually transmitted disease. Lymphoplasmacytic infiltrates may be seen in chancres caused by *Treponema pallidum*, the causative agent of syphilis. Trichomoniasis may produce small blisters or papules, but these are often self-limited and not typically recurrent.

BP7 544-545, 676-677　　BP6 595-596　　PBD7 365-366
PBD6 360-361

46 (C) These farmers are infected with *Schistosoma mansoni* or *S. japonicum*. Female worms in the portal venous system release eggs that incite a granulomatous inflammatory reaction in liver. With time, the portal granulomas undergo fibrosis, compressing the portal veins. This gives rise to severe portal hypertension, splenomegaly, and ascites. A dilated cardiomyopathy may occur with Chagas disease, in which the *Trypanosoma cruzi* organisms are transmitted through the reduviid (triatomid) bug. Elephantiasis is a complication of filariasis, which is transmitted via mosquitoes. Mucocutaneous ulcers may be seen in *Leishmania braziliensis* infection, which is transmitted via sand flies. Skin anesthesia is a feature of *Mycobacterium leprae* infection. Squamous cell carcinomas may be seen in the bladder in chronic *Schistosoma hematobium* infection. A voluminous watery diarrhea is more typical of bacterial infections such as *Vibrio cholerae*.

BP7 312　　PBD7 408-409　　PBD6 396-397

47 (E) *Pseudomonas aeruginosa* organisms secrete several virulence factors: exotoxin A, which inhibits protein synthesis; exoenzyme S, which interferes with host cell growth; phospholipase C, which degrades pulmonary surfactant; and iron-containing compounds, which are toxic to endothelial cells. These virulence factors result in extensive vasculitis with necrosis. Neutropenic patients are particularly at risk. *Coccidioides immitis* and *Histoplasma capsulatum* are fungi that can produce pulmonary disease resembling that of *Mycobacterium tuberculosis*, with granulomatous inflammation. *Pneumocystis* pneumonia is more likely to occur in patients with weak cell-mediated immunity. Pneumococcal infections produce alveolar exudates without significant vascular involvement. *Toxoplasma gondii* is a rare cause of pulmonary infection in immunocompromised patients.

BP7 319　　BP6 418　　PBD7 378-379　　PBD6 376-377

48 (D) *Vibrio cholerae* organisms are noninvasive. Instead, they produce severe diarrhea by elaboration of an enterotoxin, called cholera toxin. This toxin acts on bowel mucosal cells to cause persistent activation of adenylate cyclase and high levels of intracellular cyclic AMP that drives massive secretion of sodium, chloride, and water. The fluid loss is life threatening because of resultant dehydration. African trypanosomiasis leads to cerebral disease with sleeping sickness. Amebiasis tends to produce dysentery, with a bloody diarrhea. Aspergillosis is seen in immunocompromised patients, particularly those with neutropenia, and is a rare cause of a diarrheal illness. Filariasis involves the lymphatics and produces elephantiasis. Hydatid disease caused by *Echinococcus* produces space-occupying cystic lesions in viscera. Typhoid fever produces diarrhea and many systemic symptoms.

BP7 568-569　　BP6 495　　PBD7 835-836　　PBD6 357-358

49 (E) This patient has cysticercosis. Eating uncooked pork can result in the release of larvae that penetrate the gut wall and disseminate hematogenously, often settling in gray and white cerebral tissue, where they develop into cysts. Aspergillosis is a fungal disease in which the foci of inflammation grossly resemble granulomas, but there is often minimal inflammatory response, and the propensity for vascular invasion often produces a hemorrhagic border to the lesions. Cryptococcosis most often involves the lungs and meninges. Malaria caused by *Plasmodium falciparum* produces hemolytic anemia, splenomegaly, and cerebral thrombosis. Poliovirus infects motor neurons, producing paralysis. Toxoplasmosis can be a congenital infection. In immunocompromised adults, it can produce inflammation in multiple tissues, but most often it causes chronic abscessing inflammation in the brain. African trypanosomiasis produces sleeping sickness.

PBD7 406-407　　PBD6 395-396

50 (A) *Aspergillus*, *Candida*, and *Mucor* infections may become disseminated in the setting of neutropenia. Vascular invasion can occur with fungal infections, particularly with *Aspergillus* and *Mucor*. The branching septate hyphae are shown in the figure projecting from a fruiting body. After these organisms gain a foothold (hyphae-hold) in tissues, they are very difficult to eradicate. *Coccidioides immitis* and *Histoplasma capsulatum* are fungi that can produce pulmonary disease resembling that of *Mycobacterium tuberculosis*, with granulomatous inflammation. They do not have a propensity for vascular invasion. *Corynebacterium diphtheriae* produces upper respiratory tract disease, mainly in children who are not vaccinated against it. *Pneumocystis* pneumonia is not typically accompanied by vascular changes. Pneumococcal infections produce alveolar exudates without significant vascular involvement.

BP7 492, 494　　BP6 428　　PBD7 399-401　　PBD6 380-381

51 (C) Dengue fever, one form of hemorrhagic fever, is caused by an arbovirus of the Flavivirus group. This organism can be devastating, because it produces bone marrow suppression and because any antibodies to the virus enhance cellular viral uptake. It is transmitted by the mosquito vector, *Aedes aegypti*. The cow is in the life-cycle loop for *Taenia saginata*. Louse-borne infections include rickettsial diseases. The pig can be involved in the life cycle of *Taenia solium* and of *Trichinella spiralis*. *T. spiralis* can produce marked muscle pain, but typically not disseminated intravascular coagulopathy. Some snails can serve as an intermediate host for *Schistosoma* organisms. Ticks can transmit typhus and Lyme disease. The tsetse fly can transmit sleeping sickness, which is endemic to Africa.

PBD7 365　　PBD6 383

52 (D) These are findings of congenital syphilis. Because the spirochetes cross the placenta in the third trimester, early stillbirths do not occur. Most infants born with HIV infection have no initial gross or microscopic pathologic findings. Herpes infections in the neonate usually are not initially obvious, because most of these infections are acquired by passage through the birth canal. Congenital toxoplasmosis and cytomegalovirus produce severe cerebral disease.

BP7 321, 672-673   BP6 592   PBD7 388-390
PBD6 362-363

53 **(A)** The features are those of cutaneous and respiratory anthrax. *Bacillus anthracis* forms spores that resist environmental degradation. The spores can be transmitted by aerosols, making this organism an ideal terror weapon. Like many gram-positive organisms, *B. anthracis* produces disease via elaboration of exotoxins that have an active A subunit and a binding B subunit. None of the other choices involve outbreaks in domestic animals. Herpetic infections form clear vesicles that can rupture to shallow ulcers. *Mycobacterium leprae* can produce a faint rash early in its course, but involvement of peripheral nerves with loss of sensation predisposes to repeated trauma with deformity. *Staphylococcus aureus* can produce impetigo, typically on the face and hands. Variola major is the agent for smallpox, which is characterized by skin pustules, and pneumonia is the most likely cause of death. *Yersinia pestis* produces plague, which can have bubonic and pneumonic forms, characterized by ulcerating lymph nodes surrounded by a rosy rash.

BP7 318   PBD7 375-376   PBD6 344

54 **(A)** Gram-negative sepsis is classically mediated by endotoxins, particularly the lipopolysaccharide component of the outer cell wall. Exotoxins are typically released by gram-positive organisms such as tetanospasmin, which is released by *Clostridium tetani* organisms. Mycolic acids found in the lipid wall of mycobacteria aid in the resistance of these organisms to degradation by acute inflammatory responses, leading to granulomatous inflammation. RNA polymerase is found in negative-sense RNA viruses and produces a positive-sense mRNA that directs the host cell to produce viral components. Superantigens may produce findings similar to lipopolysaccharide-induced septic shock; the best known is toxic shock syndrome toxin, which is elaborated by some staphylococcal organisms. Tumor necrosis factor is elaborated by human inflammatory cells, not by microorganisms, but by the release of TNF by the action of endotoxins on macrophages can mimic gram-negative sepsis.

BP7 316-319   BP6 273   PBD7 350, 358   PBD6 134-136

55 **(B)** The Centers for Disease Control and Prevention has classified microbes into several categories based upon the danger they pose as agents for bioterrorism on the basis of their ease in production, dissemination, and production of serious illness. Variola major is the causative agent for small pox, and has a mortality rate of up to 30%. *Francisella tularensis* is very infectious, for only 10 to 50 organisms can cause disease. As a weapon, the bacteria can be made airborne for exposure by inhalation. Infected persons experience life-threatening pneumonia. *C. psittaci* can cause psittacosis, which can also produce pneumonitis, but the course is more variable. Hantavirus can produce a severe pneumonia, but the prodrome is longer, and the vector is the deer mouse. *M. kansasii* produces findings similar to *M. tuberculosis*. *R. typhi* is the causative agent for murine typhus with headache and rash.

PBD7 345-346

CHAPTER 9

Environmental and Nutritional Pathology

PBD7 Chapter 9: Environmental and Nutritional Pathology
PBD6 Chapter 10: Environmental and Nutritional Pathology
BP7 and BP6 Chapter 8: Environmental Diseases

1 A 55-year-old woman has been steadily gaining weight for the past 30 years. The medical history includes a cholecystectomy for cholelithiasis 5 years ago. She does not smoke. She is now 164 cm (5 ft 4 in) tall and weighs 126 kg (BMI 47). On physical examination, there is decreased range of motion with pain on movement of the knees. Laboratory studies show a serum glucose level of 176 mg/dL. This patient is at greatest risk of developing which of the following neoplasms?

- ❑ (A) Colonic adenocarcinoma
- ❑ (B) Endometrial carcinoma
- ❑ (C) Hepatocellular carcinoma
- ❑ (D) Pulmonary adenocarcinoma
- ❑ (E) Renal cell carcinoma

2 In an experiment, the effects of xenobiotic activation of the compound benzo[a]pyrene, a chemical carcinogen present in cigarette smoke, are studied in various tissues. Investigators determine that formation of a secondary metabolite, which binds covalently to DNA, increases the frequency of lung cancers. Which of the following is the most likely metabolic pathway for generation of this xenobiotic?

- ❑ (A) Biomethylation
- ❑ (B) Cytochrome P-450
- ❑ (C) Flavin-containing monooxygenase
- ❑ (D) Glucuronidation
- ❑ (E) Glutathione
- ❑ (F) Peroxidase-dependent cooxidation

3 A 50-year-old man with a history of chronic alcoholism has had increasing congestive heart failure for the past year. For the past month, he has experienced increasing confusion, disorientation, and difficulty ambulating. Physical examination shows nystagmus, ataxia of gait, and decreased sensation in the lower extremities. Laboratory studies show hemoglobin of 13.1 g/dL, hematocrit 39.3%, MCV 90 μm^3, platelet count 269,300/mm^3, and WBC count 7120/mm^3. A long-term dietary deficiency of which of the following nutrients is most likely to produce these findings?

- ❑ (A) Folate
- ❑ (B) Thiamine
- ❑ (C) Pyridoxine
- ❑ (D) Niacin
- ❑ (E) Riboflavin

4 A 9-month-old infant has failure to thrive. The examining physician elicits a history of prematurity and low birth weight. The parents, who have two other children, admit they have difficulty providing food, clothing, and medical care for their growing family. The infant is now at the 40th percentile for height and the 25th percentile for weight. He exhibits absent deep tendon reflexes, decreased vibration and pain sense, muscle weakness, and abnormalities of eye movement. Laboratory studies show hemoglobin of 9.2 g/dL, hematocrit 27.6%, MCV 86 μm³, platelet count 208,000/mm³, WBC count 6080/mm³, total protein 6.4 g/dL, albumin 3.4 g/dL, glucose 70 mg/dL, and creatinine 0.3 mg/dL. A deficiency of which of the following vitamins is most likely to contribute to these findings?

- ❑ (A) Vitamin A
- ❑ (B) Vitamin B₁
- ❑ (C) Vitamin B₃
- ❑ (D) Vitamin B₁₂
- ❑ (E) Vitamin C
- ❑ (F) Vitamin E
- ❑ (G) Vitamin K

5 A 19-year-old pregnant woman receives no prenatal care, eats a diet containing mostly carbohydrates and fats, and does not take prenatal vitamins with iron. She feels increasingly tired and weak during the third trimester. The infant is born at 35 weeks gestation and is listless during the first week of life. Laboratory studies show markedly decreased serum ferritin levels in both infant and mother. Which of the following conditions is most likely to be present in the infant and mother?

- ❑ (A) Peripheral neuropathy
- ❑ (B) Goiter
- ❑ (C) Microcytic anemia
- ❑ (D) Dermatitis
- ❑ (E) Skeletal deformities
- ❑ (F) Soft tissue hemorrhages

6 A 42-year-old woman with a chronic cough has a positive tuberculin skin test result. A chest radiograph shows several cavitary lesions in the right upper lobe. The woman is given isoniazid therapy. On physical examination 6 months later, a peripheral neuropathy is observed. Administration of which of the following with isoniazid would most likely have prevented the neuropathy?

- ❑ (A) Ascorbic acid
- ❑ (B) Calcium
- ❑ (C) Cobalamin (vitamin B₁₂)
- ❑ (D) Folate
- ❑ (E) Niacin
- ❑ (F) Pyridoxine
- ❑ (G) Riboflavin

7 A 29-year-old previously healthy man suddenly collapses at a party where legal and illicit drugs are being used. En route to the hospital, he requires resuscitation with defibrillation to establish a normal cardiac rhythm. His vital signs are temperature 40°C, respirations 30/min, heart rate 110/min, and blood pressure 175/90 mm Hg. Physical examination shows dilated pupils, a perforated nasal septum, and a prominent callus on the right thumb. CT scan of the head shows an acute right frontal lobe hemorrhage. Which of the following substances detectable in blood and urine is most likely responsible for these findings?

- ❑ (A) Ethanol
- ❑ (B) Heroin
- ❑ (C) Marijuana
- ❑ (D) Phencyclidine
- ❑ (E) Cocaine
- ❑ (F) Amphetamine
- ❑ (G) Barbiturate

8 A 26-year-old woman with a 6-month history of depression accompanied by active suicidal ideation ingests 35 g of acetaminophen. She quickly experiences nausea and vomiting. Within 1 day, she becomes progressively obtunded. On physical examination, her temperature is 36.9°C, pulse 75/min, respirations 15/min, and blood pressure 100/65 mm Hg. Which of the following laboratory findings is likely to indicate the most severe organ damage?

- ❑ (A) Hypokalemia
- ❑ (B) Elevated serum CK
- ❑ (C) Ketonuria
- ❑ (D) Elevated serum ALT
- ❑ (E) Hyperamylasemia

9 An infant born at term has Apgar scores of 8 and 9 at 1 and 5 minutes. The infant appears healthy, but 3 days after birth, there is bleeding from the umbilical cord stump, and ecchymoses are observed over the buttocks. Seizures soon develop. A deficiency of which of the following nutrients best accounts for these findings?

- ❑ (A) Iron
- ❑ (B) Vitamin E
- ❑ (C) Folic acid
- ❑ (D) Vitamin K
- ❑ (E) Iodine

10 Sir Robert Falcon Scott reaches the South Pole on January 17, 1912, barely 1 month after Roald Amundsen achieves this goal with a more experienced and prepared expeditionary party. Scott's dejected party must now make the long trip back to their base, but they are weak and running low on supplies, and the weather is unusually cold, even for Antarctica. Finally, they can go no further because of severe storms. Months later, a rescue team finds the bodies of the men. All have a hyperkeratotic, papular rash, ecchymoses, and severe gingival swelling with hemorrhages. Which of the following was most likely to be a contributing cause of death in these men?

- ❑ (A) Rickets
- ❑ (B) Beriberi
- ❑ (C) Scurvy
- ❑ (D) Kwashiorkor
- ❑ (E) Pellagra

11 For the past 3 years, a 72-year-old man has noticed a gradually enlarging nodule on the right lower eyelid. On physical examination, the 0.8-cm nodule is firm and has a small central area of ulceration. The nodule is excised, and plastic repair to the eyelid is performed. Which of the following forms of electromagnetic radiation most likely played the greatest role in the development of this lesion?

- ❏ (A) Ultraviolet rays
- ❏ (B) Infrared rays
- ❏ (C) Visible rays
- ❏ (D) X-rays
- ❏ (E) Gamma rays

12 Several children between the ages of 3 and 6 have been admitted to a local hospital because of encephalopathic crisis. They have lived in the same community all their lives. All have previously exhibited retarded psychomotor development. On physical examination, the children have diffuse abdominal pain and are experiencing nausea and vomiting. CT scans of the head show marked cerebral edema. Laboratory studies show microcytic anemia. An investigator sent to the housing project where the children live finds a run-down apartment complex with extensive water damage, poor plumbing, lack of ventilation, and peeling, flaking paint. Toxic exposure to which of the following substances best accounts for these findings?

- ❏ (A) Sodium hypochlorite
- ❏ (B) Ethylene glycol
- ❏ (C) Methanol
- ❏ (D) Kerosene
- ❏ (E) Lead

13 A 33-year-old man incurs thermal burn injuries to 40% of his total body surface area in an accidental fire while repairing a fuel storage tank. On physical examination, the skin of the trunk, neck, and face is pink, shows blister formation, and is painful to touch. The skin of the arms is white and anesthetic. Skin grafting is necessary on the arms but not on other injured areas of skin. Which of the following structures is most likely absent from the sites that required skin grafting?

- ❏ (A) Collagen fibers
- ❏ (B) Dermal appendages
- ❏ (C) Epidermal basal layer
- ❏ (D) Keratin
- ❏ (E) Macrophages
- ❏ (F) Nerves

14 While touring the grounds of the Imperial Palace in Kyoto, a 75-year-old woman collapses suddenly. She remains conscious but says that she feels weak and light-headed. On physical examination by the nurse, her temperature is 35.2°C, pulse 93/min, respirations 17/min, and blood pressure 95/50 mm Hg. The temperature in the shade is 34°C with 90% humidity. One hour after drinking cool green tea, the woman revives and is able to return to her hotel. Which of the following terms best describes these findings?

- ❏ (A) Heat cramps
- ❏ (B) Thermal inhalation injury
- ❏ (C) Heat exhaustion
- ❏ (D) Malignant hyperthermia
- ❏ (E) Heat stroke

15 A previously healthy 52-year-old man has an episode of hemoptysis with coughing. He does not smoke. On physical examination, he has wheezes and dullness to percussion over the right lung. A chest radiograph shows a 6-cm, perihilar mass in the right upper lobe. Laboratory studies include sputum cytology showing atypical squamous cells suggestive of lung cancer. Which of the following inhaled pollutants is most likely to produce these findings?

- ❏ (A) Carbon monoxide
- ❏ (B) Ozone
- ❏ (C) Radon gas
- ❏ (D) Silica
- ❏ (E) Carbonaceous dust

16 An epidemiologic study observes increased numbers of respiratory tract infections among children living in a community in which most families are at the poverty level. The infectious agents include *Streptococcus pneumoniae,* *Haemophilus influenzae,* and *Klebsiella pneumoniae*. Most of the children have had pneumonitis and rubeola infection. The study documents increased rates of keratomalacia, urinary tract calculi, and generalized papular dermatosis in these children. A deficiency of which of the following vitamins is most likely to be present in these children?

- ❏ (A) Vitamin E
- ❏ (B) Vitamin D
- ❏ (C) Vitamin K
- ❏ (D) Vitamin A
- ❏ (E) Vitamin B$_1$

17 A 22-year-old man is brought to the hospital emergency department by a friend, who found him unconscious in his apartment after trying to contact him for 3 days. On arrival, the patient is in a state of respiratory depression. He experiences convulsions for several minutes, followed by cardiac arrest. Advanced cardiac life support measures are instituted, and he is stabilized and intubated. On physical examination, there are needle tracks in the left antecubital fossa, and a loud diastolic heart murmur is audible. The patient has a temperature of 39.2°C. Use of which of the following substances most likely produced these findings?

- ❏ (A) Cocaine
- ❏ (B) Ethanol
- ❏ (C) Flurazepam
- ❏ (D) Heroin
- ❏ (E) Meperidine
- ❏ (F) Phencyclidine
- ❏ (G) Phenobarbital

18 A 20-year-old star football player suddenly collapses during practice and has a cardiac arrest and cannot be resuscitated. The medical examiner is called to investigate this sudden and unexpected death. At autopsy, there is marked coronary atherosclerosis and histologic evidence of hypertension in the renal blood vessels. Use of which of the following substances is most likely to contribute to these findings?

❑ (A) Amphetamine
❑ (B) Barbiturate
❑ (C) Benzodiazepine
❑ (D) Cocaine
❑ (E) Ethanol
❑ (F) Heroin
❑ (G) Marijuana

19 A 36-year-old man is the owner of a radiator repair shop, where he works cleaning, cutting, polishing, and welding metals. The shop is poorly ventilated. Over several months, he develops worsening malaise with headache and abdominal pains and has difficulty holding his tools. CBC indicates microcytic anemia, and basophilic stippling of RBCs is seen on the peripheral blood smear. An elevated blood level of which of the following would be most useful in determining the toxic exposure causing this illness?

❑ (A) Alanine aminotransferase
❑ (B) Creatine kinase
❑ (C) Zinc protoporphyrin
❑ (D) Sodium
❑ (E) Calcium

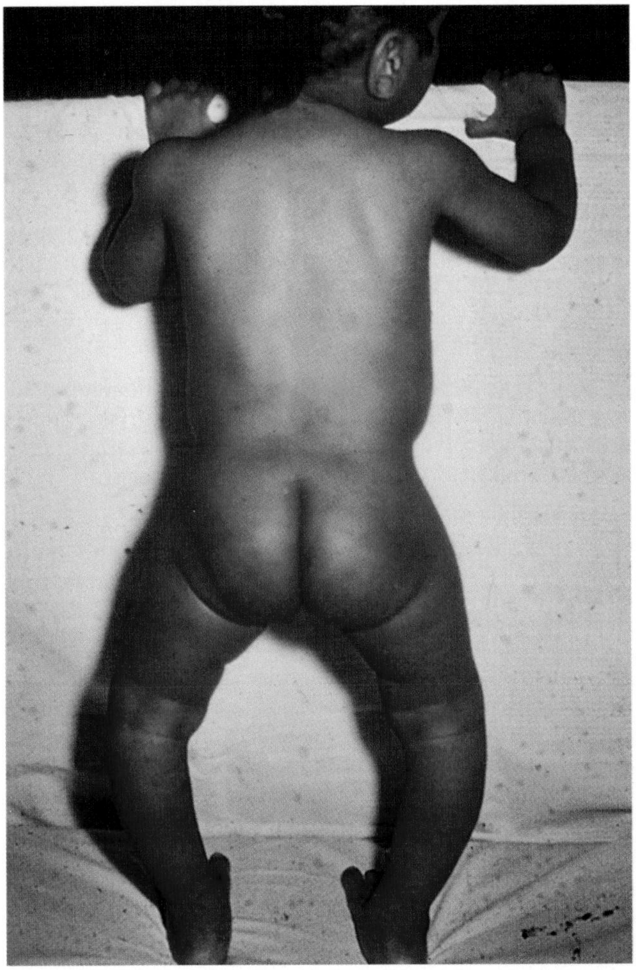

20 The parents of a 3-year-old boy are concerned because their son does not appear to be developing normally. On physical examination, the child has the appearance shown in the figure above. Vision testing is normal. There are no petechiae or areas of purpura on the skin. The abdomen is not enlarged. Which of the following is the most likely diagnosis?

❑ (A) Scurvy
❑ (B) Rickets
❑ (C) Pellagra
❑ (D) Beriberi
❑ (E) Kwashiorkor

21 A 7-year-old boy falls off his bicycle while traveling down the street at 5 km/h. The skin of his right calf and right arm scrape along the pavement, and the top layer of epidermis is removed. Which of the following terms best describes this injury?

❑ (A) Incision
❑ (B) Contusion
❑ (C) Laceration
❑ (D) Burn
❑ (E) Abrasion

22 An epidemiologic study evaluates the rate of dental caries and tooth abscesses among children living in communities within a metropolitan area. Investigators discover that the rate is high among children in an upper middle class community but low in a community of persons living below the poverty level. The levels of trace elements in the water supplies for those communities are measured. A higher level of which of the following minerals in the water is most likely to be associated with a lower rate of dental decay among children?

❑ (A) Zinc
❑ (B) Iodine
❑ (C) Selenium
❑ (D) Fluoride
❑ (E) Copper

23 A 75-year-old woman lives alone and eats sparingly because of her low fixed retirement income. For the past 2 weeks, she has noticed a pain in her right leg. On physical examination, there is marked tenderness to palpation over the lateral aspect of the right shin, a poorly healed cut on the right hand, and a diffuse hyperkeratotic skin rash. A radiograph shows a right tibial diaphyseal subperiosteal hematoma. Laboratory studies show a hemoglobin level of 11.3 g/dL. A deficiency of which of the following is most likely to explain these findings?

❑ (A) Ascorbic acid
❑ (B) Folate
❑ (C) Niacin
❑ (D) Riboflavin
❑ (E) Selenium
❑ (F) Vitamin A
❑ (G) Vitamin K
❑ (H) Zinc

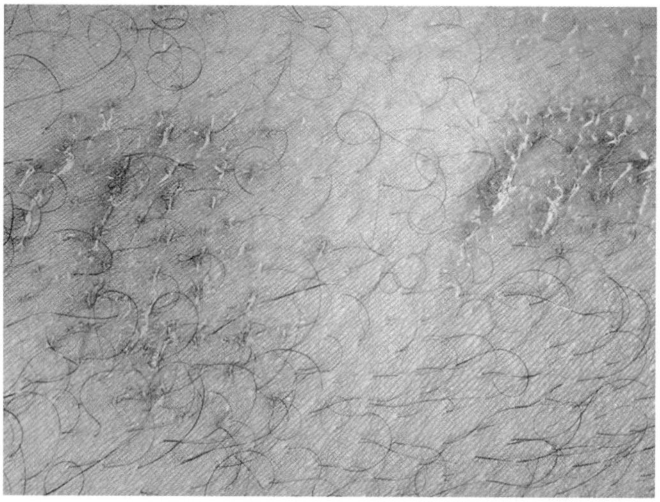

From the teaching collection of the Department of Pathology, University of Texas Southwestern Medical School, Dallas, TX.

24 A 5-year-old boy is brought to the physician for examination. A police agency suspects child abuse. On physical examination, the child's skin has the appearance shown above. Which of the following terms best describes this injury?

- ❑ (A) Abrasion
- ❑ (B) Contusion
- ❑ (C) Gunshot wound
- ❑ (D) Hypothermia
- ❑ (E) Incision
- ❑ (F) Kwashiorkor
- ❑ (G) Laceration
- ❑ (H) Thermal burn

25 Over the past 7 months, a 60-year-old woman with a 90 pack-year history of smoking cigarettes has developed a worsening cough. One week ago, she had an episode of hemoptysis. A chest radiograph shows a 7-cm infiltrative, perihilar mass in the right lung. Exposure to which of the following is most likely to be associated with these findings?

- ❑ (A) Carbon monoxide
- ❑ (B) Nicotine
- ❑ (C) Nitrous oxide compounds
- ❑ (D) Ozone
- ❑ (E) Polycyclic aromatic hydrocarbons
- ❑ (F) Silica
- ❑ (G) Sulfur dioxide

26 A 75-year-old man who lives alone in a poorly ventilated house without central heating uses a portable unvented kerosene heater to warm the house during the winter months. One morning, a neighbor finds him in an obtunded state. On physical examination, he appears cyanotic. Results of blood gas measurement on room air are PO_2 90 mm Hg, PCO_2 35 mm Hg, and pH 7.3. Pulse oximetry shows low O_2 saturation. Exposure to which of the following is most likely to have produced this man's illness?

- ❑ (A) Beryllium
- ❑ (B) Carbon monoxide
- ❑ (C) Nitrous oxide compounds
- ❑ (D) Oxygen
- ❑ (E) Ozone
- ❑ (F) Polycyclic aromatic hydrocarbons
- ❑ (G) Sulfur dioxide

27 A 3-year-old child has had a succession of respiratory infections during the past 6 months. On physical examination, the child appears chronically ill, listless, and underdeveloped. He is 50% of ideal body weight and has marked muscle wasting. Laboratory findings include hemoglobin of 9.4 g/dL, hematocrit 27.9%, MCV 75 μm^3, platelet count 182,000/mm^3, WBC count 6730/mm^3, serum albumin 4.1 g/dL, total protein 6.8 g/dL, glucose 52 mg/dL, and creatinine 0.3 mg/dL. Which of the following conditions is most likely to explain these findings?

- ❑ (A) Marasmus
- ❑ (B) Leukemia
- ❑ (C) Folate deficiency
- ❑ (D) Kwashiorkor
- ❑ (E) Bulimia
- ❑ (F) Lead poisoning

28 A 3-year-old child has erosion of a roughened corneal surface caused by xerophthalmia. Keratomalacia results in corneal scarring with eventual blindness after several years. This ocular damage could most likely have been prevented by treating a dietary deficiency of which of the following nutrients?

- ❑ (A) Protein
- ❑ (B) Vitamin K
- ❑ (C) Iron
- ❑ (D) Niacin
- ❑ (E) Vitamin A

29 A 40-year-old man with a family history of colon carcinoma asks the physician how best to reduce his risk of developing this type of cancer. Which of the following dietary practices should he be advised to follow each day?

- ❑ (A) Drink a glass of red wine
- ❑ (B) Eat a bowl of ice cream
- ❑ (C) Reduce intake of chocolate
- ❑ (D) Consume more beef
- ❑ (E) Eat more vegetables

30 In a study of lifestyle influences on health, investigators observe that sending children outside to play instead of letting them sit for hours in front of the television set can have long-term health benefits. Which of the following tissues is most likely to be in better condition by middle age from this lifestyle change?

- ❑ (A) Bones
- ❑ (B) Eyes
- ❑ (C) Skin
- ❑ (D) Lungs
- ❑ (E) Kidneys

31 A 5-year-old child is admitted to the hospital after ingesting pills he found in a cabinet at home. The child is rapidly becoming obtunded. Laboratory studies show a serum AST level of 850 U/L and ALT level of 1052 U/L. The child's respiratory and cardiac status remain stable. Which of the following drugs was most likely ingested?

- (A) Acetaminophen
- (B) Penicillin
- (C) Aspirin
- (D) Sulfamethoxazole
- (E) Codeine

32 A 45-year-old man, whose mother, father, brother, and uncle all had a history of heart disease, asks his physician about ways to reduce his risk of developing coronary artery disease. The patient is 171 cm (5 ft 6 in) tall, weighs 91 kg, and has a blood pressure of 125/80 mm Hg. His blood glucose concentration is 181 mg/dL. Which of the following is the best dietary advice to give this patient?

- (A) Reduce intake of saturated fat
- (B) Increase dietary fiber
- (C) Take vitamin A supplements
- (D) Avoid adding salt to food
- (E) Drink more water

33 A 55-year-old man with a 60 pack-year history of smoking has been diagnosed with a squamous cell carcinoma of the larynx. He receives 4000 cGy in divided doses to treat the carcinoma. One year later, endoscopy shows no gross evidence of residual carcinoma. Which of the following is most likely to be present in this patient as a result of treatment?

- (A) Hypocellular bone marrow
- (B) Absent spermatogenesis
- (C) Colonic ulceration
- (D) Vascular fibrosis
- (E) Cerebral atrophy

34 During a qualifying match for the World Cup, the goalkeeper is hit in the chest by a soccer ball kicked from 10 m away. He stays in the game. Which of the following injury patterns is most likely to be seen over the chest of the goalkeeper?

- (A) Contusion
- (B) Abrasion
- (C) Laceration
- (D) Incision
- (E) Puncture

35 While attending a party, a 19-year-old university student drinks 2 L of mixed alcoholic beverages containing 50% ethanol by volume over a period of 30 minutes. He usually does not drink much alcohol. His major use of drugs consists of acetaminophen for headaches. Which of the following complications is most likely to occur?

- (A) Hepatic cirrhosis
- (B) Acute pancreatitis
- (C) Coma and death
- (D) Wernicke disease
- (E) Massive hematemesis

36 Over the past year, a 55-year-old woman has had worsening problems with memory and the ability to carry out tasks of daily living. She has had watery diarrhea for the past 3 months. Physical examination shows red, scaling skin in sun-exposed areas. The deep tendon reflexes are normal, and sensation is intact. Which of the following is the most likely diagnosis?

- (A) Beriberi
- (B) Cheilosis
- (C) Hypothyroidism
- (D) Marasmus
- (E) Pellagra
- (F) Scurvy

37 A 72-year-old man has had increasing dyspnea for the past year. Decreased breath sounds are heard on auscultation of the right side of the chest. A chest radiograph shows a large pleural mass that nearly encases the right lung. A pleural biopsy specimen shows a malignant mesothelioma. Exposure to which of the following is most likely to be associated with these findings?

- (A) Arsenic
- (B) Asbestos
- (C) Benzidine
- (D) Chromium
- (E) Naphthylamine
- (F) Nickel

38 A 20-year-old man is trying to repair an old electrical appliance in his garage. While testing the function of the appliance, his right hand comes in contact with a frayed electrical cord carrying 120-volt, 10-ampere alternating current. Which of the following is most likely to develop as a consequence of this electrical injury?

- (A) Bronchoconstriction
- (B) Cerebral artery thrombosis
- (C) Heat stroke
- (D) Gastric hemorrhage
- (E) Ventricular fibrillation

39 A 5-year-old child has had recurrent upper respiratory infections for the past 2 months. The child is at the 55th percentile for height and the 40th percentile for weight. Physical examination shows generalized edema, ascites, muscle wasting, and areas of desquamating skin over the trunk and extremities. Laboratory studies are most likely to show which of the following findings?

- (A) Hyperglycemia
- (B) Hypoalbuminemia
- (C) Abetalipoproteinemia
- (D) Megaloblastic anemia
- (E) Hypocalcemia

40 A 48-year-old woman injured her right wrist in a fall down a flight of stairs. On physical examination, she has marked pain on palpation of the wrist and does not want to move the hand. A radiograph of the right hand and arm shows marked osteopenia and a fracture of the radial head. Which of the following underlying diseases is most likely to contribute to the risk of fracture in this patient?

- (A) Coronary atherosclerosis
- (B) Pulmonary emphysema
- (C) Primary biliary cirrhosis
- (D) Chronic lymphocytic leukemia
- (E) Atrophic gastritis

41 For the past 6 months, a 61-year-old man with a history of chronic arthritis has had pronounced tinnitus and episodes of dizziness and headache. Physical examination shows scattered petechiae over the skin of the upper extremities. There is no apparent bone conduction or nerve hearing loss. A stool guaiac test result is positive. Toxicity from which of the following drugs best explains these findings?

- (A) Penicillin
- (B) Tetracycline
- (C) Aspirin
- (D) Chlorpromazine
- (E) Quinidine

42 A 26-year-old woman has had amenorrhea for the past 8 years. She fractured her right wrist 1 year ago after a minor fall to the ground. On physical examination, she is 175 cm (5 ft 7 in) tall and weighs 52 kg (BMI 17). She has normal secondary sex characteristics. There are no abnormal findings. Radiographic measurement of bone density by dual energy x-ray absorptiometry shows a bone mineral density that is 1.5 standard deviations below the young adult reference range. Laboratory findings include anemia and hypoalbuminemia. Which of the following is the most likely diagnosis?

- (A) Kwashiorkor
- (B) Chronic alcoholism
- (C) Anorexia nervosa
- (D) Scurvy
- (E) Rickets

43 A poorly funded epidemiologic study is conducted, and the results appear in a publication available at the supermarket checkout counter. The study analyzes the diet of textbook authors. Which of the following is determined to be the most likely dietary deficiency in this population?

- (A) Iron
- (B) Calcium
- (C) Folate
- (D) Vitamin C
- (E) Chocolate

44 The firemen who initially responded to fight the fires from the Chernobyl nuclear reactor accident were exposed to high radiation levels. Some of the men received dosages exceeding 5000 cGy. Within hours, many became extremely ill. Damage to which of the following tissues most likely led to this finding?

- (A) Bone marrow
- (B) Cerebrum
- (C) Small intestine
- (D) Heart
- (E) Lungs

45 A 30-year-old woman is found dead in her hotel room 3 hours after firemen extinguish a fire on the floor below. Investigation of the scene shows no signs of fire within her room, and the medical examiner observes no external findings on the body. Which of the following injuries best explains the woman's death?

- (A) Pseudomonas aeruginosa septicemia
- (B) Pulmonary edema
- (C) Acute myocardial infarction
- (D) Cerebral edema
- (E) Malignant hyperthermia

46 A 46-year-old woman has a 25-year history of excessive ethanol consumption. She has had increasing malaise and weakness for the past 5 months. On physical examination, she appears cachectic with muscle wasting and decreased strength in all extremities. Which of the following conditions is most likely to be present?

- (A) Blindness
- (B) Carcinoma of the esophagus
- (C) Dementia
- (D) Peripheral vascular disease
- (E) Acute renal failure

47 A 23-year-old woman is delivered of a stillborn fetus at 36 weeks' gestation. The woman experienced sudden onset of lower abdominal pain several hours before delivery. An abdominal ultrasound scan showed a large retroplacental hemorrhage. Delivery was accompanied by a 1200-mL blood loss. Maternal use of which of the following agents is most likely to be associated with these findings?

- (A) Acetaminophen
- (B) Amphetamine
- (C) Cannabinoids
- (D) Cocaine
- (E) Ethanol
- (F) Heroin
- (G) Lysergic acid

48 A 4-year-old child ingests a 100-mL bottle of a clear liquid found under the kitchen sink in the home. Over the next 6 hours, he develops central nervous system depression. Laboratory studies show serum Na^+ of 141 mmol/L, K^+ 3.9 mmol/L, Cl^- 93 mmol/L, CO_2 18 mmol/L, glucose 72 mg/dL, creatinine 0.4 mg/dL, AST 29 U/L, ALT 18 U/L, and total bilirubin 0.7 mg/dL. Several weeks later, the child's visual acuity is markedly decreased. Toxic exposure to which of the following substances is most likely to explain this child's illness?

- (A) Cyanide
- (B) Ethanol
- (C) Gasoline
- (D) Lead arsenate
- (E) Mercuric chloride
- (F) Methanol
- (G) Organophosphate insecticide

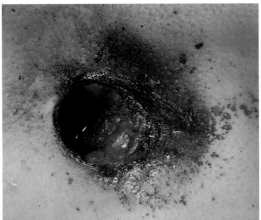

Courtesy of George Katsas, MD, forensic pathologist, Boston, MA.

49 A 14-year-old boy was taken to the emergency department of a local hospital, where he died several hours later. The principal finding on examination is shown. Laboratory studies showed that the hematocrit was 17%. Which of the following terms best describes this injury?

❏ (A) Abrasion
❏ (B) Blast injury
❏ (C) Contusion
❏ (D) Electrocution injury
❏ (E) Gunshot wound
❏ (F) Incision
❏ (G) Laceration

50 In an epidemiologic study of persons whose BMI is greater than 35, data on lifestyle and disease patterns are collected. Investigators observe that a subset of obese persons has a consistently high caloric intake, because they lack a feeling of satiety when eating. These persons have diminished responsiveness of a hypothalamic receptor to a substance elaborated by adipocytes. Which of the following receptors is most likely to be affected?

❏ (A) Adenosine
❏ (B) Glucagon
❏ (C) Glucose
❏ (D) Insulin
❏ (E) Leptin
❏ (F) LDL

51 A clinical trial involves patients with a diagnosis of cancer who have intractable nausea as a result of chemotherapy. The patients are divided into two groups; one group is given a placebo, and one group is given a drug. The group receiving the drug is found to have reduced self-reported nausea and diminished weight loss, compared with the placebo group. The patients receiving the drug appear to have no major adverse side effects. Of the following agents, classified as drugs of abuse in parts of the world, which is most likely to have the beneficial effects found in this study?

❏ (A) Barbiturate
❏ (B) Cocaine
❏ (C) Heroin
❏ (D) Marijuana
❏ (E) Methylphenidate
❏ (F) Methamphetamine
❏ (G) Phencyclidine

52 A case-control study seeks to identify long-term effects of hormone replacement therapy (HRT) in postmenopausal women receiving exogenous estrogens coupled with progestins compared with a control group not receiving this therapy. The medical records of the women in the study are reviewed after 20 years. Investigators find that the women who received HRT have a decreased incidence of osteoporosis and its complications but an increased risk of breast carcinoma. Which of the following conditions, in addition to these findings, is most likely to be observed in the women receiving HRT?

❏ (A) Cervical carcinoma
❏ (B) Chronic ulcerative colitis
❏ (C) Hepatic cirrhosis
❏ (D) Pulmonary emphysema
❏ (E) Thromboembolism

53 A 36-year-old woman has been using low dose estrogen-containing oral contraceptives for the past 20 years. She has smoked 1 pack of cigarettes per day for the past 18 years. She is G 2 P 2, and both pregnancies ended with term liveborn infants of low birth weight, but no anomalies. On physical examination no abnormal findings are noted. Her BMI is 24. She is at increased risk for developing which of the following conditions?

❏ (A) Breast carcinoma
❏ (B) Cholecystitis
❏ (C) Dementia
❏ (D) Endometrial carcinoma
❏ (E) Myocardial infarction
❏ (F) Ovarian carcinoma

54 It is 1:00 AM and a hard-working 2nd year medical student is intent on finishing her pathology reading assignment. Soon she begins to note that her concentration is fading, because 7 hours have passed since she had dinner, and she is feeling famished. Having studied the chapter on ischemic heart disease, she decides to be prudent and forgoes her favorite chocolate cookies, and instead devours 2 apples, gulping them down with a glass of low fat milk. Of the following substances, which one was most likely to have risen rapidly when she became hungry and declined promptly after she finished her healthy snack?

❏ (A) Ghrelin
❏ (B) Leptin
❏ (C) Corticotropin releasing factor (CRF)
❏ (D) α-MSH
❏ (E) Thyrotropin releasing hormone (TRH)

ANSWERS

1 **(B)** This patient is morbidly obese. The extra weight puts a strain on joints, particularly the knees. Although the overall risk of cancer increases with obesity, the relationship between endometrial carcinoma and obesity is well established. About 80% of persons with type 2 diabetes mellitus are obese. The relationship of diet and obesity to colon cancer is not as well established. Worldwide, most hepatocellular carcinomas arise in persons infected with hepatitis B; chronic alcoholism is also a risk factor. Pulmonary adenocarcinoma is the least likely bronchogenic cancer to be associated with smoking. Some renal cell carcinomas are associated with smoking.

BP7 303-305   BP6 259-261   PBD7 465   PBD6 452-454

2 **(B)** The cytochrome P-450–dependent monooxygenase, or mixed function oxidase, system is found in smooth endoplasmic reticulum and normally functions to detoxify endogenous hormones. However, it can also serve to activate xenobiotics to carcinogens. Biomethylation by environmental microorganisms of inorganic mercury dumped into bodies of water can lead to accumulation of toxic methyl mercury, which can work its way up the food chain to humans. Flavin-containing monooxygenase found in endoplasmic reticulum can oxidize nicotine. Glucuronidation can convert naphthylamine to a carcinogen that causes urinary tract cancers. Reduced glutathione helps to break down free radicals produced by oxygenase systems such as P-450; xenobiotic metabolism can deplete glutathione and enhance free radical cellular injury. The peroxidase-dependent cooxidation pathway can metabolize 2-naphthylamine to a carcinogen that causes urinary tract cancers.

PBD7 417-419   PBD6 405-408

3 **(B)** Persons with a history of chronic alcoholism are often deficient in thiamine and other nutrients (ethanol provides "empty calories"). Thiamine deficiency can lead to neuropathy, cardiomyopathy, and Wernicke disease. Alcoholic persons often have folate deficiency, with resultant macrocytic anemia. However, these findings were not described in the question. Pyridoxine or riboflavin deficiency can lead to neuropathy but do not produce cerebral findings. Niacin deficiency leads to pellagra.

BP7 302   BP6 254-255   PBD7 422-423, 456-457
PBD6 447

4 **(F)** Vitamin E deficiency is uncommon, but it may be seen in low birth weight infants with poor hepatic function and fat malabsorption. The neurologic manifestations are somewhat similar to those seen in vitamin B_{12} deficiency; affected infants may have anemia, but it is not of the megaloblastic type. Vitamin A deficiency in infants and children can lead to blindness from keratomalacia. It is the most common cause of preventable blindness in this population group. Vitamin B_1 (thiamine) deficiency can lead to beriberi. Vitamin B_3 (niacin) deficiency can lead to pellagra. Vitamin C deficiency leads to scurvy, which can be accompanied by anemia from bleeding and from decreased iron absorption. Vitamin K deficiency leads to bleeding problems.

BP7 301   BP6 231   PBD7 455-456   PBD6 414-416

5 **(C)** Iron deficiency, which gives rise to microcytic anemia, is common in women of reproductive age, because of menstrual blood loss, and in children with a poor diet. During pregnancy, women have greatly increased iron needs. Low serum ferritin is indicative of iron deficiency. Peripheral neuropathy is more characteristic of beriberi (thiamine deficiency) and deficiencies in riboflavin (vitamin B_2) and pyridoxine (vitamin B_6). Goiter results from iodine deficiency, but this is a rare occurrence today. Dermatitis can be seen in

pellagra (niacin deficiency). Bowing of the long bones and epiphyseal widening can be seen in rickets (vitamin D deficiency). Soft tissue hemorrhages can be seen in scurvy (vitamin C deficiency).

BP7 303   BP6 258   PBD7 643-646   PBD6 452

6 **(F)** Isoniazid (INH) is a pyridoxine (vitamin B_6) antagonist. Persons receiving INH therapy for tuberculosis may need supplementation to prevent vitamin B_6 deficiency. Ascorbic acid (vitamin C) is antiscorbutic. Calcium intake helps maintain bone mass and serum calcium level. Cobalamin (vitamin B_{12}) deficiency may produce a macrocytic anemia and a peripheral neuropathy, but it does not result from INH therapy. Folate deficiency leads to macrocytic anemia. Niacin deficiency causes pellagra. Riboflavin deficiency may produce neuropathy, glossitis, and cheilosis.

BP7 302   BP6 256   PBD7 458   PBD6 449

7 **(E)** Cocaine is a powerful vasoconstrictor and has a variety of vascular effects, including ischemic injury to the nasal septum following the route of administration—inhalation. Many complications result from the cardiovascular effects, which include arterial vasoconstriction with ischemic injury to the heart, arrhythmias, and central nervous system (CNS) hemorrhages. Hyperthermia is another complication. The callus is caused by flicking a lighter when using a crack cocaine pipe. Acute ethanolism may lead to CNS depression, but it does not have serious immediate cardiac effects. Opiates can depress CNS and respiratory function, and heroin may produce acute pulmonary edema. Marijuana has no serious acute toxicities. Phencyclidine (PCP) produces an acute toxicity that mimics psychosis. Amphetamines are CNS stimulants. Barbiturates are CNS depressants.

BP7 282-283   BP6 236   PBD7 424-425   PBD6 412-413

8 **(D)** Acetaminophen toxicity leads to hepatic necrosis, indicated by elevated ALT and AST levels. If death is not immediate, hyperbilirubinemia can also be seen. Hypokalemia can be a feature of renal diseases and of glucocorticoid deficiency. Elevated serum creatine kinase is seen with injury to skeletal and cardiac muscle. Ketonuria is a feature of absolute insulin deficiency in diabetes mellitus; it is also a feature of starvation. Elevated serum amylase is seen in pancreatitis.

BP7277-278   BP6 231   PBD7 426, 428   PBD6 416

9 **(D)** Coagulation factors synthesized by the liver require vitamin K for their production. Hemorrhagic disease of the newborn can occur in infants who lack sufficient intestinal bacterial flora to produce this nutrient. Iron deficiency leads to anemia, not to bleeding. Vitamin E is an antioxidant and is rarely deficient to a degree that would cause serious illness. Folic acid helps to prevent macrocytic anemia. Iodine is needed in small quantities for thyroid hormone synthesis.

BP7 301   BP6 253-254   PBD7 456   PBD6 446-447

10 **(C)** Because humans do not generate vitamin C endogenously, they must have a continuous dietary supply. The lack of fresh fruits and vegetables containing vitamin C led to scurvy in many explorers in centuries past. Rickets is seen in children who are deficient in vitamin D. Beriberi leads to heart failure and results from thiamine deficiency. Kwashiorkor results from protein deficiency. Pellagra, characterized by the

"3 Ds" of diarrhea, dermatitis, and dementia, is seen in niacin deficiency.

BP7 298-301   BP6 256-257   PBD7 458-459
PBD6 449-451

11 (A) Exposure to sunlight is a risk of developing malignancies involving the skin (basal cell carcinoma, squamous cell carcinoma, and malignant melanoma). Ultraviolet (UV) rays, mainly the UVB component, are the major causative agent of these malignancies. Infrared radiation causes mainly thermal injury. Visible light has minimal effects. The ambient x-radiation and gamma rays that filter through the earth's atmosphere are minimal and have no significant health effects.

BP7 199   BP6 711   PBD7 441-442   PBD6 430-431

12 (E) Old flaking paint that is lead-based has a sweet taste, attracting small children to ingest it. The major risk to children from lead ingestion is neurologic damage. Venous blood lead levels should normally be less than 10 μg/dL. Household bleach (sodium hypochlorite) is a local irritant and is not likely to be found in the living conditions of these children. Ethylene glycol is found in antifreeze and can produce acute renal tubular necrosis. Methanol ingestion can cause acute central nervous system depression, acidosis, and blindness. Kerosene, a hydrocarbon, can cause gastrointestinal and respiratory toxicity when ingested.

BP7 278-280   BP6 231-233   PBD7 432-433
PBD6 420-422

13 (B) The patient has a full-thickness burn injury to the arms, but only partial-thickness burns of other areas. In a full-thickness burn, all structures from which re-epithelialization could occur are lost, including dermal appendages such as sweat glands and hair follicles. Loss of only the epidermal basal layer will not prevent re-epithelialization from the skin appendages. Fibroblasts can produce more collagen, although elastic fibers do not regenerate; this is why burned skin tends to lose its elasticity, requiring additional grafting procedures in growing children. The superficial layer of keratin serves a protective function. Its loss in burns increases fluid and electrolyte loss, but it will re-form if re-epithelialization occurs. Blood monocytes can migrate into tissues to become macrophages that help in remodeling the damaged tissues. Loss of the nerve endings in full-thickness burns leads to the loss of sensation noted on physical examination in this patient, but this process does not govern re-epithelialization.

BP7 285-286   BP6 236-237   PBD7 444-445
PBD6 412-413

14 (C) Heat exhaustion results from failure of the cardiovascular system to compensate for hypovolemia caused by water depletion. It is readily reversible by replacing lost intravascular volume. Vigorous exercise with electrolyte loss can produce muscle cramping typical of heat cramps. Inhalation injury is seen when a fire occurs in an enclosed space, and hot, toxic gases are inhaled. Malignant hyperthermia occurs from a metabolic derangement such as thyroid storm or with drugs such as succinyl choline. Heat stroke is associated with organ damage when body temperatures are higher than 36°C.

BP7 286   BP6 240   PBD7 445   PBD6 434-435

15 (C) There is a natural seepage of radon gas from soil, more so in some geographic locations than in others. This gas can collect in houses and is a potential cause of lung cancer. The pollutant gases carbon monoxide and ozone are not associated with lung cancer, nor are dusts containing carbon such as coal dust. Silicosis may possibly increase the risk of lung cancer, but patients with this condition have severe, restrictive lung disease.

BP7 267, 290   BP6 242-243   PBD7 430   PBD6 418

16 (D) Vitamin A is important in maintaining epithelial surfaces. Deficiency of this vitamin can lead to squamous metaplasia of respiratory epithelium, predisposing to infection. Increased keratin buildup leads to follicular plugging and papular dermatosis. Desquamated keratinaceous debris in the urinary tract forms the nidus for stones. Ocular complications of vitamin A deficiency include xerophthalmia and corneal scarring, which can lead to blindness. Vitamin E deficiency occurs rarely; it causes neurologic symptoms related to degeneration of the axons in the posterior columns of the spinal cord. Vitamin D deficiency in children causes rickets, characterized by bone deformities. Vitamin K deficiency can result in a bleeding diathesis. Vitamin B_1 (thiamine) deficiency causes problems such as Wernicke disease, neuropathy, and cardiomyopathy.

BP7 293-295   BP6 246-248   PBD7 450-452
PBD6 439-441

17 (D) Heroin is an opiate narcotic that is a derivative of morphine. Opiates are central nervous system (CNS) depressants, and overdoses are accompanied by respiratory depression, convulsions, and cardiac arrest. The typical mode of administration is by injection; often an infection, such as an endocarditis, results from such use, because nonsterile injection technique is employed. Cocaine is most often inhaled rather than injected and acutely produces a state of excited delirium. Ethanol is typically ingested and, in excess, can lead to coma and death. Flurazepam is most often ingested; excessive use can lead to respiratory depression. Meperidine is an analgesic that can cause respiratory depression and bradycardia in overdosage. Phencyclidine (PCP) is a schizophrenomimetic and is usually ingested; users have a history of erratic behavior. Phenobarbital is usually ingested and can produce marked CNS depression.

BP7 284   BP6 237   PBD7 424, 426   PBD6 414

18 (D) Cocaine is a powerful vasoconstrictor, and the cardiac complications of its use include arterial vasoconstriction with ischemic injury and arrhythmias. Atherosclerosis, affecting small, peripheral branches of the coronary arteries, can be marked. Amphetamines may induce cardiac arrhythmias. Barbiturates are depressants and can cause respiratory failure. Benzodiazepines can produce respiratory failure. Acute ethanol poisoning can cause central nervous system depression and coma. Heroin overdoses can be accompanied by pulmonary edema and respiratory failure. Marijuana is a minor tranquilizer; no serious physiologic effects are associated with its use.

BP7 282-283   BP6 236-237   PBD7 424-425
PBD6 412-413

19 (C) This man has experienced occupational exposure to lead and shows symptoms and signs of lead toxicity. The concentration of zinc protoporphyrin is elevated in chronic lead poisoning, in anemia of chronic disease, and in iron deficiency anemia. Lead interferes with heme biosynthesis and inhibits the incorporation of iron into heme; as a result, zinc is used instead. Hepatic damage with elevation of liver enzymes ALT and AST is not a major feature of lead poisoning, but acute increases in these enzymes could be seen with acetaminophen toxicity. The level of the muscle enzyme creatine kinase is not elevated because muscle is not directly damaged by lead, although a neuropathy can occur. Lead can damage renal tubules and cause renal failure, but specific alterations in electrolytes with elevated sodium or decreased calcium are not specific for lead-induced renal failure.

BP7 278-280   BP6 232-233   PBD7 432-433
PBD6 420-422

20 **(B)** Rickets, which is caused by vitamin D deficiency, is characterized by skeletal deformity such as the bowing of the legs seen in this boy. Scurvy, resulting from vitamin C deficiency, can produce bone deformities, particularly at the epiphyses, because of abnormal bone matrix, not abnormal calcification. However, the absence of hemorrhages in this child makes this unlikely. Pellagra, resulting from niacin deficiency, is characterized by dermatitis in sun-exposed areas of skin. Beriberi, from thiamine deficiency, can result in heart failure and peripheral edema. A diet containing insufficient protein can result in kwashiorkor, characterized by areas of flaking, depigmented skin.

BP7 297-299   BP6 249-250   PBD7 452-455
PBD6 444-445

21 **(E)** A scraping injury produces an abrasion, but the skin is not broken. An incised wound is made with a sharp instrument such as a knife, leaving clean edges. A contusion is a bruise with extravasation of blood into soft tissues. Lacerations break the skin or other organs in an irregular fashion. A burn injury causes coagulative necrosis without mechanical disruption.

BP7 285   BP6 238   PBD7 443   PBD6 432

22 **(D)** Water in some areas naturally contains fluoride, and dental problems in children are fewer in these areas. Fluoride can be added to drinking water, but opposition to this practice, from ignorance or fear, is common. Zinc deficiency can produce hemorrhagic dermatitis. Iodine deficiency can predispose to goiter. Selenium deficiency can result in myopathy. Copper deficiency can produce neurologic defects. Serious illnesses from trace element deficiencies are rare.

BP7 303   BP6 258   PBD7 461   PBD6 452

23 **(A)** Signs and symptoms of scurvy can be subtle. The diet must contain a constant supply of vitamin C (ascorbic acid), because none is produced endogenously. Older persons with an inadequate diet are as much at risk as younger persons. Folate deficiency can lead to anemia, but it does not cause capillary fragility with hematoma formation or skin rash. Niacin deficiency can lead to an erythematous skin rash in sun-exposed areas but not to anemia. Riboflavin deficiency can lead to findings such as glossitis, cheilosis, and neuropathy. Selenium is a trace mineral that forms a component of glutathione peroxidase; deficiency may be associated with heart disease. Vitamin A deficiency can produce a skin rash, but it does not cause anemia. Vitamin K

is important in maintaining proper coagulation, but a deficiency state is not associated with anemia or skin rash. Zinc is a trace mineral that aids in wound healing; a deficiency state can lead to stunted growth in children and a vesicular, erythematous rash.

BP7 298-301   BP6 256-257   PBD7 458-459
PBD6 449-451

24 **(A)** The figure shows superficial tears in the epidermis, with underlying superficial dermal hemorrhage. Abrasions are made by a scraping type of injury. A contusion is a bruise characterized by breakage of small dermal blood vessels and bleeding. An exit wound from a gunshot can have an irregular appearance that resembles an incision or a laceration; it does not have a scraped appearance. Hypothermia (exposure to cold) has no characteristic appearance. An incised wound is made by a sharp instrument that produces clean-cut edges. Kwashiorkor, resulting from lack of protein in the diet, may lead to flaking of the skin and irregular pigmentation. A laceration is a cut with torn edges. Thermal burns may produce erythema, blistering, and cracking of skin but not a scraped appearance.

BP7 285   BP6 238   PBD7 443   PBD6 432

25 **(E)** The infiltrative perihilar mass suggests lung cancer. Polycyclic hydrocarbons and nitrosamines, found in tobacco smoke, are the key contributors to the development of lung cancer. The carbon monoxide levels of smokers are increased, but this promotes hypoxemia, not cancer. The nicotine in cigarette smoke has a stimulant effect on the central nervous system, but it does not play a major role in cancer development. Nitrous oxide compounds and ozone are found in smog, but they are not closely associated with risk of lung cancer. Silica dust exposure slightly increases the risk of lung cancer, most often in persons with prolonged occupational exposure. Sulfur dioxide emissions are a component of smog and promote acid rain; they may increase the risk of chronic bronchitis.

BP7 274-275   BP6 223   PBD7 419, 431-432
PBD6 408-409

26 **(B)** Heating devices that burn hydrocarbons such as petroleum products generate carbon monoxide, which can build up to dangerous levels in unventilated or poorly ventilated houses. Chronic carbon monoxide poisoning produces central nervous system damage. Carbon monoxide binds much more tightly to hemoglobin than does oxygen, resulting in hypoxia. Decreased mental functioning generally begins at carboxyhemoglobin levels greater than 20%, and death is likely at levels that exceed 60%. Acute exposure to beryllium may cause pneumonitis; chronic exposure results in a sarcoid-like pulmonary disease. Nitrous oxide compounds and ozone are found in smog and may cause respiratory discomfort with diminished respiratory function in the very young, the very old, and those with underlying respiratory diseases, but such exposure is not immediately life threatening. In very high concentrations, oxygen can be toxic to the lungs and can promote diffuse alveolar damage. Polycyclic aromatic hydrocarbons in cigarette smoke promote development of lung cancer. Sulfur dioxide emissions are a component of smog and promote acid rain; they may increase the risk of chronic bronchitis.

BP7 280   BP6 234   PBD7 428, 430   PBD6 418

27 (A) Body weight less than 60% of normal with muscle wasting is consistent with marasmus, which results from a marked decrease in total caloric intake. In kwashiorkor, protein intake is reduced more than total caloric intake, and body weight is usually 60% to 80% of normal. Hypoalbuminemia is a key laboratory finding. Malignancies can promote wasting but not to this degree. This child's problems are far more serious then a single vitamin deficiency; a lack of folate could account for the child's anemia but not for the wasting. Bulimia is an eating disorder of adolescents and adults that is characterized by binge eating and self-induced vomiting. Lead poisoning can lead to anemia and encephalopathy, but it does not cause severe wasting.

BP7 291-292   BP6 244-245   PBD7 447-448
PBD6 437-439

28 (E) Vitamin A is essential to maintain epithelia. The lack of vitamin A affects the function of lacrimal glands and conjunctival epithelium, promoting keratomalacia. Dietary protein is essential for building tissues, particularly muscle, but it has no specific effect in maintaining ocular structures. Vitamin K is beneficial for synthesis of coagulation factors by the liver to prevent bleeding problems. Iron is essential for production of heme, which is needed to manufacture hemoglobin in RBCs. Niacin is involved with nicotinamide in many metabolic pathways, and deficiency leads to diarrhea, dermatitis, and dementia.

BP7 293-295   BP6 248   PBD7 450-452   PBD6 439-441

29 (E) More fruits and vegetables are recommended in the diet to help prevent colon cancer. Vitamins C and E have an antioxidant and antimutagenic effect. Red wine in moderation may have a beneficial antiatherogenic effect. Ice cream can include animal fat that may promote cancer, as would the animal fat of beef. Chocolate includes vegetable fat that is not as harmful as animal fat.

BP7 306   BP6 261-262   PBD7 466   PBD6 455-456

30 (A) Vitamin D can be synthesized endogenously in skin with exposure to ultraviolet (UV) light. Together, vitamin D and calcium help build growing bone. Exercise helps build bone mass, which protects against osteoporosis later in life, particularly in women. There are some deleterious effects on the eye (cataracts) and the skin (cancer, elastosis) from increased exposure to UV radiation in sunlight. Increased air pollution in many cities has led to an increased incidence of pulmonary diseases, and children are particularly at risk. Renal function is not greatly affected by environment.

BP7 297-299   BP6 248   PBD7 452-454   PBD6 442-445

31 (A) Acetaminophen toxicity produces hepatic necrosis. This effect is enhanced with prior ethanol ingestion. Hepatic necrosis is indicated by extremely high levels of AST and ALT. Penicillin can cause systemic anaphylaxis in a few persons. Aspirin can produce a metabolic acidosis. Sulfa drugs may produce renal failure. Opiates, including codeine, are central nervous system and respiratory depressants.

BP7 277-278   BP6 230   PBD7 422, 428   PBD6 416

32 (A) These findings suggest a diagnosis of diabetes mellitus. The patient is obese and most likely has type 2 diabetes mellitus. Type 1 and type 2 diabetes mellitus greatly increase the risk of early and accelerated atherosclerosis. Decreasing total caloric intake, particularly saturated fat, helps reduce the risk of coronary artery disease. Vegetable and fish oils are preferable to animal fat as sources of dietary lipid for prevention of atherosclerosis. Dietary fiber helps to reduce the incidence of diverticulosis. Vitamin A has no known effect on atherogenesis. Reducing dietary sodium helps to reduce blood pressure. Increased fluid intake aids renal function.

BP7 305   BP6 261   PBD7 465   PBD6 452-454

33 (D) Therapeutic doses of radiation can cause acute vascular injury, manifested by endothelial damage and an inflammatory reaction. With time, these vessels undergo fibrosis and suffer severe luminal narrowing. There is ischemia of the surrounding tissue and formation of a scar. The radiation used in therapeutic dosages is carefully delivered in a limited field to promote maximal tumor damage while reducing damage to surrounding tissues. Whole-body irradiation affects marrow, gonads, gastrointestinal tract, and brain, but therapeutic radiation is very focused on the neoplasm to avoid widespread tissue damage.

BP7 288-289   BP6 242-243   PBD7 437   PBD6 428

34 (A) A blow with a blunt object produces soft tissue hemorrhage without breaking the skin. An abrasion scrapes away the superficial epidermis. A laceration is an irregular tear in the skin or other organ. An incised wound is made by a sharp object and is longer than a puncture, which has a rounded outline and is deeper than it is wide.

BP7 285   BP6 238   PBD7 443-444   PBD6 432-434

35 (C) The large amount of ethanol ingested over a short time can elevate blood ethanol to toxic levels, because the alcohol dehydrogenase in liver metabolizes ethanol by zero-order kinetics. Cirrhosis is a long-term complication of chronic ethanolism. Likewise, pancreatitis is a feature of chronic use of ethanol. Wernicke disease occurs rarely, even in alcoholics, and probably results from thiamine deficiency. Hematemesis from gastritis and gastric ulceration are more typically seen with chronic ethanolism, and variceal bleeding is a complication of hepatic cirrhosis. The combination of acetaminophen and ethanol increases the likelihood of hepatic toxicity.

BP7 281-282   BP6 234-235   PBD7 421-424
PBD6 410-412

36 (E) Pellagra is caused by a deficiency of niacin. The classic presentation includes the "3 Ds": diarrhea, dermatitis, and dementia. Beriberi, resulting from thiamine (vitamin B_1) deficiency leads to heart failure, neuropathy, and Wernicke disease. Cheilosis describes the fissuring at the corners of the mouth that accompanies riboflavin (vitamin B_2) deficiency. In hypothyroidism, the skin tends to be coarse and dry. Marasmus describes the severe wasting that occurs in persons with a diet that is markedly deficient in all nutrients. In scurvy, resulting from vitamin C deficiency, increased capillary fragility leads to bruises on the skin.

BP7 302   BP6 255-256   PBD7 458   PBD6 448

37 (B) Asbestos fibers can cause pulmonary interstitial fibrosis, and there is an increased risk of malignancy. Persons who have been exposed to asbestos and who smoke have a greatly increased incidence of bronchogenic carcinoma.

Mesothelioma is uncommon, even in persons with asbestos exposure, but virtually all occurrences are in persons who have been exposed to asbestos. Arsenic exposure is a risk factor for skin cancer. Benzidine exposure is a risk factor for lymphoproliferative disorders. Chromium exposure increases the risk of carcinomas of the upper respiratory tract and lung. Naphthylamine compounds can increase the risk of urinary tract cancers. Nickel exposure is associated with cancers of the respiratory tract.

BP7 272-274   BP6 227-229   PBD7 421, 430
PBD6 732-733

38 (E) Electrical current, especially alternating current, disrupts nerve conduction and electrical impulses, particularly in the heart and brain. This can lead to severe arrhythmias, especially ventricular fibrillation. These are immediate effects. The amount of tissue injury from standard (US) household current is generally not great, and there may be just a small thermal injury at the site of entry or exit of the current on the skin. The other listed options are not a direct consequence of an electrical injury.

BP7 287   BP6 240   PBD7 446   PBD6 435

39 (B) The findings are consistent with kwashiorkor, a nutritional disorder predominantly of decreased protein in the diet. Hypoalbuminemia is characteristic of this condition. Hyperglycemia occurs in diabetes mellitus; the wasting associated with this disease affects adipose tissue and muscle, and edema is not a feature. Abetalipoproteinemia is a rare disorder that causes vitamin E deficiency. Megaloblastic anemia is a feature of specific deficiencies of vitamin B_{12} or folate. Hypocalcemia can occur as a consequence of vitamin D deficiency.

BP7 291-292   BP6 244-245   PBD7 448-449
PBD6 437-439

40 (C) The osteopenia in this patient can result from osteomalacia, the adult form of vitamin D deficiency. Vitamin D is one of the fat-soluble vitamins, and it requires fat absorption, which can be impaired by chronic cholestatic liver disease, biliary tract disease, and pancreatic disease. Heart disease caused by atherosclerosis does not affect bone density. Emphysema can result in a hypertrophic osteoarthropathy but not osteopenia. Leukemias do not tend to erode bone. Atrophic gastritis affects vitamin B_{12} absorption.

BP7 297-298   BP6 251   PBD7 453-454   PBD6 444-445

41 (C) Chronic aspirin toxicity (more than 3 g/day) can result in a variety of neurologic problems. Aspirin also inhibits platelet function by suppressing the production of thromboxane A_2, thus promoting bleeding. The best known complication of penicillin therapy is systemic anaphylaxis. Tetracycline therapy may be complicated by a fatty liver. Chlorpromazine ingestion may lead to cholestatic jaundice. Quinidine therapy may lead to hemolytic anemia.

BP7 278   BP6 231-232   PBD7 428   PBD6 416

42 (C) The decreased food intake from self-imposed dieting in an adult woman can lead to changes such as hormonal deficiencies (e.g., follicle-stimulating hormone, luteinizing hormone, thyroxine). The result is diminished estrogen synthesis, which promotes osteoporosis, as in the postmenopausal state. Kwashiorkor is a disease mainly of children who have reduced protein intake. Chronic alcoholism can be accompanied by specific nutritional deficiencies, particularly of folate and thiamine, although total caloric intake may be increased (there are 7 calories per gram of ethanol). Scurvy, which results from vitamin C deficiency, does not affect hormonal function. Rickets is a specific deficiency of vitamin D that causes skeletal deformities in children.

BP7 293   BP6 246   PBD7 447, 449   PBD6 439

43 (E) This pseudoscience is just as imaginative as that appearing in many public media sources, so beware the claims and apply principles of evidence-based medicine. Some would agree that there is never quite enough chocolate, and much of the world's population must get by without it. Of course, serious dietitians would choose option A, which is a deficiency most likely to be seen in menstruating women, in pregnant women, and in children. Calcium is most important in growing children for building bones. Folate deficiency leads to macrocytic anemia and is most likely to occur in adults with an inadequate diet, such as persons with chronic alcoholism. Vitamin C deficiency occurs in persons who do not eat adequate amounts of fresh fruits and vegetables.

BP7 303   BP6 258   PBD7 643-646   PBD6 452

44 (B) The cerebral syndrome occurs within hours in persons exposed to a massive total-body radiation dose. Dosages of 200 to 700 cGy can be fatal, because of injury to radiosensitive marrow and the gastrointestinal tract; but death occurs after days to weeks, not hours. Cardiac and skeletal muscle tissue is relatively radioresistant. Early findings in radiation lung injury include edema; interstitial fibrosis develops over years in those who survive the injury.

BP7 289-290   BP6 243   PBD7 438-441   PBD6 426-427

45 (B) Fires in enclosed spaces produce hot, toxic gases. The inhalation of these gases can lead to death from pulmonary edema even when there is no injury from flames. Infections occur days to weeks after a burn injury, because of the loss of an epithelial barrier to infectious agents. An acute myocardial infarction is possible but not probable in a woman of this age. Cerebral edema is more likely to occur as a complication during recovery from a burn injury. Malignant hyperthermia, which occurs when core body temperature exceeds 40°C, is produced by metabolic disorders such as hyperthyroidism and drugs such as succinylcholine and cocaine.

BP7 285-286   BP6 239   PBD7 444-445   PBD6 434

46 (B) Excessive ethanol ingestion increases the risk of cancer in the upper aerodigestive tract, including the mouth, pharynx, and esophagus. In the stomach, it can cause acute and chronic gastritis, but there is no reported increase in gastric cancer. Chronic liver disease can lead to hepatic encephalopathy, indicated by a laboratory finding of increased blood ammonia. Dementia is not a characteristic finding, although Wernicke encephalopathy can occur rarely when thiamine deficiency is present. Blindness is an acute toxic effect of methanol ingestion. Peripheral vascular disease is usually caused by atherosclerosis. Alcohol does not increase atherosclerotic disease incidence. Acute renal failure results from ingestion of ethylene glycol.

BP7 282   BP6 234-235   PBD7 422-424, ch 17   PBD6 412

47 **(D)** Cocaine has powerful vasoactive effects, including vasoconstriction. The effects on the placenta can include decreased blood flow with fetal hypoxia and spontaneous abortion, placentae abruption, and fetal hemorrhages. Chronic maternal cocaine use results in neurologic impairment of infants. Acetaminophen overdosage can produce hepatic necrosis and encephalopathy. Amphetamines may have acute cardiovascular effects, including arrhythmias. Cannabinoids act as mild tranquilizers and have no major tissue effects. Ethanol ingestion in pregnancy can be associated with fetal alcohol syndrome, which is not fatal but results in subtle anomalies and impaired development. Heroin ingestion can lead to fetal cardiorespiratory depression but not hemorrhage. Lysergic acid (LSD) use does not cause hemorrhage.

BP7 282-283   BP6 236-237   PBD7 425   PBD6 412-413

48 **(F)** Although methanol is metabolized by the same enzymatic pathway as ethanol, it produces the toxic metabolites formaldehyde and formate, which damage the central nervous system and the retina. Acutely, a metabolic acidosis is present. Victims of cyanide poisoning die suddenly, and there are virtually no physical findings. However, the smell of "bitter almonds" may permeate the tissues at autopsy. Ethanol poisoning is one of the most common forms of overdose; victims lapse into a coma. Chronic ethanolism leads to liver disease. Gasoline is a hydrocarbon that, when ingested, is often vomited and aspirated, resulting in pneumonitis. Lead poisoning can produce anemia, abdominal pain, encephalopathy, and neuropathy. Mercury poisoning can produce encephalopathy. Organophosphates (e.g., parathion, malathion) are acetyl-cholinesterase inhibitors that do not persist in the environment but are capable of producing acute disease, including paralysis, arrhythmia, and respiratory failure.

BP6 232   PBD7 424   PBD6 412

49 **(E)** The figure shows the entry site of a gunshot wound made at close range. There is a sharply demarcated skin defect, and the surrounding skin shows some stippling of unburned gunpowder. An abrasion involves scraping of the skin surface. A blast injury can produce a variety of findings, depending on what struck the body or what the body struck, but the focal stippling seen in this figure is not likely to be present. A contusion is a bruise characterized by breakage of small dermal blood vessels and bleeding. An electrocution injury often produces very minimal findings; the site of entry of the current may be quite small. An incised wound is made by a sharp instrument that produces clean-cut edges, whereas a laceration is a cut with torn edges.

BP7 285   BP6 238   PBD7 444   PBD6 433

50 **(E)** Leptin signaling from adipocytes that have taken up an adequate supply of fatty acids ordinarily feeds back to the hypothalamus, which then decreases synthesis of neuropeptide Y. This neurotransmitter acts as an appetite stimulant and a decrease in its synthesis causes satiety. Adenosine is a nucleoside used to treat cardiac dysrhythmias. Glucagon opposes insulin by increasing hepatic glycogen storage. An increasing blood glucose level results in an increased release of insulin to promote glucose uptake into connective tissues, muscle, and adipose tissue. VLDL from the liver is transformed in adipose tissue and muscle to LDL, which is then taken up by a variety of cells with LDL receptors that need cholesterol for membrane synthesis.

BP7 303-304   PBD7 462-463   PBD6 430-431

51 **(D)** The medical uses of marijuana include intractable nausea and glaucoma. Marijuana, with the active substance tetrahydrocannabinol (THC), has a sedative effect on the central nervous system. Barbiturates are sedatives but have no effect on severe nausea. Cocaine, methylphenidate (Ritalin), and methamphetamine are stimulants. Heroin is an opioid; morphine sulfate, an opioid derivative, has a very beneficial effect in treating intractable pain in cancer patients. Phencyclidine (PCP) has a schizophrenomimetic effect.

BP7 284   BP6 237-238   PBD7 424, 426   PBD6 413

52 **(E)** Hormone replacement therapy (HRT) increases the risk of thromboembolic disease, as is the case with oral contraceptive therapy. HRT was long considered to have a protective effect against cardiovascular disease, because exogenous estrogens increase HDL and decrease LDL. However, this is not true of all women, and progestins tend to have the opposite effect. The risk of cervical carcinoma is more closely related to a lifestyle that increases the likelihood of human papillomavirus infection. Inflammatory bowel disease is not associated with HRT. Hepatic cirrhosis in men may lead to decreased degradation of circulating estrogens, with the resulting effect of testicular atrophy. Pulmonary emphysema typically is related to cigarette smoking, not to HRT.

BP7 277   PBD7 427-428

53 **(E)** With currently used low estrogen-containing oral contraceptives, there is no increase in risk for coronary atherosclerosis or myocardial infarction in non-smoking women less than 45 years of age. The risk is increased, however, in women over the age of 35 who smoke. Smoking during pregnancy increases the likelihood for low birth weight infants. Oral contraceptives do not increase the risk for breast cancer and they decrease the likelihood of ovarian and endometrial cancer; the risk for these latter two cancers is increased by postmenopausal hormone replacement therapy (HRT). The risk for cholecystitis increases with post-menopausal hormone HRT. There is no evidence for risk of dementia with oral contraceptives or HRT.

BP7 277   PBD7 420, 427

54 **(A)** Appetite and satiety are controlled by a complex system of short and long-term acting signals. The levels of ghrelin produced in the stomach rise rapidly before every meal and fall promptly after the stomach is filled. Leptin released from adipocytes exerts long-term control by activating catabolic circuits and by inhibiting anabolic circuits. α-MSH is an intermediate in leptin signaling. TRH and CRF are among the efferent mediators of leptin signaling, and they increase energy consumption.

BP7 303-304   PBD7 462-463

Diseases of Infancy and Childhood

PBD7 Chapter 10: Diseases of Infancy and Childhood

PBD6 Chapter 11: Diseases of Infancy and Childhood

BP7 and BP6 Chapter 7: Genetic and Pediatric Diseases

1 A 20-year-old woman gives birth at term to an infant weighing 1900 g. On physical examination, the infant's head size is normal, but the crown-heel length and foot length are reduced. There are no external malformations. Throughout infancy, developmental milestones are delayed. Which of the following conditions occurring during gestation would most likely produce these findings?

- ❑ (A) Pregnancy-induced hypertension
- ❑ (B) Down syndrome
- ❑ (C) Maternal diabetes mellitus
- ❑ (D) Congenital cytomegalovirus
- ❑ (E) Erythroblastosis fetalis

2 An 18-month-old African-American boy is found dead in his crib one morning. The distraught parents, both factory workers, are interviewed by the medical examiner and indicate that the child was not ill. The medical examiner finds no gross or microscopic abnormalities at autopsy, and the results of all toxicologic tests are negative. The medical examiner tells the parents that, although she cannot yet determine the cause of death, she believes that sudden infant death syndrome (SIDS) is very unlikely. This conclusion by the medical examiner is most likely based on which of the following factors?

- ❑ (A) Sex of the child
- ❑ (B) Race of the child
- ❑ (C) Age of the child
- ❑ (D) Low socioeconomic background of parents
- ❑ (E) Absence of any abnormality in the respiratory centers
- ❑ (F) Absence of prior medical conditions

3 A male newborn delivered at 28 weeks' gestation develops difficulty breathing 2 days after birth. On physical examination, there are grunting and retractions, and the newborn appears cyanotic. A chest radiograph shows a bilateral ground-glass appearance in the lungs. The newborn is treated with assisted ventilation and nutritional support. He appears to improve for 24 hours but then becomes progressively more cyanotic. He develops seizures and dies 4 days after birth. Which of the following is the most likely histologic finding in the lungs at autopsy?

- ❑ (A) Diffuse alveolar septal fibrosis
- ❑ (B) Alveolar hyaline membranes and atelectasis
- ❑ (C) Extensive alveolar transudate
- ❑ (D) Bronchiolar mucus plugging
- ❑ (E) Frothy (bubbly) alveolar exudate

4 A 12-year-old child has had increasing episodes of diarrhea for the past 3 years. The child's stools are bulky and foul smelling. The child also has a history of multiple respiratory tract infections. On physical examination, vital signs include temperature of 38.1°C, pulse 80/min, respirations 20/min, and blood pressure 90/55 mm Hg. On auscultation, diffuse crackles are heard over both lungs. Laboratory findings include quantitative stool fat of > 10 g/day. Sputum cultures have grown *Pseudomonas aeruginosa* and *Burkholderia cepacia*. Which of the following is most likely to explain the findings in this child?

- ❑ (A) Galactose-1-phosphate uridyltransferase deficiency
- ❑ (B) LDL receptor gene mutation
- ❑ (C) Abnormal fibrillin production by fibroblasts
- ❑ (D) Impaired epithelial cell transport of chloride ion
- ❑ (E) Phenylalanine hydroxylase deficiency

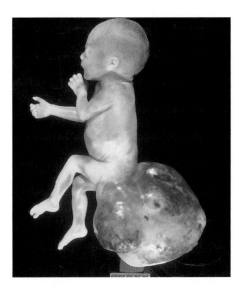

6 A 28-year-old woman, G 1, P 0, has an uncomplicated pregnancy until 28 weeks' gestation, when she develops uterine contractions and has premature rupture of membranes. An ultrasound reveals a lesion with the representative gross appearance shown in the figure above. Which of the following is the most likely diagnosis of this lesion?

- ❑ (A) Teratoma
- ❑ (B) Neuroblastoma
- ❑ (C) Hemangioma
- ❑ (D) Lymphangioma
- ❑ (E) Hamartoma

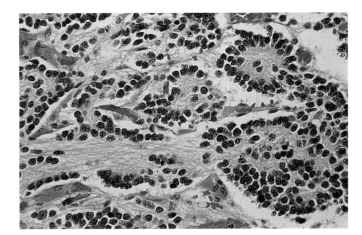

5 The mother of a 6-month-old male infant notices that he has a palpable abdominal mass. On physical examination, the infant has a temperature of 37.8°C, and he is at the 33rd percentile for weight. An abdominal CT scan shows a solid 5.5-cm mass involving the right adrenal gland. Laboratory studies show that 24-hour urine levels of homovanillic acid (HVA) and vanillylmandelic acid (VMA) are increased. The adrenal gland is excised surgically, and the histologic appearance of the mass is shown in the figure above. Which of the following features of this lesion is associated with a poor prognosis?

- ❑ (A) Age younger than 1 year
- ❑ (B) Hyperdiploidy
- ❑ (C) Presence of many ganglion cells
- ❑ (D) *N-MYC* gene amplification
- ❑ (E) Malformations of the kidney

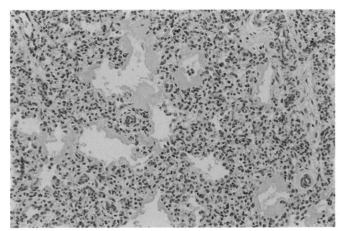

7 A 25-year-old woman gives birth at 31 weeks' gestation. The newborn girl has initial Apgar scores of 5 and 6 at 1 and 5 minutes, but within 1 hour, she experiences severe respiratory distress and dies despite resuscitative measures. At autopsy, the newborn's lungs have the microscopic appearance shown in the figure above. Which of the following conditions best accounts for these findings?

- ❑ (A) Maternal toxemia of pregnancy
- ❑ (B) Marked fetal anemia
- ❑ (C) Congenital toxoplasmosis
- ❑ (D) Immaturity of lungs
- ❑ (E) Oligohydramnios

8 A term infant has initial Apgar scores of 8 and 10 at 1 and 5 minutes. On auscultation of the chest, a heart murmur is audible. The infant is at the 30th percentile for height and weight. Echocardiography shows a membranous ventricular septal defect (VSD). Which of the following events is most likely to have resulted in the appearance of the VSD?

❏ (A) Dispermy at conception
❏ (B) Maternal thalidomide use
❏ (C) Maternal rubella infection
❏ (D) Erythroblastosis fetalis
❏ (E) Maternal folate deficiency
❏ (F) Paternal meiotic nondisjunction

9 In a study of lung maturation, the amount of surfactant at different gestational ages is measured. Investigators find that the amount of surfactant in the developing lung increases between the 26th and 32nd weeks' gestation, with progression of lung architecture to a saccular alveolar configuration. This increase in surfactant is most likely related to which of the following developmental events?

❏ (A) Differentiation of alveoli from embryonic foregut
❏ (B) Increased density of pulmonary capillaries
❏ (C) Development of ciliated epithelium in airspaces
❏ (D) Differentiation of type II alveolar epithelial cells
❏ (E) Apoptosis in interlobular mesenchymal cells

10 A 22-year-old primigravida gives birth to a male infant at 38 weeks' gestation. On physical examination, the infant appears normal except for a single midline cleft of the upper lip. The cleft lip interferes with breast-feeding, but the infant gains weight normally. The mother asks if there is any risk that future children will be born with a similar malformation. Which of the following is the most appropriate information to give her?

❏ (A) It is highly unlikely that other offspring will have a similar defect
❏ (B) There is a 2% to 7% risk that future offspring will have a cleft lip
❏ (C) It is likely that half of her offspring will have cleft lip
❏ (D) The risk of having other children with a similar defect is 1 in 4
❏ (E) Her sons, but not daughters, are at risk of having cleft lip

11 A 20-year-old woman known to have an inborn error of metabolism is planning for her first pregnancy. She is advised by her physician to begin a phenylalanine-free diet before conception and to continue this diet throughout all three trimesters of her pregnancy. This special diet is most likely to aid in preventing which of the following problems in her infant?

❏ (A) Mental retardation
❏ (B) Muscular weakness
❏ (C) Cataracts
❏ (D) Anemia
❏ (E) Congestive heart failure

12 A 38-year-old woman has premature rupture of membranes at 38 weeks' gestation, necessitating delivery. Which of the following factors is most likely to increase the risk of hyaline membrane disease in the infant?

❏ (A) Maternal corticosteroid therapy
❏ (B) Chorioamnionitis
❏ (C) Gestational diabetes
❏ (D) Oligohydramnios
❏ (E) Pregnancy-induced hypertension

13 A term infant develops vomiting and diarrhea a few days after birth. By the end of the first week of life, the infant is icteric. Cataracts develop 1 month later. At 1 year of age, developmental milestones are not being met. At age 2, the infant succumbs to *Escherichia coli* septicemia. A deficiency of which of the following substances is most likely to be present in this child?

❏ (A) Adenosine deaminase
❏ (B) α_1-Antitrypsin
❏ (C) Galactose-1-phosphate uridyltransferase
❏ (D) Globin chains
❏ (E) Glucocerebrosidase
❏ (F) Hexosaminidase
❏ (G) Spectrin

14 A neonate is born at 36 weeks' gestation. On physical examination, the neonate manifests severe hydrops fetalis, hepatosplenomegaly, generalized icterus, and scattered ecchymoses of the skin. Laboratory studies show a hemoglobin concentration of 9.4 g/dL and platelet count of 67,000/mm³. Ultrasound of the head shows ventricular enlargement. Death occurs 14 days after birth. At autopsy, there is extensive subependymal necrosis, with microscopic evidence of encephalitis. Within the areas of necrosis, there are large cells containing intranuclear inclusions. Which of the following organisms is most likely to produce these findings?

❏ (A) Cytomegalovirus
❏ (B) Herpes simplex virus
❏ (C) HIV
❏ (D) JC papovavirus
❏ (E) Parvovirus
❏ (F) Rubella virus

15 An infant is born prematurely at 32 weeks' gestation to a 34-year-old woman with gestational diabetes. At birth, the infant is at the 50th percentile for height and weight. On physical examination, there are no congenital anomalies. The infant requires 3 weeks of intubation with positive pressure ventilation and dies of sepsis at 4 months of age. At autopsy, the lungs show bronchial squamous metaplasia with peribronchial fibrosis, interstitial fibrosis, and dilation of air spaces. Which of the following conditions best explains these findings?

❏ (A) Sudden infant death syndrome
❏ (B) Ventricular septal defect
❏ (C) Cystic fibrosis
❏ (D) Bronchopulmonary dysplasia
❏ (E) Pulmonary hypoplasia

16 An 18-year-old woman gives birth to a term infant after an uncomplicated pregnancy and delivery. Over the first few days of life, the infant becomes mildly icteric. On physical examination, there are no morphologic abnormalities. Laboratory studies show a neonatal bilirubin concentration of 4.9 mg/dL. The direct Coombs test of the infant's RBCs yields a positive result. The infant's blood type is A negative and the mother's is O positive. Based on these findings, which of the following events is most likely to occur?

- ❏ (A) Kernicterus
- ❏ (B) Complete recovery
- ❏ (C) Respiratory distress syndrome
- ❏ (D) Failure to thrive
- ❏ (E) Hemolytic anemia throughout infancy

17 A 3-year-old child is brought to the physician for a routine health maintenance examination. The physician examining the child notes a large port wine stain on the left side of the child's face. This irregular, slightly raised, red-blue area is not painful, but is very disfiguring. Histologically, this lesion is most likely composed of a proliferation of which of the following tissue components?

- ❏ (A) Neuroblasts
- ❏ (B) Lymphatics
- ❏ (C) Fibroblasts
- ❏ (D) Lymphoblasts
- ❏ (E) Capillaries

18 In a study of inheritance of the cystic fibrosis gene (*CFTR*), the genetic mutations in carriers and affected individuals are documented. Based on these findings, investigators determine that there is no simple screening test to detect all carriers of mutations of the *CFTR* gene. Which of the following is most likely to be the greatest limitation to development of a screening test?

- ❏ (A) Most mutations in the *CFTR* gene cannot be detected by PCR
- ❏ (B) The fluorescence in situ hybridization technique for detecting the mutation is labor intensive and expensive
- ❏ (C) Several hundred mutations in the *CFTR* gene can give rise to cystic fibrosis
- ❏ (D) Molecular techniques can detect mutations in the *CFTR* gene only when both copies of the gene are abnormal
- ❏ (E) The frequency of heterozygotes in the population is less than 1 in 10,000

19 The mother of a 3-year-old female child notices that she has an enlarged abdomen. On physical examination, there is a palpable mass and lateral asymmetry of the abdomen. An abdominal CT scan shows bilateral adrenal enlargement and pancreatic enlargement. There is a 6-cm solid mass in the left kidney and a 3-cm cyst in the right kidney. The child later develops abdominal distention from bowel obstruction. Which of the following congenital disorders is the most likely diagnosis?

- ❏ (A) Edwards syndrome
- ❏ (B) Marfan syndrome
- ❏ (C) Beckwith-Wiedemann syndrome
- ❏ (D) McArdle syndrome
- ❏ (E) Klinefelter syndrome
- ❏ (F) Patau syndrome
- ❏ (G) Turner syndrome

20 A male neonate delivered at 38 weeks is small for gestational age. Physical examination shows microcephaly, frontal bossing, long and narrow forehead, hypotelorism, maxillary and mandibular hypoplasia, narrow palpebral fissures, thin elongated philtrum, vermillion border of the upper lip, dental malocclusion, saddle nose, tooth enamel hypoplasia, and uvular hypoplasia. Ocular problems include microphthalmia, corneal clouding, coloboma, nystagmus, strabismus, and ptosis. A systolic murmur is heard on auscultation, and echocardiography shows a membranous ventricular septal defect. Which of the following conditions is most likely to produce these findings?

- ❏ (A) Congenital rubella
- ❏ (B) Placenta previa
- ❏ (C) Maternal diabetes mellitus
- ❏ (D) Trisomy 21
- ❏ (E) Fetal alcohol syndrome

21 A 20-year-old woman, G 3, P 2, has a screening ultrasound at 18 weeks' gestation that shows hydrops fetalis but no malformations. The woman's two previous pregnancies ended at term in live births. The current pregnancy results in a live birth at 36 weeks. Physical examination shows marked hydrops of both infant and placenta. Laboratory studies show a cord blood hemoglobin level of 9.2 g/dL and total bilirubin concentration of 20.2 mg/dL. Which of the following laboratory findings best explains the pathogenesis of this infant's disease?

- ❏ (A) Positive Coombs test result on cord blood
- ❏ (B) Elevated maternal serum α-fetoprotein level
- ❏ (C) Positive maternal hepatitis B surface antigen
- ❏ (D) Diminished glucocerebrosidase activity in fetal cells
- ❏ (E) Positive placental culture for *Listeria monocytogenes*

22 A 3-month-old previously healthy infant was found dead by his mother late one evening. When she put him in his crib 1 hour earlier, he showed no signs of distress. The infant's term birth had followed an uncomplicated pregnancy, and he had been feeding well and gaining weight normally. Which of the following is the medical examiner most likely to find at autopsy?

- ❏ (A) Hyaline membrane disease
- ❏ (B) Cerebral cytomegalovirus
- ❏ (C) Tetralogy of Fallot
- ❏ (D) Adrenal neuroblastoma
- ❏ (E) No abnormalities

23 A 25-year-old woman, G 3, P 2, is in her 39th week of pregnancy. She has felt no fetal movement for 1 day. The infant is stillborn on vaginal delivery the next day. On physical examination, there are no external anomalies. Microscopic examination of the placenta shows marked acute chorioamnionitis. Which of the following infectious agents was most likely responsible for these events?

- ❏ (A) Cytomegalovirus
- ❏ (B) *Treponema pallidum*
- ❏ (C) Herpes simplex virus
- ❏ (D) *Toxoplasma gondii*
- ❏ (E) Group B *Streptococcus*

24 A 19-year-old woman, G 2, P 1, has a screening ultrasound at 20 weeks' gestation that shows no abnormalities. However, premature labor leads to an emergent vaginal delivery at 31 weeks. Soon after birth, the neonate develops respiratory distress requiring intubation with positive pressure ventilation. Which of the following prenatal diagnostic tests could have best predicted this neonate's respiratory distress?

❑ (A) Maternal serum α-fetoprotein determination
❑ (B) Phospholipid analysis of amniotic fluid
❑ (C) Chromosomal analysis
❑ (D) Coombs test on cord blood
❑ (E) Genetic analysis for cystic fibrosis gene

25 A 3-year-old light-skinned African-American child has a developmental delay characterized by mental retardation and inability to walk. The child's urine has a distinctly "mousy" odor. On physical examination, there is no lymphadenopathy or hepatosplenomegaly. Laboratory studies show hemoglobin of 14.0 g/dL, platelet count 302,700/mm³, WBC count 7550/mm³, glucose 80 mg/dL, total protein 7.1 g/dL, albumin 5.0 g/dL, and creatinine 0.5 mg/dL. A genetic mutation involving which of the following substances is most likely to be present in this child?

❑ (A) Adenosine deaminase
❑ (B) α₁-Antitrypsin
❑ (C) Galactose-1-phosphate uridyltransferase
❑ (D) Glucose-6-phosphatase
❑ (E) Lysosomal acid maltase
❑ (F) Phenylalanine hydroxylase
❑ (G) Sphingomyelinase

26 A 33-year-old woman in the 32nd week of pregnancy notices lack of fetal movement for 3 days. On physical examination, no fetal heart tones can be auscultated. The fetus is stillborn. At autopsy, scattered microabscesses are seen in the liver, spleen, brain, and placenta. No congenital anomalies are present. Similar fetal losses have occurred in the same community for the past 3 months. Congenital infection with which of the following organisms is most likely to produce these findings?

❑ (A) Cytomegalovirus
❑ (B) Group B streptococcus
❑ (C) Herpes simplex virus
❑ (D) *Listeria monocytogenes*
❑ (E) Parvovirus
❑ (F) Rubella virus
❑ (G) *Toxoplasma gondii*
❑ (H) *Treponema pallidum*

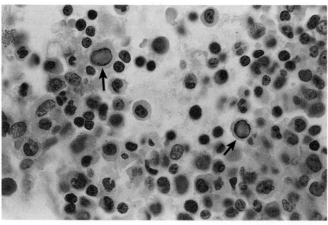

27 A 19-year-old primigravida who has had an uncomplicated pregnancy undergoes a screening ultrasound at 16 weeks' gestation that shows no abnormalities. At 18 weeks, the woman develops a mild rash on her face. She gives birth to a stillborn severely hydropic male infant at 33 weeks. At autopsy, there are no congenital malformations, but cardiomegaly is present. From the histologic appearance of the bone marrow shown in the preceding figure, which of the following is the most likely cause of these findings?

❑ (A) Maternal IgG crossing the placenta
❑ (B) Chromosomal anomaly of the fetus
❑ (C) Congenital neuroblastoma
❑ (D) Inheritance of two abnormal *CFTR* genes
❑ (E) Infection with parvovirus B19

28 A 25-year-old woman is G 5, P 0, and Ab 4. All of her previous pregnancies ended in first or second trimester spontaneous abortion. She is now in the 16th week of her fifth pregnancy and has had no prenatal problems. Laboratory findings include maternal blood type of A positive, negative serologic test for syphilis, and immunity to rubella. Which of the following laboratory studies would be most useful for determining a potential cause of recurrent fetal loss in this patient?

❑ (A) Maternal serum α-fetoprotein determination
❑ (B) Genetic analysis of the *CFTR* gene
❑ (C) Maternal serologic test for HIV
❑ (D) Amniocentesis with chromosomal analysis
❑ (E) Maternal serum antibody screening

29 A 31-year-old woman, G 3, P 2, has had an uneventful pregnancy, except for lack of any fetal movement. She has a spontaneous abortion at 20 weeks' gestation and delivers a stillborn boy. On examination at birth, the infant has an abdominal wall defect lateral to the umbilical cord insertion, a short umbilical cord, marked vertebral scoliosis, and a thin, fibrous band constricting the right lower extremity, which lacks fingers. None of the woman's other pregnancies, which ended in term births, were similarly affected. Which of the following is the most likely cause of these findings?

❑ (A) Trisomy 18
❑ (B) Oligohydramnios
❑ (C) Maternal fetal Rh incompatibility
❑ (D) Early amnion disruption
❑ (E) Congenital cytomegalovirus infection

30 In a study of potential causes of birth defects, maternal use of pharmacologic agents is analyzed. Synthetic retinoids are effective in the treatment of acne. However, pregnant women are advised against use of this medication, because retinoic acid can cause congenital malformations. The teratogenic effect of retinoic acid is most likely related to its ability to affect which of the following processes?

❑ (A) Increasing the risk of maternal infections
❑ (B) Reducing resistance of the fetus to transplacental infections
❑ (C) Increasing the likelihood of aneuploidy during cell division
❑ (D) Promoting abnormal development of blood vessels in the placenta
❑ (E) Disrupting the pattern of expression of homeobox genes

31 A 25-year-old woman, G 4, P 3, has a screening ultrasound at 18 weeks' gestation. Findings include a fetal size equivalent to 16 weeks' gestation, microcephaly, endocardial cushion defect, multicystic renal dysplasia, and bilateral clubfeet. The mother's prior pregnancies produced healthy term infants. Which of the following etiologic factors is the most common cause of the congenital malformations in this fetus?

❑ (A) Single large structural gene mutation
❑ (B) Maternal infection
❑ (C) Maternal drug use
❑ (D) Interaction of multiple genes with environmental factors
❑ (E) Chromosomal aberrations occurring early in gestation

32 An infant born at 37 weeks' gestation appears morphologically normal but weighs 1500 g. This weight is below the 10th percentile for age. Further examination indicates that the crown-heel length is below normal for gestational age, but head circumference is normal. Which of the following events is most likely to have caused this condition?

❑ (A) Transplacental spread of maternal toxoplasmosis
❑ (B) Nondisjunction of chromosomes during maternal oogenesis
❑ (C) Nondisjunction of chromosomes within the trophoblast
❑ (D) Failure of the fetal kidneys to develop
❑ (E) Mutant alleles of the *CFTR* genes from both parents

33 Examination of a fetus that was stillborn at 20 weeks shows amniotic bands that extend from amputated fingers and toes of both feet and another band in a cleft through the right aspect of the skull. Which of the following terms best describes the underlying abnormality in this fetus?

❑ (A) Disruption
❑ (B) Malformation
❑ (C) Teratogenesis
❑ (D) Inflammation
❑ (E) Deformation

34 A 16-year-old primigravida in her 18th week of pregnancy has not felt any fetal movement, and an ultrasound is performed. The amniotic fluid index is markedly decreased. Both fetal kidneys are cystic, and one is larger than the other. There is no fetal cardiac activity. The pregnancy is terminated, and a fetal autopsy is performed. Findings include multicystic renal dysplasia, hemivertebra, anal atresia, tracheoesophageal fistula, and lungs that are equivalent in size to 14 weeks' gestation. Which of the following errors in morphogenesis best accounts for the mechanism for the appearance of the lungs?

❑ (A) Agenesis
❑ (B) Aplasia
❑ (C) Deformation
❑ (D) Disruption
❑ (E) Malformation
❑ (E) Teratogenesis

35 An infant born at term develops abdominal distention in the first week of life. Meconium ileus is diagnosed. The infant has persistent steatorrhea and fails to develop normally. Later in childhood, multiple respiratory tract infections lead to widespread bronchiectasis. Which of the following laboratory findings is most likely related to this child's underlying disease?

❑ (A) Decreased serum thyroxine level
❑ (B) Positive HIV serology
❑ (C) Elevated sweat chloride level
❑ (D) Increased urine homovanillic acid level
❑ (E) Hyperbilirubinemia

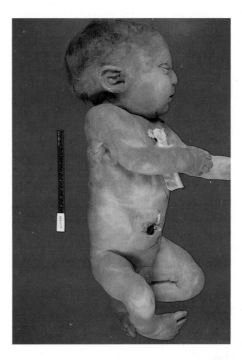

36 A 31-year-old woman, G 1, P 0, has noticed very little fetal movement during her pregnancy. At 36 weeks' gestation, she gives birth to an infant with the facial features and positioning of extremities shown. Soon after birth, the infant develops severe respiratory distress. Which of the following conditions affecting the infant best explains these findings?

❑ (A) Congenital rubella infection
❑ (B) Bilateral renal agenesis
❑ (C) Maternal diabetes mellitus
❑ (D) Hyaline membrane disease
❑ (E) Trisomy 13

37 A 17-year-old primigravida gives birth at 34 weeks' gestation to a male infant of low birth weight. The infant is given exogenous surfactant and does not develop respiratory distress. However, on the third day of life, physical examination reveals hypotension, abdominal distention, and absent bowel sounds, and there is bloody stool in the diaper. A radiograph shows pneumatosis intestinalis and free air. Which of the following conditions necessitating bowel removal is most likely to be present in this infant?

❑ (A) Duodenal atresia
❑ (B) Hirschsprung disease
❑ (C) Meckel diverticulum
❑ (D) Meconium ileus
❑ (E) Necrotizing enterocolitis
❑ (F) Pyloric stenosis

38 The parents of a 2-year-old boy are concerned because their son appears to have no vision in his right eye. On examination by the physician, there is strabismus and a whitish appearance to the pupil on the right, with tenderness to orbital palpation. Vision on the left appears to be intact. An enucleation of the right eye is performed, followed by radiation and chemotherapy. There is no recurrence on the right, but at age 5, a similar lesion develops in the left eye. At age 12, the child develops an osteosarcoma of the left distal femur. Which of the following mechanisms is most likely to produce these findings?

- ❑ (A) Aneuploidy
- ❑ (B) Chromosomal translocation
- ❑ (C) Congenital infection
- ❑ (D) Germ line mutation
- ❑ (E) Multifactorial inheritance
- ❑ (F) Teratogenesis
- ❑ (G) X-linked gene defect

39 A 13-year-old boy has had a fever and productive cough for the past 4 days. On physical examination his temperature is 38.2°C. He has passed foul-smelling stools for the past 5 years. There is a family history for cystic fibrosis; a sweat chloride test is performed and is normal. Pseudomonas aeruginosa is cultured from his sputum. Over the next 3 days he develops septicemia and dies. Notable findings at autopsy include bilateral necrotizing pneumonia, mucus plugging of pancreatic ducts with exocrine pancreatic atrophy, and bilateral absence of the vas deferens. The pancreatic lesions in this boy are most likely to be caused by which of the following mechanisms?

- ❑ (A) Failure to secrete bicarbonate ions into the pancreatic ducts
- ❑ (B) Secretion of abnormal muin into the pancreatic ducts
- ❑ (C) Vitamin A deficiency causing pancreatic ductal squamous metaplasia
- ❑ (D) Protein-energy malnutrition causing pancreatic acinar atrophy
- ❑ (E) Release of bacterial products into the circulation

ANSWERS

1 **(A)** The infant is small for gestational age because of intrauterine growth retardation. The asymmetric growth suggests a maternal or placental cause. Fetal problems such as chromosomal abnormalities, infections, and erythroblastosis are likely to produce symmetric growth retardation. Infants born to diabetic mothers are likely to be larger than normal for gestational age. Fetal hydrops can accompany congenital infections and erythroblastosis, which may artificially increase fetal weight.

BP7 242   BP6 203   PBD7 476-478   PBD6 461-462

2 **(C)** The cause of sudden infant death syndrome (SIDS) is unknown, but certain risk factors are well established. Among these is age. SIDS occurs between 1 month and 1 year of age, and 90% of SIDS deaths occur during the first 6 months of life. Although age alone cannot exclude SIDS in this case, all other factors listed increase the risk of SIDS. Male sex, African-American race, low socioeconomic background of

parents, lack of underlying medical problems, and absence of anatomic abnormality all favor the likelihood of SIDS. The only factor that argues against SIDS in this case is the age of 18 months.

BP7 245   BP6 205   PBD7 495-497   PBD6 481-482

3 **(B)** This premature newborn does not have sufficient type II alveolar cell surfactant production. As a result, the neonate has developed hyaline membrane disease. If the neonate were to survive but later develop bronchopulmonary dysplasia, fibrosis would be apparent. An alveolar transudate or exudate may accompany a variety of conditions, but it is not the key feature of hyaline membrane disease. Mucus plugging occurs in cystic fibrosis, but this is not a common finding in neonatal lungs.

BP7 242-244   BP6 204-205   PBD7 481-483
PBD6 471-472

4 **(D)** This child has cystic fibrosis. The abnormal chloride ion transport in this disease results in abnormal mucus secretions in pancreatic ducts. The secretions cause plugging with subsequent acinar atrophy and fibrosis leading to malabsorption, particularly of lipids. Galactose-1-phosphate uridyltransferase deficiency gives rise to galactosemia. Patients with this condition have liver damage but no pancreatic abnormalities. Abnormalities of the LDL receptor in familial hypercholesterolemia lead to accelerated atherogenesis. Abnormal fibrillin is a feature of Marfan syndrome. Phenylketonuria results from a deficiency of phenylalanine hydroxylase.

BP7 248-251   BP6 207-209   PBD7 489-494
PBD6 477-481

5 **(D)** Amplification of the *N-MYC* oncogene occurs in about 25% of neuroblastomas, and the greater the number of copies, the worse is the prognosis. This amplification tends to occur in neuroblastomas with a higher stage or with chromosome 1p deletions. Hyperdiploidy or near triploidy is usually associated with lack of *N-MYC* amplification, absence of 1p deletion, and high levels of nerve growth factor receptor Trk A expression. All of these are associated with good prognosis. The presence of ganglion cells is consistent with a better differentiation and better prognosis; some tumors may differentiate over time and become ganglioneuromas under the influence of Trk A. Renal malformations are not related to neuroblastomas.

BP7 253-255   BP6 211-212   PBD7 500-504
PBD6 486-487

6 **(A)** Teratomas are benign neoplasms composed of tissues derived from embryonic germ layers (ectoderm, mesoderm, or endoderm). Teratomas occur in midline locations, and the sacrococcygeal area is the most common. Less common immature or frankly malignant teratomas with neuroblastic elements can occur. Neuroblastomas are malignant childhood tumors that most often arise in the adrenal glands. Hemangiomas form irregular, red-blue skin lesions that are flat and spreading. Lymphangiomas are most often lateral head and neck lesions occurring in childhood. Hamartomas are masses composed of tissues normally found at a particular site, and they are rare.

BP7 252   BP6 210-211   PBD7 499   PBD6 484

7 **(D)** The immaturity of the fetal lungs before 35 to 36 weeks' gestation can be complicated by lack of sufficient surfactant to enable adequate ventilation after birth. This can result in hyaline membrane disease. Tests on amniotic fluid before birth, including lecithin-sphingomyelin ratio, fluorescence polarization, and lamellar body counts, are useful in predicting the degree of pulmonary immaturity. Fetal anemia leads to heart failure and pulmonary congestion. Maternal toxemia and congenital infections may lead to hyaline membrane disease if the birth occurs prematurely as a consequence of these conditions, but they do not directly affect lung maturity. Oligohydramnios may result in neonatal respiratory distress through the mechanism of pulmonary hypoplasia.

BP7 242-244   BP6 204-205   PBD7 481-483
PBD6 471-472

8 **(C)** Rubella infection in the first trimester, when organogenesis is occurring (4 to 9 weeks' gestation), can lead to congenital heart defects. Dispermy leads to triploidy, a condition that rarely results in a live birth. In the past, thalidomide use was an important cause of malformations (almost invariably prominent limb deformities). The use of thalidomide as an immunosuppressive agent is under consideration. Erythroblastosis fetalis leads to fetal anemia with congestive heart failure and hydrops but not to malformations. Folate deficiency is most likely to be associated with neural tube defects. Nondisjunctional events during meiosis in the maternal ova account for trisomies and monosomies, many of which have associated cardiac defects, including ventricular septal defect (e.g., trisomy 21). However, this mechanism is unlikely in paternal sperm, which are constantly being produced in large numbers throughout life.

BP7 241-242   BP6 201-202   PBD7 473   PBD6 466-467

9 **(D)** Surfactant is synthesized by type II pneumocytes that line the alveolar sacs. They begin to differentiate after the 26th week of gestation. These cells can be recognized on electron microscopy by the presence of lamellar bodies. Surfactant production increases greatly after 35 weeks' gestation. Other structures in the lung do not synthesize the phosphatidylcholine and phosphatidylglycerol compounds that are important in reducing alveolar surface tension.

BP7 242-244   BP6 204-205   PBD7 481-483
PBD6 471-472

10 **(B)** Most malformations, particularly those that are isolated defects, have no readily identifiable cause. They are believed to be caused by the inheritance of a certain number of genes and by the interaction of those genes with environmental factors. Their transmission follows the rules for multifactorial inheritance. The recurrence rate is believed to be 2% to 7% and is the same for all first-degree relatives, regardless of sex and relationship to the index case.

BP7 227, 240-241   BP6 201-202   PBD7 472-473
PBD6 466-467

11 **(A)** Persons with phenylketonuria (PKU) survive to reproductive age with good mental function when they are treated from infancy with a phenylalanine-free diet. After neurologic development is completed in childhood, the diet is no longer needed. However, a pregnant woman with PKU has high levels of phenylalanine, which can damage the developing fetus. Resuming a phenylalanine-free diet is a major sac-

rifice, because most foods contain phenylalanine. (Persons without PKU can find drinking even 100 mL of a liquid phenylalanine-free meal to be difficult.) PKU does not affect tissues other than those of the central nervous system and does not result in malformations.

BP7 220-221   BP6 184   PBD7 487-488   PBD6 475-476

12 **(C)** The hyperinsulinism in the fetus of a diabetic mother suppresses pulmonary surfactant production. Corticosteroids stimulate surfactant production. Infection may increase the risk of premature birth, but it does not significantly affect surfactant production. Oligohydramnios leads to constriction in utero that culminates in pulmonary hypoplasia, not decreased surfactant. Maternal hypertension may reduce placental function and increase growth retardation, but it typically does not have a significant effect on the production of surfactant.

BP7 242-244   BP6 204   PBD7 482   PBD6 471-472

13 **(C)** The infant has findings associated with galactosemia, an autosomal recessive condition that can be tested for at birth. Histologically, the liver of affected infants has marked fatty change and portal fibrosis that increases over time. In addition to hepatic lesions, these infants have diarrhea and develop cataracts. For unknown reasons, they are very susceptible to *Escherichia coli* septicemia. Adenosine deaminase deficiency is a cause of severe combined immunodeficiency, which is characterized by multiple recurrent severe infections from birth. α_1-Antitrypsin deficiency may produce cholestasis in children, but chronic liver disease develops later. An abnormality of globin chains underlies hemoglobinopathies such as the thalassemias, which are characterized by anemia. A deficiency of glucocerebrosidase leads to Gaucher disease but does not cause severe hepatic failure. A deficiency of hexosaminidase A leads to Tay-Sachs disease, which is characterized by severe neurologic deterioration. Abnormalities of the red cell membrane protein spectrin underlie hereditary spherocytosis, which causes a mild hemolytic anemia.

BP7 221   BP6 185   PBD7 488-489   PBD6 476-477

14 **(A)** About 10% of cytomegalovirus-infected neonates have extensive infection with inclusions found in many organs. Severe anemia and myocardial injury cause hydrops, and the brain is often involved. The renal tubular epithelium can be infected, and large cells with inclusions can be seen with urine microscopic examination in some cases. Cytomegalovirus manifested in neonates may have been acquired transplacentally, at birth, or in breast milk. Herpes simplex virus is usually acquired via passage through the birth canal and does not cause a periventricular leukomalacia. HIV infection in utero does not produce marked organ damage. The JC papovavirus produces multifocal leukoencephalopathy in immunocompromised adults. Parvovirus infection may cause a severe fetal anemia. Congenital rubella manifests in the first trimester, often with cardiac defects.

BP7 242   PBD7 473, 484   PBD6 376

15 **(D)** High-dose oxygen with positive pressure ventilation can cause injury to immature lungs, leading to the chronic lung disease known as bronchopulmonary dysplasia. In sudden infant death syndrome (SIDS), no anatomic abnormalities are found at autopsy. A ventricular septal defect could eventually lead to pulmonary hypertension from the left-to-right shunt. Pulmonary manifestations of cystic fibrosis are not seen at birth or in infancy. Mortality from pulmonary hypoplasia is greatest at birth.

BP7 244   BP6 205   PBD7 482-483   PBD6 472-473

16 (B) This infant has a mild hemolytic anemia. The most probable cause is an ABO incompatibility with maternal blood type O, which results in anti-A antibody coating fetal cells. Most anti-A and anti-B antibodies are IgM. However, in about 20% to 25% of pregnancies, there are also IgG antibodies, which cross the placenta in sufficient titer to produce mild hemolytic disease in most cases. The bilirubin concentration in the term infant in this case is not high enough to produce kernicterus. Respiratory distress is unlikely at term. ABO incompatibilities are not likely to have such serious consequences for subsequent pregnancies as does Rh incompatibility. As the infant matures, the level of maternal antibody diminishes, hemolysis abates, and the infant develops normally.

BP7 246   BP6 206   PBD7 485   PBD6 473

17 (E) The most common tumor of infancy is a hemangioma, and these benign neoplasms form a large percentage of childhood tumors as well. Although benign, they can be large and disfiguring. A proliferation of neuroblasts occurs in neuroblastoma, a common childhood neoplasm in the abdomen. Lymphangioma is another common benign childhood tumor seen in the neck, mediastinum, and retroperitoneum. Fibromatoses are fibromatous proliferations of soft tissues that form solid masses. Lymphoblasts as part of leukemic infiltrates or lymphomas are not likely to be seen in skin, but mediastinal masses may be seen.

BP7 251   BP6 210   PBD7 498   PBD6 483

18 (C) When a genetic disease (e.g., cystic fibrosis) is caused by many different mutations, no simple screening test that can detect all the mutations can be performed. Although 70% of patients with cystic fibrosis have a 3–base pair deletion that can be readily detected by polymerase chain reaction (the $\Delta F508$ mutation), the remaining 30% have disease caused by several hundred allelic forms of *CFTR*. To detect all would require sequencing of the *CFTR* genes. This prohibits mass screening. The other listed options do not apply.

BP7 249   BP6 207-209   PBD7 490   PBD6 478-479

19 (C) Beckwith-Wiedemann syndrome is an uncommon syndrome caused by a mutation on chromosome 11. It carries an increased risk of development of Wilms' tumor, a childhood neoplasm arising in the kidney. Renal anomalies such as horseshoe kidney can be seen in Edwards syndrome (trisomy 18) but not neoplasms. Likewise, Marfan syndrome is not associated with an increased risk of malignancy. Children with McArdle syndrome, which results from a deficiency of myophosphorylase, can have muscle cramping but are not at risk of neoplasia. The 47,XXY karyotype of Klinefelter syndrome does not carry an increased risk of renal tumors. Patau syndrome (trisomy 13) is associated with many anomalies, among them postaxial polydactyly and midline defects that include cleft lip and palate, cyclopia, and holoprosencephaly. Turner syndrome (monosomy X) occurs in females and can

be associated with multiple anomalies, including cystic hygroma, aortic coarctation, and renal anomalies.

BP7 256-257   BP6 213-214   PBD7 505   PBD6 488-489

20 (E) Alcohol is perhaps one of the most common environmental teratogens affecting fetuses, although the effects can be subtle. There is no threshold amount of alcohol consumption by the mother to produce fetal alcohol syndrome; no amount is safe. Children with this syndrome tend to be developmentally impaired throughout childhood, but the physical anomalies tend to become less apparent as the child ages. Vertebral abnormalities, including scoliosis, can be present. The liver can have fatty metamorphosis with hepatomegaly and elevated serum transaminases. The major effects of congenital rubella occur during organogenesis in the first trimester and result in more pronounced defects, including congenital heart disease. Placenta previa, a low-lying placenta at or near the cervical os, can cause significant hemorrhage at the time of delivery or uteroplacental insufficiency with growth retardation before delivery. Placental causes of intrauterine growth retardation result in asymmetric growth retardation with sparing of the brain. Maternal diabetes often results in a larger infant, and malformations may also be present. The findings of trisomy 21 are subtle at birth but typically include brachycephaly, not microcephaly.

BP7 241   BP6 202   PBD7 473   PBD6 467

21 (A) This infant has erythroblastosis fetalis, which results when maternal antibody coats fetal RBCs, causing hemolysis. The fetal anemia leads to congestive heart failure and hydrops. Hemolysis results in a very high bilirubin level. A high maternal serum level of α-fetoprotein suggests a fetal neural tube defect; such defects are not associated with hydrops. Viral hepatitis is not a perinatal infection. Diminished glucocerebrosidase activity causes Gaucher disease. This condition does not lead to perinatal liver failure or anemia. Listeriosis or other congenital infections may produce hydrops and anemia, although not of the severity described in this case.

BP7 246   BP6 206-207   PBD7 485-486   PBD6 473-475

22 (E) The events described suggest sudden infant death syndrome (SIDS). The cause is unknown and, by definition, there are no significant gross or microscopic autopsy findings. Infants with congenital anomalies or infections are unlikely to appear healthy, feed well, or gain weight normally. Hyaline membrane disease occurs at birth with prematurity. Congenital neoplasms are a rare cause of sudden death.

BP7 245   BP6 205   PBD7 495-497   PBD6 481-482

23 (E) The acute inflammation suggests a bacterial infection, and group B *Streptococcus*, which can colonize the vagina, is a common cause. The infection can develop quickly. Cytomegalovirus, syphilis, and toxoplasmosis are congenital infections that can cause stillbirth, but they are more likely to be chronic. Herpetic infections are most likely to be acquired by passage through the birth canal.

BP7 242   BP6 203   PBD7 480   PBD6 470

24 (B) The neonate most likely has hyaline membrane disease from fetal lung immaturity and lack of surfactant. Surfactant consists predominantly of dipalmitoyl phosphatidylcholine. The adequacy of surfactant production can be gauged by the phospholipid content of amniotic fluid, because fetal lung secretions are discharged into the amniotic fluid. The maternal serum α-fetoprotein level is useful to predict fetal neural tube defects and chromosomal abnormalities. Chromosomal analysis may help to predict problems after birth or the possibility of fetal loss. The Coombs test may help to determine the presence of erythroblastosis fetalis. Cystic fibrosis does not cause respiratory problems at birth.

BP7 242-244   BP6 204   PBD7 481-483   PBD6 471-472

25 **(F)** This child has phenylketonuria (PKU). The absence of phenylalanine hydroxylase genes give rise to hyperphenylalaninemia, which impairs brain development and can lead to seizures. The block in phenylalanine metabolism results in decreased pigmentation of skin and hair. It also results in the formation of intermediate compounds, such as phenylacetic acid, that are excreted in urine and impart to it a "mousy" odor. Although PKU is rare, because of the devastating consequences of this inherited disorder and because it can be treated with a phenylalanine-free diet, this is one of the diseases for which screening is performed at birth. Adenosine deaminase deficiency is a cause of severe combined immunodeficiency, which is characterized by multiple recurrent severe infections from birth. α₁-Antitrypsin deficiency may produce cholestasis in children, but chronic liver disease develops later. Galactose-1-phosphate uridyltransferase deficiency causes galactosemia, which is characterized by severe liver disease. Glucose-6-phosphatase deficiency causes type I glycogenosis (von Gierke disease), which leads to liver failure. Lysosomal acid maltase deficiency causes Pompe disease, with features that include cardiomegaly and heart failure. Sphingomyelinase deficiency causes Niemann-Pick disease; affected infants have marked hepatosplenomegaly and marked neurologic deterioration.

BP7 220-221   BP6 184-185   PBD7 487-488
PBD6 475-476

26 **(D)** Listeriosis can be a congenital infection. Although pregnant women may have only a mild diarrheal illness, the organism can prove devastating to the fetus or neonate. Miniepidemics of listeriosis are often linked to a contaminated food source, such as dairy products, chicken, or hot dogs. Neonatal meningitis can be caused by *Listeria monocytogenes*. Cytomegalovirus and toxoplasmosis are likely to produce severe central nervous system damage. Group B streptococcal infections most often infect the fetus near term or peripartum. These organisms release a factor that inhibits the neutrophilic chemotactic factor complement C5a, thus inhibiting a suppurative response. Herpetic congenital infections typically are acquired via passage through the birth canal. Parvovirus infection may cause a severe fetal anemia. Rubella infection is devastating if acquired during the first trimester and can lead to multiple congenital anomalies. *Treponema pallidum* infection is typically acquired in utero during the third trimester and leads to marked fetal and placental hydrops.

PBD7 375, 480-481   PBD6 378

27 **(E)** The erythroid precursors demonstrate large, pink, intranuclear inclusions typical of parvovirus. In adults, such an infection typically causes fifth disease, which is self-limiting. However, this is one of the "O" infections in the TORCH mnemonic describing congenital infections (*t*oxoplasmosis, *o*ther infections, *r*ubella, *c*ytomegalovirus infection, and

*h*erpes simplex infection). Parvovirus infection in the fetus can lead to a profound fetal anemia with cardiac failure and hydrops fetalis. Erythroblastosis fetalis is unlikely to occur in a first pregnancy, and only erythroid expansion is present, not erythroid inclusions. Although a variety of chromosomal anomalies—monosomy X, in particular—may lead to hydrops, malformations are typical. Congenital tumors are an uncommon cause of hydrops, and they would produce a mass lesion, which was not described in this case. Cystic fibrosis does not affect erythropoiesis.

BP7 247   PBD7 484, 486   PBD6 470,474

28 **(D)** Multiple fetal losses earlier in gestation suggest the likelihood of a chromosomal abnormality—the mother or father may be the carrier of a balanced translocation. The maternal serum level of α-fetoprotein can help identify fetal neural tube defects, but these defects are not a cause of early fetal loss. Cystic fibrosis produces problems postnatally. Maternal HIV infection is not a cause of significant fetal loss. Because the mother is blood type A positive, fetal loss with erythroblastosis fetalis is unlikely, although other blood group incompatibilities may potentially result in erythroblastosis fetalis.

BP7 240-241   BP6 214-215   PBD7 470, 472   PBD6 182

29 **(D)** This is a classic example of an embryonic disruption that leads to the appearance of congenital malformations. Fibrous bands and possible vascular insults may explain such findings, which fall within the spectrum of a limb-body wall complex that includes amniotic band syndrome. In trisomy 18 and other chromosomal abnormalities, an omphalocele is the most common abdominal wall defect. Oligohydramnios with diminished amniotic fluid leads to deformations, not disruptions. Rh incompatibility can give rise to erythroblastosis fetalis, which may manifest as hydrops fetalis. Fetuses affected by hydrops have widespread edema and intense jaundice. A variety of malformations may occur as a result of congenital infections, but amnionic bands are not among them.

BP7 238-239   BP6 200   PBD7 470-471   PBD6 465

30 **(E)** Retinoic acid embryopathy, which is characterized by cardiac, neural, and craniofacial defects, is believed to result from the ability of retinoids to affect the expression of homeobox (HOX) genes. These genes are important in embryonal patterning of limbs, vertebrae, and craniofacial structures. The other listed options do not apply to retinoic acid.

PBD7 473, 476   PBD6 469

31 **(D)** Multifactorial inheritance is the single most common known cause of congenital malformations. This information is useful when advising patients of the likelihood of recurrence. Most cases of congenital anomalies from multifactorial inheritance have a recurrence risk of 2% to 7%. All the other listed causes added together are about equal to multifactorial inheritance. Chromosomal anomalies probably account for most first trimester fetal losses; often, however, it is difficult to identify anomalies in the embryo or early fetus, or the fetus is passed via spontaneous abortion and is not recovered.

BP7 227   BP6 201-202   PBD7 473-474   PBD6 466-467

32 **(C)** The infant has asymmetric intrauterine growth retardation, which can result from placental causes. Confined placental mosaicism results from viable genetic mutations in dividing trophoblasts after zygote formation. Transplacental spread of infection to the fetus would give rise to proportionate intrauterine growth retardation (IUGR). Nondisjunction of chromosomes during maternal oogenesis would affect the fetus very early in gestation and would result in symmetric growth retardation. Failure of the kidneys to develop can cause oligohydramnios, and the fetus would be abnormal in appearance. Mutation at both alleles of the *CFTR* gene gives rise to cystic fibrosis. This condition is not associated with IUGR.

BP7 228   BP6 203   PBD7 477-478   PBD6 461-462

33 **(A)** This describes amniotic band syndrome, a subset of limb-body wall complex, which results from embryonic disruption with destruction of body regions and formation of fibrous bands. A malformation, such as congenital heart disease, results from an error in morphogenesis. Chromosomal abnormalities can be accompanied by a variety of malformations. Teratogens produce malformations but not a pattern of disruptions. Inflammation can produce malformations (e.g., congenital syphilis) or tissue destruction (e.g., congenital cytomegalovirus infection). Deformations result from mechanical forces on organs and tissues (e.g., the facial features seen in oligohydramnios).

BP7 238-239   BP6 200-201   PBD7 470-471
PBD6 464-465

34 **(C)** The lungs are hypoplastic (small) because of deformation caused by an oligohydramnios sequence. The malformation (anomaly) that initiated the sequence in this case was multicystic renal dysplasia, because the kidneys formed little fetal urine, which is passed into the amniotic cavity to form the bulk of the amniotic fluid. There was no disruption in this case. Teratogens may produce anomalies, but these are not common. The spectrum of findings in this case is consistent with the VATER association (*v*ertebral defects, imperforate *a*nus, *t*racheo*e*sophageal fistula, and *r*adial and *r*enal dysplasia).

BP7 239-240   BP6 200-201   PBD7 472   PBD6

35 **(C)** The findings are typical of cystic fibrosis, which is an inherited defect in chloride transport. Cretinism from hypothyroidism results in impaired central nervous system and skeletal development. An infant with congenital HIV infection may have a variety of opportunistic infections but not meconium ileus. Increased urine homovanillic acid level is a feature of neuroblastoma, a mass lesion that could also cause bowel obstruction but not meconium ileus. Neonatal jaundice has a variety of causes, including the inherited disorder galactosemia.

BP7 248-251   BP6 207-209   PBD7 489-495
PBD6 477-481

36 **(B)** The flattened face and deformed feet of this infant suggest oligohydramnios resulting from renal agenesis. Fetal kidneys produce urine that becomes the amniotic fluid. Pulmonary hypoplasia is the rate-limiting step to survival. Congenital rubella can lead to a variety of malformations but not deformations. Infants born to diabetic mothers have an increased risk of congenital anomalies without a specific pattern. Fetal lung maturity is typically achieved at 34 to 35 weeks' gestation, and hyaline membrane disease is unlikely at

36 weeks. Trisomy 13 is accompanied by a variety of malformations, including those affecting the kidneys. The external features, however, are quite different from those seen in this case, and affected infants almost always have midline defects such as cleft lip and palate, and microcephaly.

BP7 239-240   BP6 201   PBD7 472   PBD6 465

37 **(E)** Necrotizing enterocolitis is a complication of prematurity that is related to a variety of factors, including intestinal ischemia, bacterial overgrowth, and formula feeding. If severe, the wall of the intestine becomes necrotic and perforates, necessitating surgical intervention. Duodenal atresia is an uncommon congenital anomaly most often associated with trisomy 21; it leads to upper gastrointestinal obstruction and vomiting. Hirschsprung disease is a congenital condition resulting from an aganglionic segment of distal colon; it leads to obstruction with distention but not bloody diarrhea. A Meckel diverticulum is a common anomaly and is seen in about 2% of persons. Typically, it is an incidental finding, although later in life it may be associated with gastrointestinal tract bleeding if ectopic gastric mucosa is present within the diverticulum. Meconium ileus is seen in the setting of cystic fibrosis and can lead to obstruction, but the infant typically does not pass stool. Pyloric stenosis presents at 3 to 6 weeks of life with projectile vomiting.

BP7 244-245   BP6 497   PBD7 483   PBD6 809

38 **(D)** This child has inherited an abnormal *RB1* gene, and early in life the other allele is lost, leading to loss of tumor suppression and development of a retinoblastoma. About 60% to 70% of retinoblastomas are associated with germ line mutations. Aneuploidy usually results in fetal loss, although monosomy X and trisomies 13, 18, and 21 may occasionally lead to live births. Chromosomal translocations may be seen with other tumors, such as chronic myelogenous leukemia, acute promyelocytic leukemia, and Burkitt lymphoma. Congenital infections typically manifest at birth and are not associated with neoplasms. Multifactorial inheritance may be associated with complex diseases such as diabetes mellitus, hypertension, and bipolar disorder. Teratogens most likely produce findings manifested at birth, and neoplasia is unlikely. X-linked single gene defects are unlikely to lead to neoplasia.

BP7 255   BP6 212, 213   PBD7 500   PBD6 1372-1373

39 **(A)** This child has a classical history for cystic fibrosis (CF), but there are hundreds of known CFTR mutations, and with some mutant alleles of CFTR chloride ion secretion is normal. CFTR also controls bicarbonate transport, particularly in the pancreas. In this case, failure of bicarbonate secretion decreases the pH of the pancreatic fluid, causing increased mucus precipitation and ductal plugging. The resultant exocrine pancreatic atrophy causes steatorrhea and poor fat soluble vitamin absorption. In CF, the chemical nature of the mucin is normal. Vitamin A deficiency is the result of CF and can worsen the condition via ductal squamous metaplasia. Patients with CF can be malnourished, but this is the consequence, not the cause for pancreatic abnormalities. Bacterial products can be non-specifically toxic to many tissues. The bilateral absence of the vas deferens noted in this case is another feature of some CF cases, and azospermia occurs in 90% of cases, even when the vas deferens is patent.

BP7 248-251 PBD7 489-495

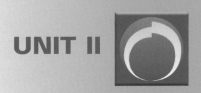

Diseases of
Organ Systems

Blood Vessels

1 The development of atheromatous plaque formation with subsequent complications is observed in an experiment. Atherosclerotic plaques are shown to change slowly but constantly in ways that can promote clinical events, including acute coronary syndromes. In some cases, however, changes occurred that were not significantly associated with acute coronary syndromes. Which of the following plaque alterations is most likely to have such an association?

- (A) Thinning of the media
- (B) Ulceration of the plaque surface
- (C) Thrombosis
- (D) Hemorrhage into the plaque substance
- (E) Intermittent platelet aggregation

2 A 60-year-old woman has reported increasing fatigue over the past year. Laboratory studies show a serum creatinine level of 4.7 mg/dL and urea nitrogen level of 44 mg/dL. An abdominal ultrasound scan shows that her kidneys are symmetrically smaller than normal. The high-magnification microscopic appearance of the kidneys is shown. These findings are most likely to indicate which of the following underlying conditions?

- (A) *Escherichia coli* septicemia
- (B) Systemic hypertension
- (C) Adenocarcinoma of the colon
- (D) Tertiary syphilis
- (E) Polyarteritis nodosa

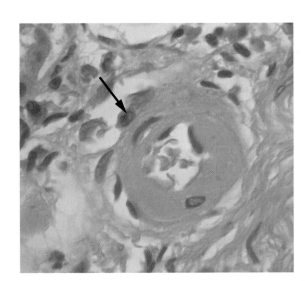

3 A 55-year-old woman visits her physician for a routine health maintenance examination. On physical examination, her temperature is 36.8°C, pulse 70/min, respirations 14/min, and blood pressure 160/105 mm Hg. Her lungs are clear on auscultation, and her heart rate is regular. She feels fine and has had no major medical illnesses or surgical procedures during her lifetime. An abdominal ultrasound scan shows that the left kidney is smaller than the right kidney. A renal angiogram shows a focal stenosis of the left renal artery. Which of the following laboratory findings is most likely to be present in this patient?

- ❏ (A) Anti–double-stranded-DNA titer 1:512
- ❏ (B) C-ANCA titer 1:256
- ❏ (C) Cryoglobulinemia
- ❏ (D) Plasma glucose level 200 mg/dL
- ❏ (E) HIV test positive
- ❏ (F) Plasma renin 15 mg/mL/h
- ❏ (G) Serologic test for syphilis positive

4 A 7-year-old child has had abdominal pain and dark urine for 10 days. Physical examination shows purpuric skin lesions on the trunk and extremities. Urinalysis shows both hematuria and proteinuria. Serologic test results are negative for P-ANCAs and C-ANCAs. A skin biopsy specimen shows necrotizing vasculitis of small dermal vessels. A renal biopsy specimen shows immune complex deposition in glomeruli, with some IgA-rich immune complexes. Which of the following is the most likely diagnosis?

- ❏ (A) Giant cell arteritis
- ❏ (B) Henoch-Schönlein purpura
- ❏ (C) Polyarteritis nodosa
- ❏ (D) Takayasu arteritis
- ❏ (E) Telangiectasias
- ❏ (F) Wegener granulomatosis

5 A 30-year-old woman has had coldness and numbness in her arms and decreased vision in the right eye for the past 5 months. On physical examination, she is afebrile. Her blood pressure is 100/70 mm Hg. Radial pulses are not palpable, but femoral pulses are strong. She has decreased sensation and cyanosis in her arms but no warmth or swelling. A chest radiograph shows a prominent border on the right side of the heart and prominence of the pulmonary arteries. Laboratory studies show serum glucose of 74 mg/dL, creatinine 1.0 mg/dL, total serum cholesterol 165 mg/dL, and negative ANA test result. Her condition remains stable for the next year. Which of the following is the most likely diagnosis?

- ❏ (A) Aortic dissection
- ❏ (B) Kawasaki disease
- ❏ (C) Microscopic polyangiitis
- ❏ (D) Takayasu arteritis
- ❏ (E) Tertiary syphilis
- ❏ (F) Thromboangiitis obliterans

6 A 61-year-old man had a myocardial infarction (MI) 1 year ago, which was the first major illness in his life. He now wants to prevent another MI and is advised to begin a program of exercise and change his diet. A reduction in the level of which of the following serum laboratory findings 1 year later would best indicate the success of this diet and exercise regime?

- ❏ (A) Cholesterol
- ❏ (B) Glucose
- ❏ (C) Potassium
- ❏ (D) Renin
- ❏ (E) Calcium

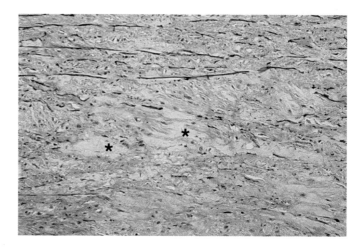

7 A 23-year-old man experiences sudden onset of severe, sharp chest pain. On physical examination, his temperature is 36.9°C, and his lungs are clear on auscultation. A chest radiograph shows a widened mediastinum. Transesophageal echocardiography shows a dilated aortic root and arch, with a tear in the aortic intima 2 cm distal to the great vessels. The representative microscopic appearance of the aorta with elastic stain is shown in the figure. Which of the following is the most likely cause of these findings?

- ❏ (A) Scleroderma
- ❏ (B) Diabetes mellitus
- ❏ (C) Systemic hypertension
- ❏ (D) Marfan syndrome
- ❏ (E) Wegener granulomatosis
- ❏ (F) Takayasu arteritis

8 A 40-year-old man has had worsening abdominal pain for the past week. On physical examination, his vital signs include a temperature of 35.9°C, pulse 77/min, respirations 16/min, and blood pressure 140/90 mm Hg. A pulsatile abdominal mass is palpated. An abdominal CT scan shows a 6-cm fusiform-shaped enlargement of the abdominal aorta. An abdominal aortic graft is surgically inserted. Which of the following is the most likely underlying disease process in this patient?

- ❏ (A) Polyarteritis nodosa
- ❏ (B) Obesity
- ❏ (C) Diabetes mellitus
- ❏ (D) Systemic lupus erythematosus
- ❏ (E) Syphilis

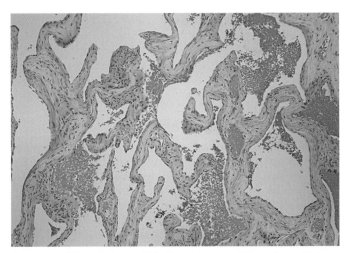

Courtesy of Tom Rogers, MD, Department of Pathology, University of Texas Southwestern Medical School, Dallas, TX.

9 A 10-year-old boy is brought to the physician for a routine health maintenance examination. The physician notes a 2-cm spongy, dull red, circumscribed lesion on the upper outer left arm. The parents state that this lesion has been present since infancy. The lesion is excised, and its microscopic appearance is shown. Which of the following is the most likely diagnosis?

- (A) Kaposi sarcoma
- (B) Angiosarcoma
- (C) Lymphangioma
- (D) Telangiectasia
- (E) Hemangioma

10 A pharmaceutical company is developing an antiatherosclerosis agent. An experiment investigates mechanisms of action of several potential drugs to determine their efficacy in reducing atheroma formation. Which of the following mechanisms of action is likely to have the most effective antiatherosclerotic effect?

- (A) Inhibits the release of platelet-derived growth factor (PDGF) and macrophage-mediated lipoprotein oxidation
- (B) Promotes the release of PDGF and inhibits macrophage-mediated lipoprotein oxidation
- (C) Inhibits the release of PDGF and promotes macrophage-mediated lipoprotein oxidation
- (D) Decreases the level of HDL and inhibits macrophage-mediated lipoprotein oxidation
- (E) Increases the level of intercellular adhesion molecule-1 (ICAM-1) and vascular cell adhesion molecule-1 (VCAM-1) on endothelial cells and increases endothelial permeability

11 A 73-year-old man who has had progressive dementia for the past 6 years dies of bronchopneumonia. Autopsy shows that the thoracic aorta has a dilated root and arch, giving the intimal surface a "tree-bark" appearance. Microscopic examination of the aorta shows an obliterative endarteritis of the vasa vasorum. Which of the following laboratory findings is most likely to be recorded in this patient's medical history?

- (A) High double-stranded DNA titer
- (B) P-ANCA positive 1:1024
- (C) Sedimentation rate 105 mm/h
- (D) Ketonuria 4+
- (E) Antibodies against *Treponema pallidum*

12 For the past 3 weeks, a 70-year-old woman has been bedridden while recuperating from a bout of viral pneumonia complicated by bacterial pneumonia. Physical examination now shows some swelling and tenderness of the right leg, which worsens when she raises or moves the leg. Which of the following terms best describes the condition involving the patient's right leg?

- (A) Lymphedema
- (B) Disseminated intravascular coagulopathy
- (C) Thrombophlebitis
- (D) Thromboangiitis obliterans
- (E) Varicose veins

13 A 49-year-old man is feeling fine when he visits his physician for a routine health maintenance examination for the first time in 20 years. On physical examination, his vital signs include a temperature of 37.0°C, pulse 73/min, respirations 14/min, and blood pressure 155/95 mm Hg. He has had no serious medical problems and takes no medications. Which of the following is most likely to be the primary factor in this patient's hypertension?

- (A) Increased catecholamine secretion
- (B) Renal retention of excess sodium
- (C) Gene defects in aldosterone metabolism
- (D) Renal artery stenosis
- (E) Increased production of atrial natriuretic factor

14 A 50-year-old man has a 2-year history of angina pectoris that occurs during exercise. On physical examination, his blood pressure is 135/75 mm Hg, and his heart rate is 79/min and slightly irregular. Coronary angiography shows a fixed 75% narrowing of the anterior descending branch of the left coronary artery. Which of the following types of cells is the initial target in the pathogenesis of this arterial lesion?

- (A) Monocytes
- (B) Smooth muscle cells
- (C) Platelets
- (D) Neutrophils
- (E) Endothelial cells

15 A study of atheroma formation leading to atherosclerotic complications evaluates potential risk factors for relevance in a population. Three factors are found to play a significant role in the causation of atherosclerosis: smoking, hypertension, and hypercholesterolemia. These factors are analyzed for their relationship to experimental models for atherogenesis. Which of the following events is the most important direct biologic consequence of these factors?

- (A) Endothelial injury and its sequelae
- (B) Conversion of smooth muscle cells to foam cells
- (C) Alterations of hepatic lipoprotein receptors
- (D) Inhibition of LDL oxidation
- (E) Alterations of endogenous factors regulating vasomotor tone

16 A 55-year-old woman has noted the increasing prominence of unsightly dilated superficial veins over both lower legs for the past 5 years. Physical examination shows temperature of 37.0°C, pulse 70/min, respirations 14/min, and blood pressure 125/85 mm Hg. There is no pain, swelling, or tenderness in either lower leg. Which of the following complications is most likely to occur as a consequence of this condition?

❑ (A) Stasis dermatitis
❑ (B) Gangrenous necrosis of the lower legs
❑ (C) Pulmonary thromboembolism
❑ (D) Disseminated intravascular coagulation
❑ (E) Atrophy of the lower leg muscles

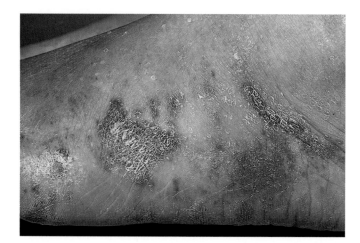

17 A 35-year-old man is known to have been infected with HIV for the past 10 years. Physical examination shows several skin lesions (as shown above). These lesions have been slowly increasing for the past year. Which of the following infectious agents is most likely to play a role in the development of these skin lesions?

❑ (A) Human herpesvirus 8
❑ (B) Epstein-Barr virus
❑ (C) Cytomegalovirus
❑ (D) Hepatitis B virus
❑ (E) Adenovirus

18 A 50-year-old man complains of a chronic cough that has persisted for the past 18 months. Physical examination shows nasopharyngeal ulcers, and the lungs have diffuse crackles bilaterally on auscultation. Laboratory studies include a serum urea nitrogen level of 75 mg/dL and a creatinine concentration of 6.7 mg/dL. Urinalysis shows 50 RBCs per high-power field and RBC casts. His serologic titer for C-ANCA is elevated. A chest radiograph shows multiple, small, bilateral pulmonary nodules. A nasal biopsy specimen shows mucosal and submucosal necrosis as well as necrotizing granulomatous inflammation. A transbronchial lung biopsy specimen shows a vasculitis involving the small peripheral pulmonary arteries and arterioles. Granulomatous inflammation is seen both within and adjacent to small arterioles. Which of the following is the most likely diagnosis?

❑ (A) Fibromuscular dysplasia
❑ (B) Glomus tumors
❑ (C) Granuloma pyogenicum
❑ (D) Hemangiomas
❑ (E) Kaposi sarcoma
❑ (F) Polyarteritis nodosa
❑ (G) Takayasu arteritis
❑ (H) Wegener granulomatosis

19 While cleaning debris out of the gate in an irrigation canal, a 50-year-old man cuts his right index finger on a sharp metal shard. The cut stops bleeding within 3 minutes, but 6 hours later he notes increasing pain in the right arm and goes to his physician. On physical examination, his temperature is 38.0°C. Red streaks extend from the right hand to the upper arm, and the arm is swollen and tender when palpated. Multiple tender lumps are noted in the right axilla. A blood culture grows group A hemolytic streptococci. Which of the following terms best describes the process that is occurring in this patient's right arm?

❑ (A) Capillaritis
❑ (B) Lymphangitis
❑ (C) Lymphedema
❑ (D) Phlebothrombosis
❑ (E) Polyarteritis nodosa
❑ (F) Thrombophlebitis
❑ (G) Varices

20 An experiment studies early atheromas. Lipid streaks on arterial walls are examined microscopically and biochemically to determine their cellular and chemical constituents and the factors promoting their formation. Early lesions show increased attachment of monocytes to endothelium. The monocytes migrate subendothelially and become macrophages; these macrophages then transform themselves into foam cells. Which of the following is most likely to produce these effects?

❑ (A) C-reactive protein
❑ (B) Homocysteine
❑ (C) Lp(a)
❑ (D) Oxidized LDL
❑ (E) Platelet-derived growth factor
❑ (F) VLDL

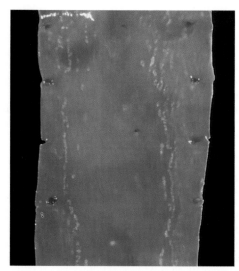

From the teaching collection of the Department of Pathology, University of Texas Southwestern Medical School, Dallas, TX.

21 A 12-year-old boy died of complications of acute lymphocytic leukemia. The gross appearance of the aorta at autopsy is shown in the preceding figure. Histologic examination of the linear pale marking is most likely to show which of the following features?

❑ (A) A core of lipid debris covered by a cap of smooth muscle cells

❑ (B) Collection of foam cells, necrotic areas, and calcification

❑ (C) A lipid core, granulation tissue, and areas of hemorrhage

❑ (D) Lipid-filled foam cells and T lymphocytes

❑ (E) Cholesterol clefts surrounded by proliferating smooth muscle cells and foam cells

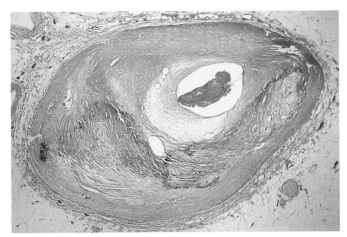

Courtesy of Tom Rogers, MD, Department of Pathology, University of Texas Southwestern Medical School, Dallas, TX.

22 A 59-year-old man has experienced chest pain at rest for the past year. On physical examination, his pulse is 80/min and irregular. The figure above shows the microscopic appearance representative of the patient's left anterior descending artery. Which of the following laboratory findings is most likely to have a causal relationship to the process illustrated?

❑ (A) Low Lp(a)

❑ (B) Positive VDRL

❑ (C) Low HDL cholesterol

❑ (D) Elevated platelet count

❑ (E) Low plasma homocysteine

23 After falling down a flight of stairs, a 59-year-old woman experiences mild intermittent right hip pain. Physical examination shows a 3-cm contusion over the right hip. The area is tender to palpation, but she has full range of motion of the right leg. A radiograph of the pelvis and right upper leg shows no fractures, but does show calcified, medium-sized arterial branches in the pelvis. This radiographic finding is most likely to represent which of the following?

❑ (A) Long-standing diabetes mellitus

❑ (B) Benign essential hypertension

❑ (C) An incidental observation

❑ (D) Increased risk for gangrenous necrosis

❑ (E) Unsuspected hyperparathyroidism

24 For more than a decade, a 45-year-old man has had poorly controlled hypertension ranging from 150/90 mm Hg to 160/95 mm Hg. Over the past 3 months, his blood pressure has increased to 250/125 mm Hg. On physical examination, his temperature is 36.9°C. His lungs are clear on auscultation, and his heart rate is regular. There is no abdominal pain on palpation. A chest radiograph shows a prominent border on the left side of the heart. Laboratory studies show that his serum creatinine level has increased during this time from 1.7 mg/dL to 3.8 mg/dL. Which of the following vascular lesions is most likely to be found in this patient's kidneys?

❑ (A) Hyperplastic arteriolosclerosis

❑ (B) Granulomatous arteritis

❑ (C) Fibromuscular dysplasia

❑ (D) Polyarteritis nodosa

❑ (E) Hyaline arteriolosclerosis

25 After a mastectomy with axillary node dissection for breast cancer 1 year ago, a 47-year-old woman has developed persistent swelling and puffiness in the left arm. Physical examination shows firm skin over the left arm and "doughy" underlying soft tissue. The arm is not painful or discolored. She developed cellulitis in the left arm 3 months ago. Which of the following terms best describes these findings?

❑ (A) Thrombophlebitis

❑ (B) Subclavian arterial thrombosis

❑ (C) Tumor embolization

❑ (D) Lymphedema

❑ (E) Vasculitis

26 A study is conducted to investigate the pathogenesis of atherosclerosis. The investigators have developed genetically modified mice that have hypercholesterolemia and spontaneously develop atherosclerosis. Next, the investigators selectively delete individual genes in order to determine the factors that are critical to the development of atherosclerosis. Deletion of the gene encoding for which of the following is most likely to reduce the experimentally observed atherosclerosis in these modified mice?

❑ (A) Von Willebrand factor

❑ (B) Homocysteine

❑ (C) T cell receptor

❑ (D) Endothelin

❑ (E) Fibrillin

❑ (F) LDL receptor

❑ (G) Factor VIII

❑ (H) Apolipoprotein

27 An 80-year-old man with a lengthy history of smoking survived a small myocardial infarction several years ago. He now reports chest and leg pain during exercise. On physical examination, his vital signs include temperature of 36.9°C, pulse 81/min, respirations 15/min, and blood pressure 165/100 mm Hg. Peripheral pulses are poor in the lower extremities. There is a 7-cm pulsating mass in the midline of the lower abdomen. Laboratory studies include two fasting serum glucose measurements of 170 mg/dL and 200 mg/dL. Which of the following vascular lesions is most likely to be present in this patient?

❑ (A) Aortic dissection
❑ (B) Arteriovenous fistula
❑ (C) Atherosclerotic aneurysm
❑ (D) Glomus tumor
❑ (E) Polyarteritis nodosa
❑ (F) Takayasu arteritis
❑ (G) Thromboangiitis obliterans

28 A 61-year-old man has smoked two packs of cigarettes per day for the past 40 years. He has experienced increasing dyspnea for the past 6 years. On physical examination, his vital signs include a temperature of 37.1°C, pulse 60/min, respirations 18/min and labored, and blood pressure 130/80 mm Hg. On auscultation, expiratory wheezes are heard over the chest bilaterally. His heart rate is regular. A chest radiograph shows increased lung volume, with flattening of the diaphragms, greater lucency to all lung fields, prominence of pulmonary arteries, and a prominent border on the right side of the heart. Laboratory studies include a blood gas measurement of PO_2 80 mm Hg, PCO_2 50 mm Hg, and pH 7.35. He dies of pneumonia. At autopsy, the pulmonary arteries have atheromatous plaques. Which of the following is most likely to have caused these findings?

❑ (A) Chronic renal failure
❑ (B) Coronary atherosclerosis
❑ (C) Cystic fibrosis
❑ (D) Diabetes mellitus
❑ (E) Familial hypercholesterolemia
❑ (F) Obesity
❑ (G) Phlebothrombosis
❑ (H) Pulmonary emphysema

29 A 75-year-old man has experienced headaches for the past 2 months. On physical examination, his vital signs include a temperature of 36.8°C, pulse 68/min, respirations 15/min, and blood pressure 130/85 mm Hg. His right temporal artery is prominent, palpable, and painful to the touch. His heart rate is regular, and there are no murmurs. A temporal artery biopsy is performed, and the segment of temporal artery excised is grossly thickened and shows focal microscopic granulomatous inflammation. He responds well to corticosteroid therapy. Which of the following complications of this disease is most likely to occur in untreated patients?

❑ (A) Renal failure
❑ (B) Hemoptysis
❑ (C) Malignant hypertension
❑ (D) Blindness
❑ (E) Gangrene of the toes

30 A 30-year-old woman has smoked 1 pack of cigarettes per day since she was a teenager. She has had painful thromboses of the superficial veins of the lower legs for 1 month and episodes during which her fingers become blue and cold. Over the next year, she develops chronic, poorly healing ulcerations of her feet. One toe becomes gangrenous and is amputated. Histologically, at the resection margin, there is an acute and chronic vasculitis involving medium-sized arteries, with segmental involvement. Which of the following is the most appropriate next step in treating this patient?

❑ (A) Hemodialysis
❑ (B) Smoking cessation
❑ (C) Corticosteroid therapy
❑ (D) Antibiotic therapy for syphilis
❑ (E) Insulin therapy

31 A 40-year-old man has experienced malaise, fever, and a 4-kg weight loss over the past month. On physical examination, his blood pressure is 145/90 mm Hg, and he has mild diffuse abdominal pain but no masses or hepatosplenomegaly. Laboratory studies include a serum urea nitrogen concentration of 58 mg/dL and a serum creatinine level of 6.7 mg/dL. Renal angiography shows right renal arterial thrombosis, and the left renal artery and branches show segmental luminal narrowing with focal aneurysmal dilation. During hemodialysis 1 week later, the patient experiences abdominal pain and diarrhea and is found to have melena. Which of the following serologic laboratory findings is most likely to be positive in this patient?

❑ (A) C-ANCA
❑ (B) ANA
❑ (C) HIV
❑ (D) HBsAg
❑ (E) Scl-70
❑ (F) RPR

32 A 30-year-old schoolteacher is known to be a strict disciplinarian in the classroom. She has angina pectoris of 6 months' duration. On physical examination, her blood pressure is 135/85 mm Hg. She is 168 cm (5 ft 5 in) tall and weighs 82 kg (BMI 29). Coronary angiography shows 75% narrowing of the anterior descending branch of the left coronary artery. Angioplasty with stent placement is performed. Which of the following is the major risk factor associated with these findings?

❑ (A) Obesity
❑ (B) Type A personality
❑ (C) Diabetes mellitus
❑ (D) Sedentary lifestyle
❑ (E) Age

33 A 46-year-old man visits his physician because he has noted increasing abdominal enlargement over the past 15 months. Physical examination shows several skin lesions on the upper chest that have central pulsatile cores. Pressing on a core causes a radially arranged array of subcutaneous arterioles to blanch. The size of the lesions, from core to periphery, is 0.5 cm to 1.5 cm. Laboratory studies show serum glucose of 119 mg/dL, creatinine 1.1 mg/dL, total protein 5.8 g/dL, and albumin 3.4 g/dL. Which of the following underlying diseases is most likely to be present in this patient?

❑ (A) Wegener granulomatosis
❑ (B) Micronodular cirrhosis
❑ (C) Marfan syndrome
❑ (D) AIDS
❑ (E) Diabetes mellitus

34 A 22-year-old woman complains of itching with burning pain in the perianal region for the past 4 months. Physical examination shows dilated and thrombosed external hemorrhoids. Which of the following underlying processes is most likely to be present in this patient?

❑ (A) Rectal adenocarcinoma
❑ (B) Pregnancy
❑ (C) Polyarteritis nodosa
❑ (D) Filariasis
❑ (E) Micronodular cirrhosis

35 A clinical study is performed that includes a group of subjects whose systemic blood pressure measurements are consistently between 145/95 mm Hg and 165/105 mm Hg. They are found to have increased cardiac output and increased peripheral vascular resistance. Renal angiograms show no abnormal findings, and CT scans of the abdomen show no masses. Laboratory studies show normal levels of serum creatinine and urea nitrogen. The subjects take no medications. Which of the following laboratory findings is most likely to be present in this group of subjects?

❑ (A) Lack of angiotensin-converting enzyme
❑ (B) Decreased urinary sodium
❑ (C) Elevated plasma renin
❑ (D) Hypokalemia
❑ (E) Increased urinary catecholamines

36 A 3-year-old child from Osaka, Japan, developed a fever and a rash and swelling of her hands and feet over a period of 2 days. On physical examination, her temperature is 37.8°C. There is a desquamative skin rash, oral erythema, erythema of the palms and soles, edema of the hands and feet, and cervical lymphadenopathy. The child improves after a course of intravenous immunoglobulin therapy. Which of the following is most likely to be a complication of this child's disease if it is untreated?

❑ (A) Asthma
❑ (B) Glomerulonephritis
❑ (C) Intracranial hemorrhage
❑ (D) Myocardial infarction
❑ (E) Pulmonary hypertension

37 An epidemiologic study seeking to determine possible risk factors for neoplasia is reviewing patient cases of neoplasms reported to tumor registries. Analysis of the data shows that one type of neoplasm is seen in two widely disparate situations: (1) the liver of persons exposed to polyvinyl chloride, and (2) the soft tissue of the arm ipsilateral to a prior radical mastectomy. The pathology reports about the neoplasms in these two groups of patients show a similar gross appearance—an irregular, infiltrative, soft reddish mass—and a similar microscopic appearance—pleomorphic spindle cells positive for CD31. Which of the following neoplasms is most likely to be described by these findings?

❑ (A) Angiosarcoma
❑ (B) Hemangioendothelioma
❑ (C) Hemangioma
❑ (D) Hemangiopericytoma
❑ (E) Kaposi sarcoma
❑ (F) Lymphangioma

ANSWERS

1 (A) Atheromatous plaques can be complicated by a variety of pathologic alterations, including hemorrhage, ulceration, thrombosis, and calcification. These processes can increase the size of the plaque and narrow the residual arterial lumen. Although atherosclerosis is a disease of the intima, in advanced disease, the expanding plaque compresses the media. This causes thinning of the media, which weakens the wall and predisposes it to aneurysm formation.

BP7 331   BP6 285-288   PBD7 516, 518-519
PBD6 507-509

2 (B) The figure shows an arteriole with marked hyaline thickening of the wall, indicative of hyaline arteriolosclerosis. Diabetes mellitus also can lead to this finding. Sepsis can produce disseminated intravascular coagulopathy with arteriolar hyaline thrombi. The debilitation that accompanies cancer tends to diminish the vascular disease caused by atherosclerosis. Syphilis can cause a vasculitis involving the vasa vasorum of the aorta. Polyarteritis can involve large to medium-sized arteries in many organs, including the kidneys; the affected vessels show fibrinoid necrosis and inflammation of the wall (vasculitis).

BP7 341   BP6 292-293   PBD7 529-530   PBD6 514-515

3 (F) This is a classic example of a secondary form of hypertension for which a cause can be determined. In this case, the renal artery stenosis reduces glomerular blood flow and pressure in the afferent arteriole, resulting in renin release by juxtaglomerular cells. The renin initiates angiotensin II–induced vasoconstriction, increased peripheral vascular resistance, and increased aldosterone, which promotes sodium reabsorption in the kidney, resulting in increased blood volume. Anti–double-stranded DNA is a specific marker for systemic lupus erythematosus. ANCAs are markers for some forms of vasculitis, such as microscopic polyangiitis or Wegener granulomatosis. Some patients with hepatitis B or C infection can develop a mixed cryoglobulinemia with a polyclonal increase in IgG. Renal involvement in such patients is common, and cryoglobulinemic vasculitis then leads to skin hemorrhages and ulceration. Hyperglycemia is a marker for diabetes mellitus, which accelerates the atherogenic process and can involve the kidneys, promoting the development of hypertension. HIV infection is not related to hypertension. Tertiary syphilis can produce endaortitis and aortic root dilation, but hypertension is not a likely sequela.

BP7 339   BP6 290-291   PBD7 526   PBD6 512-514

4 (B) In children, Henoch-Schönlein purpura is the multisystemic counterpart of the IgA nephropathy seen in adults.

The immune complexes formed with IgA produce the vasculitis that affects mainly arterioles, capillaries, and venules in skin, gastrointestinal tract, and kidney. In older adults, giant cell arteritis is seen in external carotid branches, principally the temporal artery unilaterally. Polyarteritis nodosa is seen most often in small muscular arteries and sometimes veins, with necrosis and microaneurysm formation followed by scarring and vascular occlusion. This occurs mainly in the kidney, gastrointestinal tract, and skin of young to middle-aged adults. Takayasu arteritis is seen mainly in children and involves the aorta (particularly the arch) and branches such as coronary and renal arteries, with granulomatous inflammation, aneurysm formation, and dissection. Telangiectasias are small vascular arborizations seen on skin or mucosal surfaces. Wegener granulomatosis, seen mainly in adults, involves small arteries, veins, and capillaries and causes mixed inflammation, as well as necrotizing and nonnecrotizing granulomatous inflammation with geographic necrosis surrounded by palisading epithelioid macrophages and giant cells.

BP7 525   BP6 453   PBD7 535, 541-542
PBD6 517, 961, 965

5 **(D)** Takayasu arteritis leads to "pulseless disease" because of involvement of the aorta (particularly the arch) and branches such as coronary, carotid, and renal arteries, with granulomatous inflammation, aneurysm formation, and dissection. Fibrosis is a late finding, and the pulmonary arteries can also be involved. Aortic dissection is an acute problem that, in older adults, is driven by atherosclerosis and hypertension, although this patient is within the age range for complications of Marfan syndrome, which causes cystic medial necrosis of the aorta. Kawasaki disease affects children and is characterized by an acute febrile illness, coronary arteritis with aneurysm formation and thrombosis, skin rash, and lymphadenopathy. Microscopic polyangiitis affects arterioles, capillaries, and venules with a leukocytoclastic vasculitis that appears at a similar stage in multiple organ sites (unlike classic polyarteritis nodosa, which causes varying stages of acute, chronic, and fibrosing lesions in small to medium-sized arteries). Tertiary syphilis produces an endaortitis with proximal aortic dilation. Thromboangiitis obliterans (Buerger disease) affects small to medium-sized arteries of the extremities and is strongly associated with smoking.

BP7 348-349   BP6 299   PBD7 538   PBD6 525-526

6 **(A)** Reducing cholesterol, particularly LDL cholesterol, with the same or increased HDL cholesterol level, indicates a reduced risk of atherosclerotic complications. Atherosclerosis is multifactorial, but modification of diet (i.e., reduction in total dietary fat and cholesterol) with increased exercise is the best method of reducing risk for most persons. Glucose is a measure of control of diabetes mellitus. Potassium, calcium, and renin values can be altered with some forms of hypertension, one of several risk factors for atherosclerosis.

BP7 335-336   BP6 283-284   PBD7 521-523
PBD6 504-506

7 **(D)** This is a description of cystic medial necrosis, which weakens the aortic media and predisposes to aortic dissection. In a young patient such as this, a heritable disorder of connective tissues, such as Marfan syndrome, must be strongly suspected. Scleroderma and Wegener granulomatosis do not

typically involve the aorta. Atherosclerosis associated with diabetes mellitus and hypertension are risk factors for aortic dissection, although these are seen at an older age. Takayasu arteritis is seen mainly in children and involves the aorta (particularly the arch) and branches such as the coronary and renal arteries, causing granulomatous inflammation, aneurysm formation, and dissection.

BP7 344   BP6 301   PBD7 533-534   PBD6 526-528

8 **(C)** This patient has an atherosclerotic abdominal aortic aneurysm. Diabetes mellitus, an important risk factor for atherosclerosis, must be suspected if a younger man or premenopausal woman has severe atherosclerosis. Polyarteritis nodosa does not typically involve the aorta. Obesity, a "soft" risk factor for atherosclerosis, also contributes to diabetes mellitus type 2; however, the extent of atherosclerotic disease in this patient suggests early-onset of diabetes mellitus that is more likely to be type 1. Systemic lupus erythematosus produces small arteriolar vasculitis. Syphilitic aortitis, a feature of tertiary syphilis, most often involves the thoracic aorta, but it is rare, and most thoracic aortic aneurysms nowadays are likely to be caused by atherosclerosis.

BP7 342-343   BP6 299   PBD7 530-532   PBD6 525-526

9 **(E)** The figure shows dilated, endothelium-lined spaces filled with RBCs. The circumscribed nature of this lesion and its long, unchanged course suggest its benign nature. Kaposi sarcoma is uncommon in its endemic form in childhood, and it is best known as a neoplastic complication associated with HIV infection. Angiosarcomas are large, rapidly growing malignancies in adults. Lymphangiomas, seen most often in children, tend to be more diffuse and are not blood filled. A telangiectasia is a radial array of subcutaneous dilated arteries or arterioles surrounding a central core that can pulsate.

BP7 358-359   BP6 304-305   PBD7 548-550
PBD6 532-533

10 **(A)** Atherosclerosis is considered a complex reparative response that follows endothelial cell injury. Hypercholesterolemia (high LDL cholesterol level) is believed to cause subtle endothelial injury. The oxidation of LDL by macrophages or endothelial cells has many deleterious effects. Oxidized LDL is chemotactic for circulating monocytes, causes monocytes to adhere to endothelium, stimulates release of growth factors and cytokines, and is cytotoxic to smooth muscle cells and endothelium. Smooth muscle proliferation in response to injury, important in the development of atheromas, is driven by growth factors, including platelet-derived growth factor. HDL is believed to mobilize cholesterol from developing atheromas; therefore, high HDL levels are protective. Intercellular adhesion molecule-1 (ICAM-1) and vascular cell adhesion molecule-1 (VCAM-1) are adhesion molecules on endothelial cells that promote adhesion of monocytes to the site of endothelial injury.

BP7 334-336   BP6 285-286   PBD7 520-524
PBD6 507-509

11 **(E)** This description is most suggestive of syphilitic aortitis, a complication of tertiary syphilis, with characteristic involvement of the thoracic aorta. Obliterative endarteritis is not a feature of other forms of vasculitis. High-titer double-stranded DNA antibodies are diagnostic of systemic lupus erythematosus, and the test result for P-ANCA is positive in various vasculitides, including microscopic polyangiitis. A high sedimentation rate is a nonspecific marker of inflammatory diseases. Ketonuria can occur in persons with diabetic ketoacidosis.

BP7 343   BP6 299-300   PBD7 532   PBD6 526

12 **(C)** Thrombophlebitis is a common problem that results from venous stasis. There is little or no inflammation, but the term is well established. Lymphedema takes longer than 3 weeks to develop and is not caused by bed rest alone. Disseminated intravascular coagulopathy more often results in hemorrhage, and edema is not the most prominent manifestation. Thromboangiitis obliterans is a rare form of arteritis that results in pain and ulceration of extremities. Varicose veins are superficial and can thrombose, but they are not related to bed rest.

BP7 354   BP6 302-303   PBD7 544   PBD6 530

13 **(B)** This patient has essential hypertension (no obvious cause for his moderate hypertension). Renal retention of excess sodium, which is thought to be important in initiating this form of hypertension, leads to increased intravascular fluid volume, increase in cardiac output, and peripheral vasoconstriction. Increased catecholamine secretion (as can occur in pheochromocytoma), gene defects in aldosterone metabolism, and renal artery stenosis all can cause secondary hypertension. However, hypertension secondary to all causes is much less common than essential hypertension. Increased production of atrial natriuretic factor reduces sodium retention and therefore reduces blood volume.

BP7 338-340   BP6 290-291   PBD7 526-529
PBD6 512-513

14 **(E)** Atherogenesis can be considered a chronic inflammatory response of the arterial wall to endothelial injury. The injury promotes participation by monocytes, macrophages, and T lymphocytes. Smooth muscle cells are stimulated to proliferate. Platelets adhere to areas of endothelial injury. Neutrophils are not a part of atherogenesis, although they can be seen in various forms of vasculitis. The process begins with endothelial cell alteration.

BP7 334-335   BP6 285-287   PBD7 521-523
PBD6 507-509

15 **(A)** Atherosclerosis is thought to result from a form of endothelial injury and the subsequent chronic inflammation and repair of the intima. All risk factors, including smoking, hyperlipidemia, and hypertension, cause biochemical or mechanical injury to the endothelium. Formation of foam cells occurs after the initial endothelial injury. Although lipoprotein receptor alterations can occur in some inherited conditions, these account for only a fraction of cases of atherosclerosis, and other lifestyle conditions do not affect their action. Inhibition of LDL oxidation should diminish atheroma formation. Vasomotor tone does not play a major role in atherogenesis.

BP7 331-334   BP6 284-286   PBD7 520-523
PBD6 505-508

16 **(A)** Venous stasis results in hemosiderin deposition and dermal fibrosis, with brownish discoloration and skin roughening. Focal ulceration can occur over the varicosities, but extensive gangrene similar to that seen in arterial atherosclerosis does not occur. The varicosities involve only the superficial set of veins, which can thrombose but are not the source of thromboemboli, as are the larger deep leg veins. The thromboses in superficial leg veins do not lead to disseminated intravascular coagulopathy. The varicosities do not affect muscle; however, lack of muscular support for veins to "squeeze" blood out for venous return can predispose to formation of varicose veins.

BP7 353-354   BP6 302   PBD7 543-544   PBD6 529

17 **(A)** Human herpesvirus 8 has been associated with Kaposi sarcoma and can be acquired as a sexually transmitted disease. Kaposi sarcoma is a complication of AIDS. Persons with HIV infection can be infected with a variety of viruses, including Epstein-Barr virus (EBV) and cytomegalovirus (CMV), but these have no etiologic association with Kaposi sarcoma. EBV is a factor in the development of non-Hodgkin lymphoma, and CMV can cause colitis or retinitis or can be disseminated. Hepatitis B virus can be seen in HIV-infected patients as well, particularly those with a risk factor of injection drug use. Adenovirus, which can be seen in HIV-infected persons (although not frequently), tends to be a respiratory or gastrointestinal infection.

BP7 358-359   BP6 305-307   PBD7 549-550
PBD6 535-536

18 **(H)** Wegener granulomatosis is a form of hypersensitivity reaction to an unknown antigen characterized by necrotizing granulomatous inflammation that typically involves the respiratory tract, small to medium-sized vessels, and glomeruli, though many organ sites may be affected; pulmonary and renal involvement can be life-threatening. C-ANCA are found in more than 90% of cases. Fibromuscular dysplasia is a hyperplastic medial disorder, usually involving renal and carotid arteries; on angiography, it appears as a "string of beads" caused by thickened fibromuscular ridges adjacent to less involved areas of the arterial wall. Glomus tumors are usually small peripheral masses. Granuloma pyogenicum is an inflammatory response that can produce a nodular mass, often on the gingiva or the skin. Hemangiomas are typically small, solitary, red nodules that can occur anywhere. Kaposi sarcoma can produce plaquelike to nodular masses that are composed of irregular vascular spaces lined by atypical-appearing endothelial cells; skin involvement is most common, but visceral organ involvement can occur. Polyarteritis nodosa most often involves small muscular arteries, and sometimes veins; it causes necrosis and microaneurysm formation followed by scarring and vascular occlusion, mainly in the kidney, gastrointestinal tract, and skin of young to middle-aged adults. Takayasu arteritis is seen mainly in children and involves the aorta (particularly the arch) and branches such as the coronary and renal arteries, with granulomatous inflammation, aneurysm formation, and dissection. Telangiectasias are small vascular arborizations seen on skin or mucosal surfaces.

BP7 351-352   BP6 295-296   PBD7 539, 541-542
PBD6 522-523

19 **(B)** The red streaks represent lymphatic channels through which an acute infection drains to axillary lymph nodes, and these drain to the right lymphatic duct and into the right subclavian vein (lymphatics from the lower body and left upper body drain to the thoracic duct). Capillaritis is most likely to be described in the lungs. Lymphedema occurs with blockage of lymphatic drainage and develops over a longer period without significant acute inflammation. Phlebothrombosis and thrombophlebitis describe thrombosis in veins with stasis and inflammation respectively, typically in the pelvis and lower extremities. Polyarteritis involves small to medium-sized muscular arteries, typically the renal and mesenteric branches. Varices are veins dilated from blockage of venous drainage.

BP7 354   BP6 300-302   PBD7 545   PBD6 526-528

20 **(D)** Oxidized LDL can be taken up by a special "scavenger" pathway in macrophages; it also promotes monocyte chemotaxis and adherence. Macrophages taking up the lipid become foam cells that begin to form the fatty streak. Smoking, diabetes mellitus, and hypertension all promote free radical formation, and free radicals increase degradation of LDL to its oxidized form. About one third of LDL is degraded to the oxidized form; a higher LDL level increases the amount of oxidized LDL available for uptake into macrophages. C-reactive protein is a marker for inflammation, which can increase with more active atheroma and thrombus formation and predicts a greater likelihood of acute coronary syndromes. Increased homocysteine levels promote atherogenesis through endothelial dysfunction. Lp(a), an altered form of LDL that contains the apo B-100 portion of LDL linked to apo A, promotes lipid accumulation and smooth muscle cell proliferation. Platelet-derived growth factor (PDGF) promotes smooth muscle cell proliferation. VLDL is formed in the liver and transformed in adipose tissue and muscle to LDL.

BP7 336-337   BP6 295-296   PBD7 521-523
PBD6 522-523

21 **(D)** The slightly raised, pale lesions shown are called fatty streaks and are seen in the aorta of almost all children older than 10 years. They are thought to be precursors of atheromatous plaques. T cells are present early in the pathogenesis of atherosclerotic lesions and are believed to activate monocytes, endothelial cells, and smooth muscle cells by secreting cytokines. Fatty streaks cause no disturbances in blood flow and are discovered incidentally at autopsy. All of the other lesions described are seen in fully developed atheromatous plaques. The histologic features of such plaques include a central core of lipid debris that can have cholesterol clefts and can be calcified. There is usually an overlying cap of smooth muscle cells. Hemorrhage is a complication seen in advanced atherosclerosis. Foam cells, derived from smooth muscle cells or macrophages that have ingested lipid, can be present in all phases of atherogenesis.

BP7 333   BP6 286-289   PBD7 516-518, 523
PBD6 502-503

22 **(C)** The figure shows an arterial lumen that is markedly narrowed by atheromatous plaque complicated by calcification. Hypercholesterolemia with elevated LDL and decreased HDL levels is a key risk factor for atherogenesis. Levels of Lp(a) and homocysteine, if elevated, increase the risk of atherosclerosis. Syphilis (positive VDRL test result) produces endarteritis obliterans of the aortic vasa vasorum, which weakens the wall and predisposes to aneurysms. Although platelets participate in forming atheromatous plaques, their number is not of major importance. Thrombocytosis can result in thrombosis or hemorrhage.

BP7 331-332   BP6 287-289   PBD7 517-519
PBD6 504-506

23 **(C)** Older adults with calcified arteries often have Mönckeberg medial calcific sclerosis, a benign process that is a form of arteriosclerosis with no serious sequelae. Such arterial calcification is far less likely to be a consequence of atherosclerosis with diabetes mellitus or with hypercalcemia. Hypertension is most likely to affect small renal arteries, and calcification is not a major feature, although hypertension is also a risk factor for atherosclerosis.

BP7 328   BP6 283   PBD7 516   PBD6 498

24 **(A)** This patient has malignant hypertension superimposed on benign essential hypertension. Malignant hypertension can suddenly complicate less severe hypertension. The arterioles undergo concentric thickening and luminal narrowing. A granulomatous arteritis is most characteristic of Wegener granulomatosis, which often involves the kidney. Fibromuscular dysplasia can involve the main renal arteries, with medial hyperplasia producing focal arterial obstruction. This process can lead to hypertension but not typically malignant hypertension. Polyarteritis nodosa produces a vasculitis that can involve the kidney. Hyaline arteriolosclerosis is seen with long-standing essential hypertension of moderate severity. These lesions give rise to benign nephrosclerosis. The affected kidneys become symmetrically shrunken and granular because of progressive loss of renal parenchyma and consequent fine scarring.

BP7 341   BP6 292-293   PBD7 530   PBD6 514-515

25 **(D)** A mastectomy with axillary lymph node dissection leads to disruption and obstruction of lymphatics in the axilla. Such obstruction to lymph flow gives rise to lymphedema, a condition that can be complicated by cellulitis. Thrombophlebitis from venous stasis is a complication seen more commonly in the lower extremities. An arterial thrombosis can lead to a cold, blue, painful extremity. Tumor emboli are generally small but uncommon. Vasculitis is not a surgical complication.

BP7 354-355   BP6 303   PBD7 544-545   PBD6 530-531

26 **(C)** Deletion of T cell receptor genes prevents T cell development (since engagement of T cell receptors during development in the thymus is essential for T cell survival). Early in the course of atheroma formation the T cells adhere to VCAM-1 on activated endothelial cells and migrate into the vessel wall. These T cells, activated by some unknown mechanism, secrete a variety of pro-inflammatory molecules that recruit and activate monocytes and smooth muscle cells and perpetuate chronic inflammation of the vessel wall. Hence, the loss of T cells reduces atherosclerosis. Von Willebrand factor is required for normal platelet adhesion to collagen, and its absence leads to abnormal bleeding. Homocysteine can damage endothelium, and its absence may protect against atherosclerosis, but there is no evidence that homocysteine is the major factor in initiating endothelial damage. That role, most likely, belongs to cholesterol. Endothelin is a vasoconstrictor with no known role in atherogenesis. Fibrillin loss causes weakness of the arterial media, with risk for dissection, as seen in Marfan syndrome. A reduction in LDL receptors or decreased apolipoprotein promotes atherogenesis in the disease familial hypercholesterolemia. Decreased factor VIII leads to abnormal bleeding.

PBD7 523

27 (C) Abdominal aneurysms are most often related to underlying atherosclerosis. This patient has multiple risk factors for atherosclerosis, including diabetes mellitus, hypertension, and smoking. When the aneurysm reaches this size, there is a significant risk of rupture. An aortic dissection is typically a sudden, life-threatening event with dissection of blood out of the aortic lumen, typically into the chest, without a pulsatile mass. The risk factors for atherosclerosis and hypertension underlie aortic dissection. An arteriovenous fistula can produce an audible bruit on auscultation. Glomus tumors are usually small peripheral masses. Polyarteritis nodosa can produce small microaneurysms in small arteries. Takayasu arteritis typically involves the aortic arch and branches in children. Thromboangiitis obliterans (Buerger disease) is a rare condition with occlusion of the muscular arteries of the lower extremities in smokers.

BP7 342-343   BP6 299   PBD7 531-532   PBD6 525-526

28 (H) The pulmonary vasculature is under much lower pressure than the systemic arterial circulation and is much less likely to have endothelial damage, which promotes atherogenesis. Atherosclerosis in systemic arteries is more likely to occur where blood flow is more turbulent, a situation that occurs at arterial branch points, such as in the first few centimeters of the coronary arteries or in the abdominal aorta. Factors driving systemic arterial atherosclerosis (e.g., hyperlipidemias, smoking, diabetes mellitus, and systemic hypertension) do not operate in the pulmonary arterial vasculature. Pulmonary hypertension, the driving force behind pulmonary atherosclerosis, occurs when pulmonary vascular resistance rises as the pulmonary vascular bed is decreased by either obstructive (e.g., emphysema, as in this patient) or restrictive (e.g., as in scleroderma with pulmonary interstitial fibrosis) diseases. Cystic fibrosis (CF) leads to widespread bronchiectasis, not emphysema, but CF is still an obstructive lung disease with the potential to produce pulmonary hypertension. Obesity leads to pulmonary hypoventilation, which acts as a restrictive lung disease, but pulmonary hypoventilation does not increase lung volumes, as in this patient. Phlebothrombosis affects veins and leads to possible pulmonary thromboembolism, which increases pulmonary pressures, but more acutely than in this patient.

BP7 338, 477-478   BP6 284-285   PBD7 516-517
PBD6 507-508

29 (D) This patient has clinical features suggesting giant cell (temporal) arteritis. This form of arteritis typically involves large to medium-sized arteries in the head (especially temporal arteries), but also vertebral and ophthalmic arteries. Involvement of the latter can lead to blindness. Because involvement of the kidney, lung, and peripheral arteries of the extremities is much less common, renal failure, hemoptysis,

and gangrene of toes are unusual. There is no association between hypertension and giant cell arteritis.

BP7 347-348   BP6 297   PBD7 536-538   PBD6 517-518

30 (B) This patient has features of thromboangiitis obliterans (Buerger disease). This disease, which affects small to medium-sized arteries of the extremities, is strongly associated with smoking. Renal involvement does not occur. Immunosuppressive therapy is not highly effective. Syphilis produces an aortitis. Although peripheral vascular disease with atherosclerosis is a typical finding in diabetes mellitus, vasculitis is not.

BP7 352   BP6 298-299   PBD7 539, 542   PBD6 523

31 (D) Segmental involvement of medium-sized arteries with aneurysmal dilation in the renal vascular bed and presumed mesenteric vasculitis (e.g., abdominal pain, melena) is most likely caused by polyarteritis nodosa. Polyarteritis can affect many organs at different times. Although the cause of polyarteritis is unknown, about 30% of patients have hepatitis B surface antigen in serum. Presumably, hepatitis B surface antigen–antibody complexes damage the vessel wall. Unlike the situation with microscopic polyangiitis, there is less of an association with ANCA. A collagen vascular disease with a positive ANA test result, such as systemic lupus erythematosus, may produce a vasculitis but not in the pattern seen here; the affected vessels are smaller. Vasculitis with HIV infection is uncommon. The Scl-70 autoantibody is indicative of scleroderma, which can produce renal failure. The rapid plasma reagin (RPR) is a serologic test for syphilis (STS); an endaortitis of the vasa vasorum can occur in syphilis.

BP7 349-350   BP6 293-295   PBD7 539-540   PBD6 520

32 (C) Diabetes mellitus is a significant risk factor for early, accelerated, and advanced atherosclerosis. If a premenopausal woman or a young man has severe coronary atherosclerosis, diabetes must be suspected as a predisposing factor. "Soft" risk factors that can play a lesser role in the development of atherosclerosis include obesity, stress, and lack of exercise.

BP7 334   BP6 284   PBD7 521   PBD6 504-506

33 (B) These lesions are spider telangiectasias, which are a feature of micronodular cirrhosis, typically as a consequence of chronic alcoholism. Spider telangiectasias are thought to be caused by hyperestrinism (estrogen excess) that results from hepatic damage. Vasculitis does not tend to produce skin telangiectasias. The vascular involvement in Marfan syndrome is primarily in the aortic arch with cystic medial necrosis. The most common vascular skin lesion in AIDS patients is Kaposi sarcoma, which is a neoplasm presenting as one or more irregular red-to-purple patches, plaques, or nodules. Diabetes mellitus, with its accelerated atherosclerosis, is most likely to result in ischemia or gangrene.

BP7 357   BP6 304   PBD7 547-548   PBD6 534

34 (B) The hemorrhoidal veins can become dilated from venous congestion. This situation is most common in patients with chronic constipation, but the pregnant uterus presses on pelvic veins to produce similar congestion, which promotes hemorrhoidal vein dilation. Carcinomas are not likely to obstruct venous flow. Polyarteritis does not affect veins. Filarial infections can affect lymphatics, including those in the inguinal region, and produce lymphedema. Portal hypertension with cirrhosis is most likely to dilate submucosal esophageal veins, but hemorrhoidal veins occasionally can be affected. Cirrhosis would be rare, however, at this patient's age.

BP7 354   BP6 302   PBD7 544   PBD6 530

35 **(B)** The findings in this population group suggest essential hypertension, which has several postulated theories for its cause. One theory is that there are defects in renal sodium homeostasis that reduce renal sodium excretion. The kidney then retains sodium and water, increasing intravascular fluid volume, which drives increased cardiac output (CO). CO is compensated by increasing peripheral vascular resistance, causing an increase in blood pressure. If angiotensin converting enzyme (ACE) were absent, then blood pressure would fall, because angiotensin I would not be converted to angiotensin II (drugs that act as ACE inhibitors are antihypertensives). An elevated plasma renin level is typical of renovascular hypertension, which can occur with narrowing of a renal artery. Hypertensive patients with hypokalemia can also have hyperaldosteronemia, which can be caused by an aldosterone-secreting adrenal adenoma. Increased urinary catecholamines can indicate increased catecholamine output from a pheochromocytoma.

BP7 339-340   BP6 290-292   PBD7 528-529
PBD6 511-514

36 **(D)** The child has mucocutaneous lymph node syndrome, or Kawasaki disease, which involves large, medium-sized, and small arteries. Cardiovascular complications occur in 20% of cases and include thrombosis, ectasia, and aneurysm formation of coronary arteries. Asthma can be seen in association with Churg-Strauss vasculitis. Glomerulonephritis is a feature of Wegener granulomatosis and of autoimmune diseases such as systemic lupus erythematosus. Intracranial hemorrhage can occur with septic emboli to peripheral cerebral arteries, producing mycotic aneurysms that can rupture. Pulmonary hypertension can complicate Takayasu arteritis.

BP7 350   BP6 294, 298   PBD7 540   PBD6 517, 521

37 **(A)** Angiosarcomas are very aggressive malignancies. Knowledge of the association with vinyl chloride has virtually eliminated this occupational exposure. In the past, when radical mastectomies were more common, angiosarcomas arose in the setting of chronic lymphedema of the arm; the tumor probably arose from dilated lymphatics. Most angiosarcomas are sporadic neoplasms that occur rarely in older adults. Hemangioendotheliomas demonstrate biologic behavior intermediate between the very localized, slow-growing hemangioma and the aggressive angiosarcoma; they may recur after excision. Hemangiopericytomas are rare soft tissue neoplasms that can metastasize. Kaposi sarcoma (KS) was once a rare endemic neoplasm involving the lower extremities; however, with the advent of AIDS, KS has become associated with HIV infection. KS is driven by human herpesvirus-8 infection. Lymphangiomas are benign, and when formed of capillary-like channels, are usually small and localized. Cavernous lymphangiomas, however, can be ill-defined and difficult to remove.

BP7 359-360   BP6 304, 305   PBD7 550-551
PBD6 537-538

The Heart

PBD7 Chapter 12: The Heart

PBD6 Chapter 13: The Heart

BP7 and BP6 Chapter 11: The Heart

1 A 50-year-old man experiences episodes of severe substernal chest pain every time he performs a task that requires moderate exercise. The episodes have become more frequent and severe over the past year, but they can be relieved by sublingual nitroglycerin. On physical examination, he is afebrile, his pulse is 78/min and regular, and there are no murmurs or gallops. Laboratory studies show creatinine of 1.1 mg/dL, glucose 130 mg/dL, and total serum cholesterol 223 mg/dL. Which of the following cardiac lesions is most likely to be present?

- (A) Rheumatic mitral stenosis
- (B) Serous pericarditis
- (C) Restrictive cardiomyopathy
- (D) Calcific aortic stenosis
- (E) Coronary atherosclerosis
- (F) Viral myocarditis

2 A 44-year-old woman who has rheumatic heart disease with aortic stenosis undergoes valve replacement with a bioprosthesis. She remains stable for the next 8 years and then develops diminished exercise tolerance. Which of the following complications involving the bioprosthesis has most likely occurred?

- (A) Paravalvular leak
- (B) Stenosis
- (C) Hemolysis
- (D) Embolization
- (E) Myocardial infarction

3 In a clinical study of tetralogy of Fallot, patients are examined prior to surgery to determine predictors observed on echocardiography that correlate with the severity of the disease and the need for more careful monitoring. A subset of patients is found to have more severe congestive heart failure, poor exercise tolerance, and decreased arterial oxygen saturation levels. Which of the following is most likely to predict a worse clinical presentation for these patients?

- (A) Size of the left ventricle
- (B) Degree of pulmonary stenosis
- (C) Size of the ventricular septal defect
- (D) Diameter of the tricuspid valve
- (E) Presence of an atrial septal defect

4 A 12-year-old boy was brought to the physician with a sore throat and fever 3 weeks ago, and a throat culture was positive for group A β-hemolytic *Streptococcus*. On the follow-up examination, the child is afebrile. His pulse is 85/min, respirations 18/min, and blood pressure 90/50 mm Hg. On auscultation, a murmur of mitral regurgitation is audible, and there are diffuse rales over both lungs. The child is admitted to the hospital and over the next 2 days has several episodes of atrial fibrillation accompanied by signs of acute left ventricular failure. Which of the following pathologic changes occurring in this child's heart during hospitalization is most likely to be the cause of the left ventricular failure?

- (A) Amyloidosis
- (B) Endocardial fibroelastosis
- (C) Fibrinous pericarditis
- (D) Fibrosis of mitral valve with fusion of commissures
- (E) Myocarditis
- (F) Tamponade
- (G) Verrucous endocarditis

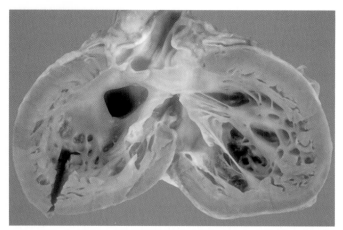

Courtesy of Arthur Weinberg, MD, Department of Pathology, University of Texas Southwestern Medical School, Dallas, TX.

5 The parents of a 5-year-old child notice that he is not as active as other children his age. During the past 9 months, the child has had several episodes of respiratory difficulty following exertion. On physical examination, his temperature is 36.9°C, pulse 81/min, respirations 19/min, and blood pressure 95/60 mm Hg. On auscultation, a loud holosystolic murmur is audible. There are diffuse crackles over the lungs bilaterally, with dullness to percussion at the bases. A chest radiograph shows a prominent border on the left side of the heart, pulmonary interstitial infiltrates, and blunting of the costodiaphragmatic recesses. The representative gross appearance of the child's heart is shown above. Which of the following additional pathologic conditions would most likely develop in this child?

- ❏ (A) Aortic regurgitation
- ❏ (B) Coronary atherosclerosis
- ❏ (C) Nonbacterial thrombotic endocarditis
- ❏ (D) Pulmonary hypertension
- ❏ (E) Restrictive cardiomyopathy

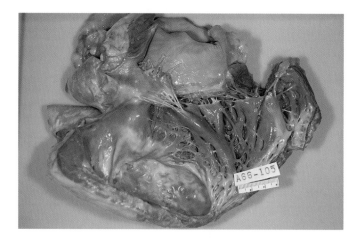

6 A 68-year-old man with a history of diabetes mellitus had chest pain and an elevated serum troponin I level 1 year ago. He was treated in the hospital with antiarrhythmic agents for 1 week. An echocardiogram showed an ejection fraction of 28%. He now has markedly reduced exercise tolerance. On physical examination, his temperature is 37°C, pulse 68/min, respirations 17/min, and blood pressure 130/80 mm Hg.

Diffuse crackles are heard on auscultation of the lungs. The representative gross appearance of the heart is shown in the preceding figure. Which of the following complications of this disease is the patient most likely to develop?

- ❏ (A) Atrial myxoma
- ❏ (B) Cardiac tamponade
- ❏ (C) Constrictive pericarditis
- ❏ (D) Hypertrophic cardiomyopathy
- ❏ (E) Infective endocarditis
- ❏ (F) Systemic thromboembolism

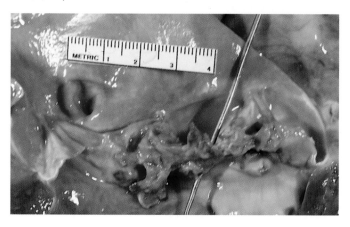

7 A 25-year-old man was found dead at home by the apartment manager, who had been called by the decedent's employer because of failure to report to work for the past 3 days. An external examination by the medical examiner showed splinter hemorrhages under the fingernails and no signs of trauma. The gross appearance of the heart at autopsy is shown above. Which of the following laboratory findings is most likely to provide evidence of the cause of the disease?

- ❏ (A) Elevated anti–streptolysin O titer
- ❏ (B) Positive ANCA determination
- ❏ (C) Increased creatine kinase-MB fraction (CK-MB)
- ❏ (D) High double-stranded DNA autoantibody titer
- ❏ (E) Positive blood culture for *Staphylococcus aureus*

8 A 10-year-old girl who is normally developed has chronic progressive exercise intolerance. Physical examination shows temperature of 37.1°C, pulse 70/min, respirations 14/min, and blood pressure 100/60 mm Hg. A chest radiograph shows cardiomegaly and mild pulmonary edema. An echocardiogram shows severe left ventricular hypertrophy and a prominent interventricular septum. The right ventricle is slightly thickened. During systole, the anterior leaflet of the mitral valve moves into the outflow tract of the left ventricle. The ejection fraction is abnormally high, and the ventricular volume and cardiac output are both low. Which of the following is the most likely cause of the cardiac abnormalities in this patient?

- ❏ (A) Mutations in β-myosin heavy chain
- ❏ (B) Autoimmunity against myocardial fibers
- ❏ (C) Excessive iron accumulation
- ❏ (D) Deposition of amyloid protein
- ❏ (E) Latent enterovirus infection

9 For the past 2 years, a 49-year-old woman has had a chronic cough that produces a small amount of whitish sputum. The sputum occasionally is blood-streaked. On physical examination, her temperature is 37.9°C, pulse 71/min, respirations 17/min, and blood pressure 125/80 mm Hg. Crackles are heard on auscultation over the upper lung fields. Heart sounds are faint, and there is a 15 mm Hg inspiratory decline in systolic arterial pressure. The chest radiograph shows prominent heart borders with a "water bottle" configuration. Pericardiocentesis yields 200 mL of bloody fluid. Infection with which of the following organisms is most likely to produce these findings?

- (A) *Mycobacterium tuberculosis*
- (B) Group A *Streptococcus*
- (C) Coxsackievirus B
- (D) *Candida albicans*
- (E) *Staphylococcus aureus*

10 A 27-year-old woman has had a fever for 5 days. On physical examination, her temperature is 38.2°C, pulse 100/min, respirations 19/min, and blood pressure 90/60 mm Hg. A cardiac murmur is heard on auscultation. The sensorium is clouded, but there are no focal neurologic deficits. Laboratory findings include hemoglobin of 13.1 g/dL, platelet count 233,300/mm³, and WBC count 19,200/mm³. Blood cultures are positive for *Staphylococcus aureus*. Urinalysis shows hematuria. An echocardiogram shows a 1.5-cm vegetation on the mitral valve. Which of the following conditions is this patient most likely to develop?

- (A) Cerebral arterial mycotic aneurysm
- (B) Dilated cardiomyopathy
- (C) Abscess of the left upper lobe
- (D) Myxomatous degeneration of the mitral valve
- (E) Polyarteritis nodosa
- (F) Polycystic kidneys

11 A 19-year-old man has had a low-grade fever for 3 weeks. On physical examination, his temperature is 38.3°C, pulse 104/min, respirations 28/min, and blood pressure of 95/60 mm Hg. A tender spleen tip is palpable. There are splinter hemorrhages under the fingernails and tender hemorrhagic nodules on the palms and soles. A heart murmur is heard on auscultation. Which of the following infectious agents is most likely to be cultured from this patient's blood?

- (A) *Streptococcus viridans* group
- (B) *Trypanosoma cruzi*
- (C) Coxsackievirus B
- (D) *Candida albicans*
- (E) *Mycobacterium tuberculosis*
- (F) *Pseudomonas aeruginosa*

12 A 50-year-old man has sudden onset of severe substernal chest pain that radiates to the neck. On physical examination, he is afebrile but has tachycardia, hyperventilation, and hypotension. No cardiac murmurs are heard on auscultation. Emergent coronary angiography shows a thrombotic occlusion of the left circumflex artery and areas of 50% to 70% narrowing in the proximal circumflex and anterior descending arteries. Which of the following complications of this disease is most likely to occur within 1 hour of these events?

- (A) Ventricular fibrillation
- (B) Pericarditis
- (C) Myocardial rupture
- (D) Ventricular aneurysm
- (E) Thromboembolism

13 One week ago, a 72-year-old woman had an episode in which she became disoriented, had difficulty speaking, and had weakness on the right side of the body. On physical examination, she is afebrile with pulse of 68/min, respirations 15/min, and blood pressure 130/85 mm Hg. On auscultation, the lungs are clear, the heart rate is irregular, and there is a midsystolic click. An echocardiogram shows nodular deposits with the density of calcium around the mitral valve. One leaflet of the mitral valve appears to balloon upward. The ejection fraction is estimated to be 55%. Laboratory findings show Na⁺ of 141 mmol/L, K⁺ 4.1 mmol/L, Cl⁻ 98 mmol/L, CO₂ 25 mmol/L, glucose 77 mg/dL, creatinine 0.8 mg/dL, calcium 8.1 mg/dL, and phosphorus 3.5 mg/dL. Which of the following is the most likely diagnosis?

- (A) Carcinoid heart disease
- (B) Hyperparathyroidism
- (C) Infective endocarditis
- (D) Infiltrative cardiomyopathy
- (E) Mitral annular calcification
- (F) Rheumatic heart disease
- (G) Senile calcific stenosis

14 An 82-year-old woman has had increasing fatigue for the past 2 years. During this time, she has experienced paroxysmal dizziness and syncope. On physical examination, she is afebrile. Her pulse is 44/min, respirations 16/min, and blood pressure 100/65 mm Hg. On auscultation, the lungs are clear and no murmurs are heard. An echocardiogram shows a normal-sized heart with normal valve motion and estimated ejection fraction of 50%. After being treated with digoxin, the heart rate slows and becomes irregular. An abnormality involving which of the following is most likely to be present in this patient?

- (A) Atrioventricular node
- (B) Bundle of His
- (C) Left bundle branch
- (D) Parasympathetic ganglion
- (E) Right bundle branch
- (F) Sinoatrial node
- (G) Sympathetic ganglion

15 A 50-year-old man with a history of infective endocarditis has increasing fatigue. On physical examination, he is afebrile. His pulse is 80/min, respirations 17/min, and blood pressure 110/70 mm Hg. On auscultation, diffuse rales are heard in the lungs. A chest radiograph shows bilateral pulmonary edema. An echocardiogram shows mitral regurgitation. He receives a bileaflet tilting disk mechanical mitral valve prosthesis. After surgery, he is stable, and an echocardiogram shows no abnormal valvular or ventricular function. Which of the following pharmacologic agents should he receive regularly following this surgical procedure?

- (A) Amiodarone
- (B) Ciprofloxacin
- (C) Warfarin
- (D) Cyclosporine
- (E) Digoxin
- (F) Propranolol

16 For the past 2 years, a 56-year-old man has experienced increased fatigue and decreased exercise tolerance. On physical examination, his temperature is 36.9°C, pulse 75/min, respirations 17/min, and blood pressure 115/75 mm Hg. On auscultation, diffuse crackles are audible. The abdomen is distended with a fluid wave, and there is bilateral pitting edema to the knees. A chest radiograph shows pulmonary edema, pleural effusions, and marked cardiomegaly. An echocardiogram shows mild tricuspid and mitral regurgitation and reduced right and left ventricular wall motion, with an ejection fraction of 30%. He suffers cerebral, renal, and splenic infarctions over the next year. Chronic use of which of the following substances is most likely to produce these findings?

❑ (A) Acetaminophen
❑ (B) Cocaine
❑ (C) Digoxin
❑ (D) Ethanol
❑ (E) Lisinopril
❑ (F) Nicotine
❑ (G) Propranolol

17 A 68-year-old man has had progressive dyspnea for the past year. On physical examination, extensive rales are heard in all lung fields. An echocardiogram shows that the left ventricular wall is markedly hypertrophied. A chest radiograph shows pulmonary edema and a prominent left-sided heart shadow. Which of the following conditions has most likely produced these findings?

❑ (A) Centrilobular emphysema
❑ (B) Systemic hypertension
❑ (C) Tricuspid valve regurgitation
❑ (D) Chronic alcoholism
❑ (E) Silicosis

18 A 73-year-old man has developed worsening congestive heart failure over the past year. On physical examination, he has pitting edema to the thighs. There is dullness to percussion at the lung bases. He develops pneumonia and dies. At autopsy, there is marked right ventricular and right atrial dilation and hypertrophy. The aorta shows minimal atherosclerosis, and the pulmonary trunk shows moderate atherosclerosis. Which of the following conditions is most likely to have produced these findings?

❑ (A) Saddle pulmonary thromboembolism
❑ (B) Ventricular septal defect
❑ (C) Chronic obstructive pulmonary disease
❑ (D) Rheumatic heart disease
❑ (E) Hypertrophic cardiomyopathy

19 During the past year, a 34-year-old woman has had palpitations, fatigue, and worsening chest pain. On physical examination, she is afebrile. Her pulse is 75/min, respirations 15/min, and blood pressure 110/70 mm Hg. Auscultation of the chest indicates a midsystolic click with late systolic murmur. A review of systems indicates that the patient has one or two anxiety attacks per month. An echocardiogram is most likely to show which of the following?

❑ (A) Aortic valvular vegetations
❑ (B) Pulmonic stenosis
❑ (C) Mitral valve prolapse
❑ (D) Patent ductus arteriosus
❑ (E) Tricuspid valve regurgitation

20 In the third match of a volleyball tournament, a 15-year-old girl jumps up for a block and collapses. Despite cardiopulmonary resuscitation, she cannot be revived. She had been healthy all her life and complained only of limited episodes of chest pain in games during the current school year. Which of the following pathologic findings of the heart is the medical examiner most likely to find?

❑ (A) Haphazardly arranged hypertrophied septal myocytes
❑ (B) Extensive myocardial hemosiderin deposition
❑ (C) Tachyzoites within foci of myocardial necrosis and inflammation
❑ (D) Mitral valvular stenosis with left atrial enlargement
❑ (E) Large, friable vegetations with destruction of aortic valve cusps

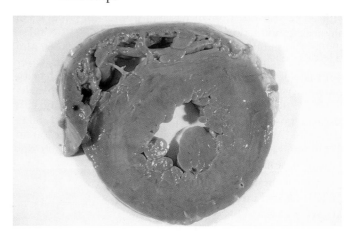

21 A 59-year-old man has experienced chronic fatigue for the past 18 months. On physical examination, he is afebrile. A chest radiograph shows bilateral pulmonary edema and a prominent border on the left side of the heart. The representative gross appearance of the heart is shown. Laboratory studies show serum glucose of 74 mg/dL, total cholesterol 189 mg/dL, total protein 7.1 g/dL, albumin 5.2 g/dL, creatinine 6.1 mg/dL, and urea nitrogen 58 mg/dL. Which of the following is the most likely diagnosis?

❑ (A) Chronic alcoholism
❑ (B) Systemic hypertension
❑ (C) Pneumoconiosis
❑ (D) Hemochromatosis
❑ (E) Diabetes mellitus

22 A 4-year-old girl who is below the 5th percentile for height and weight for age becomes easily fatigued. On physical examination, she appears cyanotic. Her temperature is 37°C, pulse 82/min, respirations 16/min, and blood pressure 105/65 mm Hg. Arterial blood gas measurement shows decreased oxygen saturation. One month later, she has fever and obtundation. A cerebral CT scan shows a right parietal, ring-enhancing, 3-cm lesion. Which of the following congenital heart diseases is the most likely diagnosis?

❑ (A) Atrial septal defect
❑ (B) Bicuspid aortic valve
❑ (C) Coarctation of the aorta
❑ (D) Patent ductus arteriosus
❑ (E) Truncus arteriosus
❑ (F) Ventricular septal defect

23 A 50-year-old man with a lengthy history of diabetes mellitus and hypertension has had pain in the left shoulder and arm for the past 12 hours. He attributes the pain to arthritis and takes acetaminophen. Over the next 6 hours, he develops shortness of breath, which persists for 2 days. On day 3, he visits the physician. On physical examination, his temperature is 37.1°C, pulse 82/min, respirations 18/min, and blood pressure 160/100 mm Hg. Laboratory studies show that the total creatine kinase (CK) activity is within reference range, but the troponin I level is elevated. The patient is admitted to the hospital and continues to experience dyspnea for the next 3 days. On day 7 after the onset of shoulder pain, he has a cardiac arrest. Resuscitative measures are unsuccessful. Postmortem examination shows a large transmural infarction of the left anterior free wall with rupture and hemopericardium. Which of the following statements is best supported by these clinical and autopsy data?

❏ (A) Infarction did not develop until day 5 or day 6 after the episode of chest pain
❏ (B) The normal CK level obtained on day 3 excludes the possibility of infarction within the preceding 72 hours
❏ (C) He had an acute infarction occurring on the day he developed shoulder pain
❏ (D) A CK-MB fraction determination would have detected acute infarction on day 3
❏ (E) A second acute infarction on day 6 or day 7 caused myocardial rupture within several hours

24 A 45-year-old man experiences crushing substernal chest pain after arriving at work one morning. Over the next 4 hours, the pain persists and begins to radiate to his left arm. He becomes diaphoretic and short of breath but waits until the end of his 8-hour shift to go to the hospital. An elevated serum value of which of the following laboratory tests would be most useful for diagnosis of this patient on admission to the hospital?

❏ (A) Lipase
❏ (B) AST
❏ (C) CK-MB fraction
❏ (D) ALT
❏ (E) LDH-1
❏ (F) C-reactive protein

25 A 60-year-old man has experienced angina on exertion for the past 6 years. A coronary angiogram performed 2 years ago showed 75% stenosis of the left anterior descending coronary artery and 50% stenosis of the right coronary artery. For the past 3 weeks, the frequency and severity of the anginal attacks have increased, and pain sometimes occurs even when he is lying in bed. On physical examination, his blood pressure is 110/80 mm Hg and pulse is 85/min with irregular beats. Laboratory studies show serum glucose of 188 mg/dL, creatinine 1.2 mg/dL, and troponin I 1.5 ng/mL. Which of the following is most likely to explain these findings?

❏ (A) Hypertrophy of ischemic myocardium with increased oxygen demands
❏ (B) Increasing stenosis of right coronary artery
❏ (C) Fissuring of plaque in left coronary artery with superimposed mural (partial) thrombosis
❏ (D) Sudden complete thrombotic occlusion of right and left coronary arteries
❏ (E) Reduction in oxygen-carrying capacity due to pulmonary congestion

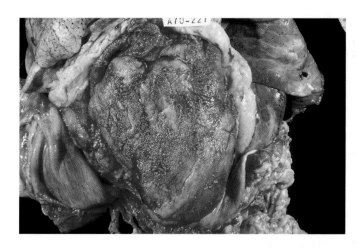

26 A 68-year-old man has become increasingly lethargic and weak for the past 7 months. On physical examination, his temperature is 36.9°C, pulse 70/min, respirations 15/min, and blood pressure 150/90 mm Hg. On auscultation, the physician notes a friction rub. There are no other remarkable findings. The representative gross appearance of the heart is shown above. Which of the following laboratory findings is most likely to be reported for this patient?

❏ (A) Positive ANA
❏ (B) Elevated anti–streptolysin O titer
❏ (C) Increased urea nitrogen level
❏ (D) Elevated renin level
❏ (E) Increased serum CK level

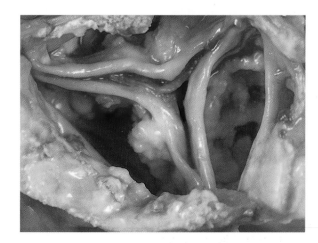

27 A 77-year-old woman sees her physician for a routine health maintenance examination. On physical examination, she is afebrile. Her pulse is 66/min, respirations 14/min, and blood pressure 125/85 mm Hg. On auscultation, a systolic ejection murmur is heard. There are a few crackles over the lung bases posteriorly. From the representative gross appearance of the aortic valve shown in the figure above, which of the following most likely contributed to the development of this lesion?

❏ (A) Chromosomal aneuploidy
❏ (B) Aging
❏ (C) Tertiary syphilis
❏ (D) Atherosclerosis
❏ (E) Systemic lupus erythematosus

28 A 32-year-old woman who lives in Pensacola, Florida, goes to the physician because of increasingly severe dyspnea, orthopnea, and swelling of the legs for the past 2 weeks. She has no previous history of serious illness or surgery. On physical examination, her temperature is 37.8 C, pulse 83/min, respirations 20/min, and blood pressure 100/60 mm Hg. An ECG shows episodes of ventricular tachycardia. An echocardiogram shows right and left ventricular dilation but no valvular deformities. An endomyocardial biopsy shows focal myocyte necrosis and lymphocytic infiltrate. Which of the following organisms most likely caused the infection?

❑ (A) *Trypanosoma cruzi*
❑ (B) *Streptococcus viridans*
❑ (C) Coxsackievirus A
❑ (D) *Toxoplasma gondii*
❑ (E) *Staphylococcus aureus*
❑ (F) *Mycobacterium kansasii*

29 While touring a 17th century European mansion, you notice that one of the antique beds was designed so that the occupant slept while sitting up. What cardiac disease in the 40-year-old wife of the mansion's owner at that time would best explain this bed design?

❑ (A) Libman-Sacks endocarditis
❑ (B) Giant cell myocarditis
❑ (C) Rheumatic heart disease
❑ (D) Atrial myxoma
❑ (E) Fibrinous pericarditis

30 One year ago, a 2-year-old child had an illness characterized by a high fever. *Staphylococcus epidermidis* was cultured from the blood. The child was given antibiotic therapy and recovered. On physical examination, a harsh, waxing and waning, machinery-like murmur is now heard on auscultation of the upper chest. A chest radiograph shows prominence of the pulmonary arteries. Echocardiography shows all valves to be normal in configuration. Laboratory studies show normal arterial oxygen saturation level. Which of the following congenital heart diseases is most likely to explain these findings?

❑ (A) Atrial septal defect
❑ (B) Tetralogy of Fallot
❑ (C) Aortic coarctation
❑ (D) Total anomalous pulmonary venous return
❑ (E) Patent ductus arteriosus
❑ (F) Aortic atresia

31 A 49-year-old previously healthy woman reports having suddenly lost consciousness four times in the past 6 months. In three instances, she was unconsciousness for only a few minutes. After the fourth episode 1 month ago, she was unconscious for 6 hours and had weakness in her left arm and difficulty speaking. On physical examination, she is afebrile and her blood pressure is normal. She has good carotid pulses with no bruits. Which of the following cardiac lesions is most likely to be present?

❑ (A) Pericardial effusion
❑ (B) Left atrial myxoma
❑ (C) Bicuspid aortic valve
❑ (D) Mitral valve stenosis
❑ (E) Left anterior descending artery thrombosis

32 A 60-year-old man visits the physician because of worsening cough and orthopnea. On physical examination, he has dullness to percussion at the lung bases and diffuse crackles in the upper lung fields. He is afebrile. Echocardiography shows marked left ventricular hypertrophy and severe aortic stenosis. The remaining cardiac valves are normal. A coronary angiogram shows no significant coronary arterial narrowing. Which of the following conditions best accounts for these findings?

❑ (A) Diabetes mellitus
❑ (B) Marfan syndrome
❑ (C) Bicuspid aortic valve
❑ (D) Systemic hypertension
❑ (E) Infective endocarditis

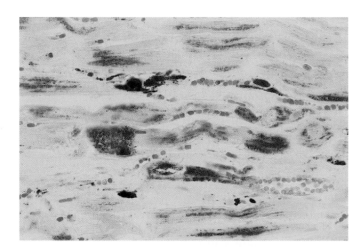

33 A 45-year-old man has had increasing fatigue, exertional dyspnea, and episodes of mild chest pain for the past 7 months. On physical examination, he is afebrile. His pulse is 79/min, respirations 15/min, and blood pressure 125/75 mm Hg. Laboratory studies show normal levels of serum troponin I, glucose, creatinine, and total cholesterol. The representative microscopic appearance of the myocardium with a Prussian blue stain is shown. Echocardiography will most likely show which of the following functional cardiac disturbances?

❑ (A) Dynamic obstruction to left ventricular outflow
❑ (B) Reduced ventricular compliance resulting in impaired ventricular filling in diastole
❑ (C) Mitral and tricuspid valvular insufficiency
❑ (D) Lack of ventricular expansion during diastole
❑ (E) Reduced ejection fraction from decreased contraction

34 A 50-year-old man has had increasing abdominal discomfort and swelling of his legs for the past 2 years. On physical examination, he has jugular venous distention, even when sitting up. The liver is enlarged and tender and can be palpated 10 cm below the right costal margin. Pitting edema is observed on the lower extremities. A chest radiograph shows bilated diaphragmatic flattening, pleural effusions, and increased lucency of lung fields. Thoracentesis on the right side yields 500 mL of clear fluid with few cells. Which of the following is most likely to produce these findings?

- [ ] (A) Tricuspid valve stenosis
- [ ] (B) Acute myocardial infarction
- [ ] (C) Pulmonary valve stenosis
- [ ] (D) Chronic obstructive pulmonary disease
- [ ] (E) Primary pulmonary hypertension

35 A 10-year-old girl develops subcutaneous nodules over the skin of her arms and torso 3 weeks after a bout of acute pharyngitis. She manifests choreiform movements and begins to complain of pain in her knees and hips, particularly with movement. A friction rub is heard on auscultation of the chest. Which of the following serum laboratory findings is most characteristic of the disease affecting this patient?

- [ ] (A) Elevated cardiac troponin I level
- [ ] (B) Positive ANA test
- [ ] (C) Elevated creatinine level
- [ ] (D) Positive rapid plasma reagin test
- [ ] (E) Elevated anti–streptolysin O level

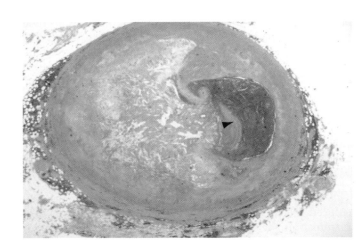

36 A 37-year-old woman dies suddenly and unexpectedly. Investigation of the scene of death in her bedroom at home and external examination of the body show no evidence of trauma. The microscopic appearance of the proximal left anterior descending artery at autopsy is shown above. Which of the following conditions is most likely to be the underlying cause of death?

- [ ] (A) Marfan syndrome
- [ ] (B) Acute leukemia
- [ ] (C) Polyarteritis nodosa
- [ ] (D) Diabetes mellitus
- [ ] (E) Chronic alcoholism

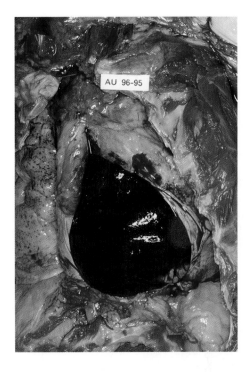

37 A 31-year-old man died suddenly after a week-long illness. He experienced chest pain and then became increasingly dyspneic and nauseated and lost consciousness multiple times. On the day of his death, he did not get up from his bed. External examination of the body by the medical examiner shows no evidence of trauma. The body is 166 cm (5 ft 5 in) in height and weighs 75 kg (BMI 27). This figure, showing the gross appearance of the chest cavity at autopsy with the pericardial sac opened, is most consistent with which of the following underlying causes of death?

- [ ] (A) Marfan syndrome
- [ ] (B) Disseminated tuberculosis
- [ ] (C) Scleroderma
- [ ] (D) Occlusive coronary atherosclerosis
- [ ] (E) Malignant melanoma
- [ ] (F) Dilated cardiomyopathy

38 A 40-year-old woman has had a 10-kg weight loss accompanied by severe nausea and vomiting of blood for the past 8 months. On physical examination, she is afebrile. Her pulse is 91/min, respirations 19/min, and blood pressure 90/50 mm Hg. Laboratory studies show hemoglobin of 8.4 g/dL, platelet count 227,100/mm³, and WBC count 6180/mm³. Biopsy specimens obtained by upper gastrointestinal endoscopy show adenocarcinoma of the stomach. CT scan of the abdomen shows multiple hepatic masses. CT scan of the head shows a cystic area in the right frontal lobe. Her condition is stable until 2 weeks later, when she develops severe dyspnea. A pulmonary ventilation-perfusion scan shows a high probability of pulmonary thromboembolism. Which of the following cardiac lesions is most likely to be present?

- [ ] (A) Epicardial metastases
- [ ] (B) Left ventricular mural thrombosis
- [ ] (C) Constrictive pericarditis
- [ ] (D) Nonbacterial thrombotic endocarditis
- [ ] (E) Calcific aortic valvular stenosis

39 A 55-year-old man undergoes orthotopic cardiac transplantation. One month later, an endomyocardial biopsy specimen shows focal myocardial cell death with scattered lymphocytes and plasma cells. Which of the following pathologic processes best accounts for the biopsy findings?

☐ (A) Autoimmunity
☐ (B) Ischemia
☐ (C) Infection
☐ (D) Rejection
☐ (E) Autophagy

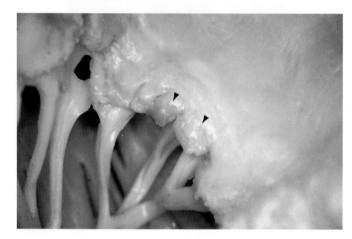

40 Two weeks after having a mild upper respiratory tract infection, a 14-year-old girl has fever and chest pain. On physical examination, her temperature is 37°C, pulse 90/min, respirations 20/min, and blood pressure 85/45 mm Hg. A friction rub is audible on auscultation of the chest. A chest radiograph shows pulmonary edema. An echocardiogram shows small vegetations at the closure line of the mitral and aortic valves. An endocardial biopsy shows focal interstitial inflammation with Aschoff nodules and Anichkov cells. Her condition improves over the next month. The representative gross appearance of the disease process 20 years later is shown. Which of the following additional complications of this illness is most likely to be seen in the patient?

☐ (A) Aortic stenosis
☐ (B) Constrictive pericarditis
☐ (C) Left ventricular aneurysm
☐ (D) Mitral valve prolapse
☐ (E) Dilated cardiomyopathy

41 A 15-year-old boy complains of pain in his legs when he runs more than 300 meters. Physical examination shows temperature of 36.8°C, pulse 76/min, respirations 22/min, and blood pressure 165/90 mm Hg. The radial pulses are 4+, and the dorsalis pedis pulses are 1+. Arterial blood gas measurement shows a normal oxygen saturation level. Which of the following lesions is most likely to be present in this patient?

☐ (A) Tricuspid atresia
☐ (B) Coarctation of the aorta
☐ (C) Aortic valve stenosis
☐ (D) Patent ductus arteriosus
☐ (E) Transposition of the great arteries

42 A 2-year-old child is brought to the physician for a routine examination. Physical examination shows a low-pitched cardiac murmur. An echocardiogram shows the presence of ostium secundum, with a 1-cm defect. Which of the following abnormalities is most likely to be found in this child?

☐ (A) Pulmonary hypertension
☐ (B) Pericardial effusion
☐ (C) Left-to-right shunt
☐ (D) Mural thrombosis
☐ (E) Cyanosis

43 A 44-year-old previously healthy man has experienced worsening exercise tolerance accompanied by marked shortness of breath for the past 6 months. On physical examination, he is afebrile. His pulse is 78/min, respirations 22/min, and blood pressure 110/70 mm Hg. He has diffuse rales in all lung fields and pitting edema to the knees. A chest radiograph shows cardiomegaly and pulmonary edema with pleural effusions. An echocardiogram shows four-chamber cardiac dilation and mitral and tricuspid valvular regurgitation, with an ejection fraction of 30%. A coronary angiogram shows no more than 10% narrowing of the major coronary arteries. Which of the following is the most likely diagnosis?

☐ (A) Rheumatic heart disease
☐ (B) Hereditary hemochromatosis
☐ (C) Chagas disease
☐ (D) Diabetes mellitus
☐ (E) Idiopathic dilated cardiomyopathy

44 A 19-year-old man suddenly collapses and is brought to the emergency department. His vital signs include temperature of 37.1°C, pulse 84/min, respirations 18/min, and blood pressure 80/40 mm Hg. Laboratory findings include hemoglobin of 13.5 g/dL, platelet count 252,000/mm³, WBC count 7230/mm³, serum glucose 73 mg/dL, and creatinine 1.2 mg/dL. The total creatine kinase (CK) level is elevated, with a CK-MB fraction of 10%. Which of the following underlying conditions is most likely to be present in this patient?

☐ (A) Hereditary hemochromatosis
☐ (B) Marfan syndrome
☐ (C) Down syndrome
☐ (D) DiGeorge syndrome
☐ (E) Familial hypercholesterolemia

45 An 86-year-old man has had increasing dyspnea and reduced exercise tolerance for the past 7 years. On physical examination, he is afebrile and has a blood pressure of 135/85 mm Hg. An irregularly irregular heart rate averaging 76/min is audible on auscultation of the chest. Crackles are heard at the bases of the lungs. A chest radiograph shows mild cardiomegaly and mild pulmonary edema. Echocardiography shows slight right and left ventricular wall thickening with reduced left and right ventricular wall motion, reduced left ventricular filling, and an ejection fraction estimated to be 25%. An endomyocardial biopsy specimen shows amorphous pink-staining deposits between myocardial fibers but no inflammation and no necrosis. Which of the following is the most likely diagnosis?

☐ (A) Cardiac amyloidosis
☐ (B) Rheumatic heart disease
☐ (C) Constrictive pericarditis
☐ (D) Mitral valve prolapse
☐ (E) Left ventricular aneurysm

46 A study of ischemic heart disease analyzes cases in which myocardial infarction was documented at autopsy. The gross and microscopic appearances of the hearts are correlated with the degree of coronary atherosclerosis and its complications, clinical symptoms, and therapies given before death. Hemorrhage and contraction bands in necrotic myocardial fibers are most likely to be seen in which of the following types of infarcts?

- ☐ (A) Subendocardial infarct resulting from diffuse narrowing of coronary arteries
- ☐ (B) Transmural infarct caused by complete thrombotic occlusion of a coronary artery
- ☐ (C) Transmural infarct complicated by mural thrombosis
- ☐ (D) Transmural infarct reperfused by thrombolytic therapy
- ☐ (E) Healing transmural myocardial infarct

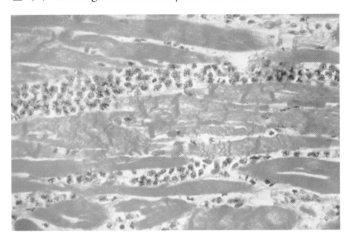

47 A 48-year-old woman has had increasing dyspnea for the past 2 days. She experiences sudden cardiac arrest and cannot be resuscitated. The light microscopic appearance of the left ventricular free wall at autopsy is shown above. Which of the following is the most likely diagnosis?

- ☐ (A) Viral myocarditis
- ☐ (B) Myocardial infarction
- ☐ (C) Acute rheumatic myocarditis
- ☐ (D) Septic embolization
- ☐ (E) Restrictive cardiomyopathy

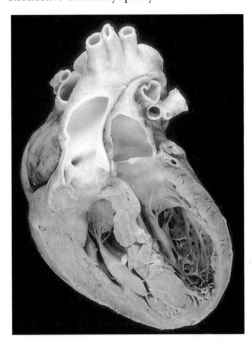

48 A 27-year-old woman gives birth to a term infant after an uncomplicated pregnancy and delivery. The infant is cyanotic at birth. Two months later, physical examination shows the infant to be at the 37th percentile for height and weight. The representative gross appearance of the infant's heart is shown in the preceding figure. Which of the following is the most likely diagnosis?

- ☐ (A) Tetralogy of Fallot
- ☐ (B) Pulmonic stenosis
- ☐ (C) Truncus arteriosus
- ☐ (D) Transposition of the great vessels
- ☐ (E) Aortic stenosis

49 A 21-year-old primigravida gives birth at term to a 2800-g infant with no apparent external anomalies. The next day, the infant develops increasing respiratory distress and cyanosis and dies. At autopsy, a slit-like left ventricular chamber, small left atrium, and atretic aortic and mitral valves are seen. Through which of the following structures could oxygenated blood most likely have reached the infant's systemic circulation?

- ☐ (A) Anomalous venous return
- ☐ (B) Foramen ovale
- ☐ (C) Patent ductus arteriosus
- ☐ (D) Right fourth aortic arch
- ☐ (E) Truncus arteriosus
- ☐ (F) Ventricular septal defect

50 A 68-year-old woman has had increasing dyspnea and orthopnea for the past year. She does not report any chest pain. On physical examination, her temperature is 36.9°C, pulse 77/min, respirations 20/min, and blood pressure 140/90 mm Hg. On auscultation of the chest, diffuse crackles are heard in all lung fields. No murmurs or gallops are heard, and the heart rate is regular. A chest radiograph shows prominent borders on the left and right sides of the heart. Coronary angiography shows 60% proximal occlusion of the right coronary and circumflex arteries, and 50% occlusion over the first 3 cm of the left anterior descending artery. Echocardiography shows no valvular abnormalities, but there is decreased left ventricular wall motion and an ejection fraction of 33%. Laboratory studies show serum glucose of 81 mg/dL, creatinine 1.6 mg/dL, total cholesterol 326 mg/dL, triglyceride 169 mg/dL, and troponin I 1 ng/mL. Which of the following pharmacologic agents is most likely to be beneficial in the treatment of this patient?

- ☐ (A) Amiodarone
- ☐ (B) Glyburide
- ☐ (C) Nitroglycerin
- ☐ (D) Propranolol
- ☐ (E) Simvastatin
- ☐ (F) Alteplase

51 A 41-year-old man has had increasing dyspnea for the past week. Physical examination shows temperature of 37.3°C, pulse 85/min, respirations 20/min, and blood pressure 150/95 mm Hg. There is dullness to percussion over the lung bases. A chest radiograph shows large bilateral pleural effusions and a normal heart size. Laboratory findings include serum creatinine of 3.1 mg/dL, urea nitrogen 29 mg/dL, troponin I 0.1 ng/mL, WBC count 3760/mm³ hemoglobin 11.7 g/dL, and positive ANA and anti–double-stranded DNA antibody test results. Which of the following cardiac lesions is most likely to be present in this patient?

❑ (A) Calcific aortic stenosis
❑ (B) Constrictive pericarditis
❑ (C) Ischemic cardiomyopathy
❑ (D) Libman-Sacks endocarditis
❑ (E) Rheumatic mitral valvulitis
❑ (F) Rhabdomyoma

52 A 70-year-old woman sees her physician because she has had episodes of chest pain during the past week. She is afebrile. Her pulse is 80/min, respirations 16/min, and blood pressure 110/70 mm Hg. On auscultation of the chest, heart sounds seem distant, but the lung fields are clear. Neck veins are distended to the angle of the jaw, even while sitting. There is a darkly pigmented, 1.2-cm skin lesion on the right shoulder. A chest radiograph shows cardiomegaly and prominent borders on the left and right sides of the heart. Pericardiocentesis yields bloody fluid. Laboratory findings include a serum troponin I level of 0.3 ng/mL. Which of the following is the most likely cause of these findings?

❑ (A) Calcific aortic stenosis
❑ (B) Coronary atherosclerosis
❑ (C) Metastases
❑ (D) Rheumatic heart disease
❑ (E) Tuberculosis

53 A 56-year-old man has experienced chest pain with exertion 3 years ago, and an angiogram showed 75% occlusion of his left anterior descending artery. He was prescribed long acting nitrates and beta blockers, and he has remained asymptomatic until the past week. He now has chest pain not relieved by resting or by his medications, and a presumptive diagnosis of unstable angina is made. Which of the following laboratory tests is most useful to assess his risk for acute myocardial infarction?

❑ (A) Homocysteine
❑ (B) C-reactive protein (CRP)
❑ (C) Lactate dehydrogenase (LDH)
❑ (D) Platelet count
❑ (E) Factor VIII activity
❑ (F) Creatine kinase-MB (CK-MB)

ANSWERS

1 (E) The patient's symptoms are typical of angina pectoris when coronary artery narrowing exceeds 75%. His risk factors include hyperglycemia (possible diabetes mellitus) and hypercholesterolemia. Persons with rheumatic heart disease

are affected by slowly worsening congestive heart failure (CHF). Pericarditis can produce chest pain, although not in relation to exercise, and it is not relieved by nitroglycerin. Cardiomyopathies result in heart failure but without chest pain. Calcific aortic stenosis leads to left-sided CHF, and the extra workload of the left ventricle may cause angina pectoris. However, calcific aortic stenosis (in the absence of a congenital bicuspid aortic valve) is rarely symptomatic at 50 years of age. Viral myocarditis may last for weeks but not for 1 year, and pain may be present at rest.

BP7 365   BP6 312   PBD7 572-576   PBD6 554

2 (B) Bioprostheses are subject to wear and tear. The leaflets may calcify, resulting in stenosis, or they may perforate or tear, leading to insufficiency. Paravalvular leaks are rare complications of the early postoperative period. Hemolysis is not seen in bioprostheses and is rare in modern mechanical prostheses. Thrombosis with embolization is an uncommon complication of mechanical prostheses, lessened by anticoagulant therapy. Myocardial infarction from embolization or from a poorly positioned valve is rare.

BP7 383   BP6 328   PBD7 600-601   PBD6 578

3 (B) The severity of the obstruction to the right ventricular outflow determines the direction of flow. If the pulmonic stenosis is mild, then the abnormality resembles a ventricular septal defect, and the shunt may be from left to right with no cyanosis. With significant pulmonary outflow obstruction, the right ventricular pressure may reach or exceed systemic vascular resistance, and the blood will be shunted from right to left, producing cyanotic heart disease. Even if pulmonic stenosis is mild at birth, the pulmonary orifice will not expand proportionately as the heart grows, and hence cyanotic heart disease supervenes.

BP7 391   BP6 335   PBD7 569   PBD6 595

4 (E) This boy developed acute left ventricular failure, an uncommon but serious complication of acute rheumatic fever. Pancarditis with pericarditis, endocarditis, and myocarditis develop during the acute phase. Dilation of the ventricle was so severe that the mitral valve became incompetent. Chronic inflammatory conditions may produce reactive systemic amyloidosis, but this is unlikely to occur given the limited and episodic nature of the streptococcal infection that causes rheumatic heart disease. Endocardial fibroelastosis is a rare disease encountered in children under the age of 2 years who may have congenital heart disease. Fibrinous pericarditis can produce an audible friction rub, but it is not constrictive and the amount of fluid and fibrin are not great, so no tamponade occurs. In fact, the myocardial necrosis with the myocarditis is patchy, and the ventricle does not rupture to produce tamponade. Fibrosis and fusion of the mitral valve leaflets develops over weeks to months and indicates chronic rheumatic valvulitis. Verrucous vegetations are small and may produce a murmur, but they do not interfere greatly with valve function and do not tend to embolize.

BP7 375-378   BP6 322-324   PBD7 593-595
PBD6 570-572

5 (D) The figure shows a large ventricular septal defect. By the age of 5 years, such an uncorrected defect causes marked shunting of blood from left to right, causing pulmonary hypertension (Eisenmenger complex). The left and right ventricular chambers undergo hypertrophy and some dilation, but the functioning of the cardiac valves is not greatly affected. In most cases, congenital heart disease is not an antecedent to ischemic heart disease. Nonbacterial thrombotic endocarditis most often occurs due to a hypercoagulable state in adults. Restrictive cardiomyopathy may occur from conditions such as amyloidosis or hemochromatosis.

BP7 390   BP6 334   PBD7 567-568   PBD6 594

6 (F) This enlarged and dilated heart has a large ventricular aneurysm. The aneurysm most likely resulted from weakening of the ventricular wall at the site of a prior healed myocardial infarction (MI). Because of the damage to the endocardial lining and stasis and turbulence of blood flow in the region of the aneurysm, mural thrombi are likely to develop. When detached, these thrombi embolize to the systemic circulation and can cause infarcts elsewhere. An atrial myxoma is the most common primary cardiac neoplasm, but it is rare and is not related to ischemic heart disease. Cardiac rupture with tamponade is most likely to occur 5 to 7 days after an acute MI. Constrictive pericarditis follows a previous suppurative or tuberculous pericarditis. Hypertrophic cardiomyopathy is not related to ischemic heart disease, but 50% of cases are familial and may be related to genetic mutations in genes encoding for cardiac contractile elements. Infective endocarditis is more likely to complicate valvular heart disease or septal defects.

BP7 370   BP6 316   PBD7 585-586   PBD6 563

7 (E) The aortic valve shown has large, destructive vegetations typical of infective endocarditis caused by highly virulent organisms such as *Staphylococcus aureus*. The verrucous vegetations of acute rheumatic fever are small and nondestructive, and the diagnosis is suggested by an elevated anti–streptolysin O titer. A positive ANCA determination suggests a vasculitis, which is unlikely to involve cardiac valves. An elevated creatine kinase-MB level suggests myocardial, not endocardial, injury. A positive double-stranded DNA finding suggests systemic lupus erythematosus, which can produce nondestructive Libman-Sacks endocarditis.

BP7 381-382   BP6 326-328   PBD7 596-597
PBD6 573-575

8 (A) These clinical and morphologic features are typical of hypertrophic cardiomyopathy, which is familial in 70% of cases and is usually transmitted as an autosomal dominant trait. The mutations affect genes that encode proteins of cardiac contractile elements. The most common mutation in the inherited forms affects the β-myosin heavy chain. Hemochromatosis can give rise to cardiomyopathy, but it occurs much later in life; amyloidosis causes restrictive cardiomyopathy. Autoimmune conditions are unlikely to involve the myocardium. Viral infections produce generalized inflammation and cardiac dilation.

BP7 386-387   BP6 331-332   PBD7 604-606
PBD6 581-583

9 (A) The clinical features are those of pericarditis with effusion, and the most common causes of hemorrhagic pericarditis are metastatic carcinoma and tuberculosis. Group A *Streptococcus* is responsible for rheumatic fever; in the acute form, it can lead to fibrinous pericarditis, and in the chronic form, it can lead to serous effusions from congestive failure. Coxsackieviruses are known to cause myocarditis. *Candida* is a rare cardiac infection in immunocompromised persons. *Staphylococcus aureus* is a cause of infective endocarditis.

BP7 393   BP6 337   PBD7 612   PBD6 588-589

10 (A) This patient is at a high risk of developing complications of infective endocarditis. The findings suggest that she developed staphylococcal septicemia followed by endocarditis of the mitral valve. The impaired functioning of the mitral valve (most likely regurgitation) would give rise to left atrial dilation. Emboli from the mitral valve vegetation could reach the systemic circulation and give rise to abscesses. Infection of an arterial wall can weaken the wall, resulting in aneurysm formation and the potential for rupture. Dilated cardiomyopathy may be due to chronic alcoholism, or it may be idiopathic, familial, or it may follow myocarditis, but it is not a direct complication of infective endocarditis. Lesions on the right side of the valve can produce septic emboli that involve the lungs, but vegetations on the left side embolize to the systemic circulation, producing lesions in the spleen, kidneys, or brain. Myxomatous degeneration of the mitral valve results from a defect in connective tissue, whether well defined or unknown. The mitral valve leaflets are enlarged, hooded, and redundant. Polyarteritis nodosa is an immunologically mediated disease that causes vasculitis of small to medium-sized arteries; it is not related to endocarditis. Septic emboli to the kidneys could produce infarctions that heal to scars, not cysts.

BP7 381-382   BP6 326-328   PBD7 596-597
PBD6 569, 574-576

11 (A) Prolonged fever, heart murmur, mild splenomegaly, and splinter hemorrhages suggest a diagnosis of infective endocarditis. The valvular vegetations with infective endocarditis are friable and can break off and embolize. The time course of weeks suggests a "subacute" form of bacterial endocarditis resulting from infection with a less virulent organism, such as *Streptococcus viridans*. *Trypanosoma cruzi* and coxsackievirus B are causes of myocarditis. *Candida* is not a common cause of infective endocarditis but may be seen in immunocompromised patients. Tuberculosis involving the heart most often manifests as pericarditis. *Pseudomonas* is more likely to cause an acute form of bacterial endocarditis that worsens over days, not weeks; this organism is more common as a nosocomial infection or in injection drug users.

BP7 381-382   BP6 326-328   PBD7 596-598
PBD6 573-575

12 (A) In the period immediately following coronary thrombosis, arrhythmias are the most important complication and can lead to sudden cardiac death. It is believed that, even before ischemic injury manifests in the heart, there is greatly increased electrical irritability. Pericarditis and rupture occur several days later. An aneurysm is a late complication of healing of a large transmural infarction; a mural thrombus may fill an aneurysm and become a source of emboli. If portions of the coronary thrombus break off and embolize, they enter smaller arterial branches in the distribution already affected by ischemia.

BP7 369-370   BP6 314-316   PBD7 573-575   PBD6 562

13 **(E)** Mitral annular calcification is often an incidental finding on chest radiograph, echocardiograph, or at autopsy. However, larger accumulations of calcium in the mitral ring can impinge on the conduction system, causing arrhythmias or disrupting the endocardium to provide a focus for thrombus formation (which can embolize and cause a "stroke," as in this patient) or infective endocarditis. Some cases are associated with mitral valve prolapse. Carcinoid heart disease leads to endocardial and valvular collagenous thickening. Hyperparathyroidism can cause metastatic calcification, which usually does not involve the heart, and deposits would not be so focal; this patient does not have hypercalcemia. Infective endocarditis is a destructive process, and healing may lead to fibrosis but not to nodular calcium deposition. The most common infiltrative cardiomyopathies are hemochromatosis and amyloidosis. Rheumatic heart disease can lead to scarring with some calcium deposition, but the valve leaflets undergo extensive scarring, with shortening and thickening of the chordae that preclude upward prolapse. Senile calcific stenosis involves the aortic valve; in this case, there is no evidence of stenosis.

BP7 375   BP6 301-302, 325-326   PBD7 590-591
PBD6 527-528, 569-570

14 **(F)** The pacemaker for the heart is the sinoatrial (SA) node, with a natural rhythm near 70/min and a normal range of 60 to 100/min. Other parts of the cardiac conduction system pass along this rate. Rates below 60/min are defined as bradycardia, and those above 100/min as tachycardia. Bradyarrhythmias less than 50/min suggest an SA node disorder. SA node dysfunction may worsen with cardioactive drugs such as cardiac glycosides, β-adrenergic blockers, calcium channel blockers, and amiodarone. Increases in sinus rate result from an increase in sympathetic tone acting via β-adrenergic receptors or a decrease in parasympathetic tone acting via muscarinic receptors, or both. Abnormalities involving the other listed options are unlikely to produce such a pronounced and consistent bradycardia.

BP7 370   BP6 325-326   PBD7 557   PBD6 569-570

15 **(C)** Anticoagulant therapy is necessary for patients with mechanical prostheses to avoid potential thrombotic complications. If the patient is unable to take anticoagulants, then use of a bioprosthesis (porcine valve) may be considered. Amiodarone is an antiarrhythmic agent used for dysrhythmias that are intractable to other agents, and this drug has a high rate of complications. Antibiotic therapy with agents such as ciprofloxacin is not indicated unless the patient has an infection or requires prophylactic antibiotic coverage for surgical or dental procedures. Cyclosporine or other immunosuppressive agents are not indicated, because allogeneic tissue was not transplanted (a bioprosthesis also is essentially "inert" immunologically). Digoxin is not indicated, because the patient's cardiac function has improved. A β-blocker is not needed in the absence of chronic cardiac failure.

BP7 383   BP6 326   PBD7 600-601   PBD6 567-577

16 **(D)** The findings point to dilated cardiomyopathy (DCM) with both right-sided and left-sided heart failure. The most common toxin producing DCM is alcohol, and persons with chronic alcoholism are more likely to have DCM than to

have ischemic heart disease. Acetaminophen ingestion can be associated with hepatic necrosis and analgesic nephropathy. Cocaine can produce ischemic effects on the heart. Digoxin is an inotropic cardiovascular agent that has been used to treat heart failure. Lisinopril is an angiotensin I–converting enzyme (ACE) inhibitor that is used to treat hypertension. Nicotine in cigarette smoke is a risk factor for atherosclerosis. Propranolol is a β-blocker that has been used to treat hypertension, and it may exacerbate bradycardia and congestive heart failure.

BP7 385-386   BP6 326-328   PBD7 601-604
PBD6 574-576

17 **(B)** Hypertension is an important cause of left ventricular hypertrophy and failure. Left-sided heart failure leads to pulmonary edema with dyspnea. Obstructive (e.g., emphysema) and restrictive (e.g., silicosis) lung diseases lead to pulmonary hypertension with right-sided heart failure from cor pulmonale. Likewise, right-sided valvular lesions (tricuspid or pulmonic valves) predispose to right-sided heart failure. Alcoholism can lead to a dilated cardiomyopathy that affects heart function on both sides.

BP7 372-374   BP6 309   PBD7 560-562, 587-588
PBD6 549

18 **(C)** This patient has evidence of pulmonary hypertension (pulmonary atherosclerosis) and right-sided heart failure. When this is secondary to lung disease, it is called cor pulmonale and is caused most often by pulmonary emphysema and other obstructive lung diseases. Restrictive lung diseases can also lead to cor pulmonale. A large pulmonary embolism can produce acute cor pulmonale, mainly with right atrial dilation. A ventricular septal defect predominantly produces left ventricular hypertrophy; however, after several years, the left-to-right shunt can cause an increase in pulmonary vascular resistance, reversing the shunt. At this stage, right ventricular hypertrophy develops. Rheumatic heart disease affects mainly mitral and aortic valves. Left ventricular function is most affected by hypertrophic cardiomyopathy.

BP7 374   BP6 320-321   PBD7 563, 588   PBD6 565-566

19 **(C)** These findings indicate a floppy mitral valve, a condition that usually is asymptomatic. When symptomatic, it can cause fatigue, chest pain, and arrhythmias. Pulmonic stenosis is most often a congenital heart disease. Valvular vegetations suggest endocarditis, and a murmur is likely to be heard with infective endocarditis causing valvular insufficiency. A patent ductus arteriosus causes a shrill systolic murmur. Tricuspid regurgitation is accompanied by a rumbling systolic murmur.

BP7 379-380   BP6 325-326   PBD7 591-592
PBD6 568-570

20 **(A)** Hypertrophic cardiomyopathy is the most common cause of sudden unexplained death in young athletes. There is asymmetric septal hypertrophy that reduces the ejection fraction of the left ventricle, particularly during exercise. Histologically, haphazardly arranged hypertrophic myocardial fibers are seen. Hemochromatosis gives rise to a restrictive cardiomyopathy in middle age. Tachyzoites of *Toxoplasma gondii* signify myocarditis, a process that may occur in immunocompromised persons. Rheumatic heart disease with chronic valvular changes would be unusual in a patient this age, and the course is most often slowly progressive. Valve destruction with vegetations is seen in infective endocarditis. This would be accompanied by signs of sepsis.

BP7 386-387   BP6 331-332   PBD7 604-606
PBD6 581-583

21 **(B)** The markedly thickened left ventricular wall is characteristic of hypertrophy due to increased pressure load from hypertension, which often is associated with chronic renal disease. Chronic alcoholism is associated with dilated cardiomyopathy. Pneumoconioses produce restrictive lung disease with cor pulmonale and predominantly right ventricular hypertrophy. Hemochromatosis leads to restrictive cardiomyopathy. Diabetes mellitus accelerates atherosclerosis, leading to ischemic heart disease and myocardial infarction.

BP7 372-374   BP6 319-320   PBD7 587-588
PBD6 564-565

22 **(E)** Cyanosis at this early age suggests a right-to-left shunt; truncus arteriosus, transposition of the great arteries, and tetralogy of Fallot are the most common causes of cyanotic congenital heart disease. The cerebral lesion suggests an abscess as a consequence of septic embolization from infective endocarditis, which can complicate congenital heart disease. Atrial septal defect, patent ductus arteriosus, and ventricular septal defect initially lead to left-to-right shunts. Coarctation is not accompanied by a shunt and cyanosis. In most cases, a bicuspid valve is asymptomatic until adulthood, and there is no shunt.

BP7 391   BP6 335-336   PBD7 569-570   PBD6 595

23 **(C)** The kinetics of creatine kinase (CK), CK-MB, and troponin I elevations following a myocardial infarction (MI) are important. Total CK activity begins to rise 2 to 4 hours after an MI, peaks at about 24 hours, and returns to normal within 72 hours. Troponin I levels begin to rise at about the same time as CK and CK-MB but remain elevated for 7 to 10 days. Total CK activity is a sensitive marker for myocardial injury in the first 24 to 48 hours. CK-MB offers more specificity but not more sensitivity. Myocardial rupture occurs 5 to 7 days after myocardial necrosis. This patient experienced an MI on the day of the shoulder pain. When he saw the physician on day 3, the CK levels had returned to normal, but troponin I levels remained elevated. Three days later, the infarct ruptured.

BP7 370-371   BP6 317   PBD7 583-584   PBD6 561

24 **(C)** This patient has symptoms of an acute myocardial infarction (MI), and of the enzymes listed, creatine kinase-MB is the most specific for myocardial injury. The levels of this enzyme begin to rise within 2 to 4 hours of ischemic myocardial injury. Lipase is a marker for pancreatitis. AST is found in a variety of tissues; therefore, elevated levels are not specific for myocardial injury. ALT elevation is more specific for liver injury. The elevation of lactate dehydrogenase (LDH)-1 compared with LDH-2 suggests myocardial injury, but LDH activity peaks 3 days after an MI. C-reactive protein is elevated with inflammatory processes but is nonspecific; it has been used as a predictor of acute coronary syndromes.

BP7 370-371   BP6 317   PBD7 583-584   PBD6 561

25 **(C)** This patient has 75% stenosis of the left anterior descending branch of the coronary artery. This degree of stenosis prevents adequate perfusion of the heart when myocardial demand is increased, which occurs during exertion. Hence, the patient had angina on exertion. The patient has recently developed unstable angina, which is manifested by increased frequency and severity of the attacks and angina at rest. In most patients, unstable angina is induced by disruption of an atherosclerotic plaque followed by a mural thrombus and possibly distal embolization, vasospasm, or both. Hypertrophy of the heart is unlikely in this case, because there is neither hypertension nor a valvular lesion. The remaining choices can theoretically give rise to a similar picture, but plaque disruption with mural thrombosis is the most common anatomic finding when the patient develops unstable angina. It is important to recognize this, because unstable angina is a harbinger of myocardial infarction.

BP7 365   BP6 312   PBD7 575   PBD6 554-555

26 **(C)** This patient has fibrinous pericarditis. The most common cause is uremia resulting from renal failure. A positive ANA test result suggests a collagen vascular disease, such as systemic lupus erythematosus. Such diseases tend to be accompanied by serous pericarditis. Elevation of the anti–streptolysin O titer accompanies rheumatic fever. Acute rheumatic fever may produce fibrinous pericarditis, but rheumatic fever is not common at this age. An elevated renin level is seen in some forms of hypertension. Elevation of serum creatine kinase occurs in myocardial infarction (MI). An acute MI may be accompanied by a fibrinous exudate over the area of infarction, not the diffuse pericarditis seen in this patient.

BP7 393   BP6 337   PBD7 611-612   PBD6 588

27 **(B)** This patient has calcific aortic stenosis of a valve with three cusps, a degenerative change that may occur in a normal aortic valve with aging. Congenital anomalies with chromosomal aneuploidies (e.g., trisomy 21) are unlikely to be associated with aortic stenosis or a bicuspid valve. In syphilis, the aortic root dilates and aortic insufficiency results. Atherosclerosis does not produce valvular disease from involvement of the valve itself. Systemic lupus erythematosus may give rise to small sterile vegetations on mitral or tricuspid valves, but these rarely cause valve disease.

BP7 379   BP6 324-325   PBD7 590-591   PBD6 567-568

28 **(C)** Focal myocardial necrosis with lymphocyte infiltrate is consistent with viral myocarditis. This is uncommon, and many cases may be asymptomatic. In North America, most cases are caused by coxsackieviruses A and B. This illness may be self-limited, end in sudden death, or progress to chronic heart failure. *Trypanosoma cruzi* is the causative agent of Chagas disease, seen most often in children. This is probably the most common infectious cause of myocarditis worldwide. Septicemia with bacterial infections may involve the heart, but the patient probably would be very ill with multiple organ failure. *Toxoplasma gondii* may cause a myocarditis in immunocompromised patients. Mycobacterial infections of the heart are uncommon, but pericardial involvement is the most likely pattern. *Streptococcus viridans* and *Staphylococcus* *aureus* are better known as causes of endocarditis with neurophilic inflammatory infiltrates.

BP7 383-384   BP6 329-330   PBD7 608-609
PBD6 584-585

29 **(C)** Paroxysmal nocturnal dyspnea is a feature of left-sided congestive heart failure, and rheumatic heart disease (RHD) most often involves the mitral, aortic, or both valves. RHD was more common before antibiotic therapy for group A β-hemolytic streptococcal infections was available. Giant cell myocarditis is a rare cause of cardiac failure. Libman-Sacks endocarditis, seen in systemic lupus erythematosus, typically does not impair ventricular function significantly. An atrial myxoma usually occurs on the left side, but the obstruction is often intermittent. Fibrinous pericarditis can produce chest pain, but the amount of accompanying fluid often is not great; hence, cardiac function is not impaired.

BP7 363, 377-378   BP6 310   PBD7 562-563   PBD6 549

30 **(E)** Although often not large, a patent ductus arteriosus can produce a significant murmur and predispose to endocarditis. The left-to-right shunt eventually results in pulmonary hypertension. An atrial septal defect is unlikely to produce a loud murmur because of the minimal pressure differential between the atria. Because pulmonic stenosis is a component of tetralogy of Fallot, no pulmonary hypertension results, and the right-to-left shunting produces cyanosis with decreased arterial oxygen saturation. Aortic coarctations by themselves produce no shunting and no pulmonary hypertension. Total anomalous pulmonary venous return is not accompanied by a murmur because of the low venous pressure. An atretic valve has no flow across it and does not produce a murmur, but there would be a murmur across a shunt around the atretic valve. Aortic atresia is not compatible with continued survival, as seen in hypoplastic left heart syndrome.

BP7 390-391   BP6 335   PBD7 567-568   PBD6 594

31 **(B)** An atrial myxoma can have a ball-valve effect that intermittently occludes the mitral valve, leading to syncopal episodes and possible strokes from embolization to cerebral arteries. Most pericardial effusions are not large and do not cause major problems. Large effusions could lead to tamponade, but this is not an intermittent problem. Calcification of a bicuspid valve can lead to stenosis and heart failure, but this condition is progressive. By the time left atrial enlargement with mural thrombosis and risk of embolization occurs from mitral stenosis, this patient would have been symptomatic for years. Coronary artery thrombosis results in an acute ischemic event.

BP7 394   BP6 338   PBD7 613-614   PBD6 589-590

32 **(C)** There is a tendency for bicuspid valves to calcify with aging, which can eventually result in stenosis. In individuals with congenitally bicuspid valves, symptoms appear by 50 to 60 years of age. By contrast, calcific aortic stenosis of tricuspid valves manifests in the seventh or eighth decade. Ischemic heart disease, expected in diabetes mellitus, does not lead to valvular stenosis. In Marfan syndrome, the aortic root dilates, producing aortic valvular insufficiency. Hypertension accounts for left ventricular hypertrophy, but the aortic valve is not affected. In infective endocarditis, the patient would

have an infection and the valve would tend to be destroyed, leading to insufficiency.

BP7 379   BP6 325   PBD7 590-591   PBD6 568

33 **(B)** The extensive iron deposition signifies hemochromatosis, which markedly reduces ventricular compliance, resulting in restrictive cardiomyopathy. Dynamic left ventricular outflow obstruction is characteristic of hypertropic cardiomyopathy. Valvular insufficiency of mitral and tricuspid valves can occur with dilated cardiomyopathy, which also reduces contractility and ejection fraction. Lack of diastolic expansion suggests constrictive pericarditis.

BP7 387-388   BP6 332   PBD7 606-607, 610
PBD6 586-587

34 **(D)** The findings point to pure right-sided congestive heart failure. This type of failure can be caused by right-sided valvular lesions such as tricuspid or pulmonic stenosis, but these are rare. Pulmonary hypertension resulting from obstructive lung diseases such as emphysema is much more common. Primary pulmonary hypertension can also cause right-sided heart failure, but it is a much less common cause than are lung diseases. Because acute myocardial infarction usually affects the left ventricle, left-sided heart failure would be more common in these patients. Chronic left-sided heart failure can eventually lead to right-sided heart failure.

BP7 362-363   BP6 309-310   PBD7 563   PBD6 549-550

35 **(E)** The findings suggest acute rheumatic fever, which can involve any or all layers of the heart. Because rheumatic fever follows streptococcal infections, the anti–streptolysin O titer is elevated. Cardiac troponin I and T are markers for ischemic myocardial injury. Although their levels may be somewhat elevated because of the acute myocarditis that occurs in rheumatic fever, this change is not a characteristic of rheumatic heart disease. The ANA level could be elevated in systemic lupus erythematosus, which is most likely to produce a serous pericarditis. The strains of group A *Streptococcus* that lead to acute rheumatic fever are not likely to cause glomerulonephritis, and an elevated creatinine level therefore is unlikely. A positive rapid plasma reagin test suggests syphilis, but the clinical features are not those of syphilis.

BP7 375-378   BP6 322-324   PBD7 593-595
PBD6 570-572

36 **(D)** The figure shows a coronary artery with marked narrowing due to atheromatous plaque, complicated by a recent thrombus. Atherosclerosis is accelerated with diabetes mellitus. When a premenopausal woman develops severe atherosclerosis, as in this case, underlying diabetes mellitus must be strongly suspected. The cystic medial necrosis that occurs in Marfan syndrome most often involves the ascending aorta and predisposes to dissection that could involve coronary arteries, although with external compression. Patients with leukemias can develop hypercoagulable states. When this occurs, there is widespread thrombosis in normal blood vessels. Polyarteritis nodosa can involve coronary arteries and give rise to coronary thrombosis. However, in these cases, the vessel wall is necrotic and inflamed. Persons with chronic alcoholism often have less atherosclerosis than do those of the same age who do not consume large amounts of alcohol.

BP7 364-365 BP6 311 PBD7 572-575 PBD6 551-552

37 **(D)** The figure shows a massive hemopericardium with pericardial tamponade. Rupture of a transmural myocardial infarction typically occurs 5 to 7 days after onset, when there is maximal necrosis before significant healing. Ischemic heart disease occurs in patients of this age, and risk factors such as obesity, smoking, diabetes mellitus, and hyperlipidemia can play a role in its development. This patient does not have a marfanoid habitus, although Marfan syndrome can cause cystic medial necrosis involving the aorta, leading to aortic dissection that can cause an acute hemopericardium. Tuberculosis can cause hemorrhagic pericarditis, typically without tamponade. Scleroderma is most likely to produce serous effusion. Metastases from melanoma and other carcinomas can produce hemorrhagic pericarditis without tamponade. Cardiomyopathies lead to ventricular hypertrophy or dilation, or both, but do not cause rupture.

BP7 368-369 BP6 337-338 PBD7 584, 611 PBD6 587

38 **(D)** These so-called marantic vegetations may occur on any cardiac valve but tend to be small and do not damage the valves. However, they have a nasty tendency to embolize. They can occur with hypercoagulable states that accompany certain malignancies, especially mucin-secreting adenocarcinomas. This paraneoplastic state is known as Trousseau syndrome. Cardiac metastases are uncommon, and they tend to involve the epicardium. Mural thromboses occur when cardiac blood flow is altered, as occurs in a ventricular aneurysm or dilated atrium. A metastatic tumor can encase the heart to produce constriction, but this is rare. Calcific aortic stenosis occurs at a much older age, usually in the eighth or ninth decade.

BP7 380 BP6 326 PBD7 597-598 PBD6 576

39 **(D)** Endomyocardial biopsies are routinely performed after cardiac transplantation to monitor rejection. This is not an autoimmune process, because the transplant is "foreign" tissue to the host. Months to years later, coronary arteriopathy characteristic of cardiac transplantations may produce ischemic changes. Infection is a definite possibility, because of the immunosuppressive drugs administered to control the rejection process, although plasma cells are not a key feature of acute infection. Turnover of cellular organelles occurs constantly by autophagy, generating lipofuscin pigment in the cells.

BP7 384 BP6 329 PBD7 615 PBD6 579

40 **(A)** This mitral valve shows shortening and thickening of the chordae typical of chronic rheumatic valvulitis, and the small verrucous vegetations are characteristic of acute rheumatic fever; scarring can follow years later. Rheumatic heart disease develops after a streptococcal infection; the immune response against the bacteria damages the heart because streptococcal antigens cross-react with the heart. The mitral and aortic valves are most commonly affected, so right ventricular dilation from tricuspid involvement is less likely. In almost all cases, the fibrinous pericarditis seen during the acute phase resolves without significant scarring, and constrictive pericarditis does not develop. A left ventricular aneurysm is a complication of ischemic heart disease. Mitral

valve prolapse can be seen in patients with Marfan syndrome, or more commonly, no antecedent disease can be identified.

BP7 377-378 BP6 321-323 PBD7 593-594
PBD6 570-572

41 **(B)** In adults, the coarctation is typically postductal, and collateral branches from the proximal aorta supply the lower extremities, leading to the pulse differential from upper to lower extremities. Diminished renal blood flow increases renin production and promotes hypertension. Tricuspid atresia affects the right side of the heart. Aortic valve stenosis causes left-sided heart failure and no pressure differential in the extremities. A patent ductus arteriosus produces a left-to-right shunt. Transposition results in a right-to-left shunt with cyanosis.

BP7 392 BP6 336 PBD7 570-571 PBD6 596-597

42 **(C)** Ostium secundum is the most common form of atrial septal defect. Because atrial pressures are low, the amount of shunting from the left atrium to the right atrium is small, and this lesion can remain asymptomatic for many years. Eventually, pulmonary hypertension can occur, with reversal of the shunt. Pericardial effusions may occur much later, if congestive heart failure develops. A dilated heart with enlarged atria predisposes to mural thrombosis. Cyanosis is a feature of a right-to-left shunt.

BP7 388-390 BP6 333-334 PBD7 567 PBD6 593-594

43 **(E)** Congestive heart failure with four-chamber dilation is suggestive of dilated cardiomyopathy; implicated in causation are myocarditis, alcohol abuse, and genetic factors (in 25–30% of cases). Many cases of dilated cardiomyopathy have no known cause. Dilation is more prominent than hypertrophy, although both are present, and all chambers are involved. Rheumatic heart disease would most often produce some degree of valvular stenosis, often with some regurgitation, and the course usually is more prolonged. Hemochromatosis produces restrictive cardiomyopathy. Chagas disease affects the right ventricle more often than the left. Coronary artery narrowing would be worse in diabetes mellitus and accelerated atherosclerosis.

BP7 385-386 BP6 330-331 PBD7 602-604
PBD6 579-581

44 **(E)** The laboratory findings suggest an acute myocardial infarction. Persons with familial hypercholesterolemia have accelerated and advanced atherosclerosis, even by the second or third decade. Hereditary hemochromatosis may result in an infiltrative cardiomyopathy with iron overload, more typically in the fifth decade. Marfan syndrome may result in aortic dissection or floppy mitral valve. DiGeorge syndrome can be associated with a variety of congenital heart defects, but survival with this syndrome is usually limited by infections due to the cell-mediated immunodeficiency.

BP7 364, 371 BP6 317 PBD7 572, 576 PBD6 561

45 **(A)** These findings suggest reduced cardiac chamber compliance with a restrictive form of cardiomyopathy. Cardiac amyloidosis may be limited to the heart (so-called "senile cardiac amyloidosis" derived from transthyretin protein) or may be part of organ involvement in systemic amyloidosis derived from serum amyloid–associated (SAA) protein or in multiple myeloma derived from light chains. Incidental isolated atrial deposits of amyloid are derived from atrial natriuretic peptide. Rheumatic heart disease may resolve with scarring of valves and focal small interstitial scars in the myocardium where Aschoff nodules were present. Constrictive pericarditis produces extensive collagenous fibrosis surrounding the heart, but this process does not typically involve the myocardium, and collagen does not have an amorphous appearance. In Marfan syndrome, mitral valve prolapse may be associated with cystic medial necrosis but not with amyloid deposition. Amyloidosis may produce a restrictive (infiltrative) form of cardiomyopathy, but aneurysm formation is a potential complication of myocardial infarction.

BP7 387-388   BP6 322-324   PBD7 601, 610
PBD6 570-572

46 (D) Reperfusion of an ischemic myocardium by spontaneous or therapeutic thrombolysis changes the morphologic features of the affected area. Reflow of blood into vasculature injured during the period of ischemia leads to leakage of blood into the tissues (hemorrhage). Contraction bands are composed of closely packed hypercontracted sarcomeres. They are most likely produced by exaggerated contraction of previously injured myofibrils that are exposed to a high concentration of calcium ions from the plasma. The damaged cell membrane of the injured myocardial fibers allows calcium to penetrate the cells rapidly. Hemorrhage would not be a prominent feature in the other listed options.

BP7 9, 368   BP6 316-317   PBD7 581-583   PBD6 561

47 (B) The figure shows deeply eosinophilic myocardial fibers with loss of nuclei, all indicative of coagulative necrosis. The deeply staining transverse bands are called contraction bands. Myocardial fibers are between neutrophils. This pattern is most likely caused by a myocardial infarction (MI) that is approximately 24 to 48 hours old. Chest pain is present in most, but not all, cases of MI. In viral myocarditis, there is minimal focal myocardial necrosis with round cell infiltrates. Rheumatic myocarditis is characterized by minimal myocardial necrosis with foci of granulomatous inflammation (Aschoff bodies). Septic emboli result in focal abscess formation. There is no significant inflammation with restrictive cardiomyopathies such as amyloidosis or hemochromatosis.

BP7 367-368   BP6 315   PBD7 579-580   PBD6 560

48 (D) The figure shows transposition of the great vessels. The aorta emerges from the right ventricle, and the pulmonic trunk exits the left ventricle. Unless there is another anomalous connection between the pulmonary and systemic circulations, this condition is not compatible with extrauterine life. The most common anomalous connections would be ventricular septal defect (VSD), patent ductus arteriosus, and patent foramen ovale (or atrial septal defect). In tetralogy of Fallot, the aorta overrides a VSD but is not transposed. In pulmonic and aortic stenosis, the great arteries are normally positioned but small. In truncus arteriosus, the spiral septum that embryologically separates the great arteries does not develop properly.

BP7 391-392   BP6 336   PBD7 569-570   PBD6 596

49 (C) These findings are compatible with hypoplastic left heart syndrome, which may have varying degrees of severity, ranging from severe (as in this case, with virtually no function on the left side of the heart), to milder degrees of hypoplasia. All blood returning to the left atrium is shunted across the foramen ovale back to the lungs, increasing pulmonary flow and decreasing oxygenation. Unoxygenated blood exiting the right ventricle can shunt through the ductus arteriosus to the aorta to supply the systemic circulation. Anomalous venous return will not generally connect to the aorta, and there still must be a connection from the lungs to the aorta. The right fourth aortic arch rarely persists. Truncus arteriosus is an anomalous, incomplete separation of the pulmonic and aortic trunks. If there is virtually no left ventricular chamber, then a ventricular septal defect will not provide any significant flow.

PBD7 571   PBD6 597

50 (E) This patient has findings suggestive of an "ischemic" cardiomyopathy from coronary atherosclerosis, but she does not appear to have an acute coronary syndrome. The major identifiable risk factor in this case is hypercholesterolemia, and the HMG-CoA reductase inhibitors (the "statin" drugs) are helpful. Amiodarone is used to treat intractable arrhythmias. Glyburide is used in the treatment of type 2 diabetes mellitus, but this patient is not hyperglycemic. Nitroglycerin is used to treat angina. Propranolol is a β-blocker that has been used to treat hypertension, and it may exacerbate bradycardia and congestive heart failure. Alteplase (tissue plasminogen activator) is used early in treatment of coronary thrombosis to help reestablish coronary blood flow.

BP7 371   BP6 317-318   PBD7 586   PBD6 564

51 (D) Libman-Sacks endocarditis is an uncommon complication of systemic lupus erythematosus (SLE) that has minimal clinical significance because the small vegetations, although they spread over valves and endocardium, are unlikely to embolize or cause functional flow problems. Calcific aortic stenosis may be seen in older persons with tricuspid valves, or it may be a complication of bicuspid valves. Although pericardial effusions are common in active SLE, along with pleural effusions and ascites from serositis, they are usually serous effusions, and no significant scarring occurs. Ischemic cardiomyopathy is unlikely in persons with autoimmune diseases, who have less atherosclerosis from the chronic, debilitating nature of their underlying disease. Rheumatic heart disease is an immunologic disease based on molecular mimicry, not autoimmunity. Cardiac rhabdomyomas are rare primary myocardial neoplasms seen in children and in persons with tuberous sclerosis.

BP7 380   BP6 106, 107   PBD7 597-599   PBD6 577

52 (C) This patient has a hemorrhagic pericardial effusion, and the two most common causes are tumor and tuberculosis. The most common neoplasm involving the heart is metastatic carcinoma, because primary cardiac neoplasms are rare. The most common primary sites are nearby: lung and breast. The skin lesion in this patient is likely to be a melanoma, which tends to metastasize widely, including to the heart. Most cardiac metastases involve the pericardium. A large effusion can cause tamponade, which interferes with cardiac motion. Calcific aortic stenosis leads to left-sided congestive heart failure, with pulmonary edema as a key finding. Coronary atherosclerosis may lead to myocardial infarction, which can be complicated by ventricular rupture and hemopericardium, but the level of troponin I in this case suggests that infarction did not occur. Rheumatic heart disease mainly affects the cardiac valves, but acute rheumatic fever can produce fibrinous pericarditis. Tuberculosis is unlikely in this case, because no pulmonary lesions were seen on the radiograph.

BP7 394   BP6 337   PBD7 611-612   PBD6 589

53 (B) Inflammation plays an important role in atherosclerosis, and CRP is a marker of acute inflammation. Active inflammation in an atherosclerotic plaque increases the risk for acute plaque change and, therefore, the likelihood for myocardial infarction. Homocysteine can injure endothelium and predispose to atherogenesis, but this is a chronic effect. LDH is a non-specific marker of tissue necrosis that, in the past, was used for diagnosis of acute myocardial infarction. CK-MB is a more specific marker of myocardial infarction, but used to diagnose the infarction once it has happened. Platelets and factor VIII are involved in hemostasis and thrombosis; but their levels or function do not predict myocardial injury.

PBD7 574

CHAPTER 13

Red Blood Cell and Bleeding Disorders

PBD7 Chapter 13: Red Blood Cell and Bleeding Disorders

PBD6 Chapter 14: Red Cells and Bleeding Disorders

BP7 and BP6 Chapter 12: The Hematopoietic and Lymphoid Systems

1 For the past 6 months, a 35-year-old woman has experienced an excessively heavy menstrual flow each month. She also has noticed increasing numbers of pinpoint hemorrhages on her lower extremities in the past month. Physical examination shows no organomegaly or lymphadenopathy. CBC shows hemoglobin of 14.2 g/dL, hematocrit 42.5%, MCV 91 μm^3, platelet count 19,000/mm^3, and WBC count 6950/mm^3. On admission to the hospital, she has melena and is given a transfusion of platelets, but her platelet count does not increase. An emergency splenectomy is performed, and her platelet count increases. Which of the following describes the most likely basis for her bleeding tendency?

- ❑ (A) Abnormalities in production of platelets by megakaryocytes
- ❑ (B) Suppression of pluripotent stem cells
- ❑ (C) Destruction of antibody-coated platelets by the spleen
- ❑ (D) Excessive loss of platelets in menstrual blood
- ❑ (E) Defective platelet-endothelial interactions

2 A 22-year-old woman has experienced malaise and a sore throat for 2 weeks. Her fingers turn white on exposure to cold. On physical examination, she has a temperature of 37.8°C, and the pharynx is erythematous. Laboratory findings include a positive Monospot test result. The direct and indirect Coombs test results are positive at 4°C, although not at 37°C. Which of the following substances on the surfaces of the RBCs most likely accounts for these findings?

- ❑ (A) IgE
- ❑ (B) Complement C3b
- ❑ (C) Histamine
- ❑ (D) IgG
- ❑ (E) Fibronectin

3 A 45-year-old woman has experienced malaise with nausea and vomiting for 3 months. On physical examination, she has scleral icterus and a yellowish hue to her skin. She has difficulty remembering three objects after 3 minutes. There are no neurologic deficits. Laboratory studies show a positive serologic test result for hepatitis C, a serum ALT of 310 U/L, AST 275 U/L, total bilirubin 7.6 mg/dL, direct bilirubin 5.8 mg/dL, alkaline phosphatase 75 U/L, and ammonia 55 μmol/L. An abnormal result of which of the following laboratory studies of hemostatic function is most likely to be reported?

- ❏ (A) Immunoassay for plasma von Willebrand factor
- ❏ (B) Platelet count
- ❏ (C) Prothrombin time
- ❏ (D) Fibrin split products
- ❏ (E) Bleeding time

4 A 25-year-old woman has a 3-year history of arthralgias. Physical examination shows no joint deformity, but she appears pale. Laboratory studies show total RBC count of 4.7 million/mm³, hemoglobin 12.5 g/dL, hematocrit 37.1%, platelet count 217,000/mm³, and WBC count 5890/mm³. The peripheral blood smear shows hypochromic and microcytic RBCs. Total serum iron and ferritin levels are within the normal range. Hemoglobin electrophoresis shows an elevated hemoglobin A₂ level of about 5.8%. Which of the following is the most likely diagnosis?

- ❏ (A) Autoimmune hemolytic anemia
- ❏ (B) β-Thalassemia minor
- ❏ (C) Infection with *Plasmodium vivax*
- ❏ (D) Anemia of chronic disease
- ❏ (E) Iron deficiency anemia

5 A 30-year-old woman has had a constant feeling of lethargy since childhood. On physical examination, she is afebrile and has a pulse of 80/min, respirations 15/min, and blood pressure 110/70 mm Hg. The spleen tip is palpable, but there is no abdominal pain or tenderness. Laboratory studies show hemoglobin of 11.7 g/dL, platelet count 159,000/mm³, and WBC count 5390/mm³. The peripheral blood smear shows spherocytosis. The circulating RBCs show an increased osmotic fragility. An inherited abnormality in which of the following RBC components best accounts for these findings?

- ❏ (A) Glucose-6-phosphate dehydrogenase
- ❏ (B) Membrane cytoskeletal protein
- ❏ (C) α-Globin chain
- ❏ (D) Heme
- ❏ (E) β-Globin chain
- ❏ (F) Carbonic anhydrase

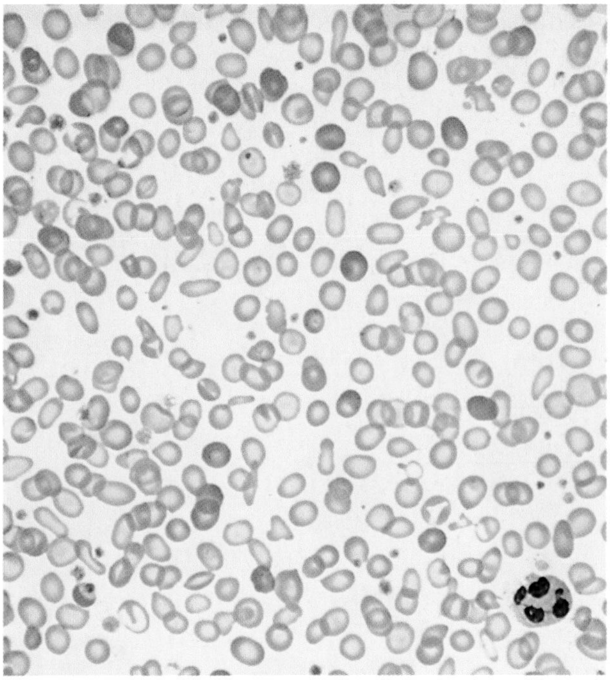

Courtesy of Dr. Robert W. McKenna, Department of Pathology, University of Texas Southwestern Medical School, Dallas, TX.

6 A 69-year-old previously healthy woman has been feeling increasingly tired and weak for 4 months. On physical examination, she is afebrile. There is no hepatosplenomegaly or lymphadenopathy. Laboratory studies show hemoglobin of 9.3 g/dL, platelet count 250,600/mm³, and WBC count 6820/mm³. The appearance of the peripheral blood smear is shown in the figure above. Which of the following conditions should be suspected as the most likely cause of these findings?

- ❏ (A) Pernicious anemia
- ❏ (B) Gastrointestinal blood loss
- ❏ (C) Aplastic anemia
- ❏ (D) β-Thalassemia major
- ❏ (E) Warm autoimmune hemolytic anemia

7 A 76-year-old woman notices that small, pinpoint-to-blotchy areas of superficial hemorrhage have appeared on her gums and on the skin of her arms and legs over the past 3 weeks. On physical examination, she is afebrile and has no organomegaly. Laboratory studies show a normal prothrombin time and partial thromboplastin time. CBC shows hemoglobin of 12.7 g/dL, hematocrit 37.2%, MCV 80 μm³, platelet count 276,000/mm³, and WBC count 5600/mm³. Platelet function studies and fibrinogen level are normal, and no fibrin split products are detectable. Which of the following conditions best explains these findings?

- ❏ (A) Macronodular cirrhosis
- ❏ (B) Chronic renal failure
- ❏ (C) Meningococcemia
- ❏ (D) Vitamin C deficiency
- ❏ (E) Metastatic carcinoma

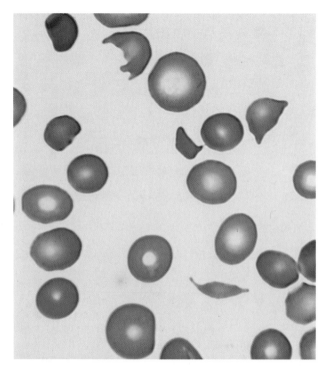

Courtesy of Dr. Robert W. McKenna, Department of Pathology, University of Texas Southwestern Medical School, Dallas, TX.

8 A 30-year-old man has had pain and burning on urination for the past week. On physical examination, he is febrile and has a pulse of 92/min, respirations 18/min, and blood pressure 80/45 mm Hg. Digital rectal examination indicates that he has an enlarged, tender prostate. Scattered ecchymoses are present over the trunk and extremities. Laboratory studies show a blood culture positive for *Klebsiella pneumoniae*. The appearance of the RBCs in a peripheral blood smear is shown in the figure above. These findings are most indicative of which of the following conditions?

- (A) Hereditary spherocytosis
- (B) Autoimmune hemolytic anemia
- (C) Microangiopathic hemolytic anemia
- (D) Iron deficiency anemia
- (E) Megaloblastic anemia

9 A 29-year-old woman has had malaise and a low-grade fever for the past week. On physical examination, she appears very pale. She has a history of chronic anemia, and spherocytes are observed on a peripheral blood smear. Her hematocrit, which normally ranges from 35% to 38%, is now 28%, and the reticulocyte count is very low. The serum bilirubin level is 0.9 mg/dL. Which of the following events is most likely to have occurred in this patient?

- (A) Development of anti-RBC antibodies
- (B) Disseminated intravascular coagulation
- (C) Accelerated extravascular hemolysis in the spleen
- (D) Reduced erythropoiesis from parvovirus infection
- (E) Superimposed iron deficiency

10 A 60-year-old man has developed widespread ecchymoses over the skin in the past month. His medical history includes a diagnosis of mucinous adenocarcinoma of the rectum. On physical examination, he appears cachectic and pale. An abdominal CT scan shows multiple hepatic masses.

Laboratory studies show prothrombin time of 30 sec, partial thromboplastin time of 55 sec, platelet count 15,200/mm³, fibrinogen level 75 mg/dL, and fibrin split product levels (D dimer) that are very elevated. Which of the following morphologic findings is most likely to be present on examination of his peripheral blood smear?

- (A) Howell-Jolly bodies
- (B) Teardrop cells
- (C) Macro-ovalocytes
- (D) Schistocytes
- (E) Target cells

11 A 30-year-old woman reports becoming increasingly tired for the past 5 months. On physical examination, she is afebrile and has mild splenomegaly. Laboratory studies show a hemoglobin concentration of 11.8 g/dL and hematocrit of 35.1%. The peripheral blood smear shows spherocytes and rare nucleated RBCs. The direct and indirect Coombs test results are positive at 37°C, although not at 4°C. Which of the following underlying diseases is most likely to be diagnosed in this patient?

- (A) Infectious mononucleosis
- (B) *Mycoplasma pneumoniae* infection
- (C) Hereditary spherocytosis
- (D) *Escherichia coli* septicemia
- (E) Systemic lupus erythematosus

12 A 23-year-old woman has had a history of bleeding problems all of her life, primarily heavy menstruation and bleeding gums. A sister and an uncle also have bleeding problems. Physical examination shows several bruises ranging in color from red to blue to purple on her arms and legs. There is no organomegaly, and no deformities are noted. Laboratory studies show hemoglobin of 9.5 g/dL, hematocrit 28.2%, platelet count 229,300/mm³, WBC count 7185/mm³, prothrombin time 12 sec, and partial thromboplastin time (PTT) 38 sec. A 1:1 dilution of the patient's plasma with normal pooled plasma corrects the PTT. Ristocetin-dependent platelet aggregation in patient plasma is markedly reduced. Factor VIII activity is 30% (reference range, 50% to 150%). Which of the following responses should the physician use when advising the patient of potential consequences of this disease?

- (A) You might need allogeneic bone marrow transplantation
- (B) Expect increasing difficulty with joint mobility
- (C) Anticoagulation is needed to prevent deep venous thrombosis
- (D) You could experience excessive bleeding after oral surgery
- (E) A splenectomy might be necessary to control the disease

13 A 12-year-old boy has a history of episodes of severe abdominal and back pain since early childhood. On physical examination, he is afebrile, and there is no organomegaly. Laboratory studies show hemoglobin of 11.2 g/dL, platelet count 194,000/mm³, and WBC count 9020/mm³. The peripheral blood smear shows occasional sickled cells, nucleated RBCs, and Howell-Jolly bodies. Hemoglobin electrophoresis shows 1% hemoglobin A₂, 6% hemoglobin F, and 93% hemoglobin S. Hydroxyurea therapy is found to be beneficial in this patient. Which of the following is the most likely basis for its therapeutic efficacy?

❑ (A) Increase in production of hemoglobin F
❑ (B) Increase in production of hemoglobin A
❑ (C) Decrease in overall globin synthesis
❑ (D) Stimulation of erythrocyte production
❑ (E) Increase in oxygen affinity of hemoglobin

14 A 73-year-old man has been healthy all his life. He takes no medications and has had no major illnesses or surgeries. However, for the past year, he has become increasingly tired and listless and appears pale. Physical examination shows no hepatosplenomegaly and no deformities. CBC shows hemoglobin of 9.7 g/dL, hematocrit 29.9%, MCV 69.7 mm3, RBC count 4.28 million/mm3, platelet count 331,000/mm3, and WBC count 5500/mm3. Which of the following is the most likely underlying condition causing this patient's findings?

❑ (A) Occult malignancy
❑ (B) Autoimmune hemolytic anemia
❑ (C) β-Thalassemia major
❑ (D) Chronic alcoholism
❑ (E) Vitamin B$_{12}$ deficiency
❑ (F) Hemophilia A

15 Three days after taking an anti-inflammatory medication that includes phenacetin, a 23-year-old African-American man passes dark reddish-brown urine. He is surprised by this, because he has been healthy all his life and has had no major illnesses. On physical examination, he is afebrile, and there are no remarkable findings. CBC shows a mild normocytic anemia, but the peripheral blood smear shows precipitates of denatured globin (Heinz bodies) with supravital staining and scattered "bite cells" in the population of RBCs. Which of the following is the most likely diagnosis?

❑ (A) α-Thalassemia
❑ (B) Sickle cell trait
❑ (C) Glucose-6-phosphate dehydrogenase deficiency
❑ (D) Autoimmune hemolytic anemia
❑ (E) β-Thalassemia minor
❑ (F) RBC membrane abnormality

16 A 50-year-old man sees his physician because he has experienced chronic fatigue and weight loss for the past 3 months. There are no remarkable findings on physical examination. Laboratory studies shows hemoglobin of 11.2 g/dL, hematocrit 33.3%, MCV 91 μm³, platelet count 240,000/mm³, and WBC count 7550/mm³. Other laboratory findings include serum iron of 80 μg/dL, total iron-binding capacity 145 μg/dL, and serum ferritin 565 ng/mL. The ANA test result is positive. Which of the following is the most likely diagnosis?

❑ (A) Iron deficiency anemia
❑ (B) Aplastic anemia
❑ (C) Anemia of chronic disease
❑ (D) Microangiopathic hemolytic anemia
❑ (E) Megaloblastic anemia
❑ (F) Thalassemia minor

17 In an epidemiologic study of anemias, the findings show that there is an increased prevalence of anemia in persons of West African ancestry. A subset of persons of this ancestry are found, by hemoglobin electrophoresis, to have increased hemoglobin S levels. The distribution of infectious illnesses is correlated with the prevalence of hemoglobin S in this population. Which of the following infectious agents is most likely to account for these observations?

❑ (A) *Cryptococcus neoformans*
❑ (B) *Borrelia burgdorferi*
❑ (C) *Treponema pallidum*
❑ (D) *Plasmodium falciparum*
❑ (E) *Clostridium perfringens*
❑ (F) *Trypanosoma gambiense*
❑ (G) *Schistosoma hematobium*

18 A 41-year-old woman sees her physician because of a 2-week history of multiple ecchymoses on her extremities after only minor trauma. She also reports feeling extremely weak. Over the previous 24 hours, she has developed a severe cough productive of yellowish sputum. On physical examination, her temperature is 38.4°C, and she has diffuse crackles on all lung fields. Laboratory studies show hemoglobin of 7.2 g/dL, hematocrit 21.4%, MCV 88 μm³, platelet count 35,000/mm³, and WBC count 1400/mm³ with 20% segmented neutrophils, 1% bands, 66% lymphocytes, and 13% monocytes. The reticulocyte count is 0.1%. Given these laboratory findings, which of the following historical findings would be most useful in determining the cause of her condition?

❑ (A) Exposure to drugs
❑ (B) Dietary history
❑ (C) Recent bacterial infection
❑ (D) Menstrual history
❑ (E) Family history of anemias

19 A 40-year-old man who has had chronic anemia since childhood is admitted to the hospital with fever and chest pain. On physical examination, his temperature is 38.7°C. A chest radiograph shows extensive patchy infiltrates. Laboratory studies include a blood culture positive for *Streptococcus pneumoniae*. Despite supportive therapy, he dies a few days later. At autopsy, there is a small, fibrotic, 5-g spleen filled with deposits of iron and calcium and prominent expansion of the marrow space in the skull. Which of the following conditions is most likely to have resulted in these findings?

❑ (A) Sickle cell anemia
❑ (B) β-Thalassemia
❑ (C) Malaria
❑ (D) Idiopathic thrombocytopenic purpura
❑ (E) Autoimmune hemolytic anemia

20 A 5-year-old boy has had a history of easy bruising and blood in his urine since infancy. Physical examination shows no organomegaly. He has several ecchymoses of the skin on the lower extremities. Laboratory studies show hemoglobin of 13.1 g/dL, hematocrit 39.3%, platelet count 287,600/mm³, WBC count 6830/mm³, prothrombin time 13 sec, partial thromboplastin time 54 sec, and less than 1% factor VIII activity measured in plasma. If he does not receive transfusions of recombinant factor VIII concentrate, which of the following manifestations of this illness is most likely to ensue?

❑ (A) Splenomegaly
❑ (B) Conjunctival petechiae
❑ (C) Hemolysis
❑ (D) Hemochromatosis
❑ (E) Hemarthroses

21 A 23-year-old woman in her 25th week of pregnancy has felt no fetal movement for the past 3 days. Three weeks later, she still has not given birth and suddenly develops dyspnea with cyanosis. On physical, examination, her temperature is 36.9°C, pulse 102/min, respirations 21/min, and blood pressure 80/40 mm Hg. She has large ecchymoses over the skin of her entire body. A stool sample is positive for occult blood. Laboratory studies show an elevated prothrombin time and partial thromboplastin time. The platelet count is decreased, plasma fibrinogen is markedly decreased, and fibrin split products are detected. A blood culture is negative. Which of the following is the most likely cause of the bleeding diathesis?

☐ (A) Increased vascular fragility
☐ (B) Toxic injury to the endothelium
☐ (C) Reduced production of platelets
☐ (D) Increased consumption of clotting factors and platelets
☐ (E) Defects in platelet adhesion and aggregation

22 A 54-year-old woman sees her physician because of sudden onset of headaches and photophobia. This condition has been worsening for the past 2 days. On physical examination, she has a temperature of 38°C and is disoriented. CBC shows hemoglobin of 11.2 g/dL, hematocrit 33.7%, MCV 94 μm³, platelet count 32,000/mm³, and WBC count 9900/mm³. The peripheral blood smear shows schistocytes. The serum urea nitrogen level is 38 mg/dL, and the creatinine level is 3.9 mg/dL. Which of the following is the most likely diagnosis?

☐ (A) β-Thalassemia major
☐ (B) Disseminated intravascular coagulation
☐ (C) Hereditary spherocytosis
☐ (D) Idiopathic thrombocytopenic purpura
☐ (E) Paroxysmal nocturnal hemoglobinuria
☐ (F) Thrombotic thrombocytopenic purpura
☐ (G) Warm autoimmune hemolytic anemia

23 A 30-year-old previously healthy man passes dark-brown urine several days after starting the prophylactic antimalarial drug primaquine. On physical examination, he appears pale and is afebrile. There is no organomegaly. Laboratory studies show that his serum haptoglobin level is decreased. Which of the following is the most likely explanation of these findings?

☐ (A) Mechanical fragmentation of RBCs
☐ (B) Increased susceptibility to lysis by complement
☐ (C) Nuclear maturation defects due to impaired DNA synthesis
☐ (D) Impaired globin synthesis
☐ (E) Hemolysis of antibody-coated cells
☐ (F) Oxidative injury to hemoglobin
☐ (G) Reduced deformability of the RBC membrane

24 A 42-year-old woman has had nosebleeds, easy bruising, and increased bleeding with her menstrual periods for the past 4 months. On physical examination, her temperature is 37°C, pulse 88/min, respirations 18/min, and blood pressure 90/60 mm Hg. She has scattered petechiae over the distal extremities. There is no organomegaly. Laboratory studies show

hemoglobin of 12.3 g/dL, hematocrit 37.0%, platelet count 21,500/mm³, and WBC count 7370/mm³. A bone marrow biopsy specimen shows a marked increase in megakaryocytes. The prothrombin and partial thromboplastin values are within the reference range. Which of the following is the most likely diagnosis?

☐ (A) Disseminated intravascular coagulation
☐ (B) Hemophilia B
☐ (C) Idiopathic thrombocytopenic purpura
☐ (D) Metastatic breast carcinoma
☐ (E) Thrombotic thrombocytopenic purpura
☐ (F) Vitamin K deficiency
☐ (G) Von Willebrand disease

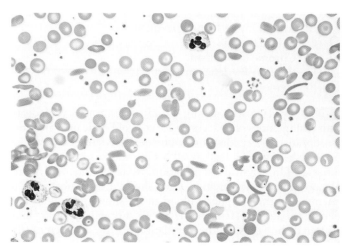

Courtesy of Dr. Robert W. McKenna, Department of Pathology, University of Texas Southwestern Medical School, Dallas, TX.

25 A 12-year-old boy experienced sudden onset of severe abdominal pain and cramping accompanied by chest pain, non-productive cough, and fever. On physical examination, his temperature is 39°C, pulse 110/min, respirations 22/min, and blood pressure 80/50 mm Hg. He has diffuse abdominal tenderness, but no masses or organomegaly. Laboratory studies show a hematocrit of 18%. The peripheral blood smear is shown in the figure above. A chest x-ray shows bilateral pulmonary infiltrates. Which of the following is the most likely mechanism for initiation of his pulmonary problems?

☐ (A) Intravascular hemolysis
☐ (B) Chronic hypoxia of the pulmonary parenchyma
☐ (C) Increased red blood cell adhesion to endothelium
☐ (D) Defects in the alternative pathway of complement activation
☐ (E) Formation of autoantibodies to alveolar basement membrane

26 A clinical study of patients who inherit mutations that reduce the level of spectrin in the RBC membrane cytoskeleton shows an increased prevalence of chronic anemia with splenomegaly. For many of these patients, it is observed that splenectomy reduces the severity of anemia. This beneficial effect of splenectomy is most likely related to which of the following processes?

❏ (A) Increase in synthesis of spectrin in RBCs
❏ (B) Increase in deformability of RBCs
❏ (C) Decrease in opsonization of RBCs
❏ (D) Decrease in trapping of RBCs in the spleen
❏ (E) Decrease in production of reactive oxygen species

27 A 39-year-old woman sees her physician because she has experienced abdominal pain and intermittent low-volume diarrhea for the past 3 months. On physical examination, she is afebrile. A stool sample is positive for occult blood. A colonoscopy is performed, and biopsy specimens from the terminal ileum and colon show microscopic findings consistent with Crohn disease. Because she has failed to respond to medical therapy, surgery is warranted, and part of the colon and terminal ileum are removed. She is transfused with 2 units of packed RBCs during surgery. Several weeks later, she appears healthy but complains of easy fatigability. On investigation, CBC findings show hemoglobin of 10.6 g/dL, hematocrit 31.6%, RBC count 2.69 million/μL, MCV 118 μm^3, platelet count 378,000/mm^3, and WBC count 9800/mm^3. The reticulocyte count is 0.3%. Which of the following is most likely to produce these findings?

❏ (A) Hemolytic anemia
❏ (B) Aplastic anemia
❏ (C) Chronic blood loss
❏ (D) Vitamin B$_{12}$ deficiency
❏ (E) Anemia of chronic disease
❏ (F) Bone marrow metastases

28 A 45-year-old man has a 3-day history of flank pain and fever. On physical examination, his temperature is 37.9°C. There is right costovertebral angle tenderness. Laboratory studies include a urine culture that is positive for *Escherichia coli*. The WBC count is 13,310/mm^3. Two days later he becomes hypotensive, and a blood culture is positive for *E. coli*. He requires increasing pressor support to maintain blood pressure. He develops a guaiac-positive stool and ecchymoses of the skin. CBC shows hemoglobin of 9.2 g/dL, hematocrit 28.1%, and platelet count 70,000/mm^3. Increased amounts of fibrin split products are identified in the blood (elevated D dimer). Which of the following conditions is most likely responsible for the low hematocrit?

❏ (A) Warm autoimmune hemolytic anemia
❏ (B) Paroxysmal nocturnal hemoglobinuria
❏ (C) Microangiopathic hemolytic anemia
❏ (D) β-Thalassemia major
❏ (E) Aplastic anemia

29 A 10-year-old child has experienced multiple episodes of pneumonia and meningitis with septicemia since infancy. Causative organisms that have been cultured include *Streptococcus pneumoniae* and *Haemophilus influenzae*. On physical examination, the child has no organomegaly and no deformities. Laboratory studies show hemoglobin of 9.2 g/dL, hematocrit 27.8%, platelet count 372,000/mm^3, and WBC count 10,300/mm^3. A hemoglobin electrophoresis shows 1% hemoglobin A$_2$, 7% hemoglobin F, and 92% hemoglobin S. Which of the following is the most likely cause of the repeated infections in this child?

❏ (A) Loss of normal splenic function from recurrent ischemic injury
❏ (B) Reduced synthesis of immunoglobulins
❏ (C) Impaired neutrophil production
❏ (D) Reduced synthesis of complement proteins by the liver
❏ (E) Reduced expression of adhesion molecules on endothelial cells

30 A healthy 19-year-old woman suffered blunt abdominal trauma in a motor vehicle accident. On admission to the hospital, her initial hematocrit was 33%, but over the next hour, it dropped to 28%. A paracentesis yielded serosanguineous fluid. She was taken to surgery, where a liver laceration was repaired and 1 L of bloody fluid was removed from the peritoneal cavity. She remained stable. A CBC performed 3 days later is most likely to show which of the following morphologic findings in RBCs in the peripheral blood?

❏ (A) Reticulocytosis
❏ (B) Leukoerythroblastosis
❏ (C) Basophilic stippling
❏ (D) Hypochromia
❏ (E) Schistocytes

31 A 32-year-old woman from Saigon, Vietnam, gives birth at 34 weeks' gestation to a markedly hydropic stillborn male infant. Autopsy findings include hepatosplenomegaly and cardiomegaly, serous effusions in all body cavities, and generalized hydrops. No congenital anomalies are noted. There is marked extramedullary hematopoiesis in visceral organs. Which of the following findings is most likely to be present on hemoglobin electrophoresis of the fetal RBCs?

❏ (A) Hemoglobin A$_1$
❏ (B) Hemoglobin A$_2$
❏ (C) Hemoglobin Bart's
❏ (D) Hemoglobin C
❏ (E) Hemoglobin E
❏ (F) Hemoglobin F
❏ (G) Hemoglobin H
❏ (H) Hemoglobin S

32 A 17-year-old boy reports passage of dark urine to his physician. He has a history of multiple bacterial infections and venous thromboses for the past 10 years, including portal vein thrombosis in the previous year. On physical examination, his right leg is swollen and tender. CBC shows hemoglobin of 9.8 g/dL, hematocrit 29.9%, MCV 92 μm^3, platelet count 150,000/mm^3, and WBC count 3800/mm^3 with 24% segmented neutrophils, 1% bands, 64% lymphocytes, 10% monocytes, and 1% eosinophils. He has a reticulocytosis, and his serum haptoglobin level is very low. A mutation affecting which of the following gene products is most likely to give rise to this clinical condition?

❏ (A) Spectrin
❏ (B) Glucose-6-phosphate dehydrogenase
❏ (C) Phosphatidylinositol glycan A (PIGA)
❏ (D) β-Globin chain
❏ (E) Factor V mutation
❏ (F) Prothrombin G20210A mutation

33 A 32-year-old man has reported easy fatigability since childhood. On physical examination, he is normally developed and is afebrile. Laboratory studies show hemoglobin of 8.8 g/dL, hematocrit 26.3%, platelet count 199,000/mm³, and WBC count 5350/mm³. α-Globin inclusions are present in erythroblasts and erythrocytes, leading to increased phagocytosis by cells of the mononuclear phagocyte system. Hemoglobin electrophoresis shows HbA2 of 6%, HbF of 1%, and HbA1 of 93%. The serum ferritin level is 3090 ng/mL. Which of the following is the most likely diagnosis?

- ❏ (A) Autoimmune hemolytic anemia
- ❏ (B) Glucose-6-phosphate dehydrogenase deficiency
- ❏ (C) Megaloblastic anemia
- ❏ (D) β-Thalassemia
- ❏ (E) Sickle cell anemia
- ❏ (F) Paroxysmal nocturnal hemoglobinuria

34 A 13-year-old child has a history of easy bruising. At the age of 10 years, he experienced hemorrhaging around the pharynx that produced acute airway obstruction. On physical examination, he has marked reduction in joint mobility of the ankles, knees, and elbows. Family history indicates that other male relatives have similar bleeding problems. Laboratory studies show hemoglobin of 13.1 g/dL, hematocrit 39.2%, platelet count 228,000/mm³, WBC count 5950/mm³, prothrombin time 13 sec, and partial thromboplastin time (PTT) 52 sec. A 1 : 1 dilution of the patient's plasma with normal pooled plasma does not correct the PTT. Which of the following is the most likely diagnosis?

- ❏ (A) Antiphospholipid syndrome
- ❏ (B) Factor V mutation
- ❏ (C) Disseminated intravascular coagulation
- ❏ (D) Hemophilia A with a factor VIII inhibitor
- ❏ (E) Idiopathic thrombocytopenic purpura
- ❏ (F) Von Willebrand disease
- ❏ (G) Vitamin K deficiency

35 A 16-year-old girl has a history of easy bruising and hemorrhages. Since menarche at the age of 14 years, she has had menometrorrhagia. On physical examination, she displays joint deformity and has decreased mobility of the ankles, knees, and wrists. Laboratory studies show hemoglobin of 11.8 g/dL, hematocrit 35.1%, platelet count 267,000/mm³, WBC count 5960/mm³, prothrombin time 13 sec, and partial thromboplastin time (PTT) 60 sec. A 1 : 1 dilution of the patient's plasma with normal pooled plasma corrects the PTT. Which of the following is the most likely diagnosis?

- ❏ (A) Antiphospholipid syndrome
- ❏ (B) Disseminated intravascular coagulation
- ❏ (C) Hemophilia A
- ❏ (D) Idiopathic thrombocytopenic purpura
- ❏ (E) Thrombotic thrombocytopenic purpura
- ❏ (F) Vitamin K deficiency
- ❏ (G) Von Willebrand disease

36 A 22-year-old woman has experienced febrile episodes over the past 2 weeks. On physical examination, her temperature is 37.5°C, pulse 82/min, respirations 18/min, and blood pressure 105/65 mm Hg. Laboratory studies show hemoglobin of 10.8 g/dL, hematocrit 32.5%, platelet count 245,700/mm³, and WBC count 8320/mm³. The serum haptoglobin level is decreased, but the direct and indirect Coombs test results are negative. The reticulocyte count is increased. The prothrombin time is 12 sec, and the partial thromboplastin time is 31 sec. The patient is observed over the next week and found to have temperature spikes to 39.1°C, with shaking chills every 48 hours. Infection with which of the following organisms is most likely to cause this patient's illness?

- ❏ (A) *Aspergillus niger*
- ❏ (B) *Babesia microti*
- ❏ (C) *Dirofilaria*
- ❏ (D) *Escherichia coli*
- ❏ (E) *Plasmodium vivax*
- ❏ (F) *Wuchereria bancrofti*

37 A 62-year-old man goes to the emergency department in an obvious state of inebriation. He is well known there, because this scenario has been repeated many times over the years. On physical examination, he is afebrile. The spleen tip is palpable, and the liver edge is firm. Laboratory studies show hemoglobin of 8.2 g/dL, hematocrit 25.1%, MCV 107 μm³, platelet count 135,000/mm³, and WBC count 3920/mm³. The peripheral blood smear shows prominent anisocytosis and macrocytosis. Polychromatophilic RBCs are difficult to find. A few of the neutrophils show six to seven nuclear lobes. Which of the following is the most likely explanation of these findings?

- ❏ (A) Mechanical fragmentation of RBCs
- ❏ (B) Increased susceptibility to lysis by complement
- ❏ (C) Nuclear maturation defects due to impaired DNA synthesis
- ❏ (D) Hemolysis of antibody-coated cells
- ❏ (E) Reduced deformability of the RBC membrane
- ❏ (F) Production of abnormal hemoglobin
- ❏ (G) Imbalance in synthesis of α- and β-globin chains

38 A 3-year-old boy of Italian ancestry is brought to the physician because he has a poor appetite and is underweight for his age and height. Physical examination shows hepatosplenomegaly. The hemoglobin concentration is 6 g/dL, and the peripheral blood smear shows severely hypochromic and microcytic RBCs. The total serum iron level is normal, and the reticulocyte count is 10%. A radiograph of the skull shows maxillofacial deformities and an expanded marrow space. Which of the following is the most likely principal cause of this child's illness?

- ❏ (A) Reduced synthesis of hemoglobin F
- ❏ (B) Imbalance in production of α- and β-globin chains
- ❏ (C) Sequestration of iron in reticuloendothelial cells
- ❏ (D) Increased fragility of erythrocyte membrane
- ❏ (E) Relative deficiency of vitamin B₁₂

39 A 28-year-old previously healthy man has noted increasing fatigue for the past 6 months and formation of bruises after minimal trauma. Over the past 2 days, he has developed a cough. On physical examination, his temperature is 38.9°C, and he has diffuse rales in both lungs. He has no hepatosplenomegaly and no lymphadenopathy. Laboratory findings include a sputum culture positive for *Streptococcus pneumoniae*, hemoglobin of 7.2 g/dL, hematocrit 21.7%, platelet count 23,400/mm³, WBC count 1310/mm³, prothrombin time 13 sec, partial thromboplastin time 28 sec, and total bilirubin 1.0 mg/dL. The ANA test result is negative. Which of the following is the most likely explanation of these findings?

❏ (A) Hemolysis of antibody-coated cells
❏ (B) Hypersplenism
❏ (C) Increased susceptibility to lysis by complement
❏ (D) Metastatic adenocarcinoma
❏ (E) Nuclear maturation defects due to impaired DNA synthesis
❏ (F) Stem cell defect
❏ (G) Varicella-zoster virus infection

40 A 55-year-old otherwise healthy man has experienced minor fatigue on exertion for the past 9 months. He has no significant previous medical or surgical history. On physical examination, there are no remarkable findings. Laboratory studies show hemoglobin of 11.7 g/dL, hematocrit 34.8%, MCV 73 μm^3, platelet count 315,000/mm^3, and WBC count 8035/mm^3. Which of the following is the most sensitive and cost-effective test that the physician should order to help to determine the cause of these findings?

❏ (A) Serum iron
❏ (B) Serum transferrin
❏ (C) Serum haptoglobin
❏ (D) Bone marrow biopsy
❏ (E) Serum ferritin
❏ (F) Hemoglobin electrophoresis

41 A 17-year-old girl has had frequent nosebleeds since childhood. Her gums bleed easily, even with routine tooth brushing. She has experienced menorrhagia since menarche at age 14. On physical examination, there are no abnormal findings. Laboratory studies show hemoglobin 14.1 g/dL, hematocrit 42.5%, MCV 90 μm^3, platelet count 277,400/mm^3, and WBC count 5920/mm^3. Her platelets fail to aggregate in response to ADP, collagen, epinephrine, and thrombin. The ristocetin agglutination test result is normal. There is a deficiency of glycoprotein IIb-IIIa. Her prothrombin time is 12 sec and her partial thromboplastin time is 28 sec. Which of the following is the most likely diagnosis?

❏ (A) Disseminated intravascular coagulation
❏ (B) Glanzmann thrombasthenia
❏ (C) Immune thrombocytopenic purpura
❏ (D) Vitamin C deficiency
❏ (E) Von Willebrand disease

42 A 78-year-old man complains of worsening malaise and fatigue over the past 5 months. On physical examination, he is afebrile and normotensive. The spleen tip is palpable. A CBC shows hemoglobin of 10.6 g/dL, hematocrit 29.8%, MCV 92 μm^3, platelet count 95,000/mm^3, and WBC count 4900/mm^3 with 67% segmented neutrophils, 4% bands, 2% metamyelocytes, 22% lymphocytes, 5% monocytes, and 3 nucleated RBCs per 100 WBCs. The peripheral blood smear shows occasional teardrop cells. An examination of the bone marrow biopsy specimen and smear is most likely to show which of the following findings?

❏ (A) Marrow packed with myeloblasts
❏ (B) Marrow fibrosis with reduced hematopoiesis
❏ (C) Replacement of marrow by fat
❏ (D) Presence of numerous megaloblasts
❏ (E) Marked normoblastic erythroid hyperplasia

43 A clinical study is performed to assess outcomes in patients who have macrocytic anemias. A comparison of laboratory testing strategies shows that the best strategy includes testing for both vitamin B$_{12}$ (cobalamin) and folate. What is the most important reason for ordering these tests simultaneously?

❏ (A) Both nutrients are absorbed similarly
❏ (B) Therapy for one deficiency also treats the other
❏ (C) The peripheral blood smear appears the same for both deficiencies
❏ (D) Aplastic anemia can result from lack of either nutrient
❏ (E) Neurologic injury must be avoided

44 A 26-year-old woman has experienced chronic fatigue since early childhood. She also has had episodes of severe pain in the abdomen, back, and legs. On physical examination, there is no organomegaly. Laboratory studies show hemoglobin of 8.9 g/dL, hematocrit 26.9%, platelet count 300,100/mm^3, and WBC count 5560/mm^3. Hemoglobin electrophoresis shows 1% hemoglobin A$_2$, 6% hemoglobin F, and 93% hemoglobin S. Which of the following is this patient most likely to develop as a complication of the underlying disease?

❏ (A) Micronodular cirrhosis
❏ (B) Chronic atrophic gastritis
❏ (C) Pigment gallstones
❏ (D) High rate of stillbirths
❏ (E) Esophageal web

45 A 9-year-old boy has developed prominent bruises on his extremities over the past week. On physical examination, he has ecchymoses and petechiae on his arms and legs. Laboratory studies show hemoglobin 13.8 g/dL, hematocrit 41.9%, MCV 93 μm^3, platelet count 22,300/mm^3, and WBC count 7720/mm^3. He had respiratory syncytial virus pneumonia 3 weeks ago. His condition improves with corticosteroid therapy. Which of the following abnormalities is most likely to cause his hemorrhagic diathesis?

❏ (A) Anti-platelet antibodies
❏ (B) Bone marrow aplasia
❏ (C) Glycoprotein IIb-IIIa dysfunction
❏ (D) Vitamin C deficiency
❏ (E) Von Willebrand factor metalloprotease deficiency

46 A 77-year-old man has experienced increasing malaise and a 6-kg weight loss over the past year. He has noted more severe and constant back pain for the past 3 months. On physical examination, his temperature is 38.7°C. His prostate is firm and irregular when palpated on digital rectal examination. There is no organomegaly. A stool sample is negative for occult blood. Laboratory studies include a urine culture positive for *Escherichia coli*, serum glucose of 70 mg/dL, creatinine 1.1 mg/dL, total bilirubin 1.0 mg/dL, alkaline phosphatase 293 U/L, calcium 10.3 mg/dL, phosphorus 2.6 mg/dL, and PSA 25 ng/mL. CBC shows hemoglobin of 9.1 g/dL, hematocrit 27.3%, MCV 94 μm^3, platelet count 55,600/mm^3, and WBC count 3570/mm^3 with 18% segmented neutrophils, 7% bands, 2% metamyelocytes, 1% myelocytes, 61% lymphocytes, 11% monocytes, and 3 nucleated RBCs per 100 WBCs. Which of the following is the most likely diagnosis?

- ❑ (A) Anemia of chronic disease
- ❑ (B) Aplastic anemia
- ❑ (C) Hemolytic anemia
- ❑ (D) Megaloblastic anemia
- ❑ (E) Myelophthisic anemia
- ❑ (F) Thalassemia

47 Soon after crossing the finish line in a 10-kilometer race, a 31-year-old man collapses. On physical examination, his temperature is 40.1°C, pulse 101/min, respirations 22/min, and blood pressure 85/50 mm Hg. He is not perspiring, and his skin shows tenting. Laboratory studies show Na$^+$ of 155 mmol/L, K$^+$ 4.6 mmol/L, Cl$^-$ 106 mmol/L, CO$_2$ 27 mmol/L, glucose 68 mg/dL, creatinine 1.8 mg/dL, hemoglobin 20.1 g/dL, hematocrit 60.3%, platelet count 230,400/mm^3, and WBC count 6830/mm^3. Which of the following is the most likely diagnosis?

- ❑ (A) Erythroleukemia
- ❑ (B) Chronic obstructive pulmonary disease
- ❑ (C) Diabetes insipidus
- ❑ (D) Hemoconcentration
- ❑ (E) Increased erythropoietin levels
- ❑ (F) Polycythemia vera

48 During the past 6 months, a 60-year-old man has noticed a malar skin rash made worse by sun exposure. He also has had arthralgias and myalgias. On physical examination, he is afebrile and has a pulse of 100/min, respirations 20/min, and blood pressure 100/60 Hg. There is erythema of skin over the bridge of the nose. No organomegaly is noted. Laboratory findings include positive serologic test results for ANA and double-stranded DNA, hemoglobin of 8.1 g/dL, hematocrit 24.4%, platelet count 87,000/mm^3, and WBC count 3950/mm^3. The peripheral blood smear shows nucleated RBCs. A dipstick urinalysis is positive for blood, but there are no WBCs, RBCs, or casts seen on microscopic examination of the urine. Which of the following serum laboratory findings is most likely to be present?

- ❑ (A) Elevated D dimer
- ❑ (B) Negative Coombs antiglobulin test
- ❑ (C) Decreased iron
- ❑ (D) Elevated prostate specific antigen
- ❑ (E) Diminished haptoglobin

49 A 45-year-old woman has experienced worsening arthritis of her hands and feet for the past 15 years. On physical examination, there are marked deformities of the hands and feet, with ulnar deviation of the hands and swan-neck deformities of the fingers. Laboratory studies show an elevated level of rheumatoid factor. CBC shows hemoglobin of 11.6 g/dL, hematocrit 34.8%, MCV 87 μm^3, platelet count 268,000/mm^3, and WBC count 6800/mm^3. There is a normal serum haptoglobin level, serum iron concentration of 20 μg/dL, total iron-binding capacity 195 μg/dL, percent saturation 10.2; and serum ferritin concentration 317 ng/mL. No fibrin split products are detected. The reticulocyte concentration is 1.1%. Which of the following is the most likely mechanism underlying this patient's hematologic abnormalities?

- ❑ (A) Poor utilization of stored iron
- ❑ (B) Space occupying lesions in the bone marrow
- ❑ (C) Mutation in the phosphatidylinositol glycan A (*PIGA*) gene
- ❑ (D) Sequestration of red blood cells in splenic sinusoids
- ❑ (E) Impaired synthesis of β-globin chains
- ❑ (F) Warm antibodies against red blood cell membranes

50 An infant is born at 34 weeks' gestation to a 28-year-old woman, G 3, P 2. At birth, the infant is observed to be markedly hydropic and icteric. A cord blood sample is taken, and the direct Coombs test result is positive for the infant's RBCs. Which of the following is the most likely diagnosis?

- ❑ (A) Mechanical fragmentation of RBCs
- ❑ (B) Nuclear maturation defects due to impaired DNA synthesis
- ❑ (C) Impaired globin synthesis
- ❑ (D) Hemolysis of antibody-coated cells
- ❑ (E) Stem cell defect
- ❑ (F) Oxidative injury to hemoglobin
- ❑ (G) Reduced deformability of the RBC membrane

51 A 65-year-old man has experienced worsening fatigue for the past 5 months. On physical examination, he is afebrile and has a pulse of 91/min, respirations 18/min, and blood pressure 105/60 mm Hg. There is no organomegaly. A stool sample is positive for occult blood. Laboratory findings include hemoglobin of 5.9 g/dL, hematocrit 17.3%, MCV 96 μm^3, platelet count 250,000/mm^3, and WBC count 7800/mm^3. The reticulocyte concentration is 3.9%. No fibrin split products are detected, and the direct and indirect Coombs test results are negative. A bone marrow biopsy specimen shows marked erythroid hyperplasia. Which of the following conditions best explains these findings?

- ❑ (A) Chronic blood loss
- ❑ (B) Iron deficiency anemia
- ❑ (C) Aplastic anemia
- ❑ (D) Metastatic prostatic adenocarcinoma
- ❑ (E) Autoimmune hemolytic anemia

52 A 21-year-old woman known to have a protein C deficiency develops recurrent pulmonary thromboembolism and is placed on anticoagulant therapy. Two weeks after initiation of this therapy, she has a sudden change in mental status and experiences difficulty speaking and swallowing. A cerebral angiogram shows a distal left middle cerebral artery occlusion. Laboratory studies show hemoglobin of 13.0 g/dL, platelet count 65,400/mm^3, WBC count 5924/mm^3, prothrombin time 12 sec, and partial thromboplastin time 51 sec. The anticoagulant therapy is discontinued. Which of the following pharmacologic agents used as an anticoagulant in this patient is most likely to have caused these findings?

- (A) Acetylsalicylic acid (aspirin)
- (B) Warfarin
- (C) Heparin
- (D) Tissue plasminogen activator
- (E) Urokinase

53 A 45-year-old woman has experienced episodes of blurred vision and headaches for the past 6 months. She has had worsening confusion with paresthesias over the past 3 days. On physical examination, she has a temperature of 39.6°C, pulse 100/min, respiratory rate 20/min, and blood pressure 80/50 mm Hg. Petechial hemorrhages are noted over her trunk and extremities. Laboratory findings include hemoglobin of 10.9 g/dL, hematocrit of 34%, MCV 96/min^3, platelet count 28,000/mm^3, and WBC count 8500/mm^3. Fragmented RBCs are noted on her peripheral blood smear. Her blood urea nitrogen is 40 mg/dL and serum creatinine 3.1 mg/dL. Which of the following is the most likely underlying cause for her findings?

- (A) Defective ADP-induced platelet aggregation
- (B) Presence of antibodies against von Willebrand factor metalloproteinase
- (C) Formation of autoantibodies to platelet glycoproteins IIb/IIIa and Ib-IX
- (D) Circulating toxin that injures capillary endothelium
- (E) Inappropriate release of thromboplastic substances into blood
- (F) Decreased factor VIII activity

54 A clinical study is performed using patients diagnosed with peptic ulcer disease, chronic blood loss, and hypochromic microcytic anemia. Their serum ferritin levels average 5 to 7 µg/mL. The rate of duodenal iron absorption in this study group is found to be much higher than in a normal control group. After treatment with omeprazole and clarithromycin, study group patients have hematocrits from 40 to 42%, MCV 82 to 85 µm^3, and serum ferritin <12 µg/mL. Measured rates of iron absorption in the study group following therapy are now decreased to the range of the normal controls. Which of the following substances derived from liver is most likely to have been increased in the study group patients prior to therapy, returning to normal following therapy?

- (A) Transferrin
- (B) Hemosiderin
- (C) Hepcidin
- (D) Divalent metal transporter-1 (DMT-1)
- (E) HLA-like transmembrane protein

ANSWERS

1 **(C)** This patient's bleeding tendency is caused by a low platelet count. She most likely has idiopathic thrombocytopenic purpura (ITP), in which platelets are destroyed in the spleen after being coated with an antiplatelet antibody. The serum contains antiplatelet antibodies that presumably coat

the patient's platelets and the transfused platelets. Because the spleen is both the source of the antibody and the site of destruction, splenectomy can be beneficial. There is no defect in the production of platelets. Suppression of pluripotent stem cells gives rise to aplastic anemia, which is accompanied by pancytopenia. Platelet functions are normal in ITP. Chronic blood loss would not lead to thrombocytopenia when normal bone marrow function is present. Abnormal platelet-endothelial interactions are more likely to cause thrombosis.
BP7 447   BP6 387   PBD7 651-652   PBD6 634-636

2 **(B)** This patient has cold agglutinin disease, with antibody (usually IgM) coating RBCs. The IgM antibodies bind to the RBCs at low temperature and fix complement; however, complement is not lytic at this temperature. With a rise in temperature, the IgM is dissociated from the cell, leaving behind C3b. Most of the hemolysis occurs extravascularly in the cells of the mononuclear phagocyte system, such as Kupffer cells in the liver, because the coating of complement C3b acts as an opsonin. Raynaud phenomenon occurs in exposed, colder areas of the body, such as the fingers and toes. The patient probably has an elevated cold agglutinin titer. IgE is present in allergic conditions, and histamine is released in type I hypersensitivity reactions. IgG is typically involved in warm antibody hemolytic anemia, which is chronic and is not triggered by cold. Fibronectin is an adhesive cell surface glycoprotein that aids in tissue healing.
BP7 408   BP6 351   PBD7 637   PBD6 620-621

3 **(C)** This patient has hepatitis C with severe hepatocyte damage. Many of the clotting factors that are instrumental in the in vitro measurement of the extrinsic pathway of coagulation, as measured by the prothrombin time, are synthesized in the liver. Von Willebrand factor is produced by endothelial cells, not hepatocytes. The platelet count is not affected directly by liver disease. Increased fibrin split products suggest a consumptive coagulopathy, such as disseminated intravascular coagulation. The bleeding time is a measure of platelet function, which is not significantly affected by liver disease.
BP7 443-444, 448   BP6 384   PBD7 649-650   PBD6 633

4 **(B)** Although β-thalassemia minor and iron deficiency anemia are characterized by hypochromic and microcytic RBCs, there is no increase in hemoglobin A$_2$ in iron deficiency states. A normal serum ferritin level also excludes iron deficiency. Unlike β-thalassemia major, there is usually a mild anemia without major organ dysfunction. Diseases that produce hemolysis and increase erythropoiesis (e.g., autoimmune hemolytic anemia, malaria) do not alter the composition of β-globin chain production. Anemia of chronic disease may mimic iron deficiency and thalassemia minor with respect to hypochromia and microcytosis; however, anemia of chronic disease is associated with an increase in the serum concentration of ferritin.
BP7 403-404   BP6 350   PBD7 632-635   PBD6 617-618

5 **(B)** Spectrin and related proteins (e.g., protein 4.1, ankyrin) are cytoskeletal proteins that are important in maintaining the RBC shape. Hereditary spherocytosis is a condition in which a mutation affects one of several membrane cytoskeletal proteins, such as ankyrin (most common) and band 4.2, which binds spectrin to the transmembrane ion transporter, band 3, and protein 4.1, which binds the "tail" of spectrin to another transmembrane protein, glycophorin A. Cells with such mutant proteins are less deformable. The abnormal RBCs appear to lack central pallor on a peripheral blood smear, and they are sequestered and destroyed in the spleen. Glucose-6-phosphate dehydrogenase deficiency is an X-linked condition that most commonly affects black males. Thalassemias with abnormal α- or β-globin chains are associated with hypochromic microcytic anemias. Iron deficiency affects the heme portion of hemoglobin, leading to hypochromia as well as to microcytosis. Carbonic anhydrase in RBCs helps to maintain buffering capacity.

BP7 399-400   BP6 343-344   PBD7 625-627
PBD6 607-609

6 **(B)** The RBCs display hypochromia and microcytosis, consistent with iron deficiency. The most common cause of this in the elderly is chronic blood loss that originates from a gastrointestinal source (e.g., carcinoma, ulcer disease). At age 69, this patient is not menstruating, and vaginal bleeding is likely to be noticed as a "red flag" for a gynecologic malignancy. Pernicious anemia from vitamin B_{12} deficiency would result in a macrocytic anemia. The RBCs are generally normocytic in persons with aplastic anemia. Microcytosis may accompany thalassemias, but the patient would be unlikely to live to the age of 69 years with β-thalassemia major. Autoimmune hemolytic anemias usually produce a normocytic anemia, or the MCV can be slightly elevated, with a brisk reticulocytosis.

BP7 398,409-411   BP6 353-354   PBD7 643-646
PBD6 629-630

7 **(D)** Platelet number and function in this case are normal, and there is no detectable abnormality in the extrinsic or intrinsic pathways of coagulation as measured by the prothrombin time (PT) or partial thromboplastin time. Petechiae and ecchymoses can result from increased vascular fragility, a consequence of nutritional deficiency (e.g., vitamin C), infection (e.g., meningococcemia), and vasculitic diseases. Liver disease would affect the PT. Chronic renal failure may depress platelet function. Meningococcemia is an acute illness. Metastatic disease does not directly affect hemostasis, although extensive marrow metastases could diminish platelet production.

BP7 444   BP6 384   PBD7 650   PBD6 634-635

8 **(C)** This patient has gram-negative sepsis in which widespread endothelial damage causes DIC. The fragmented RBCs, including "helmet cells," are typical of conditions that can produce a microangiopathic hemolytic anemia, such as disseminated intravascular coagulation, thrombocytopenia purpura, systemic lupus erythematosus, hemolytic-uremic syndrome, and malignant hypertension. Such fragmented RBCs are called schistocytes. Spherocytes may be present in hereditary spherocytosis, but the RBC destruction is extravascular, and fragmented RBCs do not appear in the peripheral blood. In autoimmune hemolytic anemia, the hemolysis is extravascular as well, and spherocytes are sometimes formed. Marked anisocytosis and poikilocytosis can occur in iron defi-

ciency and in megaloblastic anemias, but fragmentation of RBCs is not seen.

BP7 444-446   BP6 352   PBD7 656-658   PBD6 621, 640

9 **(D)** This patient has aplastic crisis, precipitated by a parvovirus infection. In adults who do not have a defect in normal RBC production, such as hereditary spherocytosis or sickle cell anemia, or who are not immunosuppressed, parvovirus infection is self-limited and often goes unnoticed. When RBC production is shut down by parvovirus, there is no reticulocytosis. Disseminated intravascular coagulation gives rise to thrombocytopenia, bleeding, and the appearance of fragmented RBCs in the blood smear. Reticulocytosis would be prominent with RBC antibodies. Iron deficiency does not occur in hemolytic anemias, because the iron that is released from hemolyzed cells is reused.

PBD7 627   PBD6 609

10 **(D)** This is an example of disseminated intravascular coagulation (DIC) with associated microangiopathic hemolytic anemia. The DIC developed in the setting of a mucin-secreting adenocarcinoma. Howell-Jolly bodies are small, round inclusions in RBCs that appear when the spleen is absent. Teardrop cells are most characteristic of myelofibrosis and other infiltrative disorders of the marrow. Macro-ovalocytes are seen in megaloblastic anemias, such as vitamin B_{12} deficiency. Target cells appear in hemoglobin C disease or severe liver disease.

BP7 444-446   BP6 343   PBD7 656-658
PBD6 640-642, 685

11 **(E)** This patient has a warm autoimmune hemolytic anemia secondary to systemic lupus erythematosus (SLE). A positive Coombs test result indicates the presence of anti-RBC antibodies in the serum and on the RBC surface. Most cases of warm autoimmune hemolytic anemia are idiopathic, but one fourth occur in persons with an identifiable autoimmune disease, such as SLE. Some are caused by drugs such as α-methyldopa. The immunoglobulin coating the RBCs acts as an opsonin to promote splenic phagocytosis. Nucleated RBCs can be seen in active hemolysis, because the marrow compensates by releasing immature RBCs. Infections such as mononucleosis and *Mycoplasma* are associated with cold autoimmune hemolytic anemia (with an elevated cold agglutinin titer). The increased RBC destruction in hereditary spherocytosis is extravascular and not immune mediated. Septicemia is more likely to lead to a microangiopathic hemolytic anemia.

BP7 407-408   BP6 351   PBD7 636-637   PBD6 620-621

12 **(D)** An inherited bleeding disorder with normal platelet count and prolonged bleeding time suggests von Willebrand disease (vWF), confirmed by the ristocetin-dependent bioassay for vWF. Von Willebrand disease is a fairly common bleeding disorder, with an estimated frequency of 1%. In most cases, it is inherited as an autosomal dominant trait. In these cases, a reduction in the quantity of vWF impairs platelet adhesion to damaged vessel walls, and hemostasis is compromised. Because vWF acts as a carrier for factor VIII, the level of this procoagulant protein (needed for the intrinsic pathway) is diminished, as in this case. However, the levels of factor VIII rarely are reduced enough to be clinically significant. Prolonged partial thromboplastin time corrected by normal plasma is a reflection of factor VIII deficiency. Because the disease is not a disorder of stem cells, transplantation is not helpful. Joint hemorrhages are a feature of hemophilia A and B, not von Willebrand disease. Patients with von Willebrand disease are not prone to thrombosis, as are persons with factor V (Leiden) mutation or other inherited disorders of anticoagulation. Splenectomy is useful in cases of idiopathic thrombocytopenic purpura, but the platelets are not consumed in von Willebrand disease.

BP7 449-450   BP6 388-389   PBD7 654-655
PBD6 638-639

13 (A) Children and adults with sickle cell anemia may benefit from hydroxyurea therapy, which can increase the concentration of HbF in RBCs, which interferes with the polymerization of HbS. However, the therapeutic response to hydroxyurea often precedes the rise in HbF levels. Hydroxyurea also has an anti-inflammatory effect, increases the mean red cell volume, and can be oxidized by heme groups to produce NO. Because HbF levels are high for the first 5 to 6 months of life, patients with sickle cell anemia do not manifest the disease during this period. Because both β-globin chains are affected, no hemoglobin$_{A1}$ is produced. Globin synthesis decreases with the thalassemias. The hemolysis associated with sickling promotes erythropoiesis, but the concentration of hemoglobin S is not changed. Hydroxyurea does not shift the oxygen dissociation curve nor change the oxygen affinity of the various hemoglobins.

BP7 403   PBD7 631-632   PBD6 612

14 (A) This patient has a microcytic anemia, which is typical of iron deficiency. Iron deficiency is the most common form of anemia worldwide. The lack of iron impairs heme synthesis. The marrow response is to "downsize" the RBCs, resulting in a microcytic and hypochromic anemia. At this patient's age, bleeding from an occult malignancy should be strongly suspected as the cause of iron deficiency. An autoimmune hemolytic anemia would appear as a normocytic anemia or as a slightly increased MCV with pronounced reticulocytosis. Thalassemias may result in a microcytosis, but β-thalassemia major causes severe anemia soon after birth, and survival to the age of 73 years is unlikely. Macrocytosis would accompany a history of chronic alcoholism, probably because of poor diet and folate deficiency. Vitamin B$_{12}$ deficiency also results in a macrocytic anemia. By this patient's age, hemophilia A would result in joint problems; because the bleeding is mainly into soft tissues without blood loss, the iron is recycled.

BP7 409-411   BP6 353   PBD7 643-646   PBD6 627-629

15 (C) Glucose-6-phosphate dehydrogenase deficiency is an X-linked disorder that affects about 10% of African-American males. The lack of this enzyme subjects hemoglobin to damage by oxidants, including drugs such as primaquine, sulfonamides, nitrofurantoin, phenacetin, and aspirin (in large doses). Infection also can cause oxidative damage to hemoglobin. Heinz bodies damage the red cell membrane, giving rise to intravascular hemolysis. The "bite cells" result from the attempts of overeager splenic macrophages to pluck out the Heinz bodies, adding an element of extravascular hemolysis.

Heterozygotes with α-thalassemia have no major problems, but in cases of α-thalassemia major, perinatal death is the rule. Likewise, β-thalassemia minor and sickle cell trait are conditions with no major problems and no relation to drug usage. Some autoimmune hemolytic anemias can be drug related, but the hemolysis is predominantly extravascular. RBC membrane abnormalities, such as hereditary spherocytosis (caused by abnormal spectrin), typically produce a mild anemia without significant hemolysis, and there is no drug sensitivity.

BP7 406-407   BP6 350   PBD7 627-628   PBD6 610-611

16 (C) The increased ferritin concentration and reduced total iron-binding capacity are typical of anemia of chronic disease, such as an autoimmune disease. Increased levels of cytokines such as interleukin-1 and tumor necrosis factor promote sequestration of storage iron, with poor utilization for erythropoiesis. Secretion of erythropoietin by the kidney is impaired. A variety of underlying diseases, including cancer, collagen vascular diseases, and chronic infections, can produce this pattern of anemia. Iron deficiency would produce a microcytic anemia, with a low serum ferritin level. The patient is unlikely to have aplastic anemia, because the platelet count and WBC count are normal. Microangiopathic hemolytic anemias are caused by serious acute conditions such as disseminated intravascular coagulation; these patients have thrombocytopenia caused by widespread thrombosis. Megaloblastic anemias are macrocytic and do not cause a large increase in iron stores. Thalassemia minor is uncommon, and is not associated with a positive ANA test result.

BP7 411   BP6 354   PBD7 646   PBD6 630

17 (D) Throughout human history, malaria has been the driving force for increasing the gene frequency of hemoglobin S. Persons who are heterozygous for hemoglobin S have the sickle cell trait. They are resistant to malaria, because the parasites grow poorly or die at low oxygen concentrations, perhaps because of low potassium levels caused by potassium efflux from red blood cells on hemoglobin sickling. Therefore, the malarial parasite cannot complete its life cycle. *Clostridium neoformans* can cause granulomatous disease in immunocompromised persons. *Borrelia burgdorferi* is the spirochete that causes Lyme disease. *Treponema pallidum* is the infectious agent causing syphilis. *Clostridium perfringens* may produce gas gangrene following soft tissue injuries. *Trypanosoma gambiense* infection causes sleeping sickness. *Schistosoma hematobium* infection leads to hematuria and iron deficiency anemia.

BP7 400   BP6 345   PBD7 402, 628-629
PBD6 389-390, 611

18 (A) The pancytopenia and absence of a reticulocytosis strongly suggest bone marrow failure. Aplastic anemia has no apparent cause in half of all cases. In other cases, drugs and toxins may be identified; drugs such as chemotherapeutic agents are best known for this effect. A preceding viral infection may be identified in some cases, but bacterial infections rarely cause aplastic anemias. Persons with pancytopenia are subject to bleeding disorders because of the low platelet count and to infections because of the low WBC count. Dietary history would not be helpful because this patient's clinical and laboratory picture is not characteristic of iron deficiency or vitamin B$_{12}$ deficiency. Menstrual history would be relevant if the patient had hypochromic microcytic anemia. The only known familial cause of aplastic anemia (Fanconi's anemia) is rare.

BP7 414   BP6 357   PBD7 647-648   PBD6 630-631

19 **(A)** This patient has so-called autosplenectomy, which results from the multiple infarctions that occur as a consequence of the sickling phenomenon. In children with sickle cell anemia, the spleen may initially be enlarged from engorgement of splenic sinusoids with the abnormal masses of sickled cells, but hypoxic tissue damage ensues. Terminally, this patient developed a vaso-occlusive crisis affecting the lung. β-Thalassemia major can lead to splenomegaly from extramedullary hematopoiesis. Some of the largest spleens occur because of malaria. With idiopathic thrombocytopenic purpura, the spleen is usually of normal size. In autoimmune hemolytic anemias, the spleen may increase in size from extravascular hemolysis or from extramedullary hematopoiesis.

BP7 402-403   BP6 346   PBD7 630-631   PBD6 614

20 **(E)** The severity of hemophilia A depends on the amount of factor VIII activity. With less than 1% activity, there is severe disease, and joint hemorrhages are common, leading to severe joint deformity and ankylosis. Mild (1% to 5%) and moderate (5% to 75%) activity is often asymptomatic, except in severe trauma. The bleeding tendency is not associated with splenomegaly. Petechiae, seen in patients with thrombocytopenia, are not a feature of hemophilia. Factor VIII deficiency does not affect the lifespan of RBCs. Because persons with factor VIII deficiency do not depend on RBC transfusions, iron overload is not a usual consequence.

BP7 450   BP6 389   PBD7 654-656   PBD6 638

21 **(D)** The presence of thrombocytopenia, increased prothrombin and partial thromboplastin values, fibrin split products, and the low fibrinogen concentration all suggest disseminated intravascular coagulation (DIC), which was most likely caused by a retained dead fetus, an obstetric complication that can lead to DIC through release of thromboplastins from the fetus. This release causes widespread microvascular thrombosis and consumes clotting factors and platelets. There is no damage to the vascular endothelium or vascular wall. Platelet production is normal, but platelets are consumed by widespread thrombosis of small vessels. There is no defect in platelet function.

BP7 444-446   BP6 385-386   PBD7 656-658
PBD6 640-642

22 **(F)** The diagnosis of thrombotic thrombocytopenic purpura (TTP) is based on finding a classic pentad: transient neurologic problems, fever, thrombocytopenia, microangiopathic hemolytic anemia, and acute renal failure. The diagnosis is confirmed by demonstration of vWF monomers in the serum. These abnormalities are produced by small platelet-fibrin thrombi in small vessels in multiple organs. The heart, brain, and kidney often are severely affected. Of the other choices, only disseminated intravascular coagulation is a microangiopathic hemolytic anemia, but the pentad of TTP is missing.

BP7 448   BP6 387-388   PBD7 652-653   PBD6 636-637

23 **(F)** This patient has glucose-6-phosphate dehydrogenase deficiency. A drug that leads to oxidative injury to the RBCs, such as primaquine, can induce hemolysis. Oxidant injury to hemoglobin produces inclusion of denatured hemoglobin within RBCs. The inclusions damage the cell membrane directly, giving rise to intravascular hemolysis. These cells have reduced membrane deformability, and they are also removed from the circulation by the spleen. The remaining mechanisms listed are not directly drug dependent. Mechanical fragmentation of RBCs is typical of microangiopathic hemolytic anemias, such as disseminated intravascular coagulation. Complement lysis is enhanced in paroxysmal nocturnal hemoglobinuria, which results from mutations in the *PIGA* gene. Impaired RBC nuclear maturation occurs as a result of vitamin B_{12} or folate deficiency. Impaired globin synthesis occurs in thalassemias. Hemolytic anemias with antibody coating RBCs can occur with autoimmune diseases, prior transfusion, and erythroblastosis fetalis. Reduced RBC membrane deformability is seen in patients with abnormalities in cytoskeletal proteins, such as spectrin; the latter causes hereditary spherocytosis.

BP7 406-407   BP6 350   PBD7 627-628   PBD6 610-611

24 **(C)** Reduced numbers of platelets can result from decreased production or increased destruction. Marrow examination in this case shows numerous megakaryocytes, which excludes decreased production. Accelerated destruction can be caused by hypersplenism, but there is no splenomegaly in this case. Peripheral platelet destruction is often immunologically mediated and can result from well-known autoimmune diseases such as systemic lupus erythematosus, or it can be idiopathic. When all known causes of thrombocytopenia are excluded, a diagnosis of idiopathic thrombocytopenic purpura (ITP) can be made. This patient seems to have no other symptoms or signs and has no history of drug intake or infections that can cause thrombocytopenia. Thus, ITP is most likely. Thrombotic thrombocytopenic purpura (TTP) is another entity to be considered, but TTP produces a microangiopathic hemolytic anemia (MAHA) that typically is associated with fever, neurologic symptoms, and renal failure. Disseminated intravascular coagulation is another form of MAHA. Hemophilia B, like hemophilia A, leads to soft tissue bleeding, and the partial thromboplastin time (PTT) is prolonged, but the platelet count is normal. Metastases can act as a space-occupying lesion in the marrow to reduce hematopoiesis, but this is unlikely to be selective with megakaryocytes, and in this case, there is a megakaryocytic hyperplasia. Vitamin K deficiency prolongs the prothrombin time initially, and the PTT if severe, but does not affect platelets. In von Willebrand disease, bleeding is due to abnormal platelet adhesion, but platelet numbers are normal.

BP7 447   BP6 387   PBD7 650-651   PBD6 634-636

25 **(E)** The crescent-shaped RBCs (sickled RBCs) are characteristic of hemoglobin SS. This disease is most common in persons of African and eastern Arabian descent. The sickled RBCs are susceptible to hemolysis (mainly vascular, in the spleen), but they also can cause microvascular occlusions anywhere in the body, but most commonly bone, lungs, liver, and brain, leading to ischemia and severe pain. Vascular occlusions in the lungs are often accompanied by infection and lead to the "acute chest syndrome." It is believed that the cell membranes of reversibly sickled cells are abnormally "sticky" and they adhere to capillary endothelium, especially in lungs. The endothelium may already be sticky due to trivial inflammation. Adhesion of RBCs to endothelium retards blood flow, creates hypoxia, and precipitates local sickling and vascular occlusion. Chronic tissue hypoxia does occur in sickle cell anemia, but it produces insidious impairment of function in organs such as heart, kidneys, and lungs. Defects in the alternative pathway of complement activation predispose to infection with encapsulated bacteria such as *Haemophilus influenzae* and *Streptococcus pneumoniae.*

BP7 400-403   BP6 345   PBD7 628-632   PBD6 612-614

26 **(D)** In patients with hereditary spherocytosis, spheroidal cells are trapped and destroyed in the spleen because the abnormal RBCs have reduced deformability. Splenectomy is beneficial because the spherocytes are no longer detained by the spleen. Splenectomy has no effect on the synthesis of spectrin or RBC deformability as a result; the RBCs in spherocytosis are not killed by opsonization. In warm antibody hemolytic anemias, opsonized RBCs are removed by the spleen. Reactive oxygen species do not play a role in anemias.

BP7 399-400   BP6 343-344   PBD7 625-627
PBD6 607-609

27 **(D)** The high MCV is indicative of a marked macrocytosis, greater than would be accounted for by a reticulocytosis alone. The two best known causes for such an anemia (also known as megaloblastic anemia when characteristic megaloblastic precursors are seen in the bone marrow) are vitamin B_{12} and folate deficiency. Because vitamin B_{12} is absorbed in the terminal ileum, its removal can cause vitamin B_{12} deficiency. Hemolytic anemia is unlikely several weeks after blood transfusion. Chronic blood loss and iron deficiency produce a microcytic pattern of anemia, as does dietary iron deficiency. Anemia of chronic disease is generally a normocytic anemia. Inflammatory bowel diseases (e.g., Crohn disease) increase the risk of malignancy, but myelophthisic anemias (from space-occupying lesions of the marrow) are usually normocytic to mildly macrocytic (from reticulocytosis).

BP7 411-413   BP6 356   PBD7 638-642   PBD6 622-623

28 **(C)** This patient has disseminated intravascular coagulation, which can result from gram-negative septicemia. This is a form of microangiopathic hemolytic anemia, in which there is deposition of fibrin strands in small vessels. The RBCs are damaged during passage between these strands. Coagulation factors and platelets are consumed, which does not occur with other forms of hemolytic anemia. Paroxysmal nocturnal hemoglobinuria and the hemolytic anemias do not typically cause a consumptive coagulopathy. Thalassemias produce chronic anemia with ineffective erythropoiesis; there is also an extravascular hemolytic component without the complication of bleeding. Aplastic anemia refers to the loss of marrow stem cell activity and therefore is associated with anemia, leukopenia, and thrombocytopenia. Aplastic anemia can follow infections, most often viral but rarely bacterial.

BP7 444-446   BP6 343   PBD7 358, 656-658
PBD6 640-642

29 **(A)** In sickle cell anemia, the cumulative damage to the spleen results in autosplenectomy, leaving behind a small

fibrotic remnant of this organ. The impaired splenic function and resultant inability to clear bacteria from the bloodstream can occur early in childhood, leading to infection with encapsulated bacterial organisms. Thus, immunodeficiency results from lack of splenic function, not from lack of immunoglobulins. There is no impairment in production or function of neutrophils. C-reactive protein is a marker of acute inflammation, and it does not help clear bacteria. Adhesion between endothelial cells and RBCs is increased in sickle cell anemia.

BP7 402-403   BP6 346-347   PBD7 630-631
PBD6 613-614

30 **(A)** The acute blood loss, in this case probably intraperitoneal hemorrhage, results in a reticulocytosis from marrow stimulation by anemia. Leukoerythroblastosis is typical of a myelophthisic process in the marrow. Basophilic stippling of RBCs suggests a marrow injury, such as with a drug or toxin. Hypochromic RBCs occur in iron deficiency and thalassemias, both associated with reduced hemoglobin synthesis. Acute blood loss does not give rise to iron deficiency. Schistocytes suggest a microangiopathic hemolytic anemia, which can accompany shock or sepsis.

BP7 397-398   BP6 342   PBD7 623-625   PBD6 605-606

31 **(C)** The infant had α-thalassemia major, which is most likely to be occur in persons of Southeast Asian ancestry, each of whose parents could have two abnormal α-globin genes on chromosome 16. A complete lack of α-globin chains precludes formation of hemoglobins A_1, A_2, and F. Only a tetramer of γ chains (Bart's hemoglobin) can be made, leading to severe fetal anemia. Inheritance of three abnormal α-globin chains leads to hemoglobin H disease, with tetramers of β chains; survival to adulthood is possible. Persons with hemoglobin S usually are asymptomatic in infancy because of hemoglobin F production. Hemoglobins C and E produce mild hemolytic anemias.

BP7 404-406   BP6 342   PBD7 635-636   PBD6 605

32 **(C)** This patient has paroxysmal nocturnal hemoglobinuria, a disorder that results from an acquired myeloid stem cell membrane defect produced by a mutation in the *PIGA* gene. A mutation in this gene prevents the membrane expression of certain proteins that require a glycolipid anchor. These include proteins that protect cells from lysis by spontaneously activated complement. As a result, RBCs, granulocytes, and platelets are exquisitely sensitive to the lytic activity of complement. The RBC lysis is intravascular; hence, patients can have hemoglobinuria (dark urine). Defects in platelet function are believed to be responsible for venous thrombosis. Recurrent infections can be caused by impaired leukocyte functions. Patients with paroxysmal nocturnal hemoglobinuria also may have acute leukemia or aplastic anemia as complications. Spectrin mutations give rise to hereditary spherocytosis. Patients with glucose-6-phosphate dehydrogenase deficiency have an episodic course from exposure to agents such as drugs that induce hemolysis. Mutations in the β-globin chain can give rise to hemoglobinopathies such as sickle cell anemia. Patients with factor V (Leiden) and prothrombin G20210A mutations can present with thromboses, but there is no anemia or leukopenia.

BP7 407   BP6 351   PBD7 636   PBD6 619-620

33 (D) The reduced β-globin synthesis results in a relative excess of α-globin chains that precipitate in RBCs and their precursors. These precipitates make the cells more susceptible to damage and removal. This intramedullary loss of RBC precursors is termed ineffective erythropoiesis. Unfortunately, it acts as a trigger for greater dietary absorption of iron by unknown mechanisms. Hemolysis of RBCs in the periphery (e.g., spleen, liver) releases iron that can be reused for hemoglobin synthesis. Hemolysis can occur in glucose-6-phosphate dehydrogenase deficiency with oxidative injury to RBCs, particularly in ingestion of certain drugs. In megaloblastic anemias, there is enough iron but not enough vitamin B_{12} or folate. In sickle cell anemia, the β-globin chains are abnormal, leading to sickling of RBCs, which are then destroyed in the spleen; however, there is no ineffective erythropoiesis. Complement lysis is enhanced in paroxysmal nocturnal hemoglobinuria, which results from mutations in the *PIGA* gene. Patients with this disorder have a history of infections.

BP7 403-405   BP6 347-348   PBD7 632-635
PBD6 615-616

34 (D) The patient's history is typical of hemophilia A caused by decreased factor VIII activity or factor VIII deficiency. The affected patient is male and has male relatives who are affected (X-linked transmission), and there is history of bleeding, especially into joints. The partial thromboplastin time (PTT) is prolonged because factor VIII is required for the intrinsic pathway; the prothrombin time (PT) is normal because the extrinsic pathway does not depend on factor VIII function. The inability to correct PTT by mixing with normal plasma is important. If the patient had a deficiency of factor VIII only, the addition of normal plasma, a source of factor VIII, would have corrected the PTT. Failure to correct PTT by normal plasma indicates the presence of an inhibitor in the patient's serum. About 15% of patients with hemophilia eventually develop an inhibitor to factor VIII. The antiphospholipid syndrome has similar PT and PTT findings because an inhibitor is present, but these patients have thromboses as well as bleeding, typically in adulthood, and without a family history. The factor V (Leiden) mutation leads to recurrent thromboses. Disseminated intravascular coagulation is an acute condition resulting from an underlying disease that triggers the coagulation mechanisms, and typically the platelets are consumed. Idiopathic thrombocytopenic purpura results from an autoimmune condition with thrombocytopenia leading to bleeding. In von Willebrand disease, the platelet count, PT, and PTT are all normal—the problem is decreased platelet adherence from decreased von Willebrand factor (vWF). Vitamin K deficiency leads to an abnormal PT.

BP7 450   BP6 389   PBD7 654-656   PBD6 639

35 (C) The history in this case is similar to that in question 34; however, the partial thromboplastin time (PTT) is corrected by normal pooled plasma. The patient has hemophilia A caused either by decreased factor VIII activity or by factor VIII deficiency, and inhibitors of factor VIII are absent from the patient's serum. How is this possible in a female patient? X-inactivation ("unfavorable Lyonization") can explain this phenomenon and could explain why female carriers of hemophilia A or B have a tendency to bleed. ("When you have eliminated the impossible, that which remains, however improbable, must be the truth," said Sherlock Holmes in *The*

Sign of Four.) An in vitro mixing study of patient and pooled plasma such as this usually corrects an abnormality caused by a deficiency of a procoagulant factor, but if there is a coagulation inhibitor in the patient's plasma, the clotting test will show an abnormal result. Thus, the mixing study excludes the antiphospholipid syndrome. Disseminated intravascular coagulation is an acute problem with consumption of platelets and coagulation factors, making the prothrombin time (PT) and PTT prolonged. Idiopathic thrombocytopenic purpura is characterized by the presence of antiplatelet antibodies and thrombocytopenia. Thrombotic thrombocytopenic purpura is a microangiopathic hemolytic anemia characterized by renal failure and central nervous system abnormalities. Vitamin K deficiency should prolong the PT. Von Willebrand disease is caused by decreased platelet adhesion and has features resembling thrombocytopenia.

BP7 450   BP6 389   PBD7 654-656   PBD6 639

36 (E) This patient has benign tertian malaria. The bite of the *Anopheles* mosquito introduces sporozoites, which travel to the liver to reproduce. The resulting merozoites are released into the bloodstream and infect RBCs. Asexual reproduction within the RBCs then yields trophozoites, and periodic hemolysis with release of the parasites produces the characteristic clinical findings. *Aspergillus* organisms invade blood vessels and cause thrombosis, but hemolysis of RBCs is inconsequential. Babesiosis is far less common than malaria, is endemic to the northeastern US, and does not produce episodic fevers. *Dirofilaria* is the heartworm found in dogs, which rarely infects humans and does not cause hemolysis. Like other gram-negative bacteria, *Escherichia coli* can release lipopolysaccharide, which causes severe sepsis and possible disseminated intravascular coagulation, a microangiopathic hemolytic anemia. *Wuchereria bancrofti* is a nematode that prefers to live in lymphatics.

BP7 408-409   BP6 388-389   PBD7 401-403, 624
PBD6 638-639

37 (C) This patient has chronic alcoholism and folate deficiency, giving rise to megaloblastic anemia. Folic acid and vitamin B_{12} act as coenzymes in the DNA synthetic pathway. A deficiency of either impairs the normal process of nuclear maturation. The nuclei remain large and primitive looking, giving rise to megaloblasts. The mature RBCs are also larger than normal (macrocytes). The nuclear maturation defect affects all rapidly dividing cells in the body, including other hematopoietic lineages. Patients can have thrombocytopenia and leukopenia, often because of secondary hypersplenism (alcoholic cirrhosis, leading to splenomegaly). Neutrophils often show defective segmentation, manifested by extra nuclear lobes. Polychromatophilic RBCs represent reticulocytes, and their number is reduced because of the failure of marrow to produce adequate numbers of RBCs despite anemia. Mechanical fragmentation of RBCs is typical of microangiopathic hemolytic anemias, such as disseminated intravascular coagulation. Complement lysis is enhanced in paroxysmal nocturnal hemoglobinuria, which results from mutations in the *PIGA* gene. Hemolytic anemias, in which antibody coats RBCs, can occur in autoimmune diseases, prior transfusion, and erythroblastosis fetalis. Reduced RBC membrane deformability is seen in patients with abnormalities of cytoskeletal proteins, such as spectrin; the latter causes hereditary spherocytosis. Hemoglobinopathies can produce a mild macrocytosis, because more reticulocytes are released. An imbalance in α- and β-globin chain synthesis, seen in thalassemias, leads to microcytosis of RBCs.

BP7 412-413   BP6 356   PBD7 642-643   PBD6 622-623

38 **(B)** This patient, of Mediterranean descent, has β-thalassemia major. In this condition, there is a severe reduction in the synthesis of β-globin chains without impairment of α-globin synthesis. The free, unpaired α-globin chains form aggregates that precipitate within normoblasts and cause them to undergo apoptosis. The death of RBC precursors in the bone marrow is called ineffective erythropoiesis. Not only does this cause anemia, but it also increases the absorption of dietary iron, giving rise to iron overload, which results in hemochromatosis with infiltrative cardiomyopathy, hepatic cirrhosis, and "bronze diabetes" from pancreatic islet dysfunction. The severe anemia triggers erythropoietin synthesis, which expands the erythropoietic marrow. The marrow expansion encroaches on the bones, causing maxillofacial deformities. Extramedullary hematopoiesis causes hepatosplenomegaly. In comparison, the hemolytic anemia is mild in β-thalassemia minor, and there is very little ineffective erythropoiesis. Hemochromatosis is particularly detrimental to the liver and heart. Patients with chronic anemia may require RBC transfusions, which adds even more iron to body stores. The other listed options do not lead to a marked expansion of hematopoiesis.

BP7 403-405   BP6 347-348   PBD7 632-635
PBD6 615-617

39 **(F)** This patient has aplastic anemia with marked pancytopenia. Many cases are idiopathic, although some can follow toxic exposures to chemotherapy drugs or to chemicals, such as benzene. Some cases may follow viral hepatitis infections. An intrinsic defect in stem cells, or T-lymphocyte suppression of stem cells, can play a role in the development of aplastic anemia. Hemolysis is unlikely, because the bilirubin is normal, and there is no history of an autoimmune disease. Sequestration of peripheral blood cells in an enlarged spleen could account for mild pancytopenia, but in this case the spleen is not enlarged. An increased susceptibility to complement lysis occurs in paroxysmal nocturnal hemoglobinuria as a result of mutations in the *PIGA* gene. It is unlikely that the patient has metastatic disease at this age, with no prior illness; metastases are more likely to produce a leukoerythroblastic peripheral blood appearance. Nuclear maturation defects are typical of megaloblastic anemias. Chickenpox (varicella-zoster virus infection) is unlikely to produce aplastic anemia; the virus becomes latent in neuronal ganglia.

BP7 414   BP6 342, 353   PBD7 647-648   PBD6 627-628

40 **(E)** This patient has a microcytic anemia, so iron deficiency anemia must be considered. The ferritin concentration is a measure of storage iron, because it is derived from the total body storage pool in the liver, spleen, and marrow. About 80% of functional body iron is contained in hemoglobin; the remainder is in muscle myoglobin. Transferrin, a serum transport protein for iron usually has about 33% iron saturation. Persons with severe liver disease can have an elevated serum ferritin level because of its release from liver stores. The serum

iron concentration or transferrin level by itself gives no indication of iron stores, because in anemia of chronic disease, the patient's iron level can be normal to low, and the transferrin levels also can be normal to low, but iron stores are increased. The serum haptoglobin level is decreased with intravascular hemolysis, but the anemia is normocytic because the iron can be recycled. A bone marrow biopsy specimen provides a good indication of iron stores, because the iron stain of the marrow shows hemosiderin in macrophages, but such a biopsy is an expensive procedure. Some patient's with hemoglobinopathies, such as β-thalassemias, can also have a microcytic anemia, but this is far less common than iron deficiency.

BP7 409   BP6 353   PBD7 643-644   PBD6 627-628

41 **(B)** Glanzmann thrombasthenia is a rare autosomal recessive disorder with defective platelet aggregation from deficiency or dysfunction of glycoprotein IIb-IIIa. Disseminated intravascular coagulation results in consumption of all coagulation factors as well as platelets, so the prothrombin time and partial thromboplastin time are elevated, with thrombocytopenia. Immune thrombocytopenic purpura is caused by antibodies to platelet membrane glycoproteins IIb-IIIa or Ib-IX. Scurvy due to vitamin C deficiency causes bleeding into soft tissues and skin from increased capillary fragility, but platelet number and function are normal. Von Willebrand disease is one of the most common bleeding disorders and results from qualitative or quantitative defects in vWF.

PBD7 127, 653-654   BP7 87

42 **(B)** Teardrop RBCs are indicative of a myelophthisic disorder (i.e., something filling the bone marrow, such as fibrous connective tissue). The leukoerythroblastosis, including immature RBCs and WBCs, is most indicative of myelofibrosis. Splenomegaly is also typically seen in myelofibrosis. A leukoerythroblastic picture also can be seen in patients with infections and metastases involving the marrow. Marrow packed with myeloblasts is typical of acute myeloid leukemia. In this condition, the peripheral blood would also show myeloblasts and failure of myeloid maturation. Replacement of marrow by fat occurs in aplastic anemia, which is characterized by pancytopenia. The presence of megaloblasts in the marrow indicates folate or vitamin B_{12} deficiency—both cause macrocytic anemia. Hyperplasia of normoblasts occurs in hemolytic anemias. Leukoerythroblastosis is not seen in hemolytic anemias.

BP7 414   BP6 357   PBD7 648-649   PBD6 632-633

43 **(E)** Although both folate and vitamin B_{12} deficiency give rise to a macrocytic anemia, a deficiency of vitamin B_{12} can also result in demyelination of the posterior and lateral columns of the spinal cord. The anemia caused by vitamin B_{12} deficiency can be ameliorated by increased administration of folate; this masks the potential neurologic injury by improving the anemia. However, treating vitamin B_{12} deficiency does not improve the anemia caused by folate deficiency. Folate has no cofactor for absorption, but vitamin B_{12} must be complexed to intrinsic factor, secreted by gastric parietal cells, and then the complex must be absorbed in the terminal ileum, so that diseases such as atrophic gastritis and Crohn disease can affect vitamin B_{12} absorption more than folate. The peripheral smear could appear the same and offers no means for distinguishing these deficiencies. An aplastic anemia is unlikely to result from a nutritional deficiency.

BP7 411-413   BP6 356   PBD7 639-642   PBD6 625

44   **(C)** The hemolysis that accompanies sickle cell anemia results in an increased indirect hyperbilirubinemia, which favors the development of gallstones containing bilirubin pigment. Cirrhosis can occur because of hemochromatosis in β-thalassemia major. Chronic atrophic gastritis leads to loss of parietal cells, and the resulting vitamin B_{12} malabsorption causes pernicious anemia. Stillbirths suggest thalassemia major. Esophageal webs occur very uncommonly in the setting of chronic iron deficiency anemia.

BP7 402-403   BP6 347   PBD7 624, 630
PBD6 613-614, 893-894

45   **(A)** Both acute immune thrombocytopenic purpura and immune thrombocytopenic purpura (ITP) are caused by antiplatelet autoantibodies, but the acute form is typically seen in children following a viral disease. If the bone marrow were aplastic, then all cell lines should be reduced. Glycoprotein IIb-IIIa dysfunction/deficiency can be seen with Glanzmann thrombasthenia and chronic ITP. Scurvy due to vitamin C deficiency leads to increased capillary fragility with ecchymoses but not to thrombocytopenia. VWF metalloprotease deficiency is a feature of thrombotic thrombocytopenic purpura (TTP).

PBD7 652

46   **(E)** This patient has findings most suggestive of prostatic adenocarcinoma that has metastasized to the bone. High alkaline phosphatase, hypercalcemia, and a leukoerythroblastic pattern in the peripheral blood (immature WBCs and RBCs) are a consequence of the tumor acting as a space-occupying lesion. Myelophthisic anemias may also be caused by infections. The anemia of chronic disease is relatively mild. Aplastic anemias are unlikely to include leukoerythroblastosis. Hemolytic anemia should be accompanied by a rise in bilirubin and no abnormalities in calcium metabolism. The MCV in this case is not in the megaloblastic range. Thalassemias can lead to ineffective erythropoiesis but not to pancytopenia.

BP7 414   BP6 349   PBD7 648-649   PBD6 616-617

47   **(D)** This man has heat stroke caused by hyperthermia and loss of perspiration from dehydration, which is producing hemoconcentration with a relative polycythemia (note the elevated serum sodium level). Erythroleukemia is quite rare, and patients with this disorder are too ill to run a race. Chronic obstructive pulmonary disease is a cause of secondary polycythemia from chronic hypoxemia, but it does not produce hemoconcentration. Diabetes insipidus can result from a lack of antidiuretic hormone release, which leads to free water loss and dehydration but not to hyperthermia. Increased erythropoietin levels are seen in secondary polycythemias, including those associated with chronic hypoxemia (high altitude or lung disease) and those associated with neoplasms secreting erythropoietin (renal cell carcinoma). Polycythemia vera is a form of myeloproliferative disorder, in which erythropoietin levels are low and there is no dehydration.

BP7 415   BP6 347   PBD7 649   PBD6 613-614

48   **(E)** Haptoglobin is a serum protein that binds to free hemoglobin. Ordinarily, circulating hemoglobin is contained within RBCs, but hemolysis can release free hemoglobin. The haptoglobin is used up as the amount of free hemoglobin increases. An elevated D dimer level suggests a microangiopathic hemolytic anemia. Systemic lupus erythematosus (SLE) is an autoimmune disease that can result in hemolysis by means of autoantibodies directed at RBCs, and the Coombs test result is often positive. Decreased iron can cause a hypochromic, microcytic anemia, but with hemolysis, the RBCs are recycled, and the iron is not lost. Prostatic adenocarcinoma could produce leukoerythroblastosis if widely metastatic to bone but not hemolysis.

BP7 398   BP6 343, 351   PBD7 624-625   PBD6 606

49   **(A)** The iron concentration and iron-binding capacity are both low; however, unlike the finding in anemia of iron deficiency, the serum ferritin level is increased. This increase is typical of anemia of chronic disease. Underlying chronic inflammatory or neoplastic diseases increase the secretion of cytokines such as interleukin-1, tumor necrosis factor, and interferon-γ. These cytokines promote sequestration of iron in storage compartments and also depress erythropoietin production. Metastases are space occupying lesions (myelophthisic process) that can lead to leukoerythroblastosis, with nucleated RBCs and immature WBCs appearing on the peripheral blood smear. Complement lysis is enhanced in paroxysmal nocturnal hemoglobinuria, which results from mutations in the *PIGA* gene. Patients with this disorder have a history of infections. Sequestration of RBCs in the spleen occur when RBC membranes are abnormal, as in hereditary spherocytosis or sickle cell anemia, or RBCs are coated by antibodies, as in autoimmune hemolytic anemias. Impaired synthesis of β-globin chains gives rise to β-thalassemias, also characterized by hemolysis. Warm autoantibody hemolytic anemias occur in several autoimmune diseases, such as SLE, but not in patients with rheumatoid arthritis, as in this case. Normal serum haptoglobin rules out intravascular hemolysis; iron is recycled at a rapid rate.

BP7 411   BP6 354   PBD7 646-647   PBD6 630

50   **(D)** The infant most likely has erythroblastosis fetalis because of the maternal antibodies coating the fetal cells. A fetal-maternal hemorrhage in utero or at the time of delivery in a previous pregnancy (or with previous transfusion of incompatible blood) can sensitize the mother, resulting in production of IgG antibodies. In subsequent pregnancies, these antibodies (unlike the naturally occurring IgM antibodies) can cross the placenta to attach to fetal cells, leading to hemolysis. In the past, most cases were caused by Rh incompatibility (e.g., Rh-negative mother, Rh-positive infant), but the use of RhoGAM administered at birth to Rh-negative mothers has eliminated almost all such cases. However, other less common blood group antigens can be involved in this process. The other conditions listed are not antibody mediated. Mechanical fragmentation of RBCs is typical of microangiopathic hemolytic anemias, such as disseminated intravascular coagulation, which is more typical of pregnant women with obstetric complications. Impaired RBC nuclear maturation occurs as a result of vitamin B_{12} or folate deficiency. Impaired globin synthesis occurs in thalassemias. A stem cell defect results in aplastic anemia and immunodeficiency. Oxidative injury to hemoglobin is typical of glucose-6-phosphate dehydrogenase deficiency. Reduced RBC membrane deformability is seen in patients with abnormalities in cytoskeletal proteins, such as spectrin; the latter causes hereditary spherocytosis.

BP7 407-408   BP6 206   PBD7 485-486, 623
PBD6 473-474

51 **(A)** The marked reticulocytosis and marrow hyperplasia indicate that the marrow is responding to a decrease in RBCs. The reticulocytes are larger RBCs that slightly increase the MCV. Iron deficiency impairs the ability of the marrow to mount a significant and sustained reticulocytosis. Iron deficiency anemia is typically microcytic and hypochromic. An aplastic marrow is very hypocellular and unable to respond to anemia; it is associated with pancytopenia. Infiltrative disorders, such as metastases in the marrow, would impair the ability to mount a reticulocytosis of this degree. The normal Coombs test results exclude an autoimmune hemolytic anemia.

BP7 397-398   BP6 342-343   PBD7 623-625
PBD6 606-607

52 **(C)** This patient has heparin-induced thrombocytopenia, which affects 3% to 5% of patients treated for 1 to 2 weeks with unfractionated heparin. These patients form IgG antibodies to heparin-platelet factor 4 complexes that bind to Fc receptors on the surface of platelets, causing platelet activation and, paradoxically, thrombosis. Aspirin has antiplatelet effects that take days to occur, and bleeding (not thrombosis) is the major risk. Warfarin (Coumadin) was avoided in this patient because of the protein C deficiency; typically the patient is switched from heparin to warfarin. Warfarin therapy prolongs the prothrombin time by interfering with vitamin K–dependent clotting factor synthesis in the liver. Both tissue plasminogen activator and urokinase are fibrinolytic agents, with the former used acutely to treat conditions such as coronary thrombosis, although the latter also may be used for venous clot lysis.

BP7 447   PBD7 652

53 **(B)** The clinical features (neurologic abnormalities, fever, thrombocytopenia, microangiopathic hemolytic anemia, renal failure) point to thrombotic thrombocytopenic purpura (TTP) in which there is an inherited or acquired defi-ciency of the von Willebrand factor (vWF) metalloproteinase (called ADAMTS-13) that normally cleaves very high molecular weight multimers of vWF. The absence of ADAMTS-13 gives rise to large multimers of vWF that promote widespread platelet aggregation, and the resulting microvascular occlusions in brain, kidney, and elsewhere produce organ dysfunction, thrombocytopenia, microangiopathic hemolytic anemia (MAHA), and bleeding. Defective aggregation of platelets in the presence of ADP and thrombin is a feature of a rare inherited disorder of platelets called Glanzmann thrombasthenia. Circulating toxins, principally endotoxins elaborated by *Enterobacteriaciae* such as *Escherichia coli* are important in causing endothelial injury in the hemolytic uremic syndrome (HUS). HUS has similar clinical findings to TTP, but has a different pathogenesis. Release of thromboplastic substances from tumor cells or a retained dead fetus can lead to disseminated intravascular coagulation (DIC) with MAHA, but this patient has no source of thromboplastins. Decreased factor VIII activity is a feature of hemophilia A, an X-linked disorder rare in women, characterized by bleeding into soft tissues such as joints, and normal platelet number and function.

BP7 448   BP6 387-388   PBD7 652-653   PBD6 636-637

54 **(C)** Iron absorption from the gut is tightly controlled. When body iron stores are adequate, absorption of dietary iron via DMT-1 in the duodenum is retarded, and release of iron from storage pools is inhibited. When body iron stores decrease, as with chronic blood loss, iron absorption increases. The liver-derived plasma peptide hepcidin has been found to be the iron absorption regulator. Hepcidin levels increase when iron stores are low, and hepatic hepcidin synthesis diminishes when body iron stores are adequate. Such fine control of iron absorption may fail, as in patients with ineffective erythropoiesis (e.g., β-thalassemia) who continue to absorb iron in spite of excess storage iron. An understanding of hepcidin actions is expected to lead to discovery of new drugs to control iron overload. Transferrin transports iron between plasma, iron stores, and developing erythroblasts. Hemosiderin is an aggregated form of ferritin that does not circulate and is found only in tissues. DMT-1 is an iron transporter that moves non-heme iron from the gut lumen to duodenal epithelium. Mutations in the *HFE* gene, which encodes an HLA-like transmembrane protein, lead to excessive absorption of dietary iron and hemochromatosis.

PBD7 644-645

CHAPTER 14

Diseases of White Blood Cells, Lymph Nodes, Spleen, and Thymus

1 A 15-year-old boy visits his physician because of high fever of 10 days' duration. Physical examination shows a temperature of 38°C. He has scattered petechial hemorrhages on the trunk and extremities. There is no enlargement of liver, spleen, or lymph nodes. The CBC indicates hemoglobin of 13.2 g/dL, hematocrit 38.9%, MCV 93 μm^3, platelet count 175,000/mm^3, and WBC count 1850/mm^3 with 1% segmented neutrophils, 98% lymphocytes, and 1% monocytes. Bone marrow biopsy examination does not show any abnormal cells. Which of the following is the most likely diagnosis?

- ❑ (A) Acute lymphoblastic leukemia
- ❑ (B) Acute myelogenous leukemia
- ❑ (C) Aplastic anemia
- ❑ (D) Idiopathic thrombocytopenic purpura
- ❑ (E) Overwhelming bacterial infection

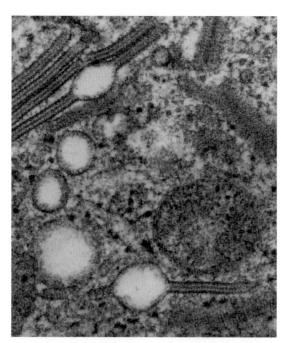

Courtesy of Dr. George Murphy, University of Pennsylvania School of Medicine, Philadelphia, PA.

2 A 9-year-old boy is taken to his pediatrician because of a generalized seborrheic skin eruption and fever. He has been diagnosed and treated for otitis media several times in the past year. On physical examination, he has mild lymphadenopathy, as well as hepatomegaly and splenomegaly. The electron micrograph shown in the preceding figure was taken from a mass lesion involving the mastoid bone. Which of the following is the most likely diagnosis?

❏ (A) Acute lymphoblastic leukemia
❏ (B) Multiple myeloma
❏ (C) Hodgkin disease, mixed cellularity type
❏ (D) Langerhans cell histiocytosis
❏ (E) Disseminated tuberculosis

3 A 67-year-old man has had increasing weakness, fatigue, and weight loss over the past 5 months. He now has decreasing vision in both eyes and has headaches and dizziness. His hands are sensitive to cold. On physical examination, he has generalized lymphadenopathy and hepatosplenomegaly. Laboratory studies indicate hyperproteinemia with a serum protein level of 15.5 g/dL and albumin concentration of 3.2 g/dL. A bone marrow biopsy is performed, and microscopic examination of the specimen shows infiltration of small plasmacytoid lymphoid cells with Russell bodies in their cytoplasm. Which of the following findings is most likely to be reported for this patient?

❏ (A) Monoclonal IgM spike in serum
❏ (B) WBC count of 255,000/mm³
❏ (C) Hypercalcemia
❏ (D) Bence Jones proteinuria
❏ (E) Karyotype with t(14;18) translocation

4 A 37-year-old woman visits her physician because of a cough and fever of 1 week's duration. On physical examination, her temperature is 38.3°C. She has diffuse crackles in all lung fields. A chest radiograph shows bilateral extensive infiltrates. CBC shows hemoglobin of 13.9 g/dL, hematocrit 42.0%, MCV 89 μm³, platelet count 210,000/mm³, and WBC count 56,000/mm³ with 63% segmented neutrophils, 15% bands, 6% metamyelocytes, 3% myelocytes, 1% blasts, 8% lymphocytes, 2% monocytes, and 2% eosinophils. The peripheral blood leukocyte alkaline phosphatase score is increased. Which of the following is the most likely diagnosis?

❏ (A) Chronic myelogenous leukemia
❏ (B) Hairy cell leukemia
❏ (C) Hodgkin disease, lymphocyte depletion type
❏ (D) Leukemoid reaction
❏ (E) Acute lymphoblastic leukemia

5 A 12-year-old boy is taken to the physician because he has had increasing abdominal distention and pain for the past 3 days. Physical examination shows lower abdominal tenderness, and the abdomen is tympanitic with reduced bowel sounds. An abdominal CT scan shows a 7-cm mass involving the region of the ileocecal valve. Surgery is performed to remove the mass. Histologic examination of the mass shows sheets of intermediate-sized lymphoid cells, with nuclei having coarse chromatin, several nucleoli, and many mitoses. A bone marrow biopsy sample is negative for this cell population. Cytogenetic analysis of the cells from the mass shows a t(8;14) karyotype. Flow cytometric analysis reveals 40% of the cells are in S-phase. The tumor shrinks dramatically in size following a course of chemotherapy. Which of the following is the most likely diagnosis?

❏ (A) Diffuse large B-cell lymphoma
❏ (B) Follicular lymphoma
❏ (C) Acute lymphoblastic leukemia
❏ (D) Plasmacytoma
❏ (E) Burkitt lymphoma

6 A 53-year-old man comes to his physician because he felt a lump near his shoulder 1 week ago. On physical examination, there is an enlarged, nontender, supraclavicular lymph node, as well as enlargement of the Waldeyer ring of oropharyngeal lymphoid tissue. There is no hepatosplenomegaly. CBC is normal except for findings of mild anemia. A lymph node biopsy specimen shows replacement by a monomorphous population of large lymphoid cells with enlarged nuclei and prominent nucleoli. Immunohistochemical staining and flow cytometry of the node indicates that most lymphoid cells are CD19+, CD10+, CD3–, CD15– and terminal deoxynucleotidyl transferase negative (TdT–). Which of the following is the most likely diagnosis?

❏ (A) Chronic lymphadenitis
❏ (B) Diffuse large B-cell lymphoma
❏ (C) Hodgkin disease
❏ (D) Lymphoblastic lymphoma
❏ (E) Small lymphocytic lymphoma

7 A 50-year-old man has had headache and dizziness for the past 3 months. He has also experienced generalized and severe pruritus, particularly when showering. He notes that his stools are dark. On physical examination, he is afebrile, and his blood pressure is 165/90 mm Hg. There is no hepatosplenomegaly or lymphadenopathy. A stool sample is positive for occult blood. CBC shows hemoglobin of 22.3 g/dL, hematocrit 67.1%, MCV 94 μm³, platelet count 453,000/mm³, and WBC count 7800/mm³. Which of the following is the most likely diagnosis?

❏ (A) Myelodysplastic syndrome
❏ (B) Essential thrombocytosis
❏ (C) Chronic myelogenous leukemia
❏ (D) Erythroleukemia
❏ (E) Polycythemia vera

8 A 50-year-old man was diagnosed with a diffuse large B-cell lymphoma. He underwent intensive chemotherapy, and a complete remission was achieved for 7 years. He now reports fatigue and recurrent pulmonary and urinary tract infections over the past 4 months. Physical examination shows no masses, lymphadenopathy, or hepatosplenomegaly. CBC shows hemoglobin of 8.7 g/dL, hematocrit 25.2%, MCV 88 μm^3, platelet count 67,000/mm^3, and WBC count 2300/mm^3 with 15% segmented neutrophils, 5% bands, 2% metamyelocytes, 2% myelocytes, 6% myeloblasts, 33% lymphocytes, 35% monocytes, and 2% eosinophils. A bone marrow biopsy specimen shows 90% cellularity with many immature cells, including ringed sideroblasts, megaloblasts, hypolobated megakaryocytes, and myeloblasts. Karyotypic analysis shows 5q deletions in many cells. Which of the following is most likely to have now occurred in this patient?

- (A) Relapse of his previous lymphoma
- (B) Transformation of the lymphoma into myeloid leukemia
- (C) Myelodysplasia related to therapy for the previous tumor
- (D) De novo acute myeloblastic leukemia
- (E) Myeloid metaplasia with myelofibrosis

9 A 63-year-old woman experiences a burning sensation in her hands and feet. Two months ago, she had an episode of swelling with tenderness in the right leg, followed by dyspnea and then right-sided chest pain. On physical examination, the spleen and liver now appear to be enlarged. CBC shows hemoglobin of 13.3 g/dL, hematocrit 40.1%, MCV 91 μm^3, platelet count 657,000/mm^3, and WBC count 17,400/mm^3. The peripheral blood smear shows abnormally large platelets. Which of the following is the most likely diagnosis?

- (A) Essential thrombocythemia
- (B) Chronic myelogenous leukemia
- (C) Myelofibrosis with myeloid metaplasia
- (D) Acute myelogenous leukemia
- (E) Polycythemia vera

10 A 9-year-old boy living in Uganda has had increasing pain and swelling on the right side of his face over the past 8 months. On physical examination, there is a large, nontender mass involving the mandible, which deforms the right side of his face. There is no lymphadenopathy and no splenomegaly, and he is afebrile. A biopsy of the mass is performed. Microscopically, the specimen is composed of intermediate-sized lymphocytes with a high mitotic rate. A chromosome analysis shows a 46,XY,t(8;14) karyotype in these cells. The hemoglobin concentration is 13.2 g/dL, platelet count 272,000/mm^3, and WBC count 5820/mm^3. Infection with which of the following is most likely to be causally related to the development of these findings?

- (A) Cytomegalovirus
- (B) Epstein-Barr virus
- (C) Hepatitis B virus
- (D) HIV
- (E) Human papillomavirus
- (F) Respiratory syncytial virus

11 A 23-year-old man undergoing chemotherapy for acute lymphoblastic leukemia has developed a fever and abdominal pain within the past week. He now has a severe cough. On physical examination, his temperature is 38.4°C. On auscultation, crackles are heard over all lung fields. Laboratory studies show hemoglobin of 12.8 g/dL, hematocrit 39.0%, MCV 90 μm^3, platelet count 221,000/mm^3, and WBC count 16,475/mm^3 with 51% segmented neutrophils, 5% bands, 18% lymphocytes, 8% monocytes, and 18% eosinophils. Infection with which of the following organisms is most likely to be complicating the course of this patient's disease?

- (A) *Cryptococcus neoformans*
- (B) Cytomegalovirus
- (C) *Helicobacter pylori*
- (D) Hepatitis C virus
- (E) *Pseudomonas aeruginosa*
- (F) *Strongyloides stercoralis*
- (G) *Toxoplasma gondii*
- (H) Varicella zoster virus

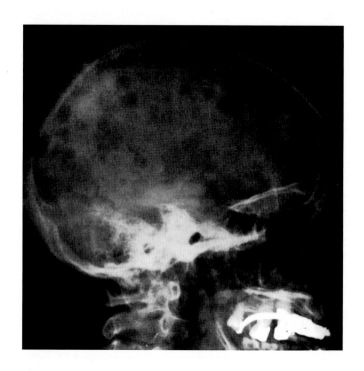

12 A 61-year-old man reports a history of back pain for 5 months. He has recently developed a cough that is productive of yellow sputum. On physical examination, he is febrile, and diffuse rales are heard on auscultation of the lungs. He has no lymphadenopathy or splenomegaly. Laboratory studies include a sputum culture that grew *Streptococcus pneumoniae*. The serum creatinine level is 3.7 mg/dL, and the urea nitrogen level is 35 mg/dL. A skull radiograph is shown. During the course of his hospitalization, a bone marrow biopsy is performed. Which of the following is the biopsy specimen most likely to show?

- (A) Scattered small granulomas
- (B) Numerous plasma cells
- (C) Nodules of small mature lymphocytes
- (D) Occasional Reed-Sternberg cells
- (E) Hypercellularity with many blasts

13 A 26-year-old man has noted lumps in his neck that have been enlarging for the past 6 months. On physical examination, he has a group of enlarged, nontender right cervical lymph nodes. A biopsy of one of the lymph nodes shows scattered Reed-Sternberg cells, as well as macrophages, lymphocytes, neutrophils, eosinophils, and a few plasma cells. Which of the following factors elaborated by the Reed-Sternberg cells has led to the appearance of the eosinophils within this lesion?

- ❑ (A) Platelet-derived growth factor
- ❑ (B) Cyclin D1
- ❑ (C) Interleukin-5
- ❑ (D) Trans-retinoic acid
- ❑ (E) Erythropoietin

14 A 53-year-old woman has experienced nausea with vomiting and early satiety for the past 7 months. On physical examination, she is afebrile and has no lymphadenopathy or hepatosplenomegaly. CBC shows hemoglobin of 12.9 g/dL, hematocrit 41.9%, platelet count 263,000/mm³, and WBC count 8430/mm³. An upper gastrointestinal endoscopy shows loss of the rugal folds of the stomach over a 4 × 8 cm area of the fundus. Gastric biopsy specimens reveal the presence of *Helicobacter pylori* organisms in the mucus overlying superficial epithelial cells. There are mucosal and submucosal monomorphous infiltrates of small lymphocytes, which are CD19+ and CD20+ but CD3−. After treatment of the *H. pylori* infection, her condition improves. Which of the following is the most likely diagnosis?

- ❑ (A) Acute lymphoblastic leukemia
- ❑ (B) Chronic lymphocytic leukemia
- ❑ (C) Diffuse large B-cell lymphoma
- ❑ (D) Follicular lymphoma
- ❑ (E) Hodgkin disease, mixed cellularity type
- ❑ (F) MALT (marginal zone) lymphoma
- ❑ (G) Waldenström macroglobulinemia

15 An 18-month-old child has developed seborrheic skin eruptions over the past 3 months. She has had recurrent upper respiratory and middle ear infections with *Streptococcus pneumoniae* for the past year. Physical examination indicates that she also has hepatosplenomegaly and generalized lymphadenopathy. Her hearing is reduced in the right ear. A skull radiograph shows an expansile, 2-cm lytic lesion involving the right temporal bone. Laboratory studies show no anemia, thrombocytopenia, or leukopenia. The mass is curetted. Which of the following is most likely to be seen on microscopic examination of this mass?

- ❑ (A) Histiocytes with Birbeck granules
- ❑ (B) Lymphoblasts
- ❑ (C) Plasma cells with Russell bodies
- ❑ (D) Reed-Sternberg cells
- ❑ (E) Ringed sideroblasts
- ❑ (F) Sézary cells

16 A 50-year-old woman sees her physician because of a 3-month history of fatigue and dizziness. She has recently experienced syncopal episodes. On physical examination, she is afebrile, with a pulse of 88/min, respirations 19/min, and blood pressure 115/75 mm Hg. She exhibits marked pallor but no hepatosplenomegaly or lymphadenopathy. Laboratory findings show hemoglobin of 6.6 gm/dL, hematocrit 19.9%, platelet count 199,800/mm³, WBC count 4780/mm³, and reticulocyte count 0.1%. The MCV, MCHC, and serum ferritin level are normal. A bone marrow biopsy specimen of aspirate shows normal cellularity, but the cells of the erythroid

series, such as pronormoblasts, normoblasts, and later stages, are greatly reduced. Other elements are normal in number and differentiation. Which of the following is the most likely diagnosis?

- ❑ (A) Breast carcinoma
- ❑ (B) Hairy cell leukemia
- ❑ (C) Hodgkin disease, mixed cellularity type
- ❑ (D) Multiple myeloma
- ❑ (E) Mycosis fungoides
- ❑ (F) Thymoma
- ❑ (G) Waldenström macroglobulinemia

17 A 46-year-old man notices that his friends have been commenting about his increasingly ruddy complexion over the past 4 months. He also has experienced increasing fatigue. On physical examination, he is afebrile, and his spleen tip is palpable. Laboratory studies show hemoglobin of 21.3 g/dL, hematocrit 63.9%, platelet count 376,000/mm³, and WBC count 9210/mm³. The serum erythropoietin level is very low. Which of the following is most likely to produce these findings?

- ❑ (A) Dehydration
- ❑ (B) Renal cell carcinoma
- ❑ (C) Polycythemia vera
- ❑ (D) Cyanotic heart disease
- ❑ (E) Living at high altitude

18 A 41-year-old man has had fevers with chills and rigors for the past 2 weeks. On physical examination, his temperature is 39.2°C. A CBC shows hemoglobin of 13.9 g/dL, hematocrit 40.5%, MCV 93 μm³, platelet count 210,000/mm³, and WBC count 13,750/mm³ with 75% segmented neutrophils, 10% bands, 10% lymphocytes, and 5% monocytes. A bone marrow biopsy specimen shows hypercellularity with a marked increase in myeloid precursors at all stages of maturation and in band neutrophils. These findings are most likely caused by which of the following conditions?

- ❑ (A) Acute viral hepatitis
- ❑ (B) Glucocorticoid therapy
- ❑ (C) Lung abscess
- ❑ (D) Vigorous exercise
- ❑ (E) Acute myelogenous leukemia

19 A 37-year-old man known to have been infected with HIV for the past 10 years is admitted to the hospital with abdominal pain of 3 days' duration. Physical examination shows abdominal distention and absent bowel sounds. An abdominal CT scan shows a mass lesion involving the ileum. He undergoes surgery to remove an area of bowel obstruction in the ileum. Gross examination of the specimen shows a firm, white mass, 10-cm long and 3 cm at its greatest depth. The mass has infiltrated through the wall of the ileum. Histologic studies show a mitotically active population of CD19+ lymphoid cells with prominent nuclei and nucleoli. Molecular analysis is most likely to show which of the following viral genomes in the lymphoid cells?

- ❑ (A) Epstein-Barr virus
- ❑ (B) HIV
- ❑ (C) Human herpesvirus type 8
- ❑ (D) Human T-cell leukemia/lymphoma virus type 1
- ❑ (E) Cytomegalovirus

20 A 70-year-old man has experienced increasing fatigue for the past 6 months. On physical examination, he has non-tender axillary and cervical lymphadenopathy, but there is no hepatosplenomegaly. The hematologic workup shows hemoglobin of 9.5 g/dL, hematocrit 28%, MCV 90 μm³, platelet count 120,000/mm³, and WBC count 42,000/mm³. The peripheral blood smear shows a monotonous population of small, round, mature-looking lymphocytes. Flow cytometry shows these cells to be CD19+, CD5+, and TdT−. Which of the following is most likely to be seen with cytogenetic and molecular analysis of the cells in the patient's blood?

❏ (A) t(9;22) leading to *BCR-ABL* rearrangement
❏ (B) Clonal rearrangement of immunoglobulin genes
❏ (C) Clonal rearrangement of T-cell receptor genes
❏ (D) t(8;14) leading to *C-MYC* overexpression
❏ (E) t(14;18) leading to *BCL2* overexpression

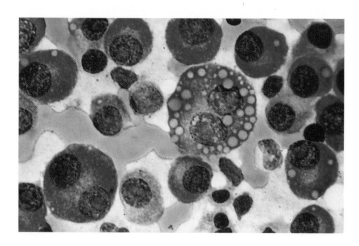

21 A 69-year-old woman complains of increasing back pain for 1 month. On physical examination, there is tenderness over the lower back but no kyphosis or scoliosis. A radiograph of the spine shows a partial collapse of T11 and several 0.5- to 1.5-cm lytic lesions with a rounded "soap-bubble" appearance in the thoracic and lumbar vertebrae. A bone marrow biopsy is performed, and a smear of the aspirate is shown. Which of the following is the most likely laboratory finding in this patient?

❏ (A) Bence-Jones proteins in the urine
❏ (B) t(9;22) in the karyotype of marrow
❏ (C) Elevated leukocyte alkaline phosphatase score
❏ (D) Decreased serum alkaline phosphatase level
❏ (E) Platelet count of 750,000/mm³
❏ (F) WBC count of 394,000/mm³

22 A 33-year-old woman reports having generalized fatigue and night sweats for 3 months. Physical examination shows nontender right cervical lymphadenopathy. Biopsy of one lymph node shows a microscopic pattern of thick bands of fibrous connective tissue with intervening lymphocytes, plasma cells, eosinophils, macrophages, and occasional Reed-Sternberg cells. An abdominal CT scan and bone marrow biopsy specimen show no abnormalities. Which of the following is the most likely subtype and stage of this patient's disease?

❏ (A) Lymphocyte predominance, stage I
❏ (B) Lymphocyte predominance, stage II
❏ (C) Nodular sclerosis, stage I
❏ (D) Mixed cellularity, stage II
❏ (E) Lymphocyte depletion, stage III

23 A 7-year-old boy has complained of worsening pain in the right side of his groin region for the past week. Physical examination shows painful, swollen lymph nodes in the right inguinal region. An inguinal lymph node biopsy is performed. Histologically, the node has large, variably sized, germinal centers containing tingible-body macrophages and numerous mitotic figures. There are numerous parafollicular and sinusoidal neutrophils. Which of the following is the most likely cause of these histologic changes?

❏ (A) Acute lymphoblastic leukemia
❏ (B) Sarcoidosis
❏ (C) Follicular lymphoma
❏ (D) Cat scratch disease
❏ (E) Acute lymphadenitis
❏ (F) Toxoplasmosis

24 A 15-year-old boy has developed a cough and a high fever over the past 4 days. On physical examination, he has a temperature of 39.2°C. Diffuse rales are heard over all lung fields. Laboratory studies show hemoglobin of 14.8 g/dL, hematocrit 44.4%, platelet count 496,000/mm³, and WBC count 15,600/mm³. Examination of the peripheral blood smear shows RBCs with marked anisocytosis and Howell-Jolly bodies. A sputum culture grows *Haemophilus influenzae*. Which of the following is the most likely diagnosis?

❏ (A) DiGeorge syndrome
❏ (B) Galactosemia
❏ (C) Gaucher disease
❏ (D) Myeloproliferative disorder
❏ (E) Prior splenectomy
❏ (F) Trisomy 21

25 A 4-year-old child has appeared listless for about 1 week. He now complains of pain when he is picked up by his mother, and he demonstrates irritability when his arms or legs are touched. In the past 2 days, several large ecchymoses have appeared on the right thigh and left shoulder. CBC shows hemoglobin of 10.2 g/dL, hematocrit 30.5%, MCV 96 μm³, platelet count 45,000/mm³, and WBC count 13,990/mm³. Examination of the peripheral blood smear shows blasts that lack peroxidase-positive granules but contain PAS-positive aggregates and stain positively for TdT. Flow cytometry shows the phenotype of blasts to be CD19+, CD3−, and sIg−. Which of the following is the most likely diagnosis?

❏ (A) Chronic myelogenous leukemia
❏ (B) Idiopathic thrombocytopenic purpura
❏ (C) Acute myelogenous leukemia
❏ (D) Chronic lymphocytic leukemia
❏ (E) Acute lymphoblastic leukemia

26 A 49-year-old woman has experienced increasing weakness and chest pain over the past 6 months. On physical examination, she is afebrile and normotensive. Motor strength is 5/5 in all extremities but diminishes to 4/5 with repetitive movement. There is no muscle pain or tenderness. Laboratory studies show hemoglobin of 14.0 g/dL, hematocrit 42%, platelet count 246,000/mm^3, and WBC count 6480/mm^3. A chest CT scan shows an irregular 10 × 12 cm anterior mediastinal mass. The surgeon has difficulty removing the mass, because it infiltrates surrounding structures. Microscopically, the mass is composed of large, spindled, atypical epithelial cells mixed with lymphoid cells. Which of the following is the most likely diagnosis of this lesion?

❑ (A) Granulomatous inflammation
❑ (B) Hodgkin disease
❑ (C) Lymphoblastic lymphoma
❑ (D) Malignant thymoma
❑ (E) Metastatic breast carcinoma
❑ (F) Organizing abscess

27 A 69-year-old man notices the presence of "lumps" in the right side of his neck that have been enlarging over the past year. Physical examination shows firm, nontender posterior cervical lymph nodes ranging from 1 to 2 cm in diameter. The overlying skin is intact and not erythematous. One of the lymph nodes is biopsied. Which of the following histologic features provides the best evidence for malignant lymphoma in this node?

❑ (A) Presence of lymphoid cells positive for kappa, but not lambda, light chains
❑ (B) Absence of a pattern of follicles with germinal centers
❑ (C) Proliferation of small capillaries in the medullary and paracortical regions
❑ (D) Presence of cells that stain with monoclonal antibody to the CD30 antigen
❑ (E) Absence of plasma cells and immunoblasts in sinusoidal spaces

28 A 62-year-old man visits his physician because of prolonged fever and a 4-kg weight loss over the past 6 months. On physical examination, his temperature is 38.6°C. He has generalized nontender lymphadenopathy, and the spleen tip is palpable. Laboratory studies show hemoglobin of 10.1 g/dL, hematocrit 30.3%, platelet count 140,000/mm^3, and WBC count 24,500/mm^3 with 10% segmented neutrophils, 1% bands, 86% lymphocytes, and 3% monocytes. A cervical lymph node biopsy specimen shows a nodular pattern of small lymphoid cells. A bone marrow specimen shows infiltrates of similar small cells having surface immunoglobulin that are CD5+ but CD10−. Cytogenetic analysis indicates t(11;14) in these cells. Which of the following is the most likely diagnosis?

❑ (A) Mantle cell lymphoma
❑ (B) Follicular lymphoma
❑ (C) Acute lymphoblastic leukemia
❑ (D) Burkitt lymphoma
❑ (E) Small lymphocytic lymphoma

29 A 45-year-old man has experienced recurrent fevers and a 6-kg weight loss over the past 5 months. On physical examination, his temperature is 37.5°C, and he has cervical lymphadenopathy. The patient reports that the adenopathy becomes very tender after he drinks a six-pack of beer. A lymph node biopsy specimen shows effacement of the nodal architecture by a population of small lymphocytes, plasma cells, eosinophils, and macrophages. Which of the following additional cell types, which stains positively for CD15, is most likely to be found in this disease?

❑ (A) Reed-Sternberg cell
❑ (B) Immunoblast
❑ (C) Epithelioid cell
❑ (D) Neutrophils
❑ (E) Mast cell

30 A 23-year-old woman has noticed that she develops a skin rash if she spends prolonged periods outdoors. She has a malar skin rash on physical examination. Laboratory studies include a positive ANA test result with a titer of 1:1024 and a "rim" pattern. An anti–double-stranded DNA test result is also positive. The hemoglobin concentration is 12.1 g/dL, hematocrit 35.5%, MCV 89 μm^3, platelet count 109,000/mm^3, and WBC count 4500/mm^3. Which of the following findings is most likely to be demonstrated by a WBC differential count?

❑ (A) Eosinophilia
❑ (B) Thrombocytosis
❑ (C) Monocytosis
❑ (D) Neutrophilia
❑ (E) Basophilia

Normal serum

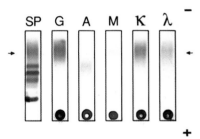

Patient serum

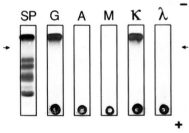

SP, serum protein electrophoresis; G, A, M, κ, and λ are gels with specific stains for IgG, IgA, IgM, kappa light chain, and lambda light chains, respectively. (Courtesy of Dr. David Sacks, Department of Pathology, Brigham and Women's Hospital, Boston, MA.)

31 A 58-year-old man reports increasing malaise over the past 8 months. On physical examination, there are no remarkable findings. Laboratory studies include serum creatinine of 4.0 mg/dL, urea nitrogen 38 mg/dL, total protein 9.3 g/dL, albumin 4.1 g/dL, and alkaline phosphatase 297 U/L. The finding on serum protein electrophoresis is shown. Which of the following laboratory findings is most likely to be reported?

❑ (A) TdT+ circulating blasts
❑ (B) Bence Jones proteinuria
❑ (C) Bone marrow karyotype with t(8;14)
❑ (D) Reactive amyloidosis
❑ (E) Hematocrit of 62%

32 In an experiment, cell samples are collected from the bone marrow aspirates of patients who were diagnosed with lymphoproliferative disorders. Cytogenetic analyses are performed on these cells, and a subset of the cases is found to have the *BCR-ABL* fusion gene from the reciprocal translocation t(9;22)(q34;11). The presence of this gene results in increased tyrosine kinase activity. Patients with which of the following conditions are most likely to have this gene?

- (A) Follicular lymphoma
- (B) Chronic myelogenous leukemia
- (C) Hodgkin disease, lymphocyte depletion type
- (D) Acute promyelocytic leukemia
- (E) Multiple myeloma

33 A 64-year-old man has inguinal, axillary, and cervical lymphadenopathy. The nodes are firm and nontender. A biopsy specimen of a cervical node shows a histologic pattern of nodular aggregates of small, cleaved lymphoid cells and larger cells with open nuclear chromatin, several nucleoli, and moderate amounts of cytoplasm. A bone marrow biopsy specimen shows lymphoid aggregates of similar cells with surface immunoglobulin that are CD10+ but CD5–. Karyotyping of these lymphoid cells indicates the presence of t(14;18). Which of the following is the most likely diagnosis?

- (A) Hodgkin disease, nodular sclerosis type
- (B) Acute lymphadenitis
- (C) Follicular lymphoma
- (D) Mantle cell lymphoma
- (E) Toxoplasmosis

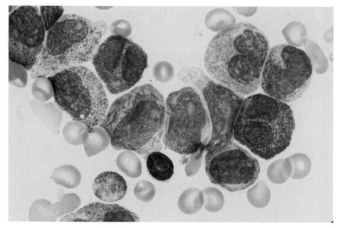

Courtesy of Dr. Robert W. McKenna, Department of Pathology, University of Texas Southwestern Medical School, Dallas, TX.

34 A 39-year-old man experiences sudden onset of a severe headache. Physical examination shows no localizing neurologic signs and no organomegaly. A stool sample is positive for occult blood. Areas of purpura appear on the skin of his extremities. Laboratory studies show hemoglobin of 9.6 g/dL, hematocrit 28.9%, platelet count 26,400/mm³, and WBC count 75,000/mm³. The peripheral blood smear has the appearance shown above, and schistocytes are also seen. The plasma D dimer level (fibrin degradation products), prothrombin time, and partial thromboplastin time are all elevated. Cytogenetic analysis of cells from a bone marrow biopsy specimen is most likely to yield which of the following karyotypic abnormalities?

- (A) t(8;21)
- (B) t(9;22)
- (C) t(14;18)
- (D) t(15;17)
- (E) t(8;14)

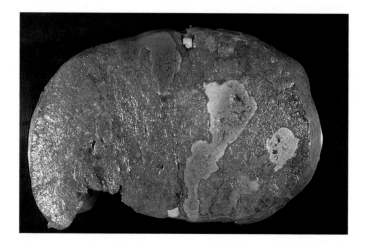

35 A 27-year-old man visits the physician because he has had a fever for the past 10 days. On physical examination, his temperature is 37.9°C, pulse 87/min, respirations 21/min, and blood pressure 100/55 mm Hg. A diastolic murmur is heard on auscultation of the chest. The tip of the spleen is palpable and tender. Laboratory studies show hemoglobin of 12.8 g/dL, hematocrit 38.4%, platelet count 231,000/mm³, and WBC count 12,980/mm³ with 70% segmented neutrophils, 6% bands, 1% metamyelocytes, 19% lymphocytes, and 4% monocytes. The representative gross appearance of the spleen is shown above. Which of the following is the most likely diagnosis?

- (A) Acute myelogenous leukemia
- (B) Disseminated histoplasmosis
- (C) Hodgkin disease
- (D) Infective endocarditis
- (E) Metastatic carcinoma
- (F) Micronodular cirrhosis
- (G) Rheumatic heart disease

36 A 29-year-old woman known to be infected with HIV has developed fever, cough, and dyspnea over the past week. On physical examination, her temperature is 37.9°C. There is dullness to percussion over lung fields posteriorly. A bronchoalveolar lavage is performed and cysts of *Pneumocystis carinii* are present. She is given trimethoprim-sulfamethoxazole. One week later, her respiratory status has improved. Laboratory studies now show hemoglobin of 7.4 g/dL, hematocrit 22.2%, MCV 98 μm³, platelet count 47,000/mm³, and WBC count 1870/mm³ with 2% segmented neutrophils, 2% bands, 85% lymphocytes, 10% monocytes, and 1% eosinophils. One week later, she experiences increasing dyspnea, and a chest CT scan shows multiple 1- to 3-cm nodules with hemorrhagic borders in all lung fields. These nodules are most likely to be caused by infection with which of the following organisms?

❏ (A) *Aspergillus fumigatus*
❏ (B) *Bartonella henselae*
❏ (C) Mycobacterium avium-complex
❏ (E) *Escherichia coli*
❏ (H) Herpes simplex virus
❏ (I) *Pneumocystis carinii*
❏ (J) *Toxoplasma gondii*

37 A 39-year-old woman felt a lump in her breast 1 week ago. She visits the physician, who palpates a firm, fixed, irregular 3-cm mass in the upper outer quadrant of the right breast and a firm, nontender lymph node in the right axilla. A lumpectomy and axillary node dissection are performed, and microscopic examination shows an infiltrating ductal carcinoma present in the breast. Flow cytometric analysis of the node shows a polyclonal population of CD3+, CD19+, CD20+, and CD68+ cells with no aneuploidy or increase in S-phase. Which of the following is most likely to be present on microscopic examination of this axillary node?

❏ (A) Acute lymphadenitis
❏ (B) Diffuse large B-cell lymphoma
❏ (C) Metastatic infiltrating ductal carcinoma
❏ (D) Necrotizing granulomas
❏ (E) Plasmacytosis
❏ (F) Sinus histiocytosis

38 A 41-year-old man has experienced several bouts of pneumonia over the past year. He now complains of vague abdominal pain and a dragging sensation. Physical examination shows marked splenomegaly. CBC shows hemoglobin of 8.2 g/dL, hematocrit 24.6%, MCV 90 μm³, platelet count 63,000/mm³, and WBC count 2400/mm³. The peripheral blood smear shows many small leukocytes with reniform nuclei and pale blue cytoplasm with threadlike extensions. A chest x-ray shows patchy infiltrates, and a culture of sputum grows *Mycobacterium Kansasii*. Which of the following laboratory findings is most characteristic of this disease?

❏ (A) CD19, CD20, and CD11c expression in leukocytes
❏ (B) Presence of Auer rods in leukocytes
❏ (C) Presence of Ph¹ chromosome
❏ (D) Presence of toxic granulations in neutrophils
❏ (E) Monoclonal IgM in serum

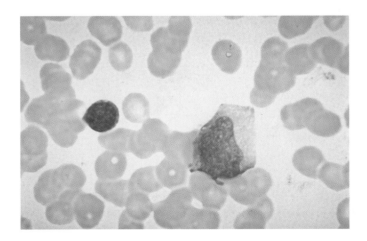

39 A previously healthy 23-year-old man has experienced malaise and a low-grade fever and sore throat for 2 weeks. On physical examination, his temperature is 37.6°C, and he has pharyngeal erythema without exudation. There is tender cervical, axillary, and inguinal lymphadenopathy. Laboratory studies show hemoglobin of 12.2 g/dL, hematocrit 36.6%, platelet count 190,200/mm³, and WBC count 8940/mm³. The peripheral blood smear is shown in the preceding figure. Which of the following is the most likely risk factor for the disease that would be diagnosed in this patient?

❏ (A) An inherited disorder of globin chain synthesis
❏ (B) Transfusion of packed RBCs
❏ (C) Close personal contact (kissing) with his date
❏ (D) Sharing infected needles for intravenous drug use
❏ (E) Ingestion of raw oysters

40 A 38-year-old woman visits her physician because she has had bleeding gums for the past 3 weeks. Physical examination shows that her gingivae are thickened and friable. She has hepatosplenomegaly and generalized nontender lymphadenopathy. CBC shows hemoglobin of 11.2 g/dL, hematocrit 33.9%, MCV 89 μm³, platelet count 95,000/mm³, and WBC count 4500/mm³ with 25% segmented neutrophils, 10% bands, 2% metamyelocytes, 55% lymphocytes, 8% monocytes, and 1 nucleated RBC per 100 WBCs. A bone marrow biopsy specimen shows 100% cellularity, with many large blasts that are peroxidase negative and nonspecific esterase positive. Which of the following is the most likely diagnosis?

❏ (A) Acute lymphoblastic leukemia
❏ (B) Acute megakaryocytic leukemia
❏ (C) Acute promyelocytic leukemia
❏ (D) Acute erythroleukemia
❏ (E) Acute monocytic leukemia

41 A 7-year-old boy has complained of a severe headache for the past week. On physical examination, there is tenderness on palpation of long bones, hepatosplenomegaly, and generalized lymphadenopathy. Petechial hemorrhages are present on the skin. Laboratory studies show hemoglobin of 8.8 g/dL, hematocrit 26.5%, platelet count 34,700/mm³, and WBC count 14,800/mm³. A bone marrow biopsy specimen shows 100% cellularity, with almost complete replacement by a population of large cells with scant cytoplasm lacking granules, delicate nuclear chromatin, and rare nucleoli. He receives a course of chemotherapy and achieves a complete remission. Which of the following combinations of phenotypic and karyotypic markers is most likely to be present in this patient?

❏ (A) Early pre-B (CD19+, CD10+, TdT+); hyperdiploidy
❏ (B) T cell (CD3+, CD2+, TdT+); normal karyotype
❏ (C) Pre-B (CD19+, CD10+, TdT+, Cμ+); t(9;22)
❏ (D) Early pre-B (CD19+, CD10+, TdT+); t(9;22)
❏ (E) Pre-B (CD19+, CD10+, TdT+, Cμ+); normal karyotype

42 A 51-year-old man visits his physician because the skin of his face, neck, and trunk has become scaly red. He also complains of intense itching and a 3-kg weight loss over the past 2 months. On physical examination, his temperature is 37.6°C, and he has a generalized exfoliative erythroderma. There is generalized nontender lymphadenopathy. Laboratory studies show hemoglobin of 12.9 g/dL, hematocrit 42.0%, platelet count 231,000/mm³, and WBC count 7940/mm³ with 57% segmented neutrophils, 3% bands, 26% lymphocytes, 5% monocytes, and 9% eosinophils. A skin biopsy specimen shows the presence of lymphoid cells in the upper dermis and epidermis. These cells have cerebriform nuclei with marked infolding of nuclear membranes. Similar cells are seen on the peripheral blood smear. Which combination of the following phenotypic markers is most likely to be expressed on his abnormal lymphocytes?

☐ (A) CD3+, CD4+
☐ (B) CD3−, CD56+
☐ (C) CD19+, sIg+
☐ (D) CD5+, CD10−, CD19+
☐ (E) CD33+, CD13+

43 A 65-year-old man sees his physician because he has experienced fatigue, a 5-kg weight loss, night sweats, and abdominal discomfort for the past year. On physical examination, he has marked splenomegaly; there is no lymphadenopathy. Laboratory studies show hemoglobin of 10.1 g/dL, hematocrit 30.5%, MCV 89 μm³, platelet count 94,000/mm³, and WBC count 14,750/mm³ with 55% segmented neutrophils, 9% bands, 20% lymphocytes, 8% monocytes, 4% metamyelocytes, 3% myelocytes, 1% eosinophils and 2 nucleated RBCs per 100 WBCs. The peripheral blood smear also shows tear-drop cells. The serum uric acid level is 12 mg/dL. A bone marrow biopsy specimen shows extensive marrow fibrosis and clusters of atypical megakaryocytes. Which of the following pathologic findings is most likely to account for the enlargement in this patient's spleen?

☐ (A) Reed-Sternberg cells mixed with many more lymphocytes, plasma cells, eosinophils, and macrophages
☐ (B) Proliferation of all hematopoietic lineages, with prominence of megakaryocytes
☐ (C) Chronic passive venous congestion and fibrosis
☐ (D) Multiple caseating granulomas, containing macrophages with *Histoplasma capsulatum*
☐ (E) Diffuse infiltration by metastatic adenocarcinoma

44 A 60-year-old man has experienced vague abdominal discomfort accompanied by bloating and diarrhea for the past 6 months. On physical examination, there is a midabdominal firm mass. The stool is positive for occult blood. An abdominal CT scan shows a 5 × 12 cm mass involving the wall of the distal ileum and adjacent mesentery. A laparotomy is performed, and the mass is removed. Microscopically, the mass is composed of sheets of large lymphoid cells with large nuclei, prominent nucleoli, and frequent mitoses. The neoplastic cells mark with CD19+ and CD20+ and have the *BCL6* gene rearrangement. Which of the following prognostic features is most applicable to this case?

☐ (A) Indolent disease with survival of 7 to 9 years without treatment
☐ (B) Aggressive disease that can be cured by aggressive chemotherapy
☐ (C) Aggressive disease that does not respond to chemotherapy and transforms to acute leukemia
☐ (D) Indolent disease that can be cured by chemotherapy
☐ (E) Indolent disease that often undergoes spontaneous remission

45 A 45-year-old man has experienced a gradual weight loss and weakness, anorexia, and easy fatigability for 7 months. Physical examination shows marked splenomegaly. CBC shows hemoglobin of 12.9 g/dL, hematocrit 38.1%, MCV 92 μm³, platelet count 410,000/mm³, and WBC count 168,000/mm³. The peripheral blood smear is depicted in part A of the figure below. Karyotypic analysis shows the Ph¹ chromosome. He undergoes chemotherapy with imatinib mesylate

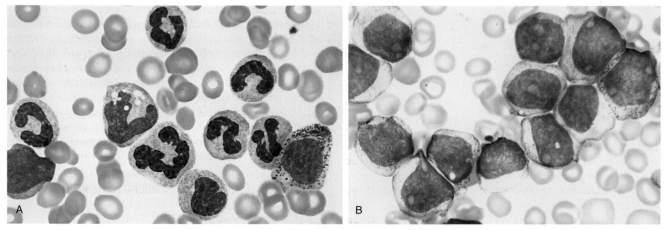

Courtesy of Dr. Robert W. McKenna, Department of Pathology, University of Texas Southwestern Medical School, Dallas, TX.
Courtesy of Dr. Jacqueline Mitus.

(tyrosine kinase inhibitor), which reduces the spleen size and brings the total leukocyte count within normal range. He remains in remission for 3 years and then begins to experience fatigue and a 10-kg weight loss. Physical examination now shows petechial hemorrhages. CBC shows hemoglobin of 10.5 g/dL, hematocrit 30%, platelet count 60,000/μL, and WBC count 40,000/μL. A peripheral blood smear is depicted in part B of the figure. Karyotypic analysis shows two Ph[1] chromosomes and aneuploidy. Flow cytometric analysis of the peripheral blood shows CD19+, CD10+, sIg−, CD3− cells. Which of the following complications of the initial disease did this patient develop following therapy?

- (A) Sézary syndrome
- (B) Myelodysplastic syndrome
- (C) Hairy cell leukemia
- (D) B-lymphoblastic leukemia
- (E) Acute myeloblastic leukemia

46 A 14-year-old boy complains of a feeling of discomfort in his chest that has worsened over the past 5 days. On physical examination, he has generalized lymphadenopathy. A chest radiograph shows clear lung fields, but there appears to be widening of the mediastinum. A chest CT scan shows a 10-cm mass in the anterior mediastinum. A biopsy specimen of the mass shows lymphoid cells with lobulated nuclei having delicate, finely stippled, nuclear chromatin. There is scant cytoplasm, and many mitoses are seen. The cells express TdT, CD1, CD3, and CD5 antigens. Which of the following is the most likely diagnosis?

- (A) Lymphoblastic lymphoma
- (B) Burkitt lymphoma
- (C) Hodgkin disease, nodular sclerosing type
- (D) Mantle cell lymphoma
- (E) Follicular lymphoma
- (F) Small lymphocytic lymphoma

47 A 60-year-old woman has had headaches and dizziness for the past 5 weeks. She has been taking cimetidine for heartburn and omeprazole for ulcers. On physical examination, she is afebrile and normotensive, and her face has a plethoric to cyanotic appearance. There is mild splenomegaly but no other abnormal findings. Laboratory studies show hemoglobin of 21.7 gm/dL, hematocrit 65%, platelet count 400,000/mm³, and WBC count 30,000/mm³ with 85% polymorphonuclear leukocytes, 10% lymphocytes, and 5% monocytes. The peripheral blood smear shows abnormally large platelets and nucleated RBCs. The serum erythropoietin level is undetectable, but the ferritin level is normal. Which of the following is most characteristic of the natural history of this patient's disease?

- (A) Death from transformation of the disease into acute B-lymphoblastic leukemia
- (B) Onset of marrow fibrosis with extensive extramedullary hematopoiesis in the spleen
- (C) Spontaneous remissions and relapses without any treatment
- (D) Gradual increase in monoclonal serum immunoglobulins
- (E) Development of a gastric lymphoma

48 A clinical study is performed in which the subjects are children from 1 to 4 years of age who have had multiple infections with viral, fungal, and parasitic diseases. Compared with a normal control group these children do not have a subpopulation of cells lacking surface immunoglobulin that mark with CD1a, CD2, CD3, CD4, and CD8. Which of the following karyotypic abnormalities is most likely to be seen in the children in this study?

- (A) +21
- (B) 22q11.2
- (C) t(9;22)
- (D) t(15;17)
- (E) X(fra)
- (F) XXY

49 A 38-year-old woman has experienced increasing dyspnea for the past 2 months. On physical examination, she is afebrile and normotensive. Inspiratory wheezes are noted on auscultation of the chest. A chest CT scan shows an 8 × 10 cm posterior mediastinal mass that impinges on the trachea and esophagus. A mediastinoscopy is performed, and the mass is biopsied. Histologically, there are scattered large multinucleated cells, with prominent nucleoli that mark with CD15, and lymphocytes and macrophages separated by dense collagenous bands. Which of the following is most likely to be seen microscopically in this biopsy?

- (A) Atypical lymphocytes
- (B) Histiocytes with Birbeck granules
- (C) Hairy cells
- (D) Lacunar cells
- (E) Lymphoblasts
- (F) Myeloblasts

50 A 30-year-old previously healthy man has had an enlarging nodular area on his arm for the past 8 months. On physical examination, there is an ulcerated, reddish-violet, 3 × 7 cm lesion on his right forearm and nontender right axillary and left inguinal lymphadenopathy. A chest radiograph shows a 4-cm nodular left pleural mass. An abdominal CT scan shows a 5-cm right retroperitoneal mass. Biopsy of an inguinal node is performed, and microscopic examination shows large anaplastic cells, some of which contain horseshoe-shaped nuclei and voluminous cytoplasm. The tumor cells cluster around venules and infiltrate sinuses. He goes into remission following chemotherapy. Which of the following immunohistochemical markers is most likely to be positive in the tumor cells?

- (A) Anaplastic lymphoma kinase protein
- (B) CD10
- (C) cKIT proto-oncogene
- (D) HTLV-1
- (E) p24 antigen

51 A 28-year-old man is brought to the emergency department with shock that developed over the past 12 hours. On physical examination, his temperature is 38.6°C, pulse 101/min, respirations 19/min, and blood pressure 80/40 mm Hg. Needle tracks are noted in the left antecubital fossa. There are crackles heard over the lower lung fields. CBC shows hemoglobin of 14.1 g/dL, hematocrit 42.6%, MCV 93 μm³, platelet count 127,500/mm³, and WBC count 12,150/mm³ with 71% segmented neutrophils, 8% bands, 14% lymphocytes, and 7% monocytes. The neutrophils show cytoplasmic toxic granulations and Döhle bodies. Which of the following is the most likely diagnosis?

☐ (A) Pulmonary *Mycobacterium tuberculosis*
☐ (B) Acute myelogenous leukemia
☐ (C) Chronic myelogenous leukemia
☐ (D) *Pseudomonas aeruginosa* septicemia
☐ (E) Infectious mononucleosis
☐ (F) *Pneumocystis carinii* pneumonia

52 A 15-year-old girl experiences sudden onset of severe dyspnea. On physical examination, her temperature is 36.9°C, pulse 92/min, respirations 22/min, and blood pressure 100/65 mm Hg. Expiratory wheezes are auscultated over both lungs. There is no lymphadenopathy. Laboratory studies show hemoglobin of 14.7 g/dL, hematocrit 43.1%, MCV 92 μm³, platelet count 233,000/mm³, and WBC count 9750/mm³ with 58% segmented neutrophils, 4% bands, 22% lymphocytes, 4% monocytes, and 12% eosinophils. Which of the following is the most likely diagnosis?

☐ (A) Bacterial septicemia
☐ (B) Bronchial asthma
☐ (C) Chronic myelogenous leukemia
☐ (D) *Pneumocystis carinii* pneumonia
☐ (E) Pulmonary *Mycobacterium tuberculosis*
☐ (F) Systemic lupus erythematosus

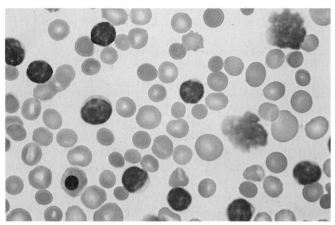

Courtesy of Dr. Robert W. McKenna, Department of Pathology,

53 A figure skater who won gold medals at the 1928, 1932, and 1936 Winter Olympic Games became progressively fatigued in her late fifties. On physical examination, she had palpable nontender axillary and inguinal lymph nodes, and the spleen tip was palpable. Laboratory studies showed hemoglobin of 10.1 g/dL, hematocrit 30.5%, MCV 90 μm³, platelet count 89,000/mm³, and WBC count 31,300/mm³. From the peripheral blood picture shown above, which of the following is the most likely diagnosis?

☐ (A) Infectious mononucleosis
☐ (B) Chronic lymphocytic leukemia
☐ (C) Iron deficiency anemia
☐ (D) Leukemoid reaction
☐ (E) Acute lymphoblastic leukemia

54 A 48-year old man visits his physician for a routine health maintenance examination. He has no complaints other than worrying about getting older and having cancer. Physical examination shows that he is afebrile and normotensive. There is no hepatosplenomegaly or lymphadenopathy. Laboratory studies show a total serum protein level of 7.4 g/dL and albumin level of 3.9 g/dL. The serum calcium and phosphorus levels are normal. Urinalysis shows no Bence Jones proteinuria. The hemoglobin is 13.6 g/dL, platelet count 301,500/mm³, and WBC count 6630/mm³. A serum protein electrophoresis shows a small (2.8-g) spike of γ-globulin, which is determined by immunoelectrophoresis to be IgG kappa. A bone marrow biopsy specimen shows normal cellularity with maturation of all cell lines. Plasma cells constitute about 4% of the marrow. A bone scan is normal, and there are no areas of increased uptake. Which of the following is the most likely diagnosis?

☐ (A) Solitary plasmacytoma
☐ (B) Waldenström macroglobulinemia
☐ (C) Monoclonal gammopathy of undetermined significance
☐ (D) Heavy-chain disease
☐ (E) Multiple myeloma
☐ (F) Reactive systemic amyloidosis

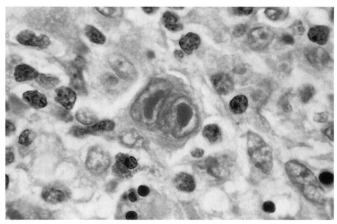

University of Texas Southwestern Medical School, Dallas, TX.

55 A 32-year-old woman visits her physician because she has experienced fatigue, fever, night sweats, and painless lumps in the right side of her neck for the past 3 months. On physical examination, her temperature is 37.5°C. She has right cervical nontender lymphadenopathy. One of the lymph nodes is biopsied, and the histologic finding is shown above at high power. Molecular analysis of large cells exemplified by the cell of the center is most likely to reveal which of the following genetic abnormalities?

- ❑ (A) Clonal rearrangement of T cell receptor genes
- ❑ (B) Clonal rearrangement of immunoglobulin genes
- ❑ (C) Polyclonal rearrangement of T cell receptor genes
- ❑ (D) Polyclonal rearrangement of immunoglobulin genes
- ❑ (E) Integration of the cytomegalovirus genome
- ❑ (F) Integration of the human herpesvirus-8 genome
- ❑ (G) Integration of the HTLV-1 genome

56 A 22-year-old university student reports easy fatigability of 2 months' duration. On physical examination, she has no hepatosplenomegaly or lymphadenopathy. Mucosal gingival hemorrhages are noted. CBC shows hemoglobin of 9.5 g/dL, hematocrit 28.2%, MCV 94 μm^3, platelet count 20,000/mm^3, and WBC count 107,000/mm^3. A bone marrow biopsy specimen shows that the marrow is 100% cellular with few residual normal hematopoietic cells. Most of the cells in the marrow are large, with nuclei having delicate chromatin and several nucleoli. The cytoplasm of these cells has azurophilic, peroxidase-positive granules. Which of the following is the most likely diagnosis?

- ❑ (A) Chronic lymphocytic leukemia
- ❑ (B) Acute myelogenous leukemia
- ❑ (C) Acute megakaryocytic leukemia
- ❑ (D) Chronic myelogenous leukemia
- ❑ (E) Acute lymphoblastic leukemia

57 A 9-year-old otherwise healthy girl has complained of pain in the right armpit for the past week. Examination by the physician shows tender lymphadenopathy of the right axillary region. There are four linear and nearly healed abrasions over a 3 × 2 cm area of the distal ventral aspect of the right forearm and a single, 0.5-cm, slightly raised erythematous nodule over one of the abrasions. No other abnormalities are noted. If a lymph node biopsy were performed, the microscopic appearance of the specimen would show a pattern of stellate, necrotizing granulomas. The lymphadenopathy regresses over the next 2 months. Infection with which of the following is most likely to have produced these findings?

- ❑ (A) *Bartonella henselae*
- ❑ (B) Cytomegalovirus
- ❑ (C) Epstein-Barr virus
- ❑ (D) *Staphylococcus aureus*
- ❑ (E) *Yersinia pestis*

ANSWERS

1 (E) The major finding in this patient is marked granulocytopenia. All that remains on the peripheral smear are mononuclear cells (remember to multiply the percentages in the differential by the total WBC count to get the absolute values; rather than one cell line being over-represented, another may be nearly missing). Accelerated removal or destruction of neutrophils could account for the selective absence of granulocytes in this case. Overwhelming infections cause increased peripheral use of neutrophils at sites of inflammation. Petechial hemorrhages also can occur in overwhelming bacterial infections, such as those caused by *Neisseria meningitidis*. Bleeding is unlikely to be caused by

thrombocytopenia, because the platelet count is normal. Normal bone marrow findings exclude acute lymphoid or myeloid leukemia. In aplastic anemia, the marrow is poorly cellular, and there is a reduction in RBCs, WBCs, and platelet production.

BP7 416   BP6 359   PBD7 662-663   PBD6 646

2 (D) Shown here are the famous rodlike tubular Birbeck granules, with the characteristic periodicity seen in Langerhans cell proliferations. In this case, the skin eruptions, organomegaly, and lesion in the mastoid suggest infiltrates in multiple organs. The diagnosis is multifocal Langerhans cell histiocytosis, a disease most often seen in children. In one half of these cases, exophthalmos occurs, and involvement of the hypothalamus and pituitary stalk leads to diabetes insipidus; these findings are then called Hand-Schüller-Christian disease. Acute lymphoblastic leukemia in children can involve the marrow but does not produce skin or bone lesions. Myeloma is a disease of adults that can produce lytic bone lesions but not skin lesions. Hodgkin disease is seen in young adults and does not produce skin lesions or bone lesions. Tuberculosis can produce granulomatous disease with bony destruction, but the macrophages present in the granulomas are epithelioid macrophages that do not have Birbeck granules.

BP7 441   BP6 383   PBD7 701-702   PBD6 685-686

3 (A) This patient has symptoms of hyperviscosity syndrome, including visual disturbances, dizziness, and headaches. He also appears to have Raynaud phenomena. His bone marrow is infiltrated with plasmacytoid lymphocytes that have stored immunoglobulins in the cytoplasm (Russell bodies). All of these findings suggest that the patient has lymphoplasmacytic lymphoma (Waldenström macroglobulinemia). In this disorder, neoplastic B cells differentiate to IgM-producing cells; hence, there is a monoclonal IgM spike in the serum. These IgM molecules aggregate and produce hyperviscosity, and some of them agglutinate at low temperatures and produce cold agglutinin disease. There is typically no leukemic phase to Waldenström macroglobulinemia. Myeloma, which is typically accompanied by a monoclonal gammopathy, most often does not cause liver and spleen enlargement, and morphologically, the cells resemble plasma cells. Hypercalcemia occurs with myeloma because of bone destruction, and punched-out lytic lesions are typical of multiple myeloma. Light chains in urine (Bence Jones proteins) are also a feature of multiple myeloma. A t(14;18) translocation is characteristic of a follicular lymphoma.

BP7 431   BP6 381   PBD7 681-682   PBD6 666-667

4 (D) Marked leukocytosis and immature myeloid cells in the peripheral blood can represent an exaggerated response to infection (leukemoid reaction), or they can be a manifestation of chronic myelogenous leukemia (CML). The leukocyte alkaline phosphatase score is high in the more differentiated cell population seen in reactive leukocytosis, whereas in CML, the leukocyte alkaline phosphatase score is low. The Philadelphia chromosome (universally present in CML) is lacking in patients with leukemoid reactions. Hairy cell leukemia is accompanied by peripheral blood leukocytes that mark with tartrate-resistant acid phosphatase. Hodgkin disease is not characterized by an increased WBC count. Acute lymphoblastic leukemia is a disease of children and young adults, and the lymphoid cells do not have leukocyte alkaline phosphatase.

BP7 59, 416 BP6 377 PBD7 665 PBD6 681

5 **(E)** Burkitt and Burkitt-like lymphomas can be seen sporadically (in young persons), in an endemic form in Africa (in children), and in association with HIV infection. All forms are highly associated with translocations of the *MYC* gene on chromosome 8. In the African form and in HIV-infected patients, the cells are latently infected with Epstein-Barr virus (EBV), but sporadic cases are negative for EBV. This form of lymphoma is typically extranodal. Diffuse large cell lymphomas are most common in adults, as are follicular lymphomas; they do not carry the t(8;14) translocation. Acute lymphoblastic lymphomas can be seen in boys this age, but the mass is in the mediastinum, and the lymphoid cells are T cells. Plasmacytomas appear in older adults and are unlikely to produce an abdominal mass. Because of the high growth fraction (40% in this case) Burkitt lymphomas respond very well to chemotherapy that includes cycle acting agents. By contrast, slow growing tumors with a low growth fraction are more indolent and less responsive to chemotherapy.

BP7 428-429 BP6 368 PBD7 677-678 PBD6 662-663

6 **(B)** Diffuse large B-cell lymphoma occurs in older persons and frequently manifests as localized disease with extranodal involvement, particularly of the Waldeyer ring. The staining pattern indicates a B-cell proliferation (CD19+, CD10+). T-cell (CD3) and monocytic (CD15) markers are absent. TdT can be expressed in B-lineage cells at an earlier stage of maturation. Small lymphocytic lymphoma is also a B-cell neoplasm, but it manifests with widespread lymphadenopathy, liver and spleen enlargement, and lymphocytosis. Lymphoblastic lymphoma is a T-cell neoplasm that occurs typically in the mediastinum of children. Hodgkin disease is characterized by Reed-Sternberg cells. In chronic lymphadenitis, the lymph node has many cell types—macrophages, lymphocytes, and plasma cells. A monomorphous infiltrate is typical of non-Hodgkin lymphomas.

BP7 427-428 BP6 366-367 PBD7 676-677
PBD6 654-656

7 **(E)** This patient has polycythemia vera, a myeloproliferative disorder characterized by an increased RBC mass, with hematocrit concentrations typically exceeding 60%. Although the increased RBC mass is responsible for most of the symptoms and signs, these patients also have thrombocytosis and granulocytosis. This occurs because, like other myeloproliferative disorders, polycythemia vera results from transformation of a multipotent stem cell. The high hematocrit concentration causes an increase in blood volume and distention of blood vessels. When combined with abnormal platelet function, this condition predisposes the patient to bleeding. Abnormal platelet function can also predispose to thrombosis. The pruritus and peptic ulceration most likely are the result of the histamine release from basophils. In some patients, the disease "burns out" to myelofibrosis. A few patients "blast out" into acute myelogenous leukemia, and other patients develop chronic myelogenous leukemia. Myelodysplastic syndromes and myeloproliferative disorders, such as essential thrombocytosis, are not accompanied by such an increase in RBC mass. Erythroleukemia typically is not accompanied by such a high

hematocrit concentration, because leukemic erythroid progenitors do not differentiate into mature RBCs.

BP7 439-440 BP6 378-379 PBD7 699-700
PBD6 682-683

8 **(C)** This patient has developed a myelodysplasia, characterized by a cellular marrow in which there are maturation defects in multiple lineages. This diagnosis is supported by the presence of ringed sideroblasts, megaloblasts, abnormal megakaryocytes, and myeloblasts in the marrow. Because the hematopoietic cells fail to mature normally, they are not released into the peripheral blood. The patient has pancytopenia and is susceptible to infections. Myelodysplasias are clonal stem cell disorders that develop de novo or after chemotherapy with alkylating agents, as in this case. The presence of chromosomal deletions such as 5q is a marker of posttherapy myelodysplasia. The morphologic abnormalities in the marrow are not seen in any of the other listed conditions.

BP7 438 BP6 376 PBD7 695-696 PBD6 678-679

9 **(A)** Essential thrombocythemia is a myeloproliferative disorder. As with all myeloproliferative diseases, the transformation occurs in a myeloid stem cell. In this form of myeloproliferative disease, the dominant cell type affected is the megakaryocyte, and hence there is thrombocytosis. However, other myeloproliferative disorders, such as chronic myelogenous leukemia, myelofibrosis, and polycythemia vera, also can be accompanied by an increased platelet count. The diagnosis of essential thrombocytosis can be made after other causes of reactive thrombocytosis are excluded, and if the bone marrow examination shows increased megakaryocytes with no evidence of leukemia. The throbbing, burning pain in the extremities is caused by platelet aggregates that occlude small arterioles. The major manifestation of this disease is thrombotic or hemorrhagic crises. The swelling in this patient's leg represents phlebothrombosis, followed by pulmonary embolism with infarction. The peripheral blood WBC count would be high in acute myelogenous leukemia, without thrombocytosis.

PBD7 700 PBD6 683

10 **(B)** This patient has the endemic African variety of Burkitt lymphoma, a B-cell lymphoma that typically appears in the maxilla or mandible of the jaw. This particular neoplasm is related to Epstein-Barr virus infection. Cytomegalovirus infection occurs in immunocompromised patients and can be a congenital infection, but it is not a direct cause of neoplasia. Hepatitis B virus infection can be a risk factor for hepatocellular carcinoma. HIV infection can be a risk factor for the development of non-Hodgkin lymphomas, but most of these are either diffuse large B-cell lymphomas or small noncleaved Burkitt-like lymphomas. Human papillomavirus infection is related to the formation of squamous dysplasias and carcinomas, most commonly those involving the cervix. Respiratory syncytial virus infection produces pneumonia in infants and young children but is not related to development of neoplasms.

BP7 428-429 BP6 368-369 PBD7 677-678
PBD6 662-663

11 **(F)** The eosinophilia suggests a parasitic infestation. Immunocompromised persons can have superinfection and dissemination with strongyloidiasis. The other organisms listed are not known to be associated with eosinophilia.

BP7 416   BP6 359   PBD7 664   PBD6 337, 648

12 **(B)** Multiple myeloma produces mass lesions of plasma cells in bone that lead to lysis and pain. The skull radiograph shows typical punched-out lytic lesions, produced by expanding masses of plasma cells. Bence Jones proteinuria can damage the tubules and give rise to renal failure. Multiple myeloma can be complicated by AL amyloid, which can also lead to renal failure. Patients with myeloma often have infections with encapsulated bacteria because of decreased production of IgG, required for opsonization. Granulomatous disease (which is not produced by pneumococcus) can involve the marrow, but usually it does not produce such sharply demarcated lytic lesions. Nodules of small lymphocytes suggest a small cell lymphocytic leukemia/lymphoma, which is not likely to produce lytic lesions. Reed-Sternberg cells suggest Hodgkin disease. Blasts suggest a leukemic process.

BP7 429-431   BP6 380-382   PBD7 678-681
PBD6 663-666

13 **(C)** Interleukin-5 acts as an eosinophilic chemotactic factor to form an eosinophilic cellular component of the mixed cellularity and nodular sclerosis types of Hodgkin lymphoma. In contrast, the transforming growth factor-β (TGF-β) secreted by eosinophils promotes the fibrosis that is part of nodular sclerosing Hodgkin disease. Platelet-derived growth factor does not play a major role in Hodgkin disease, although it may be elaborated by cells in some carcinomas and gliomas. Cyclin D1 is involved in the cell cycle and proliferation. Transretinoic acid is used in treating acute promyelocytic leukemia, in which the abnormal gene fusion product of the t(15;17) blocks myeloid maturation at the promyelocyte stage. Erythropoietin drives erythroid cell line proliferation.

PBD7 690   PBD6 674

14 **(F)** These lymphomas arise in middle-aged adults at sites of autoimmune or infectious stimulation. If the lesion is associated with lymphoid tissue, it is sometimes called a mucosa-associated lymphoid tissue tumor (MALT lymphoma, or MALToma). The most common sites are the thyroid (in Hashimoto thyroiditis), the salivary glands (in Sjögren syndrome), or the stomach (in *Helicobacter pylori* infection). Although monoclonal (like a neoplasm), these MALT lesions can regress with antibiotic therapy for *H. pylori*. A MALT lesion can transform to diffuse large B-cell lymphoma. The cells correspond to the marginal B cells found at the periphery of stimulated lymphoid follicles. The other conditions listed are neoplastic conditions that are not related to *H. pylori* and that require chemotherapy to control.

BP7 435   BP6 368   PBD7 683   PBD6 668

15 **(A)** The child has Letterer-Siwe disease, a form of Langerhans cell histiocytosis. The Birbeck granules are a distinctive feature, identified by electron microscopy, that are found in the cytoplasm of the Langerhans cells. Lymphoblasts that mark as T cells are seen in anterior mediastinal (thymic) masses in children with acute lymphoblastic leukemia/lymphoma. Plasma cells are seen in multiple myeloma, a disease of older adults accompanied by a monoclonal gammopathy. Reed-Sternberg cells are seen in Hodgkin disease, which is an

unlikely disease in children. Ringed sideroblasts can be seen in myelodysplastic syndromes. Sézary cells can be seen in peripheral T-cell lymphoma/leukemias, which often involve the skin.

BP7 441   BP6 383   PBD7 701-702   PBD6 685-686

16 **(F)** This patient has a rare disorder called pure RBC aplasia, which is characterized by selective suppression of the erythroid lineage in the bone marrow. This curious entity is sometimes associated with a thymic tumor. In about one half of such cases, removal of the thymic tumor relieves the RBC aplasia, suggesting some autoimmune mechanism as the cause of the aplasia. Carcinomas can infiltrate the marrow space, a myelophthisic process, and reduce hematopoiesis, but not the erythroid line selectively. Hodgkin disease, multiple myeloma, and Waldenström macroglobulinemia can do the same. Patients with leukemias tend to have an elevated peripheral blood WBC count, and when the leukemic cells fill the marrow, all other cell lines are reduced. Mycosis fungoides is a T-cell neoplasm involving the skin.

PBD7 648, 686, 708   PBD6 632, 693

17 **(C)** Polycythemia vera, one of the myeloproliferative disorders, is a neoplastic disorder of myeloid stem cells, which tend to differentiate predominantly along the erythroid lineage, giving rise to polycythemia. The neoplastic erythroid progenitor cells require extremely small amounts of erythropoietin for survival and proliferation; hence, the levels of erythropoietin are virtually undetectable in polycythemia vera. In patients with chronic hypoxia, erythropoietin levels are elevated, producing excess RBCs. Erythropoietin secretion is triggered by anoxia in high-altitude dwellers and in patients with chronic lung diseases or cyanotic heart disease. Renal cell carcinomas can produce erythropoietin and trigger a paraneoplastic erythrocytosis. In dehydration, hemoconcentration can cause transient polycythemia, but this does not affect normal erythropoietin secretion.

BP7 439-440   BP6 378-379   PBD7 699-700
PBD6 682-683

18 **(C)** Chronic infections and chronic inflammatory conditions, such as lung abscesses, can lead to an expansion of the myeloid precursor pool in the bone marrow. This manifests as neutrophilic leukocytosis. Acute viral hepatitis, unlike acute bacterial infections, does not cause neutrophilic leukocytosis. Glucocorticoids can increase the release of marrow storage pool cells and diminish extravasation of neutrophils into tissues. Vigorous exercise can produce neutrophilia transiently from demargination of neutrophils. In acute myelogenous leukemia, the marrow is filled with blasts, not maturing myeloid elements.

BP7 416   BP6 359   PBD7 663-665   PBD6 647-648

19 **(A)** This HIV-positive patient has an extranodal infiltrative mass, made up of B cells (CD19+), in the ileum. This is a diffuse large cell lymphoma of B cells. These tumors contain the Epstein-Barr virus (EBV) genome, and it is thought that immunosuppression allows unregulated proliferation and neoplastic transformation of EBV-infected B cells. HIV is not seen in normal or neoplastic B cells. Human herpesvirus type 8 (also called Kaposi sarcoma herpesvirus) is found in the spindle cells of Kaposi sarcoma and in body cavity B-cell lymphomas in patients with AIDS. Human

T-cell leukemia/lymphoma virus type 1 is related to HIV-1, and it causes adult T-cell leukemia/lymphoma. Cytomegalovirus is not known to cause any tumors.

BP7 157,427-428   BP6 367   PBD7 667, 676-677
PBD6 661-662

20 **(B)** The clinical history, the peripheral blood smear, and the phenotypic markers are characteristic of chronic lymphocytic leukemia, a clonal B-cell neoplasm in which immunoglobulin genes are rearranged and T-cell receptor genes are in germline configuration. The t(9;22) is a feature of chronic myeloid leukemia. The t(8;14) translocation is typical of Burkitt lymphoma; this lymphoma occurs in children at extranodal sites. The t(14;18) translocation is a feature of follicular lymphomas, which are distinctive B-cell tumors that involve the nodes and produce a follicular pattern. The lymphoma cells can be present in blood, but they do not look like mature lymphocytes.

BP7 424-426   BP6 377-378   PBD7 673-674
PBD6 658-659

21 **(A)** The characteristic "punched-out" bone lesions of multiple myeloma seen on radiographs result from bone destruction mediated by RANKL, a cytokine produced by the myeloma cells that activates osteoclasts. Excessive light chain production by the myeloma cells can be detected as Bence-Jones proteins in urine. The bone marrow aspirate shows plasma cells. The monoclonal population of plasma cells often produces a monoclonal serum "spike" seen in serum or urine protein electrophoresis. Patients can have hypercalcemia and an increased serum alkaline phosphatase level. The neoplastic cells are generally well differentiated, with features such as a perinuclear hof, similar to normal plasma cells. The t(9;22) translocation is the Philadelphia chromosome seen in chronic myelogenous leukemia (CML). CML and other myeloproliferative disorders are sometimes accompanied by a thrombocytosis but are unlikely to produce mass lesions or bony destruction. Leukemias also can fill the marrow space but generally do not destroy bone.

BP7 429-431   BP6 380-382   PBD7 679-681
PBD6 663-666

22 **(C)** The bands of fibrosis are typical of the nodular sclerosis type, which is most commonly seen in young adults, particularly female patients. Involvement of one group of lymph nodes places this in stage I. Mediastinal involvement is common. Most of such cases are stage I or II, and the prognosis of such early-stage cases is good.

BP7 432-433   BP6 369-372   PBD7 686-689
PBD6 672-675

23 **(E)** Painful and acute enlarged nodes suggest a reactive condition and not a neoplastic process such as a lymphoma or a leukemia. In children, enlarged tender nodes and acute lymphadenitis are common occurrences. There are many infectious processes that can give rise to these findings, particularly bacterial infections. Children are quite active and acquire plenty of cuts and scrapes on extremities, which can then become infected. Sarcoidosis is a chronic granulomatous process typically seen in adults and characterized by the formation of noncaseating granulomas. Follicular lymphomas are B-cell neoplasms that efface the normal architecture of the lymph nodes; these tumors do not occur in children. Cat scratch disease can produce sarcoid-like granulomas with stellate abscesses. Toxoplasmosis can be a congenital infection or can be seen in immunocompromised persons; it produces a pattern of follicular hyperplasia.

BP7 418-419   BP6 361-362   PBD7 665   PBD6 649

24 **(E)** Splenectomy in childhood reduces immunity to encapsulated bacterial organisms. The spleen recycles old RBCs and removes inclusions such as Howell-Jolly bodies (rather like getting the cherry pits out without damaging the cherry). About one third of all circulating platelets are pooled in the spleen, and granulocytes also are marginated in splenic sinusoids, so that when the spleen is absent, the WBC and platelet counts rise. DiGeorge syndrome leads to cell-mediated immunodeficiency and increased viral, fungal, and parasitic diseases. Galactosemia results from an inborn error of metabolism, leading to liver disease and fibrosis that can cause splenomegaly. Gaucher disease leads to splenomegaly without significant immunodeficiency. Myeloproliferative disorders increase the size of the spleen. The thymus, but not the spleen, is sometimes involved in patients with Down syndrome (trisomy 21).

PBD7 702-703   PBD6 687-688

25 **(E)** These findings are characteristic of a childhood acute lymphoblastic leukemia of the pre-B cell type. The rapid expansion of the marrow caused by proliferation of blasts can lead to bone pain and tenderness. Features supporting an acute leukemia are anemia, thrombocytopenia, and the presence of blasts in the peripheral blood and bone marrow. Anemia and thrombocytopenia result from suppression of normal hematopoiesis by the leukemic clone in the marrow. The phenotype of CD19+, CD3−, sIg− is typical of pre-B cells. TdT is a marker of early T- and B-cell–type lymphoid cells. Chronic myelogenous leukemia is a disease of adults, and the WBC count is quite high; the peripheral blood contains some myeloblasts, but other stages of myeloid differentiation are also detected. In idiopathic thrombocytopenic purpura, only the platelet count is reduced, because of antibody-mediated destruction of platelets. An acute myelogenous leukemia is a disease of young to middle-aged adults, and there would be peroxidase-positive myeloblasts and phenotypic features of myeloid cells. Chronic lymphocytic leukemia is a disease of older adults; patients have many small circulating mature B lymphocytes.

BP7 421-422   BP6 374-375   PBD7 670-673
PBD6 656-658

26 **(D)** Thymomas are rare neoplasms that can be benign or malignant. In one third to one half of cases, thymomas produce myasthenia gravis as an initial presentation (as in this case). Benign thymomas have a mixed population of lymphocytes and epithelial cells and are circumscribed, whereas malignant thymomas are invasive and have atypical cells. Thymic carcinomas resemble squamous cell carcinomas. Granulomas can have epithelioid macrophages and lymphocytes, but the thymus is an unusual location. Hodgkin disease involves lymph nodes in the middle or posterior mediastinum. Lymphoblastic lymphoma of the T-cell variety is seen in the thymus in children, and it has no epithelial component. Metastases to the thymus are quite unusual. An organizing abscess could have granulation tissue at its edge, with a mixture of inflammatory cell types but not atypical cells.

BP7 451-452   BP6 391   PBD7 707-708   PBD6 691-693

27 (A) All lymphoid neoplasms are derived from a single transformed cell and are therefore monoclonal. Monoclonality in B-cell neoplasms, which comprise 80% to 85% of all lymphoid neoplasms, can often be demonstrated by staining for light chains. Populations of normal or reactive (polyclonal) B cells contain a mixture of B cells expressing kappa and lambda light chains. Some lymphoid neoplasms have a follicular pattern. A normal pattern of follicles is sometimes absent if the node is involved, as in some inflammatory conditions or in immune suppression. A proliferation of capillaries is typically a benign, reactive process. The CD30 antigen is a marker for activated T and B cells. Plasma cells are variably present in reactive conditions, but their absence does not indicate malignancy.

BP7 420   BP6 362-363   PBD7 669-670   PBD6 650-653

28 (A) Of the lesions listed, lymphoblastic lymphoma and Burkitt lymphoma occur in a much younger age group. Burkitt lymphoma has a t(8;14) translocation. The remaining three occur in an older age group. Of these, small lymphocytic lymphoma presents with absolute lymphocytosis and the peripheral blood picture of chronic lymphocytic leukemia. Follicular lymphoma has a distinct and characteristic translocation t(14;18) involving the *BCL2* gene. In contrast, mantle cell lymphoma, seen in older men, has the t(11;14) translocation, which activates the cyclin D1 *(BCL1)* gene; these tumors do not respond well to chemotherapy.

BP7 426-427   BP6 366   PBD7 671, 682-683
PBD6 667-668

29 (A) The features suggest Hodgkin disease, mixed cellularity type, which tends to affect older men. As in all other forms of Hodgkin disease, the Reed-Sternberg cells and variants stain with CD15. These cells also express CD30, an activation marker on T cells, B cells, and monocytes. Clinical symptoms are common in the mixed cellularity type of Hodgkin disease, and this histologic type tends to present in advanced stages. The pain associated with alcohol consumption is a paraneoplastic phenomenon peculiar to Hodgkin disease. The Reed-Sternberg cells make up a relatively small percentage of the tumor mass, with most of the cell population consisting of reactive cells such as lymphocytes, plasma cells, macrophages, and eosinophils. Immunoblasts suggest a B-cell proliferation. Epithelioid cells are seen in granulomatous inflammatory reactions. Neutrophils accumulate at sites of acute inflammation. Mast cells are not numerous in Hodgkin disease; they participate in type I hypersensitivity responses.

BP7   BP6 370-371   PBD7 686-689   PBD6 672-676

30 (C) This patient has evidence of an autoimmune disease, most likely systemic lupus erythematosus (SLE). This can be accompanied by monocytosis. (Cytopenias also can occur in SLE because of autoantibodies against blood elements, a form of type II hypersensitivity.) Eosinophilia is a feature more often seen in allergic conditions, parasitic infestations, and chronic myelogenous leukemia (CML). Thrombocytosis usually occurs in neoplastic disorders of

myeloid stem cells, such as the myeloproliferative disorders that include CML. Neutrophilia is seen in acute infectious and inflammatory conditions. Basophilia occurs infrequently but can also be seen in CML.

PB6 359   PBD7 664   PBD6 648

31 (B) Multiple myeloma is composed of abnormal plasma cells that tend to retain the ability to secrete immunoglobulins. Heavy- and light-chain components can be produced. The light chains are excreted in the urine and are known as Bence Jones proteins. Serum protein electrophoresis (SPEP) is used to screen for the presence of a monoclonal immunoglobulin (M protein). Polyclonal IgG in normal serum (denoted by the *arrow* in the figure) appears as a broad band; in contrast, serum from a patient with multiple myeloma contains a single sharp protein band in this region. The suspected monoclonal immunoglobulin is then confirmed and characterized by immunofixation. In this procedure, the electrophoresed proteins within the gel react with specific antisera. After extensive washing, only proteins cross-linked by the antisera are retained in the gel, which is then stained for protein. The sharp band in the immunoglobulin region of the patient's serum protein is recognized by antisera against IgG heavy chain (G) and kappa light chain (κ), indicating that this band is an IgGκ M protein. The levels of polyclonal IgG, IgA (A), and lambda light chain (λ) are also decreased in the patient's serum (relative to normal serum), a common finding in multiple myeloma. The TdT-positive circulating blasts are seen in lymphoblastic leukemias. The t(8;14) translocation is typical of a Burkitt lymphoma. Amyloidosis, reactive and primary, can give rise to renal failure. In primary amyloidosis, the amyloid is derived from immunoglobulin light chains, and patients may have a monoclonal B-cell proliferation; however, reactive amyloid is made up of nonimmunoglobulin proteins. A markedly increased hematocrit may suggest polycythemia as part of a myeloproliferative process.

BP7 429-431   BP6 380-382   PBD7 678-681
PBD6 663-666

32 (B) This is the Philadelphia chromosome, or Ph[1], which is characteristic of patients with chronic myelogenous leukemia (CML). This karyotypic abnormality can be found using cytogenetic techniques, including FISH. In the few cases that appear negative by karyotyping and by FISH, molecular analysis shows *BCR-ABL* rearrangements, and the tyrosine kinase activated via this fusion gene is the target of current therapy for CML. This rearrangement is considered a diagnostic criterion for CML. CML is a disease of pluripotent stem cells that affects all lineages, but the granulocytic precursors expand preferentially in the chronic phase. Follicular lymphomas have a t(14;18) karyotypic abnormality involving the *BCL2* gene. Hodgkin disease and myelomas usually do not have characteristic karyotypic abnormalities. Acute promyelocytic leukemias often have the t(15;17) abnormality.

BP7 438-439   BP6 377   PBD7 697-698   PBD6 680-682

33 (C) This patient has follicular lymphoma, the most common form of non-Hodgkin lymphoma among adults in the US. Men and women are equally affected. The neoplastic B cells mimic a population of follicular center cells and hence produce a nodular or follicular pattern. Nodal involvement is often generalized, but extranodal involvement is uncommon.

The t(14;18) translocation, which is characteristic, causes overexpression of the *BCL2* gene; hence, the cells are resistant to apoptosis. In keeping with this, follicular lymphomas are indolent tumors that continue to accumulate cells for 7 to 9 years. In Hodgkin disease, there are few Reed-Sternberg cells, surrounded by a reactive lymphoid population. The lymphoid population in acute lymphadenitis is reactive, and there is no bone marrow involvement. Mantle cell lymphoma is also a B-cell tumor; it is more aggressive than follicular lymphoma and is typified by the t(11;14) translocation, in which the cyclin D1 gene *(BCL2)* is overexpressed. In toxoplasmosis, there would be a mixed population of inflammatory cells and some necrosis.

BP7 426   BP6 364-366   PBD7 671, 674, 676
PBD6 659-661

34 **(D)** This peripheral blood smear is characteristic of acute promyelocytic leukemia (M3 class of acute myelogenous leukemia), with many promyelocytes containing prominent azurophilic granules and short, red, cytoplasmic, rodlike inclusions called Auer rods. Release of the granules can trigger the coagulation cascade, leading to disseminated intravascular coagulation (DIC). As in this case, many patients develop DIC. The t(15;17) translocation is characteristic of this disease; it results in the fusion of the retinoic acid receptor gene on chromosome 17 with the promyelocytic leukemia gene on chromosome 15. The fusion gene results in elaboration of an abnormal retinoic acid receptor that blocks myeloid differentiation. Therapy with retinoic acid (vitamin A) can alleviate the block and induce remission in many patients. The t(8:21) abnormality is seen in the M2 variant of acute myelogenous leukemia. The t(9:22) translocation gives rise to the Philadelphia chromosome of chronic myelogenous leukemia. A t(14:18) karyotype suggests a follicular lymphoma. The t(8:14) translocation can be seen in patients with Burkitt lymphoma.

BP7 436-437   BP6 375   PBD7 692-696   PBD6 676-678

35 **(D)** The pale, tan-to-yellow, firm areas shown in the figure are infarcts. These lesions are either wedge shaped and based on the capsule or more irregularly shaped within the parenchyma. Emboli in the systemic arterial circulation can arise from vegetations on cardiac valves in a patient with infective endocarditis; these can lead to splenic infarction. Emboli exiting the aorta at the celiac axis generally take the straight route to the spleen. The kidneys and brain are other common sites for systemic emboli to lodge. Although acute myelogenous leukemia can cause enlargement of the spleen, there are typically no focal lesions—only uniform infiltration of the parenchyma. There would be scattered granulomas that are rounded and tan with granulomatous diseases of the spleen, such as histoplasmosis. In Hodgkin disease, there can be focal nodules. Metastases can enlarge the spleen somewhat, but are uncommon in the spleen and are unlikely to be accompanied by signs of infection. Similarly, the congestive splenomegaly that occurs in cirrhosis and portal hypertension does not produce focal splenic lesions. In acute rheumatic fever, the verrucous vegetations are unlikely to embolize; in chronic rheumatic valvulitis, there is scarring with valve deformity, and this increases the risk of infective endocarditis.

BP7 97   PBD7 705   PBD6 689

36 **(A)** This woman developed severe neutropenia with pancytopenia from drug toxicity, which predisposed her to sepsis. Aspergillosis is a cause of pulmonary nodules, and neutropenia is a significant risk factor. These organisms often invade blood vessels, producing hemorrhagic lesions. Bartonellosis can produce bacillary angiomatosis, which is more likely to involve the skin. Mycobacterium avium-complex is more likely to involve organs of the mononuclear phagocyte system and unlikely to produce large nodules. *Escherichia coli*, like many bacterial infections, can occur in HIV infection, but it has a pattern of acute neutrophilic infiltrates. Herpes simplex virus (either type 1 or 2) is an unlikely disseminated infection in HIV. *Pneumocystis* pneumonia rarely produces nodular lesions. Toxoplasmosis is uncommon in the lung, even in immunocompromised persons.

BP7 416   BP6 359   PBD7 399-401, 662-663
PBD6 646-647

37 **(F)** Lymph nodes draining from a cancer often demonstrate a reactive pattern, with dilated sinusoids that have endothelial hypertrophy and are filled with histiocytes (i.e., macrophages). Sinus histiocytosis represents an immunologic response to cancer antigens. Not all enlarged nodes are caused by metastatic disease in cancer patients. CD3 is a T-cell marker, CD19 and CD20 are B-cell markers, and CD68 is a macrophage (histiocyte) marker. Polyclonal proliferations are typically benign reactive processes, whereas a monoclonal proliferation suggests a neoplasm. Aneuploidy and high S-phase are characteristics of malignant neoplasms; a high S-phase mostly occurs in rapidly growing tumors such as diffuse large B cell lymphomas, and in few carcinomas such as small cell anaplastic carcinoma. Inflammation would produce pain and tenderness, and the patient may be febrile. Generalized inflammatory diseases or chronic infections can increase the numbers of plasma cells in lymph nodes.

BP7 418-419   BP6 362-363   PBD7 665-666   PBD6 650

38 **(A)** This patient has hairy cell leukemia, an uncommon neoplastic disorder of B cells. These cells infiltrate the spleen and marrow. Pancytopenia results from poor production of hematopoietic cells in the marrow and sequestration of the mature cells in the spleen. There are two characteristic features of this disease: the presence of hairy projections from neoplastic leukocytes in the peripheral blood smear and co-expression of B cell (CD19, CD20) and monocyte (CD11c) markers. In the past, staining for tartrate resistant acid phosphatase was used. Auer rods are seen in myeloblasts in acute myeloblastic leukemia. The Ph[1] chromosome is a distinctive feature of chronic myelogenous leukemia. Toxic granulations in neutrophils are seen most often in overwhelming bacterial infections. A monoclonal IgM spike is a feature of lymphoplasmacytic lymphoma (Waldenström macroglobulinemia).

BP7 435   BP6 378   PBD7 683-684   PBD6 668-669

39 **(C)** The smear shows large, "atypical" lymphocytes that are present in patients with infectious mononucleosis and other viral infections, such as those caused by cytomegalovirus. These atypical cells are large lymphocytes with abundant cytoplasm and a large nucleus with fine chromatin. Infectious mononucleosis is caused by Epstein-Barr virus (EBV) and transmitted by close personal contact. In patients with infectious mononucleosis, multiple clones of B cells are infected by EBV. The EBV genes cause proliferation and activation of B cells, and hence there is polyclonal B-cell expansion. These B cells secrete antibodies with several specificities, including those that cross-react with sheep RBCs. It is these heterophile antibodies that produce a positive Monospot test result. The atypical lymphocytes are CD8+ T cells that are activated by EBV-infected B cells. There is no increase in basophils, eosinophils, or monocytes in infectious mononucleosis. Disorders of globin chain synthesis affect RBCs, as in the thalassemias. Infectious mononucleosis is not known as a transfusion-associated disease. Likewise, intravenous drug use is typically not a risk factor for infectious mononucleosis, but persons sharing infected needles are at risk of bacterial infections, HIV infection, and viral hepatitis. Eating raw oysters is a risk factor for hepatitis A, because oysters that filter polluted seawater concentrate the virus in their tissues.

BP7 417-418   BP6 360   PBD7 370, 664   PBD6 371-373

40 **(E)** This patient has an "aleukemic" leukemia, in which the peripheral blood count of leukocytes is not high, but the leukemic blasts fill the marrow. These blasts show features of monoblasts, because they are peroxidase negative and nonspecific esterase positive. This patient has an M5 leukemia, characterized by a high incidence of tissue infiltration and organomegaly. Acute lymphoblastic leukemia is typically seen in children and young adults. Acute megakaryocytic leukemia is rare, typically is accompanied by myelofibrosis, and the blasts react with platelet-specific antibodies. The M3 variant of acute myelogenous leukemia (promyelocytic leukemia) has many promyelocytes filled with azurophilic granules, making them strongly peroxidase positive. Erythroleukemia is rare and is accompanied by dysplastic erythroid precursors.

BP7 436-437   BP6 376   PBD7 692-694   PBD6 676-679

41 **(A)** Three markers strongly favor a very good prognosis for acute lymphoblastic leukemia (ALL): early pre-B cell type, hyperdiploidy, and patient age between 7 and 10 years. Marrow infiltration by the leukemic cells leads to pancytopenia. Poor prognostic markers for acute lymphoblastic leukemia/lymphoma are T-cell phenotype, patient age younger than 2 years, presence of t(9;22), and presentation in adolescence and adulthood. In most T-cell ALL cases, a mediastinal mass arises in the thymus, and lymphoid infiltrates appear in tissues of the mononuclear phagocyte system.

BP7 421-424   BP6 374   PBD7 670-673   PBD6 657-658

42 **(A)** The involvement of skin and the presence of lymphocytes with complex cerebriform nuclei in the skin and the blood are features of cutaneous T-cell lymphomas. These are malignancies of CD4+ and CD3+ T cells that may produce a tumor-like infiltration of the skin (mycosis fungoides) or a leukemic picture without tumefaction in the skin (Sézary syndrome). Cutaneous T-cell lymphomas are indolent tumors, and patients have a median survival of 8 to 9 years. The other phenotypes provided here are those of CD3−, CD56+ NK cells, mature B cells with CD19+, sIg+; monocytes/granulocytes with CD33+, CD13+; and neoplastic B cells in chronic lymphocytic leukemia with CD19+, CD5+.

BP7 435   PBD7 671, 685   PBD6 670

43 **(B)** This patient has classic features of myelofibrosis with myeloid metaplasia. This myeloproliferative disorder is also a stem cell disorder, in which neoplastic megakaryocytes secrete fibrogenic factors leading to marrow fibrosis. The neoplastic clone then shifts to the spleen, where it shows trilineage hematopoietic proliferation (extramedullary hematopoiesis), in which megakaryocytes are prominent. The marrow fibrosis and the extramedullary hematopoiesis in the spleen fail to regulate orderly release of leukocytes into the blood. Therefore, the peripheral blood has immature RBC and WBC precursors (leukoerythroblastic picture). Tear-drop RBCs are misshapen RBCs that are seen when marrow undergoes fibrosis. Marrow injury also can be the result of other causes (e.g., metastatic tumors, irradiation). These causes can also give rise to a leukoerythroblastic picture, but splenic enlargement with trilineage proliferation usually is not seen. The other causes mentioned—Hodgkin disease and *Histoplasma capsulatum* infection—can cause splenic enlargement but not marrow fibrosis.

BP7 440-441   BP6 379-380   PBD7 696, 699-701
PBD6 683-685

44 **(B)** This patient has the clinical and morphologic features of diffuse large cell lymphoma of B cells. These tumors often involve extranodal sites, show large anaplastic lymphoid cells that involve the tissues diffusely, and contain *BCL6* gene rearrangements. Their clinical course is aggressive, and they become rapidly fatal if untreated. However, with intensive chemotherapy, 60% to 80% of patients achieve complete remission, and about 50% can be cured.

BP7 427-428   BP6 366-367   PBD7 671, 676-677
PBD6 661-662

45 **(D)** This patient came to his physician with a classic history of chronic myelogenous leukemia (CML), confirmed by the presence of different stages of myeloid differentiation in the blood and by the presence of the Philadelphia chromosome. He went into a remission and then entered a blast crisis involving B cells (CD19+). The fact that the B cells carry the original Ph[1] chromosome and some additional abnormalities indicates that the B cells and the myeloid cells belong to the same clone. The best explanation for this is that the initial transforming event affected a pluripotent stem cell, which differentiated along the myeloid lineage to produce a picture of CML. Analysis, even at this stage, indicates that the molecular counterpart of the Ph[1] chromosome—the *BCR-ABL* rearrangement—affects all lineages, including B cells, T cells, and myeloid cells. With the evolution of the disease, additional mutations accumulate in the stem cells, which then differentiate mainly along B lineages, giving rise to B-lymphoblastic leukemia; blast crisis can also affect myeloid cells, but they are not CD19+. The Sézary syndrome has a leukemic component of CD4+ cells in addition to the skin involvement (mycosis fungoides). Myelodysplastic syndromes can precede the development of acute myelogenous leukemia. Hairy cell leukemia is an indolent disease without blasts.

BP7 438-439   BP6 377   PBD7 697-698   PBD6 680-682

46 **(A)** The age and mediastinal location are typical of a lymphoblastic lymphoma involving the thymus. This lesion is within the spectrum of acute lymphoblastic leukemia or lymphoma (ALL). Most cases of ALL with lymphomatous presentation are of the pre–T-cell type. This fact is supported by the expression of the T-cell markers CD3, CD5, and CD1. TdT is a marker of pre-T- and pre-B cells. A Burkitt lymphoma is a B-cell lymphoma that also can be seen in adolescents, but usually is present in the jaw or abdomen. Nodular sclerosing Hodgkin disease does occur in the mediastinum, but it involves mediastinal nodes, not thymus. The histologic features of Hodgkin disease include the presence of Reed-Sternberg cells, and this variant has fibrous bands intersecting the lymphoid cells. Mantle cell lymphomas and follicular lymphomas are B-cell tumors usually seen in older patients, and they do not involve the thymus. Small lymphocytic lymphoma is the tissue phase of chronic lymphocytic leukemia seen in older adults.

BP7 422   BP6 367   PBD7 670-673   PBD6 645-646

47 (B) This patient has polycythemia vera. The symptoms result from the increased hematocrit and blood volume. Undetectable erythropoietin in the face of polycythemia is characteristic of polycythemia vera. Polycythemia vera is a myeloproliferative disorder in which the neoplastic myeloid cells differentiate preferentially along the erythroid lineage. However, other lineages also are affected; hence, there is leukocytosis and thrombocytosis. These patients are Ph^1-chromosome negative. Untreated, these patients die of episodes of bleeding or thrombosis—both related to disordered platelet function and the hemodynamic effects on distended blood vessels. Treatment by phlebotomy reduces the hematocrit. With this treatment, the disease in 15% to 20% of patients characteristically transforms into myelofibrosis with myeloid metaplasia. Termination in acute leukemia, unlike in chronic myeloid leukemia, is rare. When it occurs, it is an acute myeloid leukemia, not lymphoblastic leukemia.

BP7 439-440   BP6 378-379   PBD7 699-700
PBD6 682-683

48 (B) These cells mark as cortical lymphocytes in the thymus of a child. An absence of such cells can be seen in the DiGeorge anomaly with 22q11.2. Such patients also can have parathyroid hypoplasia and congenital heart disease. Patients with Down syndrome (trisomy 21) can have thymic abnormalities and the T-cell dysregulation that predisposes to acute leukemia, but the thymus is typically present. The t(9;22) gives rise to the Philadelphia chromosome, which is characteristic of chronic myelogenous leukemia. The t(15;17) is seen in patients with acute promyelocytic leukemia. Persons with fragile X syndrome usually have some form of mental retardation. Males with Klinefelter syndrome (XXY) do not have immunologic abnormalities.

BP7 146,232   BP6 360-361   PBD7 706   PBD6 371-373

49 (D) The lacunar cells and the CD15+ Reed-Sternberg cells indicate Hodgkin lymphoma, and the fibrous bands suggest the nodular sclerosis type. Lacunar cells have multilobed nuclei containing many small nucleoli. These cells have artifactual retraction of the cytoplasm around the nucleus, giving the cells their distinctive appearance. The nodular sclerosis type of Hodgkin disease is more common in women. Atypical lymphocytes are characteristic in the peripheral blood of persons with infectious mononucleosis. Histiocytes with Birbeck granules are characteristic of the Langerhans cell histiocytoses. Hairy cell leukemia often is accompanied by

splenomegaly, but not a mediastinal mass, and the leukemic cells are B cells. Lymphoblasts that mark as T cells are seen in anterior mediastinal (thymic) masses in children with acute lymphoblastic leukemia/lymphoma. Myeloblasts are characteristic of acute myelogenous leukemia, which is occasionally accompanied by soft tissue masses.

BP7 431-434   BP6 372   PBD7 696-697   PBD6 670-674

50 (A) This patient has a form of T-cell neoplasm known as anaplastic large cell lymphoma (ALCL), which most often appears in children and young adults. It is often extranodal and has a characteristic gene rearrangement on chromosome 2p23 that results in production of anaplastic lymphoma kinase (ALK) with tyrosine kinase activity. CD10 is a B cell marker. The T-cell proliferations involving skin, known as mycosis fungoides/Sézary syndrome, are CD4 positive. The *cKIT* proto-oncogene has been associated with some NK cell lymphomas. The p24 antigen is part of HIV, which is most often associated with B-cell neoplasms.

PBD7 684-686

51 (D) Toxic granulations, which are coarse and dark primary granules, and Döhle bodies, which are patches of dilated endoplasmic reticulum, represent reactive changes of neutrophils. These changes are most indicative of overwhelming inflammatory conditions, such as bacterial sepsis. The route of infection in this case is probably intravenous drug use. Leukemia, granulomatous infections, or viral infections do not cause toxic changes in neutrophils. Infectious mononucleosis is accompanied by an increase in "atypical" lymphocytes.

PBD7 664-665   PBD6 648-649

52 (B) The peripheral eosinophilia seen in this patient is a feature of allergic disorders, including type I hypersensitivity reactions. Extrinsic asthma is a commonly occurring disorder in which eosinophilia can appear. Infestations with parasites that invade tissues are also known to produce significant eosinophilia. Sepsis most commonly results in a marked neutrophilia and left shift. In chronic myelogenous leukemia (CML), the total WBC count is typically high. Although there may be increased eosinophils in CML, the peripheral blood also shows basophils, metamyelocytes, myelocytes, and a few blasts. *Pneumocystis* pneumonia typically occurs in immunocompromised patients with lymphopenia. Tuberculosis and systemic lupus erythematosus (SLE) can produce a monocytosis.

BP7 416   BP6 359   PBD7 664   PBD6 648

53 (B) Sonja Henie died from complications of chronic lymphocytic leukemia (CLL), in which there are increased numbers of circulating small, round, mature lymphocytes with scant cytoplasm seen in the peripheral blood smear. The cells express the CD5 marker and the pan B-cell markers CD19 and CD20. Most patients have a disease course of 4 to 6 years before death, and symptoms appear as the leukemic cells begin to fill the marrow. In some patients, the same small lymphocytes appear in tissues; the condition is then known as small lymphocytic lymphoma (SLL). The lymphocytes seen in infectious mononucleosis are "atypical lymphocytes," which have abundant, pale blue cytoplasm that seems to be indented by the surrounding RBCs. The RBCs in iron deficiency anemia are hypochromic and microcytic, but the WBCs are not affected. Leukemoid reactions are typically of the myeloid type, and the peripheral blood contains immature myeloid cells. The WBC count can be very high, but the platelet count is normal. Acute lymphoblastic leukemia is a disease of children and young adults, characterized by proliferation of lymphoblasts. These cells are much larger than the cells in CLL and have nucleoli.

BP7 424-426   BP6 377-378   PBD7 673-674
PBD6 658-659

54 (C) Monoclonal gammopathy of uncertain significance (MGUS) is characterized by the presence of an M protein "spike" in the absence of any associated disease of B cells. The diagnosis of MGUS is made when the monoclonal spike is small (<3 g) and the patient has no Bence Jones proteinuria. MGUS can progress to multiple myeloma in about 20% of patients over 10 to 15 years. A plasmacytoma would appear on a bone scan. Waldenström macroglobulinemia would be accompanied by an IgM spike, hepatosplenomegaly, and lymphadenopathy. Heavy-chain disease is a rare condition that can be seen in chronic lymphocytic leukemia. In multiple myeloma, the spike is greater than 3 g, and usually the patient has bone lesions. In reactive systemic amyloidosis, serum amyloid–associated (SAA) protein derived from chronic inflammatory conditions is deposited as AA amyloid in visceral organs, but there is no monoclonal gammopathy.

BP7 430   BP6 381   PBD7 679, 681   PBD6 663-666

55 (B) The cell at the center of the figure is a Reed Sternberg (RS) cell, characteristic for Hodgkin lymphoma (HL). Recent studies have conclusively established that, within most cases of HL, RS cells are derived from B cells. As such, within a given tumor, all RS cells have clonal (identical) immunoglobulin gene rearrangements. T cell receptor gene rearrangements occur in normal or neoplastic T cells (e.g., acute lymphoblastic lymphoma). In the majority of cases of HL, RS cells contain the Epstein-Barr virus (EBV) genome, but not the CMV or HHV-8 genome. This latter genome is

found in cells of Kaposi sarcoma. HTLV-1 infects CD4+ T cells and gives rise to adult T cell leukemia/lymphoma.

BP7 431-433   BP6 369-370   PBD7 686-690
PBD6 670-672

56 (B) The very high WBC count and the presence of peroxidase-positive blasts (myeloblasts) filling the marrow are characteristic of acute myelogenous leukemia. This type of leukemia is most often seen in persons between the ages of 15 and 39 years. Chronic lymphocytic leukemia is characterized by the presence of small, mature lymphocytes in the peripheral blood and bone marrow of older adults. Megakaryocytic leukemias are rare. Chronic myelogenous leukemia is also seen in adults, but this is a myeloproliferative process with a range of myeloid differentiation. Most of the myeloid cells are mature, and there are relatively few blasts. Acute lymphoblastic leukemia occurs in children and young adults. Azurophilic, peroxidase-positive granules distinguish myeloblasts from lymphoblasts.

BP7 436-437   BP6 374-376   PBD7 692-696
PBD6 657-677

57 (A) This child has cat scratch disease, a form of self-limited infectious lymphadenitis that most often is seen in children, typically "upstream" of lymphatic drainage from the site of injury, so that the axillary and cervical lymph node regions are most often involved. Cytomegalovirus infection is typically seen in immunocompromised persons and is not a common cause of lymphadenopathy. Epstein-Barr virus (EBV) infection at this age is most often associated with infectious mononucleosis and pharyngitis, and the lymphadenopathy is nonspecific. *Staphylococcus aureus* can produce suppurative inflammation with sepsis. *Yersinia pestis*, the agent that causes bubonic plague, produces lymphadenopathy that can ulcerate and a hemorrhagic necrotizing lymphadenitis; it has a high mortality rate.

BP7 419   PBD7 349, 665-666

CHAPTER 15

The Lung

PBD7 Chapter 15: The Lung
PBD6 Chapter 16: The Lung
BP7 and BP6 Chapter 13: Lungs and the Upper Respiratory Tract

1 A 63-year-old man has had progressively worsening dyspnea over the past 10 years. He has noticed a 5-kg weight loss in the past 2 years. He has a chronic cough with minimal sputum production. On physical examination, he is afebrile and normotensive. A chest radiograph shows extensive interstitial disease. Pulmonary function testing shows low FVC and a normal FEV_1/FVC ratio. Increased exposure to which of the following pollutants is most likely to produce these findings?

- ❑ (A) Silica
- ❑ (B) Tobacco smoke
- ❑ (C) Ozone
- ❑ (D) Wood dust
- ❑ (E) Carbon monoxide

2 A 50-year-old man has a history of chronic alcoholism. He is found in a stuporous condition after 3 days of binge drinking. On physical examination, his temperature is 39.2°C. A few crackles are heard on auscultation of the right lung base. A chest radiograph shows a 3-cm lesion with an air-fluid level in the right lower lobe. Which of the following organisms are most likely to be detected in bronchoalveolar lavage fluid?

- ❑ (A) *Staphylococcus aureus* and *Bacteroides fragilis*
- ❑ (B) *Mycobacterium tuberculosis* and *Aspergillus fumigatus*
- ❑ (C) *Nocardia asteroides* and *Actinomyces israelii*
- ❑ (D) Cytomegalovirus and *Pneumocystis carinii*
- ❑ (E) *Cryptococcus neoformans* and *Candida albicans*

3 A 45-year-old man has smoked two packs of cigarettes per day for 20 years. For the past 4 years, he has had a chronic cough with copious mucoid expectoration. During the past year, he has had several episodes of respiratory tract infections that were diagnosed as "viral flu," and he developed difficulty breathing, tightness of the chest, and audible wheezing. His breathing difficulty was relieved by inhalation of a β-adrenergic agonist and disappeared after the chest infection had resolved. Which of the following pathologic conditions best describes these clinical findings?

- ❑ (A) Chronic bronchitis with cor pulmonale
- ❑ (B) Chronic bronchitis with asthmatic bronchitis
- ❑ (C) Chronic bronchitis with emphysema
- ❑ (D) Bronchiectasis
- ❑ (E) Hypersensitivity pneumonitis

4 A 75-year-old woman has had worsening lower leg edema and dyspnea for the past 5 years. On physical examination, her temperature is 36.9°C, pulse 74/min, respirations 19/min, and blood pressure 110/75 mm Hg. There is dullness to percussion at the lung bases. A low rumbling heart murmur is present. An echocardiogram shows a large (4 cm) atrial septal defect. Which of the following pulmonary conditions is most likely to be present?

- ❑ (A) Pulmonary hypertension
- ❑ (B) Interstitial fibrosis
- ❑ (C) Vasculitis
- ❑ (D) Granulomatous inflammation
- ❑ (E) Pulmonary infarction

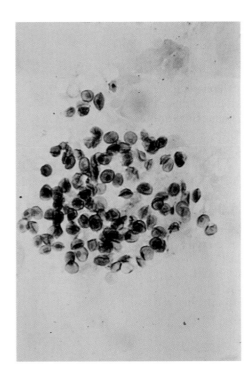

6 A 60-year-old man had a myocardial infarction 1 year ago and now has congestive heart failure. Over the past 24 hours, he has developed right-sided chest pain. On auscultation, there are lower lobe rales. He is afebrile and has a pulse of 70/min, respirations 17/min and shallow, and blood pressure 130/85 mm Hg. A section of right lower lobe representative of his disease is shown in the preceding figure. Which of the following clinical disorders is most likely to precede the appearance of this lesion?

❑ (A) Chronic obstructive pulmonary disease
❑ (B) HIV infection
❑ (C) Nonbacterial thrombotic endocarditis
❑ (D) Phlebothrombosis
❑ (E) Polyarteritis nodosa
❑ (F) Silicosis

5 A 40-year-old woman has had malaise and an 11-kg weight loss over the past 3 years. She has had fever and a nonproductive cough with increasing dyspnea for the past 3 days. On physical examination, her temperature is 37.8°C, pulse 82/min, respirations 22/min, and blood pressure 100/60 mm Hg. There is dullness to percussion over the lungs and diffuse crackles on auscultation. A chest radiograph shows extensive bilateral infiltrates. Bronchoalveolar lavage is performed, and the fluid is stained with GMS. The high-power microscopic appearance is shown above. Which of the following underlying conditions is most likely to be present?

❑ (A) Diabetes mellitus
❑ (B) Systemic lupus erythematosus
❑ (C) AIDS
❑ (D) Sarcoidosis
❑ (E) Severe combined immunodeficiency
❑ (F) Centrilobular emphysema

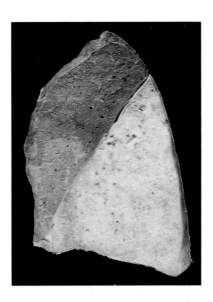

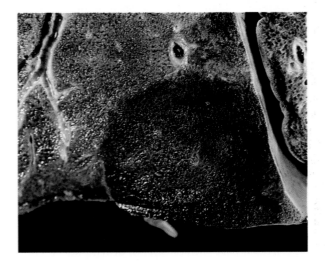

7 A 52-year-old woman has had an increasingly severe cough productive of yellowish sputum for several days. On physical examination, her temperature is 38.9°C, and diffuse crackles are heard in the left lower lung. A chest radiograph shows left lower lung consolidation. Laboratory studies show a WBC count of 11,990/mm³ with 72% segmented neutrophils, 8% bands, 16% lymphocytes, and 4% monocytes. The representative gross appearance of the lung is depicted above. Which of the following pathogens is most likely to be cultured from the patient's sputum?

❑ (A) *Mycoplasma pneumoniae*
❑ (B) *Streptococcus pneumoniae*
❑ (C) *Cryptococcus neoformans*
❑ (D) *Mycobacterium kansasii*
❑ (E) *Candida albicans*
❑ (F) *Pneumocystis carinii*
❑ (G) *Nocardia brasiliensis*

8 A 44-year-old woman has a 4-month history of mild but persistent right-sided chest pain. On physical examination, there are no remarkable findings. A chest radiograph shows a pleural mass on the right side. No pleural effusions are seen. A chest CT scan shows a localized, circumscribed 3 × 7 cm mass that appears to be attached to the visceral pleura; the lungs and chest wall appear normal. At thoracotomy, the mass is excised. On microscopic examination, the mass is composed of spindle cells resembling fibroblasts with abundant collagenous stroma. The spindle cells mark for CD34 but are cytokeratin-negative. There has been no recurrence of the lesion. The patient does not smoke. She is a research biologist specializing in marine mammals (manatees). Which of the following is the most likely diagnosis?

- (A) Bronchioloalveolar carcinoma
- (B) Hamartoma
- (C) Hodgkin disease, nodular sclerosis type
- (D) Malignant mesothelioma
- (E) Metastatic breast carcinoma
- (F) Solitary fibrous tumor

9 A 34-year-old man suddenly develops severe dyspnea with wheezing and is taken to the emergency department. On physical examination, his vital signs include temperature of 37°C, pulse 95/min, respirations 15/min, and blood pressure 130/80 mm Hg. A chest radiograph shows increased lucency in all lung fields. A sputum cytologic specimen shows Curschmann spirals, Charcot-Leyden crystals, and acute inflammatory cells in a background of abundant mucus. Many of the inflammatory cells are eosinophils. Which of the following is the most likely diagnosis?

- (A) Bronchiectasis
- (B) Aspiration
- (C) Bronchial asthma
- (D) Centrilobular emphysema
- (E) Chronic bronchitis
- (F) Obstructive sleep apnea

10 A 50-year-old man comes to the physician with gradually increasing dyspnea and a 4-kg weight loss over the past 2 years. He admits to smoking two packs of cigarettes per day for 20 years, but states that he has not smoked for the past year. Physical examination shows an increase in the anteroposterior diameter of the chest ("barrel chest"). Auscultation of the chest shows decreased lung sounds. A chest radiograph shows bilateral hyperlucent lungs; the lucency is especially marked in the upper lobes. Pulmonary function studies show that the FEV_1 is markedly decreased, but the FVC is normal, and FEV_1/FVC is decreased. Which of the following is most likely to contribute to the pathogenesis of his disease?

- (A) Impaired hepatic release of α_1-antitrypsin
- (B) Release of elastase from neutrophils
- (C) Abnormal epithelial cell chloride ion transport
- (D) Decreased ciliary motility with irregular dynein arms
- (E) Macrophage recruitment and release of interferon-γ

11 A 10-year-old girl who participated in a routine health screening program developed a 10-mm area of induration on the left forearm 3 days after intracutaneous injection of 0.1 mL of purified protein derivative (PPD). She appears healthy. A screening chest radiograph is performed. Which of the following is most likely to be seen on the radiograph?

- (A) Marked hilar adenopathy
- (B) Upper lobe calcifications
- (C) Extensive opacification
- (D) Cavitary change
- (E) Bilateral pleural effusions
- (F) Reticulonodular densities
- (G) No abnormal findings

12 A 63-year-old man worked for 20 years in a family-owned sandblasting business and used no respiratory precautions during that time. For the past 7 years, he has had increasing dyspnea without fever, cough, or chest pain. Which of the following inflammatory cell types is most crucial to the development of his underlying disease?

- (A) Plasma cell
- (B) Mast cell
- (C) Eosinophil
- (D) Macrophage
- (E) Natural killer cell

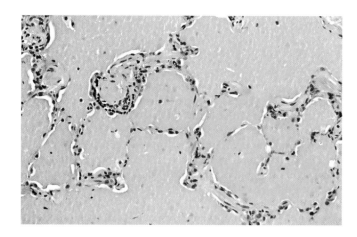

13 A 33-year-old woman has had increasing dyspnea with cough for the past 10 days. Over the past 2 days, her cough has become productive of chunks of gelatinous sputum. On physical examination, she is afebrile. There is extensive dullness to percussion over all lung fields. A chest radiograph shows diffuse opacification bilaterally. A transbronchial biopsy is performed, and light microscopic examination has the appearance shown in the figure above. On electron microscopy, there are many lamellar bodies. Antibody directed against which of the following substances is most likely to cause her illness?

- (A) α_1-antitrypsin
- (B) CFTR
- (C) DNA topoisomerase I
- (D) Glomerular basement membrane
- (E) Granulocyte macrophage colony stimulating factor
- (F) Neutrophilic myeloperoxidase

14 A 50-year-old man has developed truncal obesity, back pain, and easily bruisable skin over the past 5 months. On physical examination, he is afebrile, and his blood pressure is 160/95 mm Hg. A chest radiograph shows an ill-defined 4-cm mass involving the left hilum of the lung. Cytologic examination of bronchial washings from bronchoscopy shows round cells that have the appearance of lymphocytes but are somewhat larger. The patient is told that, although his disease is apparently localized to one side of the chest cavity, surgical treatment is unlikely to be curative. He is also advised to stop smoking. Which of the following neoplasms is most likely to be present in this patient?

- [ ] (A) Adenocarcinoma
- [ ] (B) Bronchial carcinoid
- [ ] (C) Bronchioloalveolar carcinoma
- [ ] (D) Large cell carcinoma
- [ ] (E) Metastatic renal cell carcinoma
- [ ] (F) Non-Hodgkin lymphoma
- [ ] (G) Small cell carcinoma
- [ ] (H) Squamous cell carcinoma

15 After a hemicolectomy to remove a colon carcinoma, a 53-year-old man develops respiratory distress. He is intubated and receives mechanical ventilation with 100% oxygen. Three days later, his arterial oxygen saturation decreases. A chest radiograph shows increasing opacification in all lung fields. A transbronchial lung biopsy specimen shows hyaline membranes lining distended alveolar ducts and sacs. Which of the following most likely represents the fundamental mechanism underlying these morphologic changes?

- [ ] (A) Reduced production of surfactant by type II alveolar cells
- [ ] (B) Disseminated intravascular coagulation
- [ ] (C) Aspiration of oropharyngeal contents with bacteria
- [ ] (D) Leukocyte-mediated injury to alveolar capillary endothelium
- [ ] (E) Release of fibrogenic cytokines by macrophages

16 A previously healthy 29-year-old man who has had no major illnesses experiences acute onset of hemoptysis. On physical examination, he has a temperature of 37°C, pulse 83/min, respirations 23/min, and blood pressure 150/95 mm Hg. A chest radiograph shows bilateral fluffy infiltrates. A transbronchial lung biopsy shows focal necrosis of alveolar walls associated with prominent intra-alveolar hemorrhage. Two days later, he has oliguria. The serum creatinine level is 2.9 mg/dL and urea nitrogen is 31 mg/dL. Which of the following serologic tests is most likely to be positive in this patient?

- [ ] (A) Antineutrophil cytoplasmic antibody
- [ ] (B) Anti-DNA topoisomerase I antibody
- [ ] (C) Anti–glomerular basement membrane antibody
- [ ] (D) Antimitochondrial antibody
- [ ] (E) Antinuclear antibody

17 A 49-year-old man has had increasing dyspnea for the past 4 years. He has an occasional cough with minimal sputum production. On physical examination, his lungs are hyper-resonant with expiratory wheezes. Pulmonary function testing shows increased total lung capacity (TLC) with slightly increased FVC, and decreased FEV_1 and FEV_1/FVC ratio. Arterial blood gas measurement shows pH of 7.35, PO_2 65 mm Hg, and PCO_2 45 mm Hg. Which of the following disease processes should most often be suspected as a cause of these findings?

- [ ] (A) Primary adenocarcinoma
- [ ] (B) Centrilobular emphysema
- [ ] (C) Diffuse alveolar damage
- [ ] (D) Chronic pulmonary embolism
- [ ] (E) Sarcoidosis
- [ ] (F) Pneumoconiosis

18 A 70-year-old woman is referred to an ophthalmologist because of difficulty with her right eye. She also has pain in the right upper chest. The findings on physical examination include enophthalmos, meiosis, anhidrosis, and ptosis. A chest radiograph shows right upper lobe opacification and bony destruction of the right first rib. Which of the following conditions is most likely to be present?

- [ ] (A) Bronchopneumonia
- [ ] (B) Bronchiectasis
- [ ] (C) Bronchogenic carcinoma
- [ ] (D) Sarcoidosis
- [ ] (E) Tuberculosis

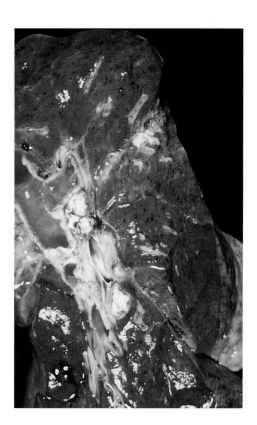

19 A previously healthy 20-year-old woman has had a low-grade fever for the past 2 weeks. On physical examination, her temperature is 37.7°C, but there are no other remarkable findings. The gross appearance of the lung shown above is representative of her disease. Which of the following studies is most likely to report a positive result?

- [ ] (A) Anticentromeric antibody
- [ ] (B) Antinuclear antibody
- [ ] (C) HIV serologic test
- [ ] (D) Rapid plasma reagin
- [ ] (E) Rheumatoid factor
- [ ] (F) Sweat chloride
- [ ] (G) Tuberculin skin test

20 A 60-year-old farmer has a 15-year history of increasing dyspnea. On physical examination, his temperature is 37.6°C. A chest radiograph shows a bilateral increase in linear markings Pulmonary function testing shows reduced FVC with a relatively normal FEV_1 value. A transbronchial lung biopsy specimen shows interstitial infiltrates of lymphocytes and plasma cells, minimal interstitial fibrosis, and small granulomas. Which of the following is the most likely cause of this clinical and pathologic picture?

- ❑ (A) Chronic inhalation of silica particles
- ❑ (B) Prolonged exposure to asbestos
- ❑ (C) Hypersensitivity to spores of actinomycetes
- ❑ (D) Infection with *Mycobacterium tuberculosis*
- ❑ (E) Autoantibodies that react with alveolar basement membranes

21 A local epidemic occurs among children at a summer camp, and they all develop upper respiratory tract infections manifested by coryza, pharyngitis, and tracheobronchitis. The children have fever and malaise but minimal sputum production. The total leukocyte count is not markedly elevated. *Mycoplasma pneumoniae* is cultured from the nasopharynx of many of the children. Which of the following histologic patterns is most likely to be found in the lungs of these children to explain these findings?

- ❑ (A) Alveolar neutrophilic exudates
- ❑ (B) Perivascular granulomatous inflammation
- ❑ (C) Hemorrhagic infarction
- ❑ (D) Hyaline membrane formation
- ❑ (E) Interstitial mononuclear cell infiltrates

22 A 6-year-old child puts the contents of a bag of peanuts in his mouth and then takes a deep breath with the idea of blowing the peanuts out all over his sister. However, he aspirates a peanut during this maneuver. One day later, he has slight dyspnea. On physical examination, his temperature is 36.8°C, pulse 70/min, respirations 17/min, and blood pressure 90/60 mm Hg. There are decreased breath sounds on auscultation and increased tympany on percussion over the right lower lung posteriorly. A chest CT scan shows a hemicircular area of density in the right lower lobe. Laboratory studies show a hemoglobin concentration of 13.6 g/dL and WBC count of 6175/mm³. Gram stain of sputum shows normal flora. Which of the following complications has this child most likely developed?

- ❑ (A) Bronchiectasis
- ❑ (B) Resorption atelectasis
- ❑ (C) Bronchopneumonia
- ❑ (D) Pneumothorax
- ❑ (E) Lung abscess

23 A 49-year-old man has sudden onset of severe lower abdominal pain with hematuria. He passes a ureteral calculus. Laboratory studies show that the calculus is composed of calcium oxalate. He is found to have a serum calcium concentration of 10.2 mg/dL, serum phosphorus level of 2.9 mg/dL, and serum albumin level of 4.6 g/dL. A chest radiograph shows a 7-cm hilar mass in the right lung. A chest CT scan shows prominent central necrosis in this mass. Which of the following neoplasms is most likely to be associated with these findings?

- ❑ (A) Metastatic colonic adenocarcinoma
- ❑ (B) Small cell anaplastic carcinoma
- ❑ (C) Bronchioloalveolar carcinoma
- ❑ (D) Squamous cell carcinoma
- ❑ (E) Large cell carcinoma

24 A 62-year-old man who has smoked one pack of cigarettes per day for the past 45 years has developed a severe cough with hemoptysis over the past month. He has experienced a 10-kg weight loss over the past year. On physical examination, he is afebrile. Laboratory studies show a serum Na^+ of 120 mmol/L, K^+ 3.8 mmol/L, Cl^- 90 mmol/L, CO_2 24 mmol/L, glucose 75 mg/dL, creatinine 1.2 mg/dL, calcium 8.1 mg/dL, phosphorus 2.9 mg/dL, and albumin 4.2 g/dL. Which of the following findings is most likely to be seen on a chest radiograph?

- ❑ (A) Bilateral fluffy infiltrates
- ❑ (B) Bilateral upper lobe cavitation
- ❑ (C) Diaphragmatic pleural calcified plaques
- ❑ (D) Left pneumothorax
- ❑ (E) Right middle lobe subpleural 2-cm nodule with hilar adenopathy
- ❑ (F) Right perihilar 4-cm mass
- ❑ (G) Right upper lung 3-cm nodule with air-fluid level

25 A 64-year-old man, who is a chain-smoker, sees his physician because he had had a cough and a 5-kg weight loss over the past 3 months. Physical examination shows clubbing of the fingers. He is afebrile. A chest radiograph shows no hilar adenopathy, but there is cavitation within a 3-cm lesion near the right hilum. Laboratory studies are unremarkable except for a calcium level of 12.3 mg/dL, phosphorus concentration of 2.4 mg/dL, and albumin level of 3.9 g/dL. Bronchoscopy shows a lesion almost occluding the right main stem bronchus. A biopsy is performed. Based on the pathologist's report and further testing, including chest and abdomen CT and bone scans, the patient is told that a surgical procedure with curative intent will be attempted. Which of the following neoplasms is most likely to be present in this patient?

- ❑ (A) Adenocarcinoma
- ❑ (B) Bronchioloalveolar carcinoma
- ❑ (C) Kaposi sarcoma
- ❑ (D) Large cell carcinoma
- ❑ (E) Metastatic renal cell carcinoma
- ❑ (F) Non-Hodgkin lymphoma
- ❑ (G) Small cell carcinoma
- ❑ (H) Squamous cell carcinoma

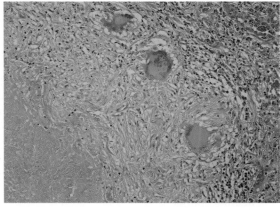

26 A 46-year-old woman goes to the physician for a routine health maintenance examination. On physical examination, there are no remarkable findings. Her BMI is 22. She does not smoke. A tuberculin skin test is positive. A chest radiograph shows a solitary, 3-cm left upper lobe mass. The mass is removed at thoracotomy by wedge resection. The microscopic appearance of this lesion is depicted in the preceding figure. Which of the following is the most likely diagnosis?

- ❑ (A) Pulmonary hamartoma
- ❑ (B) Pulmonary infarction
- ❑ (C) *Mycobacterium tuberculosis infection*
- ❑ (D) Lung abscess
- ❑ (E) Primary adenocarcinoma

27 A 3-year-old boy has had a cough, headache, and a slight fever for 5 days. His mother becomes concerned because he is now having increasing respiratory difficulty. On physical examination, his temperature is 37.8°C, pulse 81/min, respirations 25/min, and blood pressure 90/55 mm Hg. On auscultation, there are inspiratory crackles but no dullness to percussion or tympany. Respiratory syncytial virus is isolated from a sputum sample. Which of the following chest radiographic patterns is most likely to be present?

- ❑ (A) Lobar consolidation
- ❑ (B) Interstitial infiltrates
- ❑ (C) Large pleural effusions
- ❑ (D) Upper lobe cavitation
- ❑ (E) Hyperinflation
- ❑ (F) Hilar lymphadenopathy
- ❑ (G) Peripheral mass

28 A 35-year-old man comes to the nurse practitioner because of a 5-year history of episodes of wheezing and coughing. The episodes are more common during the winter months, and he has noticed that they often follow minor respiratory tract infections. In the period between the episodes, he can breathe normally. There is no family history of asthma or other allergies. On physical examination, there are no remarkable findings. A chest radiograph shows no abnormalities. A serum IgE level and WBC count are normal. Which of the following is the most likely mechanism that contributes to the findings in this illness?

- ❑ (A) Accumulation of mast cells in airspaces following viral infections
- ❑ (B) Emigration of eosinophils into bronchi
- ❑ (C) Bronchial hyperreactivity to virus-induced inflammation
- ❑ (D) Secretion of interleukin (IL)-4 and IL-5 by antiviral T cells
- ❑ (E) Hyperresponsiveness to inhaled spores of *Aspergillus*

29 A 78-year-old man has had increasing dyspnea without cough or increased sputum production for the past 4 months. On physical examination, he is afebrile. Breath sounds are reduced in all lung fields. A chest CT scan shows a dense, bright, right pleural mass encasing most of the left lung. Microscopic examination of a pleural biopsy specimen shows spindle and cuboidal cells that invade adipose tissue. Inhalation of which of the following pollutants is the most likely factor in the pathogenesis of this mass?

- ❑ (A) Asbestos
- ❑ (B) Bird dust
- ❑ (C) Silica
- ❑ (D) Cotton fibers
- ❑ (E) Coal dust
- ❑ (F) Ozone

30 An epidemiologic study is conducted in which persons with chronic lung diseases undergo pulmonary function testing and blood gas analysis. One group is found to have normal FEV_1, decreased FVC, and normal P_{CO_2}. In another group, FEV_1 is decreased more than FVC, the FEV_1/FVC ratio is 65%, and P_{CO_2} is increased. Both groups have increased bouts of pulmonary infections. Autopsy data are collected for the persons whose underlying cause of death is pulmonary disease. Which of the following morphologic changes is most likely to be seen in both groups?

- ❑ (A) Marked medial thickening of pulmonary arterioles
- ❑ (B) Destruction of elastic tissue in alveolar walls
- ❑ (C) Fibrosis of alveolar walls
- ❑ (D) Hemorrhage in alveolar lumen
- ❑ (E) Hyaline membranes lining airspaces

31 A 35-year-old woman has experienced multiple bouts of severe necrotizing pneumonia with *Haemophilus influenzae*, *Staphylococcus aureus*, *Pseudomonas aeruginosa*, and *Serratia marcescens* cultured from her sputum since childhood. She now suffers for weeks at a time with a cough productive of large amounts of purulent sputum. On physical examination, there is dullness to percussion with decreased breath sounds over the right mid to lower lung fields. A chest radiograph shows areas of right lower lobe consolidation. A bronchogram shows marked dilation of right lower lobe bronchi. Which of the following mechanisms is the most likely cause of airspace dilation in this patient?

- ❑ (A) Unopposed action of neutrophil-derived elastase
- ❑ (B) Congenital weakness of supporting structures of the bronchial wall
- ❑ (C) Diffuse alveolar damage
- ❑ (D) Destruction of bronchial walls by recurrent inflammation
- ❑ (E) Damage to bronchial mucosa by major basic protein of eosinophils

32 A 56-year-old man with ischemic heart disease undergoes a coronary artery bypass grafting procedure under general anesthesia. Two days postoperatively, he experiences increasing respiratory difficulty with decreasing arterial oxygen saturation. On physical examination, he is afebrile. His heart rate is regular at 78/min, respirations are 20/min, and blood pressure is 135/85 mm Hg. The hemoglobin concentration has remained unchanged, at 13.7 g/dL, since surgery. After he coughs up a large amount of mucoid sputum, his condition improves. Which of the following is the most likely explanation of these findings?

- ❑ (A) Resorption atelectasis
- ❑ (B) Compression atelectasis
- ❑ (C) Microatelectasis
- ❑ (D) Contraction atelectasis
- ❑ (E) Relaxation atelectasis

33 A 24-year-old man has had increasing dyspnea for the past 10 weeks. On physical examination, he is afebrile. There is dullness to percussion over the lungs posteriorly and decreased breath sounds. A chest radiograph shows large bilateral pleural effusions and widening of the mediastinum. Thoracentesis is performed on the left side and yields 500 mL of milky-white fluid. Laboratory studies of the fluid show a high protein content; microscopy shows many lymphocytes and fat globules. Which of the following is the most likely diagnosis?

- ❏ (A) Bacterial pneumonia complicated by empyema
- ❏ (B) Congenital heart disease
- ❏ (C) Marfan syndrome with aortic dissection
- ❏ (D) Micronodular cirrhosis
- ❏ (E) Miliary tuberculosis
- ❏ (F) Non-Hodgkin lymphoma

34 A 42-year-old man has suffered from chronic sinusitis for several months. He now sees his physician because of malaise and a mild fever that has persisted for 3 weeks. On physical examination, his temperature is 37.9°C. On auscultation, a few crackles are heard over the lungs. Laboratory studies show serum urea nitrogen of 35 mg/dL, creatinine 4.3 mg/dL, ALT 167 U/L, AST 154 U/L, and total bilirubin 1.1 mg/dL. The C-ANCA titer is 1 : 256. A transbronchial lung biopsy is performed, and microscopic examination shows necrotizing capillaritis with mild intra-alveolar hemorrhage. A granuloma is seen within the wall of a necrotic small artery. Which of the following is the most likely diagnosis?

- ❏ (A) Goodpasture syndrome
- ❏ (B) Hypersensitivity pneumonitis
- ❏ (C) Systemic lupus erythematosus
- ❏ (D) Wegener granulomatosis
- ❏ (E) Diffuse systemic sclerosis

35 For the past 6 years, a 45-year-old woman has had increasing respiratory difficulty that limits her activities. She does not smoke. On physical examination, she is afebrile and normotensive. Her lungs are hyperresonant. A chest radiograph shows flattening of the diaphragmatic leaves. Laboratory studies show the PiZZ phenotype of α_1-antitrypsin deficiency. Which of the following is most likely present in the lungs?

- ❏ (A) Sarcoidosis
- ❏ (B) Bronchiectasis
- ❏ (C) Interstitial fibrosis
- ❏ (D) Microatelectasis
- ❏ (E) Panacinar emphysema

36 A clinical study is conducted in which patients who have undergone surgical procedures with intubation, mechanical ventilation, and general anesthesia are followed to determine the number and type of postoperative complications. The study group is found to have a higher incidence of pulmonary infections with leukocytosis and chest radiographs showing consolidation in the 2 weeks following their surgical procedure than did patients who were not intubated and did not receive general anesthesia. Anesthesia is most likely to produce this effect via which of the following mechanisms?

- ❏ (A) Decreased ciliary function
- ❏ (B) Neutropenia
- ❏ (C) Tracheal erosions
- ❏ (D) Diminished macrophage activity
- ❏ (E) Hypogammaglobulinemia

37 A 45-year-old man has experienced a 5-kg weight loss over the past 3 months after the loss of his job. He recently developed a low-grade fever and cough with mucoid sputum production, and after 1 week, he noticed blood-streaked sputum. On physical examination, his temperature is 37.7°C. There are bilateral crackles in the upper lobe on auscultation of the chest. A chest radiograph shows bilateral upper lobe consolidations and focal cavitations. Which of the following diagnostic tests on a sputum sample is most warranted?

- ❏ (A) Acid-fast stain
- ❏ (B) GMS stain
- ❏ (C) Gram stain
- ❏ (D) Cytologic smear
- ❏ (E) Viral culture

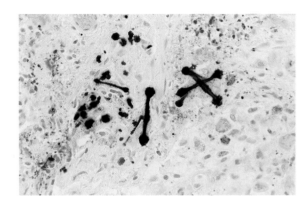

38 A 75-year-old man has experienced increasing dyspnea for the past 4 years. On physical examination, he is afebrile, with a pulse of 70/min, respirations 20/min, and blood pressure 120/75 mm Hg. A chest radiograph shows increased interstitial markings but no effusions. The right border of the heart and the pulmonary arteries are prominent. A transbronchial biopsy is performed, and the microscopic appearance with Prussian blue stain is shown. Which of the following is the most likely diagnosis?

- ❏ (A) Anthracosis
- ❏ (B) Berylliosis
- ❏ (C) Silicosis
- ❏ (D) Calcinosis
- ❏ (E) Asbestosis

39 A study is conducted of persons who smoked at least one pack of cigarettes per day for 30 years. These persons undergo pulmonary function testing, and a large subset is found to have decreased FEV_1, normal to decreased FVC, and FEV_1/FVC ratios below 70%. All persons in the study are found to have an increased risk of pulmonary bacterial infections. They are found to have increasing hypoxemia over time. Autopsy data from the subset of persons in the study with low FEV_1/FVC ratio who die of their underlying pulmonary disease are analyzed. Which of the following structures in the lungs is likely to be affected the most by the underlying disease?

❏ (A) Alveolar sac
❏ (B) Terminal bronchiole
❏ (C) Alveolar duct
❏ (D) Respiratory bronchiole
❏ (E) Capillary

40 A 40-year-old man has had an increasing cough with hemoptysis for 2 weeks. On physical examination, his temperature is 38.2°C. A chest radiograph shows an area of consolidation in the right upper lobe. His condition improves with antibiotic therapy; however, the cough and hemoptysis persist for 2 more weeks. A chest CT scan shows right upper lung atelectasis. Bronchoscopic examination shows an obstructive mass filling the bronchus of the right upper lobe. Which of the following neoplasms is most likely to produce these findings?

❏ (A) Hamartoma
❏ (B) Adenocarcinoma
❏ (C) Large cell carcinoma
❏ (D) Kaposi sarcoma
❏ (E) Carcinoid tumor

41 A 12-year-old girl is brought to the physician because of a history of coughing and wheezing and repeated attacks of difficulty breathing. The attacks are particularly common in the spring. During an episode of acute respiratory difficulty, a physical examination shows that she is afebrile. Her lungs are hyperresonant, and a chest radiograph shows increased lucency of all lung fields. Laboratory testing shows an elevated serum IgE level and peripheral blood eosinophilia. A sputum sample examined microscopically also has increased numbers of eosinophils. Which of the following histologic features is most likely to characterize the lung in this patient's acute condition?

❏ (A) Dilation of respiratory bronchiole and distention of alveoli
❏ (B) Dilation of bronchi with inflammatory destruction of walls
❏ (C) Interstitial and alveolar edema with presence of hyaline membranes that line alveoli
❏ (D) Thickening of bronchial epithelial basement membrane and hypertrophy of bronchial smooth muscle
❏ (E) Patchy areas of consolidation surrounding bronchioles and neutrophilic exudate in affected alveoli

42 A 40-year-old man comes to the physician because of a 6-year history of increasing shortness of breath and weakness. On physical examination, he is afebrile and normotensive. A radiograph of the chest shows diffuse interstitial markings. Pulmonary function tests indicate diminished FVC, decreased diffusing capacity, and a normal FEV$_1$/FVC ratio. Which of the following sets of pathologic changes is most likely to be found in the lungs?

❏ (A) Voluminous lungs with uniform dilation of air spaces distal to respiratory bronchioles
❏ (B) Chronic inflammatory cells in bronchi with a marked increase in size of mucous glands
❏ (C) Honeycomb lung with widespread alveolar septal fibrosis and hyperplasia of type II pneumocytes
❏ (D) Chronic inflammation of bronchial walls with prominence of eosinophils
❏ (E) Edematous, congested lungs with widespread necrosis of alveolar epithelial cells and prominent hyaline membranes

43 A clinical study is performed that includes patients who are hospitalized for more than 2 weeks and who were bedridden for more than 90% of that time. These patients undergo Doppler venous ultrasound examination of the lower extremities, blood gas testing, and radiographic pulmonary ventilation and perfusion scanning. A subset of patients is found who have abnormal ultrasound results suggestive of thrombosis, blood gas parameters with a lower PO$_2$, and pulmonary perfusion defects. Which of the following is most likely to be observed in the majority of patients in this subset?

❏ (A) Sudden death
❏ (B) Cor pulmonale
❏ (C) Hemoptysis
❏ (D) Dyspnea
❏ (E) No symptoms

44 A 55-year-old man has experienced increasing respiratory difficulty for the past 18 months. He can no longer pass the yearly physical examination required to maintain active status as an airline pilot, the only occupation that he has ever had. There are no remarkable findings on physical examination. Pulmonary function testing shows that the FEV$_1$ is normal, but the FVC is diminished. A chest radiograph shows diffuse interstitial disease but no masses and no hilar adenopathy. The results of ANA and anti-DNA topoisomerase I antibody testing are negative. Which of the following is the most likely diagnosis?

❏ (A) Scleroderma
❏ (B) Goodpasture syndrome
❏ (C) Silicosis
❏ (D) Diffuse alveolar damage
❏ (E) Idiopathic pulmonary fibrosis

45 A 54-year-old woman has had a mild fever with cough for the past week. Her symptoms gradually improve over the next 10 days. However, she then begins to have increasing fever, cough, shortness of breath, and malaise. On physical examination, her temperature is 37.9°C. There are inspiratory crackles on auscultation of the chest. A chest radiograph shows bilateral patchy small alveolar opacities. A chest CT scan shows small, scattered, ground-glass and nodular opacities. A transbronchial biopsy shows polypoid plugs of loose fibrous tissue and granulation tissue filling bronchioles, along with a surrounding interstitial infiltrate of mononuclear cells. She receives a course of corticosteroid therapy, and her condition improves. Which of the following is the most likely diagnosis?

❏ (A) Bronchiolitis obliterans with organizing pneumonia
❏ (B) Desquamative interstitial pneumonitis
❏ (C) Diffuse alveolar damage
❏ (D) Hypersensitivity pneumonitis
❏ (E) Pulmonary alveolar proteinosis
❏ (F) Wegener granulomatosis

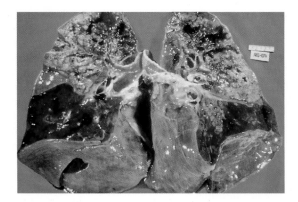

46 A 56-year-old man has had fever, night sweats, and a 3-kg weight loss over the past 4 months. In the past month, he has had episodes of hemoptysis. He dies of respiratory failure and hypoxemia. The appearance of the lungs at autopsy is shown above. Infection with which of the following organisms is most likely to have produced these findings?

- ❏ (A) *Candida albicans*
- ❏ (B) *Coccidioides immitis*
- ❏ (C) Influenza A
- ❏ (D) *Klebsiella pneumoniae*
- ❏ (E) *Legionella pneumophila*
- ❏ (F) *Mycobacterium tuberculosis*
- ❏ (G) *Mycoplasma pneumoniae*
- ❏ (H) *Nocardia asteroides*

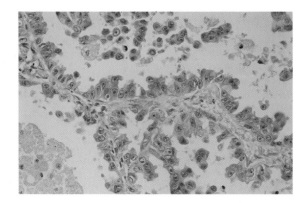

47 A 57-year-old woman comes to her physician because she has had a cough and pleuritic chest pain for the past 3 weeks. On physical examination, she is afebrile. Some crackles are audible over the left lower lung on auscultation. A chest radiograph shows an ill-defined area of opacification in the left lower lobe. After 1 month of antibiotic therapy, her condition has not improved, and the lesion is still visible radiographically. CT-guided needle biopsy of the left lower lobe of the lung is performed, and the specimen has the histologic appearance shown above. Which of the following neoplasms is most likely to be present in this patient?

- ❏ (A) Adenocarcinoma
- ❏ (B) Bronchioloalveolar carcinoma
- ❏ (C) Hamartoma
- ❏ (D) Large cell carcinoma
- ❏ (E) Mesothelioma
- ❏ (F) Metastatic breast carcinoma
- ❏ (G) Squamous cell carcinoma

48 A 65-year-old man worked in a shipyard for 10 years, and then for 5 years, he worked for a company that installed fire-retardant insulation. He experienced increasing dyspnea for several years and eventually died of progressive respiratory failure with hypoxemia. At autopsy, a firm, tan mass encased the left lung. Within the lung parenchyma adjacent to the mass, many ferruginous bodies were identified on microscopic examination. Which of the following findings is most likely to have been seen on a chest radiograph?

- ❏ (A) Bilateral fluffy infiltrates
- ❏ (B) Bilateral upper lobe cavitation
- ❏ (C) Diaphragmatic pleural calcified plaques
- ❏ (D) Left main bronchus, 1.5-cm endobronchial mass
- ❏ (E) Right middle lobe bronchial dilation

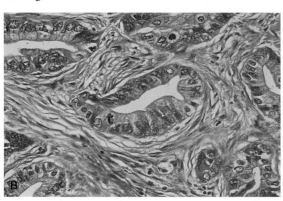

49 A 37-year-old woman comes to her physician because she has had a chronic nonproductive cough for 4 months. During this time, she has experienced loss of appetite and a 6-kg weight loss. She does not smoke. She is employed by a religious order. On physical examination, she is afebrile, and there are no remarkable findings. The chest radiograph shows a right peripheral subpleural mass. A fine-needle aspiration biopsy is performed, and the patient undergoes a right lower lobectomy. The microscopic appearance of the lesion is shown above. She remains free of symptoms for the next 10 years. Which of the following neoplasms did she most likely have?

- ❏ (A) Adenocarcinoma
- ❏ (B) Bronchial carcinoid
- ❏ (C) Bronchioloalveolar carcinoma
- ❏ (D) Hamartoma
- ❏ (E) Large cell carcinoma
- ❏ (F) Localized mesothelioma
- ❏ (G) Metastatic follicular carcinoma

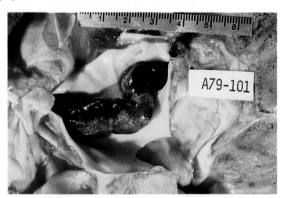

From the teaching collection of the Department of Pathology, University of Texas Southwestern Medical School, Dallas, TX.

50 A 68-year-old woman had a cerebral infarction and was hospitalized for 3 weeks. Her condition improved, and she was able to get up and move about with assistance. A few minutes after walking to the bathroom, she experienced sudden onset of severe dyspnea. Despite resuscitative measures, she died 30 minutes later. The major autopsy finding is shown in the preceding figure. Which of the following is the most likely mechanism for sudden death in this patient?

❑ (A) Atelectasis
❑ (B) Hemorrhage
❑ (C) Acute right-sided heart failure
❑ (D) Bronchoconstriction
❑ (E) Edema

51 A 61-year-old woman has experienced increasing dyspnea and a nonproductive cough for 5 months. On physical examination, her temperature is 37.7°C. A chest radiograph shows prominent hilar lymphadenopathy with reticulonodular infiltrates bilaterally. A transbronchial biopsy is performed, and the microscopic findings include interstitial fibrosis and small, noncaseating granulomas. One granuloma contains an asteroid body in a giant cell. The medical history indicates that she smoked cigarettes for 10 years but stopped 5 years ago. Which of the following is the most likely cause of her illness?

❑ (A) Delayed hypersensitivity response to an unknown antigen
❑ (B) Immune complexes formed in response to inhaled antigens
❑ (C) Diffuse alveolar damage
❑ (D) Smoke inhalation for many years
❑ (E) Infection with atypical mycobacteria

52 A 62-year-old man is a smoker with a 10-year history of cough productive of copious mucopurulent sputum. Over the past 6 months, he has developed progressive dyspnea. Physical examination shows bilateral pedal edema and a soft but enlarged liver. A chest radiograph shows bilateral pleural effusions and a prominent heart border on the right side. Arterial blood gas determinations show PO_2 of 60 mm Hg, PCO_2 55 mm Hg, pH 7.31, and HCO_3^- 28 mEq/L. The patient is intubated and placed on a ventilator, and he requires increasing amounts of oxygen. He dies 6 days later. At autopsy, which of the following microscopic findings is most likely to be characteristic of his underlying pulmonary disease?

❑ (A) Infiltrates of eosinophils
❑ (B) Extensive interstitial fibrosis
❑ (C) Granulomas in bronchovascular distribution
❑ (D) Carcinoma filling lymphatic spaces
❑ (E) Hypertrophy of bronchial submucosal glands

53 A 25-year-old woman has had progressive dyspnea and fatigue for the past 2 years. On physical examination she has pedal edema, jugular venous distension, and hepatomegaly. Lung fields are clear on auscultation. A chest CT scan shows right heart enlargement. Cardiac catheterization is performed and the pulmonary arterial pressure is increased, without gradients across the pulmonic valve, and no shunts are noted. A transbronchial biopsy is performed and microscopic examination shows plexiform lesions of peripheral pulmonary arteries, with striking smooth muscle hypertrophy causing marked luminal narrowing. A mutation in a gene encoding for

which of the following is most likely to cause her pulmonary disease?

❑ (A) Bone morphogenic receptor 2 (BMPR2)
❑ (B) Fibrillin-1
❑ (C) Lysyl hydroxylase
❑ (D) Endothelin
❑ (E) Atrial natriuretic factor
❑ (F) Renin
❑ (G) Endothelial nitric oxide synthetase (eNOS)

54 A 30-year-old man is hospitalized after a motor vehicle accident in which he sustains blunt trauma to the chest. On physical examination, there are contusions to the right side of the chest but no lacerations. Within 1 hour after the accident, he develops sudden difficulty breathing and marked pain on the right side. Vital signs now show that he is afebrile; his pulse is 80/min, respirations 23/min, and blood pressure 100/65 mm Hg. Breath sounds are not audible, and there is tympany to percussion on the right side. Which of the following radiographic findings is most likely to be present?

❑ (A) Large bilateral pleural effusions on chest radiograph
❑ (B) High probability of pulmonary embolus on ventilation/perfusion scan
❑ (C) Extensive centrilobular emphysema on chest CT scan
❑ (D) Right rib fractures with pneumothorax on chest radiograph
❑ (E) Bilateral patchy infiltrates on chest radiograph

55 A pharmaceutical company is designing pharmacologic agents to treat the recurrent bronchospasms characteristic of bronchial asthma. Several agents that are antagonistic of various mediators of bronchoconstriction are tested for efficacy in reducing the frequency and severity of acute asthmatic episodes. An antagonist of which of the following mediators is most likely to be effective in the early, acute phase of bronchial asthma?

❑ (A) Complement C3a and C3b
❑ (B) Platelet-activating factor
❑ (C) Interleukin-5
❑ (D) Leukotrienes C4 and E4
❑ (E) Histamine
❑ (F) Tumor necrosis factor and interleukin-1

56 A 59-year-old woman visits her physician because of shortness of breath that has worsened over the past 2 months. On physical examination, she is afebrile. There are diffuse rales on auscultation, with dullness to percussion up to the mid-lung fields. A chest radiograph shows bilateral pleural effusions, with effusions on the right greater than those on the left. Thoracentesis yields 700 mL of fluid from the right pleural cavity. The fluid is clear and slightly yellow tinged. A cell count performed on the fluid shows WBC $1/mm^3$ and RBC $12/mm^3$. Which of the following is the most probable cause of these findings?

❑ (A) Metastatic adenocarcinoma
❑ (B) Congestive heart failure
❑ (C) Systemic lupus erythematosus
❑ (D) Chronic renal failure
❑ (E) Mediastinal malignant lymphoma

57 A 40-year-old woman has never smoked and works as a file clerk at a university that designates all work areas as "non-smoking." She goes to the physician for a routine health maintenance examination. On physical examination, there are no remarkable findings. A routine chest radiograph shows a 3-cm sharply demarcated mass in the left upper lobe of the lung. Fine-needle aspiration of the mass is attempted, but the pathologist performing the procedure remarks, "This is like trying to biopsy a ping-pong ball." No tissue is obtained. Thoracotomy with wedge resection is performed. On sectioning, the mass has a firm, glistening, bluish-white cut surface. A culture of the mass yields no growth. Which of the following terms best describes this mass?

❑ (A) Adenocarcinoma
❑ (B) Hamartoma
❑ (C) Large cell carcinoma
❑ (D) Mesothelioma
❑ (E) Non-Hodgkin lymphoma
❑ (F) Squamous cell carcinoma

58 One day after moving into a new apartment, a 25-year-old man experiences acute onset of fever, cough, dyspnea, headache, and malaise. The symptoms subside over several days when he visits a friend in another city. On the day of his return, he visits the physician. There are no remarkable findings on physical examination. A chest radiograph also is unremarkable. Which of the following is most likely to produce these findings?

❑ (A) Antigen-antibody complex formation
❑ (B) Attachment of antibodies to basement membrane
❑ (C) Formation of mycolic acid
❑ (D) Generation of prostaglandins
❑ (E) Release of histamine
❑ (F) Release of leukotrienes
❑ (G) Toxic injury to type I pneumocytes

59 A 20-year-old man has had a mild fever with nonproductive cough, headache, and myalgia for the past week. He goes to the physician, who records a temperature of 37.9°C and notes erythema of the pharynx. Diffuse crackles are heard on auscultation of the lungs. A chest radiograph shows bilateral extensive patchy infiltrates. A sputum Gram stain shows normal flora. The cold agglutinin titer is elevated. He receives a course of erythromycin therapy, and his condition improves. Infection with which of the following organisms is most likely to produce these findings?

❑ (A) *Legionella pneumophila*
❑ (B) *Mycobacterium fortuitum*
❑ (C) *Mycoplasma pneumoniae*
❑ (D) *Nocardia asteroides*
❑ (E) Respiratory syncytial virus

60 A 26-year-old woman from East Asia developed a fever with chills over the past 4 days. Yesterday, she had increasing shortness of breath and a nonproductive cough. On physical examination, her temperature is 38.6°C. A chest radiograph shows right lower lobe infiltrates. Laboratory studies show hemoglobin of 13.4 g/dL, hematocrit 40.2%, platelet count 78,400/mm³, and WBC count 3810/mm³ with 77% segmented neutrophils, 2% bands, 5% lymphocytes, and 16% monocytes. Over the next 2 days, she has increasing respiratory distress requiring intubation and mechanical ventilation. A repeat chest radiograph shows worsening bilateral infiltrates. Her oxygen saturation has dropped to 90%. Infection with which of the following is most likely to have caused this patient's illness?

❑ (A) Coronavirus
❑ (B) Cytomegalovirus
❑ (C) Ebola virus
❑ (D) Herpes simplex virus
❑ (E) HIV
❑ (F) Paramyxovirus
❑ (G) Respiratory syncytial virus

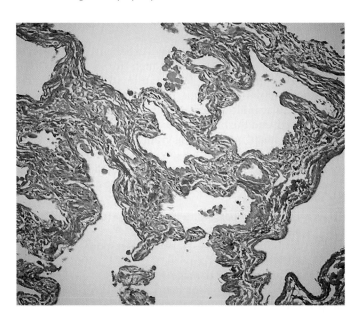

61 A 63-year-old man has had worsening dyspnea with a nonproductive cough for the past 9 months. On physical examination, he is afebrile and normotensive. His heart rate is 77/min and regular. On auscultation of the chest, diffuse dry crackles are heard in all lung fields. There are no other significant physical findings. A chest radiograph shows irregular opacifications throughout both lungs. A transbronchial biopsy specimen colored with trichrome stain is shown. Laboratory studies include negative serologic tests for ANA, anti-DNA topoisomerase I, ANCA, and anticentromere antibody. Despite glucocorticoid therapy, his condition does not improve, and he dies 2 years later. Which of the following is the most likely diagnosis?

❑ (A) Acute respiratory distress syndrome
❑ (B) Goodpasture syndrome
❑ (C) Idiopathic pulmonary fibrosis
❑ (D) Sarcoidosis
❑ (E) Scleroderma
❑ (F) Wegener granulomatosis

ANSWERS

1 (A) Silica crystals incite a fibrogenic response after ingestion by macrophages. The greater the exposure and the longer the time of exposure, the greater is the lung injury.

Tobacco smoke leads to loss of lung tissue and emphysema, not to fibrosis. Ozone, a component of smog, has no obvious pathologic effects. Particulate matter such as wood dust is mainly screened out by the mucociliary apparatus of the upper airways. Carbon monoxide readily crosses the alveolar walls and binds avidly to hemoglobin but does not directly injure the lung.

BP7 271-272, 468   BP6 224   PBD7 732-735
PBD6 731-732

2 **(A)** This patient has a lung abscess that most likely resulted from aspiration, which can occur in persons with a depressed cough reflex or in neurologically impaired persons (e.g., due to acute alcoholism, anesthesia, or Alzheimer disease). Aspiration into the right lung and the lower lobe is more common, because the mainstem bronchus to the left lung is more acutely angled. Bacterial organisms are most likely to produce abscesses. The most common pathogen is *Staphylococcus aureus*, but anaerobes such as *Bacteroides*, *Peptococcus*, and *Fusobacterium* spp may also be implicated. These anaerobes normally are found in the oral cavity and hence are readily aspirated. The purulent, liquefied center of the abscess can produce the radiographic appearance of an air-fluid level. Tuberculosis can produce granulomatous lesions with central cavitation that may be colonized by *Aspergillus*, although not over a few days. Nocardial and actinomycotic infections often lead to chronic abscesses without significant liquefaction and affect immunocompromised persons. Cytomegalovirus, *Pneumocystis*, and cryptococcal infections are seen in immunocompromised persons and do not typically form abscesses. *Candida* pneumonia is rare.

BP7 495-496   BP6 428-429   PBD7 747, 752-753
PBD6 722

3 **(B)** This patient's disease meets the clinical definition of chronic bronchitis. He has had persistent cough with sputum production for at least 3 months in 2 consecutive years. Chronic bronchitis is a disease of smokers and persons living in areas of poor air quality, which explains the chronic cough with mucoid sputum production. However, this patient's episodes of bronchoconstriction set off by viral infections suggest a superimposed element of nonatopic asthma. Cor pulmonale leads to pleural effusions, not to bronchoconstriction. Emphysema and chronic bronchitis can overlap in clinical and pathologic findings, but significant bronchoconstriction is not a feature of emphysema. Bronchiectasis results in airway dilation from bronchial wall inflammation with destruction. Hypersensitivity pneumonitis is marked by features of a restrictive lung disease, sometimes with dyspnea but without mucus production.

BP7 463-464   BP6 397   PBD7 721-723
PBD6 711-712, 715

4 **(A)** She has findings with both right and left heart failure. The left-to-right shunt produced by the atrial septal defect leads to increased pulmonary arterial pressure, thickening of the pulmonary arteries, and increased pulmonary vascular resistance. Eventually, the shunt may reverse, which is known as the Eisenmenger complex. Pulmonary fibrosis can be caused by diseases such as pneumoconioses, collagen vascular diseases, and granulomatous diseases. Pulmonary vasculitis may be seen with immunologically mediated diseases such as Wegener granulomatosis. Granulomatous inflamma-

tion does not occur from increased pulmonary arterial pressure. An infarction of the lung can occur with pulmonary embolism.

BP7 477-478   BP6 413-414   PBD7 743-745   PBD6 705

5 **(C)** Although *Pneumocystis carinii* pneumonia can be seen with a variety of acquired and congenital immunodeficient states (mainly those affecting cell-mediated immunity), it is most often associated with AIDS and is diagnostic of AIDS in HIV-infected persons. Diabetic persons are most prone to contract bacterial infections. Persons with autoimmune disease may have cytopenias that predispose to infection, and if they are treated with immunosuppressive drugs, a variety of infections are possible. Likewise, persons with sarcoidosis treated with corticosteroid therapy may have opportunistic infections. A patient with severe combined immunodeficiency is susceptible to *P. carinii* pneumonia, but it is very unlikely that without treatment she would have survived until the age of 40 years. Pulmonary emphysema predisposes to pulmonary infections, mainly caused by bacterial organisms.

BP7 497-498   BP6 430-431   PBD7 361, 747, 756
PBD6 381-382

6 **(D)** The figure shows a pleura-based "red infarct" typical of pulmonary thromboembolism that affects persons who are immobilized in the hospital, such as those with congestive heart failure. The source of the emboli is usually thrombi within pelvic or leg veins affected by phlebothrombosis. The bronchial arterial supply of blood is sufficient to produce hemorrhage but not sufficient to prevent infarction. Persons with underlying cardiac or respiratory diseases that compromise pulmonary circulation are at greater risk of infarction if thromboembolism does occur. Infarction is not a complication of smoking in patients with emphysema or asthma. HIV infection increases the risk of pulmonary infections but not of infarction. The small emboli from the small vegetations of nonbacterial thrombotic endocarditis are unlikely to produce infarction. Vasculitis of the lung typically involves arterioles, capillaries, or venules of insufficient size to produce a grossly apparent infarction. Pneumoconioses with restrictive lung disease produce pulmonary fibrosis but not a compromised vasculature or infarction.

BP7 476   BP6 411-413   PBD7 742-743   PBD6 703-704

7 **(B)** The productive cough suggests an alveolar exudate with neutrophils, and the course is compatible with an acute infection. Bacterial organisms should be suspected. Pneumococcus is the most likely agent to be cultured in persons acquiring a pneumonia outside of the hospital setting, and particularly when a lobar pneumonic pattern is present, as in this case. The atypical pneumonia of *Mycoplasma* does not produce purulent sputum, unless there is a secondary bacterial infection, which is a common complication of viral and *Mycoplasma* pneumonias. Cryptococcal and mycobacterial infections typically produce granulomatous disease. *Candida* pneumonia is rare but may occur in immunocompromised patients. *Pneumocystis* pneumonia is seen in immunocompromised patients and is unlikely to produce a lobar pattern of infection. Nocardiosis also is seen in immunocompromised persons and produces chronic abscessing inflammation.

BP7 479-482   BP6 415-416   PBD7 747-750
PBD6 718-721

8   **(F)** The solitary fibrous tumor, or localized benign mesothelioma, of pleura is a rare neoplasm that appears as a pedunculated mass. There is no relationship to asbestos exposure or other environmental pathogens. Bronchioloalveolar carcinomas are peripheral (but intraparenchymal) masses with atypical epithelial cells growing along the framework of the lung. A hamartoma is a peripheral intraparenchymal mass with a significant component of fibrous connective tissue and usually with cartilage present. Hodgkin disease is more likely to involve lymph nodes in the mediastinum. A malignant mesothelioma forms a pleural mass that is not circumscribed; the cells are atypical and cytokeratin positive. Metastases are typically multiple and often produce bloody effusions.

PBD7 768   BPD6 751

9   **(C)** Asthma, particularly extrinsic (atopic) asthma, is driven by a type I hypersensitivity response. The Charcot-Leyden crystals represent the breakdown products of eosinophil granules. The Curschmann spirals represent the whorls of sloughed surface epithelium in the mucin. There can be inflammatory cells in the sputum with bronchiectasis and chronic bronchitis, although without eosinophils as a major component. Foreign body aspiration may result in inflammation but without eosinophils. Inflammation is not a component of emphysema. There is mechanical pharyngeal obstruction with obstructive sleep apnea but without bronchoconstriction or inflammation.

BP7 455-458   BP6 397   PBD7 723-727   PBD6 715

10   **(B)** The patient's findings are predominantly those of an obstructive lung disease—emphysema—with a centrilobular pattern of predominantly upper lobe involvement. Smoking is a major cause of this disease. The inflammation that can accompany smoking leads to increased neutrophil elaboration of elastase, as well as elaboration of macrophage elastase that is not inhibited by the antiprotease action of α_1-antitrypsin. This results in a loss of lung tissue, not fibrogenesis. Fibrogenesis is typical of restrictive lung diseases, such as pneumoconioses that follow inhalation of dusts. α_1-Antitrypsin deficiency is uncommon and leads to a panlobular pattern of emphysema. Abnormal chloride ion transport is a feature of cystic fibrosis, which leads to widespread bronchiectasis. Dynein arms are absent or abnormal in Kartagener syndrome, which leads to bronchiectasis. Macrophage recruitment and activations by interferon-γ released from T cells is a feature of chronic inflammatory conditions and pneumoconioses.

BP7 458-462   BP6 400   PBD7 717-720   PBD6 710

11   **(G)** Most *Mycobacterium tuberculosis* infections are asymptomatic and subclinical. Active disease is uncommon, although a preceding illness or poor living conditions increase the risk. Calcifications and cavitation are complications most often seen after reinfection or reactivation of tuberculosis infections in adults. Lymphadenopathy or subpleural granuloma formation is more frequent in primary tuberculosis infections. A diffuse reticulonodular pattern suggests miliary tuberculosis. Extensive opacification is unlikely to occur in mycobacterial disease.

BP7 488-489   BP6 420-421   PBD7 381-386, 747
PBD6 722-725

12   **(D)** Silica is a major component of sand, which contains the mineral quartz. The small silica crystals are inhaled, and their buoyancy allows them to be carried to alveoli. There, they are ingested by macrophages, which then secrete cytokines that recruit other inflammatory cells and promote fibrogenesis. Plasma cells secrete immunoglobulins, which are not a major component of this process. Mast cells and eosinophils are prominent in the type I hypersensitivity response. Natural killer lymphocytes are more likely to be a prominent component of inflammatory processes directed against viruses.

BP7 271-272,468   BP6 226-227   PBD7 732-735
PBD6 731-732

13   **(E)** The patient has the acquired form of pulmonary alveolar proteinosis (PAP), an uncommon condition of unknown etiology characterized by autoantibodies against GM-CSF. Ten percent of PAP cases are congenital due to mutations in the granulocyte macrophage colony stimulating factor gene. Both forms of PAP have impaired surfactant clearance by alveolar macrophages. α_1-antitrypsin deficiency leads to panlobular emphysema. CFTR gene mutations lead to cystic fibrosis and widespread bronchiectasis. Anti-DNA topoisomerase I antibodies are seen in diffuse scleroderma, which produces interstitial fibrosis. Anti–glomerular basement membrane antibody is present in Goodpasture syndrome with extensive alveolar hemorrhage. Neutrophilic myeloperoxidase is a form of anti–neutrophil cytoplasmic autoantibody seen in Wegener granulomatosis.

PBD7 741   PBD6 739-740

14   **(G)** This patient has features of Cushing syndrome, a paraneoplastic syndrome resulting from ectopic corticotropin production (most often from a pulmonary small cell carcinoma), which drives the adrenal cortices to produce excess cortisol. Small cell carcinomas are aggressive tumors that tend to metastasize early. Even when they appear to be small and localized, they are not or will not remain so. Surgery is not an option for these patients. They are treated as if they have systemic disease, and some chemotherapy protocols afford benefit for 1 year or more, but cure is uncommon. Adenocarcinomas and large cell carcinomas tend to be peripheral neoplasms in the lung, and they are less likely to produce a paraneoplastic syndrome. Bronchial carcinoids tend to be small and are not likely to produce paraneoplastic effects; rarely they produce carcinoid syndrome. Renal cell carcinomas have been associated with Cushing syndrome, but the typical pattern of metastases is multiple nodules in both lungs. Non-Hodgkin lymphomas rarely occur in the lung, are not associated with smoking, and do not produce Cushing syndrome. Squamous cell carcinomas can be central and occur in smokers, but they are more likely to produce hypercalcemia.

BP7 504   BP6 434   PBD7 763-764   PBD6 746-747

15   **(D)** The clinical and morphologic picture is that of acute respiratory distress syndrome (ARDS). ARDS is characterized by diffuse alveolar damage, which is initiated in most cases by injury to capillary endothelium by neutrophils and macrophages. Leukocytes aggregate in alveolar capillaries and release toxic oxygen metabolites, cytokines, and eicosanoids. The damage to the capillary endothelium allows leakage of protein-rich fluids. Eventually, the overlying alveolar epithelium is also damaged. Reduced surfactant production causes respiratory distress syndrome with hyaline membrane disease in newborns. ARDS and disseminated intravascular coagulation (DIC) can complicate septic shock, but DIC is not the cause of ARDS. Aspiration of bacteria causes bronchopneumonia. Release of fibrogenic cytokines is an important cause of chronic diffuse pulmonary fibrosis.

BP7 466-468   BP6 405-406   PBD7 715-716
PBD6 700-703

16 (C) The patient has Goodpasture syndrome. Renal and pulmonary lesions are produced by an antibody directed against an antigen common to the basement membrane in glomerulus and alveolus. This leads to a type II hypersensitivity reaction. C-ANCA or P-ANCA are best known as markers for various forms of systemic vasculitis. The anti-DNA topoisomerase I antibody is a marker for scleroderma. Antimitochondrial antibody is associated with primary biliary cirrhosis. The ANA is used as a general screening test for a variety of autoimmune conditions, typically collagen vascular diseases such as systemic lupus erythematosus.

BP7 473-474   BP6 411   PBD7 745-746   PBD6 739

17 (B) These findings point to an obstructive lung disease, such as emphysema, that occurs from airway narrowing or from loss of elastic recoil. Adenocarcinomas, similarly to other primary lung tumors, typically involve one lung and do not produce small airway disease. Diffuse alveolar damage is an acute restrictive lung disease. Chronic pulmonary embolism does not affect FVC, because the airways are not affected, but there is a ventilation/perfusion mismatch. Sarcoidosis is a form of chronic restrictive lung disease. Pneumoconioses produce a restrictive pattern of lung disease with all lung volumes decreased, low FVC, and normal FEV_1/FVC ratio.

BP7 458-462   BP6 395   PBD7 717-719   PBD6 706-708

18 (C) This patient has Horner syndrome as a result of cervical sympathetic ganglion involvement by invasive carcinoma. Such a tumor in this location with these associated findings is called a Pancoast tumor. Infectious processes such as pneumonia are unlikely to impinge on structures outside the lung. Bronchiectasis is destructive of bronchi within the lung. Sarcoidosis can result in marked hilar adenopathy with a mass effect, but involvement of the superior cervical ganglion is unlikely. Likewise, tuberculosis is a granulomatous disease that can lead to hilar adenopathy, although usually without destruction of extrapulmonary tissues.

BP7 503   BP6 434   PBD7 763-764   PBD6 745-746

19 (G) These findings represent the so-called Ghon (or primary) complex, consisting of a small subpleural granuloma with extensive hilar nodal caseating granulomas. The Ghon complex is a feature of primary tuberculosis, which is most often a subclinical disease of younger persons. Persons who are immunocompromised, such as those with HIV infection, do not mount a good granulomatous response and have more extensive poorly formed granulomas, dissemination of tuberculosis, or both. Persons with cystic fibrosis and an elevated sweat chloride level (more often elevated in children than in adults) develop widespread bronchiectasis with infection by bacterial agents, particularly *Pseudomonas aeruginosa* and *Burkholderia cepacia*. Anticentromeric antibody is characteristic of limited scleroderma, which does not have significant

pulmonary involvement, unlike diffuse scleroderma. ANA is present in many autoimmune diseases, mainly in systemic lupus erythematosus, with pleuritis and pleural effusions. The rapid plasma reagin test is used to diagnose syphilis, which does not have significant pulmonary disease. Rheumatoid nodules may be seen in rheumatoid arthritis; these can be subpleural, but patients typically have arthritis.

BP7 487   BP6 422-423   PBD7 381-386   PBD6 723-724

20 (C) The patient has "farmer's lung," which is a form of hypersensitivity pneumonitis caused by inhalation of actinomycete spores. These spores contain the antigen that incites the hypersensitivity reaction. Because type III (early) and type IV immune hypersensitivity reactions are involved, granuloma formation can occur. The disease abates when the patient is no longer exposed to the antigen. Chronic exposure can lead to more extensive interstitial lung disease. Silicosis can produce a restrictive lung disease with fibrosis, but there are nodules of fibrosis that develop over years with minimal inflammation. Asbestosis is another pneumoconiosis that can also produce interstitial fibrosis over many years, and the risk of neoplasia is increased. Pulmonary tuberculosis can produce granulomas, but the pattern would be miliary, and it is unlikely that it would continue for 15 years. Antibodies directed against pulmonary basement membrane are a feature of Goodpasture syndrome, which mainly produces pulmonary hemorrhage.

BP7 472-473   BP6 410-411   PBD7 733, 739   PBD6 737

21 (E) Primary atypical pneumonias may result from a variety of infectious agents, including viruses, chlamydiae, and rickettsiae, although mycoplasmal infections are most common in children and young adults. About half of cases of *Mycoplasma* infection are accompanied by an increased cold agglutinin titer. Neutrophilic exudates are typical of bacterial pneumonias. Granulomatous inflammation can appear with vasculitides and infections such as tuberculosis. A hemorrhagic infarction is most often the result of a pulmonary thromboembolus, although infection with *Aspergillus* may lead to vascular invasion and thrombosis. Hyaline membranes are seen in acute lung injuries (diffuse alveolar damage).

BP7 482-484   BP6 419-420   PBD7 751   PBD6 721-722

22 (B) Complete obstruction of a bronchus can result in resorption of air and localized atelectasis. Obstruction by a foreign body can lead to localized bronchiectasis, but this takes weeks to months to develop. Distal to an obstruction, bronchopneumonia can develop, which can lead to a lung abscess. However, fever with leukocytosis would be typical. Pneumothorax is unlikely, because local obstruction does not produce enough air trapping to cause an air leak, particularly in a normal child's lung.

BP7 454   BP6 394   PBD7 713-714   PBD6 699, 751

23 (D) Most paraneoplastic syndromes involving lung carcinomas are associated with small cell anaplastic (oat cell) carcinomas, but hypercalcemia is an exception. Most commonly, it is caused by squamous cell carcinoma. Metastatic disease can also lead to hypercalcemia when bone metastases are present, but metastases to the lung usually present as multiple masses, not one large mass. Bronchioloalveolar carcinomas are not common and are not often associated with hormone-like factor production. Large cell carcinomas do not commonly cause a paraneoplastic syndrome.

BP7 206, 504   BP6 434   PBD7 763-764   PBD6 746-747

24 **(F)** The patient probably has a small cell anaplastic (oat cell) carcinoma of the lung, which is most likely to produce a paraneoplastic syndrome with the syndrome of inappropriate secretion of antidiuretic hormone. Oat cell cancers tend to be central masses, and they are strongly associated with smoking. Fluffy infiltrates suggest an infectious process. Upper lobe cavitation is suggestive of secondary tuberculosis. Diaphragmatic pleural plaques can be a feature of pneumoconioses, particularly asbestosis. Pneumothorax is most likely to occur from chest trauma, not from a neoplasm. A subpleural nodule with hilar adenopathy is the classic Ghon complex of primary tuberculosis, which is unlikely to present with hemoptysis. An air-fluid level suggests liquefaction in an abscess.

BP7 499, 503   BP6 433-434   PBD7 759-762   PBD6 746

25 **(H)** Of all lung cancers, squamous cell carcinoma is the one most likely to produce paraneoplastic hypercalcemia, and there is a strong association with smoking. These tumors can also undergo central necrosis, hence a cavity may form. Localized squamous cell carcinomas, unlike small cell carcinomas, may be cured by surgery. Adenocarcinomas, bronchioloalveolar carcinomas, and large cell carcinomas tend to produce peripheral masses and generally are not associated with paraneoplastic syndromes. Kaposi sarcoma involving visceral organs is most often seen in association with AIDS, and it is often multifocal. Renal cell carcinomas may be associated with hypercalcemia, but metastases usually appear as multiple masses (although of all metastatic tumors, renal cell carcinoma is most likely to produce solitary metastases). Non-Hodgkin lymphomas generally do not have paraneoplastic effects; they are uncommon in the lung and are not associated with smoking. Small cell carcinomas are never localized enough for curative surgery (they are usually detected at a high stage), although they often produce a variety of paraneoplastic syndromes, but not hypercalcemia.

BP7 500-501, 504   BP6 433-434   PBD7 759-763
PBD6 743-746

26 **(C)** The figure shows pink, amorphous tissue at the lower left, representing caseous necrosis. The rim of the granuloma has epithelioid cells and Langhans giant cells. Caseating granulomatous inflammation is most typical of *Mycoplasma tuberculosis* infection. A hamartoma is a benign neoplastic process, and the mass is composed of pulmonary tissue elements, including cartilage and bronchial epithelium. A pulmonary infarct should have extensive hemorrhage. A lung abscess would have an area of liquefactive necrosis filled with tissue debris and neutrophils. A carcinoma may have central necrosis, not caseation, and there would be atypical, pleomorphic cells forming the mass.

BP7 484-486   BP6 423-424   PBD7 381-386
PBD6 723-726

27 **(B)** Respiratory syncytial virus pneumonia is most common in children, and it can occur in epidemics. Viral, chlamydial, and mycoplasmal pneumonias are most often interstitial, without neutrophilic alveolar exudates. The diagnosis is often presumptive, because culture is difficult and expensive. Lobar consolidation is more typical of a bacterial process, such as can be seen in *Streptococcus pneumoniae* infection. Pleural effusions can be seen in pulmonary inflammatory processes, but they are most pronounced in heart failure. Cavitation is most likely to complicate secondary tuberculosis in adults. Hyperinflation can accompany bronchoconstriction in asthma. Marked lymphadenopathy is more characteristic of chronic processes such as granulomatous diseases or metastases. A mass lesion suggests a neoplasm or granuloma, not a viral infection.

BP7 483   BP6 419-420   PBD7 347, 747
PBD6 340-341, 721-722

28 **(C)** This history is typical of nonatopic, or intrinsic, asthma. There is no family history of asthma, no eosinophilia, and a normal serum IgE level. The fundamental abnormality in such cases is bronchial hyperresponsiveness (i.e., the threshold of bronchial spasm is intrinsically low). When airway inflammation occurs after viral infections, the bronchial muscles spasm, and an asthmatic attack occurs. Such bronchial hyperreactivity may also be triggered by inhalation of air pollutants such as ozone, sulfur dioxide, and nitrogen dioxide. Accumulation of mast cells and eosinophils is typical of atopic asthma. Secretion of interleukin (IL)-4 and IL-5 by type 2 helper T cells also occurs in cases of allergic asthma. Bronchopulmonary aspergillosis refers to colonization of asthmatic airways by *Aspergillus*, which is followed by development of additional IgE antibodies.

BP7 457-458   BP6 397   PBD7 723-727   PBD6 712-714

29 **(A)** The patient has a malignant mesothelioma. This is a rare tumor even in persons with a history of asbestos exposure. The tumor appears decades after exposure. Bronchogenic carcinoma is more common in persons with asbestos exposure, particularly when there is a history of smoking. Bird dust can lead to hypersensitivity pneumonitis. Silicosis is typified by interstitial fibrosis and causes a slight increase in the risk of bronchogenic carcinoma. Inhalation of cotton fibers (byssinosis) leads to symptoms related to bronchoconstriction. Coal dust inhalation can lead to marked anthracosis but without a significant risk of lung cancer. Ozone and nitrogen oxides in smog can cause acute respiratory discomfort but are not known to be promoters of neoplasia.

BP7 504-505   BP6 435-436   PBD7 735, 768-770
PBD6 151-153, 732-733

30 **(A)** Changes associated with pulmonary hypertension are characteristic of both restrictive and obstructive lung diseases. This explains, for example, the occurrence of cor pulmonale and right-sided congestive heart failure in persons with chronic obstructive pulmonary disease (e.g., emphysema) or with pneumoconiosis. In both cases, the pulmonary vascular bed is reduced to increase pulmonary arterial pressures. Destruction of elastic tissue in alveolar walls is seen in emphysema, and fibrosis of alveolar walls occurs in restrictive lung diseases. Alveolar hemorrhage is not a feature of restrictive or obstructive lung disease. Hyaline membranes are seen in diffuse alveolar damage (acute respiratory distress syndrome), which has characteristics of an acute restrictive lung disease

BP7 477-478   BP6 413-414   PBD7 743-745
PBD6 705-706

31 **(D)** This patient has a typical history of bronchiectasis. In this condition, irreversible dilation of bronchi results from inflammation and destruction of bronchial walls after prolonged infections or obstruction. Serious bouts of pneumonia can predispose to bronchiectasis. Unopposed action of elastases damages the elastic tissue of alveoli, giving rise to emphysema. Chondromalacia weakening the bronchial wall is rare. Diffuse alveolar damage is an acute condition that gives rise to acute respiratory distress syndrome. Bronchial mucosal damage by eosinophils occurs in bronchial asthma. It does not cause destruction of the bronchial wall.

BP7 464-465   BP6 403-404   PBD7 727-728
PBD6 716-717

32 **(A)** Resorption atelectasis is most often the result of a mucous or mucopurulent plug obstructing a bronchus. It can occur postoperatively, or it may complicate bronchial asthma. Compression atelectasis results from accumulation of air or fluid in the pleural cavity, which can happen with a pneumothorax, hemothorax, or pleural effusion. Microatelectasis can occur postoperatively, in diffuse alveolar damage, and in respiratory distress of the newborn from loss of surfactant. Contraction atelectasis occurs when fibrous scar tissue surrounds the lung. Relaxation atelectasis is a synonym for compression atelectasis.

BP7 454   BP6 394   PBD7 713-714   PBD6 699-700

33 **(F)** The pleural fluid findings are typical of chylothorax, which is uncommon but distinctive. Disruption of the thoracic duct in the posterior chest is most likely to cause chylothorax, and malignant neoplasms such as a high-grade non-Hodgkin lymphoma are most likely to do this. An empyema is composed of pus formed from neutrophilic exudation and would appear cloudy and yellow. Congenital heart disease can lead to congestive heart failure with a serous effusion. Aortic dissection is an acute condition that can produce a hemothorax. Cirrhosis is more likely associated with ascites or liver failure with hypoalbuminemia leading to hydrothorax. Miliary tuberculosis is seen as a reticulonodular pattern on a chest radiograph; tuberculosis may produce hemorrhagic effusions.

BP7 505-506   BP6 413-414   PBD7 766-767
PBD6 705-706

34 **(D)** Vasculitis is a key feature of Wegener granulomatosis. Although multiple organs can be affected, the lung and kidney are most often involved. The C-ANCA test result is often positive, whereas a positive P-ANCA result suggests microscopic polyangiitis. Renal and pulmonary disease may be present in Goodpasture syndrome; there may be a positive result for anti–glomerular basement membrane antibody but no C-ANCA or P-ANCA positivity. In hypersensitivity pneumonitis, an initial type III hypersensitivity response is followed by a type IV response, and renal disease is not expected. In systemic lupus erythematosus, renal disease is far more likely than pulmonary disease, and C-ANCA or P-ANCA positivity is not expected. Of the collagen vascular diseases, systemic sclerosis is more likely to produce significant pulmonary disease, but hemoptysis is not a prominent feature, and the C-ANCA result is unlikely to be positive.

BP7 351-352, 474   BP6 411   PBD7 535, 539, 541,
746-747   PBD6 522-523, 738-739

35 **(E)** Lack of the antielastase activity of α_1-antitrypsin promotes damage to the pulmonary elastic tissue, resulting in loss of structures throughout lung acini and causing panacinar emphysema. There is irreversible dilation of respiratory bronchioles to terminal alveoli. This is more pronounced in the lower lobes of the lung, where greater perfusion occurs. Sarcoidosis is a granulomatous, mainly interstitial disease. Bronchiectasis results from chronic and destructive inflammation of bronchi. Interstitial fibrosis results from inhalation of injurious dusts (e.g., silica, asbestos) or from lung injury in collagen vascular diseases. Microatelectasis can occur postoperatively or with loss of surfactant in diffuse alveolar damage.

BP7 461   BP6 399-400   PBD7 719-720   PBD6 709-710

36 **(A)** The anesthetic gases tend to reduce the ciliary function of the respiratory epithelium that lines the bronchi. The mucociliary apparatus helps clear organisms that are inhaled into the respiratory tree. The anesthetic gases and drugs do not typically result in marrow failure with neutropenia. The subglottic tracheal region, where the cuff of the endotracheal tube is located, can become eroded, but this is more likely to occur when intubation is prolonged for weeks. Macrophage function is not significantly affected by anesthesia. The levels of γ-globulins in serum are not reduced by the effects of anesthesia.

BP7 479   BP6 414   PBD7 727, 747   PBD6 718-719

37 **(A)** Significant adverse changes in a person's life increase the risk of illness. Upper lobe cavitation suggests reactivation or reinfection of *Mycobacterium tuberculosis* infection in adults; hence, acid-fast staining should be done. The GMS stain is helpful to identify fungi and to identify cysts of *Pneumocystis carinii*. Gram stain is most useful for determining which bacterial organisms may be present. The cytologic smear can be most helpful in screening for malignant cells. A viral illness, which typically produces an interstitial pneumonia, would not account for upper lobe cavitation.

BP7 488-490   BP6 423-425   PBD7 381-386
PBD6 722-725

38 **(E)** The ferruginous bodies shown in the figure are long, thin crystals of asbestos that have become encrusted with iron and calcium. The inflammatory reaction incited by these crystals promotes fibrogenesis and resultant pneumoconiosis. Anthracosis is a benign process seen in city dwellers as a consequence of inhaled carbonaceous dust. Berylliosis is marked by noncaseating granulomas. Silica crystals are not covered by iron and tend to result in formation of fibrous nodules (silicotic nodules). Calcium deposition may occur along alveolar walls when the serum calcium level is high (metastatic calcification).

BP7 272-274, 468   BP6 227-228   PBD7 735-736
PBD6 732-734

39 **(D)** Centrilobular emphysema results from damage to the central or proximal part of the lung acinus, with dilation that primarily affects the respiratory bronchioles. There is relative sparing of the distal acinar structures (alveolar ducts and alveolar sacs). In panacinar emphysema, the lung lobule is involved from the respiratory bronchiole to the terminal alveoli. In paraseptal emphysema, the distal acinus is involved.

BP7 459-460   BP6 398-399   PBD7 718-720
PBD6 707-709

40 (E) Most pulmonary carcinoids are central obstructing masses involving a bronchus. These neuroendocrine tumors have somewhat unpredictable behavior, but many are resectable and follow a benign course. They typically manifest with hemoptysis and the consequences of bronchial obstruction. In this case, the pneumonia in the right upper lobe probably resulted from obstruction to drainage caused by the tumor. A hamartoma is an uncommon but benign pulmonary lesion that is also located peripherally. Adenocarcinomas are common lung tumors but are typically peripheral. Large cell carcinomas are typically large, bulky, peripheral masses. Kaposi sarcoma can involve the lung in some patients with AIDS, and the tumor often has a bronchovascular distribution, but obstruction is uncommon.

BP7 504   BP6 435   PBD7 764-765   PBD6 747-748

41 (D) This child has atopic asthma, a type I hypersensitivity reaction in which there are presensitized, IgE-coated mast cells in mucosal surfaces and submucosa of airways. Contact with an allergen results in degranulation of the mast cells, with release of mediators, such as leukotrienes, histamine, and prostaglandins, that attract leukocytes, particularly eosinophils, and promote bronchoconstriction. The characteristic histologic changes in the bronchi result from the inflammation. Dilation of the respiratory bronchiole is a feature of centrilobular emphysema. Bronchial dilation with inflammatory destruction is a feature of bronchiectasis. Hyaline membranes are seen with acute diffuse alveolar damage. Neutrophilic exudates with consolidation are seen in pneumonic processes, typically from bacterial infections.

BP7 455-457   BP6 395-397   PBD7 723-727
PBD6 713-715

42 (C) The spirometric data suggest a restrictive lung disease process. The progressive pulmonary interstitial fibrosis of a restrictive lung disease such as a pneumoconiosis can eventually lead to dilation of remaining airspaces, giving a "honeycomb" appearance. The loss of lung tissue with emphysema also leads to airspace dilation but without alveolar wall fibrogenesis. The increase in mucous glands with chronic bronchitis leads to copious sputum production but not fibrogenesis. Eosinophilic infiltrates suggest atopic asthma, an episodic disease without fibrogenesis. Hyaline membranes along with edema, inflammation, and focal necrosis are features of diffuse alveolar damage (acute respiratory distress syndrome) in the acute phase; if patients survive for weeks, diffuse alveolar damage may resolve to honeycomb change.

BP7 468   BP6 395, 404   PBD7 728-729   PBD6 726-727

43 (E) The findings in this study suggest pulmonary thromboembolism, and most pulmonary emboli are small and clinically silent. Sudden death may occur with large emboli that occlude the main pulmonary arteries. Cor pulmonale can result from repeated embolization with reduction in the pulmonary vascular bed. Hemoptysis with pulmonary embolism is uncommon, although it may occur when a hem-

orrhagic infarction results from thromboembolism. Dyspnea can occur with medium to large emboli.

BP7 475-477   BP6 412-413   PBD7 742-743
PBD6 703-704

44 (E) This patient has chronic restrictive lung disease. The cause of many slowly progressive cases of restrictive lung disease is unknown. These cases must be distinguished from those with identifiable causes such as infection, collagen vascular disease, drug use, and pneumoconioses. Scleroderma may produce a progressive restrictive lung disease, but there are usually other manifestations involving the skin, and the ANA test result typically is positive. Goodpasture syndrome is a rare cause of sudden onset of severe hemoptysis. Silicosis is a progressive interstitial disease, but the patient's occupation as a pilot would tend to exclude exposure to dusts. Diffuse alveolar damage is an acute form of interstitial disease.

BP7 468   BP6 407-408   PBD7 729-731   PBD6 735-736

45 (A) Bronchiolitis obliterans with organizing pneumonia (BOOP), also called cryptogenic organizing pneumonia (COP), is an uncommon, nonspecific reaction to a lung injury such as an infection or toxic exposure. Desquamative interstitial pneumonitis (DIP) is an uncommon smoking-related interstitial disease in which monocytes gather together to form intra-alveolar macrophages; DIP is not related to idiopathic pulmonary fibrosis. Diffuse alveolar damage is an acute condition complicating an underlying lung injury; there is damage to alveolar capillary walls, followed by exudate with hyaline membrane formation. Hypersensitivity pneumonitis is a type III (and type IV) hypersensitivity response to an inhaled allergen. Pulmonary alveolar proteinosis is a rare idiopathic condition in which there are gelatinous alveolar proteinaceous exudates. Wegener granulomatosis is a form of vasculitis with pulmonary capillaritis.

BP7 475   PBD7 731, 767   PBD6 738

46 (F) The figure shows a prominent upper lobe cavitation in the tan-to-white caseating granulomas, typical of reactivation-reinfection tuberculosis in adults. *Candida* is a rare cause of lung infection. Coccidioidomycosis can produce granulomatous disease, but it is much less common than tuberculosis. Influenza viral infections have mainly interstitial mononuclear inflammation. The bacterial organisms listed, including *Legionella* and *Klebsiella*, are more likely to produce a bronchopneumonia with alveolar neutrophilic exudates. *Mycoplasma* infection produces mainly interstitial mononuclear inflammation. Nocardiosis of the lung appears mainly as chronic abscessing inflammation.

BP7 488-490   BP6 424   PBD7 381-386   PBD6 725

47 (B) Bronchioloalveolar carcinoma is a peripheral tumor that can mimic pneumonia. Most of these tumors are well differentiated. Adenocarcinomas and large cell carcinomas are also peripheral, but the former tend to produce a localized mass, whereas cells of the latter are large and pleomorphic and form sheets; sometimes it is difficult to distinguish among them. Hamartomas are uncommon, very slow-growing, benign peripheral masses composed of cartilage, epithelial cells, and fibrous connective tissue with blood vessels. Mesotheliomas almost always occur in the setting of prior asbestos exposure; they are large pleural masses.

Metastases tend to appear as multiple nodules. Squamous cell carcinomas can occasionally be peripheral (although most are central) and are composed of pink, polygonal cells that have intercellular bridges. If well differentiated, squamous cell carcinomas show keratin pearls.

BP7 502   BP6 433   PBD7 760-762   PBD6 742-745

48 (C) This patient is at occupational risk of asbestos exposure. The inhaled asbestos fibers become encrusted with iron and appear as the characteristic ferruginous bodies with iron stain. The firm, tan mass encasing the pleura is most likely a malignant mesothelioma. Asbestosis more commonly gives rise to pleural fibrosis and interstitial lung disease, like other pneumoconioses. This is seen grossly as a dense pleural plaque, which often is calcified. Asbestosis can give rise to bronchogenic carcinoma, especially in smokers. Fluffy infiltrates suggest an infectious process. Upper lobe cavitation is suggestive of secondary tuberculosis. An endobronchial mass could be a carcinoid tumor, which is not related to asbestosis. Focal bronchial dilation is a pattern seen in bronchiectasis, which is most often a complication of recurrent or chronic infection.

BP7 272-274, 468   BP6 227-229   PBD7 735-737
PBD6 732-733

49 (A) The most common primary lung malignancy in women and in nonsmokers is adenocarcinoma. Overall, lung cancers in nonsmokers are far less frequent than in smokers. Primary adenocarcinomas in the lung tend to be small, peripheral masses that are amenable to surgical excision and have a better overall prognosis than other forms of lung cancer. Bronchial carcinoids are uncommon endobronchial lesions. Bronchioloalveolar carcinomas are peripheral masses with a distinctive microscopic appearance of neoplastic cells proliferating along the alveolar and bronchiolar framework. Hamartomas are small, peripheral masses that contain benign epithelial and connective tissue elements. Large cell carcinomas are too poorly differentiated to be called adenocarcinomas or squamous cell carcinomas. Localized mesotheliomas are not related to asbestos exposure and are pedunculated masses attached to the pleura. Overall, far more metastatic adenocarcinomas involve the lung than do primary adenocarcinomas (such as thyroid follicular carcinoma), but metastases tend to be multiple, and because they denote systemic disease, surgery generally is not an option.

BP7 502   BP6 433   PBD7 758-761   PBD6 744

50 (C) The patient had a saddle pulmonary thromboembolus. Sudden death occurs from hypoxemia or from acute cor pulmonale with right-sided heart failure. Because the airways are not obstructed, the lungs do not collapse, and there is no bronchoconstriction. With such an acute course, there is not enough time for a hemorrhagic pulmonary infarction to occur. Edema is not a feature of thromboembolism.

BP7 476   BP6 412   PBD7 742-743   PBD6 703

51 (A) The clinical and morphologic features strongly suggest sarcoidosis. This granulomatous disease has an unknown cause, but the presence of granulomas and activated T cells in the lungs indicates a delayed hypersensitivity response to some inhaled antigen. Lung involvement, occurring in about one third of cases, may be asymptomatic or may

lead to restrictive lung disease. Hypersensitivity pneumonitis is an immune-complex disease that is triggered by inhaled allergens. This form of lung disease is characterized by acute dyspneic episodes. There can be granulomas in the lung, but lymph node enlargement is not seen. Diffuse alveolar damage is an acute lung injury seen in acute respiratory distress syndrome. Smoking causes chronic bronchitis and emphysema. Atypical mycobacteria cause caseating granulomas, as does *Mycobacterium tuberculosis*.

BP7 470-472   BP6 409-410   PBD7 737-739
PBD6 734-735

52 (E) This patient had chronic bronchitis complicated by pulmonary hypertension and cor pulmonale. There are few characteristic microscopic features of chronic bronchitis, so it is mainly defined clinically by the presence of a persistent cough with sputum production for at least 3 months in at least 2 consecutive years. Increased eosinophils are characteristic of bronchial asthma, which is an episodic disease unlikely to cause cor pulmonate. Chronic bronchitis does not lead to diffuse pulmonary fibrosis. Granulomatous disease is more typical of sarcoidosis or mycobacterial infection. Lymphangitic metastases may fill lymphatic spaces and produce a reticulonodular pattern on a chest radiograph, but patients tend not to live long with such advanced cancer.

BP7 463-464   BP6 405-406   PBD7 722-723, 744
PBD6 700-703

53 (A) The finding of pulmonary hypertension in a young person without any known pulmonary or cardiac disease is typical for primary pulmonary hypertension. The increased pulmonary arterial pressure leads to right heart hypertrophy. The large pulmonary arteries show atherosclerosis; the arterioles show plexogenic arteriopathy with a tuft of capillary formations producing a network, or web, that spans the lumens of dilated thin-walled arteries. BMPR2, a cell-surface protein belonging to the TGF-β receptor superfamily, causes inhibition of vascular smooth muscle cell proliferation and favors apoptosis. In the absence of BMPR2 signaling, smooth muscle proliferation occurs and pulmonary hypertension ensues. Inactivating germ-line mutations in the *BMPR2* gene are found in 50% of the familial (primary) cases of pulmonary hypertension of 26% of sporadic cases. None of the other molecules listed regulate pulmonary arterial wall structure. Fibrillin-1 gene mutation occurs in Marfan syndrome; lysyl hydroxylase is required for cross-linking collagen, and its loss gives rise to one form of Ehlers-Danlos syndrome. Endothelin and endothelial nitric oxide control vascular caliber. Renin and atrial natriuretic factor regulate sodium and water homeostasis, plasma volume, and systemic arterial pressure.

BP7   PBD7 743-745

54 (D) Blunt trauma to the chest can lead to rib fracture. The sharp bone can penetrate the pleura and produce an air leak, resulting in pneumothorax. Although pulmonary embolus and pneumonia are possible complications in hospitalized patients, they would not occur this quickly. Edema and hydrothorax are unlikely from trauma alone; hemorrhage is more likely. Although pneumothorax can complicate rupture of a bulla in emphysema, this is more likely to occur in paraseptal emphysema than in centrilobular emphysema.

BP7 506   BP6 436   PBD7 767-768   PBD6 751

55 **(D)** The early, acute phase of bronchial asthma is triggered by release of chemical mediators, whereas the late phase is mediated by recruited inflammatory cells and the cytokines they release. Among the early phase mediators, the leukotrienes C4, D4, and E4 promote intense bronchoconstriction and mucin production. Montelukast is an agent that binds to cysteinyl leukotriene (CysLT) receptors on mast cells and eosinophils to block the lipoxygenase pathway of arachidonic acid metabolism, which generates the leukotrienes. Prostaglandin D_2 is also a bronchoconstrictor, but its role is less well defined than that of leukotrienes. C3a increases vascular permeability, and C3b acts an opsonin. Platelet-activating factor (PAF) increases vascular permeability and aids in histamine release from platelet granules. Interleukin (IL)-5, as well as PAF, is chemotactic for neutrophils. Histamine acts during the early acute phase of type I hypersensitivity reactions but is far less potent, and antihistaminic agents are not useful for treating asthma. It plays very little role in chronic bronchial asthma, when the late-phase reaction takes over. Tumor necrosis factor and IL-1 mediate fever and induce acute phase responses with neutrophilia, adrenocorticotropic hormone release, and hypotension.

BP7 457   BP6 396   PBD7 717, 726   PBD6 713

56 **(B)** Congestive heart failure is far more common than the other listed conditions. The cell count and appearance indicate a transudate. Lymphoma may lead to chylothorax, and carcinomas involving the pleura tend to produce blood-tinged fluid. Systemic lupus erythematosus and renal failure tend to produce effusions with more protein or cells.

BP7 505   BP6 436   PBD7 766-767   PBD6 750-751

57 **(B)** Hamartomas are uncommon benign peripheral lesions of the lung. They are composed of benign-appearing epithelial cells and connective tissue, typically with a large component of cartilage. They are induced in the differential diagnosis of a "coin lesion" (a Susan B. Anthony dollar, not a real silver dollar) that also includes carcinoma and granuloma. Adenocarcinoma is the most common primary lung malignancy in nonsmokers, and it can present as a coin lesion, but it is composed of gland-forming, malignant cells without cartilage. It tends to be peripheral, making surgical resection an option in many cases. Large cell carcinomas are also more likely to be peripheral, but they tend to be larger masses. Malignant mesothelioma is a rare neoplasm, even in persons who have been exposed to asbestos, and it arises on the pleura. Primary non-Hodgkin lymphomas of the lung are uncommon. Some squamous cell carcinomas can be peripheral, but they are most likely to occur in persons who smoke.

BP7 167-168   BP6 433   PBD7 765   PBD6 744-745

58 **(A)** The patient has hypersensitivity pneumonitis, with acute symptoms that occur soon after exposure to an antigen, often actinomycetes or fungi (molds) growing in air conditioners. The symptoms improve when the person leaves the environment where the antigen is located. The pulmonary pathologic changes are usually minimal, with interstitial mononuclear infiltrates. This type of hypersensitivity pneumonitis is called "farmer's lung"; inhaling actinomycetes in moldy hay can cause this illness. It is mainly a type III hypersensitivity reaction, but with more chronic exposure to the antigen, there may be a component of type IV hypersensitivity with granulomatous inflammation. Attachment of antibody to basement membrane occurs in Goodpasture syndrome. Mycolic acid is a component of the cell wall of mycobacteria, and infections with these organisms are chronic, not episodic. Prostaglandins are produced by the cyclo-oxygenase pathway of arachidonic acid metabolism during acute inflammation and mediate pain and vasodilation. Histamine release is characteristic of a type I hypersensitivity reaction that more typically occurs in allergic disease. Leukotrienes are important mediators in asthma. A toxic injury is more typical of inhalation of a toxic gas such as sulfur dioxide (so-called silo-filler's disease).

BP7 472-473   BP6 410-411   PBD7 739   PBD6 737

59 **(C)** The patient has "primary atypical pneumonia" caused by *Mycoplasma pneumoniae*, a cell wall–deficient organism that is difficult to culture. Often, a diagnosis is made empirically. The findings are similar to those of other viral infections, and serologic testing shows the specific organism. *Legionella* can produce an extensive pneumonia with neutrophilic alveolar exudates, and the organisms are difficult to demonstrate—they may be revealed by Dieterle silver stain. *Mycobacterium fortuitum* is a rare infection that is most likely to be seen in very ill or immunocompromised persons. Nocardiosis produces chronic abscessing inflammation; it is mostly seen in immunosuppressed persons. Respiratory syncytial virus is typically an infection of early childhood.

BP7 482-484   BP6 419-420   PBD7 346, 349, 751
PBD6 721-722

60 **(A)** The patient has severe acute respiratory syndrome (SARS), which is caused by a strain of coronavirus that is much more virulent than the coronaviruses known to be associated with the "common cold." Cytomegalovirus is seen in immunocompromised patients and often involves multiple organs. Ebola virus is virulent and does not cause specific respiratory findings. Herpes simplex virus is a very rare cause of pneumonia, even in immunocompromised persons. HIV does not directly cause lung disease; however, HIV causes AIDS, which is associated with many pulmonary infections. Respiratory syncytial virus causes acute respiratory illness in young children.

BP7 481   PBD7 752   PBD6 721-722

61 **(C)** Idiopathic pulmonary fibrosis leads to progressive restrictive lung disease. The antigen that incites the inflammatory process with activated macrophage release of cytokines such as fibroblast growth factor and transforming growth factor–β (TGF-β) is unknown. Acute respiratory distress syndrome follows acute lung injury in very ill patients, typically those in an intensive care unit. Goodpasture syndrome is characterized by diffuse pulmonary hemorrhage. Sarcoidosis is marked by granulomatous inflammation. In this case, scleroderma is less likely because of the negative serologic test result. Wegener granulomatosis produces necrotizing granulomatous inflammation, and the ANCA test often is positive.

BP7 469-470   BP6 407-409   PBD7 729-731
PBD6 735-736

CHAPTER 16

Head and Neck

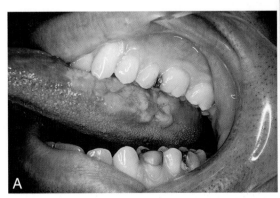

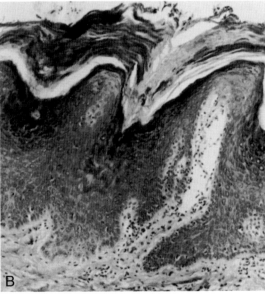

1 A 55-year-old man visited his dentist for a routine dental examination. The dentist noticed lesions with the clinical and histologic appearance shown. The past medical history showed no major medical problems. Which of the following etiologic factors most likely contributed to the development of these lesions?

- ❑ (A) Dental caries
- ❑ (B) Herpes simplex virus type 1
- ❑ (C) Eating smoked and pickled foods
- ❑ (D) Chronic sialadenitis
- ❑ (E) Smoking tobacco

2 After a bout of the "flu," a 25-year-old man notices several 0.3-cm, clear vesicles on his upper lip. The vesicles rupture, leaving shallow, painful ulcers that heal over the course of 4 weeks. Several months later, after a skiing trip, similar vesicles develop, with the same pattern of healing. Which of the following findings is most likely to be associated with these lesions?

❑ (A) Biopsy showing squamous epithelial hyperkeratosis
❑ (B) Positive serologic test for herpes simplex virus type 1
❑ (C) Peripheral blood smear showing atypical lymphocytes
❑ (D) Cytologic scraping showing budding cells with pseudohyphae
❑ (E) Biopsy showing mononuclear inflammatory infiltrate

3 For the past 4 months, a 50-year-old man has had difficulty breathing through his nose and also has experienced dull facial pain. On physical examination, there is a mass filling the right nasal cavity. CT scan of the head shows a 4-cm mass in the nasopharynx on the right that erodes adjacent bone. The mass is excised, and microscopic examination shows that it is composed of large epithelial cells with indistinct borders and prominent nuclei. Mature lymphocytes are scattered throughout the undifferentiated neoplasm. Which of the following etiologic factors most likely played the greatest role in the development of this lesion?

❑ (A) Epstein-Barr virus infection
❑ (B) Sjögren syndrome
❑ (C) Smoking tobacco
❑ (D) Allergic rhinitis
❑ (E) Wegener granulomatosis

4 Over the past 10 years, a 60-year-old man has had progressive difficulty hearing, particularly with the left ear. Audiometric testing shows that he has a bone conduction type of deafness. CT scan of the head shows no abnormal findings. The patient's brother and mother are similarly affected. Which of the following is the most likely diagnosis?

❑ (A) Otosclerosis
❑ (B) Schwannoma
❑ (C) Cholesteatoma
❑ (D) Otitis media
❑ (E) Chondrosarcoma

5 A 35-year-old man who is known to be infected with HIV complains that he has had a "bad" taste in his mouth and discoloration of his tongue for the past 6 weeks. On physical examination, there are areas of adherent, yellow-tan, circumscribed plaque on the lateral aspects of the tongue. This plaque can be scraped off as a pseudomembrane to show an underlying granular, erythematous base. Which of the following is the most likely diagnosis?

❑ (A) Aphthous ulcer
❑ (B) Cheilosis
❑ (C) Hairy leukoplakia
❑ (D) Herpetic stomatitis
❑ (E) Leukoplakia
❑ (F) Glossitis
❑ (G) Oral thrush

6 Over the past 3 years, a 65-year-old woman has noticed a slowly enlarging nodule on her face. On physical examina-

tion, a 3-cm, nontender, mobile, discrete mass is palpable on the left side of the face, anterior to the ear and just superior to the mandible. The mass is completely excised, and histologic examination shows ductal epithelial cells in a myxoid stroma containing islands of chondroid and bone. This patient is most likely to have which of the following neoplasms?

❑ (A) Acinic cell tumor
❑ (B) Mucoepidermoid carcinoma
❑ (C) Pleomorphic adenoma
❑ (D) Primitive neuroectodermal tumor (PNET)
❑ (E) Squamous cell carcinoma
❑ (F) Warthin tumor

7 A 23-year-old man has had difficulty breathing through his nose for 2 years. This problem has become progressively worse over the past 2 months. Physical examination shows glistening, translucent, polypoid masses filling the nasal cavities. Histologic examination of the excised masses shows respiratory mucosa overlying an edematous stroma with scattered plasma cells and eosinophils. Which of the following laboratory findings is most likely to be present in this patient?

❑ (A) Elevated serum hemoglobin A_{1c} level
❑ (B) Increased serum IgE level
❑ (C) Nuclear staining for Epstein-Barr virus antigens
❑ (D) Tissue culture positive for *Staphylococcus aureus*
❑ (E) Positive antinuclear antibody test result

8 A 65-year-old woman notices a lump on the right side of her face that has become larger over the past year. On physical examination, a 3- to 4-cm firm, mobile, painless mass is palpable in the region of the right parotid gland. The oral mucosa appears normal. The patient does not complain of difficulty in chewing food or talking. Which of the following conditions is most likely to account for these findings?

❑ (A) Sialolithiasis
❑ (B) Pleomorphic adenoma
❑ (C) Sjögren syndrome
❑ (D) Mucoepidermoid carcinoma
❑ (E) Malignant lymphoma

9 Over the past 3 months, a 6-year-old boy has had increased difficulty breathing, and the character of his voice has changed. Endoscopic examination shows three soft, pink excrescences on the true vocal cords and in the subglottic region. The masses are 0.6 to 1.0 cm in diameter. Microscopic examination of the excised masses shows fingerlike projections of orderly squamous epithelium overlying fibrovascular cores. Immunostaining for human papillomavirus 6 antigens is positive. Based on these findings, which of the following statements is the best advice to give the parents of this boy?

❑ (A) A total laryngectomy is necessary
❑ (B) Therapy with acyclovir is indicated
❑ (C) The boy should not overuse his voice
❑ (D) The lesions are likely to recur
❑ (E) Congenital heart disease may be present

10 A 68-year-old man goes to the physician for a routine health maintenance examination. Physical examination of the oral cavity shows that the right buccal mucosa has some discrete white patches with a leathery surface. The lesions are spread over an area of 0.7 × 2.5 cm. A biopsy sample from one of the lesions shows squamous epithelial acanthosis with marked hyperkeratosis. Which of the following risk factors is most likely to cause these lesions?

- ❑ (A) Eating chili peppers
- ❑ (B) Chewing spearmint gum
- ❑ (C) French kissing
- ❑ (D) Chewing tobacco
- ❑ (E) HIV infection

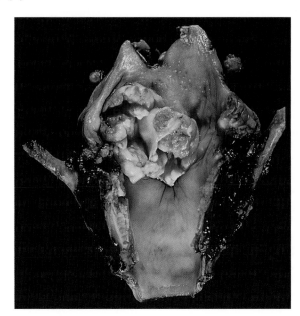

11 A 70-year-old man who experienced increasing hoarseness for almost 6 months has recently had an episode of hemoptysis. On physical examination, no lesions are noted in the nasal or oral cavity. There is a firm, nontender anterior cervical lymph node. The lesion shown in the figure above is identified by endoscopy. The patient undergoes biopsy, followed by laryngectomy and neck dissection. Which of the following etiologic factors most likely played the greatest role in the development of this lesion?

- ❑ (A) Human papillomavirus infection
- ❑ (B) Type I hypersensitivity
- ❑ (C) Smoking tobacco
- ❑ (D) Repeated bouts of aspiration
- ❑ (E) Epstein-Barr virus infection

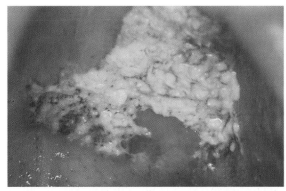

Courtesy of Drs. E.E. Vokes, S. Lippman, et al, Department of Thoracic/Head and Neck Oncology, Texas Medical Center, Houston, TX. Reprinted with permission from The New England Journal of Medicine 328:184, 1993.

12 A 49-year-old man has used chewing tobacco and snuff for many years. During a visit to his dentist, a lesion is seen on the hard palate (see preceding figure). It cannot be removed by scraping. A biopsy is performed, and microscopic examination of the lesion shows a thickened squamous mucosa. Several years later, a biopsy specimen of a similar lesion shows carcinoma in situ. Which of the following is the most likely diagnosis?

- ❑ (A) Aphthous ulcer
- ❑ (B) Oral thrush
- ❑ (C) Lichen planus
- ❑ (D) Leukoplakia
- ❑ (E) Pyogenic granuloma
- ❑ (F) Xerostomia

13 A 60-year-old woman noticed an enlarging "bump" beneath her tongue for the past year. She does not smoke or use alcohol. On physical examination, there is a 2.5-cm, movable, submucosal mass arising in the minor salivary glands on the buccal mucosa beneath the tongue on the right. Histologic examination of the excised mass shows that it is malignant and locally invasive. The tumor recurs within 1 year. Which of the following is the most likely diagnosis?

- ❑ (A) Non-Hodgkin lymphoma
- ❑ (B) Mucoepidermoid carcinoma
- ❑ (C) Primitive neuroectodermal tumor (PNET)
- ❑ (D) Pleomorphic adenoma
- ❑ (E) Squamous cell carcinoma
- ❑ (F) Warthin tumor

14 A 17-year-old girl notices a small, sensitive, gray-white area forming along the lateral border of her tongue 2 days before the end of her final examinations. On examination by the physician's assistant, the girl is afebrile. There is a shallow, ulcerated, 0.3-cm lesion with an erythematous rim. No specific therapy is given, and the lesion disappears within 2 weeks. The past history shows that the girl "does not smoke or chew tobacco and does not go out with boys who do." Which of the following is the most probable cause of this lesion?

- ❑ (A) Aphthous ulcer
- ❑ (B) Oral thrush
- ❑ (C) Herpes simplex stomatitis
- ❑ (D) Leukoplakia
- ❑ (E) Sialadenitis

15 A 5-year-old boy has had repeated bouts of earache. On examination by the physician, the bouts have been accompanied by a red, bulging tympanic membrane, either unilaterally or bilaterally, sometimes with a small amount of yellowish exudate. Laboratory studies have included cultures of *Staphylococcus aureus* and *Pseudomonas aeruginosa*. The most recent examination shows that the right tympanic membrane has perforated. The boy responds to antibiotic therapy. Which of the following complications is most likely to occur as a consequence of these events?

- ❑ (A) Otosclerosis
- ❑ (B) Labyrinthitis
- ❑ (C) Squamous cell carcinoma
- ❑ (D) Eosinophilic granuloma
- ❑ (E) Cholesteatoma

16 A 17-year-old girl is concerned about a "bump" on her neck that she has noticed for several months. It does not seem to have increased in size appreciably during that time. On physical examination, there is a discrete, slightly movable nodule in the midline of the neck just above the thyroid gland. The nodule is excised, and microscopic examination shows a cystic mass lined by squamous and respiratory epithelium. Which of the following additional histologic elements would most likely be located adjacent to this cyst?

- (A) Malignant lymphoma
- (B) Thyroid
- (C) Serous salivary glands
- (D) Squamous cell carcinoma
- (E) Noncaseating granulomas

17 A 21-year-old woman comes to the physician because she is concerned about a lump on the left side of her neck that has remained the same size for the past year. Physical examination shows a painless, movable, 2-cm nodule beneath the skin of the left lateral neck just above the level of the thyroid cartilage. There are no other remarkable findings. Fine needle aspiration of the mass is performed. The physician is less than impressed by the pathology report, which notes, "Granular and keratinaceous cellular debris." Fortunately, she has saved her Robbins pathology textbook that she used in medical school. She consults the head and neck chapter to arrive at a diagnosis, using the data from the report. Which of the following terms best describes this nodule?

- (A) Branchial cyst
- (B) Metastatic thyroid carcinoma
- (C) Mucocele
- (D) Mucoepidermoid tumor
- (E) Paraganglioma
- (F) Thyroglossal duct cyst

18 A 76-year-old man has been bothered by pain on the left side of the face for 2 weeks. On physical examination, there is a tender area of swelling 4 cm in diameter beneath the skin, anterior to the left auricle above the angle of the jaw. The patient appears somnolent and has mild muscular rigidity and expressionless facies. CT scan of the head shows cystic and solid areas in the region of an enlarged left parotid gland. After a course of antibiotic therapy, there is only minimal improvement. A parotidectomy is performed. Microscopic examination of the excised gland shows acute and chronic inflammation, with fibrosis and abscess formation, and atrophy of acini. *Staphylococcus aureus* is cultured from the tissue. Which of the following risk factors is most likely to have caused this patient's illness?

- (A) Eating chili peppers
- (B) Human papillomavirus infection
- (C) Sjögren syndrome
- (D) Smoking tobacco
- (E) Thioridazine therapy
- (F) Vitamin B₂ deficiency

19 A 55-year-old woman has noticed an enlarging lump on the right side of her neck for the past 7 months. On physical examination, there is a 3-cm nodule in the right upper neck, medial to the sternocleidomastoid muscle and lateral to the trachea at the angle of the mandible. CT scan shows a cir-

cumscribed, solid mass adjacent to the carotid bifurcation. Microscopic examination of the excised mass shows nests of round cells with pink, granular cytoplasm. Immunohistochemical markers are chromogranin and S-100. Electron microscopy shows neurosecretory granules in the tumor cell cytoplasm. The tumor recurs 1 year later and is again excised. Which of the following is the most likely diagnosis?

- (A) Metastatic squamous cell carcinoma
- (B) Metastatic thyroid medullary carcinoma
- (C) Mucoepidermoid carcinoma
- (D) Paraganglioma
- (E) Warthin tumor

20 A 28-year-old man who is a singer-songwriter has been experiencing hard times for the past 3 years. He has played at a couple of clubs a night to earn enough to avoid homelessness. He comes to the free clinic because he has noticed that his voice quality has become progressively hoarser over the past year. On physical examination, he is afebrile. There are no palpable masses in the head and neck area. He does not have a cough or significant sputum production, but he has been advised on previous visits to give up smoking. Which of the following is most likely to produce these findings?

- (A) Croup
- (B) Epiglottitis
- (C) Reactive nodule
- (D) Squamous cell carcinoma
- (E) Squamous papillomatosis

21 A 3-year-old child is brought to the physician by her parents because she has had difficulty breathing for the past 24 hours. On physical examination, the child is febrile and has a harsh cough with prominent inspiratory stridor. The lungs are clear on auscultation. An anterior-posterior neck radiograph shows subglottic edema. The child's oxygen saturation is normal with pulse oximetry. She improves over the next 3 days while taking nebulized glucocorticoids. Which of the following is the most likely causal organism?

- (A) *Corynebacterium diphtheriae*
- (B) Epstein-Barr virus
- (C) *Haemophilus influenzae*
- (D) Human papillomavirus
- (E) *Parainfluenza virus*
- (F) *Streptococcus pyogenes*, group A

22 A 20-year-old man noted progressive swelling on the left side of his face over the past year. On physical examination there is painless swelling in the region of the left posterior mandible. A head CT scan shows a circumscribed multilocular cyst of the left mandibular ramus. The lesion is surgically excised with wide bone margins. On microscopic examination the lesion shows cysts lined by stratified squamous epithelium with a prominent basal layer; no inflammation or granulation tissue is seen. Which of the following is the most likely diagnosis?

- (A) Ameloblastoma
- (B) Dentigerous cyst
- (C) Odontogenic keratocyst
- (D) Odontoma
- (E) Periapical cyst/granuloma

ANSWERS

1 **(E)** This whitish, well-defined mucosal patch on the tongue has the characteristic appearance of leukoplakia, a premalignant lesion that can give rise to squamous cell carcinoma. Pipe smoking and tobacco chewing are implicated in the development of leukoplakia. Chronic alcohol abuse is also implicated, but the association is less strong than with tobacco. Ill-fitting dentures may lead to leukoplakia but far less commonly than smoking. Dental caries is not a risk factor for leukoplakia, unless the affected tooth becomes eroded and misshapen. Infections and inflammation are not recognized risk factors for oral leukoplakia or oral squamous cell cancers. The type of food eaten has less of a correlation with cancer of the oral cavity than with cancer of the esophagus.

BP7 546   BP6 473-474   PBD7 778-780   PBD6 760-761

2 **(B)** The lesions of herpes simplex virus type 1 (HSV-1), also known as "cold sores" or "fever blisters," are common. Many people have HSV-1, and the oral and perianal lesions appear during periods of stress. Recurrence is the norm. Leukoplakia is marked by hyperkeratosis. Atypical lymphocytes are seen with infectious mononucleosis. They may be accompanied by a rash but do not produce vesicular lesions of the skin. Budding cells with pseudohyphae suggest a candidal infection with oral thrush. A mononuclear infiltrate is quite nonspecific and can be seen with aphthous ulcers.

BP7 544-545   BP6 471-472   PBD7 776-777   PBD6 757

3 **(A)** This patient has a nasopharyngeal carcinoma. There is a strong association with Epstein-Barr virus infection, which contributes to the transformation of squamous epithelial cells. Sjögren syndrome is associated with malignant lymphomas, but these typically arise in the salivary gland, not the nasal cavity. Smoking is not associated with nasopharyngeal carcinoma, although it does contribute to oral and esophageal cancers. Allergic rhinitis is associated with development of nasal polyps, but these do not become malignant. Wegener granulomatosis can involve the respiratory tract, causing granulomatous inflammation and vasculitis, but the nasopharyngeal region is not commonly affected, and there is no risk of malignant growth.

BP7 507   BP6 437   PBD7 785   PBD6 764

4 **(A)** Otosclerosis can be familial, particularly when it is severe. It results from fibrous ankylosis followed by bony overgrowth of the little ossicles of the middle ear. A schwannoma typically involves the vestibulocochlear nerve and results in a nerve conduction form of deafness. Schwannomas are usually unilateral, although familial neurofibromatosis could result in multiple schwannomas. A cholesteatoma is typically a unilateral process that complicates chronic otitis media in a child or young adult. Uncomplicated otitis media is usually self-limited and is uncommon in adults. Chondrosarcomas may involve the skull in older adults but are rare, solitary, bulky masses in the region of the jaw.

PBD7 788   PBD6 767

5 **(G)** The patient has oral thrush, a lesion resulting from oral candidiasis in persons who are immunocompromised.

The lesion is typically superficial. Microscopic examination shows the typical budding cells and pseudohyphae of *Candida*. Aphthous ulcers, or "canker sores," are very common in young persons but can appear at any age; they tend to be recurrent superficial ulcerations. Cheilosis is fissuring or cracking of the mucosa, typically at the corners of the mouth, which may be seen with vitamin B_2 (riboflavin) deficiency. Hairy leukoplakia can also be seen with HIV infection, but it is far less common than oral thrush. It occurs from marked hyperkeratosis, forming a rough "hairy" surface, and is related to Epstein-Barr virus infection. Multinucleated cells suggest a herpesvirus infection, which typically has vesicles that ulcerate. Atypical squamous epithelial cells usually arise from areas of oral leukoplakia. Glossitis may have an appearance ranging from a shiny red surface of the tongue to ulceration. It may be seen with vitamin deficiencies, including vitamin B_2, B_3, B_6, or B_{12}.

BP7 545   BP6 472   PBD7 777   PBD6 757

6 **(C)** Pleomorphic adenoma is the most common tumor of the parotid gland. These tumors are rarely malignant, although they can be locally invasive. An acinic cell tumor is composed of cells resembling the serous cells of the salivary gland; they are generally small, but about one sixth metastasize to regional lymph nodes. Mucoepidermoid tumors are less common than pleomorphic adenomas in major salivary glands. They may be high-grade and aggressive. The primitive neuroectodermal tumor (PNET), also known as an olfactory neuroblastoma, is one of the small, round, blue-cell tumors that occur in childhood. It is likely to arise in the nasopharyngeal region. Squamous cell carcinomas arise in the buccal mucosa and are invasive. Warthin tumors are uncommon and indolent, although they may be bilateral or multicentric.

BP7 548   BP6 475   PBD7 791-792   PBD6 770-771

7 **(B)** The patient has nasal polyps, which can be associated with allergic rhinitis, a form of type I hypersensitivity often called hay fever. In some patients, this inflammation results in the formation of polyps in the nasal cavity. Type I hypersensitivity is associated with high IgE levels in the serum. The elevated hemoglobin A_{1c} level is indicative of diabetes mellitus. Diabetes is not a risk factor for polyp formation, but ketoacidosis can lead to nasopharyngeal mucormycosis. Epstein-Barr virus infection can be found in nasopharyngeal carcinomas. *Staphylococcus aureus* often colonizes the nasal cavity, but it usually does not cause problems. Autoimmune diseases are not associated with nasal polyp formation.

PBD7 783   PBD6 762

8 **(B)** Pleomorphic adenoma is the most common benign salivary gland tumor and the most common tumor of the parotid gland. These tumors tend to be slow growing, and most are benign, although local invasion and recurrence are potential problems. Sialolithiasis is usually accompanied by sialadenitis and is therefore quite painful. It may produce some gland enlargement but usually is not a mass effect. Sjögren syndrome can produce some salivary gland enlargement, but the process is typically bilateral. A mucoepidermoid tumor can occur in salivary glands, but this tumor is much less common than a pleomorphic adenoma. Malignant lymphomas of the salivary gland are uncommon.

BP7 548   BP6 475   PBD7 777   PBD6 769-771

9 **(D)** The patient has juvenile laryngeal papillomatosis, which is caused by human papillomavirus (HPV) types 6 and 11. These lesions frequently recur after excision. They may regress after puberty. If laryngeal papillomas arise in adulthood, they are usually solitary and do not recur. There is no effective antiviral therapy for HPV. Although the lesions can be found throughout the airway, they are benign and do not become malignant. The occurrence of the lesions is not related to the use of the voice. This is not a congenital condition and is not part of a syndrome.

BP7 507   BP6 537   PBD7 786-787   PBD6 766

10 **(D)** The clinical and histologic features suggest leukoplakia. Oral leukoplakia may appear in various intraoral sites and on the lower lip border. Pipe smoking and tobacco chewing are implicated in the development of these white patches. Irritation from misaligned teeth or dentures may also produce leukoplakia. Transformation to dysplasia and carcinoma is possible. Foods and chewing gum are not risk factors. In some parts of the world, the chewing of betel nut is a risk factor for oral cancer. Social behavior may be a risk factor for infections such as herpes simplex. HIV infection is most often associated with oral thrush (candidiasis) and with herpes simplex virus infections.

BP7 546   BP6 472-473   PBD7 778-780   PBD6 759-760

11 **(C)** The figure shows a large, fungating neoplasm that has the typical appearance of a laryngeal squamous cell carcinoma. The most common risk factor is smoking, although chronic alcohol abuse also plays a role. About 5% of patients harbor human papillomavirus sequences. The etiologic significance of this is not clear. Allergies with type I hypersensitivity may result in transient laryngeal edema but not neoplasia. Aspiration may result in acute inflammation but not neoplasia. Epstein-Barr virus infection is associated with nasopharyngeal carcinomas.

BP7 507-508   BP6 437-438   PBD7 786-787
PBD6 765-766

12 **(D)** The raised white patches suggest leukoplakia. This is a premalignant condition. Risk factors include tobacco use, particularly tobacco chewing, and chronic irritation. Human papillomavirus infection has been implicated in some lesions. Aphthous ulcers, or "canker sores," are very common in young persons but may appear at any age; they tend to be recurrent superficial ulcerations. Oral thrush appears most often on the tongue of immunocompromised persons as a yellowish plaquelike area. Microscopic examination shows budding cells with pseudohyphae characteristic of *Candida* infection. Lichen planus in the oral cavity usually appears in conjunction with similar skin lesions; it forms whitish patches that may ulcerate. The lesions have intense submucosal chronic inflammation. A pyogenic granuloma forms a painful gingival nodule of granulation tissue. Xerostomia, or "dry mouth," is seen in Sjögren syndrome.

BP7 546   BP6 472-473   PBD7 778-780   PBD6 759-760

13 **(B)** Mucoepidermoid carcinomas can arise in major and minor salivary glands. They account for most neoplasms that arise within minor salivary glands, particularly those that are malignant. Low-grade mucoepidermoid carcinomas may

be invasive, but the prognosis is usually good, with a 5-year survival rate of 90%. High-grade mucoepidermoid carcinomas can metastasize and have a 5-year survival rate of only 50%. Non-Hodgkin lymphomas are found in adjacent cervical lymph nodes or in the Waldeyer ring of lymphoid tissue. A primitive neuroectodermal tumor (PNET), also known as an olfactory neuroblastoma, is a small, round, blue-cell tumor of childhood; it is likely to arise in the nasopharyngeal region. Pleomorphic adenomas are more common in the major salivary glands than are mucoepidermoid tumors, and they are more likely to be indolent. Squamous cell carcinomas are invasive and arise in the buccal mucosa. Warthin tumors are uncommon and indolent.

PBD7 793-794   PBD6 772

14 **(A)** An aphthous ulcer is a common lesion that is also known as a "canker sore." The lesions are never large but are annoying and tend to occur during periods of stress. Aphthous ulcers are not infectious; they probably have an autoimmune origin. Oral thrush is a superficial candidal infection that occurs in diabetic, neutropenic, and immunocompromised patients. Herpetic lesions are typically vesicles that can rupture. Leukoplakia appears as white patches of thicker mucosa from hyperkeratosis. It may be a precursor to squamous cell carcinoma in a few cases; the temperance ditty mentioned in the history is a cautionary note for all young people. Inflammation of a salivary gland (sialadenitis), typically a minor salivary gland in the oral cavity, may produce a localized, tender nodule.

BP7 544   BP6 471   PBD7 776   PBD6 757

15 **(E)** Cholesteatomas are not true neoplasms, but they are cystic masses lined by squamous epithelium. The desquamated epithelium and keratin degenerates, resulting in cholesterol formation and giant cell reaction. Although their histologic findings are benign, cholesteatomas can gradually enlarge, eroding and destroying the middle ear and surrounding structures. They occur as a complication of chronic otitis media. Otosclerosis is abnormal bone deposition in the ossicles of the middle ear that results in bone deafness in adults. Labyrinthitis typically is caused by a viral infection and is self-limited. Although cholesteatomas have a squamous epithelial lining, malignant transformation does not occur. An eosinophilic granuloma of bone occasionally may be seen in the region of the skull in young children, but it is characterized by the presence of Langerhans cells.

PBD7 788   PBD6 767

16 **(B)** The location of this nodule is classic for a thyroglossal duct (tract) cyst, which is a developmental abnormality that arises from elements of the embryonic thyroglossal duct extending from the foramen cecum of the tongue down to the thyroid gland. One or more remnants of this tract may enlarge to produce a cystic mass. Although lymphoid tissue often surrounds these cysts, malignant transformation does not occur. The cysts may contain squamous epithelium, but squamous cell carcinoma does not arise from such a cyst. If there is a cystic lesion with lymphoid tissue and squamous carcinoma in the neck, it is probably a metastasis from an occult primary tumor of the head and neck. Salivary gland choristomas are unlikely at this site. Granulomatous disease is more likely to involve lymph nodes in the typical locations in the lateral neck regions.

PBD7 789   PBD6 767-768

17 (A) Branchial cysts, also known as lymphoepithelial cysts, may be remnants of an embryonic branchial arch or a salivary gland inclusion in a cervical lymph node. They are distinguished from thyroglossal duct cysts by their lateral location, the absence of thyroid tissue, and their abundant lymphoid tissue. Occult thyroid carcinoma, often a papillary carcinoma, may present as a metastasis to a node in the neck, but the microscopic pattern is that of a carcinoma. About 5% of squamous cell carcinomas of the head and neck present initially as a nodal metastasis, without an obvious primary site. This patient, however, is quite young for such an event. Mucoceles form in minor salivary glands; mucoepidermoid tumors form in salivary glands. The nodule in this patient is in the neck. Paragangliomas are solid tumors that may arise deep in the region of the carotid body near the common carotid bifurcation.

PBD7 788-789   PBD6 767

18 (E) This patient has sialadenitis, which is more common in older persons and persons receiving phenothiazine therapy for schizophrenia. Most neuroleptic drugs are dopaminergic receptor blockers, but they have extrapyramidal and anticholinergic side effects. The dry mouth, coupled with dehydration, favors inspissation of salivary gland secretions and stone formation to block ducts and increase the risk of inflammation and infection. Chili peppers contain capsaicin, which evokes a sensation of tingling and burning pain by activating a nonselective cation channel, called VR1, on sensory nerve endings; this effect does not reach the salivary glands. Human papillomavirus infection may lead to the development of squamous dysplasias and carcinomas. Sjögren syndrome can produce xerostomia, but there is chronic fibrosing inflammation that is typically not suppurative. Smoking tobacco is associated with development of oral squamous cell carcinomas. Vitamin B_2 (riboflavin) deficiency is associated with cheilosis.

BP7 547-548   PBD7 790   PBD6 769

19 (D) Paragangliomas are neuroendocrine tumors that rarely produce sufficient catecholamines to affect blood pressure, unlike their adrenal medullary counterpart, the pheochromocytoma. The microscopic appearance of these lesions does not always correlate with their biologic behavior. There is a tendency for recurrence and metastasis in spite of the tumor's "bland" appearance. Metastases should always be considered in patients this age. About 5% of squamous cell carcinomas of the head and neck present initially as a nodal metastasis, without an obvious primary site, but the microscopic pattern here is not that of squamous cell carcinoma.

Some thyroid cancers initially may present as a nodal metastasis, but the microscopic pattern in this case fits best with paraganglioma. A mucoepidermoid carcinoma or a Warthin tumor arises in a salivary gland.

PBD7 789-790   PBD6 768-769

20 (C) Reactive nodules (vocal cord polyps, or "singer's nodules") occur most often in men who are heavy smokers or who strain their vocal cords. The nodules are generally only a few millimeters in size and have a fibrovascular core covered by hyperplastic and hyperkeratotic squamous epithelium. They are not premalignant. Croup is an acute laryngotracheobronchitis that occurs in children. It produces airway narrowing with inspiratory stridor. Epiglottitis is an acute inflammatory process that may cause airway obstruction. Squamous cell carcinomas of the pharynx and larynx are more common in smokers but generally are seen in persons older than this patient. Squamous papillomatosis usually first appears in childhood; if it is extensive, it can produce airway obstruction.

BP7 507   PBD7 786   PBD6 765

21 (E) The child has croup, a laryngotracheobronchitis that is most often caused by parainfluenza virus. The inflammation may be severe enough to produce airway obstruction. *Corynebacterium diphtheriae* is the cause of diphtheria, which produces laryngitis with a characteristic dirty-grey membrane that may slough and be aspirated. This infection is now rare because of routine childhood immunizations. Epstein-Barr virus (EBV) may be associated with infectious mononucleosis and produce pharyngitis. EBV also is associated with nasopharyngeal carcinoma. *Haemophilus influenzae* may cause an acute bacterial epiglottitis with an abrupt onset of pain and possible airway obstruction. Human papillomavirus is associated with laryngeal papillomatosis. Group A streptococci produce an exudative pharyngitis.

BP7 506   BP6 437   PBD7 363, 786   PBD6 765

22 (C) This is the typical location and histology for an odontogenic keratocyst which arises from rests of odontogenic epithelium within the jaw. They are benign but can recur if inadequately excised. Ameloblastoma and odontoma are tumors arising from odontogenic epithelium. Odontoma, the most common odontogenic tumor, shows extensive deposition of enamel and dentin. Dentigerous cysts originate around the crown of an unerupted tooth, typically the third molar, and are lined by a thin, nonkeratinizing layer of squamous epithelium; they contain a dense chronic inflammatory infiltrate in the stroma. Periapical cysts/granulomas are inflammatory lesions that develop at the apex of teeth as a complications of long-standing pulpitis.

PBD7 782

The Gastrointestinal Tract

1 A 30-year-old woman sees her physician because she has had diarrhea and fatigue and has noticed a 3-kg weight loss over the past 6 months. On physical examination, she is afebrile and has mild muscle wasting, but her motor strength is normal. Laboratory studies show no occult blood, ova, or parasites in the stool. A biopsy specimen from the upper jejunum is obtained, and microscopic findings are reviewed. The patient is placed on a special diet with no wheat or rye grain products. The change in diet produces dramatic improvement. Which of the following microscopic features is most likely to be seen in the biopsy specimen?

❑ (A) Lymphatic obstruction
❑ (B) Noncaseating granulomas
❑ (C) Villous blunting and flattening
❑ (D) Foamy macrophages within the lamina propria
❑ (E) Crypt abscesses

2 Two days after eating a chicken salad sandwich, a 35-year-old man experiences cramping abdominal pain with fever and watery diarrhea. Physical examination shows mild diffuse abdominal pain on palpation, but there are no masses. Bowel sounds are present. A stool sample is negative for occult blood. He recovers completely within a few days without therapy. Which of the following infectious organisms is most likely to produce these findings?

❑ (A) *Yersinia enterocolitica*
❑ (B) *Escherichia coli*
❑ (C) *Entamoeba histolytica*
❑ (D) *Salmonella enteritidis*
❑ (E) Rotavirus
❑ (F) *Staphylococcus aureus*
❑ (G) *Bacillus cereus*

3 A 38-year-old woman has had nausea for the past 6 months. She reports no vomiting or diarrhea. On physical examination, there are no remarkable findings. Upper gastrointestinal endoscopy shows diffuse gastric mucosal erythema with focal mucosal erosions but no ulcerations. The esophageal and duodenal mucosal surfaces appear normal. Microscopic examination of gastric biopsy specimens shows increased numbers of neutrophils, lymphocytes, and plasma cells in the mucosa, as well as edema, focal mucosal hemorrhage, and loss of the surface epithelium. No *Helicobacter pylori* organisms are seen. Laboratory studies show a normal serum gastrin level. Which of the following pharmacologic agents is most likely to produce these findings?

❑ (A) Acetylsalicylic acid (aspirin)
❑ (B) Acyclovir
❑ (C) Chlorpromazine
❑ (D) Cimetidine
❑ (E) Clindamycin
❑ (F) Omeprazole
❑ (G) Prednisone

4 One year after having an acute myocardial infarction, a 55-year-old man saw his physician because of severe abdominal pain and bloody diarrhea. On physical examination, the abdomen was diffusely tender, and bowel sounds were absent. Abdominal plain film radiographs showed no free air. Laboratory studies showed a normal CBC and normal levels of serum amylase, lipase, and bilirubin. His condition deteriorated, and he developed irreversible shock. At autopsy, which of the following lesions is most likely to be found?

❑ (A) Acute appendicitis
❑ (B) Acute pancreatitis
❑ (C) Intestinal infarction
❑ (D) Acute cholecystitis
❑ (E) Pseudomembranous colitis

❑ (A) Appendicitis
❑ (B) Collagenous colitis
❑ (C) Diverticulitis
❑ (D) Ischemic colitis
❑ (E) Pseudomembranous colitis
❑ (F) Spontaneous bacterial peritonitis
❑ (G) Typhlitis

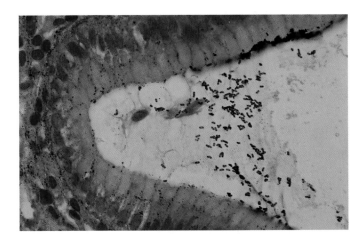

5 A 59-year-old man has had nausea and vomiting for several months. He has experienced no hematemesis. On physical examination, there is no abdominal tenderness, and bowel sounds are present. Upper gastrointestinal endoscopy shows erythematous areas of mucosa with thickening of the rugal folds in the gastric antrum. The microscopic appearance of a gastric biopsy specimen with a Steiner silver stain is shown above. Which of the following organisms is most likely to be present on the luminal surface? _Toxins_

❑ (A) Cysteine proteinase
❑ (B) Heat stable enterotoxin
❑ (C) Shiga toxin
❑ (D) Vacuolating toxin
❑ (E) Verocytotoxin

6 A 62-year-old man sees his physician because he has had fever and back pain for the past 2 days. Physical examination shows tenderness of the right costovertebral angle. Laboratory studies show leukocytosis and pyuria with WBC casts. He has been receiving antibiotic therapy with cefotaxime, clindamycin, and nafcillin for the past 16 days. He now develops lower abdominal pain and a severe diarrhea. _Clostridium difficile_ toxin is identified in a stool specimen. Which of the following conditions is he most likely to have now developed?

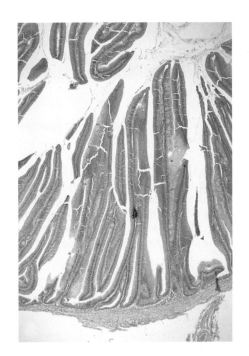

7 A 70-year-old man saw his physician for a routine health maintenance examination. On physical examination, there were no remarkable findings, but a stool sample was positive for occult blood. A colonoscopy was performed and showed a 5-cm sessile mass in the upper portion of the descending colon at 50 cm from the anal verge. The histologic appearance at low power of a biopsy specimen of the lesion is shown in the figure above. The patient refused further workup and treatment. Five years later, he sees his physician because of constipation, microcytic anemia, and a 5-kg weight loss over the past 6 months. On surgical exploration, there is a 7 cm mass encircling the descending colon. Which of the following neoplasms is he now most likely to have?

❑ (A) Adenocarcinoma
❑ (B) Non-Hodgkin lymphoma
❑ (C) Carcinoid tumor
❑ (D) Leiomyosarcoma
❑ (E) Mucinous cystadenoma
❑ (F) Squamous cell carcinoma
❑ (G) Villous adenoma

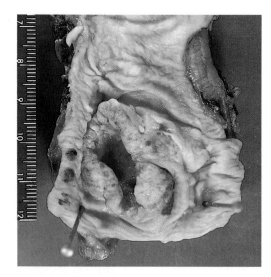

8 A 70-year-old man with a lengthy history of chronic alcoholism has had increasing difficulty swallowing and has noticed a 6-kg weight loss over the past 2 months. On physical examination, there are no remarkable findings. Upper gastrointestinal endoscopy shows a 3-cm ulcerative mass in the midesophagus that partially occludes the esophageal lumen. Esophagectomy is performed, and the gross appearance of the lesion is shown above. Which of the following is most likely to be seen on microscopic section of this mass?

☐ (A) Multinucleated cells with intranuclear inclusions
☐ (B) Squamous cell carcinoma
☐ (C) Dense collagenous scar
☐ (D) Adenocarcinoma
☐ (E) Thrombosed vascular channels

9 A 33-year-old man who lives in New York is bothered by a low-volume, mostly watery diarrhea associated with flatulence. The symptoms occur episodically, but they have been persistent for the past year. He has experienced a 5-kg weight loss. He has no fever, nausea, vomiting, or abdominal pain. On physical examination, there are no significant findings. A stool sample is negative for occult blood, ova, and parasites, and a stool culture yields no pathogens. An upper gastrointestinal endoscopy is performed. A biopsy specimen from the upper part of the small bowel shows severe diffuse blunting of villi and a chronic inflammatory infiltrate in the lamina propria. Which of the following serologic tests is most likely to be positive in this patient?

☐ (A) Anticentromeric antibody
☐ (B) Anti-DNA topoisomerase I antibody
☐ (C) Antigliadin antibody
☐ (D) Antimitochondrial antibody
☐ (E) Antinuclear antibody

10 A potluck lunch party is held at the office at noon on Thursday. A variety of meats, salads, breads, and desserts that were brought in earlier that morning are served. Everyone has a good time, and most of the food is consumed. By mid-afternoon, the single office restroom is being used by many employees who have an acute, explosive diarrhea accompanied by abdominal cramping. Which of the following infectious agents is most likely responsible for this turn of events?

☐ (A) *Escherichia coli*
☐ (B) *Staphylococcus aureus*
☐ (C) *Vibrio parahaemolyticus*
☐ (D) *Clostridium difficile*
☐ (E) *Salmonella enteritidis*
☐ (F) *Bacillus cereus*

11 During summer "Black and White Days," a week-long local community celebration of the dairy industry (Holstein cows are black and white), a 40-year-old man suffers from episodic abdominal bloating, flatulence, and explosive diarrhea. On physical examination, there are no remarkable findings. Laboratory studies show no increase in stool fat and no occult blood, ova, or parasites in the stool. A routine stool culture yields no pathogens. During the rest of the year, the patient does not consume milk shakes or ice cream sodas and is not symptomatic. Which of the following conditions best accounts for these findings?

☐ (A) Celiac sprue
☐ (B) Autoimmune gastritis
☐ (C) Cholelithiasis
☐ (D) Disaccharidase deficiency
☐ (E) Cystic fibrosis

12 For the past year, a 20-year-old man has had increasingly voluminous, bulky, foul-smelling stools and a 10-kg weight loss. There is no history of hematemesis or melena. He has some bloating but no abdominal pain. On physical examination, there are no palpable abdominal masses and bowel sounds are present. Which of the following laboratory findings is most likely to be present on examination of his stool?

☐ (A) Increased stool fat
☐ (B) *Giardia lamblia* cysts
☐ (C) Occult blood
☐ (D) *Vibrio cholerae*
☐ (E) *Entamoeba histolytica* trophozoites

13 A 68-year-old woman has had substernal pain after meals for many years. For the past year, she has had increased difficulty swallowing both liquids and solids. On physical examination, there are no remarkable findings. Upper gastrointestinal endoscopy shows a lower esophageal mass that nearly occludes the lumen of the esophagus. Biopsy of this mass is most likely to show which of the following neoplasms?

☐ (A) Adenocarcinoma
☐ (B) Leiomyosarcoma
☐ (C) Squamous cell carcinoma
☐ (D) Non-Hodgkin lymphoma
☐ (E) Carcinoid tumor

14 After an uncomplicated pregnancy, a 23-year-old woman, G 2, P 1, gave birth to a term infant boy of normal weight and length. The infant initially did well, but at 6 weeks, he began feeding poorly for 1 week, and his mother noticed that much of the milk he ingested was forcefully vomited within 1 hour. On physical examination, the infant is afebrile, and there are no external anomalies. The physician palpates a midabdominal mass. Bowel sounds are active. The medical history indicates that the mother and her first child had the same illness during infancy. Which of the following conditions is most likely to explain these findings?

❑ (A) Pyloric stenosis
❑ (B) Tracheoesophageal fistula
❑ (C) Diaphragmatic hernia
❑ (D) Duodenal atresia
❑ (E) Annular pancreas

15 A 53-year-old woman has had nausea, vomiting, and midepigastric pain for 5 months. On physical examination, there are no significant findings. An upper gastrointestinal radiographic series shows gastric outlet obstruction. Upper gastrointestinal endoscopy shows an ulcerated mass that is 2 × 4 cm at the pylorus. Which of the following neoplasms is most likely to be seen in a biopsy specimen of this mass?

❑ (A) Non-Hodgkin lymphoma
❑ (B) Neuroendocrine carcinoma
❑ (C) Squamous cell carcinoma
❑ (D) Adenocarcinoma
❑ (E) Leiomyosarcoma

16 A 60-year-old man has had increasing fatigue for the past 8 months. On physical examination, he appears pale. On digital rectal examination, no masses are palpable, but a stool sample is positive for occult blood. Physical examination of the abdomen shows active bowel sounds with no masses or areas of tenderness. Laboratory studies show hemoglobin of 8.3 g/dL, hematocrit 24.6%, MCV 73 μm3, platelet count 226,000/mm³, and WBC count 7640/mm³. A colonoscopy shows no identifiable source of the bleeding. Angiography shows a 1-cm focus of dilated and tortuous vascular channels in the mucosa and submucosa of the cecum. Which of the following is the most likely diagnosis?

❑ (A) Mesenteric vein thrombosis
❑ (B) Internal hemorrhoids
❑ (C) Angiodysplasia of the colon
❑ (D) Collagenous colitis
❑ (E) Colonic diverticulosis

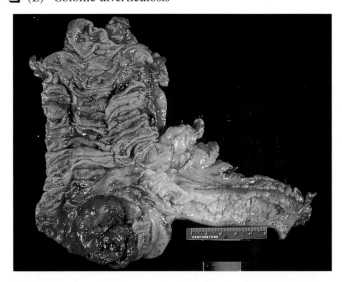

17 A 43-year-old woman has become increasingly tired and listless over the past 5 months. She has had menometrorrhagia for the past 3 months. On physical examination, there are no remarkable findings except for a positive result on stool guaiac testing. Laboratory studies show hemoglobin of 9.2 g/dL, hematocrit 27.3%, and MCV 75 μm³. Pelvic ultrasound reveals an enlarged uterus. A Pap smear shows abnor-

mal cells of probable endometrial origin. Colonoscopy is performed, followed by partial colectomy, with the gross appearance of the lesion shown in the preceding figure. Which of the following molecular abnormalities has most likely led to these findings?

❑ (A) Mutation in a DNA mismatch repair gene
❑ (B) Germ-line inheritance of an *APC* gene mutation
❑ (C) Tyrosine kinase activation due to *c-KIT* mutation
❑ (D) Homozygous loss of the *PTEN* gene
❑ (E) Inactivation of the Rb protein by HPV-16

18 A 23-year-old woman has had a bloody, mucoid, low-volume diarrhea for the past 5 weeks. She has about five stools per day. On physical examination, she is afebrile, and there is no abdominal tenderness or masses. Bowel sounds are present. Laboratory studies show no ova or parasites in the stool, only mucus and blood with few leukocytes. Colonoscopy shows friable, erythematous mucosa extending from the rectum to the middle of the descending colon. A rectal biopsy specimen shows acute mucosal inflammation with crypt abscesses and epithelial cell necrosis. Which of the following is the most likely diagnosis?

❑ (A) Shigellosis
❑ (B) Ulcerative colitis
❑ (C) Crohn disease
❑ (D) Diverticulitis
❑ (E) Ischemic colitis

19 A 52-year-old man has had a 6-kg weight loss and nausea for the past 6 months. He has no vomiting or diarrhea. On physical examination, there are no remarkable findings. Upper gastrointestinal endoscopy shows a 6-cm area of irregular pale fundic mucosa and loss of the rugal folds. A biopsy specimen shows a monomorphous infiltrate of lymphoid cells. *Helicobacter pylori* organisms are identified in mucus overlying adjacent mucosa. The patient receives antibiotic therapy for *H. pylori*, and the repeat biopsy shows a resolution of the infiltrate. Which of the following is the most likely diagnosis?

❑ (A) Chronic gastritis
❑ (B) Diffuse large B-cell lymphoma
❑ (C) Autoimmune gastritis
❑ (D) Mucosa-associated lymphoid tissue tumor
❑ (E) Crohn disease
❑ (F) Gastrointestinal stromal tumor

20 A 70-year-old man takes large quantities of nonsteroidal anti-inflammatory drugs (NSAIDs) because of chronic degenerative arthritis of the hips and knees. Recently, he has had epigastric pain with nausea and vomiting and an episode of hematemesis. On physical examination, there are no remarkable findings. A gastric biopsy specimen is most likely to show which of the following lesions?

❑ (A) Epithelial dysplasia
❑ (B) Hyperplastic polyp
❑ (C) Acute gastritis
❑ (D) Adenocarcinoma
❑ (E) *Helicobacter pylori* infection

21 A 44-year-old woman has had increasing difficulty swallowing liquids and solids for the past 6 months. On physical examination, her fingers have reduced mobility because of taut, nondeforming skin. A barium swallow shows marked dilation of the esophagus with "beaking" in the distal portion, where there is marked luminal narrowing. A biopsy specimen from the lower esophagus shows prominent submucosal fibrosis with little inflammation. Which of the following is most likely to produce these findings?

- ❑ (A) Portal hypertension
- ❑ (B) Iron deficiency
- ❑ (C) Barrett esophagus
- ❑ (D) CREST syndrome
- ❑ (E) Hiatal hernia

22 A 35-year-old man has had epigastric pain for over 1 year. The pain tends to occur 2 to 3 hours after a meal and is relieved if he takes antacids or eats more food. He has noticed a 4-kg weight gain in the past year. He does not smoke and drinks 1 glass of Johannisberg Riesling daily. The result of a urea breath test is positive, and a gastric biopsy specimen contains urease. He begins a 2-week course of antibiotics, but on day 4, he feels better and discontinues treatment. Several weeks later, the epigastric pain recurs. If the patient does not seek further treatment, which of the following complications is he most likely to develop?

- ❑ (A) Hematemesis
- ❑ (B) Fat malabsorption
- ❑ (C) Hepatic metastases
- ❑ (D) Carcinoid syndrome
- ❑ (E) Vitamin B$_{12}$ deficiency

23 A 27-year-old man has sudden onset of marked abdominal pain. On physical examination, his abdomen is diffusely tender and distended, and bowel sounds are absent. He undergoes surgery, and a 27-cm segment of terminal ileum with a firm, erythematous serosal surface is removed. The microscopic appearance of a section through the excised ileum is shown in the preceding figure. Which of the following additional complications is the patient most likely to develop as a result of this disease process?

- ❑ (A) Metastatic adenocarcinoma
- ❑ (B) Mesenteric artery thrombosis
- ❑ (C) Intussusception
- ❑ (D) Hepatic abscess
- ❑ (E) Enterocutaneous fistula

24 An 8-month-old previously healthy infant girl develops a watery diarrhea that lasts for 1 week. The infant has a mild fever during the illness but has no abdominal pain or swelling. On physical examination, her temperature is 37.7°C. A stool sample is negative for occult blood, ova, or parasites. Her parents are told to give her plenty of fluids, and she recovers fully. Which of the following organisms is most likely to produce these findings?

- ❑ (A) *Campylobacter jejuni*
- ❑ (B) *Cryptosporidium parvum*
- ❑ (C) *Escherichia coli*
- ❑ (D) *Listeria monocytogenes*
- ❑ (E) Norwalk virus
- ❑ (F) Rotavirus
- ❑ (G) *Shigella flexneri*
- ❑ (H) *Vibrio cholerae*

25 A 46-year-old woman with a lengthy history of heartburn and dyspepsia experiences sudden onset of abdominal pain. On physical examination, she has severe midepigastric pain with guarding. Bowel sounds are reduced. An abdominal plain film radiograph shows free air under the left leaf of the diaphragm. The patient is immediately taken to surgery, and a perforated duodenal ulcer is repaired. Which of the following organisms is most likely to have produced these findings?

- ❑ (A) *Campylobacter jejuni*
- ❑ (B) *Cryptosporidium parvum*
- ❑ (C) *Entamoeba histolytica*
- ❑ (D) *Giardia lamblia*
- ❑ (E) *Helicobacter pylori*
- ❑ (F) *Salmonella typhi*
- ❑ (G) *Shigella flexneri*
- ❑ (H) *Yersinia enterocolitica*

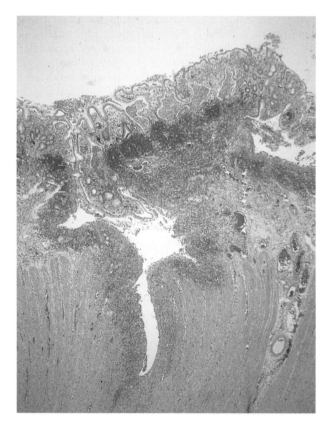

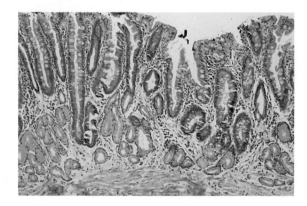

26 A 59-year-old man has had increasing difficulty swallowing during the past 6 months. There are no significant findings on physical examination. Upper gastrointestinal endoscopy shows areas of erythematous mucosa above the Z-line. A biopsy specimen from the lower esophagus has the microscopic appearance shown in the preceding figure. As a consequence of this patient's condition, which of the following complications is most likely to occur?

- (A) Hematemesis
- (B) Squamous cell carcinoma
- (C) Adenocarcinoma
- (D) Achalasia
- (E) Lacerations (Mallory-Weiss syndrome)

27 One day after a meal of raw oysters, a healthy 21-year-old woman develops a profuse, watery diarrhea. On physical examination, her temperature is 37.5°C. A stool sample is negative for occult blood. There is no abdominal distention or tenderness, and bowel sounds are present. The diarrhea subsides over the next 3 days. Which of the following organisms is most likely to produce these findings?

- (A) *Yersinia enterocolitica*
- (B) *Staphylococcus aureus*
- (C) *Cryptosporidium parvum*
- (D) *Entamoeba histolytica*
- (E) *Vibrio parahaemolyticus*

28 A 57-year-old woman has had burning epigastric pain after meals for more than 1 year. Physical examination shows no abnormal findings. Upper gastrointestinal endoscopy shows an erythematous patch in the lower esophageal mucosa. A biopsy specimen shows basal squamous epithelial hyperplasia, elongation of lamina propria papillae, and scattered intraepithelial neutrophils with some eosinophils. Which of the following is the most likely diagnosis?

- (A) Barrett esophagus
- (B) Esophageal varices
- (C) Reflux esophagitis
- (D) Scleroderma
- (E) Iron deficiency

29 A 49-year-old woman sees her physician because she has had abdominal cramps and diarrhea, with six stools per day for the past month. She has a history of similar episodes of self-limited pain and diarrhea, which have occurred several times during the past 20 years. Each episode lasts about 2 weeks and resolves without treatment. Findings on physical examination are unremarkable, but a stool sample is positive for occult blood. Laboratory studies show no ova or parasites in the stool. Colonoscopy shows diffuse and uninterrupted mucosal inflammation and superficial ulceration extending from the rectum to the ascending colon. Colonic biopsy specimens from the area show a diffuse, predominantly mononuclear, infiltrate in the lamina propria. The patient is at high risk of developing which of the following complications?

- (A) Adenocarcinoma of the colon
- (B) Diverticulitis
- (C) Primary biliary cirrhosis
- (D) Fat malabsorption
- (E) Pseudomembranous colitis
- (F) Perirectal fistula formation

30 A 41-year-old man has been HIV positive for the past 8 years and has been receiving highly active antiretroviral therapy (HAART) for the past year. For the past 2 weeks, he has experienced pain when swallowing. He has had no episodes of hematemesis and no nausea or vomiting. There are no remarkable findings on physical examination. The CD4+ lymphocyte count is now 285/μL. Which of the following conditions is most likely to produce these findings?

- (A) Esophageal squamous cell carcinoma
- (B) Achalasia
- (C) Lower esophageal fibrosis with stenosis
- (D) Herpes simplex esophagitis
- (E) Gastroesophageal reflux disease

31 A 67-year-old woman has experienced severe nausea, vomiting, early satiety, and a 9-kg weight loss over the past 4 months. On physical examination, she has mild muscle wasting. Upper gastrointestinal endoscopy shows that the entire gastric mucosa is eroded and has an erythematous, cobblestone appearance. Upper gastrointestinal radiographs show that the stomach is small and shrunken. Which of the following is most likely to be found on histologic examination of a gastric biopsy specimen?

- (A) Early gastric carcinoma
- (B) Gastrointestinal stromal tumor
- (C) Granulomatous inflammation
- (D) Chronic atrophic gastritis
- (E) Signet-ring cell adenocarcinoma

32 A 51-year-old man has sudden onset of massive emesis of bright red blood. On physical examination, his temperature is 36.9°C, pulse 103/min, respirations 19/min, and blood pressure 85/50 mm Hg. Laboratory studies show a hematocrit of 21%. The serologic test result for HBsAg is positive. He has had no prior episodes of hematemesis. The hematemesis is most likely to be a consequence of which of the following?

- (A) Esophageal varices
- (B) Barrett esophagus
- (C) *Candida albicans* infection
- (D) Reflux esophagitis
- (E) Squamous cell carcinoma
- (F) Zenker diverticulum

33 A 16-year-old boy who is receiving chemotherapy for acute lymphoblastic leukemia sees the physician because he has had pain for 1 week when he swallows food. Physical examination shows no abnormal findings. Upper gastrointestinal endoscopy shows 0.5- to 0.8-cm mucosal ulcers in the region of the middle to lower esophagus. The shallow ulcers are round, sharply demarcated, and have an erythematous base. Which of the following is most likely to produce these findings?

- (A) Aphthous ulcerations
- (B) Herpes simplex esophagitis
- (C) Gastroesophageal reflux disease
- (D) *Candida* esophagitis
- (E) Mallory-Weiss syndrome

34 An 11-month-old previously healthy infant has not produced a stool for 1 day. The mother notices that the infant's abdomen is distended. On physical examination, the infant's abdomen is very tender and bowel sounds are nearly absent. An abdominal plain film radiograph shows no free air, but there are distended loops of small bowel with air-fluid levels. Which of the following is most likely to produce these findings?

❑ (A) Meckel diverticulum
❑ (B) Duodenal atresia
❑ (C) Hirschsprung disease
❑ (D) Pyloric stenosis
❑ (E) Intussusception

35 A 22-year-old woman has had several episodes of aspiration of food associated with difficulty swallowing during the past year. On auscultation, crackles are heard at the base of the right lung. A barium swallow shows marked esophageal dilation above the level of the lower esophageal sphincter. A biopsy specimen from the lower esophagus shows an absence of the myenteric ganglia. Which of the following is the most likely diagnosis?

❑ (A) Hiatal hernia
❑ (B) Plummer-Vinson syndrome
❑ (C) Barrett esophagus
❑ (D) Systemic sclerosis
❑ (E) Achalasia

36 A 53-year-old woman comes to her physician for a routine health maintenance examination. The only abnormal finding is a stool specimen that contains occult blood. Colonoscopy shows a 1.5-cm solitary, rounded, erythematous polyp on a 0.5-cm stalk at the splenic flexure. The polyp is removed, and its histologic appearance is shown in the figure below at low (A) and high (B) magnifications. When the physician discusses these findings with the patient, which of the following statements is most appropriate?

❑ (A) You have inherited one defective copy of the *APC* gene
❑ (B) Other family members probably have colonic polyps
❑ (C) Many more polyps will appear within the next few years
❑ (D) There is a high probability that you will develop endometrial cancer
❑ (E) A detailed workup to detect metastases from this lesion is not warranted

37 A 20-year-old woman in her ninth month of pregnancy has increasing pain on defecation and notices bright red blood on the toilet paper. She has had no previous gastrointestinal problems. After she gives birth, the rectal pain subsides, and there is no more bleeding. Which of the following is the most likely cause of these findings?

❑ (A) Angiodysplasia
❑ (B) Ischemic colitis
❑ (C) Intussusception
❑ (D) Hemorrhoids
❑ (E) Volvulus

38 A neonate born at 32 weeks' gestation was in stable condition and feeding well 3 days after birth. There was no respiratory distress. On day 4, the infant's abdomen was tender and appeared distended. A stool sample is positive for occult blood. Laboratory studies showed leukocytosis and a blood culture positive for growth of *Escherichia coli*. The infant died of septic shock. Which of the following is most likely to be found at autopsy?

❑ (A) Dark red necrotic ileum and cecum
❑ (B) Markedly dilated colon above the sigmoid
❑ (C) Purulent ascitic fluid
❑ (D) Markedly enlarged mesenteric lymph nodes
❑ (E) A 5-cm mass in the retroperitoneum

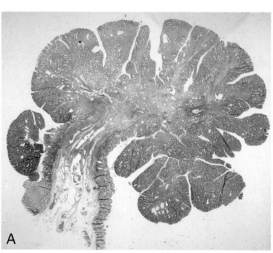
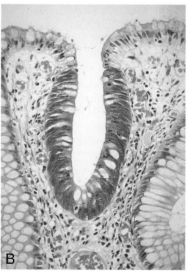

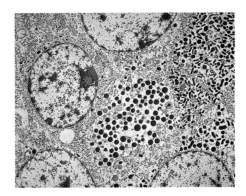

39 A 26-year-old man is brought to the emergency department after sustaining abdominal gunshot injuries. At laparotomy, while repairing the small intestine, the surgeon notices a 2-cm mass near the site of bowel perforation. The yellow-tan–colored submucosal ileal mass is removed. The electron micrograph of a neoplastic cell from the mass is shown above. Which of the following is the most likely cell of origin of this lesion?

- ❑ (A) Lipoblast
- ❑ (B) Ganglion cell
- ❑ (C) Neuroendocrine cell
- ❑ (D) Smooth muscle cell
- ❑ (E) Mucin-secreting epithelial cell

40 A 20-year-old woman has had nausea and vague lower abdominal pain for the past 24 hours, but now the pain has become more severe. On physical examination, the pain is worse in the right lower quadrant, and there is rebound tenderness. A stool sample is negative for occult blood. Abdominal plain film radiographs show no free air. The result of a serum pregnancy test is negative. Which of the following laboratory findings is most useful to aid in the diagnosis of this patient?

- ❑ (A) Hyperamylasemia
- ❑ (B) Hypernatremia
- ❑ (C) Increased serum carcinoembryonic antigen
- ❑ (D) Increased serum alkaline phosphatase
- ❑ (E) Leukocytosis
- ❑ (F) *Entamoeba histolytica* cysts in the stool

41 Over the past 3 months, a 45-year-old woman has noticed that her skin has become progressively more yellow. On physical examination, she is afebrile and has scleral icterus and generalized jaundice. Laboratory studies show total serum bilirubin of 8.9 mg/dL, direct bilirubin 6.8 mg/dL, serum ALT 125 U/L, and AST 108 U/L. A liver biopsy specimen shows histologic features of sclerosing cholangitis. Which of the following diseases of the gastrointestinal tract is most likely to coexist with the liver disease?

- ❑ (A) Chronic pancreatitis
- ❑ (B) Diverticulosis
- ❑ (C) Ulcerative colitis
- ❑ (D) Celiac sprue
- ❑ (E) Peptic ulceration

42 One week after a trip to Central America, a 31-year-old woman had an increasingly severe diarrhea. Gross examination of the stools showed mucus and streaks of blood. The diarrheal illness subsided within a couple of weeks, but now the patient has become febrile and has pain in the right upper quadrant of the abdomen. An abdominal ultrasound scan shows a 10-cm irregular, partly cystic mass in the right hepatic lobe. Which of the following infectious organisms is most likely to produce these findings?

- ❑ (A) *Giardia lamblia*
- ❑ (B) *Cryptosporidium parvum*
- ❑ (C) *Entamoeba histolytica*
- ❑ (D) *Clostridium difficile*
- ❑ (E) *Strongyloides stercoralis*

43 A 51-year-old woman has been feeling increasingly tired for the past 7 months. There are no remarkable findings on physical examination. Laboratory studies include hemoglobin of 9.5 g/dL, hematocrit 29.1%, MCV 124 μm³, platelet count 268,000/mm³, and WBC count 8350/mm³. The reticulocyte index is low. Hypersegmented polymorphonuclear leukocytes are found on a peripheral blood smear. Antibodies to which of the following are most likely to be found in this patient?

- ❑ (A) Gliaden
- ❑ (B) *Tropheryma whippelii*
- ❑ (C) *Helicobacter pylori*
- ❑ (D) Gastric H⁺, K⁺-ATPase
- ❑ (E) Intrinsic factor receptor

44 A 24-year-old woman gives birth to an infant at term after an uncomplicated pregnancy. Apgar scores are 9 and 10 at 1 and 5 minutes after birth. The infant's length and weight are at the 55th percentile. There is no significant passage of meconium. Three days after birth, the infant vomits all oral feedings. On physical examination, the infant is afebrile, but the abdomen is distended and tender and bowel sounds are reduced. An abdominal ultrasound scan shows marked colonic dilation above a narrow segment in the sigmoid region. A biopsy specimen from the narrowed region shows an absence of ganglion cells in the muscle wall and submucosa. Which of the following is most likely to produce these findings?

- ❑ (A) Hirschsprung disease
- ❑ (B) Trisomy 21
- ❑ (C) Volvulus
- ❑ (D) Colonic atresia
- ❑ (E) Necrotizing enterocolitis
- ❑ (F) Intussusception

45 A 24-year-old man sees his physician because of abdominal pain and increasing fatigue that has developed over the past 6 months. On physical examination, he is afebrile and appears pale. On palpation, there is mild pain in the right lower quadrant of the abdomen. There are no masses, and bowel sounds are active. Laboratory studies show hemoglobin of 8.9 g/dL, hematocrit 26.7%, MCV 74 μm³, platelet count 255,000/mm³, and WBC count 7780/mm³. Upper gastrointestinal endoscopy and a colonoscopy showed no lesions. One month later, the patient continues to experience the same abdominal pain. Which of the following is most likely to cause this patient's illness?

- ❑ (A) Acute appendicitis
- ❑ (B) Angiodysplasia
- ❑ (C) Celiac sprue
- ❑ (D) Diverticulosis
- ❑ (E) Giardiasis
- ❑ (F) Meckel diverticulum

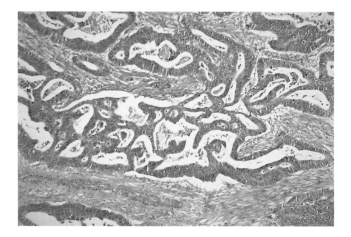

46 A 30-year-old man has a routine health maintenance examination. A stool sample is positive for occult blood. On colonoscopy, an ulcerative lesion is seen projecting into the cecum. The microscopic appearance of a section of the excised lesion is shown in the figure above. Which of the following molecular biologic events is thought to be most critical in the development of such lesions?

- [ ] (A) Overexpression of E-cadherin gene
- [ ] (B) Amplification of *ERBB2* gene
- [ ] (C) Germ-line transmission of a defective *RB* gene
- [ ] (D) A defective DNA mismatch-repair gene
- [ ] (E) Translocation of retinoic acid receptor α gene

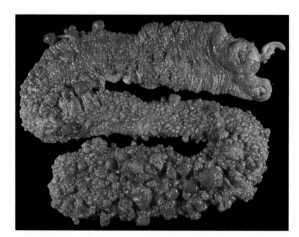

Courtesy of Dr. Tad Wieczorek, Brigham and Women's Hospital, Boston, MA.

47 A 19-year-old man is advised by other family members to see his physician because genetic screening has detected a disease in other family members. On physical examination, a stool sample is positive for occult blood. A colonoscopy is performed, followed by a colectomy. The gross appearance of the mucosal surface of the colectomy specimen is shown above. Molecular analysis of this patient's normal fibroblasts is most likely to show a mutation in which of the following genes?

- [ ] (A) *APC*
- [ ] (B) *p53*
- [ ] (C) *K-RAS*
- [ ] (D) *HNPCC*
- [ ] (E) *NOD2*

48 A 38-year-old man who has been HIV positive for 10 years has had severe nausea and vomiting for the past 2 weeks. On physical examination, he is afebrile. A stool sample is positive for occult blood. The abdomen is not distended, there are no palpable masses or organomegaly, and bowel sounds are present. The patient has oral thrush. There are several reddish-purple, 0.5- to 1-cm nodules on the skin of the trunk. Laboratory studies show a CD4+ lymphocyte count of 118/μL. Upper gastrointestinal endoscopy shows 12 reddish-purple, 0.6 to 1.8 cm, gastric mucosal nodules. A biopsy specimen of the nodules is most likely to show which of the following neoplasms?

- [ ] (A) Adenocarcinoma
- [ ] (B) Non-Hodgkin lymphoma
- [ ] (C) Carcinoid tumor
- [ ] (D) Gastrointestinal stromal tumor
- [ ] (E) Kaposi sarcoma
- [ ] (F) Peutz-Jeghers polyp
- [ ] (G) Squamous cell carcinoma
- [ ] (H) Tubular adenoma

49 A 59-year-old man with a lengthy history of chronic alcoholism has noticed increasing abdominal girth for the past 6 months. He has had increasing abdominal pain for the past 2 days. On physical examination, his temperature is 38.2°C. Examination of the abdomen shows a fluid wave and prominent caput medusae over the skin of the abdomen. There is diffuse abdominal tenderness. An abdominal plain film radiograph shows no free air. Paracentesis yields 500 mL of cloudy yellow fluid. A Gram stain of the fluid shows gram-negative rods. Which of the following is the most likely diagnosis?

- [ ] (A) Appendicitis
- [ ] (B) Collagenous colitis
- [ ] (C) Diverticulitis
- [ ] (D) Ischemic colitis
- [ ] (E) Pseudomembranous colitis
- [ ] (F) Spontaneous bacterial peritonitis

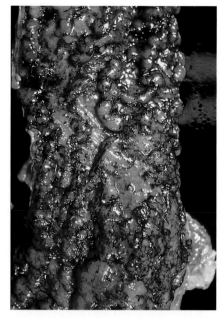

50 A 35-year-old woman has had increasing lower back pain for 5 years. At various times during the past year, she has also had arthritic pain involving the knees, hips, and wrists. A stool sample is positive for occult blood. A pelvic radiograph shows changes consistent with sacroiliitis. A colonoscopy is performed, and she undergoes a total colectomy. The gross appearance of the colectomy specimen is shown in the preceding figure. Which of the following is the most likely diagnosis?

❑ (A) Dysregulated CD4+ T-cell responses
❑ (B) Cross-reaction of antibodies against gut bacteria
❑ (C) Autoantibodies directed against tropomyosin
❑ (D) Mutations in the *NOD2* gene
❑ (E) Germ-line inheritance of the *APC* gene mutation

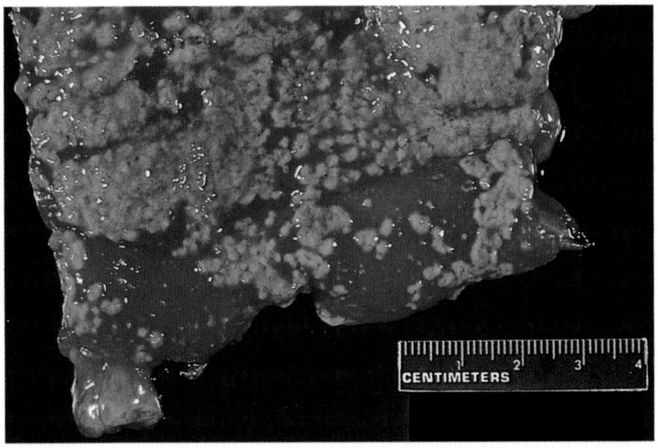

51 A 45-year-old woman is being treated in the hospital for pneumonia complicated by septicemia. She has required multiple antibiotics and was intubated and mechanically ventilated earlier in the course. On day 20 of hospitalization, she has abdominal distention. Bowel sounds are absent, and an abdominal radiograph shows dilated loops of small bowel suggestive of ileus. She has a low volume of bloody stool that is positive for *Clostridium difficile* toxin. At laparotomy, a portion of distal ileum and cecum is resected. The gross appearance of the mucosal surface is shown in the figure above. Which of the following is the most likely diagnosis?

❑ (A) Mesenteric arterial thrombosis
❑ (B) Pseudomembranous enterocolitis
❑ (C) Intussusception
❑ (D) Cecal volvulus
❑ (E) Toxic megacolon

52 A 52-year-old previously healthy man sustained an extensive thermal burn injury involving 70% of the total body surface area of his skin. He was hospitalized in stable condition. Three weeks after the initial burn injury, he had melanotic stools. His blood pressure was 80/40 mm Hg, and his hematocrit was 18%. Soon after, he experienced cardiac arrest and could not be resuscitated. At autopsy, which of the following is most likely to be found?

❑ (A) Multiple 2- to 5-mm ulcers throughout the gastric mucosa that penetrate the submucosa and the muscularis propria
❑ (B) Prominent and tortuous veins at the gastroesophageal junction with overlying irregular 0.5- to 1-cm ulcerations penetrating to submucosa
❑ (C) A single 1-cm punched-out ulcer in the gastric antrum that penetrates the submucosa and has a base filled with granulation tissue
❑ (D) Multiple 2- to 5-mm ulcers throughout the gastric mucosa that are confined to the mucosa
❑ (E) Multiple 2- to 5-mm ulcers in metaplastic columnar epithelium at the lower end of the esophagus

53 A 68-year-old woman with a history of rheumatic heart disease is hospitalized with severe congestive heart failure. Several days after admission, she develops abdominal distention. On physical examination, she is afebrile. The abdomen is tympanitic, without a fluid wave, and bowel sounds are absent. A stool sample is positive for occult blood. An abdominal plain film radiograph shows no free air. Colonoscopy shows patchy areas of mucosal erythema with some overlying tan exudate in the ascending and descending colon. No polyps or masses are found. Which of the following is the most likely diagnosis?

❑ (A) Ulcerative colitis
❑ (B) Volvulus
❑ (C) Shigellosis
❑ (D) Mesenteric vasculitis
❑ (E) Ischemic colitis

54 A 27-year-old man has had intermittent cramping abdominal pain and low-volume diarrhea for several weeks. On physical examination, he is afebrile; there is mild lower abdominal tenderness but no masses, and bowel sounds are present. A stool sample is positive for occult blood. The symptoms subside within 1 week. Six months later, the abdominal pain recurs with perianal pain. On physical examination, there is now a perirectal fistula. Colonoscopy shows many areas of mucosal edema and ulceration and some areas that appear normal. Microscopic examination of a biopsy specimen from an ulcerated area shows a patchy acute and chronic inflammatory infiltrate, crypt abscesses, and several noncaseating granulomas. Which of the following underlying disease processes best explains these findings?

❑ (A) Crohn disease
❑ (B) Amebiasis
❑ (C) Shigellosis
❑ (D) Sarcoidosis
❑ (E) Ulcerative colitis

55 A 49-year-old man has complained of "heartburn" after meals for the past decade. There are no remarkable findings on physical examination. Upper gastrointestinal endoscopy is performed, and an esophageal biopsy specimen is taken from an erythematous area of velvety mucosa just above the gastroesophageal junction. Microscopically, the mucosa shows columnar metaplasia with goblet cells. Which of the following most likely produced these findings?

❑ (A) Esophageal varices
❑ (B) Radiation therapy
❑ (C) Achalasia
❑ (D) Gastroesophageal reflux disease
❑ (E) Iron deficiency anemia

56 A 65-year-old woman goes to her physician for a routine health maintenance examination. A stool sample is positive for occult blood. CT scan of the abdomen shows numerous air-filled, 1-cm outpouchings of the sigmoid and descending colon. Which of the following complications is most likely to develop in this patient?

❑ (A) Adenocarcinoma
❑ (B) Pericolic abscess
❑ (C) Bowel obstruction
❑ (D) Malabsorption
❑ (E) Toxic megacolon

57 A 45-year-old woman has had increasing abdominal distention for the past 6 weeks. On physical examination, there is an abdominal fluid wave and bowel sounds are present. Paracentesis yields 1000 mL of slightly cloudy serous fluid. Cytologic examination of the fluid shows malignant cells consistent with adenocarcinoma. The patient's medical history indicates that she has had no major medical illnesses and no surgical procedures. Which of the following conditions is most likely to have preceded the development of the adenocarcinoma?

- ❏ (A) Angiodysplasia
- ❏ (B) Crohn disease
- ❏ (C) Diverticulosis
- ❏ (D) Hereditary nonpolyposis colon carcinoma
- ❏ (E) Hirschsprung disease
- ❏ (F) Peptic ulcer disease

58 A 32-year-old man sees the physician because he has experienced nausea and vomiting for the past week. On physical examination, he appears cachectic and says that he has noticed a 15-kg weight loss over the past 2 months. A 10-cm nontender mass is palpable in the midabdominal region. An abdominal CT scan shows that the mass involves the small intestine. Serologic tests indicate that he is HIV positive. A biopsy specimen is most likely to show which of the following microscopic features?

- ❏ (A) Blunting and flattening of villi containing increased numbers of lymphocytes and plasma cells
- ❏ (B) Densely packed tubular glands lined by dysplastic cells with hyperchromatic nuclei
- ❏ (C) Infiltrates of large monoclonal B lymphocytes
- ❏ (D) Irregular ulceration with chronic inflammation and granuloma formation
- ❏ (E) Sharply demarcated ulceration with epithelial cells containing intranuclear inclusions

59 In an epidemiologic study of infections of the gastrointestinal tract, cases of patients from whom definitive cultures were obtained are analyzed for clinical and pathologic findings that may be useful for diagnosis. A subset of patients is identified who initially had abdominal pain and diarrhea during week 1 of their illness. By week 2, these patients had splenomegaly and elevations in serum AST and ALT levels. By week 3, they were septic and had leukopenia. At autopsy, those who died were found to have ulceration of Peyer's patches. Which of the following infectious agents is most likely to produce these findings?

- ❏ (A) *Campylobacter jejuni*
- ❏ (B) *Clostridium perfringens*
- ❏ (C) *Escherichia coli*
- ❏ (D) *Mycobacterium bovis*
- ❏ (E) *Salmonella typhi*
- ❏ (F) *Shigella sonnei*
- ❏ (G) *Yersinia enterocolitica*

60 A 57-year-old man goes to the emergency department because of increasing abdominal pain with distention that developed over the past 24 hours. On physical examination, there is diffuse abdominal tenderness. The abdomen is tympanitic, without a fluid wave, and bowel sounds are nearly absent. There is a well-healed, 5-cm transverse scar in the right lower quadrant of the abdomen. There is no caput medusae.

A stool sample is negative for occult blood. An abdominal plain film radiograph shows dilated loops of small bowel with air-fluid levels, but there is no free air. At laparotomy, the surgeon notices a 20-cm portion of reddish-black ileum that changes abruptly to pink-appearing bowel on both distal and proximal margins. The patient's medical history is significant only for an appendectomy at age 25. Which of the following is most likely to have produced these findings?

- ❏ (A) Adenocarcinoma of the ileum
- ❏ (B) Adhesions
- ❏ (C) Angiodysplasia
- ❏ (D) Crohn disease
- ❏ (E) Indirect inguinal hernia
- ❏ (F) Intussusception
- ❏ (G) Volvulus

ANSWERS

1 **(C)** This patient has malabsorption that responded to dietary treatment. She probably has celiac disease (gluten sensitivity). The histologic features of celiac disease are flattening of the mucosa, diffuse and severe atrophy of the villi, and chronic inflammation of the lamina propria. There is an increase in intraepithelial lymphocytes. Lymphatic obstruction occurs in Whipple disease. In addition, foamy macrophages accumulate in the lamina propria. They contain PAS-positive granules, which, under electron microscope, show an actinomycete called *Tropheryma whippelii*. Noncaseating granulomas are found in the intestinal wall in Crohn disease. Crypt abscesses are nonspecific and can be seen in inflammatory bowel disease.

BP7 571-572   BP6 498   PBD7 843-844   PBD6 813

2 **(D)** Infection by one of several *Salmonella* species (not *S. typhi*) causes a self-limited diarrhea. This is a form of food poisoning, typically from contaminated poultry products. *Yersinia enterocolitica* is most often found in contaminated milk or pork products and may disseminate to produce lymphadenitis and further extraintestinal infection. A variety of diseases result from contamination with various strains of *Escherichia coli*, based on the characteristics of the organisms and whether they invade or produce an enterotoxin. Poultry products are usually not contaminated with *E. coli*. Amebiasis from *Entamoeba histolytica* can be an invasive, exudative infection. The stools contain blood and mucus. Rotavirus is most often seen in children; in adults, a self-limited watery diarrhea occurs. There is no particular association between rotavirus infection and a specific food product. *Staphylococcus aureus* causes an acute onset of abdominal pain, bloating, and diarrhea not by directly infecting the gastrointestinal tract but by producing an exotoxin while growing on food that is subsequently ingested. *Bacillus cereus* growing in foods such as reheated fried rice produces an exotoxin, which, upon ingestion, can produce acute onset of nausea, vomiting, and abdominal pain.

BP7 567-568   BP6 495   PBD7 834-835   PBD6 806-808

3 **(A)** These findings are consistent with an acute gastritis. Heavy consumption of ethanol is probably the most common cause, but aspirin and nonsteroidal anti-inflammatory drugs (NSAIDs), smoking, and chemotherapy agents can produce the same findings. Acyclovir (used to treat herpes simplex virus infections), chlorpromazine (used to treat nausea), and prednisone (a steroidal anti-inflammatory drug) do not have the same association. Cimetidine and omeprazole are used to treat peptic ulcer disease by reducing gastric acid production, thus increasing the serum gastrin. Cimetidine is an H₂ receptor blocker, and omeprazole is a proton pump inhibitor. Clindamycin is a broad-spectrum antibiotic that may alter flora in the lower gastrointestinal tract.

BP7 556-557   BP6 483-484   PBD7 812-813   PBD6

4 (C) The patient's history of myocardial infarction suggests that he had severe coronary atherosclerosis. Atheromatous disease most likely involved the mesenteric vessels as well, giving rise to thrombosis of the blood vessels that perfuse the bowel. The symptoms and signs suggest infarction of the gut. Acute appendicitis rarely leads to such a catastrophic illness, unless there is perforation. (The absence of free air in the radiograph argues against perforation of any viscus.) Acute pancreatitis can be a serious abdominal emergency, but the normal levels of amylase and lipase tend to exclude it. Acute cholecystitis can produce severe abdominal pain, but bloody diarrhea and absence of bowel sounds (paralytic ileus) are unlikely. Pseudomembranous colitis develops in patients receiving antibiotic therapy.

BP7 564-566   BP6 491-492   PBD7 851-853
PBD6 820-822

5 (B) *Helicobacter pylori* organisms reside in the gastric mucus and are associated with a variety of gastric disorders, from chronic gastritis with erythema and thickened rugal folds as in this case, to peptic ulcers and to adenocarcinoma. *H. pylori* orgaisms elaborate several toxic substances that injure the epithelium. Vacuolating cytotoxin (VacA) causes cell injury characterized by vacuolization, and its expression is controlled by another gene encoding cytotoxin-associated antigen (CagA). More than 80% of patients with duodenal ulcers are infected by CagA positive *H. pylori* strains also expressing VacA. Cysteine proteinases produced by *Entamoeba histolytica* aid in tissue invasion. Heat stable enterotoxin is produced by strains of *Escherichia coli* that cause traveler's diarrhea. Shiga toxin is elaborated by *Shigella flexneri* organisms that cause a form of bacillary dysentery. Verocytotoxin produced by some *E. coli* strains is associated with the hemolytic-uremic syndrome mediated by endothelial injury.

BP7 555-556   BP6 482-484   PBD7 814, 818, 834
PBD6 790-792

6 (E) Pseudomembranous colitis, caused by overgrowth of *Clostridium difficile*, occurs when the normal gut flora is altered by broad-spectrum antibiotic therapy. In this case, the patient was treated for acute pyelonephritis. Organisms other than *C. difficile*, such as *Candida*, may overgrow, but *C. difficile* is the most common organism identified with pseudomembranous colitis. The other choices are not related to antibiotic therapy. Appendicitis has a peak incidence at a younger age, and pain is more often localized in the right lower quadrant. Collagenous colitis is not common; it most often leads to watery diarrhea in middle-aged women. Diverticulitis can produce lower abdominal pain. Ischemic colitis

may produce infarction with rupture and peritonitis. Spontaneous bacterial peritonitis occurs in the setting of ascites. Typhlitis is a rare condition with cecal inflammation; it occurs in immunocompromised persons.

BP7 569   BP6 495-496   PBD7 836-837   PBD6 809-810

7 (A) This patient had a large villous adenoma, as shown in the figure. There is a high probability (>40%) that large (>4 cm) villous adenomas will progress to invasive adenocarcinoma. When they occur in the descending colon, these lesions are annular and cause obstruction. In the colon, non-Hodgkin lymphomas are far less common than adenocarcinomas, and they do not present as mucosal sessile masses. Carcinoid tumors are typically small and yellowish, and most grow slowly. Leiomyosarcomas are rare; they produce large bulky masses, but they do not arise on the mucosa. Mucinous cystadenomas are cystic and are more likely to arise in an ovary or in the pancreas. Squamous cell carcinomas can arise in the esophagus or at the anorectal junction. The original lesion in this patient was a villous adenoma.

BP7 580-581   BP6 506-507   PBD7 860-861   PBD6 830

8 (B) This large, ulcerated lesion with heaped up margins is a malignant tumor of the esophageal mucosa. There are two main histologic types of esophageal carcinomas—squamous cell carcinoma and adenocarcinoma—with distinct risk factors. Smoking and alcoholism are the most frequent risk factors for esophageal squamous cell carcinoma in the Western world. Adenocarcinoma is most likely to arise in the lower third of the esophagus and to be associated with Barrett esophagus. Intranuclear inclusions suggest infection with herpes simplex virus or cytomegalovirus, both of which are more likely to produce ulceration without a mass; both occur in immunocompromised patients. Chronic inflammation may lead to stricture and not to a localized mass. Thrombosed veins occur in sclerotherapy for esophageal varices; they do not produce an ulcerated mass. A dense, collagenous scar of the midesophagus is not common, but it may occur after injury from ingestion of a caustic liquid.

BP7 553-554   BP6 480   PBD7 806-809   PBD6 783-786

9 (C) The clinical and histologic features are most suggestive of celiac sprue. This rare chronic disease may manifest in childhood or young adulthood. Celiac sprue results from gluten sensitivity. Exposure to the gliadin protein in wheat, oats, barley, and rye (but not rice) results in intestinal inflammation. Hence, a trial of a gluten-free diet is the most logical therapeutic option. Patients usually become symptom-free, and normal histologic features of the mucosa are restored. Almost 100% of patients with active celiac disease have IgA antibodies. These antibodies generally decrease or disappear in patients on gluten-free diets. Serum tests for IgA-class endomysial antibodies in conjunction with tests for antibodies to reticulin or gliadin enable the serologic detection of virtually all cases of celiac disease. Anticentromeric antibody is most specific for limited scleroderma (CREST syndrome) with esophageal dysmotility. The anti-DNA topoisomerase I antibody is most specific for diffuse scleroderma, in which gastrointestinal tract involvement by submucosal fibrosis may be more extensive, and malabsorption may be present. Antimitochondrial antibody is more specific for primary biliary cirrhosis. Antinuclear antibody is present in a wide variety of autoimmune diseases, but it is not characteristic of celiac sprue.

BP7 571-572   BP6 498   PBD7 843-844   PBD6 813

10 **(B)** The clinical features suggest food poisoning caused by the ingestion of a preformed enterotoxin. *Staphylococcus aureus* grows in food (milk products and fatty foods are favorites) and elaborates an enterotoxin that, when ingested, produces diarrhea within hours. Some strains of *Escherichia coli* can produce a variety of diarrheal illnesses but without a preformed toxin. *Vibrio parahaemolyticus* is found in shellfish. *Clostridium difficile* can produce a pseudomembranous colitis in patients treated with broad-spectrum antibiotics. *Salmonella enteritidis* is most often found in poultry products, but the diarrheal illnesses develop within 2 days. *Bacillus cereus* is better known for growing on reheated fried rice; it produces an exotoxin that causes acute nausea, vomiting, and abdominal cramping.

BP7 567   BP6 494-495   PBD7 833-834   PBD6 809

11 **(D)** Disaccharidase (lactase) deficiency is an uncommon congenital condition (or a rare acquired condition) in which the lactose in milk products is not broken down into glucose and galactose, resulting in an osmotic diarrhea and gas production from gut flora. Affected persons do not always make the connection between diet and symptoms, or they do not consume enough milk products to become symptomatic. Celiac sprue is also diet related and results from a sensitivity to gluten in some grains. An autoimmune gastritis is most likely to result in vitamin B$_{12}$ malabsorption. Cholelithiasis can cause biliary tract obstruction with malabsorption of fats and right upper quadrant abdominal pain. Cystic fibrosis affects the pancreas and mainly produces fat malabsorption.

BP7 571   BP6 497   PBD7 844-845   PBD6 815

12 **(A)** This patient is most likely to have fat malabsorption. Smelly, bulky stools containing increased amounts of fat (steatorrhea) are characteristic. Pancreatic or biliary tract diseases are important causes of fat malabsorption. Giardiasis produces mainly a watery diarrhea. Malabsorption with steatorrhea is unlikely to be associated with bleeding. Cholera results in a massive watery diarrhea. Amebiasis can produce a range of findings from a watery diarrhea to dysentery with mucus and blood in the stool.

BP7 571-572   BP6 493   PBD7 842-843   PBD6 806

13 **(A)** Adenocarcinomas of the esophagus are typically located in the lower esophagus, where Barrett esophagus develops at the site of long-standing gastroesophageal reflux disease. Barrett esophagus is associated with a greatly increased risk of developing adenocarcinoma. Leiomyosarcoma of the esophagus is rare and is unrelated to a history of "heartburn." Squamous cell carcinomas of the esophagus are most often associated with a history of chronic alcoholism and smoking. Malignant lymphomas of the gastrointestinal tract do not commonly occur in the esophagus and are not related to reflux esophagitis. Carcinoid tumors occur in different parts of the gut, including the appendix, ileum, rectum, stomach, and colon.

BP7 552-553   BP6 480-481   PBD7 808-809   PBD6 786-787

14 **(A)** The infant's condition occurred several weeks after birth because of hypertrophy of pyloric smooth muscle. Pyloric stenosis manifests the genetic phenomenon of a "threshold of liability," above which the disease is manifested—more genetic risks are present. The incidence in males is 1/200 and in females 1/1000, reflecting the fact that more risks must be present in females for the disease to occur; thus the threshold of liability will be exceeded more easily for males born into a family with the trait. Tracheoesophageal fistula, diaphragmatic hernia, and duodenal atresia are serious conditions that are manifested at birth and are often associated with multiple anomalies. Pyloric stenosis is an isolated condition that typically occurs without other anomalies. Annular pancreas is a rare anomaly.

BP7 555   BP6 482   PBD7 812   PBD6 789

15 **(D)** The most likely cause of a large mass lesion in the stomach is a gastric carcinoma, and this lesion is an adenocarcinoma. Malignant lymphomas and leiomyosarcomas are less common and tend to form bulky masses in the fundus. Neuroendocrine carcinomas are rare. Squamous cell carcinomas appear in the esophagus.

BP7 561-563   BP6 489   PBD7 822-826   PBD6 800-801

16 **(C)** Angiodysplasia refers to tortuous dilations of mucosal and submucosal vessels, seen most often in the cecum in patients older than 50 years of age. These lesions, although not common, account for 20% of significant lower intestinal bleeding. Bleeding usually is not massive but can occur intermittently over months to years. This lesion is very difficult to diagnose and is often found radiographically. The focus (or foci) of abnormal vessels can be excised. Mesenteric venous thrombosis is rare and may result in bowel infarction with severe abdominal pain. Hemorrhoids at the anorectal junction may account for bright red rectal bleeding, but they can be seen or palpated on rectal examination. Collagenous colitis is a rare cause of a watery diarrhea that is typically not bloody. Colonic diverticulosis can be associated with hemorrhage, but the outpouchings usually are seen on colonoscopy.

BP7 566   BP6 493   PBD7 854   PBD6 823

17 **(A)** The figure shows a large, fungating mass that is typical of adenocarcinoma of the right colon. Such cancers are unlikely to obstruct, but they can bleed a small amount over months to years, causing iron deficiency anemia. This relatively young woman has evidence for an additional cancer, an endometrial cancer, and this combination is most likely due to an inherited mutation in one of the DNA mismatch repair genes such as *hMSH2* and *hMLH1*. Homozygous loss of these genes can give rise to right-sided colon cancer and endometrial cancer. Such a mutation is typically associated with microsatellite instability, in contrast to the *APC*–β-catenin pathway associated with familial adenomatous polyposis syndrome. This latter pathway is also known as the "adenoma-carcinoma sequence" since the carcinomas develop through an identifiable series of molecular and morphologic steps. Mutation with activation of *c-KIT* tyrosine kinase activity occurs in gastrointestinal stromal tumors, which respond well to treatment with imatinib mesylate, a tyrosine kinase inhibitor also used to treat chronic myelogenous leukemia. Loss of the *PTEN* tumor suppressor gene is seen in endometrial carcinomas not associated with colon carcinoma, and with some hamartomatous polyps of the colon. Infection with some strains of human papillomavirus (HPV) leads to Rb protein inactivation and development of cervical carcinoma.

PBD7 864

18 (B) The continuous mucosal involvement to a demarcated end point is more typical of ulcerative colitis than of Crohn disease, both of which are idiopathic inflammatory bowel diseases. Because the colon mainly absorbs water and concentrates stool, inflammatory conditions involving the colon tend to produce low-volume diarrhea, whereas conditions that affect the small bowel and lead to malabsorption result in high-volume diarrhea. Shigellosis causing dysentery produces many fecal leukocytes. Diverticular disease is unusual in patients of this age, as is ischemic bowel disease.

BP7 574-576   BP6 501-502   PBD7 846, 849-851
PBD6 818-820

19 (D) Certain gastrointestinal lymphomas that arise from mucosa-associated lymphoid tissue (MALT) are called MALT lymphomas. Gastric lymphomas that occur in association with *Helicobacter pylori* infection are composed of monoclonal B cells, whose growth and proliferation remains dependent on cytokines derived from T cells that are sensitized to *H. pylori* antigens. Treatment with antibiotics eliminates *H. pylori* and therefore the stimulus for B-cell growth. MALT lesions can occur anywhere in the gastrointestinal tract, although they are rare in the esophagus and appendix. In *H. pylori* chronic gastritis, which may precede lymphoma development, there are lymphoplasmacytic mucosal infiltrates. Diffuse large B-cell lymphomas and other non-Hodgkin lymphomas that are not MALT lymphomas do not regress with antibiotic therapy. Autoimmune gastritis is a risk for development of gastric adenocarcinoma. Crohn disease is rare in the stomach and is not related to *H. pylori* infection. Gastrointestinal stromal tumors are uncommon; these tumors may be proliferations of interstitial cells of Cajal, myenteric plexus cells that are thought to be the pacemaker of the gut.

BP7 587-588   BP6 513   PBD7 868   PBD6 837-838

20 (C) Prolonged use of nonsteroidal anti-inflammatory drugs is an important cause of acute gastritis. Excessive alcohol consumption and smoking are also possible causes. Acute gastritis tends to be diffuse and, when severe, can lead to significant hemorrhage that is difficult to control. Epithelial dysplasia may occur at the site of chronic gastritis. It is a forerunner of gastric cancer. Hyperplastic polyps of the stomach do not result from acute gastritis but may arise in association with chronic gastritis. Acute gastritis does not increase the risk of gastric adenocarcinoma. Infection with *Helicobacter pylori* is not associated with acute gastritis.

BP7 556-557   BP6 483-484   PBD7 812, 816, 818-819
PBD6 789-790

21 (D) Esophageal dysmotility is the "E" in CREST syndrome, the limited form of systemic sclerosis (scleroderma). Although the disease is autoimmune, little inflammation is seen by the time the patient seeks clinical attention. There is increased collagen deposition in submucosa and muscularis. Fibrosis may affect any part of the gastrointestinal tract, but the esophagus is the site most often involved. Portal hypertension gives rise to esophageal varices, not fibrosis. An upper

esophageal web associated with iron deficiency anemia might produce difficulty in swallowing, but this condition is rare. For a diagnosis of Barrett esophagus, columnar metaplasia must be seen histologically, and there is often a history of gastroesophageal reflux disease. Hiatal hernia is frequently diagnosed in persons with reflux esophagitis and can lead to inflammation, ulceration, and bleeding, but formation of a stricture is uncommon.

BP7 141-143   BP6 476, 112-113   PBD7 238, 255-256, 800
PBD6 778-779

22 (A) The clinical symptoms in this case suggest peptic ulcer disease. In most cases, peptic ulcers are associated with *Helicobacter pylori* infection. These bacteria secrete urease, which can be detected by oral administration of ^{14}C-labeled urea. After drinking the labeled urea solution, the patient blows into a tube. If *H. pylori* urease is present in the stomach, the urea is hydrolyzed, and labeled carbon dioxide is detected in the breath sample. In the biopsy urease test, antral biopsy specimens are placed in a gel containing urea and an indicator, and if *H. pylori* is present, the color changes within minutes. If not properly treated, peptic ulcers can produce many complications, including massive bleeding that can be fatal. The patient does not have fat malabsorption, because fat absorption does not occur in the stomach. Peptic ulcers rarely progress to gastric carcinoma; hence, metastases are unlikely. Carcinoid tumors can occur in the stomach, but they are rare and are not related to peptic ulcer disease, which this patient has. Vitamin B_{12} deficiency can occur with autoimmune atrophic gastritis, because intrinsic factor, which is required for vitamin B_{12} absorption, is produced in gastric parietal cells.

BP7 557-560   BP6 484-486   PBD7 816-819
PBD6 793-796

23 (E) The ileum shows chronic inflammation with lymphoid aggregates. The inflammation is transmural, affecting the mucosa, submucosa, and muscularis. A deep fissure extending into the muscularis is also seen. These histologic features are highly suggestive of Crohn disease. Extension of fissures into the overlying skin can produce enterocutaneous fistulas, although enteroenteric fistulas between loops of bowel are more common. Although the risk of adenocarcinoma is increased in Crohn disease, this complication is less common than sequelae of inflammation. Mesenteric artery thrombosis, typically a complication of atherosclerosis, is unlikely in a 27-year-old man. Intussusception may occur when there is a congenital or acquired obstruction in the bowel. Hepatic abscess can follow amebic colitis.

BP7 573-574   BP6 499-500   PBD7 846-849
PBD6 816-818

24 (F) Rotavirus is the most common cause of viral gastroenteritis in children. It is a self-limited disease that affects mostly infants and young children, who can lose a significant amount of fluid relative to their size and they can quickly become dehydrated. The death rate is less than 1%. *Campylobacter jejuni* is more often seen in children and adults as a food-borne cause of fever, abdominal pain, and diarrhea. Cryptosporidiosis most often causes a watery diarrhea in immunocompromised adults. Enterohemorrhagic strains of *Escherichia coli* can produce hemolytic-uremic syndrome in young children. Listeriosis can be a congenital infection that is present along with meningitis and sepsis at birth; in infants, children, and adults, it is a food- or water-borne infection that tends to occur in epidemics. Norwalk virus is a common cause of diarrheal illness in adults. Shigellosis produces dysentery with bloody diarrhea. Cholera results in massive loss of fluid.

BP7 567   BP6 494   PBD7 832-833   PBD6 806

25 (E) Although they are not found in the duodenum, *Helicobacter pylori* organisms alter the microenvironment of the stomach, causing both the stomach and duodenum to be susceptible to peptic ulcer disease. Virtually all duodenal peptic ulcers are associated with the presence of *H. pylori*. Ulceration can extend through the muscularis and result in perforation, as in this case. The other organisms listed are not related to peptic ulcer formation but to infectious diarrheal illnesses. *Salmonella typhi* may produce typhoid fever with more systemic symptoms; the marked ulceration of Peyer's patches may lead to perforation.

BP7 557-559   BP6 484-485   PBD7 816-819
PBD6 793-796

26 (C) The biopsy specimen shows columnar metaplasia, typical of Barrett esophagus. Patients with a focus of Barrett esophagus larger than 2 cm are at 30- to 40-fold higher risk of developing adenocarcinoma than is the general population. Squamous cell carcinomas occur in the esophagus, but they do not arise in association with Barrett esophagus. Their occurrence is related to smoking and alcohol consumption. Hematemesis is a complication of esophageal varices and other conditions such as peptic ulcers. Achalasia refers to failure of relaxation of the lower esophageal sphincter that gives rise to dilation of the proximal portion of esophagus. Mallory-Weiss syndrome is associated with vertical lacerations in the esophagus that may occur with severe vomiting and retching.

BP7 552-553   BP6 479   PBD7 804-805   PBD6 781-782

27 (E) Raw or poorly cooked shellfish can be the source of *Vibrio parahaemolyticus*, which tends to produce a milder diarrhea than *Vibrio cholerae*. *Yersinia enterocolitica* is invasive and can produce extraintestinal infection. *Staphylococcus aureus* can produce food poisoning through elaboration of an enterotoxin that causes an explosive diarrhea within 2 hours after ingestion. *Cryptosporidium* as a cause of watery diarrhea is most often found in immunocompromised persons. *Entamoeba histolytica* produces colonic mucosal invasion along with exudation and ulceration; therefore, stools contain blood and mucus.

BP7 568   BP6 495   PBD7 834   PBD6 808

28 (C) These findings indicate an ongoing inflammatory process resulting from reflux of acid gastric contents into the lower esophagus. Gastroesophageal reflux disease (GERD) is a common problem that stems from a variety of causes, including sliding hiatal hernia, decreased tone of the lower esophageal sphincter, and delayed gastric emptying. Patients may have a history of "heartburn" after eating. Barrett esophagus is a complication of long-standing GERD and is characterized by columnar metaplasia of the squamous epithelium that normally lines the esophagus. There may be inflammation and mucosal ulceration overlying varices, but this condition usually does not have heartburn as the major feature.

Progressive fibrosis with stenosis is found in scleroderma. A rare complication of iron deficiency is the appearance of an upper esophageal web (Plummer-Vinson syndrome).

BP7 552-553   BP6 478-479   PBD7 804-805
PBD6 780-781

29 (A) This patient has clinical and histologic features of ulcerative colitis. Particularly important are relapsing and remitting episodes of diarrhea containing blood and mucus and diffuse inflammation and ulceration of the rectal and colonic mucosa. One of the most dreaded complications of ulcerative colitis is the development of colonic adenocarcinoma. There is a 20- to 30-fold higher risk in patients who have had ulcerative colitis for 10 or more years compared with control populations. Diverticulitis can produce abdominal pain and blood in the stool, but there is no association with ulcerative colitis. Ulcerative colitis is associated with several extraintestinal manifestations, including sclerosing cholangitis, but it has no relationship to primary biliary cirrhosis. Fat malabsorption usually does not occur in ulcerative colitis, because the ileum often is not involved. Pseudomembranous colitis is caused by *Clostridium difficile* infections associated with antibiotic treatment. Perirectal fistula formation is more typical of Crohn disease, in which there is transmural inflammation.

BP7 574-577   BP6 502   PBD7 849-851   PBD6 818-820

30 (D) A patient who is infected with HIV and has low CD4+ cell counts is at great risk of developing infections. Herpes simplex and *Candida* are the most likely upper gastrointestinal infections involving the esophagus. Squamous cell carcinoma of the esophagus is not related to HIV infection. Achalasia, caused by a failure of relaxation of the lower esophageal sphincter, is not a feature of HIV infection or immunosuppression. Fibrosis with stenosis is a feature of gastroesophageal reflux disease (GERD) and scleroderma.

BP7 545, 551-552   BP6 125   PBD7 255-256, 805-806, 841
PBD6 782

31 (E) The endoscopy findings describe the linitis plastica ("leather bottle") appearance of diffuse gastric carcinoma. Histologically, these carcinomas are composed of gastric-type mucus cells that infiltrate the stomach wall diffusely. The individual tumor cells have a signet-ring appearance, because the cytoplasmic mucin pushes the nucleus to one side. Early gastric carcinoma is confined to the mucosa and submucosa. Gastrointestinal stromal tumors tend to be bulky masses. Granulomas are rare at this site. In chronic atrophic gastritis, the rugal folds are lost, but there is no significant scarring or shrinkage.

BP7 561-563   BP6 489   PBD7 824-825   PBD6 800-801

32 (A) Variceal bleeding is a common complication of hepatic cirrhosis, which can be an outcome of chronic hepatitis B infection. The resultant portal hypertension leads to dilated submucosal esophageal veins that can erode and bleed profusely. Barrett esophagus is a columnar metaplasia that results from gastroesophageal reflux disease (GERD). Bleeding is not a key feature of this disease. Esophageal candidiasis may be seen in immunocompromised patients, but it most often produces raised mucosal plaques and is rarely invasive. GERD may produce acute and chronic inflammation and, rarely, massive hemorrhage. Esophageal carcinomas may bleed, but not enough to cause massive hematemesis. A Zenker diverticulum is located in the upper esophagus and results from cricopharyngeal motor dysfunction; it presents a risk for aspiration but not for hematemesis.

BP7 551   BP6 478   PBD7 802-803   PBD6 783

33 (B) The "punched-out" ulcers described result from rupture of the herpetic vesicles. Herpesvirus and *Candida* infections typically occur in immunocompromised patients, and both can involve the esophagus. Candidiasis, however, has the gross appearance of tan-to-yellow plaques. Aphthous ulcers (canker sores) can also be found in immunocompromised patients, but these shallow ulcers occur most frequently in the oral cavity. Gastroesophageal reflux disease (GERD) can produce acute and chronic inflammation with some erosion, although typically not in a sharply demarcated pattern; GERD has no relationship with immune status. Mallory-Weiss syndrome results from mucosal tears of the esophagus. Such laceration of the esophagus can occur with severe vomiting and retching.

BP7 544-545, 551-552   BP6 478   PBD7 805-806
PBD6 782

34 (E) The infant has signs and symptoms of acute bowel obstruction. Intussusception occurs when one small segment of small bowel becomes telescoped into the immediately distal segment. This disorder can have sudden onset in infants and may occur in the absence of any anatomic abnormality. Almost all cases of Meckel diverticulum are asymptomatic, although in some cases functional gastric mucosa is present and can lead to ulceration with bleeding. Duodenal atresia (which typically occurs with other anomalies, particularly trisomy 21) and Hirschsprung disease (from an aganglionic colonic segment) usually manifest soon after birth. Pyloric stenosis is seen much earlier in life and is characterized by projectile vomiting.

BP7 578   BP6 490, 504   PBD7 855-856   PBD6 826

35 (E) In achalasia, there is incomplete relaxation of the lower esophageal sphincter. Most cases are "primary" or of unknown origin. They are believed to be caused by degenerative changes in neural innervation; hence, the myenteric ganglia are usually absent from the body of the esophagus. There is a long-term risk of development of squamous cell carcinoma. Reflux esophagitis may be associated with hiatal hernia, but myenteric ganglia remain intact. Plummer-Vinson syndrome is a rare condition caused by iron deficiency anemia; it is accompanied by an upper esophageal web. In Barrett esophagus, there is columnar epithelial metaplasia, but the myenteric plexuses remain intact. Systemic sclerosis (scleroderma) is marked by fibrosis with stricture.

BP7 550   BP6 477   PBD7 800-801   PBD6 778-779

36 (E) The figure shows a solitary pedunculated adenoma of the colon with no evidence of malignancy. High magnification shows a small focus of dysplastic, non–mucin-secreting epithelial cells lining a colonic crypt, giving rise to "tubular" architecture. Such a small (<2 cm), solitary, tubular adenoma is unlikely to harbor a focus of malignancy; hence, a search for metastases is unwarranted. Those who inherit a mutant *APC* gene usually develop hundreds of polyps at a young age; therefore, this patient does not need genetic testing for a somatic mutation in the *APC* gene. Patients with hereditary nonpolyposis colorectal cancer have an increased risk of endometrial cancer and develop colon cancer at a young age.

BP7 580-581   BP6 508-509   PBD7 859-861
PBD6 829-830

37 (D) This patient has hemorrhoids. This is a common problem that can stem from any condition that increases venous pressure and causes dilation of internal or external hemorrhoidal veins above and below the anorectal junction. Angiodysplasia of the colon leads to intermittent hemorrhage, typically in older persons. Ischemic colitis is rare in young persons, because the most common underlying cause (severe atherosclerotic disease involving mesenteric vessels) occurs in older patients. Intussusception and volvulus are rare causes of mechanical bowel obstruction; they occur suddenly in adults and are surgical emergencies.

BP7 566   BP6 493   PBD7 854   PBD6 823

38 (A) This infant has neonatal necrotizing enterocolitis, a complication of prematurity. Necrotizing enterocolitis is believed to result from immaturity of the immune system of the gut and is often precipitated by oral feeding. The necrotic bowel can perforate. In Hirschsprung disease with colonic dilation above an aganglionic segment, stools are absent, but there is no necrosis. A bacterial peritonitis could be seen with ascites as a consequence of necrotizing enterocolitis; however, this is a complication, not the cause. Mesenteric lymphadenitis can accompany infection and, on occasion, cause bowel obstruction, but it is not the cause of necrotizing enterocolitis. A retroperitoneal mass such as a neuroblastoma can be present at birth and can sometimes cause bowel obstruction from a mass effect, but it does not cause necrotizing enterocolitis.

BP7 244-245, 570   BP6 497   PBD7 840   PBD6 809

39 (C) The figure shows a carcinoid tumor. The cytoplasm of the tumor cell contains small, dark, round granules with a dense core (neurosecretory granules), which are characteristic of neuroendocrine cells. The gross appearance of this tumor and its location are also characteristic of carcinoid tumors. Many small carcinoids and other small, benign bowel tumors are discovered incidentally; most are 2 cm or smaller. The other listed cell types do not have neurosecretory granules.

BP7 586-587   BP6 512   PBD7 866-868, 871   PBD6 836

40 (E) These findings indicate acute appendicitis. The elevated WBC count with neutrophilia is helpful but not decisive, and the decision to operate must be based on clinical judgment. Hyperamylasemia occurs in acute pancreatitis. Diarrhea with fluid loss and dehydration can lead to hypernatremia. The serum carcinoembryonic antigen level may be increased in patients with colonic cancers; however, this test is not specific for colon cancer. The alkaline phosphatase level may be increased in biliary tract obstruction. Amebiasis is most likely associated with a history of diarrhea.

BP7 588-589   BP6 514   PBD7 870-871   PBD6 839-840

41 (C) Sclerosing cholangitis is a serious extraintestinal manifestation of idiopathic inflammatory bowel disease, most often ulcerative colitis or, less often, Crohn disease. Pancreatitis and cholangitis may be complications of biliary tract lithiasis, but they have no association with sclerosing cholangitis. Diverticulosis may be complicated by diverticulitis, but the liver is not involved. Celiac sprue may be associated with dermatitis herpetiformis but not with liver disease. Peptic ulcer disease does not lead to hepatic complications.

BP7 577   BP6 503, 543-545   PBD7 849   PBD6 818-820

42 **(C)** Diarrhea with mucus and blood in the stools can be caused by several enteroinvasive microorganisms, including *Shigella dysenteriae* and *Entamoeba histolytica*. In most cases, the diarrhea is self-limited. The initial episode of diarrhea could have been caused by one of several organisms; however, the occurrence of a liver abscess after an episode of diarrhea most likely results from infection with *E. histolytica*. Colonic mucosal and submucosal invasion by *E. histolytica* allows the organisms to gain access to submucosal veins draining to the portal system and to the liver. *Giardia* produces a self-limited, watery diarrhea. Dissemination of *Cryptosporidium* and *Strongyloides* organisms may occur in immunocompromised patients. *Clostridium difficile* causes pseudomembranous colitis after antibiotic therapy.

BP7 568   BP6 496   PBD7 839-840   PBD6 811

43 **(D)** This patient has a megaloblastic anemia with a high MCV. Delayed maturation of the myeloid cells leads to hypersegmentation of polymorphonuclear leukocytes. She most likely has pernicious anemia, resulting from autoimmune atrophic gastritis. Loss of gastric parietal cells from autoimmune injury causes a deficiency of intrinsic factor. In the absence of this factor, vitamin B_{12} cannot be absorbed in the distal ileum. Among the various "antiparietal cell" antibodies are those directed against the acid-producing "proton pump" enzyme H^+,K^+-ATPase. Antigliaden antibodies are found with celiac disease that does not affect the gastric mucosa. Infection with *Tropheryma whippelii* causes Whipple disease that may involve any organ but most often affects intestines, central nervous system, and joints; malabsorption is common. *H. pylori* causes chronic gastritis and peptic ulcer disease, but does not injure parietal cells. In pernicious anemia, no antibodies are directed against intrinsic factor receptor on ileal mucosal cells.

BP7 413-414   BP6 356, 482   PBD7 814-815
PBD6 622-625, 791

44 **(A)** This patient has Hirschsprung disease. The aganglionic segment of the bowel wall produces a functional obstruction with proximal distention. Atresias are congenitally narrowed segments of bowel (usually the small intestine) that occur with other anomalies. Patients with trisomy 21 may have intestinal (usually duodenal) atresias. Complete absence of the colonic lumen at a point of atresia is a rare congenital anomaly and is not associated with loss of ganglion cells. Volvulus is a form of mechanical obstruction that occurs from twisting of the small bowel on the mesentery or twisting of a segment of the colon (sigmoid or cecal regions). Necrotizing enterocolitis is a complication of prematurity. Intussusception is also a cause of bowel obstruction in infants, but it is not caused by an aganglionic segment of bowel.

BP7 564   BP6 490-491   PBD7 830-831   PBD6 805

45 **(F)** About 2% of persons have Meckel diverticulum, an embryologic remnant of the omphalomesenteric duct, but only a subset of these persons have ectopic gastric mucosa within it, which causes intestinal ulceration. The symptoms may mimic acute appendicitis, but appendicitis should not last for 1 month or cause significant blood loss. Angiodysplasia may be difficult to detect. It is almost always seen in patients older than 70 years of age and can cause significant blood loss. Celiac sprue can occur in young persons, but it does not produce significant hemorrhage. Diverticulosis can be associated with hemorrhage, but the diverticula are almost always in the colon. Giardiasis produces a self-limited, watery diarrhea without hemorrhage.

BP7 563-564   BP6 490   PBD7 830   PBD6

46 **(D)** The lesion is an adenocarcinoma, showing irregular glands infiltrating the muscle layer. Such a lesion in a 30-year-old man strongly indicates a hereditary predisposition. One form of hereditary carcinoma of the colon results from inheritance of a defective copy of the DNA mismatch-repair genes. A second mutation at the same locus inactivates both copies of such genes and cripples the ability to repair certain forms of DNA damage. The resultant genomic instability predisposes to early onset of colon carcinoma. This type of cancer is called hereditary nonpolyposis colorectal carcinoma (HNPCC). Unlike familial adenomatous polyposis (FAP) syndrome, HNPCC does not lead to the development of hundreds of polyps in the colon. E-cadherin is required for intercellular adhesion; its levels are reduced, not increased, in carcinoma cells. Detection of *ERBB2* (*HER2/NEU*) expression is important in breast cancers. Germ-line inheritance of the tumor suppressor gene *RB* predisposes to retinoblastoma and osteosarcoma, not colon carcinoma. Translocation of the retinoic acid receptor α gene is characteristic of acute promyelocytic leukemia.

BP7 583-584   BP6 507-508   PBD7 858, 862-864
PBD6 832-833

47 **(A)** This young patient's colon shows hundreds of polyps. This is most likely a case of familial adenomatous polyposis syndrome (FAP), which results from inheritance of one mutant copy of the *APC* tumor suppressor gene. Every somatic cell of this patient will most likely have one defective copy of the *APC* gene. Polyps are formed when the second copy of the *APC* gene is lost in many colon epithelial cells. Without treatment, colon cancers arise in 100% of these patients because of accumulation of additional mutations in one or more polyps, typically before 30 years of age. Patients with the gene for hereditary nonpolyposis colorectal carcinoma also have an inherited susceptibility to develop colon cancer, but, unlike patients with FAP, they do not develop numerous polyps. *P53* and *K-RAS* can be mutated in sporadic colon cancers, but the somatic cells of patients with these cancers do not show abnormalities of these genes. *NOD2* mutations are linked with Crohn disease.

BP7 581-583   BP6 508-509   PBD7 862-863
PBD6 831-833

48 **(E)** Kaposi sarcoma, non-Hodgkin lymphoma, and anorectal squamous carcinoma are the only neoplasms on the list that define AIDS in patients with HIV infection. Kaposi sarcoma most often involves the skin, but it can be found anywhere in the body, including the gastrointestinal tract. Kaposi sarcoma is a vascular lesion; hence the color. Non-Hodgkin lymphomas and squamous carcinomas have a white cut surface and rarely are large enough to cause obstruction. Adenocarcinoma of the stomach can produce a mass, or it can diffusely infiltrate the gastric wall. Carcinoid tumors can be multiple, but they are most common in the small and large bowel or appendix and have a yellowish appearance. Gastrointestinal stromal tumors are rare and are typically large masses that have a white cut surface. Peutz-Jeghers polyps are associated with mucocutaneous pigmentation. Tubular adenomas (adenomatous polyps) are most common in the colon in older adults.

BP7 156-157   BP6 125   PBD7 548-550, 857
PBD6 535-537

49   **(F)** Spontaneous bacterial peritonitis is an uncommon complication found in about 10% of adult patients with cirrhosis of the liver and ascites. The ascitic fluid provides an excellent culture medium for bacteria, which can invade the bowel wall or spread hematogenously to the serosa. Spontaneous bacterial peritonitis can also appear in children, particularly those with nephrotic syndrome and ascites. The most common organism cultured is *Escherichia coli*. Appendicitis has a peak incidence in younger patients, the pain is often (but not always) more localized in the right lower quadrant, and ascites is usually absent; appendicitis is not related to alcoholism. Collagenous colitis is not common; it most often leads to watery diarrhea in middle-aged women. Diverticulitis with rupture could produce peritonitis, but there is typically no ascites, and diverticulitis is not related to alcoholism. Ischemic colitis may produce infarction with rupture and peritonitis, but ascites is usually lacking, and persons with chronic alcoholism are unlikely to have marked atherosclerosis. Pseudomembranous colitis is a complication of antibiotic therapy.

PBD7 872-873   PBD6 841

50   **(A)** The segment of the colon shows the diffuse and severe ulceration characteristic of ulcerative colitis. The inflammation shown is so severe that areas of mucosal ulceration have produced pseudopolyps or islands of residual mucosa. Ulcerative colitis is a systemic disease; in some patients, it is associated with migratory polyarthritis, ankylosing spondylitis, and primary sclerosing cholangitis. The pathogenesis of UC is unclear, but is most likely mediated by a T-cell response to an unknown antigen (but not a gut infection), leading to an imbalance between T-cell activation and regulation. The CD4+ T-cells present in the lesions secrete damaging substances. Autoantibodies against tropomyosin are present but do not play a pathogenic role in UC. Mutations in the *NOD2* gene are linked to Crohn disease, not UC. Inheritance of a germ-line *APC* mutation causes familial adenomatous polyposis coli with a very high risk for colon cancer. UC also increases the risk for colon cancer, but not due to *APC* gene mutation.

BP7 574-576   BP6 502   PBD7 849-851   PBD6 818-820

51   **(B)** The opened colon shows fibrinopurulent debris attached to the mucosa. These patches are called pseudomembranes. Pseudomembranous enterocolitis is a complication of broad-spectrum antibiotic therapy, which alters gut flora to allow overgrowth of *Clostridium difficile* or other organisms that are capable of inflicting mucosal injury. This gross pattern can also appear from ischemic injury that is vascular or mechanical, but this patient's history and the time course support an iatrogenic cause. A dilated, thinned, toxic megacolon is an uncommon complication of ulcerative colitis. An ischemic colitis due to mesenteric artery thrombosis could appear similar, but it is not associated with *C. difficile*. Intussusception and volvulus are forms of mechanical bowel obstruction not related to infection.

BP7 569   BP6 495-496   PBD7 836-837   PBD6 809-810

52   **(D)** The patient has so-called stress ulcers, also known as Curling ulcers when they occur in patients with burn injuries. The ulcers are small (<1 cm) and shallow, never penetrating the muscularis propria, but they can bleed profusely. Similar lesions can occur after traumatic or surgical injury to the central nervous system (Cushing ulcers). Esophageal varices can cause massive hematemesis, but they occur in patients with portal hypertension, caused most commonly by cirrhosis. Metaplastic columnar epithelium at the lower end of the esophagus is present in Barrett esophagus, resulting from chronic gastroesophageal reflux disease. A solitary gastric ulcer is usually a feature of peptic ulcer disease.

BP7 560   BP6 487   PBD7 819-820   PBD6 796

53   **(E)** Hypotension with hypoperfusion from heart failure is a common cause of ischemic bowel in hospitalized patients. The ischemic changes begin in scattered areas of the mucosa and become confluent and transmural over time. This can give rise to paralytic ileus and bleeding from the affected regions of the bowel mucosa. Ulcerative colitis usually produces marked mucosal inflammation with necrosis, usually in a continuous distribution from the rectum upward. Volvulus is a form of mechanical obstruction caused by twisting of the small intestine on its mesentery or twisting of the cecum or sigmoid colon, resulting in compromised blood supply that can lead to infarction of the twisted segment. Shigellosis is an infectious diarrhea that causes diffuse colonic mucosal erosion with hemorrhage. A mesenteric vasculitis is uncommon but could lead to bowel infarction.

BP7 564-566   BP6 492   PBD7 851-853   PBD6 822

54   **(A)** The clinical and histologic features are consistent with Crohn disease, one of the idiopathic inflammatory bowel diseases. It is marked by segmental bowel involvement and transmural inflammation that leads to strictures, adhesions, and fistula. Ulcerative colitis has mucosal involvement extending variable distances from the rectum. Unlike Crohn disease, the mucosal involvement is diffuse and does not show "skip areas." Fissures and fistulas are not frequently seen in ulcerative colitis. The findings in Crohn disease and ulcerative colitis overlap, and in up to one sixth of cases, it may not be possible to differentiate between them on the basis of pathologic findings. In general, crypt abscesses are more typical of ulcerative colitis, and granulomas are more typical of Crohn disease, but these features are not present in most biopsy specimens from patients with either condition. A story is told of an attending physician at an academic medical center who was known to berate students and residents on rounds for not definitively diagnosing ulcerative colitis and Crohn disease. When he retired, incomplete records for patients with idiopathic inflammatory bowel disease were found in his office; the records represented about one sixth of the total cases of inflammatory bowel disease that he had seen. Amebiasis and shigellosis are infectious processes that can cause mucosal ulceration, but they do not produce granulomas or fissures. Sarcoidosis can involve many organs and give rise to noncaseating granulomas; however, involvement of the intestines is uncommon, and sarcoidosis does not give rise to ulcerative disease.

BP7 573-575   BP6 499-500   PBD7 847-849
PBD6 816-818

55 (D) Columnar metaplasia of the lower esophageal mucosa, also called Barrett esophagus, is a consequence of chronic gastroesophageal reflux disease. The metaplasia may be accompanied by inflammation. Varices result from long-standing portal hypertension; although there may be associated inflammation, columnar metaplasia is not present. Irradiation may produce inflammation and eventual fibrosis, but there is no columnar metaplasia. Achalasia refers to failure of relaxation of the lower esophageal sphincter (LES). This gives rise to progressive dilation of the esophagus above the level of LES. Upper esophageal webbing may rarely accompany iron deficiency.

BP7 562-563   BP6 479   PBD7 804-805   PBD6 781-782

56 (B) This patient has colonic diverticulosis, which may be accompanied by intermittent minimal bleeding and, rarely, by severe bleeding. One or more diverticula may become inflamed (diverticulitis) or, less commonly, may perforate to produce an abscess, peritonitis, or both. Diverticular disease is not a premalignant condition. The diverticula project outward, and even with inflammation, luminal obstruction is unlikely. Malabsorption is not a feature of diverticular disease. Toxic megacolon is an uncommon complication of inflammatory bowel disease.

BP7 577-578   BP6 503-504   PBD7 854-855
PBD6 823-824

57 (D) Of the conditions listed, the one most likely to lead to adenocarcinoma in a patient of this age is hereditary nonpolyposis colorectal carcinoma (HNPCC). Crohn disease is unlikely, because the patient has not had prior serious illness, and Crohn disease of long duration is unlikely to remain asymptomatic. Although adenocarcinoma may complicate Crohn disease, it does not occur as frequently as in ulcerative colitis. This explains why colectomy is often performed for ulcerative colitis, but bowel resections are avoided, if possible, in Crohn disease. The other conditions listed are not premalignant.

BP7 583   BP6 511   PBD7 862, 864   PBD6 826-827

58 (C) The patient has a non-Hodgkin lymphoma associated with AIDS. These lymphomas are high-grade B-cell neoplasms that have a poor prognosis. Kaposi sarcoma, non-Hodgkin lymphoma, and anorectal squamous cell carcinoma are malignancies found in the gastrointestinal tract in association with HIV infection. Lymphomas of the gastrointestinal tract may also be found in patients with sprue, which is characterized by blunting and flattening of villi. Sporadic mucosa-associated lymphoid tissue (MALT) lymphomas are associated with *Helicobacter pylori* infection. Densely packed tubular glands are characteristic of tubular adenomas (adenomatous polyps), which are far more common in the colon. Granuloma formation with ulceration is more typical of Crohn disease, and the transmural inflammation may involve loops of bowel to form an adherent mass. In AIDS, ulceration with cytomegalovirus involving the gastrointestinal tract is possible, but it is more common in the esophagus or colon, and a mass effect is unlikely.

BP7 157, 587-588   BP6 125   PBD7 257-258, 868-869
PBD6 837

59 (E) Typhoid fever begins as an intestinal infection, but it becomes a systemic illness. A chronic carrier state can occur in some infected persons, with colonization of the gallbladder. *Campylobacter jejuni* may produce dysentery, but generally not systemic disease. *Clostridium perfringens* can cause gas gangrene. Some strains of *Escherichia coli* can produce enterohemorrhagic infection (from elaboration of a Shiga-like toxin) with features of hemolytic-uremic syndrome. *Mycobacterium bovis* is now rare because of pasteurization of milk products; it was best known as a cause of bowel obstruction from circumferential ulceration and scarring of the small bowel. Shigellosis can produce dysentery, but the infection is generally limited to the colon. Infection with *Yersinia enterocolitica* can produce extra-intestinal infection with lymphadenitis but generally not dysentery.

BP7 569   BP6 495   PBD7 834-835   PBD6 356-357, 808

60 (B) The patient has acute bowel obstruction, and the findings at surgery show bowel infarction. The most common causes in developed nations are adhesions, hernias, and metastases. Adhesions are most often the result of prior surgery, as in this case, and produce "internal" hernias, where a loop of bowel becomes trapped (incarcerated) and the blood supply is compromised. Loops of bowel that become trapped in direct or indirect inguinal hernias can also infarct. When metastases are the cause, the primary site is generally known and the cancer stage is high. Primary adenocarcinomas of the small bowel are uncommon. Angiodysplasia is often difficult to detect on gross examination, and it mainly leads to blood loss. Crohn disease can be focal and present with bowel obstruction, but it is not common in patients of this age. Intussusception can be focal, but it is uncommon. Volvulus may involve the cecal or sigmoid regions of the colon (because of their mobility). When volvulus involves the small intestine, torsion about the mesentery generally occurs, and there is extensive (not segmental) small bowel infarction.

BP7 578   BP6 504   PBD7 855-856   PBD6 820-823

CHAPTER 18

Liver and Biliary Tract

PBD7 Chapter 18: Liver and Biliary Tract

PBD6 Chapter 19: The Liver and Biliary Tract

BP7 and BP6 Chapter 16: Pathology of the Liver and Biliary Tract

1 Three weeks after a meal at the Trucker's Cafe, a 28-year-old man develops malaise, fatigue, and loss of appetite. On physical examination, he has mild scleral icterus. Laboratory studies show serum AST of 62 U/L and ALT of 58 U/L. The total bilirubin concentration is 3.9 mg/dL, and the direct bilirubin concentration is 2.8 mg/dL. His symptoms abate over the next 3 weeks. On returning to the cafe, he finds that it has been closed by the city's health department. Which of the following serologic test results is most likely to be positive in this patient?

- ❑ (A) Anti-HBs
- ❑ (B) IgM anti-HDV
- ❑ (C) Anti-HCV
- ❑ (D) IgM anti-HAV
- ❑ (E) Anti-HBc

2 A 41-year-old woman who works as a tattoo artist has had increasing malaise and nausea for the past 2 weeks. On physical examination, she has icterus and mild right upper quadrant tenderness. Laboratory studies show serum AST of 79 U/L, ALT 85 U/L, total bilirubin 3.3 mg/dL, and direct bilirubin 2.5 mg/dL. She continues to have malaise for the next year. A liver biopsy is performed, and the biopsy specimen shows minimal hepatocyte necrosis, mild steatosis, and minimal portal bridging fibrosis. An infection with which of the following viruses is most likely to produce these findings?

- ❑ (A) HAV
- ❑ (B) HBV
- ❑ (C) HCV
- ❑ (D) HEV
- ❑ (E) Coinfection with HBV and HDV

3 A 17-year-old woman, G 2, P 1, gives birth to a term infant after an uncomplicated pregnancy. The infant does well for 3 weeks, but then begins to have abdominal enlargement, light-colored stools, and dark urine. On physical examination, the infant is icteric. There is hepatomegaly but no splenomegaly or lymphadenopathy. Laboratory studies show serum AST of 101 U/L, ALT 112 U/L, glucose 81 mg/dL, and creatinine 0.4 mg/dL. A liver biopsy is performed, and the biopsy specimen shows lobular disarray with focal hepatocyte necrosis, giant cell transformation, cholestasis, portal mononuclear cell infiltrates, Kupffer cell hyperplasia, and extramedullary hematopoiesis. The infant recovers in 1 month, and by the age of 1 year, all laboratory findings are normal. Which of the following is the most likely diagnosis?

- ❑ (A) Erythroblastosis fetalis
- ❑ (B) Extrahepatic biliary atresia
- ❑ (C) Galactosemia
- ❑ (D) Idiopathic neonatal hepatitis
- ❑ (E) Primary biliary cirrhosis
- ❑ (F) Von Gierke disease

4 A 48-year-old man has noticed increasing abdominal girth and a yellowish color to his skin over the past 5 months. On physical examination, he has scleral icterus and generalized jaundice. His abdomen is distended, and a fluid wave is present. Laboratory studies include total serum bilirubin of 5.2 mg/dL, direct bilirubin 4.2 mg/dL, AST 380 U/L, ALT 158 U/L, alkaline phosphatase 95 U/L, total protein 6.4 g/dL, and albumin 2.2 g/dL. The prothrombin time is 18 sec, and the partial thromboplastin time is 30 sec. The blood ammonia level is 105 mmol/L. Which of the following is the most likely cause of these findings?

- ❑ (A) Choledocholithiasis
- ❑ (B) Acute HAV infection
- ❑ (C) Metastatic adenocarcinoma
- ❑ (D) Primary biliary cirrhosis
- ❑ (E) Alcoholic liver disease

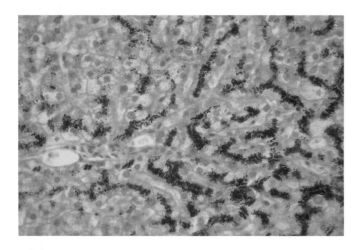

5 A 44-year-old man has developed increasing arthritis pain, swelling of the feet, and reduced exercise tolerance over the past 3 years. He has smoked 1 pack of cigarettes per day for 20 years. Laboratory studies include serum glucose of 201 mg/dL, creatinine 1.1 mg/dL, and ferritin 893 ng/mL. A chest radiograph shows bilateral pleural effusions, pulmonary edema, and cardiomegaly. He undergoes a liver biopsy, and the microscopic appearance of a biopsy specimen stained with Prussian blue is shown. Based on these findings, which of the following is the most appropriate advice to give this patient?

- ❑ (A) You need to markedly reduce your alcohol consumption
- ❑ (B) A cholecystectomy should be performed
- ❑ (C) Your siblings may be at risk of developing the same condition
- ❑ (D) You will most likely develop acute fulminant hepatitis
- ❑ (E) Smoking for many years has led to this condition

6 A 12-year-old boy with Down syndrome who lives in a residential care facility with other special needs children is brought to the physician because of listlessness, malaise, and mild fever of 3 days' duration. Dark urine is observed by one of the caregivers. On physical examination, there is mild scleral icterus and mild right upper quadrant tenderness. Laboratory studies show:

Total protein	6.5 g/dL
Albumin	4.4 g/dL
AST	337 U/L
ALT	383 U/L
Alkaline phosphatase	178 U/L
Bilirubin, total	5.0 mg/dL
Bilirubin, direct	3.1 mg/dL
HBsAg	negative
Anti-HBs	positive
Anti-HBc	positive
Anti-HBc, IgM	negative
Anti-HAV, IgM	positive
Anti-HAV, IgG	positive
Anti-HCV	negative
Anti-HDV	negative

Based on these findings, which of the following is the most likely diagnosis?

- ❑ (A) Acute HAV infection
- ❑ (B) Acute HBV infection
- ❑ (C) Acute HCV infection
- ❑ (D) Chronic HAV infection
- ❑ (E) Chronic HBV infection
- ❑ (F) Chronic HCV infection
- ❑ (G) Coinfection with HBV and HDV
- ❑ (H) Superinfection of chronic HBV with HDV

7 A 52-year-old woman has experienced malaise that has worsened during the past year. On physical examination, she now has mild scleral icterus. There is no ascites or splenomegaly. Serologic test results are positive for IgG anti-HCV and HCV RNA and negative for anti-HAV, HBsAg, ANA, and antimitochondrial antibody. The serum AST level is 88 U/L, and ALT is 94 U/L. Her condition remains stable for months. Which of the following morphologic findings is most likely to be present in this patient's liver?

- ❑ (A) Concentric "onion skin" bile duct fibrosis
- ❑ (B) Copper deposition within hepatocytes
- ❑ (C) Granulomatous bile duct destruction
- ❑ (D) Hepatic venous thrombosis
- ❑ (E) Massive hepatocellular necrosis
- ❑ (F) Microvesicular steatosis
- ❑ (G) Piecemeal hepatocellular necrosis
- ❑ (H) Nodular hepatocyte regeneration

8 A 36-year-old woman has become increasingly icteric for 1 month. In the past 3 years, she has had several bouts of colicky, midabdominal pain. On physical examination, she has generalized jaundice with scleral icterus. There is tenderness in the right upper quadrant, and the liver span is normal. A liver biopsy is performed, and microscopic examination of the specimen shows bile duct proliferation and intracanalicular bile stasis but no inflammation or hepatocyte necrosis. Which of the following serum laboratory findings is most likely to be present in this patient?

- ❑ (A) Markedly increased antimitochondrial antibody
- ❑ (B) Positive hepatitis C antibody
- ❑ (C) Markedly elevated indirect bilirubin level
- ❑ (D) Elevated alkaline phosphatase level
- ❑ (E) Increased blood ammonia level

9 A 56-year-old man from Shanghai, China, has experienced fatigue and a 10-kg weight loss over the past 3 months. Physical examination yields no remarkable findings. Laboratory test results are positive for HBsAg and negative for anti-HCV and anti-HAV. An abdominal CT scan shows a 10-cm solid mass in the left lobe of a nodular liver. A liver biopsy of the lesion indicates hepatocellular carcinoma. Which of the following mechanisms is most likely responsible for the development of this lesion?

- ❏ (A) Insertion of HBV DNA in the vicinity of the *C-MYC* oncogene
- ❏ (B) Inherited mutation in the DNA mismatch-repair genes
- ❏ (C) Repeated cycles of liver cell necrosis and regeneration caused by HBV infection
- ❏ (D) Development of a hepatic adenoma that accumulates mutations
- ❏ (E) Coinfection with *Clonorchis sinensis*

10 A 42-year-old woman has had fever, chills, and bouts of colicky right upper quadrant pain for the past week. On physical examination, her skin is icteric and there is scleral icterus. Laboratory studies show a total serum bilirubin concentration of 7.1 mg/dL and direct bilirubin concentration of 6.7 mg/dL. An abdominal ultrasound scan shows cholelithiasis, dilation of the common bile duct, and two cystic lesions, 0.8 cm and 1.5 cm, in the right lobe of the liver. Which of the following infectious agents is most likely to produce these findings?

- ❏ (A) *Clonorchis sinensis*
- ❏ (B) *Cryptosporidium parvum*
- ❏ (C) Cytomegalovirus
- ❏ (D) *Entamoeba histolytica*
- ❏ (E) *Escherichia coli*

11 Seven years ago, a 30-year-old man saw a physician because he had experienced malaise, fever, and jaundice for 2 weeks. On physical examination, there were needle tracks in the left antecubital fossa and a murmur of mitral regurgitation. Serologic test results were positive for HBsAg, HBV DNA, and IgG anti-HBc. He did not return for follow-up. Two years later, he was seen in the emergency department because of hematemesis and ascites. Serologic tests results were similar to those reported earlier. Sclerotherapy to treat esophageal varices was performed, and he was discharged. He again failed to return for follow-up. Five years after this episode, he now sees a physician because of a 5-kg weight loss, worsening abdominal pain, and rapid enlargement of the abdomen over the past month. Physical examination shows an increased liver span. Which of the following laboratory tests is most likely to be diagnostic of this last phase of his disease?

- ❏ (A) Prolonged prothrombin time
- ❏ (B) Elevated serum α-fetoprotein level
- ❏ (C) Elevated serum ALT level
- ❏ (D) Elevated serum alkaline phosphatase level
- ❏ (E) Elevated serum ferritin level
- ❏ (F) Increased blood ammonia level

12 Over the past 4 days, a previously healthy 38-year-old woman has become increasingly obtunded. On physical examination, she has scleral icterus. She is afebrile, and her blood pressure is 110/55 mm Hg. Laboratory findings show a prothrombin time of 38 sec, serum ALT 1854 U/L, AST 1621 U/L,

albumin 1.8 g/dL, and total protein 4.8 g/dL. Which of the following additional serologic test results is most likely to be reported in this patient?

- ❏ (A) Increased alkaline phosphatase level
- ❏ (B) Anti-HCV
- ❏ (C) Increased amylase level
- ❏ (D) Positive ANA
- ❏ (E) Increased ammonia level

13 A 58-year-old woman has experienced gradually increasing malaise, icterus, and loss of appetite for the past 6 months. On physical examination, she has generalized jaundice and scleral icterus. She has mild right upper quadrant tenderness; the liver span is normal. Laboratory studies show total serum bilirubin of 7.8 mg/dL, AST 190 U/L, ALT 220 U/L, and alkaline phosphatase 26 U/L. A liver biopsy is performed, and microscopic examination of the biopsy specimen shows piecemeal necrosis of hepatocytes at the limiting plate, with portal bridging fibrosis and a mononuclear infiltrate in the portal tracts. These findings are most typical of which of the following conditions?

- ❏ (A) HAV infection
- ❏ (B) Congestive heart failure
- ❏ (C) Choledocholithiasis
- ❏ (D) Hemochromatosis
- ❏ (E) HCV infection
- ❏ (F) Metastatic breast carcinoma
- ❏ (G) Sclerosing cholangitis

14 A 53-year-old man comes to the emergency department because of marked hematemesis that has continued for the past 3 hours. On physical examination, he has a temperature of 35.9°C, pulse 112/min, respirations 26/min, and blood pressure 90/45 mm Hg. He has a distended abdomen with a fluid wave, and the spleen tip is palpable. Which of the following liver diseases is most likely to be present in this patient?

- ❏ (A) Cirrhosis
- ❏ (B) Cholangiocarcinoma
- ❏ (C) Massive hepatic necrosis
- ❏ (D) Fatty change
- ❏ (E) HAV infection

15 A 40-year-old woman donates blood to help alleviate the chronic shortage of blood. Unfortunately, she is found to be positive for HBsAg and is therefore excluded as a blood donor. She feels fine. There are no significant physical examination findings. Laboratory findings for total serum bilirubin, AST, ALT, alkaline phosphatase, and albumin are normal. Further serologic test results are negative for IgM anti-HAV, anti-HBc, and anti-HCV. Repeat testing 6 months later yields the same results. Which of the following is the most appropriate statement the physician can make to this patient?

- ❏ (A) You acquired this infection through intravenous drug use
- ❏ (B) You will develop clinically overt hepatitis within 1 year
- ❏ (C) You probably have a chronic carrier state from vertical transmission
- ❏ (D) These test results are probably erroneous and need to be repeated
- ❏ (E) You should get a hepatitis B vaccination series

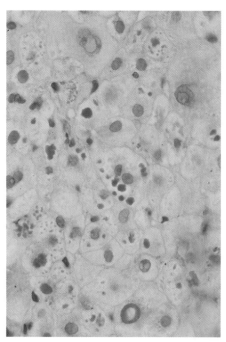

Courtesy of Dr. I. Wanless, Toronto Hospital, Toronto, Canada.

16 A 28-year-old man has had increasing shortness of breath for the past year. On physical examination, he is afebrile and normotensive. Breath sounds are decreased in all lung fields. His medical history indicates that he developed marked icterus as a neonate, but he been healthy since then. Because of a family history of liver disease, a liver biopsy is performed. The microscopic appearance of the liver biopsy specimen stained with PAS is shown above. This patient is most likely at a very high risk for development of which of the following conditions?

- (A) Diabetes mellitus
- (B) Congestive heart failure
- (C) Pulmonary emphysema
- (D) Ulcerative colitis
- (E) Systemic lupus erythematosus

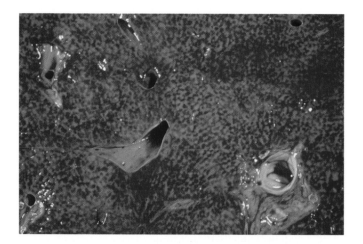

17 A 70-year-old woman has had increasing swelling of the lower legs and difficulty breathing for the past 5 years. On physical examination, she has an irregular pulse, and there is dullness to percussion at the lung bases. The liver span is increased, and her neck veins are distended. A chest radiograph shows large, bilateral pleural effusions. She dies of a cardiac dysrhythmia. The cut surface of the liver at autopsy is shown in the preceding figure. The liver is enlarged and tense with a blunted edge. Which of the following underlying conditions was most likely present?

- (A) Polyarteritis nodosa
- (B) Chronic alcoholism
- (C) Polycythemia vera
- (D) Cor pulmonale
- (E) Chronic HCV infection

18 In a clinical study, patients known to be infected with various forms of infectious hepatitis, including viral hepatitis A, B, C, D, E, F, and G, are followed for 5 years. During that time, prothrombin time, serum AST, ALT, alkaline phosphatase, total bilirubin, and ammonia are periodically measured. A liver biopsy is performed each year, and the microscopic findings are recorded. Which of the following is most likely to be the best predictor of whether a patient with viral hepatitis will develop chronic liver disease that progresses to cirrhosis?

- (A) Presence of chronic inflammatory cells in the portal tract
- (B) Degree to which hepatic transaminase enzymes are elevated
- (C) Length of time that hepatic enzymes remain elevated
- (D) Specific form of hepatitis virus responsible for the infection
- (E) Presence of inflammatory cells in the sinusoids on a liver biopsy

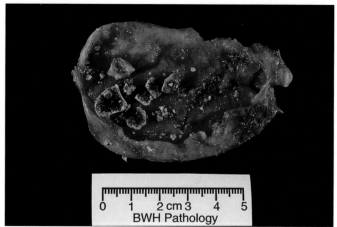

19 A 50-year-old Native-American woman comes to her physician because she has had colicky right upper quadrant pain for the past week. She has nausea, but no vomiting or diarrhea. On physical examination, she is afebrile. There is marked tenderness of the right upper quadrant. The liver span is normal. Her height is 160 cm (5 ft 3 in), and her weight is 90 kg (BMI 33). An abdominal ultrasound scan shows calculi within the lumen of the gallbladder, and the gallbladder wall appears thickened. Intrahepatic and extrahepatic bile ducts appear normal. The patient's gallbladder is removed by laparoscopic cholecystectomy and has the appearance shown above. Which of the following mechanisms is most likely to play the greatest role in development of this disease?

❏ (A) Antibody-mediated RBC lysis
❏ (B) *Ascaris lumbricoides* within bile ducts
❏ (C) Biliary hypersecretion of cholesterol
❏ (D) Decreased renal excretion of phosphate
❏ (E) Hepatocyte infection by HBV
❏ (F) Increased duodenal absorption of iron
❏ (G) Ingestion of foods rich in fat
❏ (H) Involvement of the terminal ileum by Crohn disease

20 A 60-year-old man with a 30-year history of drinking alcohol to excess sees the physician because of hematemesis. On examination, he has ascites, mild jaundice, and an enlarged spleen. He also has gynecomastia, spider telangiectasias of the skin, and testicular atrophy. Rectal examination indicates prominent hemorrhoids and a normal-sized prostate. Emergency upper endoscopy shows dilated, bleeding blood vessels in the esophagus. Sclerotherapy is performed to control the bleeding. Laboratory studies show:

Na⁺	136 mmol/L
K⁺	6.0 mmol/L
Cl⁻	92 mmol/L
CO₂	23 mmol/L
Total protein	5.8 g/dL
Albumin	3.4 g/dL
AST	137 U/L
ALT	108 U/L
Alkaline phosphatase	181 U/L
Bilirubin, total	5.4 mg/dL
Bilirubin, direct	3.0 mg/dL
Prothrombin time	20 sec
Hematocrit	25%
WBC count	12,790/mm³

Despite supportive therapy, the patient lapsed into a coma and died. Which of the following morphologic changes in the liver is most likely to be found on autopsy?

❏ (A) Liver is shrunken with a wrinkled capsular surface and microscopically shows massive irregular areas of necrosis without any obvious pattern
❏ (B) Liver is diffusely nodular with small, uniform nodules and microscopically shows diffuse fibrosis encircling nodules of regenerative hepatocytes; liver cells contain fat globules
❏ (C) Liver is diffusely nodular with small, uniform nodules and microscopically shows diffuse fibrosis encircling regenerative nodules; liver cells contain PAS-positive, globular cytoplasmic inclusions
❏ (D) Liver is markedly enlarged, yellow, and greasy and microscopically shows preservation of the architecture and marked fatty change
❏ (E) Liver is diffusely nodular and intensely green with small, uniform nodules and microscopically shows prominent bile stasis and fibrous bridging between portal areas

21 A 19-year-old mother notices that her 3-week-old neonate has increasing jaundice. The pregnancy was uncomplicated and ended in a normal term birth. On physical examination, the infant now exhibits generalized jaundice, hepatomegaly, and acholic stool. Laboratory studies show total serum bilirubin of 10.1 of mg/dL, AST 123 U/L, ALT 140 U/L, glucose 77 mg/dL, and creatinine 0.4 mg/dL. A liver biopsy is performed, and a biopsy specimen shows marked proliferation of bile ducts, portal tract edema and fibrosis, and extensive intrahepatic and canalicular bile stasis. The infant develops progressively worsening jaundice and dies of liver failure at 9 months of age. Which of the following is the most likely diagnosis?

❏ (A) α₁-Antitrypsin deficiency
❏ (B) Biliary atresia
❏ (C) Choledochal cyst
❏ (D) Congenital toxoplasmosis
❏ (E) Hepatoblastoma

22 Over the past 6 months, a 68-year-old woman has become increasingly tired and reports a 3-kg weight loss without dieting. Physical examination yields no remarkable findings except a stool sample that is positive for occult blood. Laboratory studies show total serum protein of 6.1 g/dL, albumin 3.9 g/dL, total bilirubin 1.1 mg/dL, AST 38 U/L, ALT 44 U/L, alkaline phosphatase 294 U/L, glucose 70 mg/dL, and creatinine 0.9 mg/dL. CBC shows hemoglobin of 8.9 g/dL, hematocrit 26.7%, MCV 75 μm³, platelet count 198,400/mm³, and WBC count 5520/mm³. The prothrombin time is 13 sec, and partial thromboplastin time is 25 sec. Serologic test results for hepatitis A, B, and C viruses are negative. A chest radiograph shows no abnormal findings. Which of the following is the most likely diagnosis?

❏ (A) Antiphospholipid syndrome
❏ (B) Ascending cholangitis
❏ (C) Chronic alcoholism
❏ (D) Metastatic adenocarcinoma
❏ (E) Sclerosing cholangitis

23 In a study of the mechanisms of gallstone formation, patients with cholelithiasis confirmed by radiographic imaging (ultrasound or CT) are analyzed to determine if there are underlying conditions that contribute to this process. The study identifies a subset of patients who have decreased urobilinogen excretion in urine and increased fecal bile acids. Despite normal values for serum bilirubin, albumin, haptoglobin, and calcium, many of these patients have a macrocytic anemia. Abdominal CT scans show that the liver and spleen in these patients appear normal. Which of the following conditions is most likely to be present in this subset of patients?

❏ (A) Adenocarcinoma of the gallbladder
❏ (B) Obesity
❏ (C) Hemolytic anemia
❏ (D) Crohn disease
❏ (E) Chronic hepatitis B

24 A 61-year-old man has had ascites for the past year. After paracentesis with removal of 1 L of slightly cloudy, serosanguineous fluid, physical examination shows a firm, nodular liver. Laboratory findings are positive for serum HBsAg and anti-HBc. He has a markedly elevated serum α-fetoprotein level. Which of the following hepatic lesions is most likely to be present?

❏ (A) Hepatocellular carcinoma
❏ (B) Massive hepatocyte necrosis
❏ (C) Marked steatosis
❏ (D) Wilson disease
❏ (E) Autoimmune hepatitis

25 A 50-year-old man has massive hematemesis. He has a history of chronic alcoholism, but he stopped drinking ethanol 10 years ago. He has been taking no medications. On physical examination, he is afebrile, hypotensive, and pale. The abdomen is not enlarged, and there is no tenderness. The liver span is normal. Serologic test results for hepatitis A, B, and C are negative. The hematocrit is 19%. Which of the following morphologic features is most likely to be present in this patient's liver?

☐ (A) Concentric "onion skin" bile duct fibrosis
☐ (B) Hepatic venous thrombosis
☐ (C) Massive hepatocellular necrosis
☐ (D) Macrovesicular steatosis
☐ (E) Periportal PAS-positive globules
☐ (F) Piecemeal hepatocellular necrosis at the interface of portal tracts
☐ (G) Portal bridging fibrosis with nodular hepatocyte regeneration

26 A 44-year-old woman has noticed increasingly severe generalized pruritus for the past 8 months. Serum levels of alkaline phosphatase and cholesterol are elevated; antimitochondrial antibody titer is elevated, but ANAs are not present. The serum total bilirubin concentration increases. A liver biopsy is performed, and the biopsy specimen shows nonsuppurative, granulomatous destruction of medium-sized bile ducts. Which of the following conditions is most likely to be present?

☐ (A) α₁-Antitrypsin deficiency
☐ (B) Autoimmune hepatitis
☐ (C) Choledocholithiasis
☐ (D) Hereditary hemochromatosis
☐ (E) Primary biliary cirrhosis
☐ (F) Primary sclerosing cholangitis
☐ (G) Wilson disease

27 A 36-year-old woman is in the sixth month of her first pregnancy, but she is unsure of her dates because she was taking oral contraceptives at the time she became pregnant. She experiences sudden onset of severe abdominal pain. On physical examination, she is afebrile and normotensive. There is right upper quadrant tenderness on palpation. An ultrasound scan of the abdomen shows a well-circumscribed, 7-cm subcapsular hepatic mass. Paracentesis yields bloody fluid. At laparotomy, the mass in the right lower lobe, which has ruptured through the liver capsule, is removed. The remaining liver parenchyma appears to be of uniform consistency, and the liver capsule is otherwise smooth. Which of the following lesions is the most likely diagnosis?

☐ (A) Adenocarcinoma of the gallbladder
☐ (B) Cholangiocarcinoma
☐ (C) Choledochal cyst
☐ (D) Choriocarcinoma
☐ (E) Focal nodular hyperplasia
☐ (F) Hepatic adenoma
☐ (G) Hepatoblastoma
☐ (H) Hepatocellular carcinoma

28 A 19-year-old woman is bothered by a tremor at rest, which becomes progressively worse over the next 6 months.

She begins to act strangely and is diagnosed with an acute psychosis. On physical examination, she has slight scleral icterus. A slit-lamp examination shows corneal Kayser-Fleischer rings. Laboratory findings include total serum protein of 5.9 g/dL, albumin 3.1 g/dL, total bilirubin 4.9 mg/dL, direct bilirubin 3.1 mg/dL, AST 128 U/L, ALT 157 U/L, and alkaline phosphatase 56 U/L. Which of the following additional serologic test findings is most likely to be reported in this patient?

☐ (A) Decreased serum ceruloplasmin level
☐ (B) Positive HBsAg
☐ (C) Decreased α₁-antitrypsin level
☐ (D) Increased serum ferritin level
☐ (E) Positive antimitochondrial antibody

29 A 55-year-old man has developed abdominal pain and jaundice over a period of several weeks. On physical examination, there is right upper quadrant pain but no abdominal distention. An abdominal CT scan shows a markedly thickened gallbladder wall. A cholecystectomy is performed, and sectioning shows a slightly enlarged gallbladder containing a fungating, 4 × 7 cm firm, lobulated, tan mass. Which of the following findings is most likely associated with this mass?

☐ (A) Amebic dysentery
☐ (B) Ulcerative colitis
☐ (C) *Clonorchis sinensis* infection
☐ (D) Cholelithiasis
☐ (E) Primary sclerosing cholangitis

30 A 47-year-old man has experienced intermittent upper abdominal pain for several weeks. Physical examination yields no remarkable findings. Laboratory findings show total serum protein of 7.3 g/dL, albumin 5.2 g/dL, total bilirubin 7.5 mg/dL, direct bilirubin 6.8 mg/dL, AST 35 U/L, ALT 40 U/L, and alkaline phosphatase 207 U/L. A liver biopsy is performed, and microscopic examination of the specimen shows intracanalicular cholestasis in the centrilobular regions, swollen liver cells, and portal tract edema. There is no necrosis and no fibrosis. There is no increase in stainable iron. Which of the following is the most likely diagnosis?

☐ (A) Chronic passive congestion
☐ (B) HBV infection
☐ (C) Choledocholithiasis
☐ (D) Extrahepatic biliary atresia
☐ (E) Veno-occlusive disease

31 A 42-year-old woman has had generalized pruritus for several months. The pruritus is not relieved by application of topical corticosteroid-containing creams. On physical examination, there are no remarkable findings. Laboratory findings include total serum bilirubin of 1.8 mg/dL, direct bilirubin 1.2 mg/dL, AST 55 U/L, ALT 58 U/L, alkaline phosphatase 289 U/L, total protein 6.8 g/dL, albumin 3.4 g/dL, and total cholesterol 344 mg/dL. Which of the following serologic test findings is most likely to be positive in this patient?

☐ (A) Anti–parietal cell antibody
☐ (B) Anticentromere antibody
☐ (C) Antiribonucleoprotein
☐ (D) Antimitochondrial antibody
☐ (E) Anti–double-stranded DNA antibody

32 A 35-year-old woman consults her physician because she has noticed an increasing yellowish hue to her skin for the past week. On physical examination, there is no abdominal pain or tenderness, and the liver span is normal. Laboratory findings include hemoglobin of 11.7 g/dL, hematocrit 35.2%, MCV 98 μm³, platelet count 207,600/mm³, WBC count 6360/mm³, albumin 3.5 g/dL, total protein 5.5 g/dL, total bilirubin 8.7 mg/dL, direct bilirubin 0.6 mg/dL, AST 39 U/L, ALT 24 U/L, and alkaline phosphatase 35 U/L. Which of the following is the most likely diagnosis?

- (A) Cholelithiasis
- (B) Hemolytic anemia
- (C) HAV infection
- (D) Micronodular cirrhosis
- (E) Oral contraceptive use

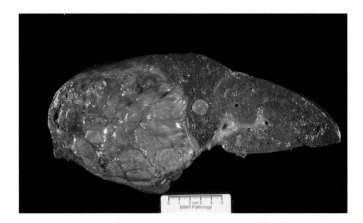

33 A 41-year-old woman experienced increasing malaise and a 10-kg weight loss in the last year of her life. She became increasingly obtunded, lapsed into a coma, and died. At autopsy, the liver has the gross appearance shown above. Ingestion of which of the following substances is most likely to have played a role in the development of this condition?

- (A) Aflatoxins
- (B) Raw oysters
- (C) Aspirin
- (D) Ferrous sulfate
- (E) Nitrites
- (F) Acetaminophen

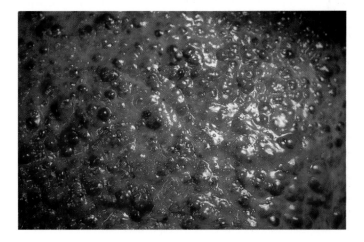

34 A 56-year-old man has had increasing abdominal enlargement for 6 months. During the past 2 days, he developed a high fever. On physical examination, his temperature is 38.5°C. The abdomen is enlarged, diffusely tender, and there is a fluid wave. Paracentesis yields 500 mL of cloudy yellowish fluid. The cell count is 532/μL with 98% neutrophils and 2% mononuclear cells. A blood culture is positive for *Escherichia coli*. The patient dies. The gross appearance of the liver at autopsy is shown in the preceding figure. Which of the following underlying diseases most commonly accounts for these findings?

- (A) α₁-Antitrypsin deficiency
- (B) HEV infection
- (C) Hereditary hemochromatosis
- (D) Primary sclerosing cholangitis
- (E) Chronic alcoholism

35 A 41-year-old man has experienced progressive fatigue, pruritus, and icterus for several months. A colectomy was performed 5 years ago for treatment of ulcerative colitis. On physical examination, he now has generalized jaundice. The abdomen is not distended; on palpation, there is no abdominal pain and no masses. Laboratory studies show a serum alkaline phosphatase level of 285 U/L. Cholangiography shows widespread obliteration of intrahepatic bile ducts and a beaded appearance in the remaining ducts. Which of the following morphologic features is most likely to be present in this patient's liver?

- (A) Concentric "onion skin" bile duct fibrosis
- (B) Copper deposition in hepatocytes
- (C) Granulomatous bile duct destruction
- (D) Periportal PAS-positive globules
- (E) Piecemeal hepatocellular necrosis at the interface of portal tracts
- (F) Portal bridging fibrosis with nodular hepatocyte regeneration

36 A 31-year-old woman has experienced increasing malaise for the past 4 months. Physical examination yields no remarkable findings. Laboratory studies show total serum protein of 6.4 g/dL, albumin 3.6 g/dL, total bilirubin 1.4 mg/dL, AST 67 U/L, ALT 91 U/L, and alkaline phosphatase 99 U/L. Results of serologic testing for hepatitis viruses A, B, and C are negative. Test results for ANA and anti–smooth muscle (ASM) antibody are positive, and the rheumatoid factor level is elevated. A liver biopsy is performed; microscopically, the specimen shows minimal portal mononuclear cell infiltrates with minimal piecemeal necrosis and mild portal fibrosis. Which of the following is the most likely diagnosis?

- (A) α₁-Antitrypsin deficiency
- (B) Autoimmune hepatitis
- (C) Chronic alcoholism
- (D) HDV infection
- (E) Isoniazid ingestion
- (F) Primary biliary cirrhosis
- (G) Wilson disease

37 An epidemiologic study is conducted of patients infected with HBV in Singapore. These patients are followed for 10 years from the time of diagnosis. Historical data is collected to determine the mode of transmission of HBV. The patients receive periodic serologic testing for HBsAg, anti-HBs, and anti-HBc, as well as serum determinations of total bilirubin, AST, ALT, alkaline phosphatase, and prothrombin time. The study identifies a subset of patients who are found to be chronic carriers of HBV. The study is most likely to show an association between the carrier state and which of the following modes of transmission of HBV?

❑ (A) Blood transfusion
❑ (B) Heterosexual transmission
❑ (C) Vertical transmission during childbirth
❑ (D) Oral transmission
❑ (E) Needle-stick injury

38 On the day of the final examination in anatomy, a 26-year-old medical student notices that her sclerae have a slight yellowish color. She has never had a major illness. On physical examination, there are no significant findings other than the mild scleral icterus. Laboratory studies show total serum protein of 7.9 g/dL, albumin 4.8 g/dL, AST 48 U/L, ALT 19 U/L, alkaline phosphatase 32 U/L, total bilirubin 4.9 mg/dL, and direct bilirubin 0.8 mg/dL. The scleral icterus resolves within 2 days. Which of the following conditions is most likely to produce these findings?

❑ (A) Choledochal cyst
❑ (B) Primary biliary cirrhosis
❑ (C) Gilbert syndrome
❑ (D) Acute HAV infection
❑ (E) Dubin-Johnson syndrome
❑ (F) Ingestion of acetaminophen

39 A 48-year-old man sees his physician because he has had nausea and colicky right upper quadrant pain for the past 2 days. On physical examination, his temperature is 38.8°C. Laboratory studies show a WBC count of 11,200/mm³ with 71% segmented neutrophils, 9% bands, 13% lymphocytes, and 7% monocytes. Which of the following is the most likely diagnosis?

❑ (A) Acute HAV infection
❑ (B) Extrahepatic biliary atresia
❑ (C) Acute cholecystitis
❑ (D) Primary sclerosing cholangitis
❑ (E) Adenocarcinoma of the gallbladder

40 A 46-year-old man has had gradually increasing abdominal distension for the past 7 months, along with decreased libido. Physical examination reveals excessive skin pigmentation in sun-exposed areas. He has an abdominal fluid wave and modest splenomegaly. Fasting serum laboratory findings include glucose 200 mg/dL, creatinine 0.8 gm/dL, ferritin 650 ng/mL, total protein 6.3 g/dL, and albumin 2.2 g/dL; his

total bilirubin, AST, ALT, and alkaline phosphatase are normal. His hemoglobin is 13.5 g/dL, hematocrit 40.6%, MCV 94 μm³, platelet count 200,000/mm³, and WBC count 6570/mm³. His prothrombin time is 20 sec and partial thromboplastin time 65 sec. A mutation in a gene leading to which of the following molecular abnormalities is most likely to explain his disease?

❑ (A) *HFE* gene, preventing the sensing of circulating iron levels by crypt enterocytes
❑ (B) *Transferrin* gene, with sequestration of iron in the liver
❑ (C) *Divalent metal transporter-1* gene, causing increased binding to intestinal luminal iron
❑ (D) *β2-microglobulin* gene, preventing the binding of β2-microglobulin to HFE
❑ (E) *β-globin* gene, with ineffective erythropoiesis and excessive absorption of iron

41 A 28-year-old woman, G 3, P 2, is in the third trimester of a previously uncomplicated pregnancy when she develops increasing lethargy with nausea, vomiting, and jaundice over a 10-day period. On physical examination, she has generalized jaundice and scattered ecchymoses over the trunk and extremities. The estimated fetal age is 35 weeks. Laboratory studies show total serum bilirubin of 5.8 mg/dL, AST 122 U/L, ALT 131 U/L, and alkaline phosphatase 125 U/L. Which of the following histologic features is most likely to be found in a liver biopsy specimen?

❑ (A) Concentric bile duct fibrosis
❑ (B) Periportal PAS-positive hepatic globules
❑ (C) Marked microvesicular steatosis
❑ (D) Extensive intrahepatic hemosiderin deposition
❑ (E) Inflammation with loss of intrahepatic bile ducts
❑ (F) Multinucleated giant cells

42 A study is conducted of patients who are infected with hepatitis virus A, B, C, D, E, F, or G. The patients are categorized according to the type of virus and are followed over the next 10 years. They receive periodic serologic testing to determine whether they are producing antibodies to the virus with which they were infected. Analysis of the data shows that a subset of patients developed antibodies but subsequently were reinfected with the same type of hepatitis virus. Which of the following forms of viral hepatitis was most likely to infect this subset of patients?

❑ (A) HAV
❑ (B) HBV
❑ (C) HCV
❑ (D) HDV
❑ (E) HEV
❑ (F) HGV

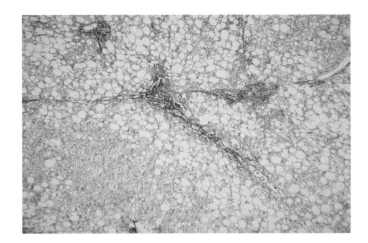

43 A 51-year-old man has had increasing malaise and swelling of the lower legs for the past 4 months. On physical examination, he is afebrile and normotensive. There is pitting edema to the knees. The abdomen is slightly distended with a fluid wave, but there is no tenderness. The liver span is increased. Laboratory studies show total serum protein of 5.0 g/dL, albumin 2.2 g/dL, AST 65 U/L, ALT 65 U/L, alkaline phosphatase 93 U/L, and total bilirubin 1.8 mg/dL. A liver biopsy is performed, and the microscopic appearance of a trichrome-stained specimen is shown above. Ingestion of which of the following is most likely to have caused this illness?

- ❑ (A) Acetaminophen
- ❑ (B) Allopurinol
- ❑ (C) Aspirin
- ❑ (D) Chlorpromazine
- ❑ (E) Ethanol
- ❑ (F) Ferrous sulfate
- ❑ (G) Isoniazid

44 After experiencing malaise and increasing icterus for 6 weeks, a 42-year-old man sees his physician. Physical examination shows jaundice, but there are no other significant findings. Serologic test results are negative for IgM anti-HAV and anti-HCV, and positive for HBsAg and IgM anti-HBc. Which of the following statements is most likely to apply to this patient's illness?

- ❑ (A) The source of the infection is a blood donation made 1 month ago
- ❑ (B) Complete recovery without sequelae is most probable
- ❑ (C) There is significant risk of development of fulminant hepatitis
- ❑ (D) There is significant risk of development of hepatocellular carcinoma
- ❑ (E) All serologic test results will be negative in 1 year

45 A 51-year-old man has a lengthy history of chronic alcoholism and comes to the physician because of increasing malaise for the past year. He was hospitalized 1 year ago because of upper gastrointestinal hemorrhage. Physical examination shows a firm nodular liver. Laboratory findings show a serum albumin level of 2.5 g/dL and prothrombin time of 28 sec. Which of the following additional physical examination findings is most likely to be present?

- ❑ (A) Splinter hemorrhages
- ❑ (B) Diminished deep tendon reflexes
- ❑ (C) Caput medusae
- ❑ (D) Papilledema
- ❑ (E) Distended jugular veins

46 A 45-year-old woman has had increasing pruritus and icterus for several months. On physical examination, she has generalized jaundice. Laboratory studies show total serum protein of 6.3 g/dL, albumin 2.7 g/dL, total bilirubin 5.7 mg/dL, direct bilirubin 4.6 mg/dL, AST 77 U/L, ALT 81 U/L, and alkaline phosphatase 221 U/L. A liver biopsy specimen shows destruction of portal tracts and loss of bile ducts as well as lymphocytic infiltrates. Which of the following additional laboratory findings is most likely to be reported?

- ❑ (A) Positive anti-HCV
- ❑ (B) Positive antimitochondrial antibody
- ❑ (C) Elevated sweat chloride level
- ❑ (D) Increased serum ferritin level
- ❑ (E) Decreased α_1-antitrypsin level

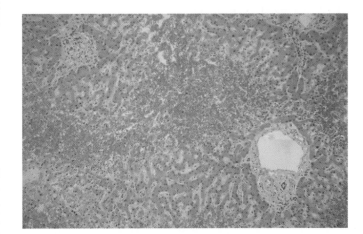

47 A 50-year-old man has increasing dyspnea as a consequence of idiopathic pulmonary fibrosis, which was diagnosed 18 months ago. Physical examination shows elevated jugular venous pressure and pedal edema. Laboratory studies show serum AST of 221 U/L, ALT 234 U/L, alkaline phosphatase 48 U/L, lactate dehydrogenase 710 U/L, total bilirubin 1.2 mg/dL, albumin 3.5 g/dL, and total protein 5.4 g/dL. The microscopic appearance of a liver biopsy specimen is shown above. Which of the following terms best describes these findings?

- ❑ (A) Apoptosis
- ❑ (B) Centrilobular congestion
- ❑ (C) Cholestasis
- ❑ (D) Hemosiderin deposition
- ❑ (E) Macrovesicular steatosis
- ❑ (F) Mallory bodies
- ❑ (G) Portal fibrosis

48 A 27-year-old man with a history of intravenous drug use is seen in the emergency department because he has experienced nausea, vomiting, and passage of dark-colored urine for the past week. Physical examination shows scleral icterus and mild jaundice. There are both recent and healed track marks in the right antecubital fossa. Neurologic examination shows a confused, somnolent man oriented only to person. He exhibits asterixis. Laboratory studies show:

Total protein	5.0 g/dL
Albumin	2.7 g/dL
AST	2342 U/L
ALT	2150 U/L
Alkaline phosphatase	233 U/L
Bilirubin, total	8.3 mg/dL
Bilirubin, direct	4.5 mg/dL
HBsAg	positive
Anti-HBs	negative
Anti-HBc	positive
Anti-HBc, IgM	negative
Anti-HAV, IgG	positive
Anti-HAV, IgM	negative
Anti-HCV	negative
Anti-HDV	positive

Based on these findings, which of the following is the most likely diagnosis?

- [ ] (A) Acute HAV infection
- [ ] (B) Acute HBV infection
- [ ] (C) Acute HCV infection
- [ ] (D) Chronic HAV infection
- [ ] (E) Chronic HBV infection
- [ ] (F) Chronic HCV infection
- [ ] (G) Coinfection with HBV and HDV
- [ ] (H) Superinfection of chronic HBV with HDV

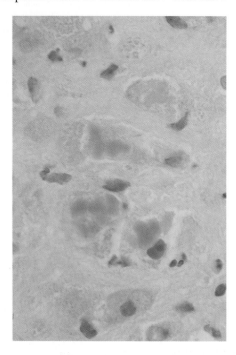

49 After a heavy bout of drinking over the weekend, a 38-year-old man feels acutely ill with nausea, upper abdominal pain, and jaundice. On physical examination, there is right upper quadrant tenderness. Laboratory studies include

a total WBC count of 16,120/mm^3 with 82% segmented neutrophils, 8% bands, 8% lymphocytes, and 2% monocytes. The total serum bilirubin is 4.9 mg/dL, AST 542 U/L, ALT 550 U/L, and alkaline phosphatase 118 U/L. A liver biopsy is performed, and the microscopic appearance of a biopsy specimen is shown in the preceding figure. Which of the following terms best describes these findings?

- [ ] (A) Apoptosis
- [ ] (B) Centrilobular congestion
- [ ] (C) Cholestasis
- [ ] (D) Hemosiderin deposition
- [ ] (E) Hepatocellular carcinoma
- [ ] (F) Mallory bodies
- [ ] (G) Periportal PAS-positive globules

ANSWERS

1 **(D)** This man developed a mild, self-limited liver disease after a meal at a restaurant. He most likely developed HAV infection by consumption of contaminated food or water. The presence of IgM anti-HAV indicates recent infection. The IgM antibody is replaced within a few months by IgG antibodies, which give lifelong immunity to reinfection. The incubation period for HAV infection is short, and the illness is short and mild, with no significant tendency to develop chronic hepatitis. The most common mode of infection for HAV is via the fecal-oral route. HBV and HCV infections have a longer incubation period and are most often acquired parenterally. HDV infection is caused by coinfection with HBV or by superinfection in a hepatitis B carrier.

BP7 600-601   BP6 525-529   PBD7 890-891
PBD6 856-857

2 **(C)** Necrosis with portal bridging suggests chronic hepatitis. Mild steatosis is seen in HCV infection. The incidence of chronic hepatitis is highest with HCV infection. More than 50% of those infected with this virus develop chronic hepatitis, and many cases progress to cirrhosis. This is in part because the IgG antibodies against HCV that develop after acute infection are not protective.

BP7 603-604   BP6 528   PBD7 894-895   PBD6 860-861

3 **(D)** Neonatal hepatitis is most often idiopathic, and most infants recover without specific therapy. Some cases are caused by α1-antitrypsin deficiency, and some are due to extrahepatic biliary atresia. However, patients with extrahepatic biliary atresia require surgery to anastomose extrahepatic ducts and prevent progressive liver damage. Patients with erythroblastosis fetalis have hydrops and icterus at birth because of maternal IgG antibody directed at fetal RBCs, leading to hemolysis. Galactosemia is an inborn error of metabolism in which deficiency of galactose 1-phosphate uridylyl transferase damages cells of the kidney, liver, and brain; there is hepatomegaly, splenomegaly, hypoglycemia, and eventual cirrhosis. Primary biliary cirrhosis affects adults. Von Gierke disease results from deficiency of glucose-6-phosphatase, and affected infants develop hypoglycemia, lactic acidosis, hyperuricemia, and hyperlipidemia.

BP7 618-619   BP6 542   PBD7 912-913, 933-934
PBD6 876-877

4 (E) This patient has liver cell injury (indicated by elevated transaminase levels), some loss of liver function (indicated by the abnormal prothrombin time), and cholestasis. These findings are not specific for a given type of liver injury. However, an AST level that is higher than the ALT level is characteristic of liver cell injury associated with chronic alcoholism. In this patient, the disease is decompensating, as evidenced by the elevated blood ammonia level. Choledocholithiasis results in a conjugated hyperbilirubinemia, but without the high ammonia level that is evidence of liver failure. HAV is typically a mild disease without a preponderance of direct bilirubin. Metastases are unlikely to obstruct all biliary tract drainage or lead to liver failure severe enough to cause elevations of blood ammonia. Primary biliary cirrhosis is rare, particularly in men, and the alkaline phosphatase level would be much higher.

BP7 592-594   BP6 522, 535, 538   PBD7 880-881
PBD6 852-853, 872-873

5 (C) This patient has clinical, histologic, and laboratory features of genetic hemochromatosis. In this condition, iron overload occurs because of excessive absorption of dietary iron. The absorbed iron is deposited in many tissues, including the heart, pancreas, and liver, giving rise to heart failure, diabetes, and cirrhosis. It appears blue with Prussian blue stain, as seen in this figure. High serum ferritin concentration is an indicator of a vast increase in body iron. Genetic hemochromatosis is an autosomal recessive condition; hence, siblings are at risk of developing the same disease.

BP7 615-616   BP6 538-540   PBD7 908-910
PBD6 873-874

6 (A) This patient has a short history of jaundice, with evidence of acute hepatitis and significant transaminase elevations. The serologic findings support a diagnosis of acute HAV, because he has anti-HAV IgM antibodies. This indicates recent infection, because these antibodies form during recovery. In contrast, the patient has antibodies against HBcAg that do not type as IgM. By inference, he has IgG antibodies against HBcAg, which are indicative of previous HBV infection. Absence of HBsAg supports this conclusion. HAV infections are acquired via the fecal-oral route and are likely to occur in institutions such as those for mentally retarded children.

BP7 600-601   BP6 525-526   PBD7 890-891
PBD6 856-857

7 (G) This patient has evidence of HCV infection and has had symptoms of liver disease for 1 year. Clinically, she has chronic hepatitis (>6 months) that may have followed an asymptomatic acute HCV infection. The anti-HCV IgG antibody is not protective. This is supported by continued HCV viremia. Approximately 85% of cases of HCV progress to chronic hepatitis, but fulminant hepatitis is uncommon. Chronic hepatitis is characterized by necrosis of hepatocytes at the interface between portal tracts and the liver lobule. This eventually leads to bridging necrosis and, finally, to cirrhosis with portal bridging fibrosis and nodular regeneration. At this time, however, the patient has no signs or symptoms of cirrhosis. Concentric bile duct fibrosis occurs in sclerosing cholangitis, which may be idiopathic or, more commonly, is associated with inflammatory bowel disease. Copper deposition is characteristic of Wilson disease, which may be associated with chronic hepatitis and cirrhosis, but it is not related

to the much more common HCV infection. Granulomatous bile duct destruction suggests primary biliary cirrhosis. The Budd-Chiari syndrome in hepatic venous thrombosis leads to hepatic enlargement and necrosis as well as to ascites. Microvesicular steatosis is more characteristic of acute fatty liver of pregnancy and of Reye syndrome in children.

BP7 603-604, 606-607   BP6 528   PBD7 894-895
PBD6 860-861

8 (D) The findings suggest obstructive jaundice from biliary tract disease (e.g., gallstones). Elevation of the serum alkaline phosphatase level is characteristic of cholestasis. The alkaline phosphatase comes from bile duct epithelium and hepatocyte canalicular membrane. Primary biliary cirrhosis with an increased antimitochondrial antibody titer eventually leads to bile duct destruction. Most cases of active HCV infection are accompanied by some degree of inflammation with fibrosis. In obstructive biliary tract disease, the direct bilirubin should be elevated, not the indirect bilirubin. The blood ammonia concentration increases with worsening liver failure. When hepatic failure is sufficient to cause hyperammonemia, mental obtundation is seen. In this case, the patient only has jaundice.

BP7 628-629   BP6 521   PBD7 887-890   PBD6 850

9 (C) There is a long-term risk of hepatocellular carcinoma in patients infected with HBV. This infection is more common (often from vertical transmission) in Asia than in North America and Europe, and it accounts for more cases of primary liver cancer worldwide than other causes such as chronic alcoholism. HBV does not encode any oncogene, nor does it integrate next to a known oncogene, such as *C-MYC*. Most likely, neoplastic transformation occurs because HBV induces repeated cycles of liver cell death and regeneration. This increases the risk of accumulating mutations during several rounds of cell division. Unlike colon carcinomas, hepatic carcinomas are not known to develop from adenomas. Hereditary nonpolyposis colon carcinoma syndrome (HNPCC) is associated with inherited DNA mismatch-repair genes. Infection with the liver fluke *Clonorchis sinensis* predisposes to bile duct carcinoma.

BP7 602, 626   BP6 548-550   PBD7 891-894
PBD6 888-889

10 (E) This patient has a history of gallstones and has developed an ascending cholangitis caused by *Escherichia coli*. These bacteria reach the liver by ascending the biliary tree. Obstruction from lithiasis is the most common risk factor. Development of cystic lesions in the right lobe of the liver suggests that the patient has developed liver abscess. *Clonorchis sinensis* is a liver fluke that is a risk factor for biliary tract cancer. Cryptosporidiosis in immunocompromised patients can occasionally occur in the biliary tract and elsewhere. Cytomegalovirus infection can also be seen in immunocompromised patients; it produces a clinical picture more like that of hepatitis but without biliary tract disease. A patient with amebiasis involving the liver is most likely to present with a history of diarrhea with blood and mucus.

BP7 631   BP6 553   PBD7 933   PBD6 898

11 (B) This intravenous drug user developed chronic HBV infection, as evidenced by the persistence of HBsAg, HBV

DNA, and IgG anti-HBc antibodies. Up to 80% to 90% of persons with a history of intravenous drug use are found to have serologic evidence of HBV or HCV infection. Ruptured varices and ascites suggest that this patient subsequently developed cirrhosis and portal hypertension. His final presentation of weight loss and rapid enlargement of the abdomen suggests that a hepatocellular carcinoma has developed. In most cases, this can be confirmed by an elevated α-fetoprotein level. The other test findings, including a prolonged prothrombin time, increased ALT level, and increased ferritin level are all indicative of chronic liver disease. Any mass lesion in the liver is associated with an elevated alkaline phosphatase level. An increasing blood ammonia level is indicative of liver failure.

BP7 601-603   BP6 548-550   PBD7 891-894
PBD6 888-890

12 (E) The patient's history points to an acute fulminant hepatitis with massive hepatic necrosis. The loss of hepatic function from destruction of 80% to 90% of the liver results in hyperammonemia from the defective hepatocyte urea cycle. An elevated alkaline phosphatase level suggests extrahepatic or intrahepatic biliary obstruction. Fulminant hepatitis from HCV is rare. An elevated amylase level suggests pancreatitis. An autoimmune hepatitis with a positive ANA finding is not likely to produce a fulminant hepatitis.

BP7 608-609   BP6 522   PBD7 881-882, 899-902
PBD6 852

13 (E) This patient has clinical evidence of liver disease that has persisted for 6 months, and histologic evidence of hepatic necrosis with portal inflammation and fibrosis. These are features of chronic hepatitis. Of all the hepatitis viruses, HCV is most likely to produce chronic hepatitis, and HAV is the least likely to produce chronic disease. Hepatic congestion with right-sided heart failure produces centrilobular necrosis, but not portal fibrosis. Choledocholithiasis leads to extrahepatic biliary obstruction and an elevated alkaline phosphatase level, but it is not likely to produce hepatocellular necrosis. Hemochromatosis can produce portal fibrosis and cirrhosis, but the liver cells show prominent accumulation of golden-brown hemosiderin pigment. Metastases produce focal obstruction, increasing the alkaline phosphatase level but not the bilirubin concentration, and there is usually no significant amount of adjacent liver necrosis or inflammation. Sclerosing cholangitis leads to inflammation and obliterative fibrosis of bile ducts.

BP7 606-608   BP6 525-528   PBD7 897-899
PBD6 856, 860-861

14 (A) The findings point to portal hypertension with bleeding esophageal varices. Cirrhosis alters hepatic blood flow to produce portal hypertension. A mass lesion, such as a cholangiocarcinoma, is unlikely to obstruct blood flow in this manner, nor does massive necrosis. Fatty change can increase liver size and can be associated with alcoholic cirrhosis, but steatosis alone does not elevate portal venous pressure. HAV infection rarely results in significant chronic liver disease.

BP7 599-600   BP6 523-524   PBD7 885, 917
PBD6 853-856

15 (C) Persistence of HBsAg in serum for 6 months or more after initial detection denotes a carrier state. Worldwide, most persons with a chronic carrier state for HBV acquired this infection in utero or at birth. Only 1% to 10% of adult HBV infections yield a chronic carrier state. The carrier state is stable in most persons, although carriers become a reservoir for infection of others.

BP7 606   BP6 530   PBD7 891-894   PBD6 864

16 (C) The PAS-positive globules in the liver seen here are characteristic of α₁-antitrypsin (AAT) deficiency. Approximately 10% of persons with the homozygous deficiency (PiZZ phenotype) of AAT deficiency will develop significant liver disease, including neonatal hepatitis and progressive cirrhosis. Deficiency of AAT also allows unchecked action of elastases in the lung, which destroys the elastic tissue and causes emphysema. Diabetes mellitus and heart failure are features of hemochromatosis, a condition of iron overload. Iron deposition in liver is detected by the Prussian blue stain. Ulcerative colitis is strongly associated with primary sclerosing cholangitis, a condition in which there is inflammation and obliterative fibrosis of bile ducts. Systemic lupus erythematosus is an immune complex disease that may affect many organs. Liver involvement, however, is uncommon.

BP7 618   BP6 541   PBD7 911-912   PBD6 875-876

17 (D) This figure shows the classic "nutmeg" appearance of the liver caused by chronic passive congestion from right-sided heart failure. Several forms of obstructive and restrictive lung diseases can cause cor pulmonale. Polyarteritis nodosa can lead to focal hepatic infarction. Chronic alcoholism results in hepatic steatosis, cirrhosis, or both. Polycythemia vera is the most common cause of Budd-Chiari syndrome. In this disease, hepatic vein thrombosis is followed by rapid hepatic congestion. This is a rare condition—far less common than cor pulmonale. Chronic HCV infection can lead to portal fibrosis and cirrhosis.

BP7 623-624   BP6 546-547   PBD7 122-123, 918
PBD6 882-883

18 (D) The most important predictor of whether a patient with viral hepatitis will develop chronic liver disease is the etiologic agent that caused the hepatitis. Of all the hepatotropic viruses, infection with HCV is the most likely to progress to chronicity and ultimately to cirrhosis. HAV, HEV, and HGV almost never cause chronic hepatitis. The pattern of histologic change, the degree of transaminase elevation, and the duration of transaminase elevation are relatively poor predictors of chronicity.

BP7 606-607   BP6 525   PBD7 894-895, 898   PBD6 856

19 (C) The figure shows cholesterol gallstones. These stones are pale yellow but acquire a variegated appearance by trapping bile pigments. In comparison, pigment stones are uniformly dark. Risk factors for such stones include Native-American descent, female sex, obesity, and increasing age. These factors cause secretion of bile that is supersaturated in cholesterol. Patients with RBC hemolysis develop pigment stones, whether the hemolysis is antibody-mediated (autoimmune hemolytic anemia) or whether it is caused by intrinsic RBC abnormalities (hemoglobinopathies such as sickle cell anemia). Infection of the biliary tract (*Escherichia coli*, *Ascaris* worms, or liver flukes) can lead to increased release of β-glucuronidases that hydrolyze bilirubin glucuronides, favoring pigment stone formation. Severe ileal dysfunction, as occurs in Crohn disease, can also predispose to pigment stones. Renal failure with phosphate retention can be a cause of secondary hyperparathyroidism with hypercalcemia, which increases the risk of gallstone formation; these stones are mixed stones. Viral hepatitis is not a risk factor for stone formation. Iron is not involved in stone formation. Fatty foods may trigger the biliary colic, but diet does not play a direct role in stone formation.

BP7 628-629   BP6 550-552   PBD7 928-931
PBD6 893-895

20 **(B)** Portal fibrosis with nodular hepatocyte regeneration and steatosis are typical features of chronic alcohol abuse. Spider telangiectasias (angiomas) refer to vascular lesions in the skin characterized by a central, pulsating, dilated arteriole from which small vessels radiate. These lesions result from hyperestrogenism (which also contributes to the testicular atrophy). The failing liver is unable to metabolize estrogens normally. Therefore, spider angiomas are a manifestation of hepatic failure. Ascites, splenomegaly, hemorrhoids, and esophageal varices are all related to portal hypertension and the resultant collateral venous congestion and dilation. Answer A describes acute fulminant hepatitis; C depicts α-1-antitrypsin deficiency; D is typical of alcoholic fatty liver; E is seen in biliary cirrhosis.

BP7 357, 597   BP6 304, 522   PBD7 883-885   PBD6 534

21 **(B)** Extrahepatic biliary atresia is a rare condition in which some or all of the bile ducts are destroyed. If the disease spares a large enough bile duct to anastomose around the obstruction, the problem may be correctable. However, in many cases, such as this, obstruction of bile ducts occurs above the porta hepatis and the only option for treatment is liver transplantation. α_1-Antitrypsin deficiency can produce a neonatal hepatitis that may clinically resemble extrahepatic biliary atresia, but most infants recover. A choledochal cyst may cause biliary colic in children; it is a congenital condition that produces dilations of the common bile duct. Congenital infections may involve the liver, and usually other organs as well; infants with these infections are ill from birth. Hepatoblastomas are rare and may be seen in infancy, but mass lesions in the hepatic parenchyma typically do not completely obstruct the biliary tree.

BP7 631   BP6 522   PBD7 933-934   PBD6 898-899

22 **(D)** An elevated alkaline phosphatase level suggests obstruction of the biliary tract, but this case must be focal, because the bilirubin is not elevated. The microcytic anemia and the blood in the stool suggest gastrointestinal tract hemorrhage, and a colonic adenocarcinoma should be suspected. Hepatic metastases from colon cancer are common. They appear as multiple masses within the hepatic parenchyma. The antiphospholipid syndrome predisposes to thrombosis with venous obstruction, in which case hepatic enzyme levels should be higher, and the partial thromboplastin time should be prolonged. Ascending cholangitis is typically caused by bacteria such as *Escherichia coli* or *Klebsiella* and presents acutely with fever, chills, jaundice, and abdominal pain. Chronic alcoholism is not accompanied by a rise in the alkaline phosphatase level, and there is often a macrocytic anemia. Sclerosing cholangitis would increase the bilirubin concentration and the alkaline phosphatase level.

BP7 625   BP6 547   PBD7 888-889   PBD6

23 **(D)** These findings indicate decreased bile acid and urobilinogen reabsorption in the ileum, which reduces the enterohepatic circulation and favors the formation of pigment stones. Crohn disease often involves the terminal ileum, and this also disturbs absorption of vitamin B_{12} complexed with intrinsic factor, leading to macrocytic anemia. Most gallbladder carcinomas occur in the setting of cholelithiasis, but the stones precede the cancer. Obesity in middle-aged women is a risk factor for cholesterol gallstones, but the enterohepatic circulation is not disrupted. Hemolysis increases the serum bilirubin (indirect component), favoring pigment stone formation, and decreases the serum haptoglobin; there is a mild macrocytosis from reticulocytosis. Viral hepatitis is not a risk factor for development of biliary tract lithiasis.

BP7 594-596   BP6 519, 551   PBD7 929   PBD6

24 **(A)** The elevated α-fetoprotein (AFP) level is most suggestive of hepatocellular carcinoma, which arises in cirrhosis. The presence of HBsAg and anti-HBc indicates chronic infection with HBV, which gave rise to cirrhosis and, ultimately, to liver cell cancer. Massive hepatocyte necrosis is unlikely late in the course of chronic hepatitis and cirrhosis. Massive liver cell necrosis gives rise to a shrunken liver, not enlarged or nodular. Steatosis is a nonspecific change that occurs in several forms of hepatocyte injury. It is found in alcoholic liver disease and in some forms of hepatitis. It does not cause an elevation of the AFP level. Cirrhosis can occur in Wilson disease or autoimmune hepatitis, but the incidence of these diseases is much lower than the incidence of HBV infection.

BP7 625-627   BP6 548-549   PBD7 924-926
PBD6 888-890

25 **(G)** Portal bridging fibrosis and nodular hepatocyte regeneration are features of cirrhosis. The massive upper gastrointestinal bleeding suggests esophageal varices as a consequence of portal hypertension from cirrhosis. If the patient is currently not drinking alcohol, no fatty change (steatosis) will be present. The architectural changes of cirrhosis persist for decades after cirrhosis develops. Concentric bile duct fibrosis is seen in primary sclerosing cholangitis, which may be idiopathic or may appear in association with inflammatory bowel disease. The Budd-Chiari syndrome in hepatic venous thrombosis leads to hepatic enlargement, and it is rare. Massive hepatocellular necrosis may occur rarely as a complication of HAV infection or ingestion of massive amounts of acetaminophen. α_1-Antitrypsin deficiency with the PAS-positive periportal globules is associated with development of cirrhosis, but this is far less common than alcoholic cirrhosis. Piecemeal necrosis is a characteristic of chronic active HBV or HCV infection.

BP7 599-600   BP6 535-538   PBD7 883-885
PBD6 869-872

26 **(E)** The presence of obstructive jaundice, granulomatous destruction of bile ducts, and elevated titers of antimitochondrial antibodies is characteristic of primary biliary cirrhosis. This is an autoimmune condition that may be associated with other autoimmune phenomena (e.g., scleroderma, thyroiditis, glomerulonephritis). Cirrhosis is a late complication of this disease that can persist for 20 years or more. α_1-Antitrypsin deficiency leads to chronic hepatitis and cirrhosis. An autoimmune hepatitis appears clinically similar to chronic viral hepatitis, but viral serologic markers are absent and a variety of autoantibodies (e.g., ANA, anti–smooth muscle antibody) may be present. Choledocholithiasis leads to extrahepatic obstruction, but bile duct granulomatous inflammation does not occur. In hereditary hemochromatosis, portal fibrosis can lead to cirrhosis. Concentric bile duct fibrosis occurs in primary sclerosing cholangitis. Wilson disease can cause an acute hepatitis, leading to chronic hepatitis and cirrhosis.

BP7 620   BP6 543   PBD7 913-915   PBD6 878-879

27 (F) This patient has a circumscribed mass in the liver, suggesting a benign tumor such as hepatic adenoma. These tumors, which may develop in young women who have used oral contraceptives, can enlarge and rupture from estrogenic stimulation during pregnancy. Gallbladder adenocarcinomas may infiltrate into the liver, but they are thus no longer circumscribed; they are rare in patients this age. Cholangiocarcinomas and hepatocellular carcinomas can be related to viral hepatitis infection and alcoholism; they are large, irregular masses that tend to occur in patients who are older than this woman. Choledochal cysts of the biliary tract are rare embryonic remnants that typically become symptomatic in childhood, along with biliary colic. Molar pregnancy can include choriocarcinoma, which can metastasize and rupture, but a solitary circumscribed metastasis is unlikely. Hepatoblastomas are rare liver neoplasms found in children.

BP7 625   BP6 548   PBD7 922-923   PBD6 887-888

28 (A) This patient has Wilson disease, an inherited disorder in which toxic levels of copper accumulate in tissues, particularly the brain, eye, and liver. The gene for Wilson disease encodes a copper-transporting ATPase in the hepatocytes. With mutations in this gene, copper cannot be secreted into plasma. Ceruloplasmin is an α_2-globulin that carries copper in plasma. Because copper cannot be secreted into plasma, ceruloplasmin levels are low. A positive HBsAg result is indicative of HBV, which infects only the liver. Chronic liver disease and panlobular emphysema may occur in α_1-antitrypsin deficiency. An increased serum ferritin may indicate hereditary hemochromatosis. A positive finding for antimitochondrial antibody can be seen in primary biliary cirrhosis.

BP7 617-618   BP6 540-541   PBD7 910-911   PBD6 875

29 (D) Almost all gallbladder carcinomas are adenocarcinomas, and most are found in gallbladders that also contain gallstones. Amebic dysentery can be complicated by amebic liver abscess; the amebae do not cause gallbladder infection. Ulcerative colitis is associated with primary sclerosing cholangitis. Infection with the biliary tree fluke *Clonorchis sinensis* is a risk factor for biliary tract cancer, not gallbladder cancer. Similarly, primary sclerosing cholangitis increases the risk of developing cholangiocarcinoma.

BP7 631-632   BP6 554-555   PBD7 934-935
PBD6 899-900

30 (C) The intermittent upper abdominal pain is a nonspecific symptom that often occurs in patients with gallstones. When a stone slips into the common bile duct, intrahepatic cholestasis occurs. This explains the conjugated hyperbilirubinemia and the increased alkaline phosphatase level. Chronic passive congestion from heart failure does not typically produce hyperbilirubinemia. Active viral hepatitis should be accompanied by some hepatocellular necrosis. Extrahepatic biliary atresia is a rare neonatal condition. Veno-occlusive

disease is rare and is accompanied by hyperbilirubinemia and cholestasis, but not by biliary tract obstruction.

BP7 631   BP6 520-521, 553   PBD7 931-933
PBD6 848-851, 898

31 (D) This patient has findings characteristic of primary biliary cirrhosis, which has a peak incidence in middle-aged women. Later in the disease, jaundice may increase with progressive destruction of intrahepatic bile ducts. Positivity for antimitochondrial antibody is a characteristic finding in most cases. Anti–parietal cell antibody is found in chronic atrophic gastritis and gives rise to pernicious anemia. Anticentromere antibody typically occurs in systemic sclerosis. Anti-ribonucleoprotein antibodies can occur in a variety of connective tissue diseases, including mixed connective tissue disease. Anti–double-stranded DNA antibodies are diagnostic of systemic lupus erythematosus.

BP7 620   BP6 543   PBD7 913-915   PBD6 878-879

32 (B) This patient has an unconjugated hyperbilirubinemia, which can result from hemolysis. With increased RBC destruction, there is more bilirubin than can be conjugated by the hepatocytes. Obstructive jaundice with biliary tract lithiasis results in mostly conjugated hyperbilirubinemia. The total bilirubin concentration may be increased in patients with viral hepatitis or cirrhosis and in persons taking drugs such as oral contraceptives. Although direct and indirect hyperbilirubinemia may occur in these conditions, conjugated hyperbilirubinemia predominates.

BP7 594-596   BP6 518-521   PBD7 885-887
PBD6 848-851

33 (A) Aflatoxin is a hepatotoxin and is the product of the fungus *Aspergillus flavus*, which grows on moldy peanuts. Aflatoxin can be carcinogenic, leading to hepatocellular carcinoma, as shown in the figure. Oysters can concentrate HAV from seawater contaminated with sewage, and eating raw oysters can result in HAV infection. Aspirin has been implicated in causing Reye syndrome in children, which results in extensive microvesicular steatosis. Prolonged and excessive intake of oral iron, rarely, can cause secondary hemochromatosis. Nitrites have been causally linked with cancers in the upper gastrointestinal tract. Ingestion of large amounts of acetaminophen leads to hepatocellular necrosis.

BP7 625-626   BP6 548-550   PBD7 924   PBD6 888-890

34 (E) The diffuse nodularity with depressed scars between the nodules is characteristic of cirrhosis, which led to his ascites complicated by spontaneous bacterial peritonitis and septicemia. The most common cause of cirrhosis in the Western world is alcohol abuse. α_1-Antitrypsin deficiency and hereditary hemochromatosis can result in cirrhosis, but both of these diseases are uncommon. In hereditary hemochromatosis, the liver has a dark brown gross appearance caused by extensive iron deposition. Of the various forms of viral hepatitis, those caused by HBV or HCV are most likely to be followed by cirrhosis. This complication is rare or nonexistent in HAV, HGV, and HEV infections. In sclerosing cholangitis, there is portal fibrosis but not much nodular regeneration, so the liver is green and hard and has a finely granular surface.

BP7 598-599   BP6 523, 535-536   PBD7 882-883
PBD6 870-871

35 **(A)** This patient has primary sclerosing cholangitis; ulcerative colitis coexists in 70% of these cases. The major targets in primary sclerosing cholangitis are intrahepatic bile ducts. They undergo a destructive cholangitis that leads eventually to periductal fibrosis and cholestatic jaundice. Eventually, cirrhosis and liver failure can occur. Copper deposition is characteristic of Wilson disease, which is associated with chronic hepatitis and cirrhosis. Granulomatous bile duct destruction occurs in primary biliary cirrhosis. α_1-Antitrypsin deficiency with PAS-positive periportal globules is associated with cirrhosis. Piecemeal hepatocellular necrosis is characteristic of chronic active viral hepatitis. Portal bridging fibrosis with nodular regeneration defines cirrhosis.

BP7 620-622   BP6 543-544   PBD7 913, 915
PBD6 879-880

36 **(B)** Autoimmune hepatitis is a chronic liver disease of unknown cause in which antibodies to hepatocyte structural components cause progressive necrosis of hepatocytes, leading to cirrhosis and liver failure. Patients tend to improve with glucocorticoid therapy. α_1-Antitrypsin deficiency and Wilson disease can lead to chronic hepatitis and cirrhosis, but autoimmune markers are absent. Chronic alcoholism is not associated with formation of autoantibodies. Because this patient does not have evidence of HBV infection, there can be no superinfection with HDV. Isoniazid may cause an acute or chronic hepatitis but without autoantibodies. Patients with primary biliary cirrhosis often have antimitochondrial antibody (which can also be seen in autoimmune hepatitis), but the bilirubin concentration and alkaline phosphatase level would be much higher in primary biliary cirrhosis.

BP7 609-610   BP6 533   PBD7 903   PBD6 868

37 **(C)** HBV infection from blood transfusion is rare because of screening of blood products. Transmission of HBV via sexual contact is not common and induces a carrier state in a minority of cases; in most cases, an immune response is elicited. Oral transmission of HAV is common (but not HBV or HCV). The risk of acquiring HBV through needlestick injury is 1% to 6%. In regions where HBV is endemic, vertical transmission produces a carrier rate of 90% to 95%. Development of viral hepatitis requires an immune response against virus-infected cells. In immunocompetent persons, HBV induces T cells specific for HBsAg that cause apoptosis of infected liver cells. During the neonatal period, immune responses are not fully developed; hence, hepatitis does not occur. The high carrier rate is medically significant, because it increases the risk of hepatocellular carcinomas 200-fold. In populations with a high carrier rate, coexistent cirrhosis may be absent in up to 50% of patients. In contrast, in Western countries, where HBV is not endemic, cirrhosis is present in 80% to 90% of patients who develop liver cancer.

BP7 606   BP6 526, 530   PBD7 891-894   PBD6 857, 864

38 **(C)** This patient has Gilbert syndrome, which results from decreased levels of uridine diphosphate glucuronosyltransferase (UGT). Up to 7% of persons in the general population may have decreased levels of this enzyme, and the condition is often never diagnosed. Stress may cause transient unconjugated hyperbilirubinemia to a point that scleral icterus is detectable, when the serum bilirubin reaches about 2 to 2.5 mg/dL. Choledochal cyst is a rare congenital anomaly producing extrahepatic biliary obstruction with conjugated hyperbilirubinemia. Primary biliary cirrhosis results in conjugated hyperbilirubinemia, as does the rare Dubin-Johnson syndrome. HAV infection can often be mild, but it is not so transient; it can be accompanied by a mild increase in conjugated and unconjugated bilirubin. Acetaminophen in small quantities can be properly detoxified, but ingestion of large quantities can produce hepatocyte necrosis.

BP7 596   BP6 520-521   PBD7 887-888   PBD6 850-851

39 **(C)** The symptoms are typical of acute calculous cholecystitis. Hepatitis is unlikely to produce acute pain and leukocytosis. Extrahepatic biliary atresia occurs in neonates and is characterized by obstructive jaundice. Sclerosing cholangitis is typically a chronic process that presents with jaundice and pruritus. Carcinomas of the gallbladder are not common and typically have a more insidious onset.

BP7 629-630   BP6 551-552   PBD7 931-932
PBD6 893-895

40 **(A)** This patient has ascites, splenomegaly, impaired liver function, diabetes mellitus, skin pigmentation, and elevated ferritin which all point to excessive hepatic iron storage and consequent hemochromatosis. Since there are no predisposing causes for increased iron absorption, the most likely diagnosis is primary, or genetic, hemochromatosis. This disease results from a mutation in the *HFE* gene that encodes for an HLA class I–like molecule that binds β2-microglobulin. HFE is expressed on the basolateral surface of the small intestinal crypt epithelial cells, where it is complexed with transferrin receptor and senses the levels of plasma transferrin. Through this sensing mechanism, HFE regulates the levels of several other proteins such as DMT-1 that are involved in iron absorption. Mutant HFE fails to exert such an influence, thereby causing excessive iron absorption and accumulation of iron in liver and other organs, leading to hemochromatosis. Since he is not anemic and has a normal MCV, a *β-globin* gene mutation with β-thalassemia is unlikely. None of the other listed mutations affect iron absorption.

BP7 615-617   PBD7 908-909

41 **(C)** This patient has acute fatty liver of pregnancy, an uncommon condition of varying severity. Accumulation of small droplets of fat in hepatocytes (microvesicular steatosis) is the typical histologic finding. This feature is not seen in any of the other conditions included in the list of options. The condition may occur because of a defect in intramitochondrial fatty acid oxidation. Extrahepatic biliary atresia is a rare neonatal disease. Concentric bile duct fibrosis is a feature of sclerosing cholangitis. PAS-positive globules are seen in α_1-antitrypsin deficiency, a condition that affects adults. Hereditary hemochromatosis manifests with complications in middle age after extensive iron deposition has occurred. The loss of intrahepatic bile ducts in primary biliary cirrhosis is also a rare disease of middle age. Multinucleated giant cells may be seen in neonatal giant cell hepatitis.

PBD7 920   PBD6 864-865

42 **(C)** Antibodies to hepatitis C do not confer protection against reinfection. HCV RNA remains in the circulation, despite the presence of neutralizing antibodies. In infections with hepatitis A, B, D, E, or G, development of IgG antibodies offers lifelong immunity. An HBV vaccine exists for this purpose.

BP7 603-604   BP6 528   PBD7 894-897   PBD6 860

43 (E) This patient has macrovesicular steatosis (fatty change) of the liver with early fibrosis. The most common cause of fatty liver and fibrosis is chronic alcoholism. In patients with no history of significant ethanol ingestion, a nonalcoholic steatohepatitis may be considered, with obesity, diabetes mellitus, or both, as possible causes. Acetaminophen ingestion in excess can cause centrilobular necrosis or diffuse necrosis. Allopurinol toxicity can cause granuloma formation. Aspirin may be associated with a microvesicular steatosis. Chlorpromazine can lead to cholestasis. Ferrous sulfate ingested in excess can promote hemochromatosis. Isoniazid use can be complicated by acute and chronic hepatitis.

BP7 612-615   BP6 517   PBD7 906-908   PBD6 869-870

44 (B) The patient has serologic markers for HBV (HBsAg positive), and the detection of IgM anti-HBc indicates acute infection. Most cases of HBV infection do not progress to chronic hepatitis, but a small number of cases are complicated by fulminant hepatitis or by progression to cirrhosis. In some patients, cirrhosis progresses to hepatocellular carcinoma, but given that most patients with HBV recover, the risk of liver cancer in a specific person is very small. Donation of blood is not a risk to the donor, but testing for HBV and HCV is performed to lessen the risk to blood recipients. After a patient recovers from HBV infection, IgG antibodies against HBsAg may persist for life. They confer protection from reinfection.

BP7 601-603   BP6 527   PBD7 898-902   PBD6 857-859

45 (C) This patient has alcoholic cirrhosis with portal hypertension. Venous collateral flow can be increased in esophageal submucosal veins, producing varices, and in the abdominal wall, producing caput medusae. The coagulopathy from decreased liver function may lead to purpuric hemorrhages, but splinter hemorrhages of the nails are most characteristic of embolization from infective endocarditis. Liver failure with cirrhosis may lead to hepatic coma, but brain swelling with papilledema is not a major feature. Hyperreflexia, but not diminution of deep tendon reflexes, can occur when hepatic encephalopathy develops. Right-sided heart failure, in which the liver may be enlarged because of passive congestion, is associated with distended jugular veins.

BP7 599-600   BP6 524   PBD7 883-885   PBD6 853-854

46 (B) This patient has primary biliary cirrhosis, an uncommon autoimmune disorder that causes progressive intrahepatic bile duct destruction. Pruritus, conjugated hyperbilirubinemia, and increased alkaline phosphatase levels are indicative of obstructive jaundice resulting from bile duct destruction. About 90% or more of patients with this disease have antimitochondrial antibodies in the serum. Chronic hepatitis C is marked by hepatocyte necrosis, not by bile duct destruction. An elevated sweat chloride level is found in cystic fibrosis, which can cause neonatal jaundice. An increased serum ferritin level is seen in patients with hereditary hemochromatosis. α_1-Antitrypsin deficiency can affect the

liver, causing chronic hepatitis and cirrhosis, and also causes panlobular emphysema.

BP7 620   BP6 543-544   PBD7 913-915   PBD6 878-879

47 (B) The restrictive lung disease leads to cor pulmonale with right-sided congestive heart failure. This causes passive venous congestion in the liver that is most pronounced in the centrilobular areas. When congestion is severe, the anoxia can cause centrilobular necrosis with transaminase elevation. The microscopic appearance is that of intense centrilobular congestion. Notice that the area around the portal tract is less congested. Apoptosis does not produce widespread necrosis, because single cells are involved, and this is most typical of viral hepatitis. Cholestasis is marked by plugs of yellow-green bile in canaliculi. Hemosiderin appears granular and brown on H&E staining, but it is blue with Prussian blue stain. Large lipid droplets fill the hepatocyte cytoplasm with macrovesicular steatosis. Mallory bodies are globular red cytoplasmic structures most characteristic of alcoholism, and acute alcoholic hepatitis in particular. Portal fibrosis begins the process of cirrhosis.

BP7 623-625   BP6 546-547   PBD7 918   PBD6 882-883

48 (H) This patient has serologic evidence of superinfection of HDV on chronic hepatitis caused by HBV. The evidence for chronic hepatitis B is the presence of HBsAg and anti-HBc IgG antibody. (Note that the presence of total anti-HBc and the absence of anti-HBc IgM antibody indicate that an anti-HBc antibody other than IgM is present. It is usually IgG.) The evidence of recent HDV infection is the presence of anti-HDV IgM antibodies. HBV and HDV infections are likely to occur in drug users who inject parenterally. HDV cannot replicate in the absence of HBV; hence, isolated HDV infection does not occur. When HDV infection is superimposed on chronic HBV, three outcomes are possible: mild HBV hepatitis may be converted to fulminant disease; acute hepatitis may occur in an asymptomatic HBV carrier; or chronic progressive disease may develop, culminating in cirrhosis.

BP7 604-605   BP6 528-529   PBD7 891, 895-896
PBD6 861-862

49 (F) This is a classic case of acute alcoholic hepatitis. The figure shows globular eosinophilic cytoplasmic inclusions called Mallory bodies. These inclusions are characteristic of, but not specific for, alcoholic hepatitis. There are also areas of hepatocyte necrosis surrounded by neutrophils. Some neutrophils can be seen in the figure. Apoptosis does not produce widespread necrosis, because single cells are involved; this is most typical of viral hepatitis. Centrilobular congestion can lead to centrilobular necrosis without inflammation or Mallory bodies. Cholestasis is marked by plugs of yellow-green bile in canaliculi. Hemosiderin appears granular and brown on H&E staining, but it is blue with Prussian blue stain. Hepatocellular carcinoma can arise in the setting of chronic alcoholism with cirrhosis, but the architecture is distorted and the cells appear atypical. Periportal PAS-positive globules are characteristic of α_1-antitrypsin deficiency; the globules tend to be smaller than Mallory bodies, and there is no acute inflammation.

BP7 612-614   BP6 535-538   PBD7 904-905
PBD6 869-871

The Pancreas

1 A study of patients recently diagnosed with type 2 diabetes mellitus follows them for 20 years to determine the prevalence and severity of complications of their disease. The records of these patients are analyzed to identify the laboratory methods used to monitor patients' ability to maintain disease control and thus reduce the potential for complications. Which of the following laboratory studies is most likely to afford the best method of monitoring disease control in these patients?

- (A) Random plasma glucose
- (B) Fasting plasma glucose
- (C) Glycosylated hemoglobin
- (D) Glycosylated serum albumin
- (E) Serum fructosamine
- (F) Microalbuminuria

2 A 33-year-old woman has had several "fainting spells" over the past 6 months. Each time, she has a prodrome of light-headedness followed by a brief loss of consciousness. After each episode, she awakens and on examination has no loss of motor or sensory function. Physical examination after the current episode shows that she is afebrile, with a pulse of 72/min, respirations 14/min, and blood pressure 120/80 mm Hg. On the basis of the microscopic finding shown in the preceding figure, which of the following disorders is most likely to be present in this patient?

- (A) Adenocarcinoma
- (B) Acute pancreatitis
- (C) Islet cell adenoma
- (D) Pseudocyst
- (E) Fatty replacement

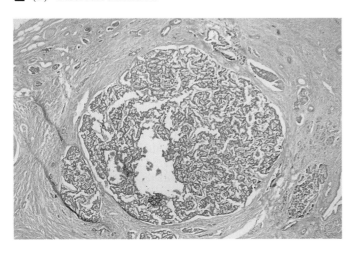

3 A 66-year-old woman has had diabetes mellitus for more than 30 years. She now has decreasing visual acuity. There is no eye pain. On physical examination, her intraocular pressure is normal. She is 160 cm (5 ft 2 in) tall and weighs 79 kg (BMI 31). Which of the following lesions is most likely to account for her visual problems?

- (A) Keratomalacia
- (B) Optic neuritis
- (C) Cytomegalovirus retinitis
- (D) Proliferative retinopathy
- (E) Glaucoma

4 The prenatal course of a 25-year-old primigravida is uncomplicated. She gives birth to a 4500-g son whose Apgar scores are 8 and 10 at 1 and 5 minutes. Shortly after birth, he develops irritability with seizure activity. On examination, the infant is normally developed with no anomalies. The lungs are clear to auscultation. Laboratory studies show serum Na^+ of 145 mmol/L, K^+ 4.2 mmol/L, Cl^- 99 mmol/L, CO_2 25 mmol/L, urea nitrogen 0.4 mg/dL, and glucose 18 mg/dL. Which of the following pathologic findings is most likely to be present in the pancreas of this infant?

❑ (A) Amyloid deposition in the islets of Langerhans
❑ (B) Extensive fibrosis and fatty replacement of the acinar parenchyma
❑ (C) Hyperplasia of the islets of Langerhans
❑ (D) Infiltration of T lymphocytes into the islets of Langerhans
❑ (E) Necrosis with circumferential granulation tissue formation comprising a 4-cm mass in the tail
❑ (F) Necrosis with neutrophilic infiltration and interstitial hemorrhage
❑ (G) Normal islets of Langerhans in a fibrous stroma containing a few lymphocytes
❑ (H) Irregular glandular structures comprising a 5-cm mass in the head
❑ (I) Small concretions within an irregularly dilated pancreatic duct
❑ (J) Islet cells comprising a 1-cm nodule in the body

5 A 28-year-old man has been using insulin injections to control his diabetes mellitus for the past 10 years. One morning, his roommate is unable to awaken him. The man is unconscious when he arrives at the emergency department. On physical examination, his temperature is 37°C, pulse 91/min, respirations 30/min and forceful, and blood pressure 90/65 mm Hg. Laboratory findings include a high plasma level of insulin and a lack of detectable C peptide. Urinalysis shows no blood, protein, or glucose, but 4+ ketonuria. Which of the following conditions is most likely to be present?

❑ (A) Acute myocardial infarction
❑ (B) Bacteremia
❑ (C) Hepatic failure
❑ (D) Hyperosmolar coma
❑ (E) Hypoglycemic coma
❑ (F) Ketoacidosis

6 A 73-year-old woman has noticed a 10-kg weight loss in the past 3 months. She is becoming increasingly icteric and has constant vague epigastric pain, nausea, and episodes of bloating and diarrhea. On physical examination, she is afebrile. There is mild tenderness to palpation in the upper abdomen, but bowel sounds are present. Her stool is negative for occult blood. Laboratory findings include a total serum bilirubin concentration of 11.6 mg/dL and a direct bilirubin level of 10.5 mg/dL. Which of the following conditions involving the pancreas is most likely to be present?

❑ (A) Islet cell adenoma
❑ (B) Chronic pancreatitis
❑ (C) Cystic fibrosis
❑ (D) Adenocarcinoma
❑ (E) Pseudocyst

7 A study is conducted of patients with type 2 diabetes mellitus. A subgroup of these patients has had poorly controlled hyperglycemia for at least 20 years, based on periodic measurements of blood glucose. As a consequence, they have had nonenzymatic glycosylation of free amino groups of proteins in body tissues. Which of the following pathologic abnormalities is most likely to be caused by this process?

❑ (A) Peripheral neuropathy
❑ (B) Amyloid replacement of islets
❑ (C) Diabetic retinopathy
❑ (D) Accelerated atherogenesis
❑ (E) Cataracts

8 A 38-year-old woman has had a low-volume watery diarrhea for the past 3 months. She now has midepigastric pain. Over-the-counter antacid medications do not relieve the pain. On physical examination, she is afebrile; on palpation, there is no abdominal tenderness and no masses. An upper gastrointestinal endoscopy shows multiple 0.5- to 1.1-cm, shallow, sharply demarcated, ulcerations in the first and second portions of the duodenum. She is given cimetidine. Three months later, repeat endoscopy shows that the ulcerations are still present. Which of the following analytes in serum or plasma is most likely to be increased in this patient?

❑ (A) Insulin
❑ (B) Somatostatin
❑ (C) Glucagon
❑ (D) Vasoactive intestinal polypeptide (VIP)
❑ (E) Gastrin

9 A clinical study is conducted in patients diagnosed with either type 1 or type 2 diabetes mellitus. The family histories and past medical histories of the patients are analyzed. Laboratory testing determines their HLA types. Their levels of plasma insulin, glucagon, C peptide, hemoglobin A_{1c}, and autoantibodies to islet cells and insulin are measured. Which of the following features common to patients with either type 1 or type 2 diabetes mellitus is most likely to be found by this study?

❑ (A) Presence of islet cell antibodies
❑ (B) Association with certain MHC class II alleles
❑ (C) Marked resistance to the action of insulin
❑ (D) Nonenzymatic glycosylation of proteins
❑ (E) Concordance rate of more than 90% in monozygotic twins

10 A 40-year-old man has been taking daily insulin injections for the past 25 years. When he does not arrive at work, a friend visits his house and finds him on the floor in an obtunded state. He is taken to the hospital by ambulance. On admission to the hospital, he cannot be aroused. He is afebrile, with a pulse of 90/min, respirations 17/min, and blood pressure 90/60 mm Hg. Laboratory studies show a hemoglobin A_{1c} concentration of 8.9%, serum glucose level of 11 mg/dL, and serum osmolality of 295 mOsm/kg. Urinalysis shows 4+ ketonuria with a specific gravity of 1.010. Which of the following statements best characterizes these findings?

(A) He is in poor glycemic control and has had an insulin overdose

(B) He is in good glycemic control but has developed ketoacidosis

(C) He is in poor glycemic control and is not taking his insulin

(D) He is in good glycemic control but has not eaten food recently

(E) He is in poor glycemic control and has developed a hyperosmolar coma

11 A previously healthy 36-year-old woman has had several "fainting spells" in the past month. During these episodes, she becomes light-headed and then collapses. She recovers within a few minutes but experiences diaphoresis and palpitations. On physical examination during the latest episode, her temperature is 36.9°C, pulse 88/min, respirations 16/min, and blood pressure 100/55 mm Hg. Which of the following laboratory findings is most likely to be reported during one of these episodes?

(A) Hypocalcemia

(B) Hypoglycemia

(C) Hypercarbia

(D) Ketonuria

(E) Hyperglycemia

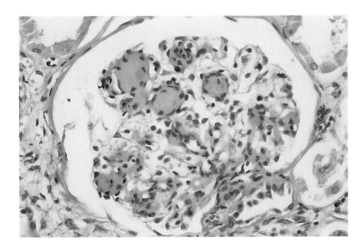

12 A 35-year-old woman is admitted to the hospital with severe anginal pain of 4 hours' duration. On physical examination, she is afebrile, with a pulse of 94/min, respirations 18/min, and blood pressure 85/45 mm Hg. An ECG shows evidence of left ventricular infarction, which is confirmed by elevated serum levels of creatine kinase (CK) and the CK-MB fraction, as well as troponin I. Additional laboratory findings include 2+ proteinuria, a blood glucose level of 210 mg/dL, and a blood urea nitrogen level of 25 mg/dL. A renal biopsy specimen is shown under high magnification in the figure above. This patient is most likely to be at greatest risk for which of the following additional complications?

(A) Gallstones

(B) Gangrene of the foot

(C) Chronic pancreatitis

(D) Uric acid stones

(E) Renal cell carcinoma

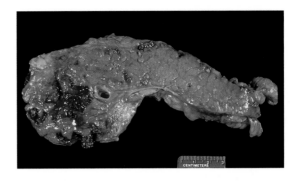

13 A 52-year-old man has had severe abdominal pain for the past 2 days. Physical examination shows boardlike rigidity of the abdominal muscles, making further examination difficult. There is no observable abdominal distention. The representative gross appearance of the disease process is shown in the figure above. Which of the following is the mechanism most likely to produce this appearance?

(A) *CFTR* gene mutation

(B) Coxsackie B virus infection

(C) Dysregulation of trypsinogen inactivation

(D) *K-RAS* gene mutation

(E) Hypertriglyceridemia

(F) Vasculitis with acute ischemia

(G) Blunt force trauma to the abdomen

14 The patient described in Question 13 is admitted to the hospital. With supportive care, his acute condition subsides within 7 days. Which of the following complications is most likely to occur in this patient?

(A) Pseudocyst formation

(B) Hemoperitoneum

(C) Small bowel infarction

(D) Gastric ulceration

(E) Hyperosmolar coma

(F) Ketoacidosis

15 A clinical study is conducted in patients diagnosed with hyperglycemia. Which of the following laboratory findings is most likely to be characteristic for those patients whose hyperglycemia is due to type 1 diabetes mellitus?

(A) Elevated hemoglobin A_{1c} level

(B) Ketonuria

(C) Glucosuria

(D) Decreased plasma insulin concentration

(E) Hyperglycemia

(F) Hypertriglyceridemia

16 A 52-year-old man has been concerned about a gradual weight gain over the past 30 years. He is 174 cm (5 ft 7 in) tall and weighs 91 kg (BMI 30). He is taking no medications. On physical examination, he has decreased sensation to pinprick and light touch over the lower extremities. Patellar reflexes are reduced. Motor strength appears to be normal in all extremities. Laboratory studies show glucose of 169 mg/dL, creatinine 1.9 mg/dL, total cholesterol 220 mg/dL, HDL cholesterol 27 mg/dL, and triglycerides 261 mg/dL. A chest radiograph shows mild cardiomegaly. Five years later, he has claudication in the lower extremities when he exercises. Based on these findings, which of the following complications is most likely to occur in this patient?

❑ (A) Systemic amyloidosis
❑ (B) Chronic pancreatitis
❑ (C) Gangrenous necrosis
❑ (D) Hypoglycemic coma
❑ (E) Ketoacidosis
❑ (F) Mucormycosis

17 Relatives of persons diagnosed with type 1 or type 2 diabetes mellitus are studied for 10 years. Laboratory testing for glucose and insulin levels and autoantibody formation is performed on a periodic basis. The HLA types of the subjects are determined. A subset of the subjects between the ages of 8 and 22 years of age has no overt clinical illnesses and no hyperglycemia; however, autoantibodies to glutamic acid decarboxylase are present. Many in this subset have the HLA-DQA1 and HLA-DQB1 alleles. Which of the following pancreatic abnormalities is most likely to be found in this subset of study subjects?

❑ (A) Amyloid deposition in the islets of Langerhans
❑ (B) Extensive fibrosis and fatty replacement of the acinar parenchyma
❑ (C) Hyperplasia of the islets of Langerhans with a normal surrounding acinar parenchyma
❑ (D) Infiltration of T lymphocytes into the islets of Langerhans
❑ (E) Necrosis with neutrophilic infiltration and interstitial hemorrhage
❑ (F) Normal islets of Langerhans in a fibrous stroma containing a few lymphocytes
❑ (G) Small concretions in an irregularly dilated pancreatic duct

18 A 72-year-old woman is admitted to the hospital in an obtunded condition. Her temperature is 37°C, pulse 95/min, respirations 22/min, and blood pressure 90/60 mm Hg. She appears to be dehydrated and has poor skin turgor. Her serum glucose level is 872 mg/dL. Urinalysis shows 4+ glucosuria but no ketones, protein, or blood. Which of the following factors is most important in the pathogenesis of this patient's condition?

❑ (A) HLA-DR3/HLA-DR4 genotype
❑ (B) Insulin resistance
❑ (C) Autoimmune insulitis
❑ (D) Severe depletion of β cells in islets
❑ (E) Virus-induced injury to β cells in islets

19 For the past 24 years, a 70-year-old man has had hemoglobin A_{1c} values between 8% and 11%. On physical examination, he has hard exudates and cotton-wool spots, as well as foci of neovascularization, seen on funduscopy. He now has increasing serum urea nitrogen and creatinine levels as well as proteinuria. Which of the following pathologic findings on renal biopsy is most likely to be present?

❑ (A) Membranous glomerulonephritis
❑ (B) Amyloid deposition
❑ (C) Diffuse glomerulosclerosis
❑ (D) Necrotizing vasculitis
❑ (E) Polycystic change

20 A 38-year-old woman with a lengthy history of gallbladder disease has a sudden onset of severe midabdominal pain. On physical examination, she has marked abdominal tenderness, particularly in the upper abdomen, and bowel sounds are reduced. An abdominal radiograph shows no free air, but there is marked soft tissue edema. An abdominal CT scan shows decreased attenuation with fluid density along with many small, bright foci of calcification involving the pancreas. She is given intravenous fluids and nasogastric suction and recovers gradually. Which of the following serum laboratory findings is most likely to be reported in this disease process?

❑ (A) Hyperammonemia
❑ (B) Increased amylase level
❑ (C) Hypoglycemia
❑ (D) Increased ALT level
❑ (E) Hypokalemia

21 A 56-year-old woman with a lengthy history of diabetes mellitus dies suddenly and unexpectedly. She was obese—about 40 kg over her ideal body weight. Her only previous serious medical problem was a poorly healing ulcer on the sole of her left foot. Which of the following lesions is most likely to be found at autopsy?

❑ (A) Subarachnoid hemorrhage
❑ (B) Pulmonary thromboembolism
❑ (C) Perforated duodenal ulcer
❑ (D) Pancreatic adenocarcinoma
❑ (E) Coronary artery thrombosis

22 For the past 35 years, a 39-year-old man has had numerous bouts of pneumonia caused by *Pseudomonas aeruginosa* and *Burkholderia cepacia*. He now has a mild- to moderate-volume diarrhea. On physical examination, he has decreased breath sounds and dullness to percussion in both lungs. His stool guaiac test is negative. Laboratory studies show the ΔF508 mutation. His quantitative stool fat is 7.5 g/day. Which of the following pathologic findings is most likely to be present in the pancreas of this patient?

❑ (A) Acute inflammation
❑ (B) Pseudocyst
❑ (C) Amyloidosis
❑ (D) Acinar atrophy
❑ (E) Adenocarcinoma

23 A 13-year-old girl collapses while playing basketball. On arrival at the emergency department, she is obtunded. On physical examination, she is hypotensive and tachycardic with deep, rapid, labored respirations. Laboratory studies show serum Na^+ of 151 mmol/L, K^+ 4.6 mmol/L, Cl^- 98 mmol/L,

CO_2 7 mmol/L, and glucose 521 mg/dL. Urinalysis shows 4+ glucosuria and 4+ ketonuria levels but no protein, blood, or nitrite. Which of the following is the most probable pathologic finding in the pancreas at the time of her collapse?

- (A) Amyloid replacement of islets
- (B) Chronic pancreatitis
- (C) Eosinophil infiltration of islets
- (D) Pancreatic duct obstruction
- (E) Loss of islets of Langerhans

24 A 50-year-old man has a 35-year history of diabetes mellitus. During this time, he has had hemoglobin A_{1c} values between 6% and 10%. He now has problems with sexual function, including difficulty attaining an erection. He is also plagued by a mild but recurrent low-volume diarrhea and difficulty with urination. These problems are most likely to originate from which of the following mechanisms of cellular injury?

- (A) Coagulative necrosis
- (B) Sorbitol accumulation
- (C) Nonenzymatic glycosylation
- (D) Leukocytic infiltration
- (E) Hyaline deposition
- (F) Apoptosis

25 A 40-year-old woman has experienced chest pain on exertion for the past 2 months. A month ago she had pneumonia with *Streptococcus pneumoniae* cultured from her sputum. On physical examination she has a BMI of 32. A random blood glucose is 132 mg/dL. The next day, a fasting blood glucose is 122 mg/dL, followed by a value of 128 mg/dL on the following day. She is given an oral glucose tolerance test, and her blood glucose is 240 mg/dL 2 hours after receiving the standard 75 g glucose dose. On the basis of these findings she is prescribed an oral thiazolidinedione (TZD) drug. After 2 months of therapy, her fasting blood glucose is 90 mg/dL. The beneficial effect of TZD in this patient is most likely related to which of the following processes?

- (A) Regeneration of β cells in islets of Langerhans
- (B) Decreased secretion of glucagon by α cells in islets of Langerhans
- (C) Increased density of insulin receptors in adipocytes
- (D) Activation of PPARγ nuclear receptor in adipocytes
- (E) Increased half-life of circulating plasma insulin
- (F) Decreased production of insulin autoantibodies

26 A 63-year-old man who had worsening congestive heart failure with cardiac dysrhythmias in the last year of his life died of pneumonia. At autopsy, his pancreas is grossly small and densely fibrotic. Microscopic examination shows extensive atrophy of the acini with abundant collagenous interstitial fibrosis, but the islets of Langerhans appear normal. Inspissated proteinaceous secretions are present in branches of the pancreatic duct. The heart weighs 500 g and all four chambers are dilated. Which of the following conditions is most likely to account for these findings?

- (A) α$_1$-Antitrypsin deficiency
- (B) Hypercholesterolemia
- (C) Chronic alcoholism
- (D) Blunt trauma to the abdomen
- (E) Cholelithiasis

ANSWERS

1 **(C)** Nonenzymatic glycosylation refers to the chemical process whereby glucose attaches to proteins without the aid of enzymes. The degree of glycosylation is proportionate to the level of blood glucose. Many proteins, including hemoglobin, undergo nonenzymatic glycosylation. Because RBCs have a life span of about 120 days, the amount of glycosylated hemoglobin is a function of the blood glucose level over the previous 120-day period. The level of glycosylated hemoglobin is not appreciably affected by short-term changes in plasma glucose levels. Random glucose testing is an immediate way for monitoring short-term adjustments with diet and medications such as insulin and oral agents. Fasting glucose testing affords a better way to initially diagnose diabetes mellitus. Measurements of glycosylated albumin and fructosamine have no value in diabetes mellitus. Microalbuminuria may presage the development of diabetic renal disease.

BP7 647   BP6 567   PBD7 1198   PBD6 919

2 **(C)** The figure shows a circumscribed cellular lesion in the pancreas, most suggestive of an islet cell adenoma. Secretion of insulin by these lesions causes hypoglycemia and the described symptoms. Many of these tumors are less than 1 cm in diameter, making them difficult to detect. Most patients who have an islet cell adenoma have only mild insulin hypersecretion. The laboratory finding of an increased insulin-to-glucose ratio is helpful. Surgical excision is necessary in patients with marked symptoms. Adenocarcinomas of the pancreas are derived from ductal epithelium and have no endocrine function. Acute pancreatitis is unlikely to increase islet cell release of insulin. Pseudocysts are complications of pancreatitis that are focal and do not produce insulin hypersecretion. Fatty replacement of the pancreas can occur with cystic fibrosis, but the number of islets also gradually diminishes.

BP7 654   BP6 559   PBD7 1205-1206   PBD6 926-927

3 **(D)** A variety of retinal lesions occur in diabetes mellitus. Retinopathy, cataracts, and glaucoma result in acquired blindness in some diabetic patients. Keratomalacia may be seen in vitamin A deficiency. Optic neuritis can be seen in systemic autoimmune diseases, in ischemia from temporal arteritis, and in toxicity resulting from methanol poisoning. Cytomegalovirus retinitis is seen in immunocompromised patients, particularly those with AIDS. Glaucoma is marked by increased intraocular pressure.

BP7 651-652   BP6 571   PBD7 1205, 1437-1439
PBD6 924, 1369-1370

4 **(C)** Maternal diabetes can result in hyperplasia of the fetal islets because of the maternal hyperglycemic environment. This can occur if gestational diabetes is present or if the mother has had diabetes mellitus prior to pregnancy. After birth, the hyperplastic islets continue to overfunction, resulting in neonatal hypoglycemia. Infants of diabetic mothers also tend to exhibit macrosomia because of the growth-promoting effects of increased insulin levels. Amyloid deposition in islets may be seen in some cases of type 2 diabetes mellitus.

Extensive fibrosis and fatty replacement of the pancreas is seen in patients with cystic fibrosis surviving for decades. Infiltration of T cells into islets occurs with the insulitis that presages overt clinical type 1 diabetes mellitus. Granulation tissue around a necrotic central region defines a pseudocyst, which can complicate pancreatitis. Neutrophilic infiltration with necrosis and hemorrhage are characteristic of acute pancreatitis. A fibrous stroma with minimal chronic inflammation and scattered normal islets is seen in chronic pancreatitis. A mass with irregular glands and abnormal nuclear features could be an adenocarcinoma. A dilated pancreatic duct with concretions can be seen in chronic pancreatitis. A mass of islet cells is an adenoma.

BP7 642   BP6 574   PBD7 1190   PBD6 927

5   (E) This patient has experienced hypoglycemic coma. He does not have detectable C peptide, which indicates that there is no endogenous insulin production, as would be expected in type 1 diabetes. The high insulin level is the result of the patient's use of exogenous insulin to treat diabetes. Because he has not eaten enough to maintain glucose at an adequate level, he has developed hypoglycemia. The lack of food intake has led to the ketosis. Acute myocardial infarction is a complication that generally occurs later in the course of diabetes when more atherosclerosis has developed. The patient has no obvious source of sepsis. Insulin is not injected into the bloodstream, and the injections are almost never complicated by infection. Hepatic failure is not a typical complication of diabetes mellitus. Hyperosmolar coma can complicate type 2 diabetes mellitus. The ketosis in this case results from decreased food intake; ketoacidosis would be accompanied by hyperglycemia.

BP7 652   BP6 572-574   PBD7 1191   PBD6 924-926

6   (D) The findings of weight loss and pain suggest a malignant tumor. The jaundice (a conjugated hyperbilirubinemia) occurs because of biliary tract obstruction by a mass in the head of the pancreas. Such a carcinoma may present with "painless jaundice" as well, but it is more likely to invade the nerves around the pancreas, causing pain. Islet cell adenoma is not as common as pancreatic carcinoma. An adenoma located near the ampulla could have an effect similar to that of carcinoma; however, weight loss with adenoma is unlikely. Chronic pancreatitis usually does not obstruct the biliary tract. In cystic fibrosis, there is progressive pancreatic acinar atrophy without a mass effect. Most pseudocysts from pancreatitis are in the region of the body or tail of the pancreas, not the head.

BP7 640-641   BP6 561-562   PBD7 948-952
PBD6 561-562

7   (D) Nonenzymatic glycosylation of collagen accelerates atherosclerosis, because it eventually leads to the formation of irreversible advanced glycosylation end products (AGEs), which accumulate over a period of time. Such changes in collagen in the arterial walls aid in trapping LDL and thus accelerate lipid deposition. The neuropathy, retinopathy, and cataracts common to diabetes mellitus result from sorbitol accumulation and subsequent osmotic cell injury. The amyloid replacement of islets is a feature in some cases of type 2 diabetes mellitus.

BP7 649-650   BP6 567   PBD7 1198   PBD6 919-920

8   (E) This patient has Zollinger-Ellison syndrome, with one or more islet cell adenomas of the pancreas secreting gastrin. This secretion leads to intractable peptic ulcer disease, with multiple duodenal or gastric ulcerations. Islet cell tumors may secrete a variety of hormonally active compounds. Insulinomas may produce hypoglycemia. Glucagonomas and somatostatinomas may produce a syndrome characterized by mild diabetes mellitus. VIPomas may be associated with marked watery diarrhea, hypokalemia, and achlorhydria.

BP7 654   BP6 574-575   PBD7 1206-1207   PBD6 927

9   (D) Nonenzymatic glycosylation of proteins is a function of the level of blood glucose rather than the cause of hyperglycemia. Type 1 and type 2 diabetes mellitus are characterized by hyperglycemia, but the underlying pathogenetic mechanisms are different. Type 1 diabetes mellitus is an autoimmune disease that is associated with certain alleles of the MHC class II molecules. It is characterized by a very high concordance rate and the presence of autoantibodies. Insulin resistance is a feature of type 2 diabetes mellitus.

BP7 647   BP6 567   PBD7 1198   PBD6 919-920

10   (A) The increased hemoglobin A_{1c} level suggests that this patient has poorly controlled hyperglycemia. The profound hypoglycemia is consistent with an overdose of insulin, and the ketonuria suggests that he has not been eating any food. If he had not been taking his insulin, the glucose level would be higher, and if this were coupled with ketonuria, a diagnosis of ketoacidosis could be made. Because the serum osmolarity and glucose level are not increased, he does not have hyperosmolar coma.

BP7 647   BP6 572-573   PBD7 1198, 1201   PBD6 924-925

11   (B) This patient has features of hypoglycemia. An islet cell tumor may be suspected as the cause of episodic hypoglycemia. Reactive hypoglycemia after meals may also be considered. Hypocalcemia gives rise to tetany, characterized by muscle spasms. Hypercarbia may result from decreased respiration. Ketonuria is a feature of type 1 diabetes mellitus and accompanies hyperglycemia.

BP7 654   BP6 574   PBD7 1205-1206   PBD6 926-927

12   (B) Nodular glomerulosclerosis is a characteristic feature of renal involvement in advanced diabetes mellitus. Myocardial infarction in this premenopausal woman strongly suggests an underlying predisposing condition such as diabetes mellitus. Proteinuria and evidence of renal failure support the likelihood of diabetes. Diabetic individuals also are prone to early and accelerated atherosclerosis of peripheral vessels. Thrombotic occlusion of arteries in the leg places these patients at a very high risk of developing gangrene. None of the other diseases has any association with diabetes.

BP7 650   BP6 569-572   PBD7 1201   PBD6 920-928

13   (C) This patient has acute hemorrhagic pancreatitis with foci of chalky white fat necrosis. Fundamental to the causation of acute pancreatitis is inappropriate activation of digestive enzymes in the acini and the consequent autodigestion of the pancreas. These enzymes are present as proenzymes in the acini and are activated by trypsin. Trypsin itself is derived from trypsinogen, and any abnormality that prevents regulated inactivation of trypsinogen can lead to excessive trypsin-mediated activation of other digestive enzymes such as lipase, amylase, and elastase. Evidence for this mechanism comes from the observation that the rare disease hereditary pancreatitis, with germ-line mutations that affect a site on the cationic trypsinogen molecule essential for the cleavage of trypsin by trypsin itself, results in trypsinogen and trypsin that become resistant to inactivation, and the abnormally active trypsin activates other digestive proenzymes, leading to development of pancreatitis. Pancreatic duct obstruction by gallstones is the most common event precipitating trypsinogen activation. A *CFTR* gene mutation can give rise to chronic pancreatitis, even in the absence of cystic fibrosis. A *K-RAS* mutation is an early event in pancreatic carcinogenesis. Viral infections, hypertriglyceridemia, vasculitis, and trauma are less common causes for pancreatitis.

BP7 636-638   BP6 558-559   PBD7 942-944
PBD6 904-907

14 (A) During acute pancreatitis, the extent of necrosis may be so severe that a liquefied area becomes surrounded by granulation tissue, forming a cystic mass. However, because there is no epithelial lining in the cyst, it is best called a pseudocyst. Although acute pancreatitis may be hemorrhagic, the hemorrhage is confined to the body of the pancreas and surrounding fibroadipose tissue. The inflammation is unlikely to compromise the blood supply to abdominal organs and produce an infarction. Although the pancreas is inferior and posterior to the stomach, spread of inflammation to the stomach does not typically occur. The islets of Langerhans usually continue to function despite marked inflammation of the parenchyma. Therefore, lack of insulin is not a typical feature of pancreatitis.

BP7 636   BP6 558   PBD7 944-947   PBD6 909

15 (B) The markedly diminished insulin levels associated with type 1 diabetes mellitus, coupled with absolute or relative increases in glucagon, result in catabolism of adipose tissue. The released fatty acids can then become oxidized to form ketone bodies and produce ketonuria and possible ketoacidosis. Patients with type 2 diabetes mellitus can have mild to moderately decreased insulin levels, but there is still sufficient insulin to prevent this complication. Elevated glucose levels occur in patients with either type 1 or type 2 diabetes mellitus, with resultant increases in the hemoglobin A_{1c} level and spillage of glucose into the urine (glucosuria). Hyperlipidemia may occur in all types of diabetes mellitus and contribute to atherogenesis.

BP7 652-654   BP6 572   PBD7 1202-1204   PBD6 924-926

16 (C) Severe peripheral atherosclerotic disease is a common complication of long-standing diabetes mellitus. Atherosclerotic narrowing of the arteries to the lower legs can cause ischemia and gangrene. The foot is often involved with gangrene, which may necessitate amputation. Diabetic neuropathy with decreased sensation increases the risk of repeated trauma, which in turn enhances the risk of ulcerations that cause infection and inflammation that promotes gangrene. Although pancreatic islets may have amyloid deposits, systemic amyloidosis and chronic pancreatitis (which involves the parenchymal acini) do not occur with type 2 diabetes mellitus. However, patients with type 2 diabetes mellitus or obesity, or both, are at increased risk of developing nonalcoholic steatohepatitis (NASH). Because this patient is not

taking medications such as insulin, it is unlikely that he could become severely hypoglycemic. Because he is overweight, it is more likely that he has type 2 diabetes mellitus; thus, ketoacidosis is unlikely. Infections with *Mucor circinelloides* are more likely to occur in ketoacidosis.

BP7 649   BP6 567-569   PBD7 1199-1200   PBD6 919-921

17 (D) The presence of HLA-DQA1 and HLA-DQB1 alleles of the MHC class II region has the strongest linkage to type 1 diabetes mellitus. Autoantibodies to islet cell antigens such as glutamic acid decarboxylase are present years before overt clinical diabetes develops. Similarly, an insulitis caused by T-cell infiltration occurs prior to the onset of symptoms or very early in the course of type 1 diabetes mellitus. The insulitis in type 1 diabetes mellitus is associated with increased expression of class I MHC molecules and aberrant expression of class II MHC molecules on the β cells of the islets. These changes are mediated by cytokines such as interferon-γ elaborated by CD4 cells (along with CD8 cells). Amyloid deposition in islets may be seen in some cases of type 2 diabetes mellitus. Extensive fibrosis and fatty replacement of the pancreas is seen in patients with cystic fibrosis surviving for decades. Islet hyperplasia occurs in infants of diabetic mothers. Neutrophilic infiltration with necrosis and hemorrhage are characteristic of acute pancreatitis. A fibrous stroma with minimal chronic inflammation and scattered normal islets is seen with chronic pancreatitis, as is a dilated pancreatic duct with concretions.

BP7 643   BP6 565   PBD7 1194   PBD6 916

18 (B) This patient has type 2 diabetes mellitus with hyperosmolar, nonketotic coma. In type 2 diabetes mellitus, there is a decrease in plasma insulin or a relative lack of insulin, but there is still enough to prevent ketosis. The fundamental defect is insulin resistance. The resulting hyperglycemia tends to produce polyuria, leading to dehydration that further increases the serum glucose level. If enough fluids are not ingested, dehydration drives the serum glucose to very high levels. The HLA-DR3/HLA-DR4 genotype is a predisposing factor for type 1 diabetes mellitus. Severe loss of β cells is a feature of autoimmune, or type 1, diabetes mellitus.

BP7 652   BP6 572   PBD7 1195, 1202-1203   PBD6 926

19 (C) Diffuse glomerulosclerosis and nodular glomerulosclerosis are changes that are characteristic of diabetic nephropathy. The nephropathy takes years to develop, and renal function gradually diminishes. The other complication of diabetes mellitus in this man is retinopathy. The hard exudates and cotton-wool spots are part of a background retinopathy, but the neovascularization is part of the more ominous proliferative retinopathy. Membranous glomerulonephritis is most often idiopathic. Amyloidosis is uncommonly associated with diabetes mellitus. Although there are progressive vascular changes in the kidney with diabetes mellitus—notably, large-artery atherosclerosis and hyaline arteriolosclerosis—vasculitis is not a feature of diabetes mellitus. Polycystic changes are most likely to appear in diabetic patients who have received long-term hemodialysis.

BP7 650   BP6 570   PBD7 1201   PBD6 923

20 (B) The clinical features, as well as the preexisting gallbladder disease, are highly suggestive of acute pancreatitis.

This is confirmed by the appearance of the pancreas at laparotomy. The serum amylase level is rapidly elevated after an attack of acute pancreatitis. Serum and urine lipase levels are also elevated. These enzymes are released from necrotic pancreatic acini. Abnormalities in liver function test results may be seen in cases of gallstone pancreatitis. Hyperammonemia is a feature of liver failure. In acute pancreatitis, the islets of Langerhans still function but do not become hyperactive. An increased ALT level is more characteristic of liver cell injury. The serum potassium concentration does not decrease in pancreatitis.

BP7 636-638   BP6 558-559   PBD7 942-945
PBD6 904-907

21 (E) The most common cause of death in diabetic patients is ischemic heart disease. Diabetic individuals have accelerated, advanced atherosclerosis. The heart, kidneys, and brain are most often affected by ischemia resulting from vascular narrowing, thrombosis, or thromboembolic disease. There can also be severe peripheral vascular disease, with poor tissue perfusion and poor wound healing. This complication would explain this woman's poorly healing foot ulcer. A diabetic patient could have a hemorrhagic cerebral infarction from a thromboembolus or a hypertensive hemorrhage, but these lesions are not known to involve the subarachnoid space. The advanced atherosclerosis of diabetes has a minimal impact on the venous system. The risk of duodenal ulcers or cancer is not appreciably greater in diabetic persons.

BP7 654   BP6 568   PBD7 1199-1200   PBD6 922

22 (D) This patient has cystic fibrosis, an autosomal recessive condition that results from an abnormal cystic fibrosis transmembrane conductance regulator (*CFTR*) gene. The most common mutation is ΔF508. The decreased bicarbonate secretion gives rise to abnormal viscid secretions affecting the pancreas. This results in ductal obstruction, and this leads to a form of chronic pancreatitis with acinar atrophy. Eventually, the exocrine function is gone. Clinically symptomatic, florid acute and chronic pancreatitis do not typically occur in this setting, nor does the complication of inflammation known as a pseudocyst. Amyloid deposition may be seen in the islets of Langerhans in a patient with type 2 diabetes mellitus, but generalized amyloid deposition of the pancreas is rare. Cystic fibrosis is not a risk factor for adenoma or carcinoma of the pancreas.

BP7 639   BP6 208-209   PBD7 489-495, 945
PBD6 479-480

23 (E) Type 1 diabetes mellitus does not become overt until the β cells are markedly depleted and insulin levels are greatly reduced. In this case, the girl has ketoacidosis. Amyloid replacement of islets is a feature of type 2 diabetes mellitus; ketoacidosis is not a feature of type 2 diabetes mellitus. Chronic pancreatitis diminishes exocrine pancreatic function but rarely destroys enough islets to cause overt diabetes mellitus. Inflammatory cells, mostly T cells, can be seen in the islets of patients with type 1 diabetes mellitus *before* the diabetes is clinically overt. Eosinophils, however, are rare. They usually are found in the islets of diabetic infants who fail to survive the immediate postnatal period. Pancreatic duct obstruction can produce an acute pancreatitis that is unlikely to affect the function of enough islets to cause diabetes mellitus.

BP7 644,653   BP6 564-565   PBD7 1192-1194
PBD6 915-917

24 (B) This patient has autonomic neuropathy caused by long-standing diabetes mellitus. It is thought that nerve cells do not require insulin for glucose uptake. In the presence of hyperglycemia, excess glucose diffuses into the cell cytoplasm and accumulates. The excess glucose is metabolized by intracellular aldose reductase enzyme to sorbitol and then to fructose. This increased amount of carbohydrate increases cellular osmolarity and free water influx, injuring the cell. Schwann cells are injured in this manner; the injury may lead to peripheral neuropathy. Coagulative necrosis in diabetic patients is most likely to be a complication of atherosclerosis. Glycosylation tends to affect vascular walls and promote atherosclerosis. Infections with inflammation are more common in diabetic patients but do not lead to the characteristic neuropathy. Hyalinization affects small blood vessels, not nerves. Apoptosis, or single-cell necrosis, is not induced by diabetes mellitus.

BP7 651-652   BP6 567   PBD7 1199, 1201   PBD6 920

25 (D) The clinical features of obesity with angina and glucose intolerance in this patient are strongly suggestive of type 2 diabetes mellitus. This is confirmed by the oral glucose tolerance test (>200 mg/dL at 2 hours), useful in this case because her fasting blood glucose levels of 122 and 128 mg/dL did not quite reach the diagnostic criterion of 126 mg/dL on two occasions. The fundamental abnormality in type 2 diabetes mellitus is insulin resistance. Several adipocyte-derived molecules, such as adiponectin and resistin, have been implicated in the causation of insulin resistance, thus establishing the link between obesity and type 2 diabetes mellitus. The nuclear receptor PPARγ has emerged as a key molecule in the regulation of insulin resistance through its actions on adipocytes hormones. TZDs bind to and activate PPARγ in adipocytes and thereby increase the levels of the insulin-sensitizing hormone adiponectin and reduce the levels of free fatty acids and resistin, both of which increase insulin resistance. β cell loss and density of insulin receptors are not major factors in the pathogenesis of type 2 diabetes mellitus. Glucagon excess worsens diabetes, but TZDs do not affect its secretion. TZDs do not affect the metabolism of insulin. Insulin autoantibodies are seen with type 1 diabetes mellitus.

BP7 646-647   PBD7 1195-1196

26 (C) This patient has chronic pancreatitis. Alcohol promotes intracellular proenzyme activation that leads to acinar cell injury. Chronic alcoholism also causes secretion of protein-rich pancreatic fluid, which is inspissated and deposited in small pancreatic ducts. Ductal obstruction predisposes to acinar injury. Ongoing or repeated injury leads to chronic pancreatitis. A dilated cardiomyopathy can also occur in chronic alcoholism, as in this case. A deficiency of α1-antitrypsin can produce liver disease with chronic hepatitis or cirrhosis, or both. Hypercholesterolemia can cause acute pancreatitis, as can cholelithiasis. Blunt abdominal trauma can produce hemorrhage, sometimes with a component of acute pancreatitis.

BP7 639-640   BP6 561   PBD7 945-946   PBD6 907-909

The Kidney and the Lower Urinary Tract

1 A 24-year-old man is diagnosed with urolithiasis after passing a small radiopaque stone. He has no underlying illnesses and has been healthy all his life. On physical examination, he is afebrile and has a blood pressure of 110/70 mm Hg. Laboratory studies show serum Na^+ of 142 mmol/L, K^+ 4.0 mmol/L, Cl^- 96 mmol/L, CO_2 25 mmol/L, glucose 74 mg/dL, creatinine 1.1 mg/dL, calcium 9.1 mg/dL, and phosphorus 2.9 mg/dL. Urinalysis shows a pH of 7, specific gravity of 1.020, and no protein, glucose, ketones, or nitrite. The patient is advised to drink more water. He likes iced tea and consumes large quantities over the course of a hot summer. However, he continues to have urinary tract calculi. Which of the following types of calculi is most likely to be identified?

☐ (A) Uric acid
☐ (B) Magnesium ammonium phosphate
☐ (C) Calcium oxalate
☐ (D) Cystine
☐ (E) Mucoprotein

2 A 47-year-old man has had a decreased urine output over the past 10 days. On physical examination, he is afebrile. Urinalysis shows 1+ proteinuria, 4+ hematuria, urobilinogen, and no glucose or ketones. Microscopic examination of the urine shows few WBCs and some RBCs with RBC casts. A renal biopsy is performed, and the light microscopic appearance of a PAS-stained specimen is shown in the following figure. Which of the following is the most likely clinical course in this patient?

☐ (A) Acute renal failure that is reversible with supportive therapy
☐ (B) Slowly developing renal failure that is unresponsive to corticosteroid treatment
☐ (C) Rapidly progressive renal failure accompanied by hemoptysis
☐ (D) Stable clinical course with intermittent hematuria
☐ (E) Fever, leukocytosis, and endotoxic shock

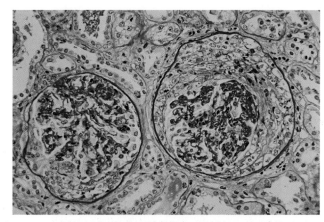

Courtesy of Dr. M.A. Ventkatachalam, Department of Pathology, University of Texas Health Sciences Center, San Antonio, TX.

3 A 3-year-old previously healthy boy has become increasingly lethargic for the past 3 weeks. On physical examination, his temperature is 36.9°C, pulse 80/min, respirations 15/min, and blood pressure 140/90 mm Hg. Periorbital edema is present. Urinalysis shows 4+ proteinuria, and no blood, ketones, or glucose. Which of the following is the best information to give the boy's parents about his disease?

❑ (A) A relative should be found to provide a renal transplant
❑ (B) A course of antibiotic therapy is indicated
❑ (C) Rapid onset of renal failure is likely
❑ (D) Corticosteroid therapy should alleviate this problem
❑ (E) Other family members are at risk for this disease

4 A 58-year-old woman dies from a cerebral infarction. Laboratory findings before death included serum urea nitrogen level of 110 mg/dL and creatinine level of 9.8 mg/dL. At autopsy, the kidneys are small (75 g) and have a coarsely granular surface appearance. Microscopic examination shows sclerotic glomeruli, a fibrotic interstitium, tubular atrophy, arterial thickening, and scattered lymphocytic infiltrates. Which of the following clinical findings was most likely reported on the patient's medical history?

❑ (A) Rash
❑ (B) Hypertension
❑ (C) Hemoptysis
❑ (D) Lens dislocation
❑ (E) Pharyngitis

5 For the past 6 months, a 72-year-old woman has noticed a slowly enlarging mass on the urethra. The mass causes local pain and irritation and is now bleeding. Physical examination shows a 2.5-cm warty, ulcerated mass protruding from the external urethral meatus. There are no lesions of the labia or vagina. A biopsy specimen of the lesion is most likely to identify which of the following?

❑ (A) Embryonal rhabdomyosarcoma
❑ (B) Leiomyoma
❑ (C) Papilloma
❑ (D) Squamous cell carcinoma
❑ (E) Syphilitic chancre

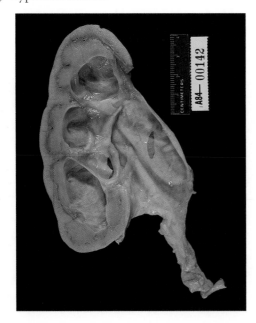

6 A 72-year-old man with Alzheimer disease succumbs to pneumonia. The gross appearance of the right kidney at autopsy is shown in the preceding figure. The left kidney is normal in size, with a smooth cortical surface and a single 0.6-cm fluid-filled cyst. The appearance of the right kidney is most suggestive of renal injury from which of the following?

❑ (A) Ureteral obstruction
❑ (B) Benign nephrosclerosis
❑ (C) Analgesic abuse
❑ (D) Chronic pyelonephritis
❑ (E) Diabetes mellitus

7 A 25-year-old man has a 5-year history of celiac sprue. Several days after a mild upper respiratory infection, he begins passing dark red-brown urine. The dark urine persists for the next 3 days and then becomes clear and yellow, only to become red-brown again 1 month later. There are no remarkable findings on physical examination. Urinalysis shows a pH of 6.5, specific gravity 1.018, 3+ hematuria, 1+ proteinuria, and no glucose or ketones. Microscopic examination of the urine shows RBCs and no WBCs, casts, or crystals. A 24-hour urine protein level is 200 mg. A renal biopsy specimen from the glomeruli of this patient is most likely to show which of the following alterations?

❑ (A) Subepithelial electron-dense deposits
❑ (B) Granular staining of the basement membrane by anti-IgG antibodies
❑ (C) Mesangial IgA staining by immunofluorescence
❑ (D) Diffuse proliferation and basement membrane thickening
❑ (E) Thrombosis in the glomerular capillaries

8 A 7-year-old boy is recovering from impetigo. Physical examination shows a few honey-colored crusts on his face. The crusts are removed, and a culture of the lesions grows group A *Streptococcus pyogenes*. He is treated with a course of antibiotics. One week later, he develops malaise with nausea and a slight fever and passes dark brown urine. Laboratory studies show a serum anti–streptolysin O (ASO) titer of 1 : 1024. Which of the following is the most likely outcome?

❑ (A) Development of rheumatic heart disease
❑ (B) Chronic renal failure
❑ (C) Lower urinary tract infection
❑ (D) Complete recovery without treatment
❑ (E) Progression to crescentic glomerulonephritis

9 A 28-year-old previously healthy man suddenly develops severe abdominal pain and begins passing red-colored urine. There are no abnormalities on physical examination. Urinalysis shows a pH of 7, specific gravity 1.015, 1+ hematuria, and no protein, glucose, or ketones. The patient is given a device to use in straining the urine for calculi. The next day, the patient recovers a 0.3-cm stone that is sent for analysis. The chemical composition is found to be calcium oxalate. Which of the following underlying conditions is most likely to be present?

❑ (A) Gout
❑ (B) Acute cystitis
❑ (C) Diabetes mellitus
❑ (D) Primary hyperparathyroidism
❑ (E) Idiopathic hypercalciuria

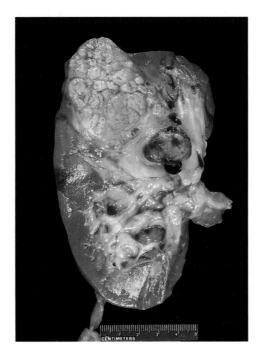

10 A 56-year-old man has had back pain and has passed dark-colored urine for the past month. On physical examination, there is right costovertebral angle tenderness. Urinalysis shows a pH of 6, specific gravity 1.015, 2+ hematuria, and no protein, glucose, or ketones. Microscopic examination of the urine shows numerous RBCs, few WBCs, and no casts or crystals. The representative gross appearance of the renal lesion is shown above. Which of the following laboratory findings is most likely to be reported?

❑ (A) Elevated serum cortisol level
❑ (B) Elevated hematocrit
❑ (C) Ketonuria
❑ (D) Decreased creatinine clearance
❑ (E) Increased plasma renin activity

11 A 15-year-old boy has been passing dark-colored urine for the past month. On physical examination, he has bilateral sensorineural hearing loss and corneal erosions. Urinalysis shows a pH of 6.5, specific gravity 1.015, 1+ hematuria, 1+ proteinuria, and no ketones, glucose, or leukocytes. The serum creatinine level is 2.5 mg/dL, and the urea nitrogen level is 24 mg/dL. A renal biopsy specimen shows tubular epithelial foam cells by light microscopy. By electron microscopy, the glomerular basement membrane shows areas of attenuation, with splitting and lamination of lamina densa in other thickened areas. Which of the following is the most likely diagnosis?

❑ (A) Acute tubular necrosis
❑ (B) Berger disease
❑ (C) Membranous glomerulonephritis
❑ (D) Diabetic nephropathy
❑ (E) Alport syndrome

12 A 32-year-old man has developed a fever and skin rash over the past 3 days. Five days later, he has increasing malaise and visits his physician. On physical examination, the maculopapular erythematous rash on his trunk has nearly faded away. His temperature is 37.1°C and blood pressure is 135/85 mm Hg. Laboratory studies show a serum creatinine level of 2.8 mg/dL and blood urea nitrogen level of 29 mg/dL. Urinalysis shows 2+ proteinuria, 1+ hematuria, and no glucose, ketones, or nitrite. The leukocyte esterase result is positive. Microscopic examination of urine shows RBCs and WBCs, some of which are eosinophils. Which of the following is the most likely cause of this patient's condition?

❑ (A) Urinary tract infection
❑ (B) Congestive heart failure
❑ (C) Antibiotic use
❑ (D) Streptococcal pharyngitis
❑ (E) Poorly cooked ground beef

13 After eating a cheeseburger, French fries, and ice cream for dinner one night, a 6-year-old girl develops nausea, mild abdominal cramping, and a slight fever. Three days later, her parents notice that she is passing dark stools and dark urine and appears fatigued and weak. On physical examination, she has a temperature of 37.9°C, pulse 88/min, respirations 18/min, and blood pressure 140/90 mm Hg. Scattered petechiae are present on the extremities. Laboratory findings show a serum creatinine level of 2.2 mg/dL and urea nitrogen level of 20 mg/dL. Urinalysis shows a pH of 6, specific gravity 1.016, 2+ hematuria, and no protein or glucose. A renal biopsy specimen shows small thrombi within glomerular capillary loops. Which of the following diseases is most likely to produce these findings?

❑ (A) Postinfectious glomerulonephritis
❑ (B) Wegener granulomatosis
❑ (C) Hereditary nephritis
❑ (D) Hemolytic-uremic syndrome
❑ (E) IgA nephropathy

14 The parents of a 6-year-old girl notice that she has become increasingly lethargic over the past 2 weeks. On examination by the physician, she has puffiness around the eyes. Her temperature is 36.9°C and blood pressure is 100/60 mm Hg. Laboratory findings show a serum creatinine level of 0.7 mg/dL and urea nitrogen level of 12 mg/dL. Urinalysis shows a pH of 6.5, specific gravity 1.011, 4+ proteinuria, and no blood or glucose. The 24-hour urine protein level is 3.8 g. The child's condition improves after a course of glucocorticoid therapy. Which of the following findings by electron microscopy is most likely to characterize this disease process?

❑ (A) Subepithelial electron-dense humps
❑ (B) Reduplication of glomerular basement membrane
❑ (C) Areas of thickened and thinned basement membrane
❑ (D) Increased mesangial matrix
❑ (E) Effacement of podocyte foot processes

15 A 25-year-old woman experiences sudden onset of fever, malaise, and nausea. On physical examination, her temperature is 38.2°C, pulse 85/min, respirations 18/min, and blood pressure 140/90 mm Hg. A routine urinalysis shows 1+ proteinuria, 4+ hematuria, and no ketones or glucose. RBC casts are seen on microscopic examination of the urine. A renal biopsy is performed, and light microscopic examination shows marked glomerular hypercellularity with neutrophils in glomerular capillary loops. Immunofluorescence microscopy shows granular deposition of IgG and C3 in glomerular capillary basement membranes. Electron microscopy shows electron-dense subepithelial "humps." Which of the following is the most likely diagnosis?

- ❑ (A) Goodpasture syndrome
- ❑ (B) Systemic amyloidosis
- ❑ (C) Membranous glomerulonephritis
- ❑ (D) Diabetes mellitus
- ❑ (E) Postinfectious glomerulonephritis

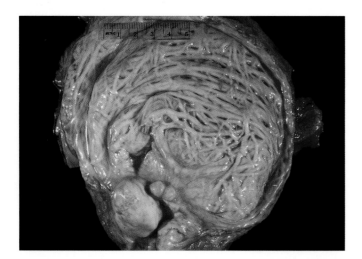

16 A 77-year-old man has had increasing difficulties with urination for the past 2 years. He has difficulty starting and stopping the urine stream. On physical examination, his temperature is 37.0°C and blood pressure is 130/85 mm Hg. The representative gross appearance of the bladder is shown. Which of the following laboratory findings is most likely to be reported in this patient?

- ❑ (A) Positive ANA test result
- ❑ (B) Urine culture positive for *Mycobacterium tuberculosis*
- ❑ (C) Hemoglobin concentration 22.5 g/dL
- ❑ (D) *Schistosoma haematobium* eggs in urine
- ❑ (E) Prostate-specific antigen level of 5 ng/mL

17 A 50-year-old woman sees her physician because she has had flank pain for the past 2 days. Physical examination shows bilateral costovertebral angle tenderness. Urinalysis shows a pH of 7, specific gravity 1.010, 2+ hematuria, and no protein, glucose, or ketones. An abdominal ultrasound scan shows bilaterally enlarged kidneys that have been replaced completely by 0.5- to 3-cm cysts. Which of the following complications is most likely to develop in this patient?

- ❑ (A) Hypertension
- ❑ (B) Renal cell carcinoma
- ❑ (C) Nephrotic syndrome
- ❑ (D) Microangiopathic hemolytic anemia
- ❑ (E) Renal infarction
- ❑ (F) Urothelial carcinoma
- ❑ (G) Cushing syndrome

18 A 26-year-old man is involved in a motor vehicle accident and sustains acute blood loss. He is hypotensive for several hours before paramedical personnel arrive. They stabilize the bleeding and transport him to a hospital, where he receives a transfusion of 3 units of packed RBCs. Over the next week, the serum urea nitrogen level increases to 48 mg/dL, the serum creatinine level increases to 5 mg/dL, and the urine output decreases. He undergoes hemodialysis for the next 2 weeks and then develops marked polyuria, with urine output of 2 to 3 L per day. His recovery is complicated by bronchopneumonia, but renal function gradually returns to normal. The patient's transient renal disease is best characterized by which of the following histologic features?

- ❑ (A) Glomerular crescents in Bowman's space
- ❑ (B) Interstitial lymphocytic infiltrates
- ❑ (C) Arteriolar fibrinoid necrosis
- ❑ (D) Nodular glomerulosclerosis
- ❑ (E) Rupture of the tubular basement membrane

19 A 60-year-old previously healthy man sees his physician because he feels feverish and weak. He reports passing dark-colored urine on several occasions during the past month but has no urinary frequency, dysuria, or nocturia. On physical examination, his temperature is 37.8°C and blood pressure is 125/85 mm Hg. A dipstick urinalysis shows 4+ hematuria, 1+ proteinuria, and no glucose or ketones. Which of the following procedures is the most appropriate in management of this patient?

- ❑ (A) Straining of urine for calculi
- ❑ (B) Urine microbiologic culture
- ❑ (C) Abdominal CT scan for renal mass
- ❑ (D) Collection of a 24-hour urine specimen for protein
- ❑ (E) Percutaneous renal biopsy

20 A 40-year-old man has experienced increasing lower extremity edema for the past 3 weeks. On physical examination, he is afebrile and has a blood pressure of 135/90 mm Hg and pitting edema to the knees. Laboratory findings show a serum creatinine level of 1.2 mg/dL and urea nitrogen level of 16 mg/dL. The 24-hour urine protein level is 7 g. Urinalysis shows 4+ protein but no blood or glucose. Serologic test results for ANA, anti–streptolysin O (ASO), HIV, and ANCA are all negative. Serum complement levels are normal. A renal biopsy is performed; light microscopy shows normal-appearing glomeruli except for diffuse, uniform thickening of the glomerular capillary basement membranes. Immunofluorescence shows granular peripheral staining of the basement membrane for IgG and C3. Given the clinical and histopathologic findings, electron microscopy of the biopsy specimen is most likely to show which of the following findings?

❏ (A) Subepithelial electron-dense deposits
❏ (B) Subendothelial electron-dense deposits with duplication of the basement membrane
❏ (C) Mesangial electron-dense deposits only
❏ (D) No deposits but marked podocyte foot process fusion
❏ (E) No abnormality

21 A 50-year-old woman has had fever and flank pain for the past 2 days. On physical examination, her temperature is 38.2°C, pulse 81/min, respirations 16/min, and blood pressure 130/80 mm Hg. Urinalysis shows no protein, glucose, or ketones. The leukocyte esterase test is positive. Microscopic examination of the urine shows numerous polymorphonuclear leukocytes and occasional WBC casts. Which of the following organisms is most likely to be found in the urine culture?

❏ (A) *Mycobacterium tuberculosis*
❏ (B) *Mycoplasma hominis*
❏ (C) *Escherichia coli*
❏ (D) Group A streptococcus
❏ (E) *Cryptococcus neoformans*

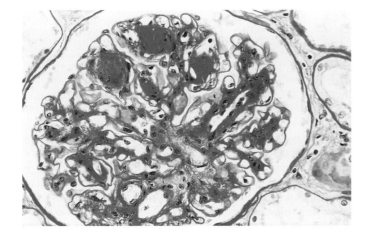

22 A 58-year-old man who is relatively healthy sees his physician for a routine health maintenance examination. Physical examination shows mild hypertension. Laboratory findings show a serum creatinine level of 2.2 mg/dL and urea nitrogen level of 25 mg/dL. Microalbuminuria is present, with excretion of 250 mg/day of albumin. Two years later, he returns for a followup visit. He is now hypertensive and has a serum creatinine level of 3.8 mg/dL, urea nitrogen level of 38 mg/dL, and 24-hour urine protein level of 2.8 g. A renal biopsy is performed, and the light microscopic appearance of a PAS-stained specimen is shown above. Which of the following laboratory findings is most likely to be abnormal in this patient?

❏ (A) Anti–glomerular basement membrane antibody
❏ (B) ANA
❏ (C) ANCA
❏ (D) Anti–streptolysin O (ASO)
❏ (E) C3 nephritic factor
❏ (F) Hemoglobin A₁c
❏ (G) Hepatitis B surface antigen

23 A 20-year-old woman, G 1, P 0, who is in the third trimester, has felt minimal fetal movement. An ultrasound scan shows a markedly decreased amniotic fluid index char-

acteristic of oligohydramnios. She gives birth to a stillborn male fetus at 33 weeks' gestation. At autopsy, there are deformations resulting from marked oligohydramnios, including flattening of the facies, varus deformities of the feet, and marked pulmonary hypoplasia. Microscopic examination of the liver shows multiple epithelium-lined cysts and a proliferation of bile ducts. Which of the following best describes the appearance of the kidneys in this fetus?

❏ (A) Bilaterally enlarged kidneys replaced by 1- to 4-cm fluid-filled cysts
❏ (B) Bilaterally shrunken kidneys with uniformly finely granular cortical surfaces
❏ (C) Decreased overall size of the right kidney and a normal-sized left kidney
❏ (D) Irregular cortical scars in asymmetrically shrunken kidneys with marked calyceal dilation
❏ (E) Marked bilateral renal pelvic and calyceal dilation with thinning of the cortices
❏ (F) Normal-sized kidneys with smooth cortical surfaces
❏ (G) Symmetrically enlarged kidneys composed of small, radially arranged cysts

24 A 65-year-old woman has experienced increasing malaise with nocturia and polyuria for the past year. On physical examination, her blood pressure is 170/95 mm Hg. Urinalysis shows a pH of 7.5, specific gravity 1.010, 1+ proteinuria, and no glucose, blood, or ketones. The tests for leukocyte esterase and nitrite yield positive results, and levels of serum urea nitrogen and serum creatinine are both elevated. Her clinical course is characterized by worsening renal failure, and she dies of bronchopneumonia. At autopsy, the kidneys are shrunken but unequal in size and have deep, irregular surface scars. On sectioning, the calyces underlying the cortical scars are blunted and deformed. Which of the following is the most likely cause of renal failure in this patient?

❏ (A) Chronic glomerulonephritis
❏ (B) Essential hypertension
❏ (C) Reflux nephropathy
❏ (D) Autosomal dominant polycystic kidney disease
❏ (E) Systemic lupus erythematosus

25 A 29-year-old woman sees her physician because she has had a fever and sore throat for the past 3 days. On physical examination, her temperature is 38.0°C. The pharynx is erythematous, with yellowish tonsillar exudate. Group A *Streptococcus pyogenes* is cultured. She is treated with ampicillin and recovers fully in 7 days. Two weeks later, she develops fever and a rash and notices a slight decrease in urinary output. Her temperature is 37.7°C, and there is a diffuse erythematous rash on the trunk and extremities. Urinalysis shows a pH of 6, specific gravity 1.022, 1+ proteinuria, 1+ hematuria, and no glucose or ketones. Microscopic examination of the urine shows RBCs and WBCs, including eosinophils, but no casts or crystals. Which of the following is the most likely cause of her disease?

❏ (A) Deposition of immune complexes with streptococcal antigens
❏ (B) Hematogenous dissemination of septic emboli
❏ (C) Renal tubular cell necrosis caused by bacterial toxins
❏ (D) Hypersensitivity reaction to ampicillin
❏ (E) Formation of antibodies against glomerular basement membrane

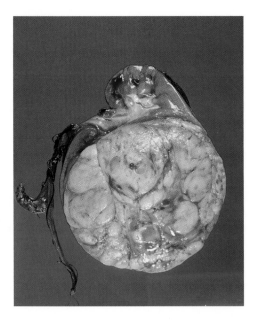

26 A 4-year-old girl has complained of abdominal pain for the past month. On physical examination, she is febrile, and palpation of the abdomen shows a tender mass on the right. Bowel sounds are present. Laboratory studies show hematuria without proteinuria. An abdominal CT scan shows a 12-cm circumscribed, solid mass in the right kidney. A right nephrectomy is performed, and the gross appearance of the mass is shown above. Which of the following is the most likely diagnosis?

❏ (A) Angiomyolipoma
❏ (B) Interstitial cell tumor
❏ (C) Renal cell carcinoma
❏ (D) Transitional cell carcinoma
❏ (E) Wilms tumor

27 One week after a mild flulike illness, a 9-year-old boy has an episode of hematuria that subsides within 2 days. One month later, he tells his parents that his urine is red again. On physical examination, there are no significant findings. Urinalysis shows a pH of 7, specific gravity 1.015, 1+ proteinuria, 1+ hematuria, and no ketones, glucose, or urobilinogen. The serum urea nitrogen level is 36 mg/dL, and the creatinine level is 3.2 mg/dL. A renal biopsy specimen shows diffuse mesangial proliferation and electron-dense deposits in the mesangium. Which of the following mechanisms is most likely to produce these findings?

❏ (A) Deposition of immune complexes containing IgA
❏ (B) Formation of antibodies against type IV collagen
❏ (C) Virus-mediated injury to the glomeruli
❏ (D) Cytokine-mediated injury to the glomerular capillaries
❏ (E) Congenital defects in the structure of glomerular basement membranes

28 A 35-year-old man is awakened at night because of severe lower abdominal pain that radiates to the groin. The pain is very intense and comes in waves. The next morning, he notices blood in his urine. On examination, there are no remarkable findings. Which of the following is the most likely diagnosis?

❏ (A) Acute cystitis
❏ (B) Renal cell carcinoma
❏ (C) Ureteral lithiasis
❏ (D) Hydronephrosis
❏ (E) Autosomal dominant polycystic kidney disease

29 A 7-year-old boy is brought to the physician by his mother, who is concerned because he has become less active over the past 10 days. On physical examination, the boy has facial puffiness. Urinalysis shows no blood, glucose, or ketones, and microscopic examination shows no casts or crystals. The serum creatinine level is normal. A 24-hour urine collection yields 3.8 g of protein. He improves after a course of corticosteroid therapy. He has two more episodes of proteinuria over the next few years, both of which respond to corticosteroid therapy. A renal biopsy is performed. Which of the following is the most likely mechanism causing his disease?

❏ (A) Immune complex-mediated glomerular injury
❏ (B) Verocytotoxin-induced endothelial cell injury
❏ (C) Cytotoxic T cell-mediated tubular epithelial cell injury
❏ (D) Cytokine-mediated visceral epithelial cell injury
❏ (E) IgA-mediated mesangial cell injury

30 A 49-year-old man saw his physician because he had increased swelling in the extremities for 2 months. Physical examination showed generalized edema. A 24-hour urine collection yielded 4.1 g of protein as well as albumin and globulins. Extensive testing did not indicate the presence of a systemic disease, such as diabetes mellitus or systemic lupus erythematosus. He did not respond to a course of corticosteroid therapy. A renal biopsy was performed, and microscopic examination showed diffuse thickening of the basement membrane. Immunofluorescence staining with antibody to the C3 component of complement was positive in a granular pattern in the glomerular capillary loops. Two years later, he experiences increasing malaise. Laboratory studies now show serum creatinine level of 4.5 mg/dL and urea nitrogen level of 44 mg/dL. Which of the following immunologic mechanisms was most likely responsible for the glomerular changes observed in the biopsy specimen?

❏ (A) Antibodies that react with basement membrane collagen
❏ (B) Antibodies against streptococci that cross-react with the basement membrane
❏ (C) Release of cytokines by inflammatory cells
❏ (D) Cytotoxic T cells directed against renal antigens
❏ (E) Deposition of immune complexes on the basement membrane

31 A 31-year-old woman experiences a bout of abdominal pain and sees her physician 1 week later after noticing blood in her urine. She has had three episodes of urinary tract infection during the past year. There are no remarkable findings on physical examination. Urinalysis shows 2+ hematuria, 1+ proteinuria, hypercalciuria, and no glucose or ketones. Microscopic examination of the urine shows numerous RBCs and oxalate crystals. An intravenous pyelogram shows linear striations radiating into the renal papillae, along with small cystic collections of contrast in dilated collecting ducts. She is advised to increase her daily intake of fluids, and her condition improves. Which of the following conditions is most likely to be associated with these findings?

- ❏ (A) Autosomal dominant polycystic kidney disease
- ❏ (B) Gout
- ❏ (C) Medullary sponge kidney
- ❏ (D) Multicystic renal dysplasia
- ❏ (E) Autosomal recessive polycystic kidney disease
- ❏ (F) Urothelial carcinoma
- ❏ (G) Vesicoureteral reflux

32 A 42-year-old man has had right flank pain for the past 2 days. On physical examination, his temperature is 37.4°C, pulse 70/min, respirations 14/min, and blood pressure 130/85 mm Hg. Laboratory studies show a serum creatinine level of 1.1 mg/dl. Urinalysis shows no blood, protein, or glucose, and microscopic examination of the urine shows no WBCs or RBCs. An abdominal CT scan shows a 7-cm eccentric lesion of the upper pole of the right kidney. The lesion is well-circumscribed and cystic with a thin wall and focal hemorrhage. Which of the following is the most likely diagnosis?

- ❏ (A) Acute pyelonephritis
- ❏ (B) Acute tubular necrosis
- ❏ (C) Diabetic nephropathy
- ❏ (D) Hydronephrosis
- ❏ (E) Simple renal cyst
- ❏ (F) Rapidly progressive glomerulonephritis
- ❏ (G) Renal cell carcinoma
- ❏ (H) Urothelial carcinoma

33 A 51-year-old woman has had recurrent urinary tract infections for the past 15 years. On many of these occasions, *Proteus mirabilis* was cultured from her urine. For the past 4 days, she has had a burning pain on urination and urinary frequency. On physical examination, her temperature is 37.9°C, pulse 70/min, respirations 15/min, and blood pressure 135/85 mm Hg. There is marked tenderness on deep pressure over the right costovertebral angle and on deep abdominal palpation. Urinalysis shows a pH of 7.5, specific gravity 1.020, 1+ hematuria, and no protein, glucose, or ketones. Microscopic examination of the urine shows many RBCs, WBCs, and triple-phosphate crystals. Which of the following renal lesions is most likely to be present?

- ❏ (A) Renal cell carcinoma
- ❏ (B) Acute tubular necrosis
- ❏ (C) Malignant nephrosclerosis
- ❏ (D) Staghorn calculus
- ❏ (E) Papillary necrosis

34 A 53-year-old woman has had dysuria and frequency of urination for the past week. On physical examination, her temperature is 38.0°C, and she has pain on palpation over the left costovertebral angle. Laboratory findings show glucose of 177 mg/dL, hemoglobin A_{1c} 9.8%, hemoglobin 13.1 g/dL, platelet count 232,200/mm³, and WBC count 11,320/mm³.

Urinalysis shows a pH of 6.5, specific gravity 1.016, 2+ glucosuria, and no blood, protein, or ketones. Microscopic examination of the urine shows numerous neutrophils, and a urine culture is positive for *Escherichia coli*. Which of the following complications is most likely to develop in this patient?

- ❏ (A) Acute tubular necrosis
- ❏ (B) Necrotizing papillitis
- ❏ (C) Crescentic glomerulonephritis
- ❏ (D) Hydronephrosis
- ❏ (E) Renal calculi

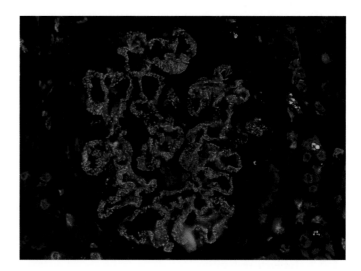

35 A 42-year-old man has experienced increasing malaise for the past month. He is bothered by increasing swelling in both hands and legs. On physical examination, there is generalized edema. He is afebrile, and his blood pressure is 140/90 mm Hg. Urinalysis shows a pH of 6.5, specific gravity 1.017, 4+ proteinuria, and no blood, glucose, or ketones. Microscopic examination of the urine shows no casts or RBCs and 2 WBCs per high-power field. The 24-hour urine protein level is 4.2 g. A renal biopsy specimen is obtained, and immunofluorescence staining with antibody to the C3 component of complement produces the pattern shown above. Which of the following underlying disease processes is most likely to be present?

- ❏ (A) Chronic hepatitis B
- ❏ (B) AIDS
- ❏ (C) Multiple myeloma
- ❏ (D) Recurrent urinary tract infection
- ❏ (E) Nephrolithiasis

36 A 58-year-old man is in stable condition after an acute myocardial infarction. Two days later, his urine output decreases, and the serum urea nitrogen level increases to 3.3 mg/dL. Oliguria persists for 5 days, followed by polyuria for 2 days. He is then discharged from the hospital. Which of the following renal lesions best explains these renal abnormalities?

- ❏ (A) Acute tubular necrosis
- ❏ (B) Benign nephrosclerosis
- ❏ (C) Acute renal infarction
- ❏ (D) Hemolytic-uremic syndrome
- ❏ (E) Rapidly progressive glomerulonephritis

37 Several members of a family developed chronic renal failure by the age of 50 years. Most are males. The affected persons also developed visual problems. Some younger family members have proteinuria and hematuria on urinalysis. A renal biopsy specimen from a 20-year-old man shows prominent tubular foam cells and glomerular basement membrane thickening and thinning. Family members with this disease are most likely to have which of the following additional manifestations?

- ❑ (A) Watery diarrhea
- ❑ (B) Nerve deafness
- ❑ (C) Presenile dementia
- ❑ (D) Dilated cardiomyopathy
- ❑ (E) Infertility

38 A 65-year-old man recently retired after many years in a job that involved exposure to aniline dyes, including β-naphthylamine. One month ago, he had an episode of hematuria that was not accompanied by abdominal pain. On physical examination, there are no abnormal findings. Urinalysis shows 4+ hematuria and no ketones, glucose, or protein. Microscopic examination of the urine shows RBCs that are too numerous to count, 5 to 10 WBCs per high-power field, and no crystals or casts. The result of a urine culture is negative. Which of the following is the most likely diagnosis?

- ❑ (A) Renal cell carcinoma
- ❑ (B) Hemorrhagic cystitis
- ❑ (C) Tubercular cystitis
- ❑ (D) Urothelial carcinoma
- ❑ (E) Squamous cell carcinoma of the urethra

39 A 55-year-old woman has had poorly controlled hyperglycemia for many years. She sees her physician after experiencing burning pain on urination for 3 days. Physical examination shows a 2-cm ulceration on the skin of the heel and reduced sensation in the lower extremities. Her visual acuity is 20/100 bilaterally. Urinalysis shows 1+ proteinuria, 2+ glucosuria, and no blood, ketones, or urobilinogen. A urine culture contains more than 100,000 colony-forming units/mL of *Klebsiella pneumoniae*. Which of the following pathologic findings is most likely to be present in both kidneys?

- ❑ (A) Deposits of IgG and C3 in the glomerular basement membrane
- ❑ (B) Effacement of podocyte foot processes
- ❑ (C) Glomerular crescents
- ❑ (D) Mesangial deposits of IgA
- ❑ (E) Necrotizing granulomatous vasculitis
- ❑ (F) Nodular hyaline mesangial masses
- ❑ (G) Thickening and thinning of the glomerular basement membrane

40 A 17-year-old girl has had arthralgias and myalgias for several months. During the past week, she has noticed a decreased output of urine, which is reddish-brown. On physical examination, her blood pressure is 160/100 mm Hg, and she has an erythematous malar skin rash. The ANA and anti–double-stranded DNA test results are both positive. The serum urea nitrogen level is 52 mg/dL. Which of the following urinalysis findings is most likely to be reported for this patient?

- ❑ (A) Eosinophils
- ❑ (B) Glucose
- ❑ (C) Ketones
- ❑ (D) Myoglobin
- ❑ (E) Oval fat bodies
- ❑ (F) RBC casts
- ❑ (G) Triple phosphate crystals
- ❑ (H) Uric acid crystals
- ❑ (I) Waxy casts

41 A 28-year-old woman has had dysuria, frequency, and urgency for the past 2 days. On physical examination, her temperature is 37.6°C. A urine culture grows > 100,000 colonies/mL of *Escherichia coli*. She is treated with antibiotic therapy. If the problem continues to recur, the patient is likely to be at greatest risk for development of which of the following renal diseases?

- ❑ (A) Diffuse glomerulosclerosis
- ❑ (B) Chronic glomerulonephritis
- ❑ (C) Amyloidosis
- ❑ (D) Membranous glomerulonephritis
- ❑ (E) Chronic pyelonephritis

42 A sexually active 26-year-old man has had pain on urination for the past 4 days. On physical examination, there are no lesions on the penis. He is afebrile. Urinalysis shows no blood, ketones, protein, or glucose. Microscopic examination of the urine shows few WBCs and no casts or crystals. Which of the following infectious agents is most likely to produce these findings?

- ❑ (A) *Chlamydia trachomatis*
- ❑ (B) *Mycobacterium tuberculosis*
- ❑ (C) Herpes simplex virus
- ❑ (D) *Candida albicans*
- ❑ (E) *Treponema pallidum*

43 A 61-year-old woman sees the physician because she has experienced increasing malaise for the past 5 years. On physical examination, there are no abnormalities other than a blood pressure of 150/95 mm Hg. One week later, she dies suddenly and unexpectedly. At autopsy, both kidneys have the external (left panel) and bisected (right panel) appearance, as shown in the figure on page 271. Which of the following conditions was the most probable cause of death?

- ❑ (A) Metastatic Wilms tumor
- ❑ (B) Ruptured berry aneurysm
- ❑ (C) Acute tubular necrosis
- ❑ (D) Disseminated intravascular coagulation
- ❑ (E) Pneumothorax

44 For the past 20 years, a 69-year-old man with chronic arthritis has taken more than 3 g of analgesics per day, including phenacetin, aspirin, and acetaminophen. He sees his physician because of increasing malaise, nausea, and diminished mentation. On physical examination, his blood pressure is 156/92 mm Hg. Laboratory findings show a serum urea nitrogen level of 68 mg/dL and a creatinine level of 7.1 mg/dL. CBC shows hemoglobin of 11.7 g/dL, hematocrit 35.1%, platelet count 188,500/mm³, and WBC count 5385/mm³. Which of the following renal diseases is this patient most likely to develop?

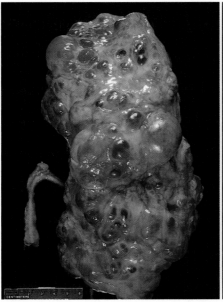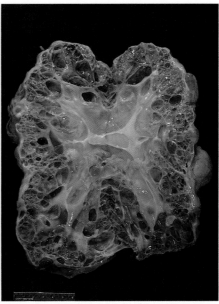

❏ (A) Hydronephrosis
❏ (B) Chronic glomerulonephritis
❏ (C) Renal papillary necrosis
❏ (D) Renal cell carcinoma
❏ (E) Acute tubular necrosis

45 A 58-year-old woman sees her physician for a routine health maintenance examination. The only abnormality on physical examination is a blood pressure of 168/109 mm Hg. Urinalysis shows a pH of 7.0, specific gravity 1.020, 1+ proteinuria, and no blood, glucose, or ketones. An abdominal ultrasound scan shows bilaterally and symmetrically small kidneys with no masses. The ANA test result is negative, the serum urea nitrogen level is 51 mg/dL, and the creatinine level is 4.7 mg/dL. The hemoglobin A_{1c} concentration is within the reference range. Which of the following is the most likely diagnosis?

❏ (A) Lupus nephritis
❏ (B) Autosomal dominant polycystic kidney disease
❏ (C) Chronic glomerulonephritis
❏ (D) Nodular glomerulosclerosis
❏ (E) Amyloidosis

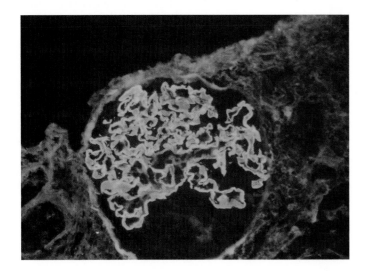

46 A previously healthy 21-year-old man sees his physician because he notices blood in his urine. He reports no dysuria, frequency, or hesitancy of urination. On physical examination, there are no abnormal findings. Laboratory findings show a serum urea nitrogen level of 39 mg/dL and creatinine level of 4.1 mg/dL. A renal biopsy specimen is obtained, and the immunofluorescence pattern of staining with antibody against human IgG is shown in the figure at the bottom of the page. Which of the following serum laboratory studies is most likely to be positive in this patient?

❏ (A) Anti–streptolysin O (ASO) antibody
❏ (B) HIV antibody
❏ (C) Anti–glomerular basement membrane antibody
❏ (D) Hepatitis B surface antibody
❏ (E) C3 nephritic factor

47 A 33-year-old woman has had fever and increasing fatigue for the past 2 months. Over the past year, she has noticed soreness of her muscles and joints and has had a 4-kg weight loss. On physical examination, her temperature is 37.5°C, pulse 80/min, respirations 15/min, and blood pressure 145/95 mm Hg. She has pain on deep inspiration, and a friction rub is heard on auscultation of the chest. Laboratory findings show glucose of 73 mg/dL, total cholesterol 160 mg/dL, total protein 5.2 g/dL, albumin 2.9 g/dL, total bilirubin 0.9 mg/dL, and creatinine 2.4 mg/dL. Serum complement levels are decreased. CBC shows hemoglobin of 9.7 g/dL, platelet count 85,000/mm³, and WBC count 3560/mm³. A renal biopsy specimen shows a diffuse proliferative glomerulonephritis with extensive granular immune deposits of IgG and C1q in capillary loops and mesangium. After being treated with immunosuppressive therapy consisting of prednisone and cyclophosphamide, her condition improves. Which of the following serologic studies is most likely to be positive in this patient?

❏ (A) Anticentromere antibody
❏ (B) Anti–double-stranded DNA antibody
❏ (C) Anti-DNA topoisomerase I antibody
❏ (D) Anti–glomerular basement membrane antibody
❏ (E) Antihistone antibody
❏ (F) ANCA
❏ (G) Antiribonucleoprotein

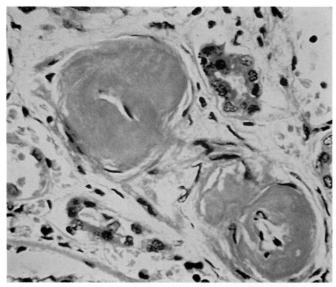

Courtesy of Dr. M.A. Ventkatachalam, Department of Pathology, University of Texas Health Sciences Center, San Antonio, TX.

48 A 66-year-old woman died of an acute myocardial infarction. At autopsy, both kidneys were decreased in size (about 120 g each) with a finely granular cortical surface. The representative appearance of the kidney under high magnification is shown above. Which of the following clinical abnormalities most likely accompanied this lesion?

- ❑ (A) Oliguria
- ❑ (B) Benign hypertension
- ❑ (C) Malignant hypertension
- ❑ (D) Hematuria
- ❑ (E) Flank pain

49 A 79-year-old man has had increasing back pain and fatigue for the past 6 months. On physical examination, there are no remarkable findings. Laboratory studies include a CBC with hemoglobin of 9.6 g/dL, platelet count 241,600/mm³, and WBC count 7160/mm³. The serum total protein is 9.8 g/dL, albumin 3.6 g/dL, glucose 72 mg/dL, creatinine 3.3 mg/dL, and urea nitrogen 30 mg/dL. A dipstick urinalysis shows a pH of 7, specific gravity 1.011, and no blood, protein, or glucose. One month later, he develops a cough with fever, and *Streptococcus pneumoniae* is cultured from his sputum. Despite antibiotic therapy, he develops sepsis and dies. At autopsy, the kidneys are normal in size, but microscopic examination shows dilated tubules filled with amorphous blue to pink casts and occasional multinucleated giant cells. Which of the following is the most likely underlying cause of this patient's death?

- ❑ (A) Cystinuria
- ❑ (B) Diabetes mellitus
- ❑ (C) Gout
- ❑ (D) Multiple myeloma
- ❑ (E) Parathyroid adenoma
- ❑ (F) Systemic lupus erythematosus

50 A 30-year-old woman with a history of recurrent urinary tract infections has had a high fever for the past 3 days. On physical examination, her temperature is 38.4°C. There is marked abdominal tenderness on deep palpation. A renal sonogram shows an enlarged right kidney with pelvic and calyceal enlargement and cortical thinning; the left kidney appears normal. A right nephrectomy is performed, and microscopic examination shows inflammatory infiltrates extending from the medulla to the cortex, with tubular destruction and extensive interstitial fibrosis. Lymphocytes, plasma cells, and neutrophils are abundant. Which of the following is most likely to produce these findings?

- ❑ (A) Benign nephrosclerosis
- ❑ (B) Vesicoureteral reflux
- ❑ (C) Lupus nephritis
- ❑ (D) Systemic amyloidosis
- ❑ (E) Congestive heart failure
- ❑ (F) Autosomal dominant polycystic kidney disease

51 A 32-year-old man with a history of intravenous drug use comes to the emergency department because he has had a high fever for the past 2 days. On physical examination, his temperature is 38.4°C. He has a palpable spleen tip, bilateral costovertebral angle tenderness, and diastolic cardiac murmur. Laboratory findings show a serum urea nitrogen level of 15 mg/dL. Urinalysis shows 2+ hematuria, and no glucose, protein, or ketones. A blood culture is positive for *Staphylococcus aureus*. Which of the following best describes the kidneys in this patient?

- ❑ (A) Bilaterally enlarged kidneys replaced by 1- to 4-cm fluid-filled cysts
- ❑ (B) Bilaterally shrunken kidneys with uniformly finely granular cortical surfaces
- ❑ (C) Irregular cortical scars in asymmetrically shrunken kidneys with marked calyceal dilation
- ❑ (D) Marked bilateral renal pelvic and calyceal dilation with thinning of the cortices
- ❑ (E) Normal-sized kidneys with smooth cortical surfaces
- ❑ (F) Scattered petechial hemorrhages in slightly swollen kidneys
- ❑ (G) Wedge-shaped regions of yellow-white cortical necrosis involving both kidneys

52 Three years ago, a 47-year-old woman had a mastectomy of the right breast to remove an infiltrating ductal carcinoma. She now has bone pain, and a radionuclide scan shows multiple areas of increased uptake in the vertebrae, ribs, pelvis, and right femur. Urinalysis shows a specific gravity of 1.010, which remains unchanged after water deprivation for 12 hours. She undergoes several courses of chemotherapy over the next year. During this time, the serum urea nitrogen level progressively increases. Which of the following abnormal laboratory findings is most likely to be reported for this patient?

- ❑ (A) Hepatitis B surface antigenemia
- ❑ (B) Hypercalcemia
- ❑ (C) Hypercholesterolemia
- ❑ (D) Hypergammaglobulinemia
- ❑ (E) Hyperglycemia
- ❑ (F) Hyperuricemia

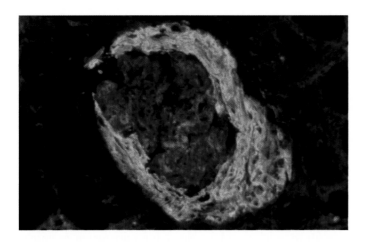

53 A 45-year-old man has experienced increasing malaise, nausea, and reduced urine output for the past 3 days. On physical examination, he is afebrile and normotensive. Laboratory findings show a serum creatinine level of 2.5 mg/dL. Urinalysis shows hematuria but no pyuria or glucosuria. A renal biopsy is performed and the immunofluorescence pattern with anti-fibrinogen is shown. Which of the following additional studies is most useful for classification and treatment of this disease?

- (A) ANA titer
- (B) Antiglomular basement membrane antibody test
- (C) HIV titer
- (D) Quantitative serum immunoglobulins
- (E) Rheumatoid factor
- (F) Urine immunoelectrophoresis

54 A 28-year-old man is diagnosed with acute myelogenous leukemia (M2). After induction with a multiagent chemotherapy protocol, he has an episode of lower abdominal pain accompanied by passage of red-colored urine. He has no fever, dysuria, or urinary frequency. On physical examination, there are no remarkable findings. Urinalysis shows a pH of 5.5, specific gravity 1.021, 2+ hematuria, and no protein, ketones, or glucose. There are no remarkable findings on an abdominal radiograph. Which of the following additional urinalysis findings is most likely to be reported for this patient?

- (A) Bence-Jones protein
- (B) Eosinophils
- (C) Myoglobin
- (D) Oval fat bodies
- (E) RBC casts
- (F) Triple phosphate crystals
- (G) Uric acid crystals
- (H) Waxy casts
- (I) WBC casts

55 A 44-year-old man has developed a fever, nonproductive cough, and decreased urine output over the past 3 days. On physical examination, his temperature is 37.7°C and blood pressure is 145/95 mm Hg. He has sinusitis. On auscultation, crackles are heard over all lung fields. A chest radiograph shows bilateral patchy infiltrates and nodules. The serum creatinine level is 4.1 mg/dL, and the urea nitrogen level is

43 mg/dL. The results of serologic testing are negative for ANA but positive for C-ANCA. A renal biopsy specimen shows glomerular crescents and granulomatous vasculitis. The result of immunofluorescence staining with anti-IgG and anti-C3 antibodies is negative. Which of the following is the most likely diagnosis?

- (A) Focal segmental glomerulosclerosis
- (B) Goodpasture syndrome
- (C) Lupus nephritis
- (D) Membranoproliferative glomerulonephritis type II
- (E) Membranous glomerulonephritis
- (F) Postinfectious glomerulonephritis
- (G) Wegener granulomatosis

56 A 65-year-old woman has recently experienced several transient ischemic attacks. On physical examination, the only abnormal finding is a blood pressure of 150/95 mm Hg. Urinalysis shows 1+ proteinuria and no glucose, blood, or ketones. Microscopic examination of the urine shows no RBCs or WBCs and few oxalate crystals. On abdominal ultrasound, the kidneys are slightly decreased in size. Which of the following renal lesions is most likely to be present in this patient?

- (A) Crescentic glomerulonephritis
- (B) Hyaline arteriolosclerosis
- (C) Mesangial cell proliferation
- (D) Arteriolar fibrinoid necrosis
- (E) Acute tubular necrosis
- (F) Interstitial nephritis

57 Over the past 72 hours, a 44-year-old man has experienced worsening headache, nausea, and vomiting. On physical examination, his blood pressure is 276/158 mm Hg, and there is bilateral papilledema. Urinalysis shows 2+ proteinuria, 1+ hematuria, and no glucose or ketones. Which of the following renal lesions is most likely to be present in this patient?

- (A) Papillary necrosis
- (B) Acute infarction
- (C) Necrotizing arteriolitis
- (D) Acute tubular necrosis
- (E) Acute pyelonephritis

58 A 35-year-old previously healthy man is found dead in his home. At autopsy, the medical examiner notices bilaterally enlarged kidneys that contain multiple, irregularly arranged cysts of different shapes and sizes. There is a 0.5-cm nonruptured intracerebral berry aneurysm of the anterior communicating artery. There are scattered 1- to 2-cm fluid-filled, liver cysts involving 10% of the parenchymal volume. Postmortem laboratory testing of the urine and blood shows markedly elevated levels of cocaine and its metabolite, benzoylecgonine. Which of the following is the most appropriate conclusion to be drawn from these findings?

- (A) He had lesions related to chronic use of cocaine
- (B) He had autosomal recessive polycystic kidney disease but survived to adulthood
- (C) His surviving family (children, siblings, and parents) should be evaluated for a similar condition
- (D) The immediate cause of death is berry aneurysm
- (E) The underlying cause of death is autosomal dominant polycystic kidney disease

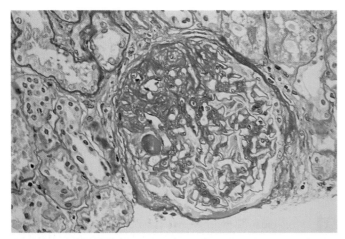

Courtesy of Dr. Helmut Rennke, Department of Pathology, Brigham and Women's Hospital, Boston, MA.

59 A 12-year-old girl has experienced increasing malaise for the past 2 weeks. There is periorbital edema on physical examination. The child is afebrile. Laboratory findings show proteinuria on dipstick urinalysis but no hematuria or glucosuria. Microscopic examination of the urine shows numerous oval fat bodies. The serum creatinine level is 2.3 mg/dL. She receives a course of corticosteroid therapy but does not improve. A renal biopsy is performed, and the biopsy specimen shows that approximately 50% of the glomeruli in the specimen are affected by the lesion shown. Which of the following is the most likely diagnosis?

☐ (A) Focal segmental glomerulosclerosis
☐ (B) Lipoid nephrosis
☐ (C) Membranoproliferative glomerulonephritis type I
☐ (D) Membranoproliferative glomerulonephritis type II
☐ (E) Nodular glomerulosclerosis
☐ (F) Postinfectious glomerulonephritis
☐ (G) Rapidly progressive glomerulonephritis

60 A 19-year-old woman has had a fever and chills accompanied by right flank pain for the past 3 days. On physical examination, her temperature is 38.3°C, blood pressure is 150/90 mm Hg, and there is right costovertebral angle tenderness. Laboratory findings show a serum glucose level of 77 mg/dL and creatinine level of 1.0 mg/dL. Urinalysis shows a pH of 6.5, specific gravity 1.018, and no protein, blood, glucose, or ketones. Microscopic examination of the urine shows many WBCs and WBC casts. Which of the following factors is most important in the pathogenesis of the renal disease affecting this patient?

☐ (A) Age
☐ (B) Sex
☐ (C) Vesicoureteral reflux
☐ (D) Blood pressure
☐ (E) Focus of infection in the lungs

61 Several days after eating a hamburger, chili, and ice cream at a home barbecue, a 5-year-old girl develops cramping abdominal pain and diarrhea. The next day, she has decreased urine output. On physical examination, there are petechial hemorrhages on the skin. Her temperature is 37.0°C, pulse 90/min, respirations 18/min, and blood pressure 90/50 mm Hg. A stool sample is positive for occult blood. Labora-

tory findings show hemoglobin of 10.8 g/dL, hematocrit 32.4%, platelet count 64,300/mm³, and WBC count 6480/mm³. The peripheral blood smear shows schistocytes, and the serum D dimer level is elevated. Which of the following is the most likely causative organism?

☐ (A) *Candida albicans*
☐ (B) *Proteus mirabilis*
☐ (C) *Clostridium difficile*
☐ (D) *Escherichia coli*
☐ (E) *Staphylococcus aureus*

62 A 17-year-old boy is involved in a motor vehicle accident in which he sustains severe blunt trauma to the extremities and abdomen. Over the next 3 days, he develops oliguria and dark brown-colored urine. The urine dipstick analysis is positive for myoglobin and for blood, but microscopic examination of the urine shows no RBCs. His serum urea nitrogen level rises to 38 mg/dL, and he undergoes hemodialysis for 3 weeks. His condition improves, but the urine output remains in excess of 3 L per day for 1 week before the urea nitrogen returns to normal. Which of the following renal lesions was most likely present in this patient?

☐ (A) Malignant nephrosclerosis
☐ (B) Renal vein thrombosis
☐ (C) Membranous glomerulonephritis
☐ (D) Acute pyelonephritis
☐ (E) Acute tubular necrosis

63 A 45-year-old man has had headaches, nausea, and vomiting that have worsened over the past 5 days. He has started "seeing spots" before his eyes. On physical examination, his blood pressure is 268/150 mm Hg. Urinalysis shows 1+ proteinuria, 2+ hematuria, and no glucose, ketones, or leukocytes. The serum urea nitrogen and creatinine level are both elevated. Which of the following histologic findings is most likely to be seen in this patient's kidneys?

☐ (A) Nodular glomerulosclerosis
☐ (B) Segmental tubular necrosis
☐ (C) Hyperplastic arteriolosclerosis
☐ (D) Mesangial IgA deposition
☐ (E) Glomerular crescents

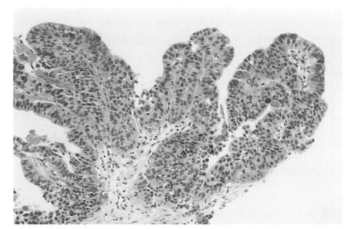

Courtesy of Dr. Christopher Corless, University of Oregon, Eugene, OR.

64 A 62-year-old man has had several episodes of hematuria over the past week. He has not experienced increased urinary frequency or dysuria. On physical examination, there are no remarkable findings. Urinalysis shows 4+ hematuria. The urine culture is negative. A cystoscopy is performed, and a 2-cm sessile, friable mass is seen on the right bladder wall. A biopsy specimen is obtained, and the microscopic appearance is shown in the preceding figure. Which of the following risk factors is most important in the pathogenesis of this bladder lesion?

- ❏ (A) Smoking cigarettes
- ❏ (B) Schistosomiasis
- ❏ (C) Diabetes mellitus
- ❏ (D) Chronic bacterial cystitis
- ❏ (E) Nodular prostatic hyperplasia

65 A 38-year-old woman sees her physician because she has been feeling tired and lethargic for several months. On physical examination, she is afebrile, and her blood pressure is 140/90 mm Hg. Laboratory findings show hemoglobin of 10.3 g/dL, hematocrit 30.9%, platelet count 310,700/mm^3, and WBC count 5585/mm^3. The serum creatinine level is 5.8 mg/dL. C3 nephritic factor is present in serum, and the ANA test result is negative. Urinalysis shows 2+ proteinuria. A renal biopsy is performed, and microscopic examination shows hypercellular glomeruli and prominent electron-dense deposits along the lamina densa of the glomerular basement membrane. Which of the following forms of glomerulonephritis is most likely to be present in this patient?

- ❏ (A) Postinfectious glomerulonephritis
- ❏ (B) Rapidly progressive glomerulonephritis
- ❏ (C) Membranoproliferative glomerulonephritis
- ❏ (D) Chronic glomerulonephritis
- ❏ (E) Membranous glomerulonephritis

66 A 60-year-old man presents with a feeling of fullness in his abdomen and a 5 kg weight loss over the past 6 months. Physical examination is entirely normal. Laboratory studies show hemoglobin 8.2 g/dL, hematocrit 24%, and MCV 70 μm^3. Urinalysis shows 3+ hematuria but no protein, glucose, or leukocytes. An abdominal CT scan shows an 11 cm mass in the upper pole of the right kidney. A right nephrectomy is performed and on gross examination the mass invades the renal vein. Microscopic examination of the mass shows cells with abundant clear cytoplasm. Which of the following molecular abnormalities is most likely to be found in tumor cell DNA?

- ❏ (A) Homozygous loss of the *von Hippel Lindau (VHL)* gene
- ❏ (B) Mutational activation of the *MET* protooncogene
- ❏ (C) Trisomy of chromosome 7 associated genes
- ❏ (D) Integration of human papillomavirus-16 (HPV-16)
- ❏ (E) Microsatellite instability

67 A 45-year-old Hispanic man has had increasing malaise with headaches and easy fatigability for the past 3 months. Physical examination reveals his blood pressure is 200/100 mm Hg. There are no palpable abdominal masses and no costovertebral tenderness. Laboratory studies show hemoglobin 9.5 g/dL, hematocrit 28.3%, MCV 92 μm^3, creatinine 4.5 mg/dL, and urea nitrogen 42 mg/dL. Urinalysis reveals 3+ hematuria and 3+ proteinuria but no glucose or leukocytes. A renal biopsy is performed and on light microscopic examination shows that approximately 50% of the glomeruli appear normal, but the rest show that a portion of the capillary tuft is sclerotic. Immunofluorescence staining shows IgM and C3

deposition in these sclerotic areas. Past history is significant for repeated episodes of passing dark brown urine, which failed to respond to corticosteroid therapy. Which of the following mechanisms is most likely responsible for his disease?

- ❏ (A) Deposition of immune complexes containing microbial antigens
- ❏ (B) Dysfunction of the podocyte slit diaphragm apparatus
- ❏ (C) Deposition of antiglomerular basement membrane antibodies
- ❏ (D) Inherited defect in the basement membrane collagen
- ❏ (E) Deposition of C3 nephritic factor (C3NeF)

ANSWERS

1 **(C)** About 75% of all renal stones are composed of calcium oxalate crystals. Patients with these stones tend to have hypercalciuria without hypercalcemia. Uric acid stones and cystine stones are radiolucent and tend to form in acidic urine. Cystine stones are rare. Triple phosphate stones tend to occur in association with urinary tract infections, particularly those caused by urease-positive bacteria such as *Proteus*.

BP7 536-537   BP6 465   PBD7 1014-1015   PBD6 989-990

2 **(C)** The figure shows glomeruli with epithelial crescents that are the morphologic correlates of rapidly progressive glomerulonephritis. Patients with this condition rapidly develop renal failure. One cause of rapidly progressive renal failure is Goodpasture syndrome, in which anti–glomerular basement membrane antibodies damage both the glomeruli and the pulmonary alveoli. Damage to the alveoli results in hemoptysis. Acute tubular necrosis is potentially reversible. Focal segmental glomerulosclerosis is typically nonresponsive to corticosteroids. IgA nephropathy can have intermittent hematuria. Acute pyelonephritis is accompanied by fever and leukocytosis.

BP7 523-524   BP6 452-453   PBD7 976-978
PBD6 951-952

3 **(D)** The most likely cause of nephrotic syndrome in a child is minimal change disease. For this reason, a course of corticosteroids is indicated, and 90% of patients respond. If there is no response, further workup, including a renal biopsy, can be performed. Few cases progress to chronic renal failure requiring dialysis or transplantation. The cause of minimal change disease is unknown. Children with minimal change disease do not develop rapid renal failure, and there is no genetic tendency associated with the disease.

BP7 518-519   BP6 447   PBD7 978-979, 981-982
PBD6 954-956

4 **(B)** These findings describe end-stage renal disease, the appearance of which is similar regardless of the cause (e.g., vascular disease or glomerular disease). With advanced renal destruction, hypertension almost always supervenes, even if it was absent at the onset of renal disease. Many such cases are referred to as "chronic glomerulonephritis" for want of a better term. A rash might have preceded the postinfectious glomerulonephritis. Hemoptysis occurs in Goodpasture syndrome. Lens dislocation is a feature of Alport syndrome. Pharyngitis with group A streptococcal infection may precede postinfectious glomerulonephritis.

BP7 526   BP6 454-455   PBD7 960-961   PBD6 963-964

5 **(D)** Carcinoma of the urethra is uncommon. It tends to occur in older women and is locally aggressive. An embryonal rhabdomyosarcoma (sarcoma botryoides) is a rare tumor that occurs in children. Benign tumors such as a leiomyoma or papilloma are typically well circumscribed and do not ulcerate. Syphilis produces indurated, painless lesions rather than ulcerated, warty masses.

BP 547   PBD7 1034   PBD6 1009

6 **(A)** The ureteral, pelvic, and calyceal dilation results from long-standing obstruction leading to hydroureter and hydronephrosis. With benign nephrosclerosis, the kidneys become smaller and develop granular surfaces, but there is no dilation. The scarring that accompanies analgesic nephropathy or chronic pyelonephritis can be marked; it is associated with significant loss of renal parenchyma but not with pelvic dilation. There are many renal complications of diabetes mellitus, mostly from vascular, glomerular, or interstitial injury, but there is no obstruction. In some patients, diabetes is complicated by a neurogenic bladder, and this can lead to functional obstruction. However, in such cases, both kidneys and ureters would be affected.

BP7 537-538   BP6 465-466   PBD7 1012-1014
PBD6 988-989

7 **(C)** IgA nephropathy, also known as Berger disease, can explain the presence of recurrent hematuria in a young adult. Nephrotic syndrome is not present, and mesangial IgA deposition is characteristic. The initial episode of hematuria usually follows an upper respiratory infection. IgA nephropathy occurs with increased frequency in patients with celiac disease. Granular staining of basement membrane with IgG antibodies denotes immune complex deposition, which may occur in postinfectious glomerulonephritis. The subepithelial deposits are seen on electron microscopy. Patients with these changes have nephritic syndrome. Diffuse proliferation and basement membrane thickening denote membranoproliferative glomerulonephritis. In this condition, IgG and C3 are deposited in the glomeruli. Glomerular capillary thrombosis is typical of the hemolytic-uremic syndrome.

BP7 524-525   BP6 453   PBD7 986-988   PBD6 961-962

8 **(D)** These findings are characteristic of poststreptococcal glomerulonephritis. The strains of group A streptococci that cause poststreptococcal glomerulonephritis are different from those that give rise to rheumatic fever. Most children with poststreptococcal glomerulonephritis recover, although perhaps 1% develop a rapidly progressive glomerulonephritis. Progression to chronic renal failure may occur in 10% to 15% of affected adults. A urinary tract infection is not likely to accompany poststreptococcal glomerulonephritis, because the organisms that caused the immunologic reaction are no longer present when symptoms of glomerulonephritis appear.

BP7 522-523   BP6 451-452   PBD7 974-976
PBD6 949-951

9 **(E)** Calcium oxalate stones are the most common type of urinary tract stone. Approximately 50% of patients with calcium oxalate stones have increased excretion of calcium without hypercalcemia. The basis of hypercalciuria is not clear. Most uric acid stones are formed in acidic urine and are not related to gout. It is thought that these patients have an unexplained tendency to excrete acidic urine. At low pH, uric acid is insoluble, and stones form. Infections can predispose to the formation of magnesium ammonium phosphate stones. Diabetes mellitus is not a common cause of urinary tract lithiasis; although infections are more common in diabetic persons, most are not caused by urea-splitting bacteria. Hyperparathyroidism predisposes affected persons to form stones containing calcium, but few patients with urinary tract stones have this condition.

BP7 536-537   BP6 464-465   PBD7 1014-1015
PBD6 989-990

10 **(B)** The figure shows a renal cell carcinoma. About 5% to 10% of these tumors secrete erythropoietin, giving rise to polycythemia. Other substances can be secreted—among them corticotropin (adrenocorticotropic hormone), resulting in hypercortisolism in Cushing syndrome—but these cases are encountered less frequently than polycythemia. Ketonuria is a feature of type 1 diabetes mellitus, which is not associated with the development of renal neoplasms. Renal cell carcinomas are usually unilateral, and typically they do not destroy all of a kidney. There is no significant loss of renal function, and the serum urea nitrogen and creatinine levels are not elevated. Hypertension from hyperreninemia can occur in patients with some renal cell carcinomas, although this is not common. Ketonuria is seen in patients with decreased caloric intake and with type 1 diabetes mellitus. Renal cell carcinomas are usually unilateral and involve part of the kidney; thus renal failure is unlikely.

BP7 539-541   BP6 466-467   PBD7 1016-1018
PBD6 991-993

11 **(E)** Alport syndrome is a form of hereditary nephritis. Hematuria is the most common presenting feature, but proteinuria is often present and may be in the nephrotic range. Patients progress to chronic renal failure in adulthood. Most patients have an X-linked dominant pattern of inheritance, but autosomal dominant and autosomal recessive pedigrees also exist. The foamy change in the tubular epithelial cells and ultrastructural alterations of the basement membrane are characteristic features. The genetic defect results from mutation in the gene for the α-5 chain of type IV collagen. Acute tubular necrosis follows ischemic or toxic injuries to the kidney and does not involve glomeruli. Berger disease, or IgA nephropathy, is a form of glomerulonephritis that does not produce tubular epithelial changes. Membranous glomerulonephritis generally produces a nephrotic syndrome and deposition of immune complexes in glomerular basement membrane. Nodular and diffuse glomerulosclerosis are typical changes in diabetic nephropathy.

BP7 525-526   BP6 454   PBD7 988   PBD6 962-963

12 **(C)** These findings are typical of drug-induced interstitial nephritis. A variety of drugs can cause this condition, including sulfonamides, penicillins, cephalosporins, the fluoroquinolone antibiotics ciprofloxacin and norfloxacin, and the antituberculous drugs isoniazid and rifampin. Acute tubulointerstitial nephritis can also occur with use of thiazide and loop diuretics, cimetidine, ranitidine, omeprazole, and nonsteroidal anti-inflammatory drugs. The disease appears about 2 weeks after the patient begins to use the drug. Elements of type I (increased IgE) and type IV (skin test positivity to drug haptens) hypersensitivity are present. WBCs, but not eosinophils, may be present in the urine of a patient with a urinary tract infection. Congestive heart failure can lead to acute tubular necrosis, but it is not associated with a rash or proteinuria. Poststreptococcal glomerulonephritis could account for the proteinuria and hematuria seen in this patient, but not for the rash, because the strains of group A β-hemolytic streptococci that cause a skin infection precede by weeks the development of glomerulonephritis. Hemolytic-uremic syndrome can occur after ingestion of strains of *Escherichia coli* that may be present in ground beef.

BP7 530   BP6 458   PBD7 1002   PBD6 977-978

13 **(D)** Hemolytic-uremic syndrome is one of the most common causes of acute renal failure in children. It most commonly occurs after ingestion of meat infected with verocytotoxin-producing *Escherichia coli*, most often serotype O157 : H7 The toxin damages endothelium, reducing nitric oxide, promoting vasoconstriction and necrosis, and promoting thrombosis. With supportive therapy, most patients recover in a few weeks, although perhaps one fourth progress to chronic renal failure. Postinfectious glomerulonephritis occurs several weeks after an infection, usually with group A β-hemolytic streptococci. Wegener granulomatosis is a vasculitis that most often occurs in adults. Hereditary nephritis may occur in childhood; it is progressive and is not related to vascular disease. An IgA nephropathy most often occurs in young adults; it is not accompanied by vascular changes.

BP7 534-535   BP6 463   PBD7 1009-1010   PBD6 985-986

14 **(E)** A child with nephrotic syndrome and no other clinical findings is most likely to have lipoid nephrosis, also called minimal change disease. The term "minimal change disease" reflects the paucity of pathologic findings. There is fusion of foot processes, which can be seen only by electron microscopy. Subepithelial electron-dense humps represent immune complexes and are seen in postinfectious glomerulonephritis. Variability of basement membrane thickening may be seen in Alport syndrome. The mesangial matrix is expanded in some forms of glomerulonephritis (e.g., IgA nephropathy) and other diseases, such as diabetes mellitus, but not in minimal change disease.

BP7 518-519   BP6 447   PBD7 981-982   PBD6 954-956

15 **(E)** Postinfectious glomerulonephritis is one of many causes of a nephritic syndrome characterized by hematuria and RBC casts. Most children recover completely, but one in six adults may progress to chronic renal failure. Some cases may occur after a streptococcal pharyngitis (poststreptococcal glomerulonephritis). In other cases such as this one, the preceding infection is so mild that patients give no history. Goodpasture syndrome may also produce a nephritic syndrome, but there is linear deposition of antibody in the glomerular basement membrane. Amyloidosis of the kidney mainly produces proteinuria without hematuria, as does

membranous glomerulonephritis. Nodular and diffuse glomerulosclerosis are characteristic of diabetic nephropathy.

BP7 522-523   BP6 451   PBD7 974-976   PBD6 949-951

16 **(E)** This patient has bladder hypertrophy resulting from outlet obstruction. In an older man, this type of obstruction is most often caused by prostatic enlargement resulting from hyperplasia or carcinoma. Mild elevations in the prostate-specific antigen (PSA) level may occur in patients with prostatic hyperplasia, and greater increases in PSA suggest carcinoma. Autoimmune conditions may be associated with interstitial cystitis, but cystitis does not cause bladder neck obstruction. Bladder outlet obstruction can increase the risk of infection, typically with bacterial organisms such as *Escherichia coli*, not *Mycobacterium tuberculosis*. Polycythemia can be the result of a paraneoplastic syndrome, but urothelial malignancies are unlikely to produce this finding; renal cell carcinoma is a more likely cause. Schistosomiasis leads to chronic inflammation and scarring.

PBD7 1033   PBD6 1008

17 **(A)** This woman has an autosomal dominant form of polycystic kidney disease. Hypertension and infection are the most frequent complications of this disorder. The risk of renal cell carcinoma is increased in persons with dialysis-acquired cysts but not in those with polycystic kidney disease. Although some proteinuria is present in many forms of chronic renal disease, nephrotic syndrome is not common in polycystic kidney disease. A microangiopathic hemolytic anemia may be seen in hemolytic-uremic syndrome. Vascular changes with resultant infarction are not seen in polycystic kidney disease. Transitional cell carcinomas are not related to polycystic kidney diseases. Cushing syndrome may complicate renal cell carcinoma, but it is not a complication of polycystic kidney disease.

BP7 535-536   BP6 463-464   PBD7 962-964
PBD6 937-940

18 **(E)** This patient's history is typical of ischemic acute tubular necrosis, which is often accompanied by rupture of the basement membrane (tubulorrhexis). An initiating phase that lasts approximately 1 day is followed by a maintenance phase during which progressive oliguria and rising blood urea nitrogen levels occur, with salt and water overload. This is followed by a recovery phase during which there is a steady increase in urinary output and hypokalemia. Eventually, tubular function is restored. Treatment of this acute renal failure results in recovery of nearly all patients. Crescents suggest a rapidly progressively glomerulonephritis that is unlikely to resolve. Interstitial infiltrates suggest a chronic tubulointerstitial process. Fibrinoid necrosis in arterioles is a feature of malignant nephrosclerosis, a serious condition that produces significant renal damage. Nodular glomerulosclerosis is a feature of diabetic nephropathy and is a progressive condition that leads to chronic renal failure.

BP7 531-533   BP6 460-461   PBD7 993-996
PBD6 969-971

19 **(C)** Painless hematuria in an older adult suggests a renal neoplasm. The additional presence of constitutional symptoms, such as fever and weakness, should raise the suspicion of a renal cell carcinoma. Urinary tract calculi usually cause severe, colicky pain when they are passed. Urinary tract infections are not characterized by recurrent hematuria without fever or other signs of acute inflammation. Nephrotic syndrome, which manifests with proteinuria, typically is not associated with hematuria. A renal biopsy has a low yield in a patient without an acute-onset renal disease, and it is an ineffective way of diagnosing tumors.

BP7 539-541   BP6 468-469   PBD7 1016-1018   PBD6 994

20 **(A)** This patient with nephrotic syndrome has clinical and histologic features of membranous glomerulonephritis. In most cases, this is an idiopathic disease caused by immune complex deposition on the glomerular basement membranes. Granular immunofluorescence with IgG and C3 supports this diagnosis. Under the electron microscope, electron-dense immune complexes are seen on the epithelial side of the basement membrane. Subendothelial electron-dense deposits with duplication of the basement membrane are a feature of type I membranoproliferative glomerulonephritis. Electron-dense deposits limited to the mesangium are seen in IgA nephropathy. Podocyte foot process fusion without any other abnormality occurs in lipoid nephrosis.

BP7 518-520   BP6 447-449   PBD7 979-981
PBD6 953-955

21 **(C)** The clinical features in this patient are typical of urinary tract infection, and *Escherichia coli* is the most common cause. The WBCs are characteristic of an acute inflammatory process. The presence of WBC casts indicates that the infection must have occurred in the kidney, because casts are formed in renal tubules. Most infections of the urinary tract begin in the lower urinary tract and ascend to the kidneys. Hematogenous spread is less common. *Mycobacterium tuberculosis* causes the rare "sterile pyuria"; however, renal tuberculosis typically does not present as an acute febrile illness. *Mycoplasma* and *Cryptococcus* are rare urinary tract pathogens. Group A streptococcus is best known as an antecedent infection to poststreptococcal glomerulonephritis, an immunologically mediated disease in which the organisms are not present at the site of glomerular injury.

BP7 527-529   BP6 455-456   PBD7 996-1000
PBD6 974-975

22 **(F)** The figure shows nodular and diffuse glomerulosclerosis, a classic lesion in diabetes mellitus. Patients with diabetes mellitus have an elevated level of glycosylated hemoglobin (Hgb A_{1c}). Patients with type 1 diabetes mellitus may initially have microalbuminuria, which predicts development of future overt diabetic nephropathy. There is progressive loss of renal function. These patients are often hypertensive and have hyaline arteriolosclerosis. The presence of overt proteinuria suggests progression to end-stage renal disease within 5 years. Anti–glomerular basement membrane antibody is seen in Goodpasture syndrome, which manifests as a rapidly progressive glomerulonephritis. The ANA test is positive in a wide variety of autoimmune diseases, most typically systemic lupus erythematosus, which can be accompanied by glomerulonephritis. The ANCA test is positive in some forms of vasculitis, such as Wegener granulomatosis, which can involve the kidneys. The anti–streptolysin O (ASO) titer is elevated following streptococcal infections, which may cause postinfectious glomerulonephritis. The C3 nephritic factor may be present in type II membranoproliferative glomerulonephritis (dense deposit disease). Some patients with membranous

glomerulonephritis have a positive serologic test result for HBsAg.

BP7 650   BP6 570   PBD7 991-992   PBD6 966-968

23 **(G)** This fetus has features of autosomal recessive polycystic kidney disease (RPKD) involving the liver. RPKD is a disease that occurs in children; by contrast, autosomal dominant polycystic kidney disease (DPKD) leads to presentation with renal failure in adults. Some less common forms of RPKD are accompanied by survival beyond infancy, and these patients develop congenital hepatic fibrosis. Enlarged kidneys with 1- to 4-cm cysts are characteristic of DPKD in adults. Perhaps the most common renal cystic disease seen in fetuses and infants is multicystic renal dysplasia (multicystic dysplastic kidney), in which the cysts and kidneys are variably sized. This disease can be focal, unilateral, or bilateral; however, congenital hepatic fibrosis is not present. Small, shrunken, granular kidneys typify end-stage renal diseases in adults. For oligohydramnios to be present, both kidneys must be affected, not just one. Irregular cortical scars with pelvicaliceal dilation may represent hydronephrosis complicated by infection in chronic pyelonephritis, a process that occurs in adults. Dilation with calyceal thinning can occur with obstructions in utero, such as posterior urethral valves in males or urethral atresia in either males or females; liver lesions are not present in these cases. A cause of oligohydramnios other than abnormalities of the urinary tract (e.g., leakage of amniotic fluid with premature and prolonged rupture of membranes) could be present if the kidneys appear normal, but in this case the distinctive finding of congenital hepatic fibrosis points to RPKD.

BP7 536   PBD7 964-965   PBD6 940

24 **(C)** This description of the gross appearance of the kidney is characteristic of chronic pyelonephritis, caused most often by reflux nephropathy. Typical features include coarse and irregular scarring resulting from ascending infection, blunting and deformity of calyces, and asymmetric involvement of the kidneys. The loss of tubules from scarring gives rise to reduced renal concentrating ability; hence, the patient had polyuria with a low specific gravity of the urine. Chronic glomerulonephritis, benign nephrosclerosis (caused by essential hypertension), and systemic lupus erythematosus produce bilateral symmetric involvement, and the affected kidneys are shrunken and finely granular. Autosomal dominant polycystic kidney disease is characterized by large cysts that replace the renal parenchyma and greatly increase the size of the kidneys bilaterally.

BP7 529-530   BP6 457-458   PBD7 1000-1001
PBD6 975-977

25 **(D)** These findings point to an acute drug-induced interstitial nephritis caused by ampicillin. This is an immunologic reaction, probably caused by a drug acting as a hapten. Poststreptococcal glomerulonephritis is unlikely to be accompanied by a rash or by eosinophils in the urine. Acute pyelonephritis is an ascending infection; only uncommonly is it caused by hematogenous spread of bacteria from other sites. Acute tubular necrosis can give rise to acute renal failure. It is caused by hypoxia resulting from shock or from toxic injury caused by chemicals such as mercury, and only rarely if ever by bacterial toxins. Anti-GBM antibodies occur in Goodpasture syndrome, with hemorrhages in lungs as well.

BP7 530   BP6 458   PBD7 1002   PBD6 977-978

26 **(E)** Wilms tumor is the most common renal neoplasm in children, and one of the most common childhood neoplasms. A complex staging, grading, and molecular analysis formula, as well as surgery, chemotherapy, and radiation, result in a high cure rate. The microscopic pattern of Wilms tumor (nephroblastoma) resembles the fetal kidney nephrogenic zone. Angiomyolipomas may be sporadic or part of the genetic syndrome of tuberous sclerosis. They may be multiple and bilateral and have well-differentiated muscle, adipose tissue, and vascular components. Renomedullary interstitial cell tumors ("medullary fibromas") are generally less than 1 cm and are incidental findings. Renal cell carcinoma is rare in children, and the most common patterns are clear cell, papillary, and chromophobe. Transitional cell carcinomas arise in the urothelium in adults and microscopically resemble urothelium.

BP7 256-257, 541   BP6 212-214   PBD7 504-506
PBD6 487-489

27 **(A)** Development of recurrent hematuria following a viral illness in a child or young adult is typically associated with IgA nephropathy. In these patients, some defect in immune regulation causes excessive mucosal IgA synthesis in response to viral or other environmental antigens. IgA complexes are deposited in the mesangium and initiate glomerular injury. Antibodies against type IV collagen are formed in Goodpasture syndrome. Although viruses induce IgA synthesis, they do not cause direct glomerular damage. Cytokine-mediated injury can occur in transplant rejection. Defects in the structure of glomerular basement membrane are a feature of hereditary nephritis.

BP7 524-525   BP6 453-454   PBD7 986-988
PBD6 961-962

28 **(C)** This patient has ureteral colic from the passage of a stone down the ureter. Dysuria may accompany acute cystitis, but not colicky pain. Flank pain may accompany a renal cell carcinoma, but the pain is usually dull. Renal carcinoma is rare in patients this age. Hydronephrosis is typically a "silent" disease that develops slowly and painlessly over years. A rupture of one of the many cysts in adult polycystic kidney disease can cause acute pain, but it is usually not colicky, and hematuria may not be present.

BP7 537   BP6 464-465   PBD7 1013, 1025   PBD6 989-990

29 **(D)** Steroid-responsive proteinuria in a child is typical of minimal change disease in which the kidney looks normal by light microscopy but there is foot process fusion by electron microscopy. The most likely cause of foot process fusion is a primary injury to visceral epithelial cells caused by T-cell derived cytokines. Immune complex deposition in membranous glomerulopathy can give rise to nephrotic syndrome, but is less common in children than adults and is not steroid-responsive. Certain verocytotoxin-producing *Escherichia coli* strains can cause hemolytic-uremic syndrome by injury to capillary endothelium. Acute cellular renal transplant rejection is mediated by T cell injury with tubulitis. IgA nephropathy with mesangial IgA deposition and consequent glomerular injury gives rise to recurrent gross or microscopic hematuria and far less commonly to nephrotic syndrome.

BP7 518-519   BP6 447   PBD7 981-982   PBD6 954-956

30 **(E)** This patient has idiopathic membranous glomerulopathy, producing nephrotic syndrome. Diffuse basement membrane thickening, in the absence of proliferative changes, and granular deposits of IgG and C3 are typical of this condition. It is caused by the deposition of immune complexes on the basement membrane, which activates complement. Antibodies that react with basement membrane give rise to a linear immunofluorescence pattern, as in Goodpasture syndrome. Membranous glomerulopathy has no association with streptococcal infections. There is also no evidence of cytokine- or T-cell–mediated damage in this disease. In 85% of patients with membranous glomerulopathy, the cause of immune complex deposition is unknown. In the remaining 15%, an associated systemic disease (e.g., systemic lupus erythematosus) or some known cause of immune complex formation (e.g., drug reaction) exists.

BP7 518-520   BP6 447-449   PBD7 979-981
PBD6 953-954

31 **(C)** The congenital disorder known as medullary sponge kidney (MSK) is present to some degree in up to 1% of adults. In MSK, cystic dilation of 1 to 5 mm is present in the inner medullary and papillary collecting ducts. MSK is bilateral in 70% of cases. Not all papillae are equally affected, although calculi are often present in dilated collecting ducts. Patients usually develop kidney stones, infection, or recurrent hematuria in the third or fourth decade. More than 50% of patients have stones. Autosomal dominant polycystic kidney disease produces much larger cysts that involve the entire kidney, eventually leading to massive renomegaly. Uric acid crystals are present in gout and may be deposited in the medulla, but cysts do not form. Multicystic renal dysplasia may occur sporadically or as part of various genetic syndromes, such as Meckel-Gruber syndrome, in fetuses and newborns. Autosomal recessive polycystic kidney disease is rare and leads to bilateral, symmetric renal enlargement manifested in utero, with renal failure evident at birth. Transitional cell carcinoma may be multifocal, but it produces masses, not cysts. Vesicoureteral reflux can lead to hydroureter, hydronephrosis, and an increased risk of infection.

PBD7 962, 965   PBD6 940-941

32 **(E)** Simple cysts are common in adults, and multiple cysts also may occur. The cysts are not as numerous as those occurring in autosomal dominant polycystic kidney disease (DPKD), and there is no evidence of renal failure. Simple cysts may be as large as 10 cm, and hemorrhage sometimes occurs into a cyst. Multiple cysts sometimes develop in patients receiving long-term hemodialysis. Acute pyelonephritis is unlikely in this patient because of the absence of fever and WBCs in the urine. Acute pyelonephritis may be associated with small abscesses but not with cysts, although in patients with DPKD, cysts may become infected. Acute tubular necrosis follows ischemic or toxic injury, and there is evidence of renal failure. Diabetic nephropathy includes vascular and glomerular disease but not cysts. Hydronephrosis may produce a focal obstruction of a calyx with dilation, but it does not produce an eccentric cyst. Glomerulonephritis is not associated with cyst formation. Neoplasms usually produce solid masses, although sometimes a renal cell carcinoma is cystic. The latter, however, is much less common than a simple cyst.

BP7 535   BP6 463   PBD7 962, 966   PBD6 942

33 **(D)** Recurrent urinary tract infections with urea-splitting organisms such as *Proteus* can lead to formation of magnesium ammonium phosphate stones. These stones are large, and they fill the dilated calyceal system. Because of their large size and projections into the calyces, such stones are sometimes called "staghorn calculi." Infections are not a key feature of renal cell carcinoma. Cases of acute tubular necrosis typically occur from toxic or ischemic renal injuries. Malignant nephrosclerosis is primarily a vascular process that is not associated with infection. Papillary necrosis can complicate diabetes mellitus.

BP7 537   BP6 465   PBD7 1014-1015   PBD6 989-990

34 (B) This patient has laboratory findings consistent with diabetes mellitus and clinical features of acute pyelonephritis caused by *Escherichia coli* infection. Necrotizing papillitis with papillary necrosis is a complication of acute pyelonephritis, and diabetic patients are particularly prone to this development. In the absence of diabetes mellitus, papillary necrosis develops when acute pyelonephritis occurs in combination with urinary tract obstruction. Papillary necrosis also can occur with chronic use of analgesics. Acute tubular necrosis typically occurs in acute renal failure caused by hypoxia (e.g., shock) or toxic injury (e.g., mercury). Crescentic glomerulonephritis causes rapidly progressive renal failure. Hydronephrosis occurs when urinary outflow is obstructed in the renal pelvis or in the ureter. Renal calculi can complicate conditions such as gout, but they do not complicate diabetes mellitus.

BP7 527-529   BP6 457   PBD7 990, 998-999   PBD6 979

35 (A) One of the most common cause of nephrotic syndrome in adults is membranous glomerulopathy, caused by immune complex deposition, shown here as granular deposits with C3. About 85% of cases are idiopathic, but some cases follow infections (e.g., hepatitis, malaria) or are associated with causes such as malignancies or autoimmune diseases. In some cases of AIDS, a nephropathy resembling focal segmental glomerulosclerosis occurs. Multiple myeloma can be complicated by systemic amyloidosis, which can involve the kidney. Recurrent urinary tract infection can cause chronic pyelonephritis. Nephrolithiasis may lead to interstitial nephritis, but it does not cause glomerular injury.

BP7 518-520   BP6 447-449   PBD7 978-981
PBD6 953-955

36 (A) The most common cause of acute tubular necrosis is ischemic injury. The hypotension that develops after myocardial infarction causes decreased renal blood flow. Benign nephrosclerosis takes years to develop and is associated with benign essential hypertension. Emboli from mural thrombosis after myocardial infarction could reach the kidney, causing renal infarction, but these infarctions are small and focal. Hemolytic-uremic syndrome is a thrombotic microangiopathy that most often occurs in children following infection with enterotoxigenic *Escherichia coli*. A rapidly progressive glomerulonephritis does not follow ischemic injury and would not resolve as quickly as in this patient.

BP7 531-533   BP6 459-460   PBD7 993-996
PBD6 969-971

37 (B) These findings are characteristic of Alport syndrome, a form of hereditary nephritis. Most cases are inherited in an X-linked dominant pattern, but autosomal dominant and autosomal recessive patterns of inheritance also are seen. Most commonly, males are severely affected. Vision, hearing, and renal function are affected, but other organ systems are not affected.

BP7 525-526   BP6 454   PBD7 988   PBD6 962-963

38 (D) Exposure to arylamines markedly increases the risk of bladder cancer, which can occur decades after the initial exposure. After absorption, aromatic amines are hydroxylated into an active form, which is detoxified by conjugation with glucuronic acid and then excreted. Urinary glucuronidase then splits the nontoxic conjugated form into the active carcinogenic form. Renal cell carcinomas also may present as painless hematuria, but exposure to aniline dyes is not a risk factor. Hemorrhagic cystitis occurs after radiation injury or treatment with cytotoxic drugs such as cyclophosphamide. Tubercular cystitis is typically a complication of renal tuberculosis. Squamous cell carcinoma is the most common malignancy of the urethra, but it is rare and has no relation to carcinogens.

BP7 541-542   BP6 468-469   PBD7 1032   PBD6 1007

39 (F) This patient has diabetes mellitus. Nodular and diffuse glomerulosclerosis often occur in patients with long-standing diabetes mellitus. Infections with bacterial organisms also occur more frequently in patients with diabetes mellitus. Deposits of IgG and C3 in the glomerular basement membrane occur with forms of glomerulonephritis caused by immune complex deposition, including lupus nephritis and membranous glomerulonephritis. The only abnormality observed in minimal change disease (MCD) is effacement of podocyte foot processes, but this change is not specific for MCD and may be seen in other disorders that produce proteinuria. Crescentic glomerulonephritis is not typically seen in diabetes mellitus. IgA deposition in the mesangium occurs in IgA nephropathy (Berger disease). A necrotizing granulomatous vasculitis can be present in the kidneys of patients with Wegener granulomatosis. Thickening and thinning of glomerular basement membranes occurs in Alport syndrome.

BP7 650   BP6 570   PBD7 991-992   PBD6 966-967

40 (F) This patient has findings of systemic lupus erythematosus, an autoimmune disease that often manifests with renal involvement. There are several forms of lupus nephritis, and they tend to produce a nephritic pattern of involvement. Because these patients have leakage of RBCs from damaged glomeruli, as well as proteinuria, RBC casts are found in the urine. Eosinophils may appear in the urine as a result of drug-induced interstitial nephritis. Glucosuria and ketonuria are features of type 1 diabetes mellitus. Myoglobinuria results most often from rhabdomyolysis, which can occur after severe crush injuries. Oval fat bodies are sloughed tubular cells containing abundant lipid that are characteristic of nephrotic syndromes. Triple phosphate crystals are typical findings in patients with infections caused by urease-positive bacteria, such as *Proteus*. Uric acid crystals form in acidic urine when uricosuria is present; this is a characteristic feature in some patients with gout. Waxy casts form in dilated, damaged tubules.

BP7 134-136   BP6 106-108   PBD7 231-233, 990
PBD6 220-222, 965

41 **(E)** Most cases of pyelonephritis result from ascending bacterial infections, which are more common in women. Recurrent urinary tract infections complicated by vesicoureteral reflux cause progressive interstitial damage and scarring, which can lead to chronic pyelonephritis with renal failure. Diffuse glomerulosclerosis is a feature of diabetes mellitus. Glomerular injury is not the major consequence of renal infections. Some cases of membranous glomerulonephritis are preceded by chronic infections such as hepatitis B or malaria, but recurrent urinary tract infections alone are unlikely antecedents. Some chronic infections (e.g. lung abscess, pulmonary tuberculosis) can lead to reactive systemic amyloidosis that may involve the kidney. However, recurrent urinary tract infections do not cause amyloidosis.

BP7 527-529   BP6 455-457   PBD7 997-1000
PBD6 972-975

42 **(A)** This patient has urethritis. The most common cause of nongonococcal urethritis in males is *Chlamydia trachomatis*. The condition is a nuisance; however, the behavior that led to the infection can place the patient at risk of other sexually transmitted diseases. Tuberculosis of the urinary tract is uncommon. Herpes simplex can produce painful vesicles on the skin. *Candida* infections typically occur in immunocompromised patients or in those receiving long-term antibiotic therapy. A syphilitic chancre on the penis is an indicator of *Treponema pallidum* infection.

BP7 675   PBD7 1034   PBD6 1009

43 **(B)** These findings are characteristic of autosomal dominant polycystic kidney disease (DPKD). As seen in the figure, several large cysts have completely replaced the kidney. In autosomal recessive polycystic kidney disease, which typically presents in fetal and neonatal life, the kidneys have a smooth external appearance. On cut section, many small cysts give the kidney a spongelike appearance. About 10% to 30% of affected patients with DPKD have an intracranial berry aneurysm, and some of these can rupture without warning. Wilms tumor does not arise in a polycystic kidney. Acute tubular necrosis is the result of ischemic or toxic renal injuries. Disseminated intravascular coagulation may complicate hemolytic-uremic syndrome. Pulmonary disease does not accompany adult polycystic kidney disease.

BP7 535-536   BP6 463-464   PBD7 962-964
PBD6 937-940

44 **(C)** This patient has analgesic nephropathy, which damages the renal interstitium and can give rise to papillary necrosis. Hydronephrosis is unlikely to develop, because there is no urinary tract obstruction in analgesic nephropathy. However, there is an increased risk of transitional cell carcinoma of the renal pelvis. The toxic injury that occurs with analgesic use is slowly progressive and not acute, in contrast to the course of acute tubular necrosis.

BP7 531   BP6 458-459   PBD7 1003-1004   PBD6 978-979

45 **(C)** Chronic glomerulonephritis may follow specific forms of acute glomerulonephritis. In many cases, however, it develops insidiously with no known cause. With progressive glomerular injury and sclerosis, both kidneys become smaller, and their surfaces become granular. Hypertension often develops because of renal ischemia. Regardless of the initiating cause, these "end-stage" kidneys appear morphologically identical. They have sclerotic glomeruli, thickened arteries, and chronic inflammation of interstitium. Because the patient's ANA test result is negative, lupus is unlikely. Polycystic kidney disease and amyloidosis would cause the kidney size to increase, not decrease. The normal hemoglobin A_{1c} concentration indicates that the patient does not have diabetes mellitus. Nodular glomerulosclerosis is typical of diabetes mellitus with an elevated hemoglobin A_{1C}.

BP7 526   BP6 454-455   PBD7 1000-1002   PBD6 963-964

46 **(C)** The linear pattern of staining shown in the figure indicates the presence of anti–glomerular basement membrane antibodies. Such antibodies are typically seen in Goodpasture syndrome. The anti–streptolysin O (ASO) titer is increased in poststreptococcal glomerulonephritis, which typically has a granular pattern of immune complex deposition. HIV infection can lead to a nephropathy that resembles focal segmental glomerulosclerosis, in which IgM and C3 are deposited in the mesangial areas of affected glomeruli. Some cases of membranous glomerulonephritis are associated with hepatitis B virus infection, but the immune complex deposition is granular, not linear. The C3 nephritic factor can be a marker for type II membranoproliferative glomerulonephritis.

BP7 513-514, 523-524   BP6 444   PBD7 968, 975
PBD6 943-944

47 **(B)** This patient has findings characteristic of systemic lupus erythematosus (SLE) with lupus nephritis. Systemic problems include fever, arthralgias, myalgias, pancytopenia, and serositis with pericarditis and pleuritis. Renal disease is common in SLE, and a renal biopsy helps to determine the severity of involvement and the appropriate therapy. Anticentromere antibody is most specific for limited scleroderma (CREST syndrome), which is unlikely to have renal involvement. Anti-DNA topoisomerase I antibody is more specific for diffuse scleroderma, which does have renal involvement, although usually this manifests as vascular disease and not as glomerulonephritis. Anti–glomerular basement membrane antibody is characteristic of Goodpasture syndrome, in which IgG antibody is deposited in a linear fashion along glomerular capillary basement membranes. Antihistone antibody may be present in drug-induced lupus. ANCAs can be seen in some forms of vasculitis, such as Wegener granulomatosis or microscopic polyangiitis. Antiribonucleotide protein is present in mixed connective tissue disease, which has some features of SLE but usually does not include severe renal involvement.

BP7 134-136   BP6 106-108   PBD7 231-233, 990
PBD6 220-222, 965

48 **(B)** The figure shows hyaline arteriolosclerosis, which typically occurs in patients with benign hypertension. Similar changes also can be seen with aging in the absence of hypertension. Oliguria is a sign of acute renal failure that does not complicate benign essential hypertension, a slowly progressive disease that is often clinically silent. Blood pressure screening is an important method that can identify patients with hypertension before significant organ damage has occurred. Malignant hypertension causes distinctive renal vascular lesions that include fibrinoid necrosis and hyperplastic arteriosclerosis. Hematuria may be present in malignant hypertension from vascular injury, but it is not a feature of benign hypertension. Flank pain is a symptom of acute pyelonephritis and some renal neoplasms.

BP7 533   BP6 461   PBD7 1006-1007   PBD6 981-982

49 **(D)** This patient has a high serum globulin level from the presence of a monoclonal protein, and the back pain is probably caused by lytic lesions in the spine. Patients with myeloma often have Bence-Jones proteinuria (not detected by the standard dipstick urinalysis), and some have cast nephropathy (as in this case), which can cause acute or, more commonly, chronic renal failure (as in this case). Cystinuria is an uncommon condition arising from defective transport of the amino acids cystine, lysine, arginine, and ornithine by the brush borders of renal tubule and intestinal epithelial cells. Excessive amounts of these amino acids are lost in the urine, leading to stone formation (the distinctive crystals look like miniature "stop" signs). Diabetic nephropathy can take many forms, but cast nephropathy is not one of them. Gouty deposits in the kidney are not in the form of casts, and uric acid crystals form at acidic pH. Hypercalcemia from a parathyroid adenoma can increase urine calcium excretion, favoring formation of stones but not casts. Systemic lupus erythematosus is more likely to cause glomerulonephritis.

BP7 430-431   BP6 380-382   PBD7 993, 1005-1006
PBD6 980-981

50 **(B)** These changes are characteristic of chronic pyelonephritis. Urinary tract obstruction favors recurrent urinary tract infection. Vesicoureteral reflux propels infected urine from the urinary bladder to the ureters and renal pelvis and predisposes to infection. Benign nephrosclerosis is a vascular disease that does not carry a risk of infection. Lupus nephritis is associated with extensive inflammatory changes of glomeruli that are noninfectious. Amyloidosis can lead to progressive renal failure as a result of amyloid deposition in the glomeruli; however, amyloid does not evoke an inflammatory response. Congestive heart failure may predispose to acute tubular necrosis. Autosomal dominant polycystic kidney disease is a bilateral process; patients usually are not symptomatic until middle age.

BP7 529-530   BP6 457-458   PBD7 1000-1002
PBD6 975-976

51 **(G)** This patient is septic, and the heart murmur strongly suggests infective endocarditis. Cardiac lesions are the source of emboli (from valvular vegetations or mural thrombi) that can lodge in renal artery branches, producing areas of coagulative necrosis. These areas of acute infarction typically are wedge-shaped on cut section because of the vascular flow pattern. Bilaterally enlarged, cystic kidneys are typical of autosomal dominant polycystic kidney disease. Small, shrunken kidneys represent an end stage of many chronic renal diseases. Irregular cortical scars with pelvicaliceal dilation may represent hydronephrosis complicated by infection in chronic pyelonephritis, whereas dilation alone points to obstructive uropathy, such as occurs with nodular prostatic hyperplasia. This patient's kidneys may well have been normal-sized and smooth-surfaced prior to this event. Petechiae and edema may be seen in hyperplastic arteriolosclerosis associated with malignant hypertension.

BP7 97-98   PBD7 997, 1012   PBD6 987-988

52 **(B)** This patient has findings characteristic of nephrocalcinosis resulting from hypercalcemia. One of the most common causes of hypercalcemia in adults is metastatic disease. The hypercalcemia produces a chronic tubulointerstitial disease of the kidneys that is initially manifested by loss of concentrating ability. With continued hypercalcemia, there is progressive loss of renal function. Urinary tract stones formed of calcium oxalate may also be present. Some patients with membranous glomerulonephritis have a positive serologic test result for hepatitis B surface antigen. Hypercholesterolemia may be seen in some cases of minimal change disease, which can occur in Hodgkin disease and other lymphoproliferative malignancies. Hypergammaglobulinemia with a monoclonal protein (M protein) may be present in multiple myeloma but not in breast cancer. Hyperglycemia can occur in diabetes mellitus, but patients with cancer are not at increased risk of developing diabetes mellitus. Hyperuricemia occurs in some cases of gout. It also can occur in patients with neoplasms (particularly lymphomas and leukemias) that have a high proliferation rate and are treated with chemotherapy. In these cases, extensive cell death (lysis syndrome) causes acute elevations in uric acid levels, leading to urate nephropathy.

PBD7 1005   PBD6 980

53 **(B)** The renal biopsy specimen shows glomerular crescents, indicative of rapidly progressive glomerulonephritis. Crescentic glomerulonephritis is divided into three groups on the basis of immunofluorescence: type I (anti–glomerular basement membrane [GBM] disease); type II (immune-complex disease); and type III (characterized by absence of anti-GBM antibodies or immune complexes). Each type has a different cause and treatment. The presence of anti-GBM antibodies suggests Goodpasture syndrome; patients with this disorder require plasmapheresis. Type II crescentic glomerulonephritis can occur in systemic lupus erythematosus, in Henoch-Schönlein purpura, and after infections. Causes of type III crescentic glomerulonephritis include Wegener granulomatosis and microscopic polyangiitis. Immunofluorescence studies are critical for the classification and treatment of crescentic glomerulonephritis. A positive ANA test result may be reported in patients with lupus nephritis, which uncommonly manifests with glomerular crescents. HIV nephropathy has features similar to those of focal segmental glomerulosclerosis, which is not rapidly progressive. Quantitative serum immunoglobulins are not helpful, because the important consideration is the pattern of immune deposits in the kidney. Rheumatoid factor is present in rheumatoid arthritis, which is not associated with renal complications. Urine immunoelectrophoresis is useful in categorizing a monoclonal gammopathy.

BP7 523-524   BP6 452-453   PBD7 976-978
PBD6 951-952

54 **(G)** The rapid cell turnover in acute leukemias, and cell death from treatment, causes the release of purines from the cellular DNA breakdown. The resulting hyperuricemia can predispose to the formation of uric acid stones. Renal stones can produce colicky pain when they pass down the ureter and through the urethra, and the local trauma to the urothelium can produce hematuria. Uric acid stones form in acidic urine. Unlike stones containing calcium, uric acid stones are radiolucent and are not visible on a plain radiograph. The urine dipstick is sensitive to albumin, but not to globulins; therefore, a separate test for Bence-Jones protein may be positive, although the dipstick protein result is negative. However, Bence-Jones proteinuria is characteristic of multiple myeloma, not of leukemias or lymphomas. Eosinophils may appear in the urine in drug-induced interstitial nephritis. Myoglobin can cause the dipstick reagent for blood to become positive in the absence of RBCs or hemoglobin. Myoglobinuria results most often from rhabdomyolysis, which can occur after severe crush injuries. Oval fat bodies are sloughed tubular cells containing abundant lipid; they are characteristic of nephrotic syndromes. RBC casts appear in nephritic syndromes as a result of glomerular injury. Triple phosphate crystals are typical of infections with urease-positive bacteria, such as *Proteus*. Waxy casts form in dilated, damaged tubules. WBC casts alone are most indicative of acute pyelonephritis, but they can appear in conjunction with other cellular elements in severe glomerular injury.

BP7 537, 774   BP6 465   PBD7 1004-1005   PBD6 990

55 **(G)** Wegener granulomatosis causes rapidly progressive glomerulonephritis characterized by epithelial crescents in Bowman's space. Several features differentiate Wegener granulomatosis from other forms of crescentic glomerulonephritis (e.g., Goodpasture syndrome). These are the presence of granulomatous vasculitis, the absence of immune complexes or anti–glomerular basement membrane-(GBM) antibodies, and the presence of C-ANCA. Focal segmental glomerulosclerosis does not affect renal vessels and is unlikely to produce crescents with a rapidly progressive presentation. Goodpasture syndrome is a form of rapidly progressive glomerulonephritis with crescent formation, but a granulomatous vasculitis is not present, and there is anti-GBM antibody, not C-ANCA. Lupus nephritis, membranoproliferative glomerulonephritis, and postinfectious glomerulonephritis can occasionally have a rapidly progressive course with crescent formation, but they do not produce granulomatous vasculitis. In patients with lupus, the ANA test result is often positive. Membranous glomerulonephritis is most likely to produce nephrotic syndrome without crescents.

BP7 351-352, 524   BP6 452-453   PBD7 541-542, 977
PBD6 951-952

56 **(B)** Hyaline arteriosclerosis, characterized by thickening and hyalinization of small arteries and arterioles, is typically seen in patients with long-standing benign hypertension. Such a change also occurs with aging. Vascular narrowing causes ischemic changes that are slow and progressive. There is diffuse scarring and shrinkage of the kidneys. RBCs and RBC casts are a feature of crescentic glomerulonephritis, which typically is a rapidly progressive form of renal failure. Mesangial proliferation is a feature of some forms of glomerulonephritis. Fibrinoid necrosis in arterioles is seen in malignant hypertension. Acute tubular necrosis results from anoxic or toxic injury to the renal tubules. In interstitial nephritis, more cells would be seen in the urine sediment.

BP7 533   BP6 461   PBD7 1006-1007   PBD6 981-982

57 **(C)** This patient has malignant hypertension. Necrotizing arteriolitis and hyperplastic arteriolosclerosis are the distinctive vascular lesions of malignant hypertension. Papillary necrosis is more likely to complicate diabetic nephropathy or

analgesic nephropathy. Infarction of the kidney may result from emboli originating in the systemic circulation. However, malignant hypertension does not damage the large systemic vessels. Acute tubular necrosis is seen in hypoxic or toxic injury to the renal tubules. Acute pyelonephritis is a febrile illness, without severe blood pressure elevation.

BP7 533-534   BP6 461-462   PBD7 1007-1008
PBD6 982-984

58 **(C)** The combination of cysts in the kidney and berry aneurysms in the brain is characteristic of adult autosomal dominant polycystic kidney disease (DPKD). The cysts also may appear in the liver and pancreas. Because of the autosomal dominant pattern of inheritance, with high penetrance of the gene, first-degree relatives are at risk of having the same disorder and should be evaluated by ultrasound or other imaging techniques. This is particularly important, because many patients remain asymptomatic until the onset of renal failure as adults. Cocaine use can increase the risk of hemorrhages, but no hemorrhage was found in this case. The cause of death was cocaine intoxication. Autosomal recessive polycystic kidney disease is unlikely to remain asymptomatic from birth. Because the berry aneurysm had not ruptured, it was not the cause of death. About 1% of all persons have a berry aneurysm, whereas at least 10% of persons with DPKD have such an aneurysm. Most berry aneurysms, however, do not rupture. The patient did not die as a consequence of DPKD; had he lived, he might have developed complications from renal failure, leading to death decades later.

BP7 535-536   BP6 463-464   PBD7 962-964
PBD6 937-940

59 **(A)** The biopsy specimen shows sclerosis of only a segment of the glomerulus (segmental lesion), and because only 50% of the glomeruli are affected, this is focal disease. Focal segmental glomerulosclerosis manifests clinically with nephrotic syndrome that does not respond to corticosteroid therapy. In contrast, corticosteroid-responsive nephrotic syndrome in children is typically caused by minimal change disease (lipoid nephrosis); this disease is not associated with any glomerular change seen under the light microscope. Membranoproliferative glomerulonephritis of either type I or type II is more likely to produce a nephritic syndrome in adults. A diabetic patient with nephrotic syndrome is likely to have nodular glomerulosclerosis or diffuse thickening of the basement membrane. Sore throat (pharyngitis) followed by nephritic syndrome is the typical clinical history of acute proliferative poststreptococcal (postinfectious) glomerulonephritis. A rapidly progressive glomerulonephritis is associated with hematuria, and glomerular crescents are present.

BP7 520-521   BP6 449   PBD7 982-984   PBD6 956-958

60 **(C)** This patient has acute pyelonephritis. Vesicoureteral reflux, acquired or congenital, is extremely important in the pathogenesis of ascending urinary tract infections, because it allows bacteria to ascend from the urinary bladder into the ureter and the pelvis. In general, urinary tract infections are more common in females because of their shorter urethra, but in the absence of vesicoureteral reflux, the infections tend to remain localized in the urinary bladder. Older women and sexually active women are at increased risk of urinary tract infections. Hypertension can cause renal vascular narrowing and ultimately impair renal function, but it does not predispose to infections. Foci of infection in the lungs can seed the kidney hematogenously, but this route is far less common than ascending infection.

BP7 527-529   BP6 455-456   PBD7 997-998
PBD6 974-975

61 (D) This girl has hemolytic-uremic syndrome. Some strains of *Escherichia coli*, which can contaminate ground beef products, may elaborate a toxin that damages endothelium, causing this syndrome. Hemolytic-uremic syndrome most often occurs in children and is one of the most common causes of acute renal failure in children. Candidal urinary tract infections typically affect the urinary bladder. *Proteus* is a common cause of bacterial urinary tract infections. *Clostridium difficile* is best known for causing a pseudomembranous enterocolitis, not renal lesions. *Staphylococcus aureus* can cause urinary tract infections.

BP7 534-535   BP6 462-463   PBD7 1009-1011
PBD6 985-986

62 (E) This patient suffered muscle injury that resulted in myoglobinemia and myoglobinuria. The large amount of excreted myoglobin produces a toxic acute tubular necrosis. With supportive care, the tubular epithelium can regenerate, and renal function can be restored. During the recovery phase of acute tubular necrosis, patients excrete large volumes of urine, because the glomerular filtrate cannot be adequately reabsorbed by the damaged tubular epithelium. Trauma is not a cause of malignant hypertension. A bilateral renal vein thrombosis is not common. Glomerulonephritis does not occur as a result of trauma. An infection with pyelonephritis is unlikely to be characterized by such a short course or such a marked loss of renal function.

BP7 531-533   BP6 459-460   PBD7 993   PBD6 969-971

63 (C) This patient has malignant hypertension, which may follow long-standing benign hypertension. Two types of vascular lesions are found in malignant hypertension. Fibrinoid necrosis of the arterioles may be present; in addition, there is intimal thickening in interlobular arteries and arterioles, caused by proliferation of smooth muscle cells and collagen deposition. The proliferating smooth muscle cells are concentrically arranged, and these lesions, called hyperplastic arteriolosclerosis, cause severe narrowing of the lumen. The resultant ischemia elevates the renin level, which further promotes vasoconstriction to potentiate the injury. Nodular glomerulosclerosis is a feature of diabetes mellitus that slowly progresses over many years. Segmental tubular necrosis occurs in ischemic forms of acute tubular necrosis. An IgA nephropathy involves glomeruli but not typically the interstitium or vasculature. Glomerular crescents are a feature of a rapidly progressive glomerulonephritis; however, the blood pressure elevation is not as marked as that seen in this patient.

BP7 533-534   BP6 461-462   PBD7 1007-1008
PBD6 982-984

64 (A) The figure shows a high-grade transitional cell carcinoma of the bladder. Cigarette smoking is the greatest risk factor in half of all men with such cancers. Schistosomiasis is also a risk factor for bladder cancer, although typically for squamous cell carcinoma. The increased risk of infection that occurs in both diabetes mellitus and prostatic hyperplasia, with the resultant acute and chronic cystitis, does not predispose to transitional cell carcinoma.

BP7 541-542   BP6 468-469   PBD7 1028-1032
PBD6 1004-1007

65 (C) This patient has type II membranoproliferative glomerulonephritis, or dense-deposit disease, which usually leads to chronic renal failure. Postinfectious glomerulonephritis is often characterized by a hypercellular glomerulus with infiltration of polymorphonuclear leukocytes but no basement membrane thickening. A rapidly progressive glomerulonephritis is marked by crescents. The term "chronic glomerulonephritis" often is used when sclerosis of many glomeruli is present with no clear cause. Membranous glomerulonephritis is characterized by thickening of only the basement membrane and small electron-dense deposits.

BP7 521-522   BP6 450-451   PBD7 984-986
PBD6 958-960

66 (A) Clear cell carcinoma, the most common form of kidney cancer, often presents with painless hematuria, most often in persons in the 6th or 7th decade. Approximately 80% of sporadic clear cell carcinomas show loss of both alleles of the *VHL* gene. Germ-line inheritance of the *VHL* mutation can give rise to von Hippel Lindau syndrome, with peak incidence of renal cell carcinoma in the 4th decade, and they may have other tumors including cerebellar and retinal hemangioblastomas and adrenal pheochromocytomas. Mutation of the *MET* gene on chromosome 7 is associated with the papillary variant of renal cell carcinoma. HPV-16 infection is associated with carcinomas of the uterine cervix. Microsatellite instability is a feature of the Lynch syndrome, also called hereditary non-polyposis colon cancer (HNPCC) syndrome characterized by right-sided colon cancer and, in some cases, endometrial cancer.

BP7 539-540   PBD7 1016-1018

67 (B) Corticosteroid-resistant hematuria and proteinuria in a Hispanic male leading to hypertension and renal failure is typical for focal segmental glomerulosclerosis (FSGS). FSGS is now the most common cause of nephrotic syndrome in adults in the U.S. Specialized extracellular areas overlying the glomerular basement membrane between adjacent foot processes of podocytes are called slit diaphragms, and these exert control over glomerular permeability. Mutations in genes affecting several proteins including nephrin and podocin have been found in inherited cases of FSGS, and their dysfunction, possibly caused by cytokines or unknown toxic factors, is believed to be responsible for the acquired cases of FSGS. FSGS is also seen in patients with HIV-associated nephropathy. Immune complexes containing microbial antigens give rise to postinfectious glomerulonephritis. Anti-GBM antibodies are responsible for Goodpasture syndrome. Inherited defects in basement membrane collagen give rise to Alport syndrome, also characterized by hematuria, but other congenital abnormalities such as deafness are often present, and nephrotic syndrome is uncommon. C3NeF is an autoantibody directed against C3 convertase, and it is seen in MPGN type II.

PBD7 959, 973

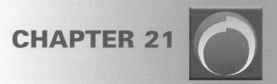

The Male Genital Tract

1 A 30-year-old man comes to his physician because he has noticed increasing enlargement and a feeling of heaviness in his scrotum for the past year. On physical examination, the right testis is twice its normal size, and it is firm and slightly tender. An ultrasound examination shows a 3.5-cm solid mass in the right testis. An abdominal CT scan shows enlargement of the para-aortic lymph nodes. Multiple lung nodules are seen on a chest radiograph. Laboratory findings include markedly increased serum levels of chorionic gonadotropin and α-fetoprotein. Which of the following testicular neoplasms is the most likely diagnosis?

❏ (A) Leydig cell tumor
❏ (B) Mixed germ cell tumor
❏ (C) Pure spermatocytic seminoma
❏ (D) Choriocarcinoma
❏ (E) Metastatic adenocarcinoma of the prostate gland
❏ (F) Large diffuse B-cell lymphoma

2 For the past year, a 65-year-old man has had multiple, recurrent urinary tract infections. *Escherichia coli* and streptococcal organisms have been cultured from his urine during several of these episodes, with bacterial counts of more than 10^5/mL. He has difficulty with urination, including starting and stopping the urinary stream. Over the past week, he has again developed burning pain with urination. Urinalysis shows a pH of 6.5 and specific gravity of 1.020. No blood or protein is present in the urine. Tests for leukocyte esterase and nitrite are positive. Microscopic examination of the urine shows numerous WBCs and a few WBC casts. Which of the following is the most likely diagnosis?

❏ (A) *Neisseria gonorrhoeae* infection
❏ (B) Prostatic nodular hyperplasia
❏ (C) Phimosis
❏ (D) Epispadias
❏ (E) Adenocarcinoma of the prostate gland
❏ (F) Vesicoureteral reflux

3 A 35-year-old man has noticed a slight enlargement of the right testis over the past 3 months. He has also noticed bilateral breast enlargement over the past 6 months. On physical examination, the right testis is about 1.5 times larger than the left testis. Both testes are firm and normal to the touch. An ultrasound scan shows a discrete, rounded 2-cm mass in the body of the right testis, and a right orchiectomy is performed. The mass has a grossly uniform, brown cut surface. Ten years later, the patient is healthy. Which of the following descriptions best explains the microscopic appearance of this testicular mass?

- ❑ (A) Back-to-back irregular glands lined by cells with nuclei containing prominent nucleoli
- ❑ (B) Large monomorphic lymphoid cells with scant cytoplasm, clumped chromatin, and prominent nucleoli
- ❑ (C) Diffuse suppurative inflammation with gram-negative rods identified on Gram-stained smear
- ❑ (D) Full-thickness epithelial dysplasia with an intact underlying basement membrane
- ❑ (E) Islands of cartilage, squamous epithelial pearls, and glands lined by tall columnar epithelium
- ❑ (F) Nests of large polyhedral cells with watery cytoplasm and large nuclei with prominent nucleoli, surrounded by a lymphoid stroma
- ❑ (G) Rounded cells with abundant granular eosinophilic cytoplasm containing crystalloids of Reinke
- ❑ (H) Syncytiotrophoblast and cytotrophoblast arranged in sheets, with extensive hemorrhage and necrosis

4 A 23-year-old sexually active man has been treated for *Neisseria gonorrhoeae* infection several times during the past 5 years. He now comes to the physician because of the increasing number and size of warty lesions on his external genitalia. The lesions have enlarged slowly during the past year. On physical examination, there are multiple 1- to 3-mm sessile, nonulcerated, papillary excrescences over the inner surface of the penile prepuce. These lesions are excised, but 2 years later, similar lesions appear. Which of the following descriptions best explains the microscopic appearance of the lesions?

- ❑ (A) Edema with inflammatory infiltrates composed of neutrophils, macrophages, and lymphocytes
- ❑ (B) Diffuse suppurative inflammation with gram-negative rods identified by Gram-stained smear
- ❑ (C) Full-thickness epithelial dysplasia with an intact underlying basement membrane
- ❑ (D) Rounded cells with abundant granular eosinophilic cytoplasm containing crystalloids of Reinke
- ❑ (E) Syncytiotrophoblast and cytotrophoblast arranged in sheets, with extensive hemorrhage and necrosis
- ❑ (F) Thickened squamous epithelium with acanthosis, koilocytosis, and overlying hyperkeratosis

5 A 55-year-old man has dysuria, increased frequency, and urgency of urination for the past 6 months. He has sometimes experienced mild lower back pain. On physical examination, he is afebrile. There is no costovertebral angle tenderness. The prostate gland feels normal in size; no nodules are palpable. Laboratory studies show that expressed prostatic secretions contain 30 leukocytes per high-power field. Which of the following is the most likely diagnosis?

- ❑ (A) Benign prostatic hyperplasia
- ❑ (B) Acute bacterial prostatitis
- ❑ (C) Syphilitic prostatitis
- ❑ (D) Chronic abacterial prostatitis
- ❑ (E) Metastatic prostatic adenocarcinoma

6 A 32-year-old man has noticed an increased feeling of heaviness in his scrotum for the past 10 months. On physical examination, the left testis is three times the size of the right testis and is firm on palpation. An ultrasound scan shows a 6-cm solid mass within the body of the left testis. Laboratory studies include an elevated serum α-fetoprotein level. Which of the following cellular components is most likely to be present in this mass?

- ❑ (A) Yolk sac cells
- ❑ (B) Leydig cells
- ❑ (C) Seminoma cells
- ❑ (D) Cytotrophoblasts
- ❑ (E) Embryonal carcinoma cells
- ❑ (F) Lymphoblasts

7 A 25-year-old man has occasionally felt pain in the scrotum for the past 3 months. On physical examination, the right testis is more tender than the left but does not appear to be appreciably enlarged. An ultrasound scan shows a 1.5-cm mass. A right orchiectomy is performed, and gross examination shows the mass to be hemorrhagic and soft. A retroperitoneal lymph node dissection is performed. In sections of the lymph nodes, a neoplasm is seen with grossly extensive necrosis and hemorrhage. Microscopic examination shows that areas of viable tumor are composed of cuboidal cells intermingled with large eosinophilic syncytial cells containing multiple dark, pleomorphic nuclei. Immunohistochemical staining of the tumor is most likely to show which of the following antigenic components in the syncytial cells?

- ❑ (A) Human chorionic gonadotropin
- ❑ (B) α-Fetoprotein
- ❑ (C) Vimentin
- ❑ (D) CD20
- ❑ (E) Testosterone
- ❑ (F) Carcinoembryonic antigen
- ❑ (G) Cancer antigen 125

8 A 70-year-old man comes to his physician for a routine health examination. On palpation, his prostate is normal in size. However, laboratory studies show a serum prostate-specific antigen (PSA) level of 17 ng/mL, four times the upper limit of normal and twice the value reported 1 year ago in this patient. A routine urinalysis shows no abnormalities. The patient is healthy, with no history of major illnesses. Which of the following histologic findings in a subsequent biopsy of the prostate is most likely to account for the patient's current status?

- ❑ (A) Hyperplastic nodules of the stroma and glands lined by two layers of epithelium
- ❑ (B) Poorly differentiated glands lined by a single layer of epithelium and packed back to back
- ❑ (C) Foci of chronic inflammatory cells in the stroma and in normal-appearing glands
- ❑ (D) Areas of liquefactive necrosis filled with neutrophils
- ❑ (E) Multiple caseating granulomas

9 A 35-year-old man and his 33-year-old wife are childless. They have tried to conceive a child for 12 years and believe that time is running out for them. They undergo an infertility workup. On physical examination, neither spouse has any remarkable findings. Laboratory studies show that the man has a sperm count in the low-normal range. On microscopic examination of the seminal fluid, the sperm have a normal morphologic appearance. A testicular biopsy is performed. The biopsy shows patchy atrophy of seminiferous tubules, but the remaining tubules show active spermatogenesis. Which of the following disorders is the most likely cause of these findings?

- (A) Mumps virus infection
- (B) Cryptorchidism
- (C) Hydrocele
- (D) Klinefelter syndrome
- (E) Prior chemotherapy

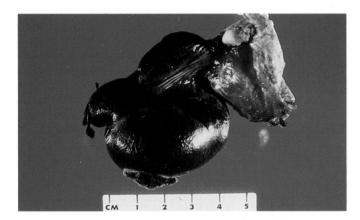

10 A 25-year-old previously healthy man suddenly develops severe pain in the scrotum. The pain continues unabated for 6 hours, and he goes to the emergency department. On physical examination, he is afebrile. There is exquisite tenderness of a slightly enlarged right testis, but there are no other remarkable findings. The gross appearance of the right testis is shown in the figure above. Which of the following conditions is most likely to cause these findings?

- (A) Local invasion by a testicular tumor
- (B) Parasitic infestation of the scrotum
- (C) Obstruction of blood flow
- (D) Obstruction of lymph flow
- (E) Dissemination of tuberculosis from the lungs to the testis

11 The mother of a 2-year-old child notices that he has had increasing asymmetric enlargement of the scrotum over the past 6 months. On physical examination, there is a well-circumscribed 2.5-cm mass in the left testis. Histologic examination of this mass shows sheets of cells and ill-defined glands composed of cuboidal cells, some of which contain eosinophilic hyaline globules. Microcysts and primitive glomeruloid structures also are seen. Immunohistochemical staining shows α-fetoprotein in the cytoplasm of the neoplastic cells. Which of the following is the most likely diagnosis?

- (A) Choriocarcinoma
- (B) Seminoma
- (C) Yolk sac tumor
- (D) Teratoma
- (E) Leydig cell tumor

12 A 19-year-old man comes to his physician complaining of worsening local pain and irritation with difficult urination over the past 3 years. He has become more sexually active during the past year and describes his erections as painful. Physical examination shows that he is not circumcised. The prepuce (foreskin) cannot be easily retracted over the glans penis. Which of the following is the most likely diagnosis?

- (A) Epispadias
- (B) Bowenoid papulosis
- (C) Phimosis
- (D) Genital candidiasis
- (E) Paraphimosis

13 A 19-year-old man comes to his physician for a routine health maintenance examination. On physical examination, there is no left testis palpable in the scrotum. The patient is healthy, has had no major illnesses, and has normal sexual function. In counseling this patient, which of the following statements regarding his condition would be most appropriate?

- (A) You will be unable to father children
- (B) You are at increased risk of developing a testicular tumor
- (C) This is a common finding in more than half of all men
- (D) This is an outcome of childhood mumps infection
- (E) This is an inherited disorder

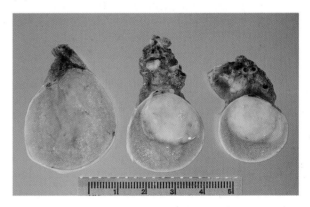

14 A 29-year-old man complains of a vague feeling of heaviness in the scrotum, but he has had no increase in pain for the past 5 months. He is otherwise healthy. Physical examination shows that the right testis is slightly larger than the left testis. An ultrasound scan shows the presence of a solid, circumscribed, 1.5-cm mass in the body of the right testis. The representative gross appearance of the mass is shown above. A biopsy is performed, and microscopic examination of the mass shows uniform nests of cells with distinct cell borders, glycogen-rich cytoplasm, and round nuclei with prominent nucleoli. There are aggregates of lymphocytes between these nests of cells. Which of the following features is most characteristic of this lesion?

- (A) Excellent response to radiation therapy
- (B) Likelihood of extensive metastases early in the course of disease
- (C) Elevation of human chorionic gonadotropin levels in the serum
- (D) Elevation of α-fetoprotein levels in the serum
- (E) Elevation of serum testosterone levels
- (F) Association with 46,X(fra)Y karyotype
- (G) Association with 46,XXY karyotype

15 A 5-year-old boy has a history of recurrent urinary tract infections. Urine cultures have grown *Escherichia coli, Proteus mirabilis*, and enterococcus. Physical examination now shows an abnormal constricted opening of the urethra on the ventral aspect of the penis, about 1.5 cm from the tip of the glans penis. There is also a cryptorchid testis on the right and an inguinal hernia on the left. Which of the following terms best describes the child's penile abnormality?

❑ (A) Hypospadias
❑ (B) Phimosis
❑ (C) Balanitis
❑ (D) Epispadias
❑ (E) Bowen disease

16 A 46-year-old man with a history of poorly controlled diabetes mellitus comes to the physician because he has had painful, erosive, markedly pruritic lesions on the glans penis, scrotum, and inguinal regions of the skin for the past 2 months. Physical examination shows irregular, shallow 1- to 4-cm erythematous ulcerations. Scrapings of the lesions are examined under the microscope. Which of the following microscopic findings in the scrapings is most likely to be reported?

❑ (A) Eggs and excrement of *Sarcoptes scabiei*
❑ (B) Budding cells with pseudohyphae
❑ (C) Atypical cells with hyperchromatic nuclei
❑ (D) Enlarged cells with intranuclear inclusions
❑ (E) Spirochetes under darkfield examination

17 A clinical trial of two pharmacologic agents compares one agent that inhibits 5α-reductase and diminishes dihydrotestosterone (DHT) synthesis in the prostate with another agent that acts as an α₁-adrenergic receptor. The subjects are 40 to 80 years of age. The study will determine whether symptoms of prostate disease are ameliorated in the persons who take these drugs. Which of the following diseases of the prostate is most likely to benefit from one or both of these drugs?

❑ (A) Acute prostatitis
❑ (B) Adenocarcinoma
❑ (C) Leiomyoma
❑ (D) Chronic prostatitis
❑ (E) Nodular hyperplasia

18 A 33-year-old man has noted asymmetric enlargement of the scrotum over the past 4 months. On physical examination, the right testis is twice its normal size and has increased tenderness to palpation. The right testis is removed. The epididymis and the upper aspect of the right testis have extensive granulomatous inflammation with epithelioid cells, Langhans giant cells, and caseous necrosis. Which of the following is the most likely cause of these findings?

❑ (A) Mumps
❑ (B) Syphilis
❑ (C) Tuberculosis
❑ (D) Gonorrhea
❑ (E) Sarcoidosis

19 A 48-year-old man has noticed a reddish area on the penis for the past 3 months. He has had no episodes of sexual intercourse for more than 1 month. On physical examination, there is a solitary 0.8-cm plaquelike, erythematous area on the distal shaft of the penis. A routine microbiologic culture with a Gram-stained smear of the lesion shows normal skin flora. Microscopic examination of a biopsy specimen of the lesion shows dysplasia involving the full thickness of the epithelium. Which of the following is the most likely diagnosis?

❑ (A) Primary syphilis
❑ (B) Balanitis
❑ (C) Soft chancre
❑ (D) Bowen disease
❑ (E) Condyloma acuminatum

20 An 85-year-old man comes to the physician because he had had urinary hesitancy and nocturia for the past year. He has had increasing back pain for the past 6 months. On digital rectal examination, there is a hard, irregular prostate gland. A bone scan shows increased areas of uptake in the thoracic and lumbar vertebrae. Laboratory studies show a serum alkaline phosphatase level of 300 U/L, serum prostatic acid phosphatase level of 8 ng/mL, and serum prostate-specific antigen (PSA) level of 72 ng/mL. The blood urea nitrogen concentration is 44 mg/dL, and the serum creatinine level is 3.8 mg/dL. Transrectal biopsies of all lobes of the prostate are performed. Microscopic examination shows that over 90% of the tissue has a pattern of cords and sheets of cells with hyperchromatic pleomorphic nuclei, prominent nuclei, and scant cytoplasm. Which of the following is the best classification for this patient's disease?

	Stage	Gleason grade
❑ (A)	A1	1,1
❑ (B)	A2	1,2
❑ (C)	B1	2,3
❑ (D)	B2	3,3
❑ (E)	C1	3,4
❑ (F)	C2	4,4
❑ (G)	D1	4,5
❑ (H)	D2	5,5

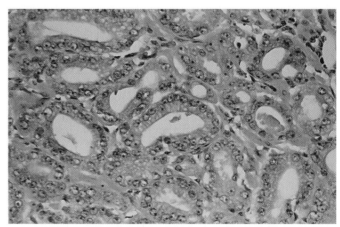

Courtesy of Dr. Kyle Molberg, Department of Pathology, University of Texas Southwestern Medical Center, Dallas, TX.

21 A 63-year-old man comes to the physician for a routine health maintenance examination. On physical examination, there are no remarkable findings. Laboratory findings include serum creatinine of 1.1 mg/dL, urea nitrogen 17 mg/dL, glucose 76 mg/dL, alkaline phosphatase 89 U/L, and prostate-specific antigen (PSA) 8 ng/mL. The patient is referred to a urologist, who performs transurethral prostate biopsies. The high-power microscopic appearance of a biopsy specimen is shown in the preceding figure. Which of the following complications is most likely to develop if the disease is untreated?

- ❏ (A) Destructive vertebral lesions
- ❏ (B) Recurrent urinary tract infections
- ❏ (C) Hydronephrosis
- ❏ (D) Gram-negative bacteremia
- ❏ (E) Sterility

22 A 59-year-old man notices gradual enlargement of the scrotum over the course of 1 year. The growth is not painful but produces a sensation of heaviness. He has no problems with sexual function. Physical examination shows no lesions of the overlying scrotal skin and no obvious masses, but the scrotum is enlarged, boggy, and soft bilaterally. The transillumination test result is positive. Which of the following is the most likely diagnosis?

- ❏ (A) Varicocele
- ❏ (B) Elephantiasis
- ❏ (C) Orchitis
- ❏ (D) Seminoma
- ❏ (E) Hydrocele

23 An otherwise healthy 72-year-old man has had increasing difficulty with urination for the past 10 years. He now has to get up several times each night because of a feeling of urgency, but each time the urine volume is not great. He has difficulty starting and stopping urination. On physical examination, the prostate is enlarged to twice its normal size but is not tender to palpation. One year ago, his serum prostate-specific antigen (PSA) level was 6 ng/mL, and it is still at that level when retested. Which of the following findings is most likely to be seen microscopically in a biopsy specimen of the prostate gland?

- ❏ (A) Hyperplastic nodules of stroma and glands lined by two layers of epithelium
- ❏ (B) Poorly differentiated glands lined by a single layer of epithelium and packed back to back
- ❏ (C) Foci of chronic inflammatory cells in the stroma and in normal-appearing glands
- ❏ (D) Areas of liquefactive necrosis filled with neutrophils
- ❏ (E) Multiple areas of caseating granulomatous inflammation

24 Over the past 9 months, a 30-year-old man has noticed increased heaviness with enlargement of the scrotum. On physical examination, there is an enlarged, firm left testis but no other remarkable findings. An ultrasound scan shows a 5-cm solid mass within the body of the left testis. An orchiectomy of the left testis is performed. Microscopic examination of the mass shows areas of mature cartilage, keratinizing squamous epithelium, and colonic glandular epithelium. Laboratory findings include elevated levels of serum human chorionic gonadotropin (hCG) and α-fetoprotein (AFP). Despite the appearance of the cells in the tumor, the surgeon tells the patient that he probably has a malignant testicular tumor. The surgeon's conclusion is most likely to be based on which of the following factors?

- ❏ (A) Size of the tumor
- ❏ (B) Age of the patient
- ❏ (C) Presence of colonic glandular epithelium
- ❏ (D) Elevation of hCG and AFP levels
- ❏ (E) Location of the mass in the left testis

25 A 71-year-old currently healthy man comes to his physician for a checkup because he is worried about his family history of prostate cancer. Physical examination does not indicate any abnormalities. Because of the patient's age and family history, his prostate-specific antigen (PSA) level is immediately measured, and the PSA level is 5 ng/mL. Six months later, the PSA test yields 6 ng/mL. A urologist performs transrectal biopsies, and microscopic examination shows multifocal areas of prostatic intraepithelial neoplasia as well as glandular hyperplasia. Based on these findings, which of the following is the most appropriate course of management for this patient?

- ❏ (A) Antibiotic therapy
- ❏ (B) Monitoring PSA levels
- ❏ (C) Multiagent chemotherapy
- ❏ (D) Radiation therapy
- ❏ (E) Radical prostatectomy
- ❏ (F) Transurethral prostate resection

ANSWERS

1 **(B)** Although a modest elevation of the human chorionic gonadotropin (hCG) concentration can occur when a seminoma contains some syncytial giant cells, significant elevation of the α-fetoprotein (AFP) level never occurs with pure seminomas. Elevated levels of AFP and hCG effectively exclude the diagnosis of a pure seminoma and indicate the presence of a nonseminomatous tumor of the mixed type. The most common form of testicular neoplasm combines multiple elements; thus the term "teratocarcinoma" is sometimes used to describe tumors with elements of teratoma, embryonal carcinoma, and yolk sac tumor. The yolk sac element explains the high AFP level. Mixed tumors may include seminoma. Leydig cell tumors are non–germ cell tumors derived from the interstitial (Leydig) cells; they may elaborate androgens. Choriocarcinomas secrete high levels of hCG but no AFP. It is unusual for a tumor to metastasize to the testis; this patient is of an age at which a primary cancer of the testis should be considered when a testicular mass is present. Lymphomas may involve the testis, usually when there is systemic involvement by a high-grade lesion. Lymphomas do not elaborate hormones.

BP7 661-664   BP6 583-584   PBD7 1041-1042, 1046
PBD6 1018-1023

2 **(B)** Of the diseases listed, prostatic nodular hyperplasia is the most common in older adult men. When it causes obstruction of the prostatic urethra, it can predispose to bacterial infections. Gonorrhea is more likely to be seen in younger, sexually active males, and obstruction is not a key feature. Phimosis can occur in uncircumcised males. It may be congenital or acquired from inflammation, usually at a much younger age. Epispadias is a congenital condition, observed at birth. Prostatic adenocarcinomas are less likely than hyperplasia to cause obstructive symptoms. Vesicoureteral reflux is more likely to be present at an earlier age, and it does not account for the obstructive symptoms the patient has on urination.

BP7 665-666   BP6 585-586   PBD7 1048-1050
PBD6 1028-1029

3 **(G)** The patient has a Leydig cell tumor of the testis. These tumors are most often small benign masses that may go unnoticed. Some patients, however, have gynecomastia caused by androgenic or estrogenic hormone production (or both) by the tumor. Most patients are young to middle-aged men; sexual precocity may occur in the few boys who have such tumors. A back-to-back glandular pattern is seen in prostatic adenocarcinomas. A monomorphous proliferation of large lymphoid cells characterizes a non-Hodgkin lymphoma. Diffuse suppurative inflammation indicates an infection, which should make the mass very tender; acute orchitis is uncommon. Epithelial dysplasia may be seen involving transitional or squamous epithelial surfaces. Elements of the three primary germ layers, with cartilage, squamous epithelium, and glands, are seen in teratomas. The polyhedral cells in a lymphoid stroma are seen in a seminoma. Syncytiotrophoblast and cytotrophoblast are elements of choriocarcinoma.

PBD7 1046   PBD6 1024

4 **(F)** The patient's lesions are characteristic of condyloma acuminata, which is typical of human papillomavirus (HPV) infection. A condyloma acuminatum is a benign, recurrent squamous epithelial proliferation resulting from infection with HPV, one of many sexually transmitted diseases that can occur in sexually active persons. Koilocytosis is particularly characteristic of HPV infection. Recurrent gonococcal infection indicates that the patient is sexually active. Gonococcal infection causes suppurative lesions in which there may be liquefactive necrosis and a neutrophilic exudate or mixed inflammatory infiltrates with chancroid. Epithelial dysplasia is not present in a condyloma acuminatum. Rounded cells with crystalloids of Reinke typify a Leydig cell tumor of the testis. Syncytiotrophoblast and cytotrophoblast are elements of choriocarcinoma of the testis.

BP7 677   BP6 596   PBD7 1035-1036   PBD6 1012-1013

5 **(D)** The patient has more than 10 leukocytes per high-power field, indicating prostatitis. Chronic abacterial prostatitis is the most common form of the disorder. Patients typically do not have a history of recurrent urinary tract infections. Nodular prostatic hyperplasia by itself is not an inflammatory process. Patients with acute bacterial prostatitis, most often caused by *Escherichia coli* infection, have fever, chills, and dysuria; on rectal examination, the prostate is very tender. Syphilis is a disease of the external genitalia, although the testis may be involved. Prostate carcinomas generally do not have a significant amount of acute inflammation, and metastases are most often associated with pain; most prostatic conditions causing dysuria are benign.

BP7 664-665   BP6 584-585   PBD7 1047-1048
PBD6 1026

6 **(A)** α-Fetoprotein (AFP) is a product of yolk sac cells that can be demonstrated by immunohistochemical testing. Pure yolk sac tumors are rare in adults, but yolk sac components are common in mixed nonseminomatous tumors.

Leydig cells produce androgens. Pure seminomas do not produce AFP. Cytotrophoblasts do not produce a serum marker, but they may be present in a choriocarcinoma along with syncytiotrophoblasts, which do produce human chorionic gonadotropin. Embryonal carcinoma cells by themselves do not produce any specific marker. However, embryonal carcinoma cells are common in nonseminomatous tumors and are often mixed with other cell types. Lymphoblasts may be seen in high-grade non-Hodgkin lymphomas, which do not produce hormones.

BP7 661-664   BP6 584   PBD7 1043, 1045
PBD6 1020-1021

7 **(A)** This patient has a choriocarcinoma, the most aggressive testicular carcinoma. It often metastasizes widely. The primitive syncytial cells mimic the syncytiotrophoblast of placental tissue and, therefore, stain for human chorionic gonadotropin. α-Fetoprotein is a marker that is more likely to be found in mixed tumors with a yolk sac component. Vimentin is more likely to be seen in sarcomas, which are rare in the testicular region. CD20 is a lymphoid marker for B cells. Testosterone is found in Leydig cells. Carcinoembryonic antigen (CEA) is found in a variety of epithelial neoplasms, particularly adenocarcinomas. Cancer antigen 125 (CA-125) is best known as a marker for ovarian epithelial malignant tumors.

BP7 661-664   BP6 581-584   PBD7 1043-1044, 1046
PBD6 2021

8 **(B)** The prostate-specific antigen (PSA) level is significantly elevated in this patient. The increase over time is more likely to be indicative of carcinoma. Typically, prostatic carcinomas are adenocarcinomas that form small glands packed back to back; unlike hyperplastic glands, malignant glands are lined by a single layer of epithelium. Many adenocarcinomas of the prostate do not produce obstructive symptoms and may not be palpable on digital rectal examination. Hyperplasias can increase the PSA level, although not to a high level that increases significantly over time. Prostatitis, like hyperplasia, can elevate the PSA level slightly.

BP7 667-669   BP6 586-588   PBD7 1054-1056
PBD6 1022-1023

9 **(A)** Mumps is a common childhood infection that can produce parotitis. Adults who have this infection more often develop orchitis. The orchitis is usually not severe, and its involvement of the testis is patchy; therefore, infertility is not a common outcome. Cryptorchidism results from failure of the testis to descend into the scrotum normally; the abnormally positioned testis becomes atrophic throughout. A hydrocele is a fluid collection outside the body of the testis that does not interfere with spermatogenesis. Klinefelter syndrome and estrogen therapy can cause tubular atrophy, although it is generalized in both cases. Patchy loss of seminiferous tubules indicates a local inflammatory process. Many chemotherapeutic agents are particularly harmful to rapidly and continuously proliferating testicular germ cells, but the effect would not be patchy within the testicular parenchyma. Patients who wish to father children may want to store sperm in a sperm bank before undergoing chemotherapy.

BP7 660   BP6 580   PBD7 1039   PBD6 1017

10 **(C)** The markedly hemorrhagic appearance results from testicular torsion that obstructs venous outflow to a greater extent than the arterial supply. Doppler ultrasound shows reduced or no vascular flow in the affected testis. An abnormally positioned or anchored testis in the scrotum is a risk factor for this condition. Testicular cancers do not obstruct the blood flow. Parasitic infestation, typically filariasis, obstructs the flow of lymph, leading to gradual enlargement of the scrotum with thickening of the overlying skin. Tuberculosis can spread from the lung through the bloodstream, producing miliary tuberculosis, seen as multiple pale, millet-sized lesions. Isolated spread to the epididymis or testis can also occur, but it does not cause vascular obstruction.

PBD7 1040   PBD6 1017

11 **(C)** Yolk sac tumors are typically seen in boys younger than 3 years of age. The primitive glomeruloid structures are known as Schiller-Duval bodies. Choriocarcinomas contain large, hyperchromatic, syncytiotrophoblastic cells. Seminomas have sheets and nests of cells resembling primitive germ cells, often with an intervening lymphoid stroma. Teratomas contain elements of mature cartilage, bone, or other endodermal, mesodermal, or ectodermal structures. Embryonal carcinomas with yolk sac cells contain α-fetoprotein, but they are seen in adults. They are composed of cords and sheets of primitive cells. Leydig cell tumors may produce androgens or estrogens, or both.

BP7 661-664   BP6 581-584   PBD7 1043-1044
PBD6 1019-1021

12 **(C)** Phimosis can be congenital but is more often a consequence of multiple episodes of balanitis (inflammation of the glans penis or foreskin). Balanitis leads to scarring that prevents retraction of the foreskin. Forcible retraction may result in vascular compromise, with further inflammation and swelling (paraphimosis). Epispadias is a congenital condition in which the penile urethra opens onto the dorsal surface of the penis. Bowenoid papulosis is a premalignant lesion of the penile shaft resulting from viral infection. Candidiasis is most likely to produce shallow ulcerations that are intensely pruritic.

BP7 658   BP6 578   PBD7 1035   PBD6 1012

13 **(B)** This patient has cryptorchidism, which results from failure of the testis to descend from the abdominal cavity into the scrotum during fetal development. One or both testes may be involved. It is associated with an increased risk of testicular cancer. An undescended testis eventually atrophies during childhood. Unilateral cryptorchidism usually does not lead to infertility, but it may be associated with atrophy of the contralateral descended testis. Mumps infection tends to produce patchy testicular atrophy, usually without infertility. Isolated cryptorchidism is a developmental defect that is usually sporadic and is not inherited in the germ line.

BP7 659-660   BP6 580   PBD7 1037-1038
PBD6 1015-1016

14 **(A)** This is the most common form of "pure" testicular germ cell tumor that may remain confined to the testis (stage I). The prognosis is good in most cases, even with metastases, because seminomas are radiosensitive. The human chorionic gonadotropin (hCG) levels may be slightly elevated in about 15% of patients with seminoma. Elevated hCG levels suggest a component of syncytial cells; very high levels suggest choriocarcinoma. α-Fetoprotein levels are elevated in testicular tumors with a yolk sac component, and many tumors with an embryonal cell component also contain yolk sac cells. Testosterone is a product of Leydig cells, not germ cells. Fragile X syndrome is associated with mental retardation. The testes are enlarged bilaterally. Klinefelter syndrome is associated with decreased testicular size and reduced fertility.

BP7 661-664   BP6 581-583   PBD7 1040-1042
PBD6 1018-1020

15 **(A)** Hypospadias is a congenital condition seen in about 1 in 300 male infants. The inguinal hernia and the cryptorchidism are abnormalities that may accompany this condition. Phimosis is a constriction preventing retraction of the prepuce. It can be congenital but more likely is the result of inflammation of the foreskin of the penis (e.g., balanitis, a form of local inflammation of the glans penis). Epispadias is a congenital condition in which the urethra opens on the dorsal aspect of the penis. Bowen disease, which is squamous cell carcinoma in situ of the penis, occurs in adults.

BP7 658   BP6 578   PBD7 1035   PBD6 1012

16 **(B)** Genital candidiasis can occur in persons without underlying illnesses, but it is far more common in those with diabetes mellitus. Warm, moist conditions at these sites favor fungal growth. Scabies mites are more likely to be found in linear burrows in epidermis scraped from the extremities. Neoplasms may ulcerate, but such lesions are unlikely to be shallow or multiple without a mass lesion present. Intranuclear inclusions suggest a viral infection; however, diabetes is not a risk factor for genital viral infections. These lesions are too large and numerous to be syphilitic chancres.

BP7 658   BP6 578   PBD7 1035   PBD6 1012

17 **(E)** Androgens are the major hormonal stimuli of glandular and stromal proliferation resulting in nodular prostatic hyperplasia. Although testosterone production decreases with age, prostatic hyperplasia increases, probably because of an increased expression of hormonal receptors that enhance the effect of any dihydrotestosterone (DHT) that is present. The 5α-reductase inhibitors, such as finasteride, diminish the prostate volume, specifically the glandular component, leading to improved urine flow. However, the $α_1$-adrenergic receptor blockers, such as tamsulosin, cause smooth muscle in the bladder neck and prostate to relax, which relieves symptoms and improves urine flow immediately. The other listed conditions are not amenable to therapy with these drugs.

BP7 665-666   BP6 585   PBD7 1048-1049   PBD6 1027

18 **(C)** Tuberculosis is an uncommon infection in the testes, but it can occur with disseminated disease. The infection typically starts in the epididymis and spreads to the body of the testis. Mumps produces patchy orchitis with minimal inflammation, which heals with patchy fibrosis. Syphilis involves the body of the testis, and there can be gummatous inflammation with neutrophils, necrosis, and some mononuclear cells. Gonococcal infections produce acute inflammation. Sarcoidosis produces noncaseating granulomas that are not likely to be found in the testis.

BP7 660   BP6 580   PBD7 1039   PBD6 1016-1017

19 **(D)** Bowen disease is a form of squamous cell carcinoma in situ. Like carcinoma in situ elsewhere, it has a natural history of progression to invasive cancer if untreated. Poor hygiene and infection with human papillomavirus (particularly types 16 and 18) are factors that favor development of dysplasias and cancer of the genital epithelia. Syphilis is a sexually transmitted disease that produces a hard chancre, which heals in a matter of weeks. Balanitis is an inflammatory condition without dysplasia. A soft chancre may be seen with *Haemophilus ducreyi* infections. Condylomas are raised, whitish lesions.

BP7 658   BP6 578   PBD7 1036   PBD6 1013-1014

20 **(H)** The presence of a hard irregular nodule, along with the extremely high prostate-specific antigen (PSA) level, points most clearly to prostate carcinoma. Modest elevations of the PSA concentration can occur in nodular hyperplasia of the prostate and prostatitis. Symptoms of urinary obstruction are more prominent in nodular hyperplasia because the nodules are in the periurethral region, but this sign is not sufficient to distinguish cancer from hyperplasia. Similarly, renal failure due to obstruction or infiltration is most common with nodular hyperplasia but can occur with cancer as well. Levels of alkaline phosphatase are elevated when prostate carcinoma gives rise to osteoblastic metastases. Although staging and grading schemes for malignant disease appear daunting, they are applied intuitively. The lowest stage is the smallest, most localized tumor; higher stages represent larger tumors or spread of the disease inside or outside of the primary organ site. Grading schemes also start with the lowest, most well differentiated tumor, as seen with the microscope. Higher-grade tumors have increasingly abnormal-appearing cells and structures so poorly differentiated that they hardly resemble their site of origin. In this case, the prostate cancer has the highest grade (it does not have glandular structures) and the highest stage (it has metastasized to the spine).

BP7 667-669   BP6 586-588   PBD7 1050-1056
PBD6 1031-1032

21 **(A)** The prostate-specific antigen (PSA) level is twice the upper limit of normal. This is worrisome but not an absolute indication of prostate cancer. Elevated PSA levels can occur with nodular hyperplasia or prostatitis. A higher level or a level that increases over time is more suggestive of carcinoma. The back-to-back glands shown indicate prostatic adenocarcinoma. The neoplasm shown is moderately well differentiated, and the nucleoli are prominent. Without treatment, prostatic carcinomas, particularly those of higher grade, may metastasize, often to the vertebrae, where they can produce osteolytic or, more commonly, osteoblastic lesions. Recurrent urinary tract infections and hydronephrosis are complications of obstruction produced most commonly by nodular prostatic hyperplasia. Acute bacterial prostatitis can cause bacteremia. Sterility is rarely a complication of any prostatic lesion, benign or malignant. Impotence may follow radical surgery for prostate carcinoma.

BP7 667-669   BP6 587-588   PBD7 1055
PBD6 1030-1031

22 **(E)** Hydrocele is one of the most common causes of scrotal enlargement. It consists of a fluid collection within the tunica vaginalis. Most cases are idiopathic, although some may result from local inflammation. A varicocele is a collection of dilated veins (pampiniform plexus) that may produce increased warmth, which inhibits spermatogenesis. Elephantiasis is a complication of parasitic filarial infections involving the inguinal lymphatics. Orchitis involves the body of the testis without marked enlargement but with tenderness. A seminoma is typically a firm unilateral mass.

BP7 659   BP6 579-580   PBD7 1047   PBD6 1025

23 **(A)** The clinical features are typical of nodular hyperplasia of the prostate. Slight elevation of the PSA level can occur with nodular hyperplasia. A PSA level that remains unchanged for a year, as in this case, is unlikely to be found with a prostate cancer. The area of the prostate most often involved in nodular hyperplasia producing significant obstruction is the inner (transitional and periurethral) zone. The hyperplastic nodules consist of proliferating glands, lined by two layers of cells, and the intervening fibromuscular stroma. Prostatitis may cause dysuria and increased frequency because of inflammation, but it is less common than hyperplasia in older males and is less likely to produce obstructive symptoms. Adenocarcinomas of the prostate are common in older men, but they arise in the posterior zone of the prostate and are less likely to produce obstructive symptoms than is hyperplasia. Acute prostatitis (abscesses with neutrophils) produces much more dysuria, and the symptoms are of shorter duration. Tuberculosis can affect the prostate, but it does not produce symptoms of obstruction.

BP7 665-666   BP6 584-585   PBD7 1047-1050
PBD6 1028

24 **(D)** The tumor has elements of all three germ layers and is a teratoma. It is uncommon for teratomas in adult men to be completely benign. The most common additional histologic component is embryonal carcinoma. The elevated levels of human chorionic gonadotropin and α-fetoprotein indicate that this is a mixed tumor with elements of choriocarcinoma and yolk sac cells. The size of the tumor, age of the patient, location of the tumor (e.g., right, left, cryptorchid), and differentiation of the glandular epithelium are not markers of malignancy. Upon examining more histologic sections from the mass, the pathologist will find the malignant elements.

BP7 661-664   BP6 580-582   PBD7 1044-1045
PBD6 1019-1022

25 **(B)** Prostatic intraepithelial neoplasia (PIN) is a potential precursor of prostatic adenocarcinoma. By itself it does not warrant therapy, because only about one third of patients diagnosed with PIN develop invasive cancer within 10 years. Conversely, in about 80% of cases in which prostate cancer is present, PIN can be found in the surrounding tissue. PIN usually does not increase the PSA levels. In this case, the elevation in PSA levels was probably caused by the coexistent hyperplasia. Thus, following the patient with PSA tests can aid in determining if cancer has developed. Antibiotic therapy is appropriate in the treatment of an infectious process, not for PIN. Radiation and chemotherapy are reserved for malignancies, not for a preneoplastic condition. Surgical resection of the prostate gland is considered, once a diagnosis of adenocarcinoma is established.

BP7 668   PBD7 1053   PBD6 1031

The Female Genital Tract

PBD7 Chapter 22: The Female Genital Tract

PBD6 Chapter 24: The Female Genital Tract

BP7 and BP6 Chapter 19: Female Genital System and Breast

1 A 24-year-old woman experiences sudden onset of severe lower abdominal pain. Physical examination shows no masses, but there is severe tenderness in the right lower quadrant. A pelvic examination shows no lesions of the cervix or vagina. Bowel sounds are detected. An abdominal ultrasound shows a 4-cm focal enlargement of the proximal right fallopian tube. A dilation and curettage procedure shows only decidua from the endometrial cavity. Which of the following laboratory findings is most likely to be reported for this patient?

- ❏ (A) Cervical culture positive for *Neisseria gonorrhoeae*
- ❏ (B) 69,XXY karyotype on decidual tissue
- ❏ (C) Positive result of serum pregnancy test
- ❏ (D) Positive result of serologic testing for syphilis
- ❏ (E) Pap smear showing *Candida*

2 A 30-year-old sexually active woman has had a mucopurulent vaginal discharge for 1 week. On pelvic examination, the cervix appears reddened around the os, but no erosions or mass lesions are present. A Pap smear shows numerous neutrophils but no dysplastic cells. Cervical biopsy shows marked follicular cervicitis. Which of the following infectious agents is most likely to produce these findings?

- ❏ (A) *Chlamydia trachomatis*
- ❏ (B) *Candida albicans*
- ❏ (C) *Gardnerella vaginalis*
- ❏ (D) Herpes simplex virus
- ❏ (E) Human papillomavirus
- ❏ (F) *Neisseria gonorrhoeae*
- ❏ (G) *Trichomonas vaginalis*

3 A 36-year-old woman has had menorrhagia and pelvic pain for several months. She had a normal, uncomplicated pregnancy 10 years ago. She has been sexually active with one partner for the past 20 years and has had no dyspareunia. On physical examination, she is afebrile. A pelvic examination shows a symmetrically enlarged uterus, with no apparent nodularity or palpable mass. A serum pregnancy test result is negative. Which of the following is the most likely diagnosis?

- ❏ (A) Endometriosis
- ❏ (B) Leiomyoma
- ❏ (C) Endometrial hyperplasia
- ❏ (D) Adenomyosis
- ❏ (E) Chronic endometritis

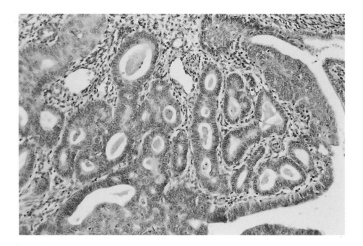

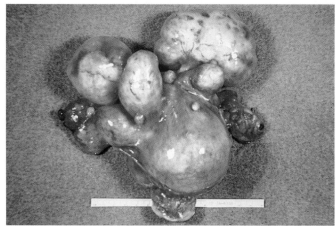

Courtesy of Dr. Kyle Molberg, Department of Pathology, University of Texas Southwestern Medical School, Dallas, TX.

4 A 45-year-old woman has had menometrorrhagia for the past 3 months. On physical examination, there are no remarkable findings. The microscopic appearance of an endometrial biopsy specimen is shown in the figure above. The patient then undergoes a dilation and curettage, and the bleeding stops, with no further problems. Which of the following conditions is most likely to produce these findings?

- ❏ (A) Ovarian mature cystic teratoma
- ❏ (B) Chronic endometritis
- ❏ (C) Failure of ovulation
- ❏ (D) Pregnancy
- ❏ (E) Use of oral contraceptives

6 A healthy 52-year-old woman has had a feeling of pelvic heaviness for the past 11 months. There is no history of abnormal bleeding, and her last menstrual period was 8 years ago. Her physician palpates an enlarged nodular uterus on bimanual pelvic examination. A Pap smear shows no abnormalities. Pelvic CT imaging shows multiple solid, uterine masses; there is no evidence of necrosis or hemorrhage. A total abdominal hysterectomy is performed. Based on the gross appearance of the mass shown above, which of the following is the most likely diagnosis?

- ❏ (A) Metastases
- ❏ (B) Endometriosis
- ❏ (C) Infiltrative leiomyosarcoma
- ❏ (D) Multiple leiomyomas
- ❏ (E) Adenomyosis

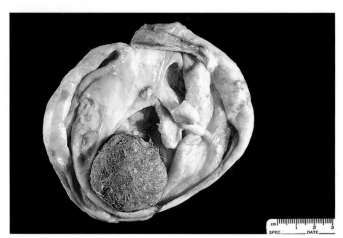

Courtesy of Dr. Christopher Crum, Brigham and Women's Hospital, Boston, MA.

5 A 31-year-old woman has had dull, constant, abdominal pain for 6 months. On physical examination, the only finding is a right adnexal mass. CT scan of the pelvis shows a 7-cm circumscribed mass that involves the right ovary and contains irregular calcifications. The right fallopian tube and ovary are surgically excised. The gross appearance of the ovary, which has been opened, is shown in the figure above. Which of the following is the most likely diagnosis?

- ❏ (A) Mucinous cystadenoma
- ❏ (B) Choriocarcinoma
- ❏ (C) Dysgerminoma
- ❏ (D) Serous cystadenoma
- ❏ (E) Mature cystic teratoma

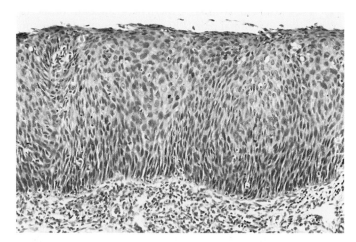

7 A 33-year-old woman comes to the physician for a routine health maintenance examination. On physical examination, there are no abnormal findings. A Pap smear shows abnormalities; colposcopy and a biopsy are performed. The microscopic appearance of the biopsy specimen is shown above. Which of the following factors is likely to have contributed most to the development of this lesion?

❑ (A) Diethylstilbestrol (DES) exposure
❑ (B) Recurrent *Candida* infections
❑ (C) Early age at first intercourse
❑ (D) Multiple pregnancies
❑ (E) Postmenopausal estrogen therapy

8 A 62-year-old obese nulliparous woman had an episode of vaginal bleeding, which produced only about 5 mL of blood. On pelvic examination, there appears to be no enlargement of the uterus, and the cervix appears normal. A Pap smear shows cells consistent with adenocarcinoma. Which of the following conditions is most likely to have contributed to the development of this malignancy?

❑ (A) Endometrial hyperplasia
❑ (B) Chronic endometritis
❑ (C) Use of oral contraceptives
❑ (D) Human papillomavirus infection
❑ (E) Adenomyosis

9 A 36-year-old primigravida developed peripheral edema late in the second trimester. On physical examination, her blood pressure was 155/95 mm Hg. Urinalysis showed 2+ proteinuria but no blood, glucose, or ketones. At 36 weeks, the patient gives birth to a normal viable, but low-birth-weight, infant. Her blood pressure then returns to normal, and she no longer has proteinuria. Which of the following is most likely to be found on examination of the placenta?

❑ (A) Chronic villitis
❑ (B) Partial mole
❑ (C) Hydrops
❑ (D) Multiple infarcts
❑ (E) Choriocarcinoma

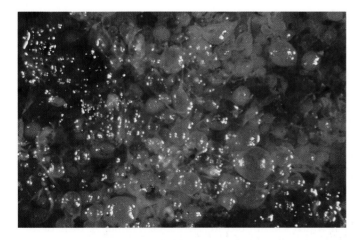

10 A 22-year-old woman, G 2, P 1, is in the early second trimester. She has noted a small amount of vaginal bleeding for the past week and has had marked nausea and vomiting for several weeks. On physical examination, the uterus measures large for dates. Ultrasound shows intrauterine contents with a "snowstorm appearance," and no fetus is identified. The gross appearance of tissue obtained by dilation and curettage is shown above. Which of the following substances is most likely to be increased in the serum?

❑ (A) α-Fetoprotein
❑ (B) Thyroxine (T₄)
❑ (C) Estradiol
❑ (D) Lactate dehydrogenase
❑ (E) Human chorionic gonadotropin
❑ (F) Human placental lactogen
❑ (G) Acetylcholinesterase

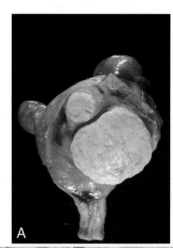

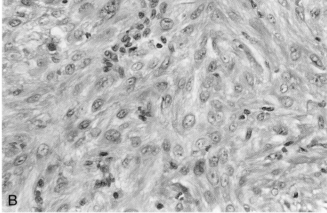

11 A 46-year-old perimenopausal woman has had pelvic discomfort for 5 months. On physical examination, the uterus appears slightly enlarged, and there are no adnexal masses. The cervix and vagina appear normal. A total abdominal hysterectomy is performed. The gross (A) and microscopic (B) features of the uterus are shown. Which of the following is most likely prevented by the hysterectomy performed on this patient?

❑ (A) Iron deficiency
❑ (B) Malignant transformation
❑ (C) Endometriosis
❑ (D) Osteoporosis
❑ (E) Invasive mole
❑ (F) Preeclampsia

12 A 62-year-old childless woman noticed a blood-tinged vaginal discharge twice during the past month. Her last menstrual period was 14 years ago. Bimanual pelvic examination shows that the uterus is normal in size, with no palpable adnexal masses. There are no cervical erosions or masses. Her BMI is 33. Her medical history indicates that for the past 30 years she has had hypertension and type 2 diabetes mellitus. An endometrial biopsy is most likely to show which of the following?

❏ (A) Adenomyosis
❏ (B) Leiomyosarcoma
❏ (C) Adenocarcinoma
❏ (D) Squamous cell carcinoma
❏ (E) Choriocarcinoma
❏ (F) Malignant mixed müllerian tumor

13 A 23-year-old woman, G 3, P 2, has a spontaneous abortion at 15 weeks' gestation. The male fetus is small for gestational age and is malformed and has syndactyly of the third and fourth digits of each hand. The placenta is also small and shows 0.5-cm grapelike villi scattered among morphologically normal villi. Chromosomal analysis of placental tissue is most likely to show which of the following karyotypes?

❏ (A) 69,XXY
❏ (B) 46,XX
❏ (C) 23,Y
❏ (D) 45,X
❏ (E) 47,XXY
❏ (F) 47,XY, + 18

14 A 54-year-old woman has had weight loss accompanied by abdominal enlargement for the past 6 months. She is concerned because of a family history of ovarian carcinoma. On physical examination, there are no lesions of the cervix, and the uterus is normal in size, but there is a left adnexal mass. An abdominal ultrasound scan shows a 10-cm cystic mass in the left adnexal region, with scattered 1-cm peritoneal nodules. Cytologic studies of peritoneal fluid show malignant cells consistent with a cystadenocarcinoma. Which of the following mutated genes is most likely a factor in the development of this neoplasm?

❏ (A) *RAS*
❏ (B) *BRCA1*
❏ (C) *ERBB2 (HER2)*
❏ (D) *MYC*
❏ (E) *RB1*

15 A 4-year-old girl is brought to the physician by her parents, who noticed blood-stained underwear and "something" protruding from her external genitalia. On physical examination, there are polypoid, grapelike masses projecting from the vagina. Histologic examination of a biopsy specimen from the lesion shows small, round tumor cells, some of which have eosinophilic strap-like cytoplasm. Immunohistochemical staining shows desmin in these cells. Which of the following is the most likely diagnosis?

❏ (A) Neuroblastoma
❏ (B) Embryonal rhabdomyosarcoma
❏ (C) Condyloma acuminatum
❏ (D) Vulvar intraepithelial neoplasm
❏ (E) Infiltrating squamous cell carcinoma

16 A 42-year-old woman has had menometrorrhagia for the past 2 months. She has no history of irregular menstrual bleeding, and she has not yet reached menopause. On physical examination, there are no vaginal or cervical lesions, and the uterus appears normal in size, but there is a right adnexal mass. An abdominal ultrasound scan shows the presence of a 7-cm solid right adnexal mass. Endometrial biopsy shows hyperplastic endometrium but no cellular atypia. Which of the following is the most likely diagnosis?

❏ (A) Mature cystic teratoma
❏ (B) Endometrioma
❏ (C) Corpus luteum cyst
❏ (D) Metastasis
❏ (E) Granulosa-theca cell tumor
❏ (F) Struma ovarii

17 A 19-year-old woman has had pelvic pain for 1 week. A pelvic examination shows mild erythema of the ectocervix. A Pap smear shows many neutrophils but no dysplastic cells. A cervical culture grows *Neisseria gonorrhoeae*. If the infection is not adequately treated, the patient will be at increased risk for which of the following complications?

❏ (A) Ectopic pregnancy
❏ (B) Dysfunctional uterine bleeding
❏ (C) Cervical carcinoma
❏ (D) Endometrial hyperplasia
❏ (E) Endometriosis
❏ (F) Placenta previa

18 A 28-year-old sexually active woman comes to her physician for a routine health maintenance examination. There are no abnormal findings on physical examination. The patient has been taking oral contraceptives for the past 10 years. A Pap smear shows a moderate dysplasia, or cervical intraepithelial neoplasia (CIN) II. Which of the following is the major significance of this finding?

❏ (A) A cervicitis needs to be treated
❏ (B) The patient has an increased risk of cervical carcinoma
❏ (C) Condyloma acuminata are probably present
❏ (D) An endocervical polyp needs to be excised
❏ (E) The patient should stop taking oral contraceptives

19 A 50-year-old woman has noticed vaginal bleeding for the past month. Her last menstrual period was 5 years ago. On physical examination, there are no abnormal findings. An endometrial biopsy shows endometrial adenocarcinoma. The patient undergoes a total abdominal hysterectomy. The uterus is normal in size, but sectioning shows a single 1.5-cm firm, tan-white, circumscribed subserosal nodule. Which of the following is the most likely diagnosis?

❏ (A) Metastasis
❏ (B) Leiomyoma
❏ (C) Choriocarcinoma
❏ (D) Endometrioma
❏ (E) Malignant mixed müllerian tumor
❏ (F) Adenomyosis

20 A 25-year-old woman has experienced discomfort during sexual intercourse for the past month. On physical examination, there are no lesions of the external genitalia. Pelvic examination shows a focal area of swelling on the left posterolateral inner labium that is very tender on palpation. A 3-cm cystic lesion filled with purulent exudate is excised. In which of the following structures is this lesion most likely to develop?

- ❏ (A) Bartholin's gland
- ❏ (B) Gartner duct
- ❏ (C) Hair follicle
- ❏ (D) Urogenital diaphragm
- ❏ (E) Vestibular bulb

21 A 58-year-old woman has had dull pain in the lower abdomen for the past 6 months and minimal vaginal bleeding on three occasions. Her last menstrual period was 14 years ago. Pelvic examination shows a right adnexal mass, and the uterus appears normal in size. An abdominal ultrasound scan shows an 8-cm solid mass. A total abdominal hysterectomy is performed, and the mass is diagnosed as an ovarian granulosa-theca cell tumor. Which of the following additional lesions is most likely to be found in the excised specimen?

- ❏ (A) Condyloma acuminata of the cervix
- ❏ (B) Endometrial hyperplasia
- ❏ (C) Metastases to the uterine serosa
- ❏ (D) Bilateral chronic salpingitis
- ❏ (E) Partial mole of the uterus

22 A 43-year-old woman has had postcoital bleeding for 6 months. She experienced menarche at age 11 and has had 12 sexual partners during her life. She continues to have regular menstrual cycles without abnormal intermenstrual bleeding. Pelvic examination shows a focal, slightly raised area of erythema on the cervix at the 5 o'clock position. A Pap smear shows high-grade cervical intraepithelial neoplasia (CIN III). In situ hybridization performed on cells from the cervix shows the presence of human papillomavirus type 16. If the cervical lesion is not treated, which of the following malignancies is she at greatest risk of developing?

- ❏ (A) Clear cell carcinoma
- ❏ (B) Immature teratoma
- ❏ (C) Krukenberg tumor
- ❏ (D) Leiomyosarcoma
- ❏ (E) Papillary serous cystadenocarcinoma
- ❏ (F) Sarcoma botryoides
- ❏ (G) Squamous cell carcinoma

23 An 18-year-old woman has had pelvic discomfort for several months. On pelvic examination, there is a 10-cm right adnexal mass. An abdominal CT scan shows the mass to be solid and circumscribed. On surgical removal, the mass is solid and white, with small areas of necrosis. Microscopically, it contains mostly primitive mesenchymal cells along with some cartilage, muscle, and foci of neuroepithelial differentiation. Which of the following is the most likely diagnosis?

- ❏ (A) Brenner tumor
- ❏ (B) Dysgerminoma
- ❏ (C) Granulosa cell tumor
- ❏ (D) Immature teratoma
- ❏ (E) Leiomyosarcoma
- ❏ (F) Malignant mixed müllerian tumor
- ❏ (G) Sarcoma botryoides

24 A 32-year-old woman has cyclic abdominal pain that coincides with her menses. Attempts to become pregnant have failed over the past 5 years. There are no abnormal findings on physical examination. Laparoscopic examination shows numerous hemorrhagic 0.2- to 0.5-cm lesions over the peritoneal surfaces of the uterus and ovaries. Which of the following ovarian lesions is most likely to be visualized during the laparoscopic procedure?

- ❏ (A) Fibroma
- ❏ (B) Brenner tumor
- ❏ (C) Endometriotic cyst
- ❏ (D) Krukenberg tumor
- ❏ (E) Mature cystic teratoma
- ❏ (F) Mucinous cystadenocarcinoma

25 A 21-year-old woman who is sexually active has noticed multiple warty lesions on the perineum over the past 3 years. On physical examination, the lesions are slightly raised, soft pink to white color, and 0.2 to 1 cm in diameter. A scraping from one of the lesions yields cells with cytologic features consistent with koilocytotic atypia. There is no necrosis or acute inflammation. Which of the following infectious agents is most likely to produce these findings?

- ❏ (A) *Neisseria gonorrhoeae*
- ❏ (B) *Chlamydia trachomatis*
- ❏ (C) Human papillomavirus
- ❏ (D) *Trichomonas vaginalis*
- ❏ (E) Herpes simplex virus type 2

26 A 31-year-old woman has had a whitish, globular, vaginal discharge for the past week. On pelvic examination, the cervix appears erythematous, but there are no erosions or masses. A Pap smear shows budding cells and pseudohyphae. No dysplastic cells are present. Which of the following infectious agents is most likely to produce these findings?

- ❏ (A) *Trichomonas vaginalis*
- ❏ (B) *Ureaplasma urealyticum*
- ❏ (C) *Candida albicans*
- ❏ (D) *Chlamydia trachomatis*
- ❏ (E) *Neisseria gonorrhoeae*

27 A 57-year-old woman comes to the physician because she recently noticed a pale area of discoloration on the labia. Pelvic examination shows the presence of a 0.7-cm flat, white area on the right labia majora. A biopsy specimen shows dysplastic cells that occupy about half the thickness of the squamous epithelium, with minimal underlying chronic inflammation. In situ hybridization shows human papillomavirus type 16 DNA in the epithelial cells. Which of the following is the most likely diagnosis?

- ❏ (A) Lichen sclerosus et atrophicus
- ❏ (B) Condyloma acuminatum
- ❏ (C) Squamous hyperplasia
- ❏ (D) Vulvar intraepithelial neoplasia
- ❏ (E) Chronic vulvitis
- ❏ (F) Contact dermatitis

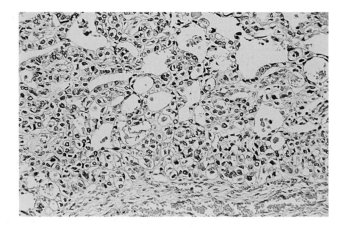

28 A 19-year-old sexually active woman has had dyspareunia followed by vaginal bleeding for the past month. On pelvic examination, a red, friable 2.5-cm nodular mass is seen on the anterior wall of the upper third of the vagina. The microscopic appearance of a biopsy specimen is shown above. Which of the following conditions is likely to have contributed most to the origin of this neoplasm?

- (A) Diethylstilbestrol (DES) exposure
- (B) *Trichomonas vaginitis*
- (C) Polycystic ovaries
- (D) Human papillomavirus infection
- (E) Congenital adrenal hyperplasia

29 A 33-year-old woman has had dyspareunia and dysuria for several years. Each time she visits a physician, a pelvic examination reveals no gross abnormalities in the vulva, vagina, or cervix. A recent Pap smear also shows no abnormalities. She is referred to a psychiatrist, who finds no psychiatric problems or evidence of neurologic disease, but he does elicit a history of severe dysmenorrhea and pelvic pain on defecation. He refers the patient to a gynecologist. Which of the following lesions is the gynecologist most likely to find on laparoscopic examination?

- (A) Tubo-ovarian adhesions
- (B) Red-blue to brown 0.3-cm implants on the uterine serosa
- (C) Multiple 0.7- to 1.5-cm firm white peritoneal nodules
- (D) Papillations on the surface of an enlarged right ovary
- (E) Subserosal 3-cm uterine leiomyoma

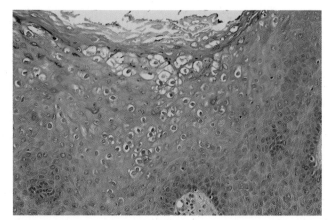

Courtesy of Dr. Jag Bhawan, Boston University School of Medicine, Boston, MA.

30 A 36-year-old woman has noticed that warty vulvar lesions have been increasing in size and number over the past 5 years. On physical examination, there are several 0.5- to 2-cm red-pink, flattened lesions with rough surfaces present on the vulva and perineum. One of the larger lesions is excised, and its microscopic appearance is shown in the preceding figure. Which of the following infectious agents is most likely to produce these lesions?

- (A) Human papillomavirus
- (B) *Chlamydia trachomatis*
- (C) *Treponema pallidum*
- (D) *Haemophilus ducreyi*
- (E) *Candida albicans*

31 A 35-year-old woman has a routine Pap smear for the first time. The results indicate that dysplastic cells are present, and the lesion is consistent with cervical intraepithelial neoplasia (CIN) III. The patient is referred to a gynecologist, who performs colposcopy and takes several biopsy specimens that all show CIN III. Conization of the cervix shows a focus of microinvasion at the squamocolumnar junction. Based on these findings, which of the following is the next step in treating this patient?

- (A) Course of radiation therapy
- (B) Hysterectomy
- (C) Bone scan for metastatic lesions
- (D) Pelvic exenteration
- (E) No further therapy is indicated at this time

32 A 20-year-old woman experienced menarche at age 14 and had fairly regular menstrual cycles for several years. For the past year, she has had oligomenorrhea and has developed hirsutism. She has noticed a 10-kg weight gain in the past 4 months. On pelvic examination, there are no vaginal or cervical lesions, the uterus is normal in size, and the adnexa are prominent. A pelvic ultrasound scan shows that each ovary is about twice normal size, whereas the uterus is normal in size. Which of the following conditions is most likely to be present?

- (A) Immature teratomas
- (B) Polycystic ovaries
- (C) Krukenberg tumors
- (D) Tubo-ovarian abscesses
- (E) Ovarian cystadenocarcinomas

33 A 28-year-old woman sees her physician because she has had fever, pelvic pain, and a feeling of pelvic heaviness for the past week. Pelvic examination shows a palpable left adnexal mass. Laparoscopy shows an indistinct left fallopian tube that is part of a 5-cm circumscribed, red-tan mass involving the left adnexal region. Which of the following infectious agents is most likely to produce these findings?

- (A) Human papillomavirus
- (B) *Mycobacterium tuberculosis*
- (C) *Treponema pallidum*
- (D) *Chlamydia trachomatis*
- (E) *Candida albicans*
- (F) Herpes simplex virus
- (G) *Haemophilus ducreyi*

34 A 42-year-old woman has a Pap smear as part of a routine health maintenance examination. Her previous Pap smear was obtained 10 years ago. There are no remarkable findings on physical examination. The current Pap smear shows findings consistent with cervical intraepithelial neoplasia (CIN) III. A cervical biopsy is performed, and microscopic examination shows dysplastic cells that occupy the full thickness of the epithelium above the basement membrane, and intense chronic inflammation with squamous metaplasia is seen in the endocervical canal. Which of the following is the most likely explanation for proceeding with cervical conization for this patient?

- ❑ (A) She has a high risk of invasive carcinoma
- ❑ (B) Human papillomavirus infection cannot be treated
- ❑ (C) She is perimenopausal
- ❑ (D) She has chronic cervicitis
- ❑ (E) Her reproductive years are over

35 A 20-year-old woman notices a bloody, brownish vaginal discharge. The next day, she sees a physician because of shortness of breath. On physical examination, a 3-cm red-brown mass is seen on the lateral wall of the vagina. A chest radiograph shows numerous 2- to 5-cm nodules in both lungs. A biopsy specimen of the vaginal mass shows malignant cells resembling syncytiotrophoblasts. Which the following proteins is most likely to be elevated in the serum?

- ❑ (A) Human chorionic gonadotropin
- ❑ (B) α-Fetoprotein
- ❑ (C) Estradiol
- ❑ (D) Testosterone
- ❑ (E) Thyroxine
- ❑ (F) Carcinoembryonic antigen

36 A 14-year-old girl began menstruation 1 year ago. She now has abnormal uterine bleeding, with menstrual periods that are 2 to 7 days long and 2 to 6 weeks apart. The amount of bleeding varies considerably, from minimal spotting to a very heavy flow. On physical examination, there are no remarkable findings. A pelvic ultrasound scan shows no abnormalities. Which of the following is most likely to produce these findings?

- ❑ (A) Endometrial polyp
- ❑ (B) Anovulatory cycles
- ❑ (C) Ectopic pregnancy
- ❑ (D) Uterine leiomyomata
- ❑ (E) Endometrial carcinoma

37 A 51-year-old woman is concerned about pale areas on her labia that have been slowly enlarging for the past year. The areas cause discomfort and become easily irritated. Physical examination shows pale gray to parchment-like areas of skin that involve most of the labia majora, labia minora, and introitus. The introitus is narrowed. A biopsy specimen shows thinning of the squamous epithelium, a dense band of upper dermal hyaline collagen, and scattered upper dermal mononuclear inflammatory cells. Which of the following is the most likely diagnosis?

- ❑ (A) Pelvic inflammatory disease
- ❑ (B) Lichen sclerosus et atrophicus
- ❑ (C) Vulvar intraepithelial neoplasia
- ❑ (D) Extramammary Paget disease
- ❑ (E) Human papillomavirus infection

38 A 57-year-old nulliparous woman has had vaginal bleeding for the past 2 months. She went through menopause 7 years ago and has had no menstrual periods since then. On physical examination, there are no cervical lesions or adnexal masses, and the uterus is normal in size. The patient is 155 cm (5 ft 1 in) tall and weighs 74.5 kg (BMI 38). A Pap smear shows atypical glandular cells of uncertain significance. The

hemoglobin A_{1c} concentration is 9.8%. The patient is at greatest risk of developing which of the following conditions?

- ❑ (A) Adenomyosis
- ❑ (B) Endometrial adenocarcinoma
- ❑ (C) Krukenberg tumor
- ❑ (D) Ovarian mature cystic teratoma
- ❑ (E) Ovarian papillary serous cystadenocarcinoma
- ❑ (F) Ovarian infarction
- ❑ (G) Uterine malignant mixed müllerian tumor

39 A 35-year-old woman has had increasing abdominal enlargement for the past 6 months. She states that she feels like she is pregnant, but results of a pregnancy test are negative. On physical examination, there is abdominal distention with a fluid wave. A pelvic ultrasound scan shows bilateral cystic ovarian masses, 10 cm on the right and 7 cm on the left. The masses are surgically removed. On gross examination, the excised masses are unilocular cysts filled with clear fluid, and papillary projections extend into the central lumen of the cyst. Microscopic examination shows that the papillae are covered with atypical cuboidal cells that invade underlying stroma. Psammoma bodies are present. Which of the following is the most likely diagnosis?

- ❑ (A) Endometrioid tumor
- ❑ (B) Clear cell carcinoma
- ❑ (C) Cystadenocarcinoma
- ❑ (D) Dysgerminoma
- ❑ (E) Granulosa cell tumor
- ❑ (F) Malignant mixed müllerian tumor
- ❑ (G) Mature cystic teratoma
- ❑ (H) Sertoli-Leydig cell tumor

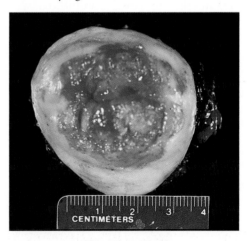

40 A 45-year-old woman has had a small amount of vaginal bleeding and a brownish, foul-smelling discharge for the past month. On pelvic examination, there is a 3-cm lesion on the ectocervix, shown in the figure. Microscopic examination of the lesion is most likely to show which of the following?

- ❑ (A) Dysplastic changes affecting the lower third of the cervical epithelium
- ❑ (B) Dysplastic changes affecting the full thickness of the epithelium
- ❑ (C) Nests and sheets of epithelial cells with squamous differentiation in the subepithelial region
- ❑ (D) Multiple irregular mucus-secreting glands in the subepithelial region
- ❑ (E) Dense mononuclear infiltrate with a normally differentiating cervical epithelium

41 A healthy 30-year-old woman comes to the physician for a routine health maintenance examination. No abnormalities are found on review of systems or physical examination, but a screening Pap smear shows cells consistent with cervical intraepithelial neoplasia (CIN) I. Which of the following is most likely related to the Pap smear findings?

- ❏ (A) Intake of oral contraceptives
- ❏ (B) Diethylstilbestrol (DES) exposure
- ❏ (C) Vitamin B₁₂ (cobalamin) deficiency
- ❏ (D) Treated squamous cell carcinoma
- ❏ (E) Multiple sexual partners

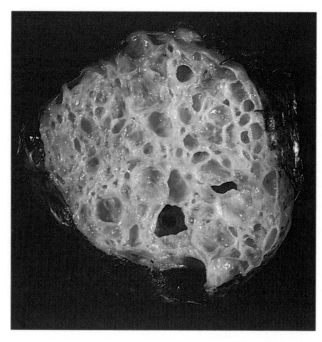

42 A 24-year-old woman has had lesions of the external genitalia that first appeared several years ago, after she vacationed at a resort near Negril, Jamaica, where she goes every year. The gross appearance of the external genitalia (A) and histologic features (B) of an excised lesion are shown below. Which of the following factors is likely to have contributed most to the development of these lesions?

- ❏ (A) Lack of menstrual cycles
- ❏ (B) Inheritance of a faulty tumor suppressor gene
- ❏ (C) Poorly controlled diabetes mellitus
- ❏ (D) Exposure to ultraviolet light
- ❏ (E) Sexual intercourse

43 A 40-year-old woman has noticed progressive enlargement of the abdomen over the past 5 months, although her diet has not changed and she has been exercising more. Physical examination shows no palpable masses, but a fluid wave is present. Paracentesis yields 500 mL of slightly cloudy fluid. Cytologic examination of the fluid shows malignant cells. An abdominal ultrasound scan shows a 15-cm multilobular mass that involves the right adnexal region. The uterus is normal in size. The mass is surgically removed, and the gross features of a section of the excised mass are shown above. Which of the following is the most likely diagnosis?

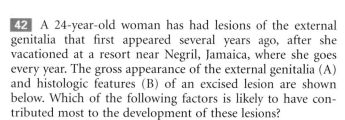

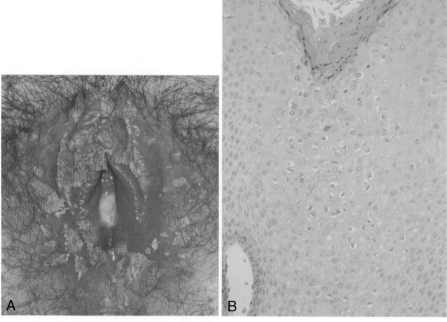

Courtesy of Dr. Alex Ferenczy, McGill University, Montreal, Quebec, Canada.

- ❏ (A) Immature teratoma
- ❏ (B) Mucinous cystadenocarcinoma
- ❏ (C) Granulosa cell tumor
- ❏ (D) Choriocarcinoma
- ❏ (E) Dysgerminoma

44 A 35-year-old primigravid woman is in the 7th month of an otherwise unremarkable pregnancy when she develops worsening headaches and a 3 kg weight gain over the past week. On physical examination she is afebrile but her blood pressure is 190/110 mm Hg (it was 120/80 mm Hg at a pre-natal visit a month ago). She has edema involving her head and all extremities. Fetal heart tones and movement are present. Laboratory studies show hemoglobin 12.5 g/dL, hematocrit 37.6%, MCV 92 μm^3, platelet count 199,000/mm^3, serum creatinine 1.0 mg/dL, urea nitrogen 17 mg/dL, glucose 101 mg/dL, Na$^+$ 137 mmol/L, K$^+$ 4.1 mmol/L, Cl$^-$ 99 mmol/L, and CO$_2$ 24 mmol/L. Urinalysis shows 2+ proteinuria but no hematuria, RBCs, WBCs, or casts. She is placed at bed rest and given antihypertensive medications. Which of the following is the most likely underlying factor in the causation of her disease?

- ❏ (A) Gestational trophoblastic disease
- ❏ (B) Disseminated intravascular coagulation
- ❏ (C) Adrenal cortical hyperplasia
- ❏ (D) Placenta ischemia
- ❏ (E) Ovarian neoplasm producing estrogen

ANSWERS

1 (C) The patient has an ectopic pregnancy. Conditions predisposing to ectopic pregnancy include chronic salpingitis (which may be caused by gonorrhea, but a culture would be positive only with acute infection), intrauterine tumors, and endometriosis. In about half of cases, there is no identifiable cause. Gestational trophoblastic disease associated with a triploid karyotype, such as a complete or partial mole developing outside the uterus, is rare. Syphilis is not likely to produce a tubal mass with acute symptoms (a gumma is a rare finding). *Candida* produces cervicitis and vaginitis and is rarely invasive or extensive in immunocompetent patients.

BP7 701   BP6 620   PBD7 1105   PBD6 1079-1080

2 (A) The redness of the cervix, the inflammatory cells in the cervical discharge, and the biopsy findings indicate that the patient has cervicitis. *Chlamydia trachomatis* is the most common cause of cervicitis in sexually active women. Candidiasis, gonorrhea, and trichomoniasis are also common. However, candidiasis often produces a scant, white, curdlike vaginal discharge; gonorrhea may have an associated urethritis; and *Trichomonas* may produce a profuse homogeneous, frothy, and adherent yellow or green vaginal discharge. *Gardnerella* is found in bacterial vaginosis, a common condition caused by overgrowth of bacteria. *Gardnerella* infection produces a moderate, homogeneous, low-viscosity, adherent vaginal discharge that is white or gray and has a characteristic "fishy" odor; "clue" cells are seen on a wet mount. Herpetic infections are more likely to manifest as clear vesicles on the skin in the perineal region. Infection with human papillomavirus is associated with condyloma, dysplasias, and carcinoma.

BP7 685   BP6 603   PBD7 1062-1063, 1072-1073
PBD6 1038-1039

3 (D) In adenomyosis, endometrial glands extend from the endometrium down into the myometrium. The process may be superficial, but occasionally it is extensive and the uterus becomes enlarged two to four times its normal size because of a reactive thickening of the myometrium. In endometriosis, endometrial glands and stroma are found outside the uterus in such sites as peritoneum, ovaries, and ligaments. A leiomyoma is a myometrial tumor mass that, if large, produces an asymmetric mass. Endometrial hyperplasias do not increase the size of the uterus. Chronic endometritis does not extend to the myometrium and does not increase uterine size.

BP7 689-690   BP6 608   PBD7 1083   PBD6 1057

4 (C) This patient has endometrial hyperplasia, which results from excessive estrogenic stimulation. This lesion often occurs with failure of ovulation about the time of menopause. Estrogen-secreting ovarian tumors may also produce endometrial hyperplasia, but teratomas are not known for this phenomenon. Hyperplasias do not develop from endometritis. A secretory pattern of the endometrium is seen in pregnancy, not the proliferative pattern shown in the figure. Oral contraceptives contain small doses of estrogenic compounds that do not lead to hyperplasia.

BP7 691   BP6 610   PBD7 1085-1086   PBD6 1059-1060

5 (E) This patient has a cystic tumor with a mass of hair in the lumen. This is the typical appearance of a mature cystic teratoma. This tumor is also known as a dermoid cyst, because it is cystic and filled with hair and sebum derived from ectodermal structures. Dermoid cysts are benign tumors of germ cell origin, and they can contain various ectodermally, endodermally, and mesodermally derived tissues. A mucinous cystadenoma is often multiloculated and filled with mucoid fluid, but it does not contain hair or calcifications. A choriocarcinoma is gestational in origin and is an aggressive neoplasm that usually has a hemorrhagic appearance. A dysgerminoma is a solid, lobulated, tan-white mass; it is the female equivalent of a male testicular seminoma. A serous cystadenoma is usually a unilocular cyst filled with clear fluid and little else.

BP7 698-700   BP6 617-619   PBD7 1099-1100
PBD6 1073-1075

6 (D) The masses shown are well-circumscribed, suggesting the presence of multiple benign tumors. Leiomyomas are the most common benign tumors of the uterus; perhaps one third to one half of all women have them. After menopause, they generally do not continue to enlarge. Metastases of this size and location are unlikely to occur in a healthy-appearing person. The small implants of endometriosis rarely exceed 1 to 2 cm in diameter; when a large mass forms, it is cystic and filled with "old" blood ("chocolate cyst"). A leiomyosarcoma is a rare tumor and is usually a large, solitary mass. Endometrial glands and stroma that extend into the myometrium constitute adenomyosis, a process that tends to enlarge the uterus diffusely, without nodularity.

BP7 692-693   BP6 611   PBD7 1089-1090
PBD6 1063-1064

7   **(C)** The figure shows cervical intraepithelial neoplasia (CIN) III, because the dysplasia involves the full thickness of the cervical epithelium. Such lesions arise more frequently among women who have had first intercourse at an early age, have multiple sexual partners, or a male partner with multiple sexual partners. These factors are believed to increase the risk of infection with human papillomavirus (HPV), particularly types 16 and 18. HPV-16 and HPV-18 are associated with dysplasias and carcinomas of the cervix. Diethylstilbestrol (DES) exposure in utero is strongly associated with clear cell adenocarcinomas of the vagina and cervix. Recurrent *Candida* infections are a nuisance, but they are not premalignant. Pregnancy does not play a role in the development of cervical neoplasia. Most cervical dysplasias occur in premenopausal women. Estrogen therapy and the use of oral contraceptives do not increase the risk of cervical dysplasia.

BP7 686-688   BP6 604-605   PBD7 1073-1076
PBD6 1048-1051

8   **(A)** The patient has an endometrial carcinoma. Estrogenic stimulation from anovulatory cycles, nulliparity, obesity, and exogenous estrogens (in higher amounts than found in birth control pills) gives rise to endometrial hyperplasia and can progress to endometrial carcinoma if the estrogenic stimulation continues. Atypical endometrial hyperplasias progress to endometrial cancer in about 25% of cases. Chronic endometritis does not give rise to cancer, nor does human papillomavirus infection (which is associated with squamous epithelial dysplasias and neoplasia). Adenomyosis increases the size of the uterus and is not a risk for endometrial carcinoma.

BP7 693-694   BP6 612   PBD7 1086-1088
PBD6 1061-1062

9   **(D)** This patient has toxemia of pregnancy. Her condition is best classified as pre-eclampsia, because she has hypertension, proteinuria, and edema but no seizures. The placenta tends to be small because of reduced maternal blood flow and uteroplacental insufficiency; infarct and retroplacental hemorrhages can occur. Microscopically, the decidual arterioles may show acute atherosis and fibrinoid necrosis. A chronic villitis is characteristic of a congenital infection such as cytomegalovirus. In a partial mole, a fetus is present, but it is malformed and rarely liveborn. Placental hydrops often accompanies fetal hydrops in conditions such as infections and fetal anemias. A fetus is not present in a choriocarcinoma.

BP7 704-705   BP6 622-623   PBD7 1106-1110
PBD6 1082-1084

10   **(E)** The figure shows a hydatidiform mole, or complete mole, with enlarged, grapelike villi that form the tumor mass in the endometrial cavity. These trophoblastic tumors secrete human chorionic gonadotropin. Molar pregnancies result from abnormal fertilization. In a complete mole, only paternal chromosomes are present. α-Fetoprotein is a marker for some germ cell tumors that contain yolk sac elements. Thyroxine can be produced by the rare struma ovarii, which is a teratoma composed predominantly of thyroid tissue. Estrogens can be elaborated by a variety of ovarian stromal tumors, including thecomas and granulosa cell tumors. More ominously, a drop in maternal serum estriol suggests incipient abortion. Lactate dehydrogenase may be increased in many conditions, such

as liver and cardiac disease, but it is not known as a marker for genital tract lesions. Human placental lactogen is produced in small quantities in the developing placenta, and serum levels typically are not measured. Neural tube defects can be distinguished from other fetal defects (e.g., abdominal wall defects) by use of the acetylcholinesterase test on amniotic fluid obtained by amniocentesis. If acetylcholinesterase and maternal serum α-fetoprotein (MSAFP) are elevated, a neural tube defect is likely. If the acetylcholinesterase is not detectable, then another fetal defect is suggested.

BP7 702-703   BP6 620-622   PBD7 1110-1112
PBD6 1085-1086

11   **(A)** The figure shows a uterus with two well-circumscribed gray-white masses in the myometrium. Microscopically, the lesions show spindle-shaped cells in whorled bundles. The cells are uniform in size and shape, and mitotic figures are scarce. These features are characteristic of a benign neoplasm—a leiomyoma. A leiomyosarcoma is are not as well demarcated, and its cut surface is not as homogeneous as that of a leiomyoma. Though leiomyomas are often asymptomatic, those that are submucosal in location may produce menometrorrhagia and chronic blood loss leading to iron deficiency anemia. A leiomyosarcoma arises de novo, not from a leiomyoma, and is usually a larger, more irregular mass composed of more pleomorphic spindle cells with many mitoses. Endometriosis may cause pelvic pain, but usually has an onset at an earlier age, and the hemorrhagic lesions are located outside the uterus. Decreased ovarian function following menopause accelerates bone loss, which may be severe enough to be termed osteoporosis, but this process is not related to female genital tract neoplasia. About 10% of complete moles are complicated by invasive mole, which is unlikely to produce a large, circumscribed mass. Preeclampsia with hypertension and proteinuria is associated with abnormal decidual vascularization and placental ischemia.

BP7 692-693   BP6 611   PBD7 1089-1090
PBD6 1064-1065

12   **(C)** Postmenopausal vaginal bleeding is a "red flag" for endometrial carcinoma. Such carcinomas often arise in the setting of endometrial hyperplasia. Increased estrogenic stimulation is thought to drive this process, and risk factors include obesity, type 2 diabetes mellitus, hypertension, and infertility. Adenomyosis is an extension of endometrial glands and stroma into the myometrium, generally resulting in symmetric uterine enlargement. A submucosal leiomyosarcoma could produce vaginal bleeding, but the uterus would be enlarged, because leiomyosarcomas tend to be large masses. Squamous carcinomas of the endometrium are rare. Choriocarcinomas are gestational in origin. Malignant mixed müllerian tumors are much less common than endometrial carcinomas, but they could produce similar findings.

BP7 693-694   BP6 612   PBD7 1086-1088
PBD6 1061-1062

13   **(A)** This patient has a partial hydatidiform mole, which results from triploidy (69 chromosomes). Unlike a complete mole, in which no fetus is present, a partial mole has a fetus, because maternal chromosomes are present. Survival of the fetus to term is rare. A partial mole may contain some grapelike villi or none. The fetus is usually malformed. A 46,XX karyotype could be present in a complete mole or a normal male fetus. The 23,Y karyotype is typical of a sperm. A fetus with Turner syndrome has a 45,X karyotype. Most female fetuses with loss of an X chromosome undergo spontaneous abortion. Klinefelter syndrome has a 47,XXY karyotype, and male infants are liveborn. A 47,XY, + 18 karyotype of trisomy 18 is associated with multiple congenital malformations but not with a partial mole.

BP7 702-703   BP6 620-621   PBD7 1110-1112
PBD6 1085-1086

14 **(B)** Some familial cases of ovarian carcinoma (usually serous cystadenocarcinoma) are associated with the homozygous loss of the *BRCA1* gene. This tumor suppressor gene also plays a role in the development of familial breast cancers. However, familial syndromes account for less than 5% of all ovarian cancers. Mutations of the *RAS* and *MYC* oncogenes occur sporadically in cancers. The *ERBB2* gene may be overexpressed in ovarian cancers; however, mutations of this gene do not give rise to familial tumors. The *RB1* gene can be involved in familial forms of retinoblastoma and osteosarcoma.

BP7 696   BP6 614   PBD7 1093   PBD6 1067

15 **(B)** Embryonal rhabdomyosarcoma is an uncommon vaginal tumor found in girls younger than 5 years of age. Because it forms polypoid, grapelike masses, it is sometimes called sarcoma botryoides. Histologically, it is a small, round, blue-cell tumor that shows skeletal muscle differentiation in the presence of muscle-specific proteins such as desmin. Neuroblastomas are also small blue-cell tumors, but they occur in the adrenal glands or extra-adrenal sympathetic chain. Condyloma acuminata are caused by sexually transmitted human papillomavirus and hence rarely occur in such young patients. Vulvar intraepithelial neoplasm is a carcinoma in situ of the vulvar skin. It occurs in older patients. Invasive squamous cell carcinomas are rare in very young patients, and they show histologic evidence of squamous epithelial differentiation.

BP7 786   BP6 602   PBD7 1071-1072   PBD6 1046-1047

16 **(E)** The mass is probably producing estrogen, which has led to endometrial hyperplasia. Estrogen-producing tumors of the ovary are typically sex cord tumors, such as a granulosa-theca cell tumor or a thecoma-fibroma, the former more often being functional. Teratomas can contain a variety of histologic elements, but not estrogen-producing tissues. Endometriosis can give rise to an adnexal mass called an endometrioma, which enlarges over time. Endometrial glands are hormonally sensitive, but they do not produce hormones. Corpus luteum cysts are relatively common, but they are unlikely to produce estrogens. Metastases to the ovary do not cause increased estrogen production. A struma ovarii is a variant of a teratoma in which more than half the mass is thyroid tissue, which may be functional and cause hyperthyroidism.

BP7 691   BP6 610, 618   PBD7 1085, 1102-1104
PBD6 1076-1077

17 **(A)** Gonorrheal infections can lead to salpingitis and pelvic inflammatory disease with scarring. This predisposes to ectopic pregnancy. Gonorrhea and other genital tract infections do not cause dysfunctional bleeding. Gonorrhea does not carry the risk of dysplasias or carcinomas that human papillomavirus infection does. Gonorrhea and other infections do not contribute to endometrial hyperplasia. The actual cause of endometriosis is unknown, but infection does not appear to play a role in this process. Placenta previa results from low-lying implantation of the placenta and is not related to sexually transmitted diseases.

BP7 673-675,685   BP6 620   PBD7 1064-1065
PBD6 1079-1080

18 **(B)** Dysplasias of the cervix should not be ignored, because they naturally progress to more severe dysplasias and to invasive carcinomas. Although not all cases progress, the physician should not take this chance. Dysplasias are strongly related to human papillomavirus (HPV) infections, and HPV DNA can be found in about 90% of cases. In about 10% to 15% of cases, there is no evidence of HPV, and other factors may play a role in the development of the dysplasia. A condyloma acuminatum is also an HPV-associated lesion, but it is usually caused by a distinct, low-risk type of HPV. With such HPV infection, the Pap smear may show changes of cervical intraepithelial carcinoma (CIN) I. Cervicitis usually is due to bacterial or fungal organisms and is not a significant risk of dysplasia or carcinoma. Endocervical polyps may produce some bleeding but typically show no dysplasia. Oral contraceptive use does not significantly increase the risk of dysplasia.

BP7 686-688   BP6 604-605   PBD7 1073-1076
PBD6 1048-1051

19 **(B)** Leiomyomas ("fibroids") can be present in one third to one half of all women. They tend to enlarge during the reproductive years and then stop growing or involute after menopause. Most are asymptomatic. They are a common incidental finding in a uterus removed for another reason. A solitary metastasis to the serosa is unusual. A choriocarcinoma is unlikely in a postmenopausal woman. A "chocolate cyst" (endometrioma) represents a focus of endometriosis in the ovary and develops because of recurrent hemorrhage. It is typically a cystic lesion, and its center is filled with chocolate-brown sludge. A malignant mixed müllerian tumor is typically a large, bulky mass. Adenomyosis tends to be a diffuse process without formation of a focal mass lesion.

BP7 692-693   BP6 611   PBD7 1089-1090
PBD6 1063-1064

20 **(A)** Bartholin's glands may become obstructed, inflamed, and cystic because of abscess formation. A Gartner duct cyst may form in the lateral vaginal wall from the remnant of a wolffian duct; the cyst is filled with fluid and is not inflamed. Hair follicles are not present at the inner labia. The Bartholin's gland lies just inferior to the fascia of the urogenital diaphragm and just anterior to the vestibular bulb, which is not glandular and does not become cystic.

PBD7 1065   PBD6 1040

21 **(B)** Most granulosa-theca cell tumors are hormonally active and secrete estrogens that can lead to endometrial hyperplasia or carcinoma. Most of these tumors are also benign and do not metastasize. A condyloma acuminatum is related to infection with human papillomavirus and is more likely to occur in younger, sexually active persons. In most cases, chronic salpingitis is related to sexually transmitted infections, such as gonorrhea. A partial mole is an uncommon form of gestational trophoblastic disease and occurs only in women of reproductive age.

BP7 699   BP6 618   PBD7 1085, 1102   PBD6 1076-1077

22 (G) This woman has several risk factors for the development of cervical squamous cell carcinoma. These include multiple sexual partners, documented infection of the cervix with high-risk human papillomavirus (HPV) type 16, and diagnosis of a high-grade squamous intraepithelial neoplasm. The remaining choices are not related to HPV infection. Clear cell carcinomas of the cervix are uncommon; some are associated with maternal use of diethylstilbestrol (DES) in pregnancy. An immature teratoma arises in the ovary. A Krukenberg tumor is a form of metastasis to the ovary. Leiomyosarcomas are rare and typically arise in the myometrium, although they can form in the cervix. Cystadenocarcinomas arise in the ovary. Sarcoma botryoides is a vaginal lesion that typically occurs in young girls.

BP7 686-688   BP6 604-605   PBD7 1076-1079
PBD6 1048-1049

23 (D) Immature teratomas are not cystic like mature teratomas. Tissues derived from multiple germ cell layers are present, however, as in all teratomas. The presence of neuroectodermal tissues in immature teratomas is typical. The less differentiated and more numerous the neuroepithelial elements, the worse is the prognosis. Brenner tumors of the ovary are uncommon solid tumors that contain epithelial nests resembling transitional cells of the urinary tract; most are benign. Dysgerminomas are the female equivalent of male testicular seminomas. Granulosa cell tumors have cells that resemble those in ovarian follicles and may secrete estrogens. Leiomyosarcomas are solid tumors of smooth muscle origin that are found most often in the myometrium. Malignant mixed müllerian tumors are typically uterine neoplasms that have glandular and stromal elements; the malignant stromal component can be "heterologous" and may resemble mesenchymal cells not ordinarily found in the myometrium, such as cartilage. Sarcoma botryoides resembles an embryonal rhabdomyosarcoma and is typically a vaginal tumor of young girls.

BP7 700   BP6 617   PBD7 1100-1101   PBD6 1074-1075

24 (C) This woman has endometriosis, a condition in which functional endometrial glands are found outside the uterus. Common sites include ovaries, uterine ligaments, rectovaginal septum, and pelvic peritoneum. These glands respond to ovarian hormones; hence, cyclic abdominal pain coincides with menstruation. Recurrent hemorrhages are followed by scarring and the formation of fibrous adhesions in the pelvis. This may cause distortion of the ovaries and fallopian tubes and may lead to infertility. One common variation is formation of an endometrioma, or "chocolate cyst," which represents a focus of endometriosis that becomes a cystic lesion, its center filled with chocolate-brown sludge from the recurrent hemorrhage. The remaining choices are not associated with endometriosis, although endometrioid tumors may form in foci of endometriosis.

BP7 690   BP6 608-609   PBD7 1083-1084
PBD6 1057-1058

25 (C) Infection with human papillomavirus results in squamous epithelial changes marked by nuclear hyperchromatism and a clear perinuclear halo. These changes, called koilocytosis, occur in condyloma acuminata. Gonococci can cause acute cervicitis, characterized by an acute inflammatory infiltrate. *Chlamydia trachomatis* and *Trichomonas vaginalis* cause cervicitis and produce a discharge containing inflammatory cells. Infection with herpes simplex virus causes vesicles that may rupture and form herpetic ulcers; microscopic findings include inclusion-bearing, multinucleated syncytia, a viral cytopathic effect.

BP7 681-682   BP6 604-605   PBD7 1067
PBD6 1049-1050

26 (C) The presence of pseudohyphae is indicative of a fungal infection. Candidal (monilial) vaginitis is common, because this organism is present in about 5% to 10% of adult women. The inflammation tends to be superficial, and there is typically no invasion of underlying tissues. Infection with *Trichomonas vaginalis* can produce a purulent vaginal discharge, but the organisms are protozoa and do not produce hyphae. *Ureaplasma* is a bacterial agent, as is *Chlamydia*, and both can produce cervicitis. *Neisseria gonorrhoeae*, a gram-negative diplococcus, is the causative agent of gonorrhea.

BP7 685   BP6 602   PBD7 1062-1063   PBD6 1038-1039

27 (D) The presence of dysplastic cells occupying half of the thickness of the epithelium suggests vulvar intraepithelial neoplasia (VIN). The incidence of these lesions has been increasing, probably because of more cases of human papillomavirus (HPV) infections. Some VIN lesions may progress to invasive cancers. Lichen sclerosus is a vulvar dystrophy characterized by thinning of the squamous epithelium and sclerosis of the dermis. A condyloma is usually a raised, nodular lesion. It is also caused by HPV, principally HPV-6 and HPV-11. Like VIN, squamous hyperplasia, another form of vulvar dystrophy, can appear as an area of leukoplakia, but no dysplastic changes are present. Chronic inflammation does not produce dysplasia. A contact dermatitis typically produces reddish "bumps" of various sizes, with irritation and itching that may persist for days or as long as 2 weeks.

BP7 682-683   BP6 600   PBD7 1067-1068
PBD6 1042-1044

28 (A) The microscopic appearance is that of a malignant tumor containing cells with a clear cytoplasm. Vaginal clear cell carcinomas are associated with exposure of the patient's mother to diethylstilbestrol (DES) during pregnancy. These tumors are generally first diagnosed in the late teenage years. Trichomonal infections do not give rise to neoplasia. Polycystic ovary disease can lead to hormonal imbalances from excess androgen production, but vaginal neoplasms do not arise in this setting. Infection with human papillomavirus is associated with squamous epithelial dysplasias and malignancies, not with clear cell adenocarcinomas. Congenital adrenal hyperplasia can produce masculinization in girls, manifesting in early childhood.

BP7 684   BP6 602   PBD7 1071   PBD6 1046

29 (B) These findings point to a diagnosis of endometriosis, in which endometrial glands and stroma are found outside the uterus. The small implants of endometriosis bleed with menstrual cycles, causing local irritation and pain. The process is chronic and can be difficult to diagnose. Tubo-ovarian adhesions can be part of pelvic inflammatory disease, in which the pain tends to be more constant. The presence of peritoneal nodules suggests metastases, which are usually not painful. An enlarged ovary with papillations suggests a cystadenocarcinoma, often associated with ascites. A subserosal leiomyoma of this size is generally asymptomatic.

BP7 690   BP6 608-609   PBD7 1083-1084
PBD6 1057-1058

30 (A) The epithelium shows typical features of infection with human papillomavirus; specifically, prominent perinuclear vacuolization (koilocytosis) and angulation of nuclei. These lesions, called condyloma acuminata, may occur anywhere on the anogenital surface, as single lesions or, more commonly, as multiple lesions. They are not precancerous. Chlamydial infections may produce urethritis, cervicitis, and pelvic inflammatory disease. *Treponema pallidum* is the infectious agent of syphilis, characterized by the gross appearance of a "hard" chancre. *Haemophilus ducreyi* is the agent that produces the "soft" chancre of chancroid. Candidal infections produce a vaginitis or cervicitis with exudate and erythema.

BP7 681-682   BP6 599   PBD7 1067   PBD6 1042

31 (E) Microinvasive squamous cell carcinomas of the cervix are stage I lesions that have a survival rate similar to that of in situ lesions. Such minimal invasiveness does not warrant more aggressive therapies. The likelihood of metastasis or recurrence is minimal.

BP7 686-688   BP6 606-607   PBD7 1076-1079
PBD6 1051-1053

32 (B) Polycystic ovarian disease is a disorder of unknown origin that is typically associated with oligomenorrhea, obesity, and hirsutism. It is thought to be caused by abnormal regulation of androgen synthesis. Teratomas are mass lesions that can be bilateral but usually are not symmetric. Krukenberg tumors represent metastatic disease involving the ovaries, usually from a primary site in the gastrointestinal tract, and are rare among patients of this age. Abscesses are usually unilateral and do not account for the hormonal changes seen in this patient. Cystadenocarcinoma can be bilateral; however, androgen production by ovarian tumors is very uncommon, except by the rare Sertoli-Leydig cell tumors.

BP7 695   BP6 614   PBD7 1092-1093   PBD6 1066

33 (D) Sexually transmitted diseases are the most common cause of inflammation of the fallopian tube. When the incidence of gonorrhea caused by *Neisseria gonorrhoeae* decreases in a population, the proportion of cases of salpingitis caused by *Chlamydia* and *Mycoplasma* increases. The fallopian tube can become distended and adherent to the ovary and may even form a tubo-ovarian abscess. These are features of pelvic inflammatory disease. Infection with human papillomavirus is associated with squamous epithelial dysplasia and neoplasia of the genital tract. *Mycobacterium tuberculosis* is an uncommon cause of salpingitis. *Treponema pallidum* infection causes syphilis, which does not produce florid inflammation with mass effect. *Candida* infections are typically limited to

the vagina and cervix and are superficial, without invasion. Herpes simplex virus most often involves the external genitalia, but it may produce vaginal or cervical lesions; it is unlikely to advance farther. *Haemophilus ducreyi* causes chancroid, which can produce erythematous papules of the external genitalia or vagina, but grossly visible lesions may not be present in women.

BP7 694   BP6 613   PBD7 1063, 1091   PBD6 1065

34 (A) The patient has cervical intraepithelial neoplasia (CIN) III, or carcinoma in situ, which may progress to invasive carcinoma in several years if not treated. Infection with human papillomavirus (HPV) often drives this process, but the presence of HPV alone does not determine therapy. HPV infection cannot be eradicated, but the goal of eradication is not the reason to treat dysplasias. Chronic cervicitis with squamous metaplasia is not a malignant lesion, and conization should be done with or without microinvasion. The conization can preserve fertility in women who are of childbearing age.

BP7 686-688   BP6 604-605   PBD7 1075-1076
PBD6 1049-1051

35 (A) This patient has a choriocarcinoma, an aggressive malignant trophoblastic tumor. Some of these tumors can arise without evidence of pregnancy. Metastases in the vaginal wall and lungs and a hemorrhagic appearance are characteristic. The syncytiotrophoblastic cells produce human chorionic gonadotropin. The α-fetoprotein level is elevated in yolk sac tumors; estrogens are elevated in granulosa-theca cell tumors; androgens such as testosterone are elevated in Leydig cell tumors; and thyroxine can be elevated in specialized teratomas that contain thyroid tissue (e.g., struma ovarii). Carcinoembryonic antigen is a tumor marker that is more characteristic of visceral malignancies such as colonic adenocarcinoma.

BP7 703-704   BP6 622   PBD7 1101-1102, 1113-1114
PBD6 1087-1088

36 (B) Anovulatory cycles are a common cause of dysfunctional uterine bleeding in young women who are beginning menstruation and in women approaching menopause. There is prolonged estrogenic stimulation that is not followed by secretion of progesterone. Polyps are more common in older women. An ectopic pregnancy has acute findings and does not have a prolonged course. Submucosal leiomyomas are a cause of less-variable bleeding and are more likely to be seen in older women. Endometrial carcinomas are rare in patients this age.

BP7 691   BP6 609   PBD7 1081-1082   PBD6 1056

37 (B) This patient has lichen sclerosus et atrophicus, which is most common in postmenopausal women. It is not premalignant, but 1 to 4% of women with this condition develop a carcinoma. Pelvic inflammatory disease results from infection of internal genital organs with organisms such as *Neisseria gonorrhoeae* and *Chlamydia trachomatis*. Vulvar intraepithelial neoplasia is marked by dysplastic squamous epithelial changes. Extramammary Paget's disease is rare; it produces reddish areas of scaling and is caused by the presence of adenocarcinoma-like cells at the dermal-epidermal junction. Human papillomavirus infection is associated with the condyloma acuminata and with squamous epithelial dysplasias.

BP7 681   BP6 599   PBD7 1066   PBD6 1041

38 **(B)** This woman has multiple risk factors for the development of endometrial cancer; these include obesity, diabetes, and nulliparity. All of these factors are thought to contribute to the development of endometrial hyperplasias and carcinomas caused by hyperestrinism. The remaining choices of primary ovarian tumor (D, E, and G) are not related to hyperestrinism. Adenomyosis is caused by the presence of endometrial glands and stroma within the myometrium. A Krukenberg tumor is a form of metastasis to the ovary. Ovaries have a rich blood supply, and torsion is the only likely cause of infarction.

BP7 693-694   BP6 612   PBD7 1086-1088   PBD6 1061

39 **(C)** Cystadenocarcinomas are common ovarian tumors that are often bilateral. The serous variety occurs more frequently than the mucinous type and is typically unilocular, whereas the mucinous tumors are multilocular. Serous cystadenocarcinomas account for more than half of ovarian cancers. As the name indicates, they are cystic in appearance. They may be benign, borderline, or malignant. Benign tumors have a smooth cyst wall with small or absent papillary projections. Borderline tumors have increasing amounts of papillary projections. Endometrioid tumors resemble endometrial carcinomas and may arise in foci of endometriosis. Clear cell carcinomas are uncommon malignancies of the vagina and cervix. Dysgerminomas are solid tumors of germ cell origin. Granulosa cell tumors can be solid and cystic and may produce estrogens. Malignant mixed müllerian tumors are, typically, uterine neoplasms that have glandular and stromal elements; the malignant stromal component can be "heterologous" and may resemble mesenchymal cells that are not ordinarily found in the myometrium, such as cartilage. Mature cystic teratomas typically contain abundant hair and gooey sebaceous fluid within the cystic cavity; surrounding tissues are formed from various germ layers. Sertoli-Leydig cell tumors are rare, yellow-brown, solid masses; they may secrete androgens or estrogens.

BP7 697-699   BP6 615-616   PBD7 1095-1097   PBD6 1068-1070

40 **(C)** The lesion shown in the figure is large and ulcerative and projects into the vagina. It is most likely an invasive squamous cell carcinoma that has infiltrated into the subepithelial region. Dysplastic changes confined to the epithelium represent cervical intraepithelial neoplasms. Glandular invasive lesions indicate an adenocarcinoma, which is much less common than squamous cell carcinoma of the cervix. Mononuclear infiltrates indicate chronic cervicitis.

BP7 684   BP6 606-607   PBD7 1076-1079
PBD6 1051-1053

41 **(E)** Cervical intraepithelial neoplasia (CIN) I represents minimal (mild) dysplasia and is a potentially reversible process. Dysplasias are preneoplastic and may progress to carcinomas if not treated. Risk factors for cervical dysplasias and carcinoma include early age at first intercourse, multiple sexual partners, and a male partner with multiple previous sexual partners. These factors all increase the potential for infection with human papillomavirus. Use of oral contraceptives does not cause cervical dysplasia or carcinoma. Diethylstilbestrol (DES) exposure is a factor in the development of clear cell carcinomas of the vagina and cervix. A vitamin B$_{12}$ deficiency may produce some megaloblastic epithelial changes but not dysplasia. Treatment of carcinomas does not result in dysplasia.

BP7 686-688   BP6 604-605   PBD7 1075-1076
PBD6 1049-1051

42 **(E)** The lesions shown are condyloma acuminata, which are often multiple and can become several centimeters in diameter. They are also known as genital or venereal warts and are the result of infection with human papillomavirus (HPV) acquired during sexual intercourse. The presence of HPV-infected cells is indicated by koilocytotic change. These cells have cytoplasmic vacuolation. Anovulatory cycles can lead to irregular menstrual periods but not to vulvar skin changes. The best-known association of a faulty tumor suppressor gene and a genital tract cancer is the *BRCA1* gene and ovarian carcinoma. Diabetic patients are more prone to infections, typically bacterial or fungal, that do not produce nodular masses. Portions of this data are best left to the imagination of the reader to interpret.

BP7 681-682   BP6 599-600   PBD7 1067   PBD6 1042

43 **(B)** Mucinous tumors of the ovary are of epithelial origin, are less common than serous tumors, and tend to be multiloculated. The appearance of ascites suggests metastases, which is most common with surface epithelial neoplasms of the ovary. Immature teratomas tend to be solid masses, as do granulosa cell tumors and dysgerminomas. Choriocarcinomas rarely reach this size, because they metastasize early; they are typically hemorrhagic.

BP7 697-699   BP6 616-617   PBD7 1097
PBD6 1070-1071

44 **(D)** This woman has classical features of preeclampsia defined by hypertension, edema, and proteinuria, typically with onset in the third trimester. The addition of convulsions or coma defines eclampsia. Primigravid women are at greater risk. There is no evidence in this case that primary renal disease could cause her hypertension, and the onset was sudden. While the precise cause of preeclampsia is not known, placental ischemia is believed to be the underlying mechanism. This is associated with shallow placentation and incomplete conversion of decidual vessels into high volume channels required to adequately perfuse the placenta. Untreated patients may go on to develop eclampsia and DIC. Gestational trophoblastic disease predisposes patients to preeclampsia, but hydatidiform mole is excluded by the presence of a fetus, and a partial mole would be unlikely to persist into the third trimester. Cushing syndrome with adrenal cortical hyperplasia could lead to hypertension with sodium retention, but she does not have hypokalemia or hyperglycemia. Functional ovarian tumors, most commonly estrogen-secreting, such as a granulosa cell tumor or thecoma, do not produce hypertension and proteinuria.

BP7 704-705   PBD7 1106-1110

The Breast

PBD7 Chapter 23: The Breast

PBD6 Chapter 25: The Breast

BP7 and BP6 Chapter 19: Female Genital System and Breast

1 A 36-year-old woman has noticed a bloody discharge from the nipple of her right breast for the past 3 days. On physical examination, the skin of the breasts appears normal, and no masses are palpable. There is no axillary lymphadenopathy. The patient has regular menstrual cycles and is using oral contraceptives. Excisional biopsy is most likely to show which of the following lesions?

☐ (A) Fibroadenoma
☐ (B) Phyllodes tumor
☐ (C) Acute mastitis
☐ (D) Intraductal papilloma
☐ (E) Sclerosing adenosis

2 A 28-year-old woman in the third trimester of her third pregnancy discovered a lump in her right breast. The physician palpated a 2-cm discrete, freely movable mass beneath the nipple. After the birth of a term infant, the mass appears to decrease slightly in size. The infant breast-feeds without difficulty. Which of the following is the most likely diagnosis?

☐ (A) Intraductal papilloma
☐ (B) Phyllodes tumor
☐ (C) Lobular carcinoma in situ
☐ (D) Fibroadenoma
☐ (E) Medullary carcinoma

3 A 30-year-old woman suffered a traumatic blow to the right breast. Initially, there was a 3-cm contusion that resolved within a few weeks, but she then felt a firm lump below the site of the bruise. Which of the following is the most likely diagnosis?

☐ (A) Fibroadenoma
☐ (B) Sclerosing adenosis
☐ (C) Fat necrosis
☐ (D) Intraductal carcinoma
☐ (E) Mammary duct ectasia

4 A 55-year-old man has developed bilateral breast enlargement over the past year. On physical examination, the enlargement is symmetric and is not painful to palpation. There are no masses. The patient is not obese and is not taking any medications. Which of the following underlying conditions best accounts for these findings?

☐ (A) Micronodular cirrhosis
☐ (B) Chronic glomerulonephritis
☐ (C) Choriocarcinoma of the testis
☐ (D) ACTH-secreting pituitary adenoma
☐ (E) Rheumatoid arthritis

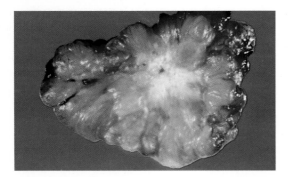

5 A 44-year-old woman sees her physician because she felt a lump in her left breast 1 week ago. The physician palpates a firm, irregular mass in the upper outer quadrant of the left breast. There are no overlying skin lesions. The gross appearance of the excisional biopsy specimen is shown in the figure above. Which of the following additional findings is most likely to be present on physical examination?

❑ (A) Axillary lymphadenopathy
❑ (B) Bloody discharge from the nipple
❑ (C) Painful breast enlargement
❑ (D) Mass in the opposite breast
❑ (E) Cushingoid face

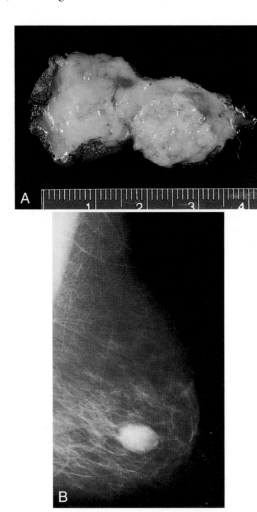

Courtesy of Dr. Jack G. Meyer, Brigham and Women's Hospital, Boston, MA.

6 A 25-year-old woman sees her physician because she has noticed a lump in her right breast. The physician palpates a 2-cm firm, circumscribed mass in the lower outer quadrant. The excised mass (A) and the mammogram (B) are shown. Which of the following is the most likely diagnosis?

❑ (A) Phyllodes tumor
❑ (B) Fibrocystic changes
❑ (C) Fibroadenoma
❑ (D) Fat necrosis
❑ (E) Infiltrating ductal carcinoma
❑ (F) Mastitis

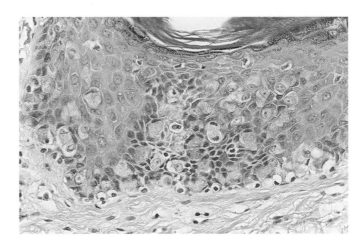

7 A 47-year-old woman has noticed a red, scaly area of skin on her left breast that has grown slightly larger over the past 4 months. On physical examination, there is a 1-cm area of eczematous skin just lateral to the areola. The microscopic appearance of the skin biopsy specimen is shown in the figure. Which of the following is the most likely diagnosis?

❑ (A) Apocrine metaplasia
❑ (B) Paget disease of the breast
❑ (C) Inflammatory carcinoma
❑ (D) Lobular carcinoma in situ
❑ (E) Fat necrosis

8 Three weeks after giving birth to a normal term infant, a 24-year-old woman is breast-feeding the infant and notices fissures in the skin around her left nipple. Over the next few days, the region around the nipple becomes erythematous and tender. Purulent exudate from a small abscess drains through a fissure. Which of the following organisms is most likely to be cultured from the exudate?

❑ (A) *Listeria monocytogenes*
❑ (B) *Streptococcus viridans*
❑ (C) *Candida albicans*
❑ (D) *Staphylococcus aureus*
❑ (E) *Lactobacillus acidophilus*

9 A 27-year-old woman feels a lump in her right breast. The physician palpates a 2-cm irregular, firm area beneath the lateral edge of the areola. A biopsy specimen shows microscopic evidence of an increased number of ducts, which are compressed because of proliferation of fibrous connective tissue. Dilated ducts with apocrine metaplasia are also present. Which of the following is the most likely diagnosis?

- (A) Traumatic fat necrosis
- (B) Fibrocystic changes
- (C) Mammary duct ectasia
- (D) Fibroadenoma
- (E) Infiltrating ductal carcinoma

10 Two months ago, a 44-year-old woman noticed several lumps in her right breast. The lumps have not decreased in size since then. A mammogram shows several 0.5- to 1-cm foci of irregular density in both breasts. Fine-needle aspirates of lesions in both breasts contain malignant cells. Which of the following breast carcinomas is most likely to produce these findings?

- (A) Infiltrating ductal carcinoma
- (B) Malignant phyllodes tumor
- (C) Colloid carcinoma
- (D) Medullary carcinoma
- (E) Infiltrating lobular carcinoma

11 A 56-year-old woman sees her physician for a routine health examination. There are no remarkable findings on physical examination. A mammogram shows a 0.5-cm irregular area of increased density with scattered microcalcifications in the upper outer quadrant of the left breast. Excisional biopsy shows atypical lobular hyperplasia. The patient has been on postmenopausal estrogen-progesterone therapy for the past 10 years. She has smoked 1 pack of cigarettes per day for the past 35 years. Which of the following conclusions is most pertinent to these findings?

- (A) She has the *BRCA1* gene mutation
- (B) The postmenopausal estrogen replacement therapy should be stopped
- (C) Her risk of breast carcinoma is increased
- (D) She should undergo bilateral simple mastectomies
- (E) She should stop smoking

12 A 54-year-old woman sees her physician after feeling a lump in her left breast. The physician palpates a firm, irregular mass in the lower outer quadrant just beneath the lateral margin of the areola. A mammogram shows a 2-cm density with focal microcalcifications. Excisional biopsy shows both intraductal and invasive components of a breast carcinoma. Immunohistochemical staining shows that the cells are positive for *ERBB2* (*HER2/neu*) expression but negative for estrogen receptor and progesterone receptor expression. Flow cytometry shows a small aneuploid peak and a low S-phase. When combined with doxorubicin, which of the following drugs is most likely to be useful in treating this patient?

- (A) Hydroxyurea
- (B) Celecoxib
- (C) Raloxifene
- (D) Tamoxifen
- (E) Trastuzumab

13 A 35-year-old woman feels a poorly defined lump in her right breast. The physician palpates an irregular 1-cm mass in the upper inner quadrant. The mass is not painful and does

not feel firm. There are no lesions of the overlying skin and no axillary lymphadenopathy. The patient has normal menstrual cycles. She is G 3, P 3, and her last child was born 5 years ago. Which of the following is the most likely diagnosis?

- (A) Fibrocystic changes
- (B) Lobular carcinoma
- (C) Acute mastitis
- (D) Fibroadenoma
- (E) No pathologic diagnosis

14 A 51-year-old woman has noticed an area of swelling with tenderness in her right breast that has worsened over the past 2 months. On physical examination, the 7-cm area of erythematous skin is tender and firm. There is swelling of the right breast, nipple retraction, and right axillary lymphadenopathy. Excisional biopsy is most likely to show which of the following lesions?

- (A) Atypical epithelial hyperplasia
- (B) Phyllodes tumor
- (C) Fat necrosis
- (D) Sclerosing adenosis
- (E) Infiltrating ductal carcinoma

15 A 39-year-old woman has noticed an enlarging mass in her left breast for the past 2 years. The physician palpates a 4-cm firm mass. A simple mastectomy is performed with axillary lymph node sampling and plastic reconstruction of the breast. On gross sectioning, the mass has a soft, tan, fleshy surface. Histologically, the mass is composed of large cells with vesicular nuclei and prominent nucleoli. There is a marked lymphocytic infiltrate within the tumor, and the tumor has a discrete, noninfiltrative border. No axillary node metastases are present. The tumor cells are negative for estrogen receptor and progesterone receptor. Which of the following is the most likely diagnosis?

- (A) Colloid carcinoma
- (B) Fibroadenoma
- (C) Infiltrating ductal carcinoma
- (D) Infiltrating lobular carcinoma
- (E) Intraductal papilloma
- (F) Medullary carcinoma
- (G) Papillary carcinoma
- (H) Phyllodes tumor

16 A 47-year-old woman has a routine health examination. There are no remarkable findings except for a barely palpable mass in the right breast. A mammogram shows an irregular 1.5-cm area of density in the upper outer quadrant. Scattered microcalcifications are present in the density. A biopsy specimen from this area shows atypical ductal hyperplasia. Which of the following is the most appropriate advice to give to this patient?

- (A) There is a risk of cancer in the opposite breast
- (B) A mastectomy should be performed
- (C) These changes are related to smoking cigarettes
- (D) Antibiotic therapy is indicated to treat the lesion
- (E) The *BRCA1* oncogene has been inherited

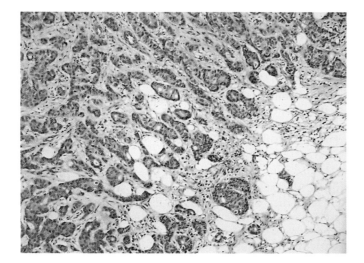

17 A 25-year-old Jewish woman sees her physician after finding a lump in her right breast. On physical examination, a 2-cm firm, nonmovable mass is palpated in the upper outer quadrant. There are no overlying skin lesions and no axillary lymphadenopathy. An excisional biopsy specimen is shown. The family history indicates that the patient's mother, maternal aunt, and maternal grandmother have had similar lesions. Her 18-year-old sister has asked a physician to determine whether she is genetically at risk of developing a similar disease. The physician is most likely to order an analysis of which of the following genes?

❑ (A) *HER2/neu (ERBB2)*
❑ (B) *MYC*
❑ (C) *BRCA1*
❑ (D) *RB*
❑ (E) Estrogen receptor gene

18 A study of women with breast carcinoma is performed to determine the presence and amount of estrogen receptor (ER) and progesterone receptor (PR) in the carcinoma cells. Large amounts of ER and PR are found in the carcinoma cells of some patients. These receptors are not present in the cells of other patients. The patients with positivity for ER-PR are likely to exhibit which of the following traits?

❑ (A) Higher response to therapy
❑ (B) Increased immunogenicity
❑ (C) Greater risk of familial breast cancer
❑ (D) Higher tumor stage
❑ (E) Greater likelihood of metastases
❑ (F) Greater aneuploidy with flow cytometry
❑ (G) Higher tumor grade

19 A 50-year-old woman has a routine health examination. There are no remarkable findings on physical examination, but a mammogram shows a 1-cm irregular density in the right breast. A fine-needle aspirate of the lesion contains malignant cells. The mass is excised, and axillary lymph node sampling is performed. The microscopic features of the neoplasm are consistent with ductal carcinoma in situ. There are no lymph node metastases. She receives radiation therapy. Which of the following statements provides the most appropriate advice to the patient?

❑ (A) You will probably survive less than 5 years
❑ (B) Another cancer is probably present in the opposite breast
❑ (C) Distant metastases are unlikely to be found
❑ (D) Your family members should be screened for *BRCA1* and *BRCA2* mutations
❑ (E) Flow cytometry can determine whether chemotherapy is warranted

20 A 79-year-old previously healthy woman feels a lump in her right breast. The physician palpates a 2-cm firm mass in the upper outer quadrant. Nontender right axillary lymphadenopathy is present. A lumpectomy with axillary lymph node dissection is performed. Microscopic examination shows that the mass is an infiltrating ductal carcinoma. Two of 10 axillary nodes contain metastases. Flow cytometry on the carcinoma cells shows a small aneuploid peak and high S-phase. Immunohistochemical tests show that the tumor cells are positive for estrogen receptor, negative for *ERBB2* (*HER2/neu*) expression, and positive for cathepsin D expression. Which of the following is the most important prognostic factor for this patient?

❑ (A) Age
❑ (B) Histologic subtype of carcinoma
❑ (C) DNA content in the carcinoma
❑ (D) Presence of lymph node metastases
❑ (E) Expression of stromal proteases in the carcinoma
❑ (F) Estrogen receptor positivity
❑ (G) Lack of *ERBB2* (*HER2/neu*) expression in the carcinoma.

21 A 29-year-old woman and her 32-year-old sister were diagnosed with infiltrating ductal carcinoma of the breast, and both had bilateral mastectomies. Which of the following risk factors is most significant for this type of cancer?

❑ (A) Oral contraceptive use
❑ (B) Inheritance of a mutant p53 allele
❑ (C) Obesity
❑ (D) Multiparity
❑ (E) Smoking cigarettes

22 A 63-year-old woman feels a small lump in her right breast. The physician palpates a firm area that has a cordlike feel. No lesions of the overlying skin are present, and there is no axillary lymphadenopathy. A mammogram shows a density that contains microcalcifications. An excisional biopsy specimen contains soft, white material that is extruded from small ducts when pressure is applied. Microscopic examination shows ducts that contain large, atypical cells in a cribriform pattern. Which of the following is the most likely diagnosis?

❑ (A) Colloid carcinoma
❑ (B) Infiltrating ductal carcinoma
❑ (C) Infiltrating lobular carcinoma
❑ (D) Comedocarcinoma
❑ (E) Medullary carcinoma
❑ (F) Paget disease of the breast
❑ (G) Papillary carcinoma
❑ (H) Phyllodes tumor

23 An epidemiologic study is conducted with male subjects who have been diagnosed with breast carcinoma. Their demographic data, past medical histories, family histories, and laboratory data are examined to identify factors that increase the risk of cancer. Which of the following factors is most likely to significantly increase the risk of developing male breast carcinoma?

- ❏ (A) Gynecomastia
- ❏ (B) Age >70 years
- ❏ (C) Asian ancestry
- ❏ (D) Chronic alcoholism
- ❏ (E) *BRCA1* gene mutation

24 A clinical study is performed on postmenopausal women living in Tampa, Florida, who are between the ages of 45 and 70 years. All have been diagnosed with infiltrating ductal carcinoma positive for estrogen receptor (ER) and progesterone receptor (PR), which has been confirmed by biopsy and microscopic examination of tissue. None has the *BRCA1* or *BRCA2* mutation. Which of the following is most likely to indicate the highest relative risk of developing the carcinomas seen in this group of women?

- ❏ (A) Age at menarche of greater than 16 years
- ❏ (B) Age at menopause younger than 45 years
- ❏ (C) First-degree relative with breast cancer
- ❏ (D) Smoking cigarettes, >40 pack years
- ❏ (E) Multiparity
- ❏ (F) Prior diagnosis of mastitis

25 A 26-year-old woman has felt a breast lump for the past month and is worried because she has a family history of early onset and bilateral breast cancers. On physical examination there is a firm 2 cm mass in the upper outer quadrant of her left breast. A biopsy is performed and microscopically shows carcinoma. Genetic analysis shows that she is a carrier of the *BRCA1* gene mutation, as are her mother and sister. Which of the following histologic types of breast carcinoma has the highest incidence in families such as hers?

- ❏ (A) Lobular carcinoma
- ❏ (B) Tubular carcinoma
- ❏ (C) Metaplastic carcinoma
- ❏ (D) Papillary carcinoma
- ❏ (E) Medullary carcinoma

ANSWERS

1 (D) Intraductal papillomas are usually solitary and smaller than 1 cm. They are located in large lactiferous sinuses or ducts and have a tendency to bleed. Fibroadenomas contain ducts with stroma and are not highly vascular; these lesions are not located in ducts. Phyllodes tumors also arise from intralobular stroma and can be malignant. They do not invade ducts to cause bleeding. Abscesses complicating mastitis organize with a fibrous wall. Sclerosing adenosis, a lesion occurring with fibrocystic changes, has abundant collagen, not vascularity.

BP7 710   BP6 629   PBD7 1129   PBD6 1104-1105

2 (D) Fibroadenomas are common and may enlarge during pregnancy or late in each menstrual cycle. Most intraductal papillomas are smaller than 1 cm and are not influenced by hormonal changes. Phyllodes tumors are uncommon and tend to be larger than 4 cm. Lobular carcinoma in situ is typically an ill-defined lesion without a mass effect. Medullary carcinomas tend to be large; they account for only about 1% of all breast carcinomas.

BP7 709-710   BP6 628   PBD7 1149-1150
PBD6 1102-1103

3 (C) Fat necrosis is typically caused by trauma to the breast. The damaged, necrotic fat is phagocytosed by macrophages, which become lipid laden. The lesion resolves as a collagenous scar within weeks to months. A fibroadenoma is a neoplasm, and tumors are not induced by trauma. Sclerosing adenosis is a feature of fibrocystic changes, a common cause of nontraumatic breast lumps. An intraductal carcinoma may not be palpable. Mammary duct ectasia from inspissated secretions can induce chronic inflammation and fibrosis, which mimic a carcinoma.

BP7 709   BP6 628   PBD7 1126   PBD6 1097-1098

4 (A) Micronodular cirrhosis is most often a consequence of chronic alcoholism and impairs hepatic estrogen metabolism, which can lead to gynecomastia. Chronic renal failure is not likely to have this consequence. Choriocarcinomas of the testis produce human chorionic gonadotropin, not estrogens. ACTH-secreting pituitary adenomas cause truncal obesity because of Cushing syndrome. Rheumatoid nodules can appear in various locations along with rheumatoid arthritis, but they rarely occur in the breast and are unlikely to be bilateral.

BP7 716   BP6 635   PBD7 1151-1152   PBD6 1117

5 (A) This irregular, infiltrative mass is an infiltrating ductal carcinoma, the most common form of breast cancer. Breast carcinomas are most likely to metastasize to regional lymph nodes. By the time a breast cancer becomes palpable, lymph node metastases are present in more than 50% of patients. A bloody discharge from the nipple most often results from an intraductal papilloma. Pain with breast enlargement suggests inflammation. Lobular carcinomas are more often bilateral, but they are less common than infiltrating ductal carcinomas. Breast cancers are associated in rare cases with ectopic corticotropin secretion or Cushing syndrome.

BP7 713-714   BP6 631-633   PBD7 1142-1144
PBD6 1110

6 (C) Both grossly and radiographically she has a discrete mass that in a patient of this age is most likely a fibroadenoma. Phyllodes tumors are typically much larger and are far less common. Fibrocystic changes are generally irregular lesions, not discrete masses. Fat necrosis and infiltrating cancers are masses with irregular outlines. Mastitis has a more diffuse involvement, without mass effect.

BP7 709-710   BP6 628   PBD7 1149-1150
PBD6 1102-1103

7 (B) Paget cells are large cells that have clear, mucinous cytoplasm and infiltrate the skin. They are malignant and extend to the skin from an underlying breast carcinoma. Apocrine metaplasia affects the cells lining the cystically dilated ducts in fibrocystic change. "Inflammatory carcinoma" does not refer to a specific histologic type of breast cancer; rather, it describes the involvement of dermal lymphatics by infiltrating carcinoma. In lobular carcinoma in situ, terminal ducts or acini are filled with neoplastic cells. The overlying skin is unaffected. The macrophages in fat necrosis do not infiltrate the skin and do not have the atypical nuclei seen in the figure.

BP7 713   BP6 632   PBD7 1140-1141   PBD6 1108-1109

8 (D) Staphylococcal acute mastitis typically produces localized abscesses, whereas streptococcal infections tend to spread throughout the breast. Listeriosis can be spread by contaminated food, including milk products, not by human milk. *Candida* may cause some local skin irritation but is likely to become invasive only in immunosuppressed patients. *Lactobacillus acidophilus* is the organism used to produce fermented nonhuman milk.

BP7 708-709   BP6 627   PBD7 1125   PBD6 1096

9 **(B)** Fibrocystic changes account for the largest category of breast lumps. They are characterized by ductal proliferation, ductal dilation (sometimes with apocrine metaplasia), and fibrosis. Fat necrosis may produce a localized, firm lesion that mimics carcinoma, but histology shows macrophages and neutrophils surrounding necrotic adipocytes, and healing leaves a fibrous scar. Inspissated duct secretions may produce duct ectasia with a surrounding lymphoplasmacytic infiltrate. A fibroadenoma is a discrete mass formed by a proliferation of fibrous stroma with compressed ductules. Carcinomas have proliferations of atypical neoplastic cells that fill ducts and can invade stroma.

BP7 705-708   BP6 626   PBD7 1127-1129
PBD6 1098-1100

10 **(E)** Among primary malignancies of the breast, lobular carcinoma in situ (LCIS) is most likely to be bilateral. LCIS may precede invasive lesions by several years. Lobular carcinoma may be mixed with ductal carcinoma, and it may be difficult to distinguish them histologically.

BP7 714   BP6 633   PBD7 1141-1142   PBD6 1110-1111

11 **(C)** Both atypical lobular hyperplasia and atypical ductal hyperplasia increase the risk of breast cancer fivefold; the risk affects both breasts and is higher in those women who are premenopausal or have a family history of breast cancer. The *BRCA1* mutation accounts for about 10% to 20% of familial breast carcinomas and only a few percent of all breast cancers. Mastectomies are probably not warranted at this time, but close follow-up is needed. Smoking and exogenous estrogen therapy are not well-established risk factors for breast cancer.

BP7 707   BP6 629-630   PBD7 1129   PBD6 1105-1106

12 **(E)** The expression of *ERBB2* (*HER2/neu*) suggests that biotherapy with trastuzumab may have some effectiveness. Drug names with the suffix *-mab* are monoclonal antibodies that target a specific biochemical component of cells. This form of biotherapy is useful, because normal breast cells do not have *ERBB2* (*HER2/neu*) expression. Doxorubicin is a standard chemotherapeutic agent that is part of various multi-agent protocols. Hydroxyurea is a cycle-acting agent that is not useful in breast cancer. Celecoxib is an inhibitor of cyclooxygenase 2 in the arachidonic acid pathway that forms prostaglandins as part of an inflammatory reaction. Tamoxifen is an antiestrogenic compound that has effectiveness in the treatment of breast cancers positive for estrogen receptor.

BP7 711-712   BP6 634   PBD7 1136-1137, 1148
PBD6 1115-1116

13 **(A)** Statistically, the largest category of breast "lumps" (40% of all masses) comprises fibrocystic changes. These lesions are probably related to cyclic breast changes that occur during the menstrual cycle. In about 30% of cases, no specific pathologic diagnosis can be made. Carcinomas often produce palpable masses and represent about 10% of lumps. Fibroade-nomas constitute 7% of lumps, but they are usually discrete, firm masses. Acute mastitis does not usually manifest as a lump and is most often a complication of lactation.

BP7 705-708   BP6 624   PBD7 1122-1124   PBD6 1096

14 **(E)** The gross appearance of the skin is consistent with invasion of dermal lymphatics by carcinoma—the so-called inflammatory carcinoma. Nipple retraction and axillary lymphadenopathy also suggest invasive ductal carcinoma. Atypical ductal hyperplasia may increase the risk of carcinoma, but it does not produce visible surface skin changes. A phyllodes tumor can be large and sometimes tender, but the overlying skin is typically not affected, and spread to lymph nodes is uncommon. The feel of fat necrosis on palpation can mimic that of carcinoma, but the skin is not involved. Sclerosing adenosis is a feature of benign fibrocystic changes and has no skin involvement.

BP7 714   BP6 633   PBD7 1142, 1146   PBD6 1114

15 **(F)** Medullary carcinomas account for about 1% to 5% of all breast carcinomas. They tend to occur in women at younger ages than do most other breast cancers. Despite poor prognostic indicators, such as absence of estrogen receptors and progesterone receptors (ER-PR), medullary carcinomas have a better prognosis than most other breast cancers. Perhaps the infiltrating lymphocytes are helpful. Colloid carcinomas are about as frequent as medullary carcinomas, but they are often positive for ER-PR, and the prognosis is better than average. Fibroadenomas are small benign lesions that tend to stop enlarging after menopause, once hormonal stimulation has ceased. Infiltrating ductal and infiltrating lobular carcinomas tend not to produce large, localized lesions, because they are more invasive, and they lack a distinct lymphoid infiltrate. Intraductal papillomas are unlikely to be larger than 1 cm. True papillary carcinomas are quite rare, although other types of breast carcinoma may have a papillary component. The phyllodes tumor is typically large, but it has both stromal and glandular components.

BP7 714   BP6 633   PBD7 1145   PBD6 1111

16 **(A)** Fibrocystic changes without epithelial hyperplasia do not suggest an increased risk of breast cancer. Moderate to florid hyperplasia increases the risk twofold, and atypical ductal or lobular hyperplasias increase the risk fivefold. The risk in this patient is not great enough to suggest radical or simple mastectomy at this time. Breast cancers are not associated with tobacco use. These changes are not the result of infection. The *BRCA1* gene accounts for a small percentage of breast cancers, primarily in families in which cancer onset occurs at a young age.

BP7 706-708   BP6 626-627   PBD7 1127-1129
PBD6 1099-1100

17 **(C)** The biopsy shows an invasive breast cancer. Given the young age of the patient and the strong family history of breast cancer, it is reasonable to assume that she has inherited an altered gene that predisposes to breast cancer. There are two known breast cancer susceptibility genes: *BRCA1* and *BRCA2*. Both are cancer suppressor genes. Specific mutations of *BRCA1* are common in some ethnic groups, such as Ashkenazi Jews. *ERBB2* (*HER2/neu*) is a growth factor receptor gene that is amplified in certain breast cancers and is a marker of poor prognosis, not susceptibility. Inheritance of *RB1* mutations predisposes to retinoblastoma and osteosarcomas, not breast carcinomas. Estrogen receptors are expressed in 50% to 75% of breast cancers. Their presence bodes well for therapy with receptor antagonists. There is no known relationship between the structure of the estrogen receptor gene and susceptibility to breast cancer.

BP7 710-714   BP6 630-631   PBD7 1131-1134
PBD6 1106-1107, 1110

18 **(A)** The estrogen receptor and progesterone receptor (ER-PR) status helps predict whether chemotherapy with antiestrogen compounds such as tamoxifen will be effective; however, the correlation is not perfect. The ER and PR do not affect immunogenicity and are not targets for immunotherapy. In contrast, immunotherapy targeted to the overexpressed *ERBB2* (*HER2/neu*) gene is being used. The overall prognosis may be predicted from several factors, including histologic type, histologic grade, presence of metastases, degree of aneuploidy, and tumor stage. A family history and the presence of specific mutations such as *BRCA1* or *BRCA2* correlate with familial risk of breast cancer.

BP7 716   BP6 634   PBD7 1136-1137   PBD6 1115

19 **(C)** At least half of mammographically detected breast cancers are ductal carcinoma in situ (DCIS). This in situ carcinoma is highly unlikely to metastasize, because the cells lack the ability to invade basement membrane. Thus, with surgical excision and radiotherapy, the 5-year survival rate is high, although some tumors may progress to invasive lesions over time. Lobular carcinomas are most likely to be present in the opposite breast. Patients with *BRCA1* or *BRCA2* mutations can have familial breast carcinomas. In these patients, there is usually a strong family history, and the age of onset may be early. The occurrence of a sporadic breast cancer in a racial group that is not at high risk of familial cancer does not warrant mutational analysis of *BRCA1* and *BRCA2*. Flow cytometry is useful to suggest prognosis, not treatment.

BP7 712-713   BP6 633-635   PBD7 1139-1141
PBD6 1107-1109, 1113-1115

20 **(D)** Many factors affect the course of breast cancer. The involvement of axillary lymph nodes is the most important prognostic factor. If there is no spread to axillary nodes, the 10-year survival rate is almost 80%. It falls to 35% to 40% with one to three positive nodes and to 15% with more than 10 positive nodes. Increasing age is a risk of breast cancer, but age alone does not indicate a prognosis, and treatment of cancers in the elderly can be successful. Some histologic types of breast cancer have a better prognosis than others, but staging is a more important factor than histologic type. An increased DNA content with aneuploidy and a high S-phase suggests a worse prognosis, but staging is still a more important determinant of prognosis. The expression of stromal proteases, such as cathepsin D, predicts metastases, but in this case "the horse is out of the barn" and metastasis has occurred. Estrogen receptor positivity suggests a better response to hormonal manipulation of the tumor, whereas expression of *ERBB2* (*HER2/neu*) suggests responsiveness to biotherapy with the monoclonal antibody trastuzumab.

BP7 716   BP6 634   PBD7 1146-1148   PBD6 1115-1116

21 **(B)** Bilateral breast cancer in very young women in the same family suggests a germ-line mutation in a tumor sup-

pressor gene. The affected genes may be *BRCA1*, *BRCA2*, or *p53*. The *BRCA1* and *BRCA2* genes account for most hereditary breast cancers. Establishment of other risk factors is not as secure. Multiparity actually reduces the risk of breast cancer.

BP7 711-712   BP6 630   PBD7 1133-1135   PBD6 1105

22 **(D)** An intraductal carcinoma, or ductal carcinoma in situ (DCIS), may not produce a palpable mass. The necrosis of the neoplastic cells in the ducts leads to calcification, and the necrotic cells can be extruded from the ducts, giving rise to the term comedocarcinoma. Such intraductal carcinomas represent about one fourth of all breast cancers. If not excised, such lesions become invasive. Intraductal carcinoma has several other histologic patterns, including noncomedo DCIS and Paget disease of the nipple, in which extension of the malignant cells to the skin of the nipple and areola produces the appearance of a seborrheic dermatitis. Colloid carcinomas occur about as frequently as medullary carcinomas, but they are often positive for estrogen receptor and progesterone receptor, and the prognosis is better than average. Infiltrating ductal carcinomas tend to produce irregular, firm, mass lesions, because they are more invasive. Infiltrating lobular carcinomas can have a diffuse pattern without significant mass effect. Medullary carcinomas tend to be large masses; microscopically, they have nests of large cells with a surrounding lymphoid infiltrate. True papillary carcinomas are rare, although a papillary component may be present in other types of breast carcinoma. The phyllodes tumor is typically large, but it has both stromal and glandular components.

BP7 712-713   BP6 631   PBD7 1138-1141
PBD6 1107-1108

23 **(B)** Male breast cancers are rare, and they occur primarily among the elderly. Additional risk factors include first-degree relatives with breast cancer, decreased testicular function, exposure to exogenous estrogens, infertility, obesity, prior benign breast disease, exposure to ionizing radiation, and residency in Western countries. Gynecomastia does not appear to be a risk factor. Four per cent to 14% of cases in males are attributed to germ-line *BRCA2* mutations.

BP7 717   BP6 635   PBD7 1152   PBD6 1118

24 **(C)** The relative risk of breast cancer increases with a variety of factors, but family history is one of the strongest. A history of bilateral breast disease and earlier age of onset of cancer increase the risk. The earlier age of onset increases the risk of *BRCA1* or *BRCA2*. A longer reproductive life, with early menarche (younger than 12 years) and late menopause (older than 55 years), and nulliparity increase the risk of breast cancer, probably because of increased estrogen exposure. "Soft" risk factors include exogenous estrogens, obesity, and smoking. Mastitis does not affect the risk of breast cancer.

BP7 710-712   BP6 629-630   PBD7 1130-1133
PBD6 1106

25 **(E)** Patients with the *BRCA1* gene mutation have a high incidence of medullary carcinomas that are poorly differentiated, do not express the *HER2/neu* (*ERBB2*) protein, and are negative for estrogen and progesterone receptors.

PBD7 1134, 1145

CHAPTER 24

The Endocrine System

PBD7 Chapter 24: The Endocrine System

PBD6 Chapter 26: The Endocrine System

BP7 and BP6 Chapter 20: The Endocrine System

1 A 2-year-old child is brought to the family physician because of failure to thrive. Physical examination shows that the child is short and has coarse facial features, a protruding tongue, and an umbilical hernia. Profound mental retardation becomes apparent as the child matures. A deficiency of which of the following hormones is most likely to explain these findings?

- ❑ (A) Cortisol
- ❑ (B) Norepinephrine
- ❑ (C) Somatostatin
- ❑ (D) Thyroxine (T_4)
- ❑ (E) Insulin

2 The parents of a 5-year-boy notice that he has developed features suggestive of puberty over the past 6 months. On physical examination, the boy has secondary sex characteristics, including pubic hair and enlargement of the penis. Which of the following morphologic features is most likely to be seen in his adrenal glands?

- ❑ (A) Bilateral adrenal cortical hyperplasia
- ❑ (B) Bilateral adrenal cortical atrophy
- ❑ (C) Nodule in the adrenal medulla
- ❑ (D) Normal size and architecture
- ❑ (E) Nodule in the adrenal cortex

3 A 40-year-old woman has experienced increasing intolerance to cold for the past 18 months. She wears a jacket in the office while her coworkers keep turning down the thermostat. She reports a 4-kg weight gain and has become constipated over the past year. Physical examination shows no remarkable findings. Which of the following is the most appropriate initial diagnostic test?

- ❑ (A) Total thyroxine (T_4) level
- ❑ (B) Total triiodothyronine (T_3) level
- ❑ (C) Thyroid-stimulating hormone (TSH) level
- ❑ (D) Fine-needle aspiration biopsy
- ❑ (E) Radioiodine scan

4 A 47-year-old woman visits her physician because she noticed a "lump" in her neck 1 week ago. On physical examination, there is a 2-cm nodule in the right lobe of the thyroid gland. A fine-needle aspiration biopsy is performed, and microscopic examination of the specimen shows cells consistent with a follicular neoplasm. She undergoes a subtotal thyroidectomy. Which of the following laboratory tests should be performed on this patient in the immediate postoperative period?

- ❑ (A) Calcitonin
- ❑ (B) TSH
- ❑ (C) Parathyroid hormone
- ❑ (D) Antithyroglobulin antibody
- ❑ (E) Calcium

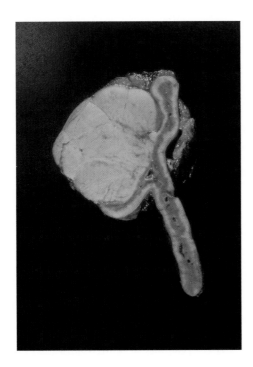

5 A 28-year-old otherwise healthy man sees his physician because he has had headaches for the past 2 weeks. Physical examination yields no remarkable findings except for a blood pressure of 170/110 mm Hg. An abdominal CT scan shows an enlarged right adrenal gland. A right adrenalectomy is performed, and the gross appearance of the specimen is shown. Which of the following laboratory findings was most likely reported in this patient?

❑ (A) Hyponatremia
❑ (B) Hyperglycemia
❑ (C) Low serum renin level
❑ (D) Hyperkalemia
❑ (E) Low serum corticotropin level

6 A 60-year-old woman has felt a "lump" on the right side of her neck for several months. On physical examination, she has a firm 3-cm mass in the right lobe of the thyroid gland. There is no palpable lymphadenopathy. Laboratory studies show a serum TSH level of 3 mU/L and a T₄ level of 8.8 μg/dL. A fine-needle aspiration biopsy is performed, and she undergoes a thyroidectomy. A 3-cm solid mass is present within the right thyroid lobe. Six months later, she visits her physician again because of pain in the right thigh. A radiograph shows a fracture of the right femur in an area of lytic bone destruction. A radioiodine scan shows uptake localized to the region of the fracture. Which of the following was most likely to have been present in the patient's thyroid gland?

❑ (A) Anaplastic carcinoma
❑ (B) Follicular carcinoma
❑ (C) Granulomatous thyroiditis
❑ (D) Hashimoto thyroiditis
❑ (E) Medullary carcinoma
❑ (F) Non-Hodgkin lymphoma

7 A 40-year-old man sees his physician because of weight loss, increased appetite, and double vision. On physical examination, his temperature is 37.7°C, pulse 106/min, respirations 15/min, and blood pressure 140/80 mm Hg. A fine tremor is observed in his outstretched hands. He has bilateral proptosis and corneal ulceration. Laboratory findings include a serum TSH level of 0.1 μU/mL. A radioiodine scan indicates increased diffuse uptake throughout the thyroid. He receives propylthiouracil therapy, and his condition improves. Which of the following best describes the microscopic appearance of the patient's thyroid gland?

❑ (A) Destruction of follicles, lymphoid aggregates, and Hürthle cell metaplasia
❑ (B) Papillary projections in thyroid follicles and lymphoid aggregates in the stroma
❑ (C) Follicular destruction with inflammatory infiltrates containing giant cells
❑ (D) Nodules with nests of cells separated by hyaline stroma that stains with Congo red
❑ (E) Enlarged thyroid follicles lined by flattened epithelial cells

8 A 40-year-old man sees his physician because he has had headache, weakness, and a 5-kg weight gain over the past 3 months. On physical examination, his face is puffy. His temperature is 36.9°C, pulse 79/min, respirations 15/min, and his blood pressure is 160/75 mm Hg while lying down. Laboratory findings show a fasting plasma glucose level of 200 mg/dL, serum Na⁺ 150 mmol/L, and serum K⁺ 3.1 mmol/L. The plasma cortisol level is 38 μg/dL at 8:00 AM and 37 μg/dL at 6:00 PM. Administration of low and high doses of dexamethasone fails to suppress the plasma cortisol level and excretion of urinary 17-hydroxycorticosteroids. The plasma corticotropin level is 0.8 pg/mL. Which of the following lesions is most likely to be present in this patient?

❑ (A) Adenoma of the right adrenal cortex with atrophy of the contralateral adrenal cortex
❑ (B) Small cell carcinoma of the lung with bilateral hyperplasia of the adrenal cortex
❑ (C) Corticotroph adenoma of the anterior pituitary with bilateral hyperplasia of the adrenal cortex
❑ (D) Adenoma of the right adrenal cortex without atrophy of contralateral adrenal cortex
❑ (E) Corticotroph adenoma of the anterior pituitary, medullary carcinoma of thyroid, and bilateral nodular hyperplasia of the adrenal cortex

9 A 69-year-old man has become progressively obtunded over the past week. On physical examination he is afebrile and normotensive. A head CT scan shows no intracerebral hemorrhages. Laboratory findings include serum Na⁺ of 115 mmol/L, K⁺ 4.2 mmol/L, Cl⁻ 85 mmol/L, and bicarbonate 23 mmol/L. The serum glucose is 80 mg/dL, urea nitrogen 19 mg/dL, and creatinine 1.7 mg/dL. Which of the following neoplasms is most likely to be present?

❑ (A) Pituitary adenoma
❑ (B) Adrenal cortical carcinoma
❑ (C) Renal cell carcinoma
❑ (D) Pheochromocytoma
❑ (E) Pulmonary small cell carcinoma

10 A 40-year-old man visits the physician because of weakness and easy fatigability of 2 months' duration. Physical examination yields no remarkable findings. Laboratory studies show serum calcium of 11.5 mg/dL, inorganic phosphorus 2.4 mg/dL, and serum parathyroid hormone level near the top of the reference range, at 58 pg/mL. A radionuclide bone scan fails to show any areas of increased uptake. Which of the following is the most likely cause of these findings?

❑ (A) Chronic renal failure
❑ (B) Parathyroid adenoma
❑ (C) Parathyroid carcinoma
❑ (D) Parathyroid hyperplasia
❑ (E) Hypervitaminosis D
❑ (F) Medullary thyroid carcinoma

11 A 23-year-old previously healthy woman died suddenly and unexpectedly after complaining of a mild sore throat the previous day. At autopsy, her adrenal glands are enlarged, and there are extensive bilateral cortical hemorrhages. Infection with which of the following organisms best accounts for these findings?

❑ (A) *Mycobacterium tuberculosis*
❑ (B) *Streptococcus pneumoniae*
❑ (C) *Neisseria meningitidis*
❑ (D) *Histoplasma capsulatum*
❑ (E) Cytomegalovirus

12 A 45-year-old woman reports a feeling of fullness in her neck but has no other complaints. The enlargement has been gradual and painless for more than 1 year. Physical examination confirms diffuse enlargement of the thyroid gland without any apparent masses. Laboratory studies of thyroid function show a normal free T₄ level and a slightly increased TSH level. Which of the following is the most likely cause of these findings?

❑ (A) Toxic multinodular goiter
❑ (B) Papillary carcinoma
❑ (C) Subacute granulomatous thyroiditis
❑ (D) Hashimoto thyroiditis
❑ (E) Diffuse nontoxic goiter
❑ (F) Follicular adenoma

13 A 37-year-old woman complains that she has had difficulty swallowing, accompanied by a feeling of fullness in the anterior neck for the past week. She reports recovering from a mild upper respiratory tract infection 1 month ago. On physical examination, her temperature is 37.4°C, pulse 74/min, respirations 14/min, and blood pressure 125/80 mm Hg. Palpation of her diffusely enlarged thyroid elicits pain. Laboratory studies show an increased serum free T₄ level and a decreased TSH level. She is seen by an endocrinologist 2 months later and no longer has these complaints. The free T₄ level is now normal. Which of the following conditions is most likely to have produced these findings?

❑ (A) Medullary carcinoma
❑ (B) Subacute thyroiditis
❑ (C) Toxic multinodular goiter
❑ (D) Toxic follicular adenoma
❑ (E) Hashimoto thyroiditis

14 A 40-year-old woman has had an increasing feeling of fullness in her neck for the past 7 months. On physical

examination, her thyroid gland is enlarged and nodular. There is no lymphadenopathy. A fine-needle aspiration biopsy of the thyroid is performed, and she undergoes thyroidectomy. Gross examination of the thyroid shows a multicentric thyroid neoplasm; microscopically, the neoplasm is composed of polygonal to spindle-shaped cells forming nests and trabeculae. There is a prominent, pink hyaline stroma that stains positively with Congo red. Electron microscopy shows varying numbers of intracytoplasmic, membrane-bound, electron-dense granules. Which of the following immunohistochemical stains is most likely to be useful in corroborating the diagnosis of this neoplasm?

❑ (A) Calcitonin
❑ (B) Cathepsin D
❑ (C) Parathormone
❑ (D) Vimentin
❑ (E) Cytokeratin
❑ (F) Estrogen receptor

15 Over the past 6 months, a 42-year-old man has experienced increasing fatigue and a 6-kg weight gain, predominantly in a truncal distribution. On physical examination, his temperature is 37.1°C, pulse 77/min, respirations 14/min, and blood pressure 165/105 mm Hg. He exhibits proximal muscle weakness. Laboratory findings include a fasting serum glucose level of 155 mg/dL, an 8:00 AM serum cortisol level that is elevated at 54 µg/dL, and an elevated serum corticotropin level at 63 pg/mL. Which of the following tests is most likely to be helpful in establishing the diagnosis?

❑ (A) MR imaging of the brain
❑ (B) Abdominal CT scan of the adrenals
❑ (C) Serum assay for glycosylated hemoglobin
❑ (D) Biopsy of the gastrocnemius
❑ (E) Assay for urinary catecholamine metabolites

16 A 27-year-old woman experienced sudden severe abdominal pain. On physical examination, she had marked abdominal tenderness and guarding. Laboratory studies showed serum glucose of 76 mg/dL, calcium 12.2 mg/dL, phosphorus 2.6 mg/dL, creatinine 1.1 mg/dL, and parathormone level 62 pg/mL (normal range, 9 to 60 pg/mL). During surgery, four enlarged parathyroid glands were found and excised, with reimplantation of one half of one gland. After the surgery, her serum calcium concentration returned to normal. Three years later, she had an episode of upper gastrointestinal hemorrhage. An endoscopy and biopsy showed multiple benign gastric ulcerations. Abdominal MR imaging indicated multiple 1- to 2-cm mass lesions in the pancreas. She underwent surgery, and multiple gastrinomas were found. Two years later, she now has galactorrhea. Which of the following lesions is now most likely to be present?

❑ (A) Medullary carcinoma of the thyroid
❑ (B) Adrenal pheochromocytoma
❑ (C) Small cell anaplastic carcinoma of the lung
❑ (D) Endometrial carcinoma
❑ (E) Pituitary adenoma

17 An infant is born at term to a 41-year-old woman after an uncomplicated pregnancy. Soon after birth, the neonate develops hypotension. Physical examination shows no anomalies. Laboratory studies show Na⁺ of 131 mmol/L, K⁺ 5.1 mmol/L, Cl⁻ 93 mmol/L, CO₂ 18 mmol/L, glucose

65 mg/dL, creatinine 0.4 mg/dL, testosterone 50 mg/dL (normal < 30 mg/dL), and cortisol 2 μg/dL. An abdominal ultrasound scan shows bilaterally enlarged adrenal glands. Which of the following enzyme deficiencies is most likely to be present in this infant?

- (A) Aromatase
- (B) 11-Hydroxylase
- (C) 21-Hydroxylase
- (D) 17α-Hydroxylase
- (E) Oxidase

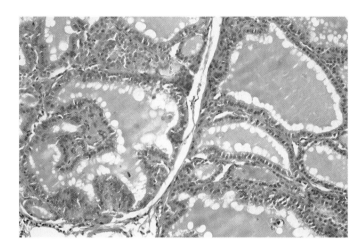

18 A 22-year-old woman has experienced increasing fatigue and a 7-kg weight loss without dieting over the past 4 months. She also has experienced increasing anxiety and nervousness with no apparent changes in her job or home life. She now has diarrhea. Physical examination shows a diffusely enlarged thyroid gland. Her temperature is 37.6°C, pulse 103/min, respirations 17/min, and blood pressure 135/75 mm Hg. A radionuclide scan of the thyroid shows a diffuse increase in uptake. The representative microscopic appearance of the thyroid gland is shown at high power. Which of the following is most likely to produce these findings?

- (A) Antibodies against TSH receptor
- (B) Dietary deficiency of iodine
- (C) Mutation in the *RET* protooncogene
- (D) Maternal deficiency in T₄
- (E) Irradiation of the neck

19 A 43-year-old man felt a small "bump" on the left side of his neck 1 month ago, and it has not changed since then. Physical examination shows a 1-cm nodule palpable in the right lower pole of the thyroid gland. There is no lymphadenopathy. A fine-needle aspiration biopsy of the nodule is performed, and the nodule has the cytologic features of a follicular neoplasm. Radionucleotide scanning shows that the nodule does not absorb radioactive iodine, and no other nodules are present. Based on these findings, which of the following is most likely to be present in this patient?

- (A) Anti–TSH receptor immunoglobulins
- (B) High free T₄ and low TSH
- (C) Normal free T₄ and TSH
- (D) Low free T₄ and elevated TSH
- (E) Antimicrosomal (thyroid peroxidase) antibody

20 A 10-year-old boy has been bothered by frequent headaches for the past 5 months. Physical examination yields no specific findings. Laboratory studies show normal electrolyte levels. CT scan of the head shows no bony abnormalities and no intracranial hemorrhage. MR imaging of the brain shows a 2-cm solid mass without calcifications or cystic change in the area inferior to the splenium of the corpus callosum, superior to the collicular plate, and between the right and left thalamic pulvinar regions. Because of the location, the mass is difficult to remove completely. Which of the following neoplasms is most likely to be present in this child?

- (A) Craniopharyngioma
- (B) Hypothalamic glioma
- (C) Lymphoblastic lymphoma
- (D) Metastatic carcinoma
- (E) Pineoblastoma
- (F) Prolactinoma

21 A 20-year-old woman and her twin sister both experience increasing diplopia. Their conditions develop within 3 years of each other. On physical examination, they have exophthalmos and weak extraocular muscle movement. The thyroid gland is diffusely enlarged but painless in each sister, and there is no lymphadenopathy in either woman. Which of the following laboratory findings is most likely to be reported in these sisters?

- (A) Decreased serum free T₄ level
- (B) Increased urinary free catecholamine level
- (C) Decreased serum thyroid-stimulating hormone level
- (D) Increased serum parathormone level
- (E) Increased serum thyrotropin-releasing hormone level
- (F) High titer serum antimicrosomal antibody

22 A 32-year-old woman with systemic lupus erythematosus has been treated with corticosteroid therapy for several years because of recurrent lupus nephritis. While on vacation, she undergoes an emergency appendectomy for acute appendicitis. On postoperative day 2, she becomes somnolent and develops severe nausea and vomiting. She then becomes hypotensive. Blood cultures are negative, and laboratory studies now show Na⁺ of 128 mmol/L, K⁺ 4.9 mmol/L, Cl⁻ 89 mmol/L, CO₂ 19 mmol/L, glucose 52 mg/dL, and creatinine 1.3 mg/dL. Which of the following morphologic findings in the adrenal glands is most likely to be present in this patient?

- (A) Bilateral caseating granulomas
- (B) Bilateral cortical atrophy
- (C) Bilateral hemorrhagic necrosis
- (D) Bilateral cortical nodular hyperplasia
- (E) Solitary 1-cm adenoma without atrophy of the contralateral adrenal cortex
- (F) Solitary 2-cm adenoma with atrophy of the contralateral adrenal cortex
- (G) Solitary 4-cm mass arising in the adrenal medullae
- (H) Solitary 12-cm cortical mass with extensive necrosis and hemorrhage

23 A 55-year-old man has experienced increasing lethargy for the past 7 months. Physical examination shows hyperpigmentation of the skin. Vital signs include temperature of 36.9°C, pulse 70/min, respirations 14/min, and blood pressure 95/65 mm Hg. Laboratory studies include a serum cortisol level of 3 µg/mL at 8:00 AM with a serum corticotropin level of 65 pg/mL. Which of the following diseases is most likely to accompany this disorder?

- (A) Systemic lupus erythematosus
- (B) Hashimoto thyroiditis
- (C) Diabetes mellitus type 2
- (D) Ulcerative colitis
- (E) Polyarteritis nodosa

24 A 40-year-old woman has experienced lethargy, weakness, and constipation for the past 6 months. On physical examination, she is afebrile and normotensive, and her heart rate is slightly irregular. There is pain on palpation of the left third proximal finger. An ECG shows a prolonged QT (corrected) interval. Laboratory studies show Na^+ of 142 mmol/L, K^+ 4.0 mmol/L, Cl^- 95 mmol/L, CO_2 24 mmol/L, glucose 73 mg/dL, creatinine 1.2 mg/dL, calcium 11.6 mg/dL, phosphorus 2.8 mg/dL, total protein 7.1 g/dL, albumin 5.3 g/dL, alkaline phosphatase 202 U/L, and total bilirubin 0.9 mg/dL. A radiograph of the left hand shows focal expansion by a cystic lesion of the third proximal phalanx. A radionuclide scan shows a 1-cm area of increased uptake in the right lateral neck. Which of the following mutations is most likely to precede the development of these findings?

- (A) GNAS1
- (B) MEN1
- (C) NF1
- (D) RET
- (E) RB1
- (F) p53
- (F) VHL

25 A 20-year-old woman visits her physician with a 4-month history of chronic headache and visual problems. On physical examination, she has defects in lateral visual fields but no loss of visual acuity. CT scan of the head shows an expansion of the sella turcica with no significant bony destruction. Laboratory studies show a serum prolactin level of 70 ng/mL; serum calcium and blood glucose concentrations are normal. Transsphenoidal resection of a sellar mass is performed. Histologic examination of the mass shows a monomorphous population of cells that fails to demonstrate immunohistochemical staining for growth hormone, thyroid-stimulating hormone, follicle-stimulating hormone, corticotropin, or prolactin. Which of the following lesions is most consistent with these clinical and laboratory findings?

- (A) Nonsecretory adenoma with "stalk effect"
- (B) Multiple endocrine neoplasia type I (MEN I)
- (C) Chronic renal failure
- (D) Craniopharyngioma
- (E) Multiple endocrine neoplasia type II (MEN II)

26 A 45-year-old otherwise healthy man feels a small lump on the left side of his neck. His physician palpates a firm, painless, 1.5-cm cervical lymph node. The thyroid gland is not enlarged. A chest radiograph is unremarkable. Laboratory findings include serum glucose of 83 mg/dL, creatinine 1.2 mg/dL, calcium 9.1 mg/dL, phosphorus 3.3 mg/dL, thyroxine 8.7 µg/dL, and TSH 2.3 mU/L. The hemoglobin is 14.0 g/dL, platelet count 240,400/mm³, and WBC count 5830/mm³. A fine-needle aspiration biopsy of the thyroid gland is performed, and the cells are examined microscopically. Which of the following is the most likely diagnosis?

- (A) Papillary carcinoma
- (B) Parathyroid carcinoma
- (C) Medullary carcinoma
- (D) Follicular carcinoma
- (E) Anaplastic carcinoma
- (F) Small lymphocytic lymphoma

27 A 23-year-old man has experienced headaches, polyuria, and visual problems for the past 3 months. On physical examination, he has bilateral temporal visual field defects. CT scan of the head shows a large, partially calcified, cystic mass in the sellar and suprasellar areas. Laboratory findings show a serum prolactin concentration of 60 ng/mL and serum sodium level of 152 mEq/L. Serum calcium, phosphate, and glucose levels are normal. The mass is excised, and histologic examination shows a mixture of squamous epithelial elements and lipid-rich debris containing cholesterol crystals. Which of the following lesions is most consistent with the clinical laboratory findings in this patient?

- (A) Craniopharyngioma that has destroyed the posterior pituitary
- (B) Prolactin-secreting adenohypophyseal macroadenoma
- (C) Multiple endocrine neoplasia I (MEN I)
- (D) Metastases from a lung neoplasm in the sella and brain
- (E) Multiple endocrine neoplasia II (MEN II)

28 A 25-year-old woman has noted breast secretions for the past month. She is not breast-feeding and has never been pregnant. She has not menstruated for the past 5 months. Physical examination yields no abnormal findings. MR imaging of the brain shows a 0.7-cm mass in the adenohypophysis. Which of the following additional complications is most likely to be present in this patient?

- (A) Infertility
- (B) Hyperthyroidism
- (C) Acromegaly
- (D) Cushing disease
- (E) Syndrome of inappropriate antidiuretic hormone

29 A 60-year-old woman has experienced back pain for the past month. She also has experienced mental depression for the past 3 months and has been prescribed antidepressants. On physical examination, her vital signs include temperature of 37°C, pulse 81/min, respirations 15/min, and blood pressure 150/95 mm Hg. She has cutaneous striae over the lower abdomen and ecchymoses scattered over the extremities. A radiograph of the spine shows a compressed fracture of T11. An abdominal CT scan shows that the adrenal glands are atrophic bilaterally. CT scan of the head shows a normal-sized sella turcica. Which of the following conditions is most likely to explain these findings?

- □ (A) Addison disease
- □ (B) Corticosteroid therapy
- □ (C) 21-Hydroxylase deficiency
- □ (D) Cushing disease
- □ (E) Waterhouse-Friderichsen syndrome

30 A 45-year-old woman had frequent headaches for about 1 month. She suddenly suffered a generalized seizure and became obtunded. She is taken to the emergency department, where a physical examination indicates no abnormalities. Laboratory findings include serum calcium of 15.4 mg/dL, serum phosphorus 1.9 mg/dL, and albumin 4.2 g/dL. A chest radiograph shows multiple lung masses, and there are lytic lesions of the vertebral column. Which of the following conditions best accounts for these findings?

- □ (A) Parathyroid carcinoma
- □ (B) Renal failure
- □ (C) Metastatic breast cancer
- □ (D) Vitamin D toxicity
- □ (E) Tuberculosis

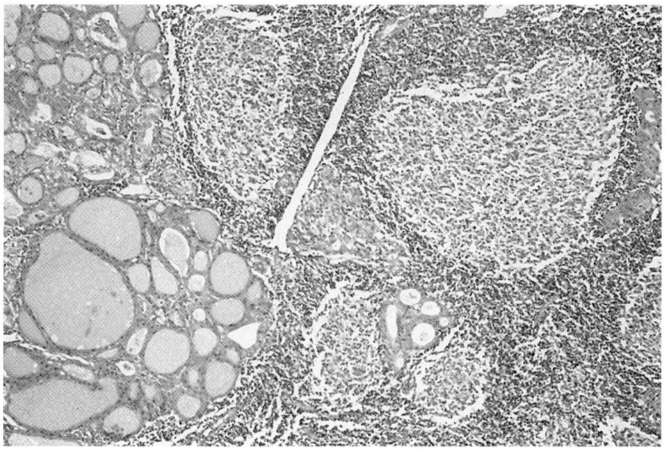

31 A 46-year-old woman has experienced a feeling of fullness in her neck for the past year. Her energy level is decreased, and she has difficulty concentrating at work. On physical examination, the thyroid gland is enlarged diffusely and symmetrically and is not tender on palpation. She has dry, coarse skin and alopecia. The figure shows the microscopic appearance of the thyroid gland. Which of the following autoantibodies is most likely to be present in the serum of this patient?

- □ (A) Antithyroid peroxidase
- □ (B) Antimitochondrial
- □ (C) Antiribonucleoprotein
- □ (D) Anti–double-stranded DNA
- □ (E) Anti–gastric parietal cell
- □ (F) Anticentromere
- □ (G) Anti–Jo-1

32 An infant is born at term to a 25-year-old woman. On newborn physical examination, the infant is found to have an enlarged abdomen, but there are no other abnormal findings except for slightly elevated blood pressure. An abdominal

ultrasound scan shows a right retroperitoneal mass in the adrenal gland. Which of the following laboratory findings is most likely to be reported in this neonate?

- □ (A) Increased urinary homovanillic acid (HVA) level
- □ (B) Decreased serum calcium level
- □ (C) Increased urinary free catecholamine level
- □ (D) Increased serum corticotropin level
- □ (E) Increased serum growth hormone level
- □ (F) Increased serum prolactin level
- □ (G) Increased serum cortisol level

33 A 27-year-old man sees his physician for evaluation of headaches that have occurred frequently for the past 3 months. On physical examination, he is afebrile, and his blood pressure is 140/85 mm Hg. There are no neurologic abnormalities and no visual defects; however, he has a right thyroid mass. Laboratory studies show that his serum calcitonin level is elevated. A total thyroidectomy is performed, and on sectioning, the thyroid has multiple tumor nodules in both lobes. Microscopically, the thyroid nodules are composed of nests of neoplastic cells separated by amyloid-rich stroma. The endocrinologist says that the patient's family members could be at risk for development of similar tumors and advises that they undergo genetic screening. Which of the following morphologic findings in the adrenal glands is most likely to be present in this patient?

- □ (A) Bilateral caseating granulomas
- □ (B) Bilateral cortical atrophy
- □ (C) Bilateral hemorrhagic necrosis
- □ (D) Bilateral cortical nodular hyperplasia
- □ (E) Solitary 1-cm adenoma without atrophy of the contralateral adrenal cortex
- □ (F) Solitary 2-cm adenoma with atrophy of the contralateral adrenal cortex
- □ (G) Solitary 4-cm mass arising in the adrenal medullae
- □ (H) Solitary 12-cm cortical mass with extensive necrosis and hemorrhage

34 A 40-year-old woman notices that her gloves from the previous winter no longer fit her hands. Her friends remark that her facial features have changed in the past year and that her voice seems deeper. On physical examination, she is afebrile. Her blood pressure is 140/90 mm Hg. She has course facial features. There is decreased sensation to pinprick over the palms in the distribution of her thumb and first two fingers. A radiograph of the foot shows an increased amount of soft tissue beneath the calcaneus. A chest radiograph shows cardiomegaly. Laboratory studies indicate a fasting serum glucose level of 138 mg/dL and hemoglobin A_{1c} level of 8.6%. Which of the following additional test results is most likely to indicate the cause of these physical and laboratory findings?

- □ (A) Elevated serum prolactin level
- □ (B) Failure of growth hormone suppression
- □ (C) Increased serum cortisol level
- □ (D) Abnormal glucose tolerance test result
- □ (E) Increased serum TSH level

35 For the past 7 months, a 44-year-old woman has become increasingly listless and weak and has had chronic diarrhea and a 5-kg weight loss. She also notices that her skin seems darker, although she rarely goes outside because she is too tired to participate in her usual outdoor activities. On physical examination, she is afebrile, and her blood pressure is 85/50 mm Hg. A chest radiograph shows no abnormal findings. Laboratory findings include serum Na^+ of 120 mmol/L, K^+ 5.1 mmol/L, glucose 58 mg/dL, urea nitrogen 18 mg/dL, creatinine 0.8 mg/dL. The serum corticotropin level is 82 pg/mL. Which of the following is most likely to account for these findings?

- [ ] (A) Adenohypophyseal adenoma
- [ ] (B) Autoimmune destruction
- [ ] (C) Islet cell adenoma
- [ ] (D) Metastatic carcinoma
- [ ] (E) *Neisseria meningitidis* infection
- [ ] (F) Sarcoidosis

36 A term infant is born to a 15-year-old mother whose pregnancy was uncomplicated. A newborn physical examination shows no abnormalities. However, 1 day later, the neonate has neuromuscular irritability and seizures. Laboratory findings include a serum calcium level of 6.6 mg/dL and a phosphorus level of 3.8 mg/dL. During the first year of life, the infant experiences multiple fungal and viral infections. FISH analysis of the infant's cells shows del 22q11.2. Which of the following mechanisms is most likely to cause this disease?

- [ ] (A) Autoimmune destruction of the adrenal cortices
- [ ] (B) Mutational inactivation of the *21-hydroxylase* gene
- [ ] (C) Mutational activation of the *aldosterone synthetase* gene
- [ ] (D) Congenital malformation of the 4th pharyngeal pouches
- [ ] (E) Mutational inactivation of the *MEN1* gene
- [ ] (F) Mutational activation of the *RET receptor* gene

37 A 67-year-old woman has experienced malaise and a 10-kg weight loss over the past 4 months. She also has developed a chronic cough during this time. Physical examination shows muscle wasting and 4/5 motor strength in all extremities. An abdominal CT scan shows bilaterally enlarged adrenal glands. A chest radiograph shows a 6-cm perihilar mass on the right and prominent hilar lymphadenopathy. Laboratory studies show Na^+ of 118 mmol/L, K^+ 6.0 mmol/L, Cl^- 95 mmol/L, CO_2 21 mmol/L, and glucose 49 mg/dL. Her 8:00 AM serum cortisol level is 9 ng/mL. Which of the following is the most likely diagnosis?

- [ ] (A) Meningococcemia
- [ ] (B) Pituitary adenoma
- [ ] (C) Amyloidosis
- [ ] (D) Metastatic carcinoma
- [ ] (E) Ectopic corticotropin syndrome

38 A 42-year-old man sees his physician because he has had polyuria and polydipsia for the past 4 months. His medical history shows that he fell off a ladder and hit his head just prior to the onset of these problems. On physical examination, there are no specific findings. Laboratory findings include serum Na^+ 155 mmol/L, K^+ 3.9 mmol/L, Cl^- 111 mmol/L, CO_2 27 mmol/L, glucose 84 mg/dL, creatinine 1.0 mg/dL, and osmolality 350 mOsm/mL. The specific

gravity of his urine is 1.002. This patient is most likely to have a deficiency of which of the following hormones?

- [ ] (A) Oxytocin
- [ ] (B) Antidiuretic hormone
- [ ] (C) Corticotropin
- [ ] (D) Prolactin
- [ ] (E) Melatonin

39 A 37-year-old woman states that, although most of the time she feels fine, she has experienced episodes of palpitations, tachycardia, tremor, diaphoresis, and headache over the past 3 months. When her symptoms are worse, her blood pressure is in the range of 155/90 mm Hg. She collapses suddenly one day and is brought to the hospital, where her ventricular fibrillation is converted successfully to sinus rhythm. On physical examination, there are no remarkable findings. Which of the following laboratory findings is most likely to be reported in this patient?

- [ ] (A) Increased urinary homovanillic acid (HVA) level
- [ ] (B) Decreased serum potassium level
- [ ] (C) Increased serum free T_4 level
- [ ] (D) Increased urinary free catecholamines
- [ ] (E) Decreased serum glucose level

40 A 60-year-old woman has been feeling tired and sluggish for over 1 year. On physical examination, her thyroid gland is not palpable; there are no other remarkable findings. Laboratory studies show a serum T_4 level of 1.6 μg/dL and a TSH level of 7.9 mU/L. Which of the following is most indicative of the pathogenesis of this patient's disease?

- [ ] (A) Irradiation of the neck during childhood
- [ ] (B) Antithyroid peroxidase antibodies
- [ ] (C) Prolonged iodine deficiency
- [ ] (D) Mutations in the *RET* protooncogene
- [ ] (E) Recent viral upper respiratory tract infection

41 A 68-year-old man has experienced increasing malaise for 3 years. Physical examination shows no remarkable findings. Laboratory findings include a serum creatinine level of 4.9 mg/dL and urea nitrogen level of 45 mg/dL. An abdominal CT scan shows bilaterally enlarged cystic kidneys. DNA analysis shows a *polycystin-1* gene mutation. Which of the following lesions is the most likely complication of this man's disease?

- [ ] (A) Multinodular goiter
- [ ] (B) Islet cell hyperplasia
- [ ] (C) Adrenal atrophy
- [ ] (D) Parathyroid hyperplasia
- [ ] (E) Pituitary microadenoma

42 A 44-year-old man with no previous illnesses sees his physician because he has had progressive hoarseness, shortness of breath, and stridor for the past 3 weeks. On physical examination, he has a firm, large, tender mass involving the entire right thyroid lobe. CT scan shows that this mass extends posterior to the trachea and into the upper mediastinum. A fine-needle aspiration biopsy of the mass is performed, and the specimen shows pleomorphic spindle cells. Surgery is performed to resect the mass, which has infiltrated the adjacent skeletal muscle. Four of seven cervical lymph nodes have metastases. Pulmonary metastases also are identified on a chest radiograph. Which of the following neoplasms is most likely to be present in this patient?

- ❑ (A) Non-Hodgkin lymphoma
- ❑ (B) Follicular carcinoma
- ❑ (C) Medullary carcinoma
- ❑ (D) Papillary carcinoma
- ❑ (E) Anaplastic carcinoma

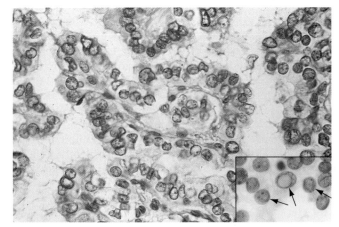

Courtesy of Dr. Edmund Cibas, Brigham and Women's Hospital, Boston, MA.

43 A 44-year-old man sees his physician because he felt a "lump" on the left side of his neck. Physical examination shows a nontender nodule on the left lobe of the thyroid gland. A cervical node is enlarged and nontender. Laboratory studies show no thyroid autoantibodies in his serum, and the T₄ and TSH levels are normal. A thyroidectomy is performed, and the high-power microscopic appearance of the nodule is shown. Which of the following is most likely to contribute to the development of the thyroid nodule in this patient?

- ❑ (A) Chronic dietary iodine deficiency
- ❑ (B) Tyrosine kinase receptor gene mutation
- ❑ (C) Consumption of goitrogens
- ❑ (D) Adrenal medullary pheochromocytoma
- ❑ (E) Viral infection

44 A 21-year-old woman delivers a term infant after an uncomplicated pregnancy. However, the placenta cannot be delivered, and there is substantial hemorrhage, requiring transfusion of 10 units of packed RBCs. She must undergo a hysterectomy. Over the next 3 months, she is unable to produce sufficient breast milk to breast-feed her infant, and she becomes increasingly fatigued. Laboratory studies show Na⁺ of 134 mmol/L, K⁺ 5.2 mmol/L, Cl⁻ 88 mmol/L, CO₂ 23 mmol/L, glucose 59 mg/dL, calcium 9.3 mg/dL, phosphorus 3.5 mg/dL, and creatinine 0.9 mg/dL. Over the next 5 months, her menstrual cycles do not return. Which of the following laboratory findings is now most likely to be reported?

- ❑ (A) Decreased oxytocin
- ❑ (B) Elevated dopamine
- ❑ (C) Failure of growth hormone stimulation
- ❑ (D) Increased antidiuretic hormone
- ❑ (E) Increased corticotropin
- ❑ (F) Lack of corticotropin-releasing hormone

45 A 39-year-old woman, G 2, P 2, whose last pregnancy was 14 years ago, has had regular menstrual cycles until 6 months ago, when the cycles ceased. She also reports expression of milk from her breasts. On physical examination, she is afebrile and normotensive. She is 150 cm (4 ft 11 in) tall and weighs 63 kg (BMI 28). Secondary sex characteristics are normal. Laboratory testing indicates that her β-human chorionic gonadotropin level is normal. She has a normal growth hormone stimulation test. CT scan of the head shows no abnormalities of bone and no hemorrhage. Brain MR imaging shows fluid density within a normal-sized sella turcica. Which of the following is the most likely diagnosis?

- ❑ (A) Craniopharyngioma
- ❑ (B) Empty sella syndrome
- ❑ (C) Hereditary hemochromatosis
- ❑ (D) Prader-Willi syndrome
- ❑ (E) Prolactinoma
- ❑ (F) Sheehan syndrome

46 A 51-year-old man has noted increasing weakness and weight gain over the past 5 months. He has experienced low back pain for the past week. On physical examination, vital signs include temperature of 37.3°C, pulse 80/min, respirations 15/min, and blood pressure 155/95 mm Hg. He has bilateral breast enlargement, testicular atrophy, and a prominent fat pad in the posterior neck and back. There are abdominal cutaneous striae. Laboratory findings include Na⁺ 139 mmol/L, K⁺ 4.1 mmol/L, Cl⁻ 96 mmol/L, CO₂ 23 mmol/L, glucose 163 mg/dL, creatinine 1.3 mg/dL, calcium 8.9 mg/dL, and phosphorus 4.1 mg/dL. His serum ACTH level is low. A radiograph of the spine shows decreased bone density with a compression fracture at T9. Which of the following radiographic findings is most likely to be present in this patient?

- ❑ (A) Decreased radionuclide uptake in a thyroid gland nodule
- ❑ (B) Left adrenal 10-cm solid mass with abdominal CT scan
- ❑ (C) Pulmonary 6-cm right hilar mass on chest radiograph
- ❑ (D) Retroperitoneal 5-cm mass at the aortic bifurcation on pelvic MR imaging scan
- ❑ (E) Sella turcica enlargement with erosion on head CT scan

47 A 30-year-old woman comes to her physician with a 6 month history of weight loss (3 kg), hand tremors, mild watery diarrhea, and heat intolerance. On physical examination, vital signs include temperature 37.3°C, pulse 103/min with sinus rhythm, respirations 17/min, and blood pressure 125/85 mm Hg. She has a 1 cm firm, painless nodule palpable on the left side of her neck. There is no lymphadenopathy. No other abnormal findings are noted. Laboratory findings include a total serum T4 of 11.6 µg/dL with TSH of 0.2 mU/mL. A scintigraphic scan shows more uptake of radioactive iodine into the nodule than the surrounding thyroid. Fine needle aspiration biopsy is performed and no malignant cells are seen cytologically. A partial thyroidectomy is performed and microscopic examination of the excised nodule shows well-differentiated thyroid follicles without vascular or capsular invasion. Molecular analysis of this nodule is most likely to reveal which of the following changes?

- ❑ (A) Fusion gene formed by *PAX8* and *PPARγl* genes
- ❑ (B) Mutational activation of RET tyrosine kinase receptor
- ❑ (C) Overexpression of the *cyclin D1* gene
- ❑ (D) Gain of function mutation of the *TSH receptor* gene
- ❑ (E) Mutation of the GNAS1 gene
- ❑ (F) Mutation of the *autoimmune receptor* (*AIRE*) gene

ANSWERS

1 **(D)** The child has cretinism, a condition that is uncommon when there is routine testing and treatment at birth for hypothyroidism. Hypothyroidism that develops in older children and adults is known as myxedema. A lack of cortisol from primary adrenal failure leads to Addison disease, or a 21-hydroxylase deficiency could produce congenital adrenal hyperplasia. There is no deficiency caused by a lack of norepinephrine or somatostatin. An absolute deficiency of insulin leads to type 1 diabetes mellitus.

BP7 728   BP6 645   PBD7 1168   PBD6 1133

2 **(A)** This patient has precocious puberty, most likely caused by the adrenogenital syndrome, which in turn is caused most commonly by a deficiency of 21-hydroxylase. The lack of this enzyme reduces cortisol production, driving corticotropin production, which leads to adrenal hyperplasia and production of sex steroid hormones. This condition is rare. Bilateral adrenal cortical atrophy is typically seen in cases of Addison disease or after exogenous glucocorticoid therapy. A nodule in the adrenal medulla, if functional, produces catecholamines, and older patients with such nodules have hypertension. A nodule in the adrenal cortex that has zona glomerulosa cells produces primary hyperaldosteronism; if it has fasciculata cells, it produces Cushing syndrome.

BP7 746-748   BP6 659   PBD7 1211-1214
PBD6 1157-1159

3 **(C)** The TSH level is an indication of whether there is a primary disease in the thyroid. If the patient appears hypothyroid and a primary thyroid disease (e.g., Hashimoto thyroiditis) is suspected, the TSH level is elevated. If the patient appears hyperthyroid and a primary thyroid disease (e.g., Graves disease) is suspected, the TSH level is decreased. The total T_4 level is low in hypothyroidism and high in most forms of hyperthyroidism, but it does not necessarily implicate the thyroid gland as the cause. Hyperthyroidism due to an elevated T_3 level is much less common than that due to an elevated T_4 level. Fine-needle aspiration biopsy and isotopic scans are employed to study mass lesions of the thyroid, which typically do not alter thyroid function. Hyperfunction or hypofunction of the thyroid because of diseases of the pituitary gland is uncommon.

BP7 728   BP6 643-645   PBD7 1165, 1167-1168
PBD6 1130-1133

4 **(E)** Inadvertent removal of or damage to the parathyroid glands during thyroid surgery can cause hypocalcemia due to hypoparathyroidism. This is the most common cause of hypoparathyroidism. Persons with hypocalcemia exhibit neuromuscular irritability, carpopedal spasm, and sometimes seizures. Calcitonin quantitation is not a useful measure to determine the status of calcium metabolism. The TSH concentration can increase if the patient becomes hypothyroid after surgery and is not receiving thyroid hormone replacement, but this is not an immediate problem. Parathyroid hormone levels decrease if the parathyroid glands are inadvertently removed during thyroid surgery, but the calcium level is the best immediate indicator of hypoparathyroidism,

and this test is more readily available in the laboratory. Antithyroglobulin antibody levels are of no use in diagnosing surgical diseases of the thyroid.

BP7 742   BP6 655   PBD7 1188   PBD6 1151

5 **(C)** The gross specimen shows a tumor in the adrenal cortex. In young, otherwise healthy persons who are hypertensive, a surgically curable cause of hypertension must be sought. This patient had an adrenal cortical adenoma that secreted aldosterone (Conn syndrome). Hyperaldosteronism reduces the synthesis of renin by the juxtaglomerular apparatus in the kidney. Adrenal adenomas can be nonfunctional or can secrete glucocorticoids or mineralocorticoids. Had this been a glucocorticoid-secreting adenoma, the patient could be hypertensive, but he also would have some clinical features of Cushing syndrome. Aldosterone does not exhibit feedback suppression of the anterior pituitary, and corticotropin levels therefore are not affected. Patients with hyperaldosteronism have low serum potassium levels and sodium retention. There is no effect on blood glucose.

BP7 745-746   BP6 658-659   PBD7 1210-1211
PBD6 1155-1157

6 **(B)** This patient has a follicular carcinoma, which can be difficult to differentiate from follicular adenoma unless there is microscopic evidence of invasion. Follicular carcinomas are often indolent, but they can metastasize and then are easily distinguished from follicular adenomas. Follicular carcinomas are much less likely than papillary carcinomas to involve lymph nodes, but they are more likely to metastasize to distant sites such as bone, lung, and liver. If the metastatic lesions are functional, they will absorb radioactive iodine. An anaplastic carcinoma of the thyroid is an uncommon but very aggressive neoplasm that is unlikely to be confined to the thyroid gland. Thyroiditis is unlikely to present as a mass, because the entire gland is typically involved. Medullary carcinoma is less common than follicular carcinoma. Medullary carcinomas can be multicentric and tend to invade locally before metastases are evident. There is an increased risk of non-Hodgkin B-cell lymphoma in patients with Hashimoto thyroiditis, but lymphomas are unlikely to destroy bone, although they can be present in the marrow.

BP7 736-737   BP6 651-652   PBD7 1180-1181
PBD6 1144-1145

7 **(B)** The clinical findings in this case point to hyperthyroidism, and the increased, diffuse uptake corroborates Graves disease as a probable cause, because the TSH level is quite low. The thyroid-stimulating immunoglobulins that appear in this autoimmune condition result in diffuse thyroid enlargement and hyperfunction, as well as papillary projections lined by tall columnar epithelial cells. Destruction of thyroid follicles with lymphoids aggregates and Hürthle cell metaplasia is characteristic of Hashimoto thyroiditis. Follicular destruction, as well as the presence of giant cells, occurs in granulomatous thyroiditis. Nests of cells in a Congo red–positive hyaline stroma characterize a medullary carcinoma, which can be multifocal but is not diffuse and does not lead to hyperthyroidism. A goiter has enlarged follicles and flattened epithelial cells; most of these patients are euthyroid.

BP7 728-730   BP6 645-646   PBD7 1166-1167, 1172-1173
PBD6 1136-1137

8 **(A)** The clinical and laboratory features of this case point to Cushing syndrome. The dexamethasone suppression test is used to localize the source of excess cortisol. When low- and high-dose dexamethasone trials fail to suppress cortisol secretion, a pituitary corticotropin-secreting adenoma as the source of excess glucocorticoids is unlikely. The choice then is an ectopic source of corticotropin, such as a lung cancer, or a tumor of the adrenal cortex that is secreting glucocorticoids. The plasma corticotropin level distinguishes between these two possibilities. Corticotropin levels are high if there is an ectopic source, whereas glucocorticoid secretion from an adrenal neoplasm suppresses corticotropin production by the pituitary, leading to atrophy of the contralateral adrenal cortex. An adrenal cortical adenoma that secretes aldosterone does not cause atrophy of the contralateral adrenal cortex.

BP7 743-745   BP6 656-657   PBD7 1207-1210
PBD6 1152-1154

9 **(E)** This man has syndrome of inappropriate antidiuretic hormone (SIADH) secretion, which results in increased free water resorption by the kidney and hyponatremia. SIADH is most often a paraneoplastic effect, and oat cell carcinoma of the lung is the most likely candidate among probable malignant neoplasms. Anterior pituitary adenomas do not produce antidiuretic hormone (ADH). Adrenal cortical carcinomas can secrete cortisol or sex steroids but not ADH. Renal cell carcinomas are known for a variety of paraneoplastic effects, but SIADH is not a high probability. Pheochromocytomas secrete catecholamines.

BP7 726   BP6 643   PBD7 1164   PBD6 1129

10 **(B)** When a patient presents with hypercalcemia, a disorder of the parathyroid glands or a malignancy at a visceral location must be considered. Hypercalcemia from malignancy can be caused by osteolytic metastases or a paraneoplastic syndrome from secretion of parathyroid hormone (PTH)–related protein by the tumor. If the possibility of a malignant neoplasm can be excluded, an intrinsic abnormality of the parathyroid glands must be sought. The most common cause of primary hyperparathyroidism is a parathyroid adenoma. Secondary hyperparathyroidism, most commonly resulting from renal failure, is excluded when the serum inorganic phosphate level is low, because phosphate is retained with renal failure. Hypervitaminosis D can cause hypercalcemia because of increased calcium absorption, but in these cases, the PTH levels are expected to be near the low end of the reference range because of feedback suppression. Serum PTH levels near the high end of the reference range indicate autonomous PTH secretion unregulated by hypercalcemia. Although medullary carcinomas of the thyroid often have positive immunohistochemical staining for calcitonin, and plasma levels are sometimes increased, there is no major reduction in serum calcium.

BP7 739-741   BP6 653-655   PBD7 1185-1188
PBD6 1148-1150

11 **(C)** This is the typical adrenal finding in Waterhouse-Friderichsen syndrome, and meningococcemia is the most likely cause of such a rapid course. Chronic adrenocortical insufficiency can result from disseminated tuberculosis and from fungal infections, such as histoplasmosis, that involve the adrenal glands. *Streptococcus pneumoniae* can produce sep-

ticemia, but it is unlikely to involve the adrenal glands specifically. Cytomegalovirus infections of the adrenals can be seen in immunocompromised states and can be severe enough to produce diminished adrenal function, although not acute failure.

BP7 749   BP6 661-662   PBD7 1214-1215   PBD6 1160

12 **(E)** Diffuse nontoxic goiter is most often caused by dietary iodine deficiency. This condition is endemic in regions of the world where there is a deficiency of iodine (e.g., inland mountainous areas), and it also may occur sporadically. As in this case, the patients are typically euthyroid. Plummer syndrome, or toxic multinodular goiter, occurs when there is a hyperfunctioning nodule in a goiter. Papillary carcinomas most often produce a mass effect or metastases and do not affect thyroid function. Subacute granulomatous thyroiditis can lead to diffuse enlargement, and transient hyperthyroidism can occur, but the disease typically runs a course of no more than 6 to 8 weeks. A lymphocytic thyroiditis, such as Hashimoto thyroiditis, initially can produce thyroid enlargement, but atrophy eventually occurs. A follicular adenoma rarely functions to produce thyroid hormone and rarely causes hypothyroidism; most are "cold," nonfunctioning nodules that do not involve the thyroid diffusely.

BP7 727-728, 730   BP6 646-647   PBD7 1167, 1173-1174
PBD6 1138-1139

13 **(B)** Subacute thyroiditis is a self-limited condition that can be of viral origin, because many cases are preceded by an upper respiratory infection. The transient hyperthyroidism results from inflammatory destruction of the thyroid follicles and release of thyroid hormone. The released colloid acts as a foreign body, producing florid granulomatous inflammation in the thyroid. Thyroid neoplasms are not typically associated with signs and symptoms of inflammation. A toxic goiter likewise produces no signs of inflammation. Hashimoto thyroiditis can enlarge the thyroid transiently, but there is usually no pain or hyperthyroidism.

BP7 732   BP6 649   PBD7 1170-1171   PBD6 1135-1136

14 **(A)** This patient has a medullary carcinoma, which is derived from the C cells, or parafollicular cells, of the thyroid, which synthesize calcitonin. An amyloid stroma is a common feature of this tumor. These tumors occur sporadically in about 80% of cases, but they can be part of multiple endocrine neoplasia (MEN) types IIA and IIB. Cathepsin D is a useful marker for some breast carcinomas. Staining for parathyroid hormone (PTH) is useful to determine if a parathyroid carcinoma is present. Vimentin is a marker for sarcomatous neoplasms, and cytokeratin is a useful marker to determine if a neoplasm is epithelial. Although a variety of tissues may show positivity for estrogen receptors, this finding has no clinical significance.

BP7 737-738   BP6 652   PBD7 1182-1183
PBD6 1146-1147

15 **(A)** This patient has Cushing disease. If the cortisol concentration and the corticotropin level increase, the pituitary is producing cortisol, or there is an ectopic source such as a lung carcinoma. An MR imaging scan to determine the size of the pituitary is the logical investigation, because more than 70% of patients with endogenous Cushing syndrome have a pituitary adenoma. If the source of cortisol is primary adrenal hyperplasia or an adrenal neoplasm, the corticotropin level should be suppressed. A CT scan to determine adrenal size is therefore of no value. Because the patient has hyperglycemia, the glycosylated hemoglobin level is increased. This finding can confirm diabetes mellitus but cannot indicate the cause of hyperglycemia. Muscle changes are not specific in determining the cause of Cushing syndrome. Measuring urinary catecholamine levels is useful to determine the diagnosis of pheochromocytoma. Although patients with pheochromocytoma can be hypertensive, they do not exhibit the other changes noted in Cushing syndrome.

BP7 743-745   BP6 656-658   PBD7 1207-1210
PBD6 1153-1154

16 (E) This patient has multiple endocrine neoplasia (MEN) type I, also known as Wermer syndrome. (Remember the "three Ps" in neoplasia or hyperplasia: *p*ancreas, *p*ituitary, and *p*arathyroids.) Endometrial carcinomas can arise in patients who have unopposed estrogen secretion, which can occur in estrogen-producing ovarian tumors. These are not part of MEN I. Medullary carcinomas are part of MEN IIA or IIB. Small cell carcinomas of the lung are known for a variety of paraneoplastic syndromes, but not usually hypercalcemia. It is also very doubtful that this patient would have lived 5 years with a small cell carcinoma. If her hypercalcemia had been a paraneoplastic syndrome, the parathyroid glands would not have been enlarged, nor would the serum calcium level have returned to normal after surgery.

BP7 753   BP6 664-665   PBD7 1221-1222
PBD6 1166-1167

17 (C) A deficiency of 21-hydroxylase leads to a salt-wasting form of adrenogenital syndrome, because the enzyme deficiency blocks formation of aldosterone and cortisol. A deficiency of 11-hydroxylase blocks cortisol and aldosterone production as well, although intermediate metabolites with some glucocorticoid activity also are synthesized. Aromatase is involved with conversion of androstenedione to estrone, a pathway of steroid synthesis that does not affect cortisol production. A deficiency of 17α-hydroxylase would lead to reduction of cortisol and sex steroid synthesis. Oxidase is the final enzyme in the pathway to aldosterone production.

BP7 746-748   BP6 659-660   PBD7 1212-1214
PBD6 1157-1159

18 (A) The tall columnar epithelium with papillary infoldings and scalloping of the colloid is characteristic of Graves disease, which leads to hyperthyroidism. This disease is caused by autoantibodies that bind to the TSH receptor and mimic the action of TSH. Dietary iodine deficiency can cause diffuse compensatory enlargement of thyroid, but it does not cause hyperthyroidism. Mutations in the *RET* protooncogene occur in papillary carcinoma of the thyroid and in medullary carcinomas of the thyroid. These neoplasms do not cause diffuse enlargement of the gland, hyperthyroidism, or diffuse increase in radioiodine uptake. Tumors usually produce "cold nodules" on radioiodine scans. Irradiation of the neck is a predisposing factor for papillary carcinoma of the thyroid.

BP7 728-730   BP6 644   PBD7 1172-1173
PBD6 1236-1238

19 (C) Most solitary cold thyroid nodules in younger persons are likely to be neoplastic, and most are benign follicular adenomas that do not affect thyroid function. If the nodule were hyperfunctioning, and produced hyperthyroidism, it would appear "hot" on the scan. Anti-TSH receptor immunoglobulins can be seen in Graves disease, as may high T_4 and low TSH levels, but this is a diffuse disease of the thyroid. Antimicrosomal and antithyroglobulin antibodies are seen in Hashimoto thyroiditis, but thyroiditis is a diffuse process and unlikely to produce a solitary nodule. As Hashimoto thyroiditis progresses, decreasing function of the thyroid can lead to decreasing T_4 level and increasing TSH level, typical of primary thyroid failure.

BP7 733-734   BP6 649-650   PBD7 1175-1177
PBD6 1140-1142

20 (E) The anatomic location of the mass is the pineal gland. In children, the most common pineal tumor is a pineoblastoma, whereas in adults, it is a pineocytoma. Both are quite rare, and their location makes them difficult to remove completely. Craniopharyngiomas are aggressive neoplasms that are often suprasellar and difficult to remove. Hypothalamic gliomas are also suprasellar. Central nervous system lymphomas are uncommon in children and rare at this site. Metastatic carcinoma is rare in any location in children, because children do not have many malignancies, and the malignancies that they do have are often not carcinomas. A prolactinoma occurs in the sella turcica.

PBD7 1223-1224   PBD6 1168

21 (C) Exophthalmos is a feature seen in about 40% of persons with Graves disease. The hyperfunctioning thyroid gland leads to an increased T_4 level, with positive feedback from the pituitary to decrease TSH secretion. There is about 50% concordance of Graves disease among identical twins. The autoimmune character of this disorder is evidenced by an association with HLA-DR3. The autoimmune character of this disorder is evidenced by the presence of an autoantibody against TSH receptor that activates T_4 secretion. Increased urinary free catecholamines are seen in pheochromocytomas. An increased parathormone level is seen in parathyroid adenomas and carcinomas. An increased thyrotropin-releasing hormone (TRH) level would increase the TSH level and increase the T_4, but feedback typically occurs at the level of both the pituitary and the hypothalamus, and abnormal increases in TRH are uncommon. Antithyroid peroxidase antibodies can be seen in Hashimoto thyroiditis and in Graves disease, but the highest titers occur in Hashimoto thyroiditis.

BP7 728-730   BP6 645-646   PBD7 1167, 1172
PBD6 1136-1138

22 (B) This woman has findings of acute adrenocortical insufficiency (acute addisonian crisis). Chronic corticosteroid therapy shuts off corticotropin stimulation to the adrenal glands, leading to adrenal atrophy. When this history is not elicited and the patient is not continued on the corticosteroid therapy, a crisis ensues, in this case made worse by the stress of surgery. Many years ago, when tuberculosis was more prevalent and more severe without current drug therapy, Addison disease from granulomatous destruction of the adrenals was more common. Hemorrhagic necrosis suggests Waterhouse-Friderichsen syndrome, which can complicate septicemia with organisms such as *Neisseria meningitidis*. Cortical nodular hyperplasia can be driven by an ACTH-secreting pituitary adenoma, or it can be idiopathic; in either case, hypercortisolism ensues, not Addison disease. An adrenal cortical adenoma without atrophy of the contralateral adrenal cortex could be a nonfunctioning adenoma or an aldosterone-secreting adenoma. If the contralateral cortex is grossly atrophic, then the adenoma on the opposite side is secreting excess glucocorticoids. An adrenal medullary mass in an adult is most likely a pheochromocytoma, which secretes catecholamines. A large mass with hemorrhage and necrosis in the adrenals suggests a cortical carcinoma.

BP7 748-749   BP6 661-662   PBD7 1214-1216
PBD6 1159

23 **(B)** Addison disease (primary chronic adrenocortical insufficiency) most often results from an idiopathic autoimmune condition (in areas of the world where the incidence of active tuberculosis is low). Autoimmune adrenalitis is associated with the appearance of other autoimmune diseases in about one half of all cases. Such autoimmune phenomena are frequently seen in other endocrine organs, such as the thyroid gland. Other presumed autoimmune diseases, such as systemic lupus erythematosus, ulcerative colitis, and the vasculitides, are usually not forerunners to adrenal failure, although treatment of these conditions with corticosteroids can lead to iatrogenic adrenal atrophy.

BP7 748-749   BP6 661   PBD7 1214-1217
PBD6 1160-1162

24 **(B)** This patient has a parathyroid neoplasm, most likely an adenoma, with hypercalcemia complicated by osteitis fibrosa cystica of her finger. The *MEN1* mutation is the second most common mutation in parathyroid tumors, after the *PRAD1* mutation with overexpression of *cyclin D1*. *MEN1* is a tumor suppressor gene, the loss of which occurs not only in sporadic parathyroid tumors but also in multiple endocrine neoplasia (MEN) type I. *GNAS1* mutations are seen in 40% of cases of somatotroph (growth hormone–producing) pituitary adenomas. *NF1* is seen in neurofibromatosis type 1. The *RET* gene mutation is seen in cases of medullary thyroid carcinoma. The *RB1* mutation is unlikely to be seen in endocrine tumors. The *p53* mutation can be seen in anaplastic thyroid carcinomas. The *VHL* mutation can be seen in some pheochromocytomas in patients with von Hippel-Lindau disease.

BP7 740-741   BP6 653-654   PBD7 1185-1186
PBD6 1148-1150

25 **(A)** The hyperprolactinemia is a "stalk section" effect, with loss of a hypothalamic-inhibiting factor for prolactin secretion. This can occur from an enlarging sellar mass that also produces headache and visual disturbances, caused by pressure on the optic chiasm. There is generally enough residual adenohypophysis to prevent panhypopituitarism. Patients with multiple endocrine neoplasia (MEN) type I can have pituitary adenomas, as well as lesions in the pancreas and parathyroid. Chronic renal failure can cause hyperprolactinemia but not a sellar mass. A craniopharyngioma is a destructive sellar mass. MEN II does not involve the pituitary.

BP7 725   BP6 643   PBD7 1158-1160, 1162   PBD6 1126

26 **(A)** Some patients with papillary carcinomas may initially present with metastases, and local lymph nodes are the most common sites for metastases. The primary site may not be detectable as a palpable nodule. Papillary carcinoma is the most common thyroid malignancy. Metastases to the thyroid are uncommon. Both medullary and follicular carcinomas tend to spread hematogenously. Anaplastic carcinomas are uncommon but are very aggressive, locally invasive lesions. A parathyroid carcinoma is also a locally infiltrative mass, and the serum calcium level is usually quite high in such patients. A small lymphocytic lymphoma, which is the tissue form of chronic lymphocytic leukemia, is uncommon at this patient's age, usually involves multiple nodes, and is accompanied by an elevated WBC count.

BP7 735-736   BP6 650-651   PBD7 1178-1180
PBD6 1143-1144

27 **(A)** Craniopharyngiomas are uncommon neoplasms, usually suprasellar in location and found in young persons. They are thought to arise from embryologic remnants of the Rathke pouch in the region of the pituitary. These are aggressive neoplasms that infiltrate and destroy surrounding tissues, making complete excision difficult. Despite their aggressive behavior, they are composed of benign-appearing squamoid or primitive tooth structures. The rise in prolactin occurs as a "stalk section" effect, and the hypernatremia results from diabetes insipidus caused by destruction of the hypothalamus, posterior pituitary, or both. Prolactinomas, similar to pituitary adenomas, can enlarge the sella but are not typically suprasellar or destructive of surrounding structures. Multiple endocrine neoplasia (MEN) type I includes pituitary adenomas but not craniopharyngiomas. A metastasis to this location in a young person is highly unlikely. MEN II does not involve the pituitary.

PBD7 1164   PBD6 1129

28 **(A)** Prolactinomas are more common than the other hormone-secreting pituitary adenomas. In addition to her galactorrhea and infertility, she may also have decreased libido and amenorrhea from the excessive prolactin secretion. Microadenomas might not be detected because pressure effects on surrounding structures do not occur, but they can be discovered because of their hormonal effects. A TSH-secreting pituitary adenoma is uncommon, but it could account for elevated levels of T_4 and TSH in a hyperthyroid patient. Acromegaly results from a growth hormone–secreting pituitary adenoma in an adult. Cushing disease occurs when there is an ACTH-secreting pituitary adenoma. Syndrome of inappropriate diuretic hormone is most often a paraneoplastic syndrome caused by a small cell anaplastic lung carcinoma.

BP7 723   BP6 639-641   PBD7 1160-1161
PBD6 1125-1126

29 **(B)** This patient has evidence of Cushing syndrome, and the accompanying adrenal atrophy suggests an exogenous source of cortisol. Corticosteroid therapy has many side effects, including immunosuppression, osteoporosis, depression, and reduced collagen synthesis. Deficiency of 21-hydroxylase is a rare congenital condition seen in children and associated with adrenal hyperplasia. Cushing disease results from a pituitary adenoma that is secreting corticotropin, and the adrenals would be large in such a case. Acute adrenal failure in patients with Waterhouse-Friderichsen syndrome is accompanied by massive adrenal hemorrhage and most often results from severe infection, typically with meningococcemia. Addison disease is associated with bilateral adrenal cortical atrophy, most often because of autoimmunity; patients with this disease show symptoms and signs of adrenal failure that are not present in this case.

BP7 743-745   BP6 656-662   PBD7 1208-1209
PBD6 1153-1155

30   (C) The most common cause of clinically significant hypercalcemia in adults is a malignancy. Metastatic disease from common primary sites, such as the breast, lung, and kidney, is much more common than parathyroid carcinoma, which tends to be local but aggressive. Parathyroid carcinomas are an uncommon cause of hyperparathyroidism, and bone metastases from parathyroid carcinomas are rare. Chronic renal failure causes phosphate retention, which tends to depress the serum calcium level and leads to secondary hyperparathyroidism; therefore, the serum calcium level is maintained at near normal levels. Vitamin D toxicity theoretically can lead to hypercalcemia, but this condition is uncommon. Tuberculosis is another granulomatous disease that can be associated with hypercalcemia, but lytic bone lesions from tuberculosis are uncommon.

BP7 741   BP6 654-655   PBD7 334-335, 1184
PBD6 1148-1149

31   (A) Notice the lymphoid follicles and the large, pink Hürthle cells in this photomicrograph. This patient has Hashimoto thyroiditis. The antithyroid peroxidase (antimicrosomal) and antithyroglobulin antibody titers typically are increased in patients with Hashimoto thyroiditis when thyroid enlargement is still present. In the later, "burnt-out" phase of Hashimoto thyroiditis, the antibodies are sometimes undetectable—only the hypothyroidism is. Increased antimitochondrial antibody is indicative of primary biliary cirrhosis. Antiribonucleoprotein antibodies are seen in some of the collagen vascular diseases, such as mixed connective tissue disease. Anti–double-stranded DNA antibody is very specific for systemic lupus erythematosus. Anti–parietal cell antibody occurs in atrophic gastritis, which gives rise to pernicious anemia. Although pernicious anemia can coexist with Hashimoto thyroiditis and other endocrinopathies, this is uncommon. Anticentromere antibody is characteristic of limited scleroderma (CREST syndrome). Anti–Jo-1 antibody can be seen in polymyositis.

BP7 731-732   BP6 648   PBD7 1169-1170
PBD6 1134-1135

32   (A) Neuroblastomas are neoplasms that occur in children and may be congenital. They arise most commonly in the retroperitoneum in the adrenal glands or in extra-adrenal paraganglia. They are primitive "small blue cell" tumors that can produce high levels of catecholamine precursors and their metabolites. HVA is most often detected. Adult pheochromocytomas are more likely to be detected by increased urinary free catecholamines. Neuroblastomas do not affect serum calcium, prolactin, or growth hormone levels. A newborn with

tetany and hypocalcemia could have the DiGeorge anomaly. Because neuroblastomas are usually unilateral, abnormalities of ACTH or cortisol production are unlikely.

BP7 253-255   BP6 211   PBD7 500-504, 1221
PBD6 485-487, 1166

33   (G) These findings suggest multiple endocrine neoplasia (MEN) type II (Sipple syndrome) or possibly type IIB (William syndrome). These patients have medullary carcinomas of the thyroid, pheochromocytomas, and parathyroid adenomas. This patient's headaches could be caused by hypertension from a pheochromocytoma arising in the adrenal medulla. More than 70% of cases of pheochromocytomas are bilateral when familial. This patient's thyroid mass is a medullary carcinoma, which also tends to be multifocal in this syndrome. This syndrome is associated with germ-line mutations in the *RET* protooncogene. Family members who inherit the same mutation are at increased risk of developing similar cancers. Genetic screening followed by increased surveillance of affected family members is advised. Granulomatous destruction of the adrenal glands suggests disseminated tuberculosis as a cause of Addison disease, which leads to adrenal insufficiency. Bilateral cortical atrophy from autoimmune destruction of the adrenals, leading to bilateral cortical atrophy, is now the most common cause of Addison disease. Hemorrhagic necrosis suggests Waterhouse-Friderichsen syndrome, which can complicate septicemia with organisms such as *Neisseria meningitidis*. Cortical nodular hyperplasia can be driven by an ACTH-secreting pituitary adenoma, or it can be idiopathic; in either case hypercortisolism ensues, not Addison disease. An adrenal cortical adenoma without atrophy of the contralateral adrenal cortex could be a nonfunctioning adenoma or an aldosterone-secreting adenoma. If the contralateral cortex is grossly atrophic, then the adenoma on the opposite side is secreting excess glucocorticoids. A large mass with hemorrhage and necrosis in the adrenals suggests a cortical carcinoma.

BP7 753   BP6 665   PBD7 1222-1223   PBD6 1167

34   (B) Failure to suppress growth hormone (GH) levels by glucose infusion suggests autonomic GH production. The patient's symptoms suggest acromegaly, and a GH-secreting adenoma is most likely. Acromegaly causes an overall increase in soft tissue in adults because of the anabolic effects of the increase in GH. Because the epiphyses of the long bones are closed in adults, there is not the increase in height, or gigantism, that would be seen in children with a pituitary adenoma that is secreting excessive GH. Instead, an increase in soft tissue mass occurs, which can manifest as increasing shoe or glove size, carpal tunnel syndrome, and coarse facial features. A prolactinoma would cause amenorrhea and galactorrhea. Cushing syndrome from an adrenal tumor could be accompanied by glucose intolerance, hypertension, and truncal obesity, but there is no overall increase in soft tissues. This woman probably has an abnormal glucose tolerance test result, but this does not indicate the underlying cause of diabetes mellitus. A TSH-secreting adenoma of the pituitary can give rise to hyperthyroidism. The increased metabolic rate found in hyperthyroidism is most likely to lead to weight loss, and glucose intolerance is not a feature of hyperthyroidism. Functional pituitary tumors can be detected clinically before they become large enough to cause pressure symptoms such as visual disturbances.

BP7 723-724   BP6 641   PBD7 1161-1162   PBD6 1126

35 (B) This woman has chronic adrenal insufficiency (Addison disease) with decreased cortisol production and decreased mineralocorticoid activity. The skin hyperpigmentation results from increased corticotropin precursor hormone production, which stimulates melanocytes. The most common cause of Addison disease, in areas where tuberculosis is not endemic, is autoimmune adrenalitis. This process causes gradual destruction of the adrenal cortex, mediated most likely by infiltrating lymphocytes. Sarcoidosis may also involve the adrenals, but this is less common, and in this woman's case, the normal chest radiograph helps to eliminate this possibility, because hilar adenopathy is almost always present in sarcoid. An islet cell adenoma secreting insulin could account for hypoglycemia, but not for the other metabolic changes. Metastases can occasionally destroy enough adrenal cortex to cause adrenal insufficiency, but the most common primary site is the lung, and there is no lung mass in her chest radiograph. Bilateral hemorrhages and resultant destruction of the adrenal glands are typically caused by meningococcemia, and this presents as acute adrenocortical insufficiency.

BP7 748-749   BP6 662   PBD7 1214-1217
PBD6 1160-1162

36 (D) This patient has DiGeorge syndrome, a developmental defect that results from failure of development of the third and fourth pharyngeal pouches. The fourth pharyngeal pouches give rise to the thymus, the parathyroids, and some clear cells of the thyroid. Congenital anomalies in the nearby esophagus and heart may also occur. These patients have a T-cell immunodeficiency and hypoparathyroidism. Hypocalcemia is responsible for the neuromuscular irritability and seizures, and 90% of these patients have deletion of chromosome 22q11.2. In Addison disease caused by autoimmune adrenalitis, there is adrenal cortical insufficiency, as well as hyponatremia, hyperkalemia, and hypoglycemia, but the serum calcium level is not directly affected. There can also be salt wasting from the adrenogenital syndrome. Conn syndrome is caused by overactivity of the aldosterone synthetase gene, and there is an aldosterone-secreting adrenal cortical adenoma, and the classic findings are hypertension and hypokalemia. Sipple syndrome is multiple endocrine neoplasia (MEN) type IIA with parathyroid hyperplasia, pheochromocytoma, and thyroid medullary carcinoma, with the *RET* gene mutation. Wermer syndrome is MEN I, with *p*ituitary, *p*arathyroid, and *p*ancreatic lesions (the "three Ps").

BP7 742   BP6 655   PBD7 243, 1188   PBD6 1151

37 (D) The lung mass suggests a primary carcinoma, and the bilaterally enlarged adrenal glands can be explained by adrenal metastases. Destruction of the adrenal cortex is responsible for malaise and the low serum cortisol concentration as well as the electrolyte disturbances. Waterhouse-Friderichsen syndrome, caused by *Neisseria meningitidis* infection, can increase the adrenal size from marked hemorrhage (two to three times the normal size), but this does not explain the lung mass. This syndrome has an abrupt onset. A pituitary adenoma that is secreting corticotropin could increase adrenal

size bilaterally, but hypercortisolism would occur. Amyloidosis can increase adrenal size but does not produce a lung mass. In the ectopic corticotropin syndrome, a lung cancer is a likely finding, and typically the adrenal glands are enlarged, but hypercortisolism would also be present.

BP7 748   BP6 658   PBD7 1214-1217   PBD6 1161

38 (B) This patient has developed diabetes insipidus with a lack of antidiuretic hormone. There is failure of resorption of free water in the renal collecting tubules—hence the diluted urine. Oxytocin is involved in lactation. Corticotropin stimulates the adrenal glands, mainly with the effect of increasing cortisol secretion. Prolactin and melatonin deficiencies have no identifiable specific clinical effect in men.

BP7 725-726   BP6 643   PBD7 1163-1164   PBD6 1129

39 (D) These findings suggest a pheochromocytoma of the adrenal medulla. This is a rare neoplasm, but in cases of episodic hypertension, this diagnosis should be considered. Screening for urinary free catecholamines, metanephrine, and vanillylmandelic acid (VMA) can help to determine the diagnosis. The level of HVA is increased in a neuroblastoma, which is a tumor that occurs in children. The serum potassium level can be decreased with aldosterone-secreting adrenal adenomas. An increased T_4 level occurs in patients with Graves disease; this disease can cause tachycardia, tremors, and cardiac arrhythmia. Episodic hypertension is not a feature of thyrotoxicosis. Hypoglycemia can occur in Addison disease and islet cell tumors.

BP7 751-752   BP6 663-664   PBD7 1219-1221
PBD6 1164-1165

40 (B) This patient has hypothyroidism, most likely Hashimoto thyroiditis. Autoantibodies are present in the serum. Many of these cases are not diagnosed as Hashimoto thyroiditis, but patients simply present with hypothyroidism, which is the late, "burnt-out" phase of this autoimmune inflammatory condition. It is one of the most common causes of hypothyroidism in adults. An iodine deficiency can lead to hypothyroidism, but a goiter would be present. Irradiation of the thyroid gland can give rise to hypothyroidism, but it is unlikely that irradiation in childhood would give rise to hypothyroidism at the age of 60 years. Irradiation can also predispose to the development of papillary carcinoma, but these tumors do not affect thyroid hormone secretion. Mutations in the *RET* protooncogene are associated with papillary carcinoma and medullary carcinoma of the thyroid. A history of a viral infection sometimes precedes subacute thyroiditis, which is typically a self-limited disease that lasts for weeks to 2 months.

BP7 731-732   BP6 648   PBD7 1167-1170
PBD6 1134-1135

41 (D) This patient has autosomal dominant polycystic kidney disease with secondary hyperparathyroidism resulting from decreased phosphate excretion by the kidneys. The resultant hyperphosphatemia depresses the serum calcium level and stimulates parathyroid gland activity. Because of reduced renal parenchymal function, there is also less active vitamin D, which leads to decreased dietary calcium absorption. Renal failure does not lead to any other endocrine lesions.

BP7 742   BP6 655   PBD7 1187-1188   PBD6 1150-1151

42 **(E)** The large size, histologic features, and aggressive nature of this neoplasm are consistent with anaplastic carcinoma. The prognosis is poor. Malignant lymphomas do not have spindle cells and do not tend to be infiltrative. Other thyroid malignancies tend to form solitary or multifocal (in papillary and medullary carcinomas) masses without spindle cells; they are less likely to be extensively invasive, although metastases can occur, particularly to local lymph nodes in the case of papillary carcinoma.

BP7 738   BP6 652   PBD7 1183   PBD6 1147

43 **(B)** The nodule shows a papillary architecture, with cells that have clear nuclei; this pattern is typical of a papillary carcinoma. There is no such thing as a papillary adenoma. The enlarged clear nuclei are typical of papillary carcinoma. These nuclear changes, even if the pattern is follicular, confirm the diagnosis of papillary carcinoma. About 30% of all papillary thyroid carcinomas have mutational activation of *RET* or *NTRK1* protooncogenes, which belong to the family of receptor tyrosine kinases that transduce extracellular signals for cell growth and differentiation and exert many of their downstream effects through the ubiquitous MAP kinase signaling pathway. Iodine deficiency gives rise to uniform thyroid enlargement, because the secretion of TSH increases when there is reduced synthesis of T_4. Goitrogens interfere with thyroid hormone synthesis and have an effect similar to that of iodine deficiency. An adrenal pheochromocytoma can occur with medullary carcinoma of the thyroid in multiple endocrine neoplasia (MEN) type II or type III. Viral infections can cause a subacute thyroiditis, not carcinoma.

BP7 735-736   BP6 651   PBD7 1178-1180
PBD6 1143-1144

44 **(C)** This patient has Sheehan syndrome, or postpartum pituitary necrosis. The pituitary enlarges during pregnancy, causing its blood supply to be more tenuous, so that hypotension with obstetric bleeding complications (e.g., the placenta accreta in this patient) predisposes to infarction. The anterior pituitary is at greater risk than the posterior pituitary. The laboratory findings in this patient suggest adrenal insufficiency, and her inability to breast-feed is caused by lack of prolactin; loss of menstrual cycles suggests that follicle-stimulating hormone and luteinizing hormone levels are deficient. Thus, oxytocin release from the posterior pituitary is probably not affected. She does not have syndrome of inappropriate antidiuretic hormone, which is usually a consequence of a paraneoplastic syndrome or head trauma. Dopamine production is not affected. If she were to have primary adrenal failure, the corticotropin (ACTH) level then would be increased, but in her case, ACTH is low because of anterior pituitary failure. Because the hypothalamus is unaffected, corticotropin-releasing hormone would still be present.

BP7 724-725   BP6 386, 642   PBD7 1163   PBD6 1127

45 **(B)** Empty sella syndrome is a rare condition, seen most frequently in obese women, and results from herniation of the arachnoid through the diaphragma sella. Although the increased pressure can lead to reduction in pituitary tissue through compression atrophy, there is typically adequate functional anterior pituitary to prevent hypopituitarism. However, this herniation can cause a "stalk section" effect, with loss of prolactin inhibition and hyperprolactinemia. A craniopharyngioma is a destructive tumor mass that is usually seen at a younger age. Hemochromatosis can interfere with organ function, including hypopituitarism; onset usually occurs later in women than in men (in the sixties in women compared with the forties in men), due to differences in physiologic iron losses (e.g., menstrual blood loss). Prader-Willi syndrome is an example of genomic imprinting with hypothalamic dysfunction seen in prepubertal boys. A prolactinoma could be a microadenoma, but the MR imaging in this case rules this out, because of the fluid density in the sella (seen with T_2 weighting). If she were to have had Sheehan syndrome following her pregnancy, she would have manifested hypopituitarism within months, not years.

BP7 725   BP6 642   PBD7 1163   PBD6 1128

46 **(B)** This patient has clinical findings of both Cushing syndrome and femininization, suggesting an adrenal cortical carcinoma. The low ACTH level helps to rule out the possibility of a pituitary adenoma or ectopic ACTH from a neoplasm such as lung carcinoma. A "cold" nodule of the thyroid gland can represent a thyroid medullary carcinoma seen in multiple endocrine neoplasia (MEN) type II in association with adrenal pheochromocytomas, but Cushing syndrome is not part of this complex. The location of a mass at the aortic bifurcation could be the "infamous" extra-adrenal pheochromocytoma of the obscure organ of Zuckerkandl, which explains hypertension with excess catecholamine release, but not the other features of Cushing syndrome.

BP7 745, 750   BP6 657, 662   PBD7 1217-1218
PBD6 1155, 1162-1163

47 **(D)** This patient has a thyroid nodule that is well-differentiated, non-invasive, and hyperfunctioning, all features of a "toxic" follicular adenoma, and a large proportion of these adenomas have activating mutations of the TSH receptor signaling pathway involving the TSH receptor or associated G-protein. A *PAX8-PPARγl* fusion gene is found in certain follicular carcinomas of the thyroid. Activation of the *RET* gene occurs in papillary thyroid carcinomas. Overexpression of the *cyclin D1* gene is characteristic of parathyroid adenomas. Mutation of the GNAS1 gene is seen in some pituitary adenomas. The *AIRE* gene regulates expression of self-antigens in the thymus, and mutation in this gene causes autoimmune polyendocrinopathy affecting adrenals, parathyroids, gonads, and gastric parietal cells with destruction of these tissues and consequent hypofunction

PBD7 1175-1177

The Skin

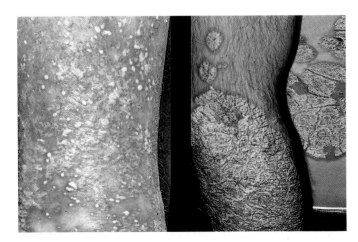

1 For the past decade, a 29-year-old man has had waxing and waning of the lesions shown. The scalp, lumbosacral region, and glans penis are also affected. For the past 2 years, he has had chronic arthritis in the hips and knees. Which of the following physical findings would most likely be present in this patient?

- ❏ (A) Guaiac-positive stool
- ❏ (B) Friction rub
- ❏ (C) Hyperreflexia
- ❏ (D) Damage to the nails
- ❏ (E) Hypertension

2 An epidemiologic study is conducted to identify factors that increase the risk of skin cancer. The study documents subjects reported to tumor registries with a diagnosis of malignant melanoma and the incidence of melanoma worldwide over the past 25 years. Demographic information is collected. Analysis of the data is most likely to show the greatest increase in incidence of malignant melanoma in which of the following locations?

- ❏ (A) Edinburgh, Scotland
- ❏ (B) Cairo, Egypt
- ❏ (C) Brisbane, Australia
- ❏ (D) Tahiti, French Polynesia
- ❏ (E) Hong Kong, China

3 A 64-year-old man has noted changes in the texture and color of skin in his armpit and groin over the past 3 months. On physical examination, there is thickened, darkly pigmented skin in the axillae and flexural areas of the neck and groin. These areas are neither painful nor pruritic. A punch biopsy specimen of axillary skin shows undulating epidermal acanthosis with hyperkeratosis and basal layer hyperpigmentation. Which of the following underlying diseases is most likely to be present in this patient?

- ❏ (A) Systemic lupus erythematosus
- ❏ (B) Mastocytosis
- ❏ (C) AIDS
- ❏ (D) Colonic adenocarcinoma
- ❏ (E) Langerhans cell histiocytosis

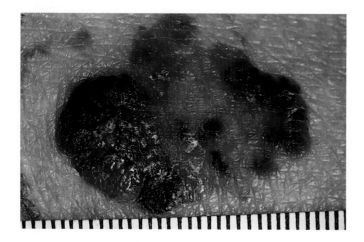

4 A 51-year-old man noticed a change in the skin lesion shown on the upper, outer area of his right arm. The lesion has enlarged during the past month. Physical examination yields no other remarkable findings. Which of the following occupations is this man most likely to have had earlier in life?

❑ (A) Chemist
❑ (B) Lifeguard
❑ (C) Miner
❑ (D) Auto mechanic
❑ (E) Radiation oncologist

5 A 35-year-old man has had an outbreak of pruritic lesions over the extensor surfaces of the elbows and knees during the past month. He has a history of malabsorption that requires him to eat a special diet, but he has had no previous skin problems. On physical examination, the lesions are 0.4- to 0.7-cm vesicles. A 3-mm punch biopsy of one of the lesions over the elbow is performed. Microscopic examination of the biopsy specimen shows accumulation of neutrophils at the tips of dermal papillae and formation of small blisters due to separation at the dermoepidermal junction. Immunofluorescence studies performed on this specimen show granular deposits of IgA localized to tips of dermal papillae. Laboratory studies show serum anti-gliadin antibodies. Which of the following is the most likely diagnosis?

❑ (A) Bullous pemphigoid
❑ (B) Contact dermatitis
❑ (C) Dermatitis herpetiformis
❑ (D) Discoid lupus erythematosus
❑ (E) Erythema multiforme
❑ (F) Impetigo
❑ (G) Lichen planus
❑ (H) Pemphigus vulgaris

6 Over the course of 1 week, a 6-year-old boy develops 1- to 2-cm erythematous macules and 0.5- to 1.0-cm pustules on his face. During the next 2 days, some of the pustules break, forming shallow erosions covered by a honey-colored crust. New lesions then form around the crust. The boy's 40-year-old uncle develops similar lesions after visiting for 1 week during the child's illness. Removal of the crusts from the boy's face is followed by healing within 1 week. The uncle does not

seek medical care, and additional pustules form at the periphery of the crusts. Which of the following conditions most likely explains these findings?

❑ (A) Acne vulgaris
❑ (B) Bullous pemphigoid
❑ (C) Contact dermatitis
❑ (D) Erythema multiforme
❑ (E) Impetigo
❑ (F) Lichen planus
❑ (G) Pemphigus vulgaris
❑ (H) Psoriasis

7 A 50-year-old woman has been bothered by a discolored area of skin on her forehead that has not faded during the past 3 years. On physical examination, there is a 0.8-cm red, rough-surfaced lesion on the right forehead above the eyebrow. A biopsy specimen examined microscopically shows hyperkeratosis and thinning of the epidermis with atypical basal cells. The upper dermal collagen and elastic fibers show homogenization with elastosis. Which of the following is the most appropriate advice to give this patient?

❑ (A) Reduce intake of dietary fat
❑ (B) Wear a hat outdoors
❑ (C) Stop taking aspirin for headaches
❑ (D) Apply hydrocortisone cream to your face
❑ (E) This condition is related to aging

8 A 10-year-old girl is brought to the physician by her mother because multiple excoriations have appeared on the skin of her hands over the past week. The child reports that she scratches her hands because they itch. Physical examination shows several 0.2- to 0.6-cm linear streaks in the interdigital regions. Treatment with a topical lindane lotion resolves the condition. Which of the following organisms is most likely responsible for these findings?

❑ (A) *Ixodes scapularis*
❑ (B) *Tinea corporis*
❑ (C) *Staphylococcus aureus*
❑ (D) Molluscum contagiosum
❑ (E) *Sarcoptes scabiei*

9 A 35-year-old man has noted a bump on his upper trunk for the past 6 weeks. On physical examination, there is a solitary 0.4-cm flesh-colored nodule on the upper trunk. The dome-shaped lesion is umbilicated, and a curdlike material can be expressed from the center. This material is smeared on a slide, and Giemsa stain shows many pink, homogenous, cytoplasmic inclusions. The lesion regresses over the next 2 months. Which of the following infectious agents most likely produced this lesion?

❑ (A) Human papillomavirus
❑ (B) *Staphylococcus aureus*
❑ (C) Molluscum contagiosum
❑ (D) *Histoplasma capsulatum*
❑ (E) Varicella-zoster virus

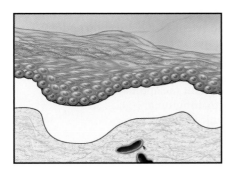

❑ (A) *Borrelia burgdorferi*
❑ (B) Group A β-hemolytic *Streptococcus*
❑ (C) Herpes simplex virus
❑ (D) Varicella-zoster virus
❑ (E) Human papillomavirus
❑ (F) Molluscum contagiosum
❑ (G) *Propionibacterium acnes*
❑ (H) *Sarcoptes scabiei*
❑ (I) *Staphylococcus aureus*
❑ (J) *Trichophyton rubrum*

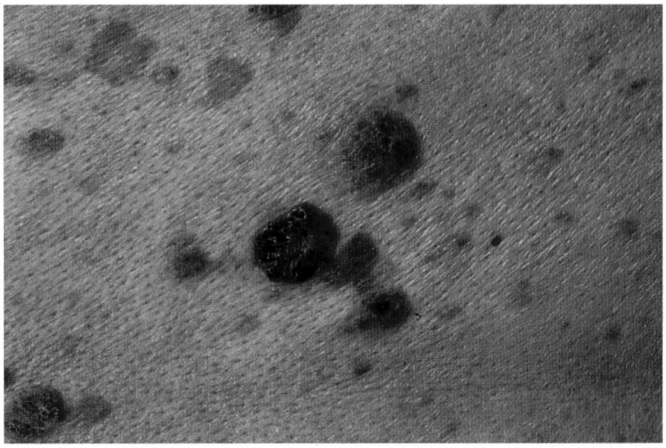

10 Many skin disorders give rise to vesicles or bullae (blisters) in the skin. The location of the bulla often aids in the diagnosis. Which of the following disorders is most likely to produce the type of blister that is schematically illustrated?

❑ (A) Impetigo
❑ (B) Pemphigus vulgaris
❑ (C) Bullous pemphigoid
❑ (D) Acute eczematous dermatitis
❑ (E) Urticaria

11 A 39-year-old woman has a nodule on her back that has become larger over the past 2 months. On physical examination, there is a 2.1-cm pigmented lesion with irregular borders and an irregular brown to black color. An excisional biopsy with wide margins is performed, and microscopic examination of the biopsy specimen shows a malignant melanoma composed of epithelioid cells that extends 2 mm down to the reticular dermis. There is a band of lymphocytes beneath the melanoma. Which of the following statements is most appropriate to make to this patient regarding these findings?

❑ (A) Your immune system will prevent metastases
❑ (B) The prognosis is poor
❑ (C) Other family members are at risk for this condition
❑ (D) The primary site for this lesion is probably the eye
❑ (E) Nevi elsewhere on your body may become malignant

12 A 39-year-old woman goes to her dentist for a routine dental examination. The dentist notes that she has 0.2- to 1.5-cm scattered, white, reticulated areas on the buccal mucosa. The woman says that these lesions have been present for 1 year. She also has some 0.3-cm purple, pruritic papules on each elbow. A biopsy specimen of a skin lesion shows a bandlike infiltrate of lymphocytes at the dermal-epidermal junction as well as degeneration of basal keratinocytes. Which of the following is the best advice to give this patient regarding these lesions?

❑ (A) A squamous cell carcinoma is likely to develop
❑ (B) You may develop chronic renal disease
❑ (C) A skin test for tuberculosis needs to be performed
❑ (D) You should stop taking all medications
❑ (E) These lesions will probably resolve over time

13 A 22-year-old man and other members of his racquetball club have noticed more itching of their feet in the past 2 months. On physical examination, the man has diffuse, erythematous, scaling skin lesions between the toes of both feet. There are no other remarkable findings. These findings are most likely the result of infection with which of the following organisms?

14 Over the past 20 years, a 75-year-old man has noticed slowly enlarging lesions (similar to those shown) on his trunk. One of the lesions is excised, and microscopic examination shows sheets of lightly pigmented basaloid cells that surround keratin-filled cysts. This lesion is sharply demarcated from the surrounding epidermis. Which of the following is the most likely diagnosis?

❑ (A) Basal cell carcinoma
❑ (B) Condyloma acuminatum
❑ (C) Intradermal nevus
❑ (D) Keratoacanthoma
❑ (E) Melanoma
❑ (F) Seborrheic keratosis
❑ (G) Squamous cell carcinoma
❑ (H) Verruca vulgaris

15 A 30-year-old man is known for his large appetite. At a luncheon meeting, he notices that all the cookies contain nuts, which the other diners have ordered knowing that he will not eat them because he will develop blotchy erythematous, slightly edematous, pruritic plaques on his skin. These plaques will form and then fade within 2 hours. If the man eats the cookies, which of the following sensitized cells will release a mediator that produces these skin lesions?

❑ (A) Mast cell
❑ (B) Neutrophil
❑ (C) Natural killer cell
❑ (D) CD4 lymphocyte
❑ (E) Plasma cells

16 A 17-year-old girl has hundreds of skin lesions on her body that have been forming since childhood. On physical examination, 0.4- to 1.7-cm macular to slightly raised, plaque-like, dark brown pigmented lesions are present on sun-exposed and non–sun-exposed areas of skin. The lesions have irregular contours, and there is variability in pigmentation. She says that her 15-year-old brother has similar lesions. Which of the following molecular changes are most likely to be present in the DNA from this patient?

- ❑ (A) Deletion of the *von Hippel Lindau* (*VHL*) gene
- ❑ (B) Mutation of the *PTCH* gene
- ❑ (C) Integration of the human papillomavirus-16 (HPV-16) genome
- ❑ (D) Deletion of the *p16INK4A* (*CDNK2*) gene
- ❑ (E) Microsatellite instability
- ❑ (F) Ultraviolet light-induced damage from pyrimidine dimers

17 A 60-year-old man has noted the appearance of a nodule on his ear during the past month. On physical examination, there is a 1.2-cm flesh-colored, dome-shaped nodule on his right ear lobe. The nodule has a central keratin-filled crater surrounded by proliferating epithelium. The lesion regresses and disappears within 1 month. Which of the following is the most appropriate diagnosis of this lesion?

- ❑ (A) Squamous cell carcinoma
- ❑ (B) Basal cell carcinoma
- ❑ (C) Seborrheic keratosis
- ❑ (D) Actinic keratosis
- ❑ (E) Keratoacanthoma
- ❑ (F) Verruca vulgaris

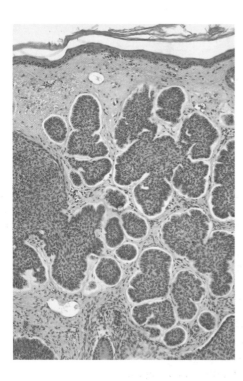

18 A 68-year-old man comes to the physician because of a slowly enlarging nodule on his right eyelid. On physical examination, there is a 0.3-cm pearly nodule on the upper eyelid near the lateral limbus of the right eye. The lesion is excised,

but multiple frozen sections are made during the surgery to minimize the extent of the resection and preserve the eyelid. The microscopic appearance of the lesion is shown at low magnification in the preceding figure. Which of the following is the most likely diagnosis?

- ❑ (A) Malignant melanoma
- ❑ (B) Dermatofibroma
- ❑ (C) Actinic keratosis
- ❑ (D) Nevocellular nevus
- ❑ (E) Basal cell carcinoma

19 A 5-year-old girl is brought to the physician by her parents for a routine health checkup. On physical examination, she has scattered 1- to 3-mm light brown macules on her face, trunk, and extremities. The parents state that these macules become more numerous in the summer months but fade over the winter. The lesions do not itch, bleed, or hurt. Which of the following is the most likely diagnosis?

- ❑ (A) Vitiligo
- ❑ (B) Lentigo
- ❑ (C) Freckle
- ❑ (D) Nevus
- ❑ (E) Melasma

20 A 19-year-old man has facial and upper back lesions that have waxed and waned for the past 6 years. On physical examination, there are 0.3- to 0.9-cm comedones, erythematous papules, nodules, and pustules most numerous on the lower face and posterior upper trunk. Other family members have been affected by this condition at a similar age. The lesions worsen during a 5-day cruise to the Caribbean. Which of the following organisms is most likely to play a key role in the pathogenesis of these lesions?

- ❑ (A) *Staphylococcus aureus*
- ❑ (B) Herpes simplex virus type 1
- ❑ (C) Group A β-hemolytic *Streptococcus*
- ❑ (D) *Mycobacterium leprae*
- ❑ (E) *Propionibacterium acnes*

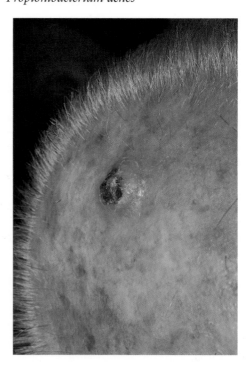

21 A 53-year-old man with idiopathic dilated cardiomyopathy underwent orthotopic heart transplantation. During the next 5 years, he had two episodes of minimal cellular rejection, which were adequately treated by an increase in immunosuppressive therapy. He has developed multiple skin lesions on the face and upper trunk over the past 6 months. On physical examination, the lesions are similar to that shown in the preceding figure. Some of the larger lesions have ulcerated. A biopsy specimen is most likely to identify which of the following lesions?

❑ (A) Psoriasis
❑ (B) Lichen planus
❑ (C) Dermatofibroma
❑ (D) Squamous cell carcinoma
❑ (E) Erythema multiforme

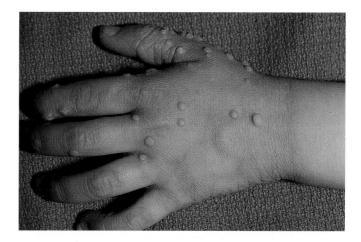

22 A 39-year-old woman comes to her physician because she has developed vesicular skin lesions over the past week. On physical examination, she has multiple 0.2- to 1-cm vesicles and bullae on the skin of her scalp, in both axillae, in the groin, and on the knees. Many lesions appear to have ruptured, and a shallow erosion with a dried crust of serum remains. A biopsy specimen of an axillary lesion examined microscopically shows epidermal acantholysis and formation of an intraepidermal blister. The basal cell layer is intact. Which of the following additional tests is most likely to explain the pathogenesis of the patient's disease?

❑ (A) Immunofluorescent staining of skin with anti-IgG
❑ (B) Viral culture of fluid from a skin vesicle
❑ (C) Determination of serum IgE level
❑ (D) Cytokeratin immunohistochemical staining
❑ (E) Darkfield microscopy of vesicular fluid

24 A 28-year-old man has noticed slowly enlarging lesions on his hands for the past 3 years. On physical examination, the lesions appear similar to those shown above. There are no other remarkable findings. The lesions have not changed in color, do not itch or bleed, and are not associated with pain. Which of the following is the most likely diagnosis?

❑ (A) Basal cell carcinoma
❑ (B) Condyloma acuminatum
❑ (C) Dermatofibroma
❑ (D) Intradermal nevus
❑ (E) Keratoacanthoma
❑ (F) Molluscum contagiosum
❑ (G) Seborrheic keratosis
❑ (H) Squamous cell carcinoma
❑ (I) Verruca vulgaris

23 For the past 3 days, a 25-year-old man known to be infected with HIV has had increasing fever, cough, and dyspnea, which has culminated in acute respiratory failure. On admission to the hospital, his temperature is 37.8°C. On physical examination, there are no significant findings. He undergoes a bronchoalveolar lavage that yields *Pneumocystis jirovecii* by direct fluorescent antigen testing. Within 1 week after initiation of therapy, he develops "target lesions" composed of red macules with a pale, vesicular center. The 2- to 5-cm lesions are distributed symmetrically over the upper arms and chest. Which of the following drugs is most likely to be implicated in the development of these lesions?

❑ (A) Ritonavir
❑ (B) Pentamidine
❑ (C) Sulfamethoxazole
❑ (D) Zidovudine
❑ (E) Dapsone
❑ (F) Adefovir
❑ (G) Nevirapine

25 A 32-year-old woman has noticed depigmented areas on her trunk that have waxed and waned for several months. She says that they do not itch or bleed and are not painful. Physical examination shows variably sized 0.3- to 1.2-cm macules over her upper trunk. The macules are lighter colored than the surrounding skin and have a fine, peripheral scale. Infection with which of the following organisms is most likely to produce these findings?

❑ (A) *Epidermophyton* sp.
❑ (B) Herpes simplex virus
❑ (C) Human papillomavirus
❑ (D) *Malassezia furfur*
❑ (E) Molluscum contagiosum
❑ (F) *Mycobacterium leprae*
❑ (G) *Propionibacterium acnes*
❑ (H) *Sarcoptes scabiei*
❑ (I) *Staphylococcus aureus*
❑ (J) *Streptococcus pyogenes*

26 After being hospitalized 1 week for treatment of an upper respiratory infection complicated by pneumonia, a 43-year-old woman develops a rash on her trunk and extremities. On physical examination, the 2- to 4-mm lesions are red, papulovesicular, oozing, and crusted. The lesions begin to disappear after she is discharged from the hospital 1 week later. Which of the following is the most likely pathogenesis of these lesions?

- ❑ (A) Type I hypersensitivity
- ❑ (B) Drug reaction
- ❑ (C) Bacterial septicemia
- ❑ (D) Photosensitivity
- ❑ (E) Human papillomavirus infection

27 A 58-year-old farmer has had a lesion on his face that has been enlarging for the past 3 years. On physical examination, a conical "cutaneous horn" projects 0.5 cm from a 0.7-cm base on the left lateral cheek. This lesion is excised, and microscopic examination shows basal cell hyperplasia. Some of the basal cells show nuclear atypicality associated with marked hyperkeratosis and parakeratosis. Which of the following lesions best accounts for these findings?

- ❑ (A) Verruca vulgaris
- ❑ (B) Keratoacanthoma
- ❑ (C) Dysplastic nevus
- ❑ (D) Actinic keratosis
- ❑ (E) Seborrheic keratosis

28 A 31-year-old man comes to his physician because of a bump on the skin of the lower abdomen that has enlarged over the past 4 years and has become more painful in the past week. On physical examination, there is a subcutaneous, movable, soft nodule at the belt line anteriorly that elicits pain with pressure. The overlying skin is intact. The patient states that the nodule began hurting about 1 day after he vigorously squeezed it. The lesion is excised and does not recur. Which of the following is the most likely diagnosis of this lesion?

- ❑ (A) Acne vulgaris
- ❑ (B) Epidermal inclusion cyst
- ❑ (C) Fibroepithelial polyp
- ❑ (D) Intradermal nevus
- ❑ (E) Trichoepithelioma
- ❑ (F) Xanthoma

29 A 9-year-old girl is brought to the physician by her parents because she has been scratching a group of small bumps on the skin of her forearm for the past month. On physical examination, there are five 0.4- to 0.9-cm small, flat to slightly papular, pale brown lesions on the volar surface. The lesions become more pruritic with swelling and erythema when rubbed. A biopsy specimen of one of the lesions examined microscopically shows an upper dermal infiltrate of large cells with abundant pink cytoplasm that stains an intense purple color with toluidine blue. Which of the following cell types is most likely to form these lesions?

- ❑ (A) CD4 lymphocyte
- ❑ (B) CD8 lymphocyte
- ❑ (C) Langerhans cell
- ❑ (D) Macrophage
- ❑ (E) Mast cell
- ❑ (F) Melanocyte
- ❑ (G) Merkel cell

30 A 50-year-old man notes several small, baglike lesions that have appeared on the skin in front of his armpits over the past 2 years. On physical examination, five small, soft papules in the anterior axillary line are covered by wrinkled skin and attached to the skin surface by a thin pedicle. They are 0.5 to 0.8 cm in length and about 0.3 cm in diameter. One lesion has undergone torsion and is more erythematous and painful to touch than the others. Which of the following is the most likely diagnosis?

- ❑ (A) Fibroepithelial polyp
- ❑ (B) Hemangioma
- ❑ (C) Lentigo
- ❑ (D) Melasma
- ❑ (E) Pilar cyst
- ❑ (F) Xanthoma

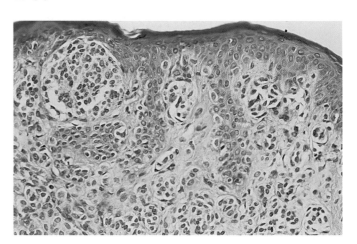

31 A 10-year-old child is brought to the physician by her parents because of an earache. On physical examination, the physician notices a flat, uniformly brown, 2-cm skin lesion, just above the right buttock. Her parents state that the lesion has been present since birth and has not changed in appearance. The representative microscopic appearance of the lesion is shown. Which of the following is the most likely diagnosis of this lesion?

- ❑ (A) Acanthosis nigricans
- ❑ (B) Basal cell carcinoma
- ❑ (C) Dysplastic nevus
- ❑ (D) Lentigo
- ❑ (E) Malignant melanoma
- ❑ (F) Nevocellular nevus
- ❑ (G) Seborrheic keratosis

ANSWERS

1 **(D)** This patient has psoriasis, a chronic skin condition with marked epithelial hyperplasia and parakeratotic scaling. Nail changes such as yellow-brown discoloration, pitting, dimpling, and separation of the nail plate from the nail bed (onycholysis) affect about one third of patients. Other manifestations of psoriasis include arthritis (resembling rheumatoid arthritis), myopathy, enteropathy, and spondylitic heart disease. Gastrointestinal mucosal involvement with hemorrhage is not a feature of psoriasis. A friction rub from fibrinous pericarditis does not occur in psoriasis, because mesothelial surfaces are not involved. Joint laxity with hyperreflexia is a feature of Ehlers-Danlos syndrome. Renal disease and hypertension are not typically the result of psoriasis.

BP7 793-794   BP6 701   PBD7 1256-1257   PBD6 1198-1199

2 **(C)** The driving force behind a worldwide increase in melanoma has been increased sun exposure. The Australian population is mainly derived from light-skinned Europeans who migrated to Australia. Indigenous, dark-skinned populations do not have the same risk.

BP7 805   BP6 711   PBD7 436-438, 1234-1236 PBD6 1177

3 **(D)** The patient has findings typical of acanthosis nigricans, a cutaneous marker for benign and malignant neoplasms. The skin lesions often precede signs and symptoms of associated cancers. They are believed to arise from the action of epidermal growth-promoting factors produced by neoplasms. The rashes that develop in systemic lupus erythematosus are the result of antigen-antibody complex deposition and often exhibit photosensitivity. Skin lesions of mastocytosis in adults often exhibit urticaria. Various skin lesions are associated with AIDS, including disseminated infections and papulosquamous dermatoses, although not pigmented lesions. Involvement of the skin in Langerhans cell histiocytoses typically occurs in children and produces reddish papules or nodules or erythematous scaling plaques because of the histiocytic infiltrates in the dermis.

PBD7 1237-1238   PBD6 1180

4 **(B)** The figure shows a malignant melanoma with irregular borders and variability of pigmentation. Any change in a pigmented lesion suggests the possibility of melanoma. Some melanomas are familial, arising from such conditions as dysplastic nevus syndrome. However, most melanomas occur sporadically and are related to sun exposure, as may occur in a lifeguard.

BP7 805-806   BP6 711-712   PBD7 1234-1236 PBD6 1177-1179

5 **(C)** The clinical and histologic findings are typical of celiac disease with dermatitis herpetiformis. The IgA or IgG antibodies formed against the gliadin protein in gluten that is ingested cross-react with reticulin. Reticulin is a component of the anchoring fibrils that attach the epidermal basement membrane to the superficial dermis. This explains the localization of the IgA to the tips of dermal papillae and the site of inflammation. A gluten-free diet may relieve the symptoms. Bullous pemphigoid can occur in older persons, with antibody directed at keratinocytes to produce flaccid bullae, but there is no association with celiac disease. Contact dermatitis is most likely to be seen on the hands and forearms. It is a type IV hypersensitivity reaction without immunoglobulin deposition and would not persist for 1 month. Discoid lupus erythematosus is seen on sun-exposed areas and has the appearance of an erythematous rash. Erythema multiforme is a hypersensitivity response to infections and drugs; it produces macules and papules with a red or vesicular center, but it is probably mediated by cytotoxic lymphocytes and not by

immunoglobulin deposition. Impetigo produced by infection with staphylococci and streptococci produces pustules and crusts, mainly on the hands and face. Lichen planus appears as violaceous papules and plaques. Pemphigus vulgaris is an autoimmune disease in which IgG deposited in acantholytic areas forms vesicles that rupture to form erosions; it is not related to celiac disease.

BP7 798   BP6 704   PBD7 1262-1263   PBD6 1204-1205

6 **(E)** Impetigo is a superficial infection of skin that produces shallow erosions. These erosions are covered with exuded serum that dries to give the characteristic honey-colored crust. Cultures of the lesions of impetigo usually grow coagulase-positive *Staphylococcus aureus* or group A β-hemolytic *Streptococcus*. The lesions are highly infectious. Acne vulgaris is typically seen during adolescence and produces pimples and pustules, but not crusts. Bullous pemphigoid can occur in older persons, with antibody directed at keratinocytes to produce flaccid bullae. Contact dermatitis is most likely to be seen on the hands and forearms. Erythema multiforme is a hypersensitivity response to infections and drugs that produces macules and papules with a red or vesicular center. Lichen planus appears as violaceous papules and plaques. Pemphigus vulgaris is an autoimmune disease in which IgG deposited in acantholytic areas forms vesicles that rupture to form erosions. Psoriasis produces patches of silvery, scaling lesions.

PBD7 1267   PBD6 1210

7 **(B)** Actinic keratoses are premalignant lesions associated with sun exposure. Decreasing dietary fat is always a good idea, but it does not have much effect on the skin of the face. Many drugs can cause acute eczematous dermatitis and erythema multiforme. Hydrocortisone can alleviate the symptoms of many dermatologic conditions, but it cannot reverse actinic damage. Older persons are more likely to have actinic keratoses because of greater cumulative sun exposure, not because of aging alone.

BP7 800-801   BP6 707   PBD7 1240-1242   PBD6 1184

8 **(E)** The small scabies mites burrow through the stratum corneum to produce the linear lesions, and the mites along with their eggs and feces produce intense pruritus. Scabies is easily transmitted by contact and typically occurs in community outbreaks. *Ixodes scapularis* is the tick that is the vector for *Borrelia burgdorferi* organisms, which cause Lyme disease and erythema chronicum migrans. *Tinea corporis* is a superficial fungal infection that can produce erythema and crusting. The erythematous macules and pustules of impetigo in children are often caused by staphylococcal and group A streptococcal infection. Molluscum contagiosum is a poxvirus that produces a localized, firm nodule.

PBD7 1268-1269   PBD6 1211-1212

9 **(C)** The pink cytoplasmic inclusions, called "molluscum bodies," are characteristic of this lesion. Immunocompromised persons may have multiple, larger lesions. The infectious agent is a poxvirus. Human papillomavirus (not a toad) is implicated in the appearance of verruca vulgaris, or the common wart. *Staphylococcus aureus* is implicated in the formation of the lesions of impetigo. Disseminated fungal infections are uncommon except in immunocompromised patients. Varicella-zoster virus causes "shingles," characterized by a dermatomal distribution of clear, painful vesicles.

PBD7 1267   PBD6 1209

10 **(C)** The figure shows a subepidermal bulla. Bullous pemphigoid results from antibody-mediated damage to the basal cell–basement membrane attachment plaques (hemidesmosomes). The bulla formed is subepidermal. In contrast, the antibodies in pemphigus vulgaris attack the desmosomes that attach the epidermal keratinocytes. Loosening of these junctions leads to acantholysis, and an intraepidermal blister is formed just above the basal layer (suprabasal). In impetigo, there is infection of the superficial layer of the skin, and the blister is just under the stratum corneum (subcorneal). Acute eczematous dermatitis has spongiotic vesicles, not bullae. In urticaria, the allergic reaction causes increased vascular permeability in dermal capillaries. This produces superficial dermal edema, not a bulla.

BP7 796-797   BP6 702-704   PBD7 1261-1262
PBD6 1201-1204

11 **(B)** Extension deep into the reticular dermis is indicative of vertical (nodular) growth. When a melanoma exhibits a nodular growth pattern, rather than a radial pattern, there is increased likelihood that a clone of neoplastic cells has arisen that is more aggressive and is more likely to metastasize. Although there has been a lymphocytic response to this tumor, it is not sufficient to destroy or contain it completely. Most melanomas are sporadic, nonfamilial, and related to sun exposure. Melanomas of the eye are much less common than melanomas of the skin. Benign skin nevi do not have a tendency to become malignant.

BP7 805-806   BP6 711-712   PBD7 1234-1236
PBD6 1177-1179

12 **(E)** This patient has the classic "pruritic, purple, polygonal papules" of lichen planus, with the distinctive bandlike infiltrate of lymphocytes at the dermal-epidermal junction. The lesions of lichen planus are typically self-limited, although the course can run for several years. Oral lesions may persist longer. There is no risk of malignancy. Although a lymphocytic infiltrate is present, an infection or autoimmunity is not implicated. A drug eruption would not last this long. Lesions of erythema multiforme are more likely to follow infections, drugs, autoimmune diseases, and malignancies.

BP7 794-795   BP6 702   PBD7 1258   PBD6 1199-1200

13 **(J)** "Athlete's foot" is a common disorder resulting from superficial dermatophyte infection by a variety of fungal species, including *Trichophyton*, *Epidermophyton*, and *Microsporum*. Those that involve the foot produce the condition known as tinea pedis. *Borrelia burgdorferi* causes Lyme disease, which may include a skin lesion called erythema chronicum migrans around the original tick bite. Streptococcal and staphylococcal organisms cause impetigo, which is more common on the face and hands. Herpetic infections first produce crops of clear vesicles, which may burst and form painful shallow ulcers. Varicella-zoster virus is the reactivation, in adults, of childhood chickenpox in the form of vesicles in a dermatomal distribution of the nerve in whose ganglion the virus lay dormant for years. Human papillomavirus is best known as the cause of genital warts (condyloma acuminatum) and as a driving force behind cervical and anal squamous cell dysplasias. Molluscum contagiosum is

caused by a poxvirus and produces an umbilicated nodule. *Propionibacterium acnes* is a factor in the development of acne. The little eight-legged critters known as *Sarcoptes scabiei* crawl around in the stratum corneum, usually between the fingers, and cause itching, a process called scabies.

PBD7 1267-1268   PBD6 1210

14 **(F)** These flat, round, pigmented, sharply demarcated lesions are benign tumors called seborrheic keratoses. They are composed of pigmented basaloid cells. Seborrheic keratoses are common in older persons. The lesions gradually enlarge, but they are not painful and do not ulcerate. They mainly are a cosmetic problem. Basal cell carcinomas are nodular, slowly enlarging lesions most common on the head and trunk and are related to sun exposure. Condylomata acuminata, or genital warts, are caused by a sexually transmitted type of human papillomavirus; the lesions tend to be pink to white. An intradermal nevus can produce a pigmented nodule, but microscopically it is composed of nests of small nevus cells, and the lesions increase minimally in size over time. Keratoacanthoma may resemble squamous cell carcinoma and grow rapidly to form an ulcerative nodule but typically regresses in several months; squamous cell carcinoma continues to grow. Melanomas have very atypical spindle to epithelioid cells that invade the dermis; they tend to change in appearance over weeks to months, not years. A verruca vulgaris, or wart, also has a rough surface, but such lesions are more common on the hands and feet, and they may regress after several years. The cells in a squamous cell carcinoma are atypical and may invade the dermis.

BP7 798-799   BP6 705-706   PBD7 1237
PBD6 1179-1180

15 **(A)** If the man eats the cookies, he will have "hives," or urticaria, from an allergy to an antigen in nuts. This causes a type I hypersensitivity reaction in which IgE antibodies are bound to the IgE receptor on mast cells. IgE-sensitized mast cells degranulate when the antigen is encountered. Neutrophils may become attracted to this site, but they are not the sensitized cells. Natural killer cells mediate antibody-dependent cell-mediated cytotoxicity and lyse major histocompatability complex class I–deficient target cells. Plasma cells secrete the IgE antibodies but do not release the mediators for allergic reactions.

BP7 791   BP6 698-699   PBD7 1252-1254   PBD6 1194

16 **(D)** The clinical appearance, distribution, and occurrence in two siblings suggest that these lesions represent the dysplastic nevus syndrome. Dysplastic nevi are precursors of malignant melanoma. The most important gene in cases of familial melanoma is *p16INK4A* (also known as cyclin-dependent kinase inhibitor 2, or *CDNK2*) on chromosome 9p21. Patients have a germ-line mutation in one *p16INK4A* allele, and as with other tumor suppressor genes, the second allele is lost in the tumor cells. The *PTCH* gene is implicated in the pathogenesis of both sporadic basal cell carcinomas and the familial nevoid basal cell carcinoma syndrome. HPV-16 infection is important in the pathogenesis of squamous epithelial dysplasias and carcinomas, particularly involving the uterine cervix. HPV-16 DNA is integrated into the host cell genome and its protein product inactives host cell *RB* and *p53* genes. The neoplasms in von Hippel Lindau disease include renal cell carcinoma, pheochromocytoma, and hemangioblastomas of the central nervous system. Microsatellite instability is a manifestation of the loss of DNA mismatch repair genes, as occurs in the hereditary nonpolyposis colon carcinoma (HNPCC) syndrome. A defect in nucleotide excision repair is present in xeroderma pigmentosa, an autosomal recessive condition in which sun exposure is associated with mutations in the *PTCH* and *p53* genes.

BP7 804-805   BP6 710   PBD7 1233-1234, 1244-1245
PBD6 1176-1177

17 (E) The gross and microscopic appearance is typical of keratoacanthoma. Keratoacanthomas are self-limited lesions that often regress on their own. Those that do not regress should be suspected of being squamous cell carcinomas, which typically do not regress. Basal cell carcinomas may also be raised lesions, but they also do not regress. A seborrheic keratosis tends to be a flatter (although raised), rough-surfaced, pigmented lesion that slowly enlarges over time. An actinic keratosis tends to be a flat, pigmented lesion that is tan to brown to red. A verruca vulgaris (wart) usually occurs on the hands and feet, has a rough upper surface, and usually comes and goes over several years' time.

BP7 799   BP6 705-706   PBD7 1240-1241   PBD6 1181

18 (E) Basal cell carcinomas arise as pearly papules on sun-exposed areas of the skin, particularly the face. They slowly infiltrate surrounding tissues, gradually enlarging. Although it rarely metastasizes, a basal cell carcinoma can have serious local effects, particularly in the area of the eye. Melanomas are usually pigmented, and they are composed of polygonal or spindle cells that tend to grow in sheets and infiltrate to produce a grossly irregular border to the lesion. A dermatofibroma is a benign lesion of the dermis composed of cells resembling fibroblasts. An actinic keratosis is a premalignant lesion of the epidermis that does not invade surrounding tissue. A nevus is a small, localized, benign lesion.

BP7 802-803   BP6 709   PBD7 1242-1244
PBD6 1186-1187

19 (C) Freckles are relatively common. Persons with a light complexion or red hair are more likely to have freckles. These lesions may be a cosmetic problem, but they have no other significance. Areas of skin with vitiligo are depigmented. A lentigo is a brown macule whose pigmentation is not related to sun exposure. Nevi do not wax and wane with sun exposure. Melasma is most often a masklike area of facial hyperpigmentation associated with pregnancy.

PBD7 1231   PBD6 1174

20 (E) This man has acne vulgaris. Teenagers and young adults are more often affected by acne than other age groups, and males are more often affected than females. *Propionibacterium acnes* breaks down sebaceous gland oils to produce irritative fatty acids, and this may promote the process. Did the food on the cruise play a role? Probably not, but stress causes the lesions to worsen. *Staphylococcus aureus* and group A streptococci are implicated in the inflammatory skin condition known as impetigo, which can include pustules and a characteristic pale yellow-brown crust. Herpes simplex virus produces vesicular skin eruptions, most often in a perioral or genital distribution. *Mycobacterium leprae* causes leprosy, which is a chronic condition that can produce focal depigmentation and areas of skin anesthesia.

PBD7 1263-1265   PBD6 1206-1207

21 (D) Risk factors for squamous cell carcinoma include ultraviolet light exposure, scarring from burn injury, irradiation, and immunosuppression. This patient was immunosuppressed to prevent graft rejection. Squamous cell carcinomas also arise in rare disorders of DNA repair, such as xeroderma pigmentosum. Psoriasis is an inflammatory dermatosis that can be associated with underlying arthritis, myopathy, enteropathy, or spondylitic heart disease. Lichen planus is a self-limited inflammatory disorder that manifests as "purple, pruritic, polygonal papules," not as elevated ulcerated lesions. A dermatofibroma is typically solitary, firm, and dermally located. Erythema multiforme is a hypersensitivity response to infections or drugs; the lesions have multiple forms, including papules, macules, vesicles, and bullae.

BP7 801-802   BP6 708   PBD7 1242-1246
PBD6 1184-1186

22 (A) These lesions are probably pemphigus vulgaris, a rare type II hypersensitivity reaction. In this disorder, IgG autoantibodies to the intercellular cement substance are formed. They disrupt intercellular bridges, causing the epidermal cells to detach from each other (acantholysis). This action then causes the formation of an intraepidermal blister. Staining with anti-IgG illuminates intercellular junctions at sites of incipient acantholysis. Herpes simplex viral infections can produce crops of vesicles, but such a wide distribution would be unusual. Type I hypersensitivity with urticaria does not produce an acantholytic vesicle. Keratinocytes are epithelial and are always positive for cytokeratin. Darkfield microscopy is used almost exclusively to identify spirochetes in cases of syphilis.

BP7 795-796   BP6 702-703   PBD7 1260-1261
PBD6 1201-1202

23 (C) The patient has erythema multiforme, a hypersensitivity response to certain infections and drugs, such as sulfonamides and penicillin. Other inciting factors include herpes simplex virus, mycoplasmal and fungal infections, malignant diseases, and collagen vascular diseases such as systemic lupus erythematosus. The other listed antiretroviral drugs or antimicrobials are far less likely to cause skin reactions. Acetaminophen and dapsone are less likely to produce erythema multiforme, but many drugs can cause skin rashes and eruptions.

BP7 793   BP6 700   PBD7 1255-1256   PBD6 1197-1198

24 (I) The "warts" in this patient are a common problem and result from infection with one of many types of human papillomavirus (HPV). They do not become malignant and tend to regress after several years. Basal cell carcinomas are nodular, slowly enlarging lesions usually seen on the head and trunk and are related to sun exposure. Condylomata acuminata, or genital warts, are caused by a type of HPV that is sexually transmitted; the lesions tend to be pink to white. A dermatofibroma forms a subcutaneous nodule, as does an intradermal nevus. A keratoacanthoma may resemble squamous cell carcinoma and grow rapidly to form an ulcerative nodule, but the keratoacanthoma typically regresses in several months; squamous cell carcinoma continues to grow. Likewise, molluscum contagiosum is a self-limited condition with a nodular appearance. Seborrheic keratoses are pale brown to dark brown, slowly enlarging lesions with a rough surface that are most commonly found on the trunk and face of older persons.

BP7 799-800   BP6 705-707   PBD7 1266-1267
PBD6 1208-1209

25 **(D)** Tinea versicolor is a relatively common condition caused by a superficial fungal infection of *Malassezia furfur*. The lesions can be lighter or darker than the surrounding skin. *Epidermophyton, Trichophyton,* and *Microsporum* genera are dermatophytic fungi best known as the cause of athlete's foot and "jock itch." Herpes simplex virus presents initially with crops of clear vesicles that may burst and form painful shallow ulcers. Human papillomavirus is best known as the cause of genital warts (condyloma acuminatum) and as a driving force behind cervical and anal squamous cell dysplasias. Molluscum contagiosum is caused by a poxvirus and produces an umbilicated nodule. *Mycobacterium leprae* is the cause of Hansen disease, which can manifest with areas of skin anesthesia that predispose to repeated trauma. *Propionibacterium acnes* is a factor in the development of acne. *Sarcoptes scabiei* is the cause of scabies, which appears as pruritic reddish lesions. Staphylococcal infections may manifest as impetigo, as a complication of acne, or as wound infections. *Streptococcus pyogenes* may cause impetigo, erysipelas, or scarlet fever.

PBD7 1268   PBD6 1210

26 **(B)** The time course of this case suggests a drug reaction producing an acute erythematous dermatitis. Urticaria in type I hypersensitivity is not as severe or as long lasting. Sepsis rarely involves the skin in an erythematous dermatitis. Photosensitivity may be enhanced by drugs, but ultraviolet light is the key component in light that produces photodermatitis. Photosensitivity is not likely to be encountered with indoor lighting in the hospital room, and most organizations will not buy light bulbs that mimic daylight, thereby increasing the prevalence of seasonal affective disorder and decreasing productivity by staff. Human papillomavirus infection is associated with formation of verruca vulgaris, the common wart.

BP7 791-792   BP6 699   PBD7 1252-1254
PBD6 1194-1196

27 **(D)** Actinic keratosis occurs on sun-exposed areas and is considered a precursor of squamous cell carcinoma. When the atypical basal cells occupy the entire thickness of the epidermis, the lesion becomes a carcinoma in situ. The presence of a hyperkeratotic layer is characteristic. Occasionally, so much keratin is produced that a "cutaneous horn" is formed. A verruca vulgaris may also be a raised lesion, but it is usually more pebbly, and there is no squamous atypia. Superficial epidermal cells show vacuolation or koilocytosis. A keratoacanthoma is a dome-shaped nodule with a central keratin-filled crater that is surrounded by epithelial cells. Microscopically, it may mimic a squamous cell carcinoma. A dysplastic nevus is typically a flat, pigmented lesion. A seborrheic keratosis can be raised, but it usually appears as a coinlike plaque.

BP7 800-801   BP6 707   PBD7 1240-1242
PBD6 1184-1185

28 **(B)** The epidermal inclusion cyst is the most common form of epithelial cyst, or wen, which is a cystic structure formed from downward growth of epithelium or expansion of a hair follicle and is lined by squamous epithelium that desquamates keratinaceous debris in the center of the expanding cyst. Rupture of the cyst produces a local inflammatory reaction. Acne produces comedones, most typically on the face and upper trunk of adolescents and young adults. A fibroepithelial polyp is a skin tag that projects from the surface of the skin on a narrow pedicle. An intradermal nevus forms a pale to pigmented nodule that tends not to change much in size. A trichoepithelioma is a form of a benign adnexal tumor, which is uncommon; it is a subcutaneous nodule usually seen on the head, neck, and upper trunk. Xanthomas are soft, yellow nodules that may form in the dermis from collections of lipid-laden macrophages in persons with hyperlipidemia.

PBD7 1238   PBD6 1181

29 **(E)** This patient has urticaria pigmentosa, a localized form of mastocytosis. The cutaneous lesions often show the characteristic Darier sign on rubbing. Some patients may have systemic mastocytosis. Point mutations in the *C-KIT* oncogene may be present. Lymphocytes, Langerhans cells, and macrophages participate in inflammatory reactions, such as contact dermatitis. Macrophages and Langerhans cells are antigen-presenting cells. Melanocytes contain melanin granules, which they pass on to keratinocytes to increase skin pigmentation. Merkel cells are derived from neural crest and can form the obscure Merkel cell tumor, which resembles a small cell carcinoma.

PBD7 1250-1251   PBD6 1192-1193

30 **(A)** A fibroepithelial polyp is also known as an acrochordon or skin tag. These common lesions are composed of a central core of fibrovascular connective tissue covered by normal-appearing squamous epithelium. They may become irritated but are otherwise incidental findings. A hemangioma forms a red nodule that is composed of vascular spaces in the upper dermis. A lentigo is a focus of melanocyte hyperplasia that produces a brown macule; in older persons, they are known as senile lentigines or "age spots" and are commonly found on the hands. Melasma is most often a masklike area of facial hyperpigmentation associated with pregnancy. A pilar (trichilemmal) cyst is an epithelial cyst that forms on the scalp. A xanthoma is a localized dermal collection of lipid-laden macrophages associated with hyperlipidemia.

PBD7 1238   PBD6 1181

31 **(F)** The figure shows a form of nevocellular nevus known as a congenital nevus. Larger nevi do have an increased risk of a melanoma to arise within them; however, the lack of additional lesions and the bland microscopic appearance argue against dysplastic nevus syndrome. Acanthosis nigricans is an uncommon condition with hyperpigmented areas in skinfolds; it may occur in association with endocrinopathies or with neoplasms. Basal cell carcinomas occur in sun-exposed skin of adults, and the cells have darker nuclei with scant cytoplasm. A lentigo is a common focal pigmented lesion that can appear at any age; it is a melanocyte hyperplasia. Melanoma occurs in adults and shows signs of rapid growth and change, with very atypical cells invading the dermis. Seborrheic keratoses are seen in older adults and are raised, pigmented lesions of thickened epidermis.

BP7 803-804   BP6 709-710   PBD7 1232-1233
PBD6 1174-1176

Bones, Joints, and Soft Tissue Tumors

PBD7 Chapter 26: Bones, Joints, and Soft Tissue Tumors

PBD6 Chapter 28: Bones, Joints, and Soft Tissue Tumors

BP7 and BP6 Chapter 21: The Musculoskeletal System

1 A 60-year-old woman comes to her physician because she has had lower back pain for 1 month. On physical examination, there are no remarkable findings except for pain on deep palpation of the abdomen. Findings from a routine urinalysis, CBC, and serum electrolyte panel are all unremarkable. Twenty years earlier, she was treated for Hodgkin disease with abdominal irradiation and chemotherapy, and there has been no evidence of recurrence during regular follow-up visits. MR imaging now shows a 10 × 15 cm ovoid mass of the left retroperitoneum. Which of the following is most likely to be found in the patient's retroperitoneum?

- (A) Desmoid tumor
- (B) Recurrent Hodgkin disease
- (C) Rhabdomyosarcoma
- (D) Leiomyosarcoma
- (E) Malignant fibrous histiocytoma

2 A 60-year-old man with a diagnosis of chronic myeloid leukemia is treated with intensive chemotherapy. He goes into remission but develops pain in the left wrist. On physical examination, there is swelling and warmth on palpation of the wrist. Polarized light microscopy of fluid aspirated from the wrist joint shows needle-shaped crystals that display negative birefringence. Which of the following

processes most likely played an important role in the pathogenesis of the patient's wrist pain?

- (A) Damage to the articular cartilage by chemotherapeutic agents
- (B) Infiltration of the synovium by leukemic cells
- (C) Synovial proliferation from cytokine secretion by leukemic cells
- (D) Excessive production of uric acid from dying leukemic cells
- (E) Hemorrhages into the joint as a result of deranged platelet function

3 A 42-year-old man on holiday is involved in a skiing accident in which he sustains a right tibial diaphyseal fracture. The fracture is set with open reduction and internal fixation for proper alignment. The holiday period is not over, and 1 week later he is in the ski lodge, sitting by the fire with drink in hand. There are now more osteoclasts in the region of the fracture. Which of the following is the most likely function of these osteoclasts?

- (A) Form collagen
- (B) Resorb bone
- (C) Synthesize osteoid
- (D) Elaborate cytokines
- (E) Divide

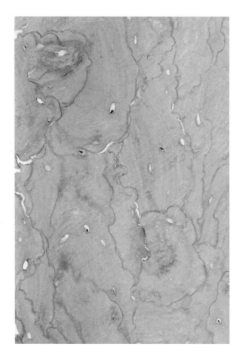

☐ (A) Osteochondroma
☐ (B) Vitamin D deficiency
☐ (C) Degenerative osteoarthritis
☐ (D) Hyperparathyroidism
☐ (E) Paget disease of bone

5 A 35-year-old woman has experienced malaise, fatigue, and joint pain for the past 5 months. She has had progressive loss of joint motion, making it more difficult to walk and to use her hands. On physical examination, the joint involvement is symmetric, and most of the affected joints are in the hands and feet. The involved joints are swollen and warm to the touch. The right second and third digits have a "swan neck" deformity, and there is ulnar deviation of both hands. Reconstructive surgery is performed on her right hand. Microscopic views of the excised joint capsule tissue are shown below. Which of the following laboratory findings is most likely to be reported in this patient?

☐ (A) Positive *Borrelia burgdorferi* serologic test
☐ (B) Positive acid-fast stain of joint tissue
☐ (C) Serum positive for rheumatoid factor
☐ (D) Hyperuricemia
☐ (E) Calcium pyrophosphate crystals in a joint aspirate

4 A 70-year-old man complains of right hip and thigh pain of several months' duration. On physical examination, he has reduced range of motion in both hips, but there is no tenderness or swelling on palpation. Radiographs of the pelvis and right leg show sclerotic, thickened cortical bone with a narrowed joint space near the acetabulum. Laboratory studies show a serum alkaline phosphatase level of 173 U/L, calcium 9.5 mg/dL, and phosphorus 3.4 mg/dL. A bone biopsy is performed, and the microscopic appearance of the specimen is shown above. Which of the following conditions is most likely to produce these findings?

6 A 79-year-old man has had progressively worsening lower back, bilateral hip, and right shoulder pain for the past 6 years. He reports that he has had to buy larger hats. On physical examination, there is no joint swelling, erythema, warmth, or tenderness, but the range of motion is reduced. Radiographs of the affected joints show narrowing of joint spaces with adjacent bony sclerosis. A skull radiograph shows thickening of the skull bone. A bone biopsy at the iliac crest shows a loss of normal trabeculae, with a mosaic pattern and increased numbers of osteoclasts and osteoblasts. Which of the following complications is the patient most likely to suffer as a result of this condition?

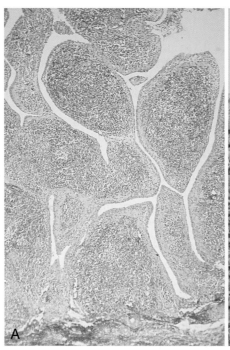

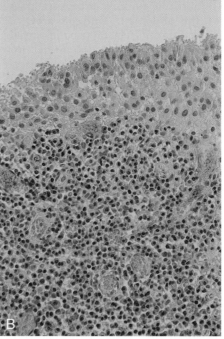

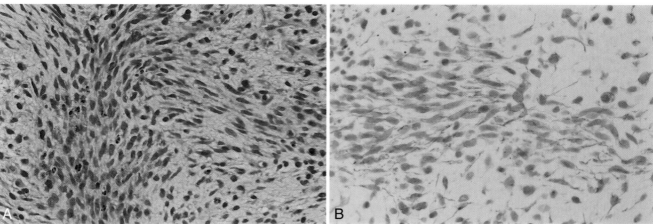

Courtesy of Jorgé Albores-Saavedra, MD, Department of Pathology, University of Texas Southwestern Medical School, Dallas, TX.

❑ (A) Ankylosing spondylitis
❑ (B) Osteoid osteoma
❑ (C) Fibrous dysplasia
❑ (D) Osteosarcoma
❑ (E) Enchondroma

7 A 6-year-old boy complains of discomfort in the right upper neck that has worsened over the past 6 months. On physical examination, a 5-cm firm mass is palpable in the right lateral neck. The mass is not painful or warm. The histologic appearance of this mass is shown above. Which of the following immunohistochemical stains is most likely to be positive in the cells of this lesion?

❑ (A) Vimentin
❑ (B) Neuron-specific enolase
❑ (C) Cytokeratin
❑ (D) Factor VIII
❑ (E) CD3

8 A 26-year-old man is struck in the left arm by a swinging steel beam at a construction site. On physical examination, a 4-cm area of the lateral upper left arm exhibits swelling and redness with pain on palpation. A radiograph of the left arm shows no fracture. Three weeks later, there now is a 2-cm painful, well-circumscribed, subcutaneous mass at the site of the original injury. A radiograph shows a solid soft tissue mass. Which of the following lesions is most likely to be present?

❑ (A) Malignant fibrous histiocytoma
❑ (B) Organizing abscess
❑ (C) Nodular fasciitis
❑ (D) Superficial fibromatosis
❑ (E) Lipoma

9 Several days after an episode of urethritis, a 28-year-old man develops acute pain and swelling of the left knee. On physical examination, the knee is swollen and is warm and tender to the touch. No other joints appear to be affected. Laboratory examination of fluid aspirated from the left knee joint shows numerous neutrophils. A Gram stain of the fluid shows gram-negative intracellular diplococci. No crystals are seen. Which of the following infectious agents is most likely responsible for this condition?

❑ (A) *Borrelia burgdorferi*
❑ (B) *Treponema pallidum*
❑ (C) *Neisseria gonorrhoeae*
❑ (D) *Staphylococcus aureus*
❑ (E) *Haemophilus influenzae*

10 A 75-year-old woman trips on the carpet in his home and falls to the floor. She immediately has marked pain in the right hip. On physical examination, there is shortening of the right leg and marked pain with any movement. A radiograph shows a right femoral neck fracture. The fracture is repaired. Six months later, a dual energy x-ray absorptiometry (DEXA) scan of the patient's left hip and lumbar vertebrae shows a bone mineral density two standard deviations below the young adult reference range. Which of the following processes contributes most to development of these findings?

❑ (A) Decreased osteoprotegerin production
❑ (B) Decreased sensitivity of osteoblasts to dihydroxy-cholecalciferol
❑ (C) Decreased secretion of interleukins 1 and 6 and tumor necrosis factor-α by monocytes
❑ (D) Increased sensitivity of bone to the effects of parathyroid hormone
❑ (E) Mutation in the fibroblast growth factor receptor 3 gene
❑ (F) Synthesis of chemically abnormal osteoid

11 A 47-year-old man sees the physician because he has had dull, constant pain in the mid-section of the right thigh for the past 4 months. On physical examination, there is pain on palpation of the anterior right thigh, which worsens slightly with movement. The right thigh appears to have a larger circumference than the left thigh. A radiograph of the right upper leg and pelvis shows no fracture, but there is an ill-defined soft tissue mass anterior to the femur. MR imaging shows a $10 \times 8 \times 7$ cm solid mass deep to the quadriceps, but it does not involve the femur. Which of the following is the most likely diagnosis?

❑ (A) Nodular fasciitis
❑ (B) Liposarcoma
❑ (C) Osteosarcoma
❑ (D) Rhabdomyosarcoma
❑ (E) Hemangioma
❑ (F) Chondrosarcoma

12 A 66-year-old man has experienced pain in the area around the left knee for the past 6 weeks. He can recall no trauma to the leg. On physical examination, no mass is palpable; there is no warmth or swelling, and there is no loss of range of motion. MR imaging shows a fairly well-circumscribed, 4-cm mass superior and inferior to the patella. The mass is within soft tissue, without bony erosion. A biopsy of the mass is performed; microscopically, the specimen shows a biphasic pattern of spindle cells and epithelial cells forming glands. Karyotypic analysis of tumor cells shows a t(X;18) translocation. Which of the following is the most likely diagnosis?

❑ (A) Leiomyosarcoma
❑ (B) Synovial sarcoma
❑ (C) Desmoid tumor
❑ (D) Mesothelioma
❑ (E) Osteoblastoma

13 A 63-year-old woman loses her balance and falls to the ground. She is unable to get up because of pain. On physical examination, there is marked tenderness to palpation and no range of motion because of pain in the right hip. A radiograph of the right leg shows a right femoral intertrochanteric fracture. Which of the following conditions is likely to be the single most important factor contributing to the fracture?

❑ (A) Chronic osteomyelitis
❑ (B) Vitamin D deficiency
❑ (C) Postmenopausal bone loss
❑ (D) Parathyroid adenoma
❑ (E) Monoclonal gammopathy
❑ (F) Chronic renal failure
❑ (G) Malabsorption

14 A 51-year-old man has experienced aching pain in the right knee, lower back, right distal fifth finger, and neck over the past 10 years. He notices that the joints feel a bit stiff in the morning, but this quickly passes. The pain is worse toward the end of the day. On physical examination, there is no joint swelling, warmth, or deformity. Some joint crepitus is audible on moving the knee. Laboratory studies show normal levels of serum calcium, phosphorus, alkaline phosphatase, and uric acid. Which of the following is the most likely diagnosis?

❑ (A) Paget disease of bone
❑ (B) Osteoarthritis
❑ (C) Gout
❑ (D) Multiple myeloma
❑ (E) Rheumatoid arthritis

15 A 30-year-old man sees his physician because he has had abdominal cramping pain and bloody diarrhea for the past 4 days. On physical examination, there is diffuse tenderness on palpation of the abdomen. Bowel sounds are present. There are no masses and no organomegaly. A stool culture is positive for *Shigella flexneri*. The episode resolves spontaneously within 1 week after onset. Six weeks later, the patient sees his physician because of increasingly severe lower back pain. Physical examination now shows stiffness of the lumbar joints and tenderness affecting the sacroiliac joints. He is treated with ibuprofen. Several months later the back pain recurs, and he complains of redness of the right

eye and blurred vision. Serologic testing for which of the following is most likely to be positive in this patient?

❑ (A) Rheumatoid factor
❑ (B) *Chlamydia trachomatis*
❑ (C) Epstein-Barr virus
❑ (D) HLA-B27
❑ (E) *Borrelia burgdorferi*

16 A 7-year-old boy sustained an open compound fracture of the right tibia and fibula in a fall from a barn loft to the floor below. On physical examination, the lower tibia and fibula can be seen protruding from the lower leg. The fracture is set by external manipulation, and the skin wound is sutured, but nothing more is done. One year later, he continues to have pain in the right leg, and a draining sinus tract has developed in the lateral lower right leg. A radiograph of the lower right leg is now most likely to show which of the following?

❑ (A) Osteolysis with osteosclerosis
❑ (B) Bone mass with bony destruction
❑ (C) Cortical nidus with surrounding sclerosis
❑ (D) Involucrum and sequestrum
❑ (E) Soft tissue hemorrhage and swelling

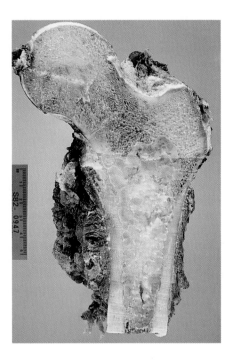

17 A 45-year-old man has experienced pain in the area of the left hip and upper thigh for the past 7 months. On physical examination, there is tenderness on deep palpation of the left side of the groin. There is a reduction in the range of motion at the left hip. There is no swelling or warmth to the touch. Pelvic and left leg radiographs show an upper femoral mass lesion arising in the metaphyseal region and eroding the surrounding bone cortex. The proximal femur is excised and on sectioning has the gross appearance shown. Which of the following cell types is most likely to be proliferating in this mass?

- ❑ (A) Osteoblasts
- ❑ (B) Chondroblasts
- ❑ (C) Osteoclasts
- ❑ (D) Primitive neuroectodermal cells
- ❑ (E) Plasma cells

18 An 18-year-old man sees the physician because he has had pain around the right knee for the past 3 months. There are no physical findings, except for local pain over the area of the distal right femur. A radiograph of the right leg shows an ill-defined mass involving the metaphyseal area of the distal right femur, and there is elevation of the adjacent periosteum. A bone biopsy specimen shows large, hyperchromatic, pleomorphic spindle cells forming an osteoid matrix. Which of the following is the most likely diagnosis?

- ❑ (A) Ewing sarcoma
- ❑ (B) Chondrosarcoma
- ❑ (C) Giant cell tumor of bone
- ❑ (D) Fibrous dysplasia
- ❑ (E) Osteosarcoma

19 A 38-year-old man who is otherwise healthy has experienced chronic leg pain for the past 4 months. On physical examination, there is local swelling with tenderness just below the right patella. A radiograph of the right lower leg shows a 4-cm cystic area in the right tibial diaphysis without erosion of the cortex or soft tissue mass. A biopsy specimen shows increased numbers of osteoclasts in this lesion, as well as fibroblast proliferation. Which of the following underlying conditions is most likely to account for these findings?

- ❑ (A) Secondary hyperparathyroidism
- ❑ (B) Paget disease of bone
- ❑ (C) Chronic osteomyelitis
- ❑ (D) Parathyroid adenoma
- ❑ (E) Giant cell tumor of bone

20 A 9-year-old boy has had pain in the area of the right hip for the past 3 weeks. On physical examination, his temperature is 38.2°C. There is swelling with marked tenderness to palpation in the area of the right hip, pain, and reduced range of motion. Radiographs of the pelvis and legs show areas of osteolysis and cortical erosion involving the femoral metaphysis, with adjacent soft tissue swelling extending from the subperiosteal region, and apparent abscess formation. Which of the following organisms is most likely to produce these findings?

- ❑ (A) *Staphylococcus aureus*
- ❑ (B) *Haemophilus influenzae*
- ❑ (C) *Salmonella enteritidis*
- ❑ (D) Group B *Streptococcus*
- ❑ (E) *Neisseria gonorrhoeae*

21 A 37-year-old woman has noticed increasing deformity and difficulty with movement involving her left hand over the past 6 months. On physical examination, there is a contracture involving the third digit of her left hand that prevents her from fully extending this finger. A firm, hard, cordlike, 1 × 3 cm area is palpable beneath the skin of the left palm. Microscopically, which of the following is most likely to be seen in greatest abundance composing this lesion?

- ❑ (A) Atypical spindle cells
- ❑ (B) Granulation tissue
- ❑ (C) Lipoblasts
- ❑ (D) Collagen
- ❑ (E) Dystrophic calcification

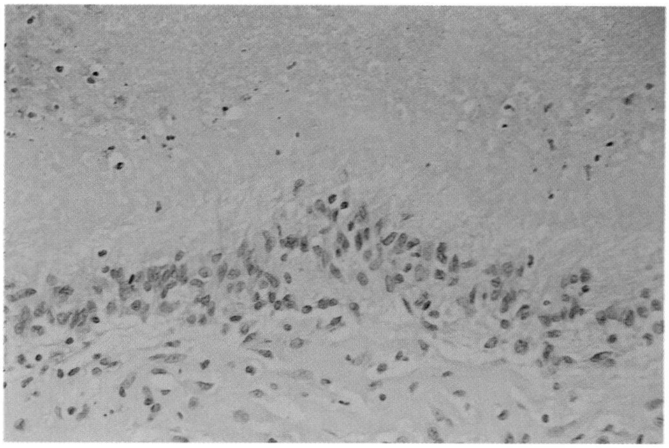

22 A 57-year-old woman has had increasing pain and deformities in her hands for the past 10 years. On physical examination, she has bilateral ulnar deviation, as well as "swan-neck" deformities of several fingers. There is a subcutaneous nodule on the ulnar aspect of the right forearm. A biopsy specimen of the nodule shows the microscopic appearance depicted in the figure. She improves with adalimumab therapy. Which of the following mechanisms plays the most important role in the causation of joint injury in her disease?

- ❑ (A) Activation of neutrophils by phagocytosis of urate crystals
- ❑ (B) Inflammation of synovium caused by infection with *Borrelia burgdorferi*
- ❑ (C) Inflammation of the synovium caused by TNF
- ❑ (D) Synthesis of antibodies against HLA-B27 antigen
- ❑ (E) Granulomatous response to long-standing *Treponema pallidum* infection

23 A 12-year-old girl has complained of sudden onset of severe pain in her left knee that has awakened her from sleep on several occasions during the past 6 weeks. For each episode, her mother has given her acetylsalicylic acid (aspirin), and the pain has been relieved. On physical examination, there are no remarkable findings. A radiograph of the left knee shows a well-defined, 1-cm lucent area surrounded by a thin rim of bony sclerosis located in the proximal tibial cortex. The patient undergoes curettage of the lesion, and the pain does not recur. Which of the following is the most likely diagnosis of this lesion?

- ❑ (A) Enchondroma
- ❑ (B) Ewing sarcoma
- ❑ (C) Fibrous dysplasia
- ❑ (D) Giant cell tumor
- ❑ (E) Osteoblastoma
- ❑ (F) Osteochondroma
- ❑ (G) Osteoid osteoma
- ❑ (H) Osteosarcoma

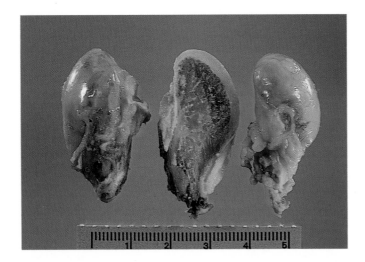

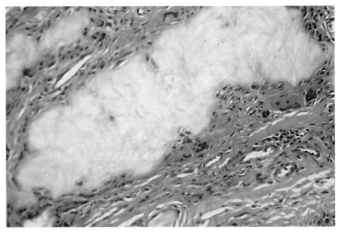

24 A 23-year-old man has had pain in the area of the right knee for the past year. On physical examination, there is mild tenderness over a 2-cm focal area just below the patella laterally over the tibia. A radiograph of the right leg shows a 3-cm broad-based excrescence projecting from the metaphyseal region of the upper tibia. The lesion is excised. The gross appearance of the sectioned lesion is shown above. Which of the following is the most likely diagnosis?

- ❏ (A) Brown tumor of bone
- ❏ (B) Enchondroma
- ❏ (C) Ewing sarcoma
- ❏ (D) Fibrous dysplasia
- ❏ (E) Giant cell tumor
- ❏ (F) Osteoblastoma
- ❏ (G) Osteochondroma
- ❏ (H) Osteosarcoma

25 A 13-year-old previously healthy boy has been complaining of pain in the right leg for the past month. His parents note that he has become less active. There is no history of trauma or recent illness. On physical examination, there is tenderness to palpation of the right lower thigh anteriorly, and the circumference of the right thigh is slightly larger than that of the left. A radiograph of the right leg shows a 6-cm expansile mass in the diaphyseal region of the right lower femur. A biopsy of the mass is performed, and microscopic examination of the specimen shows sheets of closely packed primitive cells with small, fairly uniform nuclei and only scant cytoplasm. Karyotypic analysis of the tumor cells shows a t(11;22) translocation. Which of the following is the most likely diagnosis?

- ❏ (A) Chondrosarcoma
- ❏ (B) Enchondroma
- ❏ (C) Ewing sarcoma
- ❏ (D) Fibrous dysplasia
- ❏ (E) Giant cell tumor
- ❏ (F) Metastatic carcinoma
- ❏ (G) Osteosarcoma
- ❏ (H) Plasmacytoma

26 For the past 4 months, a 51-year-old man has noticed episodes of intense local pain involving his left foot. Each episode follows a meal in which he consumes a bottle of wine (Merlot), and the pain may last hours to several days. Physical examination identifies the right metatarsophalangeal (MP) joint as the focus of this pain. There is tenderness and swelling but minimal loss of joint mobility. A painless 2-cm nodule with overlying ulcerated skin is present on the lateral aspect of the MP joint. Beneath the eroded skin is a chalky white deposit of soft material surrounded by erythematous soft tissue. A firm, 1-cm subcutaneous nodule is present on the extensor surface of the left elbow. The nodule is excised and has the microscopic appearance shown above. Which of the following mechanisms is most important in the causation of joint injury in his disease?

- ❏ (A) Activation of neutrophils by phagocytosis of urate crystals
- ❏ (B) Chronic inflammation caused by *Borrelia burgdorferi* infection
- ❏ (C) Release of TNF causing acute joint inflammation
- ❏ (D) Deposition of serum cholesterol into the synovium
- ❏ (E) Granulomatous inflammation caused by *Mycobacterium tuberculosis* infection
- ❏ (F) Reduced metabolism of homogentisic acid

27 An epidemiologic study of postmenopausal women is performed. The subjects undergo periodic examination by dual energy x-ray absorptiometry (DEXA) scan performed on the hip and lumbar vertebrae to evaluate bone mineral density over the next 10 years. They respond to a survey regarding their past and present use of drugs, diet, activity levels, history of bone fractures, and medical conditions. A subset of the subjects is identified whose bone mineral density is closest to that of the young adult reference range and in whom no bone fractures have occurred. The survey data from this subset of women are analyzed. Which of the following strategies is most likely to be supported by the study data to provide the best overall long-term reduction in risk of fracture in postmenopausal women?

- ❏ (A) Supplement the diet with calcium and vitamin D after menopause
- ❏ (B) Begin estrogen replacement therapy after a fracture
- ❏ (C) Avoid corticosteroid therapy for any inflammatory condition
- ❏ (D) Increase bone mass with exercise during childhood and young adulthood
- ❏ (E) Limit alcohol use, and avoid use of tobacco

28 A 15-year-old boy experiences severe pain in the right leg after performing a gymnastic floor exercise. On physical examination, there is marked pain on palpation of the right lower thigh just above the knee. Radiographs show a pathologic fracture across a discrete, 3-cm lower femoral diaphyseal lesion that has central lucency with a thin sclerotic rim. The lesion is completely intramedullary and well circumscribed. A bone biopsy of the affected region shows trabeculae of woven bone scattered in a background of fibroblastic proliferation. Which of the following is the most likely diagnosis?

❑ (A) Osteoid osteoma
❑ (B) Enchondroma
❑ (C) Osteogenic sarcoma
❑ (D) Ewing sarcoma
❑ (E) Monostotic fibrous dysplasia

29 A male infant of normal birth weight is born at term to a 28-year-old woman, G 4, P 3, whose pregnancy was uncomplicated. No congenital anomalies are identified on a newborn physical examination. Two weeks later, the neonate becomes septic. On physical examination, his temperature is 38.9°C, and he exhibits irritability when his left leg is moved. A radiograph of the left leg shows changes suggesting acute osteomyelitis in the proximal portion of the left femur. Culture of the infected bone is most likely to grow which of the following organisms?

❑ (A) *Staphylococcus aureus*
❑ (B) *Neisseria gonorrhoeae*
❑ (C) Group B *Streptococcus*
❑ (D) *Salmonella enteritidis*
❑ (E) *Streptococcus pneumoniae*

30 A 43-year-old woman had chronic arthritis pain involving the left shoulder and right hip for 8 months. The pain resolved within 1 month. Two months later, she developed pain in the right knee and ankle, which resolves within 6 weeks. On physical examination, she is afebrile. There is pain on movement of the left shoulder and right hip. A radiograph of the left arm shows extensive bony erosion of the humeral head. Biopsy of synovium shows a marked lymphoplasmacytic infiltrate and arteritis with endothelial proliferation. Which of the following infectious agents is most likely responsible for these findings?

❑ (A) Group B *Streptococcus*
❑ (B) *Neisseria gonorrhoeae*
❑ (C) *Treponema pallidum*
❑ (D) *Borrelia burgdorferi*
❑ (E) *Mycobacterium tuberculosis*

31 A 49-year-old woman has been bothered for at least 20 years by recurring skin lesions that are most prominent over the elbows and knees and also sometimes on the scalp and lumbosacral area. These skin lesions are silvery to salmon-colored 1- to 4-cm plaques with scaling. The lesions seem to form more readily at sites of minor trauma, such as a superficial abrasion. She has had increasing pain in her left hand and in her hips, more prominent on the left, over the past 2 years. On physical examination, she has yellow-brown discoloration with pitting of the fingernails. The distal interphalangeal joints of digits two and three of the left hand are slightly swollen and tender. There is minimal reduction in left hip mobility and no swelling or warmth to the touch. A radiograph of the left hip shows minimal joint space narrowing and surface erosion. Bone density is not markedly reduced. During the next 10 years, the joint pain persists, but there is no joint destruction or deformity. She continues to have the same skin lesions. Which of the following is most likely to be seen on biopsy of these skin lesions?

❑ (A) Bandlike upper dermal infiltrate of lymphocytes
❑ (B) Epidermal spongiosis with dermal edema and eosinophils
❑ (C) Focal keratinocyte apoptosis
❑ (D) Epidermal hyperkeratosis, parakeratosis, elongation of rete ridges, and microabscesses
❑ (E) IgG deposited at the dermal-epidermal junction

32 A 32-year-old man comes to the physician because he has noticed a lump over his right flank. The lump is not painful and has enlarged only slowly over the past 3 years. On physical examination, a soft 2-cm nodule is palpable in the subcutis of the right flank above the iliac crest. The lesion is excised. Grossly, it is circumscribed and has a uniformly yellow cut surface. Which of the following is the best advice to give the patient regarding these findings?

❑ (A) This mass is benign and will not recur
❑ (B) More lesions will develop over time
❑ (C) Metastases to regional lymph nodes are likely
❑ (D) Other members of your family should be examined for similar lesions
❑ (E) Antibiotic therapy will be needed

33 A 30-year-old man has experienced pain in the area of the left knee for more than 1 month. On physical examination, there is tenderness to palpation of the distal left thigh and knee. The area is firm, but there is no erythema or warmth. A radiograph of the left leg shows a 7-cm mass in the distal femoral epiphyseal area, with a "soap bubble" appearance. Microscopic examination of a biopsy specimen of the lesion shows multinucleated cells in a stroma predominantly composed of spindle-shaped mononuclear cells. Which of the following is the most likely diagnosis?

❑ (A) Ewing sarcoma
❑ (B) Osteoblastoma
❑ (C) Enchondroma
❑ (D) Osteitis fibrosa cystica
❑ (E) Giant cell tumor

34 A 55-year-old previously healthy man has had episodes of pain and swelling of the right first metatarsophalangeal (MP) joint for the past year. These flare-ups usually occur after consumption of alcohol, typically port wine (six grapes). On physical examination, there is exquisite tenderness with swelling and erythema of the right first MP joint. A joint aspiration is performed, and laboratory studies of the fluid obtained show needle-shaped crystals and many neutrophils in a small amount of fluid. Which of the following laboratory findings is most likely to be reported in this man?

❑ (A) Increased serum parathyroid hormone level
❑ (B) Elevated serum urea nitrogen level
❑ (C) Hyperuricemia
❑ (D) Markedly elevated levels of serum transaminases
❑ (E) Elevated rheumatoid factor titer

35 A 39-year-old man has experienced back pain for several months. On physical examination, there is tenderness to palpation over the lumbar vertebrae. A radiograph of the spine shows a compressed fracture at the L2 level. CT scan of the abdomen shows an abscess involving the right psoas muscle. Infection with which of the following microbial agents is most likely to produce these findings?

- ❏ (A) *Treponema pallidum*
- ❏ (B) *Mycobacterium tuberculosis*
- ❏ (C) *Streptococcus pyogenes*
- ❏ (D) *Borrelia burgdorferi*
- ❏ (E) *Cryptococcus neoformans*
- ❏ (F) *Salmonella enteritidis*

36 A 10-year-old girl has developed worsening pain in the knees and ankles for the past 3 months and now has difficulty walking. On physical examination, these joints are swollen and warm to the touch. She has a temperature of 39.2°C. There is an erythematous skin rash across the bridge of her nose and on the dorsa of her hands. A joint aspirate is obtained from the left knee. Laboratory studies, including a microbiologic culture of the fluid, are negative. The joint fluid has increased numbers of lymphocytes but few neutrophils. Her condition improves over the next year, and she has no residual joint deformity. Which of the following laboratory findings is most characteristic of this disease process?

- ❏ (A) Serum ANA titer 1:1024
- ❏ (B) Positive serologic test result for *Borrelia burgdorferi*
- ❏ (C) Positive urine culture for *Chlamydia trachomatis*
- ❏ (D) Serum ferritin level 7245 ng/mL
- ❏ (E) Hemoglobin S concentration 96% on hemoglobin electrophoresis
- ❏ (F) Serum rheumatoid factor titer 1:512
- ❏ (G) Positive serologic test result for syphilis
- ❏ (H) Serum uric acid level 15.8 mg/dL

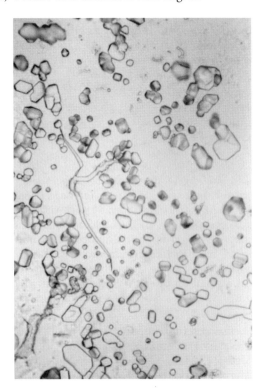

37 A 48-year-old man has had increasing pain in the left knee for the past 4 years, but the pain has become worse in the past week. On physical examination, the left knee is slightly swollen and warm to the touch. The cell count of a joint aspirate shows increased neutrophils. A smear preparation of the fluid is shown in the preceding figure. The patient experiences reduced knee joint mobility over the next 5 years. He also develops congestive heart failure, diabetes mellitus, and hepatic cirrhosis. Which of the following laboratory findings is most characteristic of this disease process?

- ❏ (A) Serum ANA titer 1:1024
- ❏ (B) Positive serologic test result for *Borrelia burgdorferi*
- ❏ (C) Serum calcium level 14.5 mg/dL
- ❏ (D) Positive urine culture for *Chlamydia trachomatis*
- ❏ (E) Serum ferritin level 7245 ng/mL
- ❏ (F) Hemoglobin S concentration 96% on hemoglobin electrophoresis
- ❏ (G) Serum parathyroid hormone level 72 pg/mL
- ❏ (H) Serum rheumatoid factor titer 1:512
- ❏ (I) Positive serologic test result for syphilis
- ❏ (J) Serum urea nitrogen level 110 mg/dL
- ❏ (K) Serum uric acid level 15.8 mg/dL

38 A 75-year-old woman sees her physician because of pain and limitation of movement affecting the right hip joint. These symptoms have been present for the past 15 years but have become disabling within the past year. Physical examination shows tenderness and swelling of the distal interphalangeal joints of the right hand. A nodular bony outgrowth can be felt in the distal interphalangeal joint of the right index finger. All other joints are normal. There is no evidence of systemic disease, and cardiovascular and respiratory findings are unremarkable. A radiograph of the affected hip shows narrowing of the joint space and subchondral sclerosis. Laboratory studies do not show rheumatoid factor or ANA. The serum uric acid level is 5 mg/dL. Which of the following factors is most important in the pathogenesis of the patient's disease?

- ❏ (A) Infiltration of the synovial membrane by activated CD4+ T cells
- ❏ (B) Partial deficiency of hypoxanthine-guanine phosphoribosyltransferase (HGPRT)
- ❏ (C) Inheritance of HLA-B27
- ❏ (D) Defects in the function of chondrocytes of the articular cartilage
- ❏ (E) Inherited defects in the synthesis of type I collagen

39 A 15-year-old boy has been hospitalized many times since childhood as a result of painful abdominal crises. He has had pain in his right hip region for the past week. On physical examination, there is marked tenderness and swelling to palpation over the right hip. Laboratory studies show hemoglobin of 8.5 g/dL, hematocrit 25.7%, platelet count 199,900/mm³, and WBC count 12,190/mm³. Examination of the peripheral blood smear shows sickled erythrocytes, spherocytes, Howell-Jolly bodies in erythrocytes, and nucleated RBCs. A radiograph of the pelvis and right upper leg shows changes of acute osteomyelitis in the femoral head and metaphysis of the right proximal femur. Which of the following infectious agents is most likely responsible for these findings?

- ❏ (A) *Staphylococcus aureus*
- ❏ (B) *Neisseria gonorrhoeae*
- ❏ (C) Group B *Streptococcus*
- ❏ (D) *Salmonella enteritidis*
- ❏ (E) *Klebsiella pneumoniae*
- ❏ (F) *Mycobacterium tuberculosis*

40 A 26-year-old previously healthy man sustains blunt force trauma to the left upper arm. On physical examination, there is focal swelling and redness. Three weeks later, the superficial contusion has resolved, but now a slightly tender mass is palpated in the outer aspect of the upper left arm. A radiograph of the left arm shows a 5-cm mass in the soft tissue. There is a radiolucent center and surrounding irregular bone formation. One month later, the mass is now 3 cm and painless. CT scan of the arm shows a well-circumscribed mass within muscle with areas of bright calcification throughout. Which of the following is the most likely diagnosis?

- ❏ (A) Gouty tophus
- ❏ (B) Hemarthrosis
- ❏ (C) Myositis ossificans
- ❏ (D) Osteochondroma
- ❏ (E) Osteosarcoma
- ❏ (F) Polymyositis

41 A 75-year-old woman has experienced increasing pain in the back, right chest, left shoulder, and left upper thigh for the past 6 months. The pain is dull but constant. She has now developed a sudden, severe, sharp pain in the left thigh. On physical examination, she is afebrile. She has intense pain on palpation of the upper thigh, and the left leg is shorter than the right. A radiograph of the left leg shows a fracture through the upper diaphyseal region of the femur in a 5-cm lytic area that extends through the entire thickness of the bone. A bone scan shows multiple areas of increased uptake in the left femur, pelvis, vertebrae, right third and fourth ribs, upper left humerus, and left scapula. Laboratory studies show serum Na$^+$ of 140 mmol/L, K$^+$ 4.1 mmol/L, Cl$^-$ 99 mmol/L, CO$_2$ 26 mmol/L, glucose 78 mg/dL, creatinine 0.9 mg/dL, total protein 6.7 g/dL, albumin 4.5 g/dL, total bilirubin 1.0 mg/dL, AST 28 U/L, ALT 22 U/L, and alkaline phosphatase 202 U/L. Which of the following is the most likely diagnosis?

- ❏ (A) Metastatic carcinoma
- ❏ (B) Multiple myeloma
- ❏ (C) Osteochondromatosis
- ❏ (D) Osteomyelitis
- ❏ (E) Paget disease of bone
- ❏ (F) Polyostotic fibrous dysplasia

42 A 10-year-old boy has complained of pain in his left leg for the past 2 months. Physical examination reveals a mass in

the left mid-thigh with overlying warmth and tenderness. His temperature is 39°C. Laboratory studies show hemoglobin 11.5 g/dL, hematocrit 34.5%, MCV 92 μm^3, and WBC count 15,200/mm^3 with WBC differential count of 85% neutrophils, 10% lymphocytes, and 5% monocytes. Radiographs of his left leg show a 7 cm lytic lesion of the lower femoral diaphysis that extends into the soft tissue and is covered by layers of reactive bone. Which of the following laboratory investigations is most likely to establish the diagnosis in this case?

- ❏ (A) Blood culture positive for *Staphylococcus aureus*
- ❏ (B) PCR analysis of the mass for the *EWS-FLI* fusion gene
- ❏ (C) Mutational analysis of the mass for the *COL1A* gene
- ❏ (D) Serologic test for syphilis
- ❏ (E) Serum level of ionized calcium
- ❏ (F) Serum level of lead

43 A 26-year-old woman sees the physician because she has had malaise, arthralgias, and myalgias for the past 2 months. On physical examination, there is no joint swelling or deformity. Laboratory studies show a serum creatinine level of 3.9 mg/dL. Serologic tests for ANA and double-stranded DNA are strongly positive. A renal biopsy shows a proliferative glomerulonephritis. She receives glucocorticoid therapy for 3 months. She now has left hip pain with movement. On physical examination, there is no swelling or deformity. A radiograph of the left leg and pelvis shows patchy radiolucency and density of the femoral head with flattening of the bone. A total replacement of the left hip is performed, and gross examination of the sectioned femoral head shows collapse of articular cartilage over a pale, wedge-shaped, subchondral area. Which of the following is the most likely diagnosis?

- ❏ (A) Avascular necrosis
- ❏ (B) Enchondroma
- ❏ (C) Osteoarthritis
- ❏ (D) Osteomyelitis
- ❏ (E) Renal osteodystrophy

44 A 33-year-old woman comes to the physician because she has been bothered by a bump on the dorsum of her left wrist for the past 4 months. On physical examination, there is a 1-cm firm but fluctuant subcutaneous nodule over an extensor tendon of the left wrist. The nodule is painful on palpation and movement. Mucoid fluid is aspirated from the nodule. Which of the following is the most likely diagnosis?

- ❏ (A) Ganglion
- ❏ (B) Lipoma
- ❏ (C) Nodular fasciitis
- ❏ (D) Rheumatoid nodule
- ❏ (E) Tophus
- ❏ (F) Villonodular synovitis

45 A 13-year-old girl who was normal at birth has bilateral hearing loss. Audiometry indicates mixed conductive and sensorineural hearing loss on both the right and the left sides. CT scan of the head shows maldevelopment of both middle ears with deficient ossification. She learns to use hearing aids. Further history indicates that her dentist has tried various whiteners to diminish the yellow-brown color of her teeth, which have a slight bell-shaped appearance. The optometrist noted that her sclerae have a peculiar steel-gray color, and her vision is 20/40. At age 30, she falls when getting out of her car and fractures the left femur. A radiograph shows that the femur is osteopenic. Bone densitometry reveals osteopenia of all measured sites. Which of the following is most likely to produce these findings?

- (A) Abnormal development of type I collagen
- (B) Absence of hypoxanthine-guanine phosphoribosyltransferase (HGPRT)
- (C) Decreased absorption of vitamin D in the small intestine
- (D) Decreased binding of osteoprotegerin to macrophage RANK receptor
- (E) Dominant mutation in the fibroblast growth factor receptor 3 gene
- (F) Increased interleukin-6 production by osteoblasts

46 After an uncomplicated pregnancy, a 29-year-old woman, G 3, P 2, gives birth to an infant less than the fifth percentile for height. On physical examination, the infant's torso and head size are normal, but the extremities are short. The forehead appears prominent. Radiographs show short, slightly bowed long bones but no osteopenia. The other two children in the family are of normal height. The affected child has no difficulty with activities of daily living, once modifications are made in the home and school for short stature, and later becomes a physician. Which of the following conditions is likely to be present in this child?

- (A) Achondroplasia
- (B) Hurler syndrome
- (C) Juvenile rheumatoid arthritis
- (D) Osteogenesis imperfecta
- (E) Rickets
- (F) Scurvy
- (G) Thanatophoric dysplasia

ANSWERS

1 (E) Although sarcomas generally are uncommon, malignant fibrous histiocytoma is one of the more common varieties of soft tissue sarcoma in adults, and it is the most common type of postirradiation soft tissue sarcoma. A desmoid tumor is deep fibromatosis of the abdomen or extremities that can be locally aggressive or recur after excision. However, it is not a true neoplasm and does not metastasize. Hodgkin disease is unlikely to recur after 20 years and is unlikely to arise in soft tissue. Rhab-

domyosarcomas generally occur in children. A leiomyosarcoma is more likely to arise in the uterus or gastrointestinal tract.

BP7 785   BP6 693   PBD7 1301, 1320-1321
PBD6 1264-1265

2 (D) This patient has secondary gout. When patients with leukemia, especially those with a high leukocyte count (as occurs in chronic myeloid leukemia), are treated with chemotherapeutic agents, there is massive lysis of nuclei, and large amounts of urate are produced. The hyperuricemia leads to deposition of crystals in the joint space that triggers a local inflammatory response. Articular cartilage damage can be seen in any form of chronic arthritis but is a prominent feature of osteoarthritis. Synovial proliferation is also a nonspecific change that is prominent in rheumatoid arthritis. Joint hemorrhages can be seen in patients with thrombocytopenia, but they typically occur in patients with hemophilia.

BP7 774-776   BP6 683   PBD7 1311-1314   PBD6 1254

3 (B) Bone remodeling is accomplished when osteoblasts produce new bone and osteoclasts resorb it. This is an ongoing process in all bones, but the process is speeded up in fracture callus. Collagen is produced by fibroblasts. Osteoid is produced by osteoblasts. Cytokines can be elaborated by macrophages and other inflammatory cells within the callus. Osteoprogenitor cells give rise to osteoblasts. Osteoclasts are derived from the same hematopoietic progenitor cells that give rise to macrophages and monocytes.

PBD7 1288-1289   PBD6 1216-1218

4 (E) The figure shows a mosaic pattern of lamellar bone characteristic of osteitis deformans (Paget disease of bone). This disease has three phases. Early in the course, there is a lytic phase, followed by the more classic mixed phase of osteosclerosis and osteolysis, leading to the appearance of a "mosaic" of irregular bone. A sclerotic "burnt-out" phase then ensues. An osteochondroma is a tumorlike projection of bone capped by cartilage that protrudes from the metaphyseal region of a long bone. Osteomalacia results in osteopenia from vitamin D deficiency in an adult. Osteoarthritis produces chronic pain from joint erosion. Osteitis fibrosa cystica is seen in hyperparathyroidism.

BP7 763-765   BP6 673-674   PBD7 1284-1286
PBD6 1225-1227

5 (C) The patient has rheumatoid arthritis, a form of autoimmune disease. The immunologically mediated damage leads to chronic inflammation with pannus formation that gradually erodes and destroys the joints, resulting in joint deformity. Typically, the joint involvement is bilateral and symmetric, and small joints are often involved. Lyme disease, caused by *Borrelia burgdorferi* infection, can produce a chronic arthritis that can destroy cartilage, but larger joints are usually involved. Tuberculous arthritis is rare. Hyperuricemia gives rise to gout. In gout, joint destruction and deformity are caused by tophaceous deposits of sodium urate crystals in a granulomatous inflammatory reaction. Calcium pyrophosphate crystal deposition disease (CPPD), also known as pseudogout, may occasionally result in large, chalky, crystalline deposits, but usually there is a neutrophilic response.

BP7 136-139, 773   BP6 109-111   PBD7 1305-1309
PBD6 1248-1251

6 **(D)** In 5% to 10% of patients with severe polyostotic Paget disease, osteosarcomas can arise years later in bone affected by the disease. Ankylosing spondylitis involves the spine and carries no risk of malignancy. An osteoid osteoma is a small cortical bone lesion that can produce severe pain in children and young adults. Fibrous dysplasia is a focal developmental defect of bone seen at a younger age. An enchondroma does not arise in the setting of Paget disease.

BP7 765   BP6 675   PBD7 1286, 1294, 1298
PBD6 1225-1227

7 **(A)** This patient has a rhabdomyosarcoma, the most common sarcoma in children. Sarcomas mark with antibody to vimentin, an intermediate cytoplasmic filament, by immunoperoxidase staining. Neuron-specific enolase is a marker of neoplasms with neural differentiation. Cytokeratin is a marker for tumors of epithelial origin (e.g., carcinomas). Factor VIII marks endothelial cells and related neoplasms. CD3 is a T-lymphocyte marker.

BP7 785-786   BP6 694   PBD7 1321-1322
PBD6 1265-1266

8 **(C)** Nodular fasciitis is a reactive fibroblastic proliferation that is seen in the upper extremities and trunk of young adults, sometimes occurring after trauma. Malignant fibrous histiocytoma is a sarcoma of retroperitoneum and deep soft tissues of extremities in older adults. A contusion is unlikely to lead to abscess formation, because there is no disruption of the skin to allow entry of infectious agents. Superficial fibromatosis is a deforming lesion of fascial planes that develops over a long period. A lipoma is a common benign soft tissue tumor that is not painful and does not follow trauma.

BP7 784   BP6 692   PBD7 1318   PBD6 1261-1262

9 **(C)** Gonorrhea should be considered the most likely cause of an acute suppurative arthritis in sexually active persons. *Borrelia burgdorferi* causes Lyme disease, characterized by chronic arthritis that may mimic rheumatoid arthritis. Syphilitic gummas in the tertiary phase of syphilis may produce joint deformity. However, there is no preceding urethritis. Tertiary syphilis may be preceded years earlier by a syphilitic chancre. *Staphylococcus aureus* is the most common cause of osteomyelitis, but the Gram stain would show gram-positive cocci. *Haemophilus influenzae* is a short, gram-negative rod that can cause osteomyelitis in children.

BP7 777   BP6 686   PBD7 1310   PBD6 1232-1233

10 **(A)** With advancing age, the ability of osteoblasts to divide and to lay down osteoid is reduced as osteoclast activity increases, giving rise to accelerated bone loss known as osteoporosis. Differentiation of macrophages into osteoclasts requires binding of RANK ligand on osteoblasts to RANK receptor on macrophages, and osteoprotegerin is a "decoy receptor" for RANK ligand that slows osteoclast formation and action. When osteoblasts produce less osteopro-

tegerin, bone loss is accelerated. Postmenopausal osteoporosis is characterized by hormone-dependent acceleration of bone loss. Estrogen deficiency results in increased secretion of interleukins 1 and 6 and tumor necrosis factor-α by monocytes-macrophages. These cytokines in turn act by increasing the levels of RANK and RANK-L, and decreasing the levels of osteoprotegrin. In older women, therefore, bone loss is accelerated by both reduced synthesis and increased resorption. Nonhormonal drugs such as alendronate are designed to reduce osteoclast resorption of bone. There are no age-associated changes in the sensitivity to vitamin D or parathyroid hormone action or composition of osteoid. Fibroblast growth factor receptor 3 gene mutations occur in dwarfism syndromes such as achondroplasia.

BP7 757-761   BP6 669-670   PBD7 1282-1284
PBD6 1223-1224

11 **(B)** A large soft tissue mass suggests cancer, most likely a sarcoma. Liposarcomas are located in deep soft tissues, can be indolent, and can reach a large size. They are the most common sarcomas of adulthood. Osteosarcomas generally occur in persons younger than 20 years of age and typically arise in the metaphysis. Nodular fasciitis is a reactive fibroblastic lesion of young adults, usually on the upper extremities and trunk, and can develop several weeks after local trauma. A rhabdomyosarcoma occurs in children and is most often a tumor of the head and neck, genitourinary tract, or retroperitoneum. Hemangiomas, when present in the extremities of adults, tend to be small, circumscribed lesions on the skin. Chondrosarcomas can be seen over a wide age range, but they arise within bone.

BP7 783   BP6 692   PBD7 1317-1318   PBD6 1261

12 **(B)** Synovial sarcomas account for 10% of all adult sarcomas and can be found around a joint or in deep soft tissues, because they arise from mesenchymal cells, not synovium. Most synovial sarcomas show the t(X;18) translocation. Leiomyosarcomas do not have a biphasic pattern microscopically and are rarely seen in soft tissues. A desmoid tumor is a fibromatosis composed of fibroblasts and collagen. A mesothelioma can be biphasic, but it more typically arises in the pleura. An osteoblastoma is a bone neoplasm that arises in the epiphyseal region.

BP7 787   BP6 695   PBD7 1323   PBD6 1266-1267

13 **(C)** Osteoporosis is the most common cause of fractures in postmenopausal women. The most significant bone loss occurs in the first decade after onset of menopause, but bone loss continues relentlessly with age. Chronic osteomyelitis is not a common cause of fractures. Vitamin D deficiency may lead to osteomalacia in adults, but this condition is much less common than osteoporosis. Metabolic bone disease from hyperparathyroidism is uncommon. The lytic lesions of multiple myeloma, the most common form of monoclonal gammopathy, can occur anywhere, but they occur most often in the vertebrae, where they may cause compression fractures. Chronic renal failure may lead to secondary hyperparathyroidism. Malabsorption of calcium and vitamin D is not common.

BP7 757-761   BP6 669-670   PBD7 1282-1284
PBD6 1222-1224

14 (B) Osteoarthritis is a common problem of aging, and a variety of joints, from large, weight-bearing joints to small joints, can be involved. Joint stiffness in the morning is a common feature. Paget disease does not cause arthritis and is marked by an increase in the alkaline phosphatase concentration. Gouty arthritis occurs in patients with elevated serum levels of uric acid. Multiple myeloma can produce lytic lesions in bone but does not typically involve joints. Rheumatoid arthritis can involve large or small joints. It is typically associated with symmetric involvement of small joints of the hands and feet.

BP7 772-773   BP6 681-682   PBD7 1304-1305
PBD6 1246-1248

15 (D) This patient developed arthritis affecting the lumbar and sacroiliac joints several weeks after *Shigella* dysentery. He subsequently developed conjunctivitis and, most likely, uveitis. This symptom complex is classic of a cluster of related disorders called seronegative spondyloarthropathies. This cluster includes ankylosing spondylitis, Reiter syndrome, psoriatic arthritis, and enteropathic arthritis (as in this case). A common feature is a very strong association with the HLA-B27 genotype. Despite some similarities with rheumatoid arthritis, these patients are invariably negative for rheumatoid factor. Urethritis caused by *Chlamydia trachomatis* can trigger Reiter syndrome, another form of seronegative spondyloarthropathy. However, such infection precedes the onset of arthritis. There is no relation between infection with *Borrelia burgdorferi*, the causative agent of Lyme disease, and reactive arthritis in HLA-B27–positive individuals. Similarly, Epstein-Barr virus infection is not a trigger for these disorders.

BP7 139-140   BP6 111   PBD7 1309   PBD6 1252

16 (D) This patient has chronic osteomyelitis. The most likely sequence of events is the occurrence of a compound fracture that became infected by direct extension of bacteria into the bone. The subsequent care for this patient was inadequate, and he developed chronic osteomyelitis. Infection of the bone and the associated vascular compromise caused bone necrosis, giving rise to a dead piece of bone, called sequestrum. With chronicity, a shell of reactive new bone, called involucrum, is formed around the dead bone. Osteolysis and osteosclerosis are features of bone remodeling with Paget disease of bone. A mass suggests a malignancy, and the most common neoplasm to develop in a sinus tract draining from osteomyelitis is squamous cell carcinoma, but this is uncommon. A nidus with surrounding sclerosis suggests an osteoid osteoma. Soft tissue hemorrhage and swelling should be minimal and resolve soon after the fracture is stabilized.

BP7 761-763   BP6 672   PBD7 1290-1291
PBD6 1232-1233

17 (B) The glistening, gray-blue appearance shown in the figure is typical of cartilage, and this lesion most likely represents neoplastic proliferation of chondroblasts. The tumor has infiltrated the medullary cavity and invaded the overlying cortex and hence is malignant. This is a chondrosarcoma. Most chondrosarcomas are low grade. They occur in a broad age range, unlike many other bone tumors that tend to occur in children or in young adults. Most chondrosarcomas arise toward central portions of the skeleton. Osteosar-

comas are derived from osteoblasts. They are usually seen in younger persons and do not have a bluish-white appearance, because they are marked by osteoid production. Giant cell tumors arise during the third to fifth decades; they involve epiphyses and metaphyses. Grossly, they are large, red-brown, cystic tumors. Giant cells resembling osteoclasts are present in giant cell tumors of bone. These tumors are believed to arise from cells of monocyte-macrophage lineage. Primitive neuroectrodermal cells are present in Ewing sarcoma. Atypical plasma cells appear with multiple myeloma. Myelomas are dark red, rounded, lytic lesions that are often multiple.

BP7 768-769   BP6 678   PBD7 1298-1299
PBD6 1240-1241

18 (E) The osteoid production by a sarcoma is diagnostic of osteosarcoma. The metaphyseal location in a long bone, particularly in the region of the knee, is consistent with osteosarcoma, as is presentation in a young person. Ewing sarcoma is composed of small, round, blue cells without osteoid production, and these neoplasms are typically diaphyseal in location. A chondrosarcoma does not produce osteoid. Most chondrosarcomas occur at an older age. Giant cell tumors of bone are most common between the ages of 20 and 40 years; they are composed of giant cells and a mononuclear cell stroma without osteoid production. Fibrous dysplasia is a localized "developmental arrest" of bone formation with irregular woven bone spicules in a fibroblastic stroma.

BP7 766-767   BP6 676-677   PBD7 1294-1296
PBD6 1236-1237

19 (D) Parathyroid adenomas secrete parathyroid hormone (PTH) and cause primary hyperparathyroidism. Excessive secretion of PTH activates osteoclastic resorption of bone. Microfractures within the areas of bone resorption give rise to hemorrhages. This causes an influx of macrophages and, ultimately, reactive fibrosis. These lesions are cystic, and they are sometimes called "brown tumor of bone." Because they contain osteoclasts and fibroblasts, these lesions can be confused with primary bone neoplasms such as giant cell tumor of bone. Giant cell tumors, however, occur in the epiphys or metaphysis, and they contain plump stromal cells, not fibroblasts. Secondary hyperparathyroidism is seen in persons with chronic renal failure. This patient is too young to have Paget disease of bone, which may be osteolytic in its early phase. Chronic osteomyelitis rarely produces such a discrete lesion.

BP7 740, 761   BP6 672   PBD7 1287-1288   PBD6 1228

20 (A) Pyogenic osteomyelitis may arise from hematogenous dissemination of an infection. In children with no history of previous illnesses, *Staphylococcus aureus* is the most common causative organism. *Haemophilus influenzae* and group B streptococcal infections are most common in the neonatal period. Salmonella infection involving bone is more common in persons with sickle cell anemia. Gonorrhea may occasionally disseminate and involve the bones (osteomyelitis) or joints (septic arthritis) of sexually active persons.

BP7 761-763   BP6 672   PBD7 1290-1291
PBD6 1232-1233

21 (D) The patient has superficial fibromatosis that has produced a lesion best known as a Dupuytren contracture. These lesions contain mature fibroblasts surrounded by dense collagen. A hard, firm lesion of this size is unlikely to be malignant. Granulation tissue from an injury would give rise to a stable scar without such severe retraction. Dystrophic calcification occurs in necrotic tissues; it is not commonly a localized mass.

BP7 784   BP6 692-693   PBD7 1319-1320
PBD6 1262-1263

22 (C) This patient has classic features of chronic rheumatoid arthritis. These include bilateral symmetric involvement of joints, destruction of joints with characteristic deformities, and presence of rheumatoid nodules. Subcutaneous rheumatoid nodules such as this are typically found over extensor surfaces. Although the pathogenesis of rheumatoid arthritis is complex, it is believed that the tissue injury is mediated by an autoimmune reaction in which CD4+ T cells secrete cytokines that have a cascade of effects on B cells, macrophages, and endothelial cells. B cells are driven to form rheumatoid factors that form immune complexes in the joint; macrophages secrete cytokines such as TNF and IL-1 that activate cartilage cells, fibroblasts, and synovial cells; and endothelial cell activation promotes accumulation of inflammatory cells in the synovium. Together, these processes form a pannus and eventually cause joint destruction. The central role of TNF in orchestrating joint destruction is the basis for the highly successful treatment of rheumatoid arthritis with anti-TNF therapy (adalimumab). Activation of neutrophils by urate crystals is involved in the pathogenesis of gouty arthritis. Infection by *Borrelia burgdorferi* causes Lyme disease. Although this can mimic rheumatoid arthritis, symmetric involvement of small joints and rheumatoid nodules are not seen. HLA-B27 has no association with rheumatoid arthritis. Infectious granulomatous inflammation involving bone and joints is uncommon and unlikely to be symmetric. Tertiary syphilis may produce gummatous necrosis.

BP7 136-139, 773   BP6 109-110   PBD7 1305-1309
PBD6 1248-1250

23 (G) This patient has an osteoid osteoma, a benign tumor of the bone that occurs in children and young adults. Pain disproportionate to the size of the tumor is characteristic. If such a lesion is larger than 2 cm, it is classified as an osteoblastoma. It can be treated effectively by curettage. The acute pain is mediated by release of prostaglandins, so aspirin is an effective analgesic. An enchondroma is a benign tumor of hyaline cartilage that arises in the medullary space in young adults. Ewing sarcoma is a diaphyseal lesion composed of primitive, small, round blue cells. Fibrous dysplasia is a localized area of developmental arrest of bone formation. A giant cell tumor is a benign but locally aggressive lesion that arises in the epiphysis of the long bones of young adults and has a "soap bubble" radiographic appearance. An osteochondroma is a projection of the cartilaginous growth plate to form an exostosis. An osteosarcoma is an infiltrative, destructive metaphyseal lesion.

BP7 765-766   BP6 676   PBD7 1293-1294   PBD6 1235

24 (G) The figure shows an osteochondroma. Notice the glistening cartilaginous cap. This tumorlike condition, also called exostosis, is benign and, when solitary, is essentially an incidental finding, because a sarcoma rarely arises from an osteochondroma. However, multiple osteochondromas can be part of an inherited syndrome, and onset can be in childhood, accompanied by bone deformity and an increased risk of development of a sarcoma. An osteochondroma is a projection of the cartilaginous growth plate with proliferation of mature bone capped by cartilage. When skeletal growth ceases, osteochondromas tend to cease proliferation as well. They may produce local irritation and pain. A brown tumor of bone arises in the setting of hyperparathyroidism. An enchondroma is a benign tumor of hyaline cartilage that arises in the medullary space of young adults. Ewing sarcoma is a diaphyseal lesion composed of primitive, small, round blue cells. Fibrous dysplasia is a localized area of developmental arrest of bone formation. A giant cell tumor is a benign but locally aggressive lesion that arises in the epiphysis of the long bones of young adults and has a "soap bubble" radiographic appearance. An osteoblastoma is a large osteoid osteoma, which can arise in epiphyseal lesions and cause intense pain. An osteosarcoma is an infiltrative, destructive metaphyseal lesion.

BP7 767-768   BP6 677   PBD7 1296   PBD6 1237-1238

25 (C) The diaphyseal location, histologic appearance, and t(11;22) translocation are characteristic of a Ewing sarcoma. This tumor usually occurs in patients between the ages of 10 and 15 years. The t(11;22) translocation is present in about 85% of Ewing sarcomas and the related primitive neuroectodermal tumors (PNETs). A chondrosarcoma can occur across a wide age range, unlike most primary malignancies arising in bone, which occur most often in the first two decades, and most are sufficiently differentiated so that a cartilaginous matrix is apparent on microscopic examination. An enchondroma is a benign tumor of hyaline cartilage that arises in the medullary space of young adults. Fibrous dysplasia is a localized area of developmental arrest of bone formation. A giant cell tumor is a benign but locally aggressive lesion that arises in the epiphysis of the long bones of young adults and has a "soap bubble" radiographic appearance. Metastatic carcinoma is the most common tumor of adults involving bone, because there are far more carcinomas than primary bone malignancies; childhood bone metastases are rare. An osteosarcoma typically arises in the metaphyseal region, and the malignant spindle cells produce an osteoid matrix. A plasmacytoma produces a focal lytic lesion within bone, and microscopically there are recognizable plasma cells.

BP7 769-770   BP6 679-680   PBD7 1301-1302
PBD6 1244

26 (A) The histologic picture is that of a central amorphous aggregate of urate crystals surrounded by reactive fibroblasts and mononuclear inflammatory cells. This is a gouty tophus. Tophi are large collections of monosodium urate crystals that can appear in joints or soft tissues of persons with gout. Large superficial tophi can erode the overlying skin. Precipitation of urate crystals into the joints produces an acute inflammatory reaction in which neutrophils and monocytes can be found. Neutrophils phagocytize urate crystals, which cannot be digested but cause release of destructive neutrophilic lysosomal enzymes and oxygen free radicals. Release of crystals from the neutrophils perpetuates this cycle of inflammatory response. *B. burgdorferi* infection causes Lyme disease in which there is arthritis that can mimic rheumatoid arthritis, but there are no subcutaneous nodules containing crystals. Inflammation of the joints involves different mechanisms depending on the etiology. In rheumatoid arthritis, release of TNF by macrophages plays a central role, as evidenced by the dramatic relief provide by anti-TNF agents such as adalimumab currently in clinical use. Marked hypercholesterolemia, as occurs in familial hypercholesterolemia, can lead to deposition of cholesterol in tendons and elsewhere, and when deposited in tendons, the yellowish lesions are called xanthomas, and microscopically the cholesterol crystals appear as clefts in the tissue. Extrapulmonary *M. tuberculosis* injection can cause granulomatous inflammation and chronic arthritis and skin lesions, but there is caseous necrosis with epithelioid cells and no urate crystals. Tuberculous arthritis, unlike gouty arthritis, almost never begins in the metatarsophalangeal joint. Reduced metabolic breakdown of homogentisic acid occurs in the inborn error of metabolism known as alkaptonuria, and deposition of homogentisic acid (ochronosis) in cartilage causes an arthritis that typically affects large joints such as knees, intervertebral disks, hips, and shoulders, but small joints of the hands and feet are spared.

BP7 774-777   BP6 682-686   PBD7 1311-1314
PBD6 1253-1257

27 (D) The total bone mass is an important determinant of the subsequent risk of osteoporosis and its complications. A proactive regimen of exercise that puts stress on bones to increase mass before the inevitable loss after age 30 is most likely to reduce the subsequent risk of osteoporosis. Dietary supplements after menopause are not harmful, but at best only partially slow the loss of bone that accompanies aging. Likewise, postmenopausal estrogen or raloxifene therapy can help preserve bone mass. By the time a fracture has occurred, there has already been significant bone loss. Corticosteroid therapy is just one of many risk factors for osteoporosis, but short courses of corticosteroids have minimal effects on bone formation. Alcohol and tobacco use are not major risks for osteoporosis.

BP7 757-760   BP6 669-670   PBD7 1282-1284
PBD6 1222-1224

28 (E) This patient has a single focus of fibrous dysplasia. This benign tumorlike condition is uncommon. The histologic appearance of woven bone in the middle of benign-looking fibroblasts is characteristic. Seventy percent of cases are monostotic, and the ribs, femur, tibia, mandible, and calvarium are the most frequent sites of involvement. Local deformity and, occasionally, fracture can occur. Polyostotic fibrous dysplasia may involve craniofacial, pelvic, and shoulder girdle regions, leading to severe deformity and fracture. An osteoid osteoma has a small central nidus with surrounding sclerosis. An enchondroma typically appears in more distal bones and is composed of cartilage. An osteosarcoma is typically a large destructive lesion without central lucency. Ewing sarcoma usually occurs in the diaphyseal region of the long bones and is identified histologically by sheets of small, round cells.

BP7 770-771   BP6 680   PBD7 1300-1301
PBD6 1242-1243

29 (C) Infections with group B *Streptococcus* and *Escherichia coli* are common in the neonatal period. Both can cause congenital infections. *Staphylococcus aureus* is the most common cause of osteomyelitis, but patients are usually adults. Gonorrhea as a cause of acute osteomyelitis should be considered in sexually active adults. *Salmonella* osteomyelitis is most characteristic of persons with sickle cell anemia. Pneumococcal osteomyelitis is uncommon.

BP7 761-763   BP6 672   PBD7 1290-1291
PBD6 1232-1233

30 (D) This woman has a form of chronic arthritis that is the late, or stage 3, manifestation of Lyme disease that, as in this case, tends to be remitting and migratory, involving primarily the large joints. The presence of a lymphoplasmacytic infiltrate with endothelial proliferation is characteristic (but not diagnostic) of Lyme arthritis. The infectious agent, *Borrelia burgdorferi*, is a spirochete that is spread by the deer tick. This stage is reached about 2 to 3 years after the initial tick bite, and joint involvement can appear in about 80% of patients. Group B *Streptococcus* may produce an acute osteomyelitis or arthritis in neonates. *Neisseria gonorrhoeae* can cause an acute suppurative arthritis. In both conditions, the inflammatory infiltrate contains a preponderance of neutrophils. *Treponema pallidum* may produce gummatous necrosis that can involve large joints, and there can be lymphoplasmacytic infiltrates with end arteritis, but syphilitic arthritis is quite rare. Tuberculous arthritis may involve large, weight-bearing joints, and it can be progressive, giving rise to ankylosis. The histologic features of tuberculous arthritis include caseating granulomas.

BP7 777   BP6 686-687   PBD7 392-393, 1310   PBD6 1253

31 (D) The patient has psoriasis with psoriatic arthritis, which has features of rheumatoid arthritis but without significant joint destruction. Psoriasis is common, affecting 1% to 2% of persons, and about 5% of these have psoriatic arthritis. For the remaining choices, there is no significant association with arthritis. A bandlike dermal infiltrate is typical of lichen planus, which produces pruritic violaceous plaques or papules but tends to abate in 1 to 2 years. Epidermal spongiosis with eosinophilic infiltrates can be seen in acute eczematous dermatitis as part of a drug reaction. Focal keratinocyte apoptosis is seen in graft-versus-host disease. IgG deposition can be seen in systemic lupus erythematosus and in bullous pemphigoid.

BP7 140   BP6 112   PBD7 1310
PBD6 1198-1199; 1252-1253

32 (A) The mass is a lipoma, the most common benign soft tissue neoplasm. Such masses are extremely well differentiated and discrete. Multiple lipomas may be seen in some familial cases, but these are rare. These benign tumors do not metastasize; moreover, mesenchymal neoplasms do not often metastasize through lymphatics. Recurrence of some atypical lipomas or liposarcomas is possible, but benign lipomas do not recur. Secondary infection of this uncomplicated excision procedure is unlikely.

BP7 782-783   BP6 691-692   PBD7 1317
PBD6 1260-1261

33 (E) Most cases of giant cell tumor arise in the epiphyses of long bones of persons between the ages of 20 and 40 years; there is a slight female predominance. The tumors may recur after curettage. Although most are histologically and biologically benign, in rare cases, a sarcoma can arise in a giant cell tumor of bone. Ewing sarcoma is seen in the diaphyseal region and usually manifests within the first two decades of life. An osteoblastoma usually involves the spine. Enchondromas are most often peripheral skeletal lesions involving the metaphyseal region of small tubular bones of the hands and feet. Osteitis fibrosa cystica is a complication of hyperparathyroidism.

BP7 769   BP6 679   PBD7 1302   PBD6 1244-1245

34 (C) Acute inflammation of the first metatarsophalangeal joint, caused by precipitation of uric acid crystals in the joint space, is typical of gout. Hyperuricemia is a sine qua non for the development of gout. However, all patients with hyperuricemia do not develop gout. Other, ill-defined factors play a role in pathogenesis. Involvement of the big toe is classic, but other joints may be involved. An increased parathyroid hormone level indicates primary hyperparathyroidism, which is unlikely to produce joint disease. Elevated serum urea nitrogen is present in renal failure, which may produce secondary hyperparathyroidism. Although attacks of gout are often precipitated by a heavy bout of alcohol consumption, liver damage (marked by elevated transaminases) is not a feature of gouty arthritis. Gout is not associated with rheumatoid arthritis.

BP7 774-777   BP6 682-686   PBD7 1311-1314
PBD6 1253-1257

35 (B) The presence of a destructive lesion in the vertebrae with extension of the disease along the psoas muscle is characteristic of tuberculous osteomyelitis. Tuberculosis of bones usually results from hematogenous spread of an infection in the lung. Long bones and vertebrae are the favored sites for tuberculosis involving the skeletal system. *Treponema pallidum* may produce gummatous necrosis in the tertiary stage, but this involves soft tissues more than bone. Streptococcal osteomyelitis is uncommon. *Borrelia burgdorferi* is the causative agent of Lyme disease, which produces arthritis. Dissemination of *Cryptococcus neoformans* infection from the lungs occurs most commonly in immunocompromised patients but infrequently produces osteomyelitis. *Salmonella* species are most likely to cause osteomyelitis in patients with sickle cell anemia.

BP7 763   BP6 673   PBD7 1291-1292   PBD6 1233

36 (A) The patient has findings typical of juvenile rheumatoid arthritis (JRA), which, unlike the adult type of rheumatoid arthritis, is more likely to be self-limited and nondeforming. JRA typically is rheumatoid factor negative but ANA positive. The juvenile form is more likely than the adult form to have systemic manifestations such as myocarditis, pericarditis, uveitis, and glomerulonephritis. A positive serologic test for *Borrelia burgdorferi* is seen in Lyme disease, which tends to be associated with migratory arthritis of large joints. Like JRA, Lyme disease produces a chronic deforming arthritis in only about 10% of cases. *Chlamydia trachomatis* is typically the agent that produces the nongonococcal urethritis seen in Reiter syndrome which, like other spondy-

loarthropathies, most commonly involves the sacroiliac joint. Ferritin levels are markedly increased in hereditary hemochromatosis, in which iron deposition in joints can produce a chronic arthritis similar to osteoarthritis or pseudogout. Sickle cell disease can lead to aseptic necrosis, often of the femoral head, and to bone infarcts. Rheumatoid arthritis tends to be recurrent and causes progressive joint deformities, typically of hands and feet. Congenital syphilis can produce periosteitis and osteochondritis with bone deformities; tertiary syphilis in adults can produce gummatous necrosis with joint destruction or loss of sensation, particularly in the lower extremities, leading to repeated trauma that deforms joints (Charcot joint). Some cases of gouty arthritis are accompanied by hyperuricemia; gouty arthritis tends to manifest as an acute attack in older persons.

BP7 139   BP6 111   PBD7 1309   PBD6 1251-1252

37 (E) The figure shows calcium pyrophosphate crystals that have been deposited in the articular matrix. In progression of the disease, the crystals can seed the joint space and give rise to pseudogout, or calcium pyrophosphate dihydrate deposition disease (CPPD), which can be primary (hereditary) or more commonly secondary to a variety of systemic diseases such as hemochromatosis or, in the elderly, with pre-existing joint damage from other conditions. Secondary forms of the disease can be associated with systemic diseases such as hemochromatosis. This patient shows evidence of hemochromatosis-caused skin pigmentation, heart failure, diabetes, and cirrhosis. In most autoimmune diseases with a positive ANA result, such as systemic lupus erythematosus, there are arthralgias but no arthritis, and little or no joint swelling, destruction, or deformity occurs. A positive serologic test for *Borrelia burgdorferi* is seen in Lyme disease, which tends to be associated with a migratory arthritis of the large joints. Like juvenile rheumatoid arthritis, Lyme disease produces a chronic deforming arthritis in only about 10% of cases. Hypercalcemia is unlikely to be associated with acute arthritis. *Chlamydia trachomatis* is typically the agent that produces the nongonococcal urethritis seen in Reiter syndrome, which, like other spondyloarthropathies, most commonly involves the sacroiliac joint. Sickle cell disease can lead to aseptic necrosis, often of the femoral head, and bone infarcts. Hyperparathyroidism is associated with bone lesions, not with arthritis. Rheumatoid arthritis tends to be recurrent and causes progressive joint deformities, typically of the hands and feet. Congenital syphilis can produce periosteitis and osteochondritis with bone deformities; tertiary syphilis in adults can produce gummatous necrosis with joint destruction or loss of sensation, particularly in the lower extremities, leading to repeated trauma that deforms joints (Charcot joint). Chronic renal failure with uremia does not cause arthritis. Some cases of gouty arthritis are accompanied by hyperuricemia; gouty arthritis tends to manifest as acute attacks in older persons.

PBD7 1314   PBD6 873, 1257

38 (D) The progressive involvement of large, weight-bearing joints, as well as osteophytes in the interphalangeal joints in an elderly woman, is characteristic of osteoarthritis. The absence of rheumatoid factor and the asymmetric joint involvement render the diagnosis of rheumatoid arthritis unlikely. Osteoarthritis is a disease of unknown cause in which chondrocytes play a primary role. In early stages, chondrocytes proliferate. This is accompanied by changes in the cartilage matrix due to secretion of interleukin-1 and tumor necrosis factor-α by chondrocytes. Eventually, the osteoarthritic cartilage is degraded. The loss of articular cartilage causes reactive subchondral sclerosis. Infiltration of the synovium with CD4+ T cells is seen in rheumatoid arthritis. A partial deficiency of HGPRT gives rise to hyperuricemia and gout. HLA-B27 is associated with ankylosing spondylitis and other seronegative spondyloarthropathies. Inherited defects in type I collagen give rise to a group of rare disorders called osteogenesis imperfecta, which may be lethal in utero or in some cases give rise to premature osteoarthritis.

BP7 772-773   BP6 681-682   PBD7 1304-1305
PBD6 1246-1248

39 (D) *Staphylococcus aureus* infection is responsible for 80% to 90% of all cases of osteomyelitis in which an organism can be cultured. However, *Salmonella* osteomyelitis is especially common in patients with sickle cell anemia. Gonorrhea can cause acute osteomyelitis in sexually active young adults. Group B streptococcal infections causing osteomyelitis are most common in neonates. *Klebsiella pneumoniae* osteomyelitis may rarely be seen in adults with urinary tract infections caused by this organism. Tuberculosis is a rare cause of osteomyelitis in adults who have had active pulmonary disease with dissemination, most likely because of a poor immune response.

BP7 761-763   BP6 672   PBD7 1290-1291
PBD6 1232-1233

40 (C) Myositis ossificans is an uncommon, exuberant repair reaction following soft tissue trauma to muscle in which there is metaplastic bone formation. The keys to diagnosis are the location within soft tissue, calcification beginning at the periphery, and decrease in size over time. Gouty tophi can form in soft tissues, but there is typically a history of gouty arthritis first, and the lesions do not calcify. A hemarthrosis forms with joint trauma and hemorrhage in and around the joint capsule but does not involve calcification. An osteochondroma is a bony exostosis projecting from bone into soft tissue. An osteosarcoma that rarely arises in soft tissue must be distinguished from myositis ossificans; the latter is characterized by the mature shell of bone, lack of enlargement, and lack of bone or soft tissue destruction. Polymyositis involves inflammation with degeneration and regeneration of muscle fibers, but there is no mass effect and no calcification.

BP7 21   BP6 20   PBD7 1319   PBD6 1262

41 (A) An elevated alkaline phosphatase level in an older adult should raise the suspicion of bone metastases, particularly when there is a "pathologic" fracture due to a bone lesion rather than from trauma. Likely primary sites include the breast (in women), prostate (in men), lung (in smokers), kidney, and thyroid. Multiple myeloma can produce lytic bone lesions, but the patient's serum gamma globulin level is not elevated. Osteochondromas are exostoses and do not produce lytic bone lesions. Osteomyelitis is usually more limited without such discrete areas of lysis. Paget disease of bone is characterized by osteolysis coupled with bone formation but without lytic lesions. Fibrous dysplasia coupled with café-

au-lait spots on skin and with endocrinopathies is known as McCune-Albright syndrome; this is a rare condition that occurs in young girls.

BP7 765   BP6 675   PBD7 1302-1303   PBD6 1245-1246

42 (B) The radiologic appearance of the mass in this child is typical for a malignant tumor, with bone destruction and soft tissue extension. The two most common malignant bone tumors in children are osteosarcoma and Ewing sarcoma. Osteosarcomas typically arise in the metaphyseal region, whereas Ewing sarcoma arises in the diaphyseal region of long tubular bones, as seen in this case. Ewing sarcoma and the related primitive neuroectodermal tumors (PNETs) belong to the "small round cell" tumors of childhood that can be difficult to distinguish microscopically. A distinctive molecular feature of Ewing sarcoma/PNET is a t(11;22) translocation, present in 85% of cases, that gives rise to the *EWS-FLI1* fusion gene, now considered the definitive test for the diagnosis of these tumors. Ewing sarcomas often produce tender masses and can also produce fever and leukocytosis, thus mimicking acute osteomyelitis. Mutations in the *COL1A* gene give rise to various forms of osteogenesis imperfecta. Tertiary syphilis can cause bone involvement, by this is quite uncommon since the disease is readily diagnosed and bone involvement is a late complication. Congenital syphilis also affects multiple bones, but the lesions are manifest before 10 years of age. Vitamin D deficiency in children can impair calcium absorption and give rise to rickets that may cause bowing deformities of long bone, but not lytic lesions. Lead is concentrated in bones of growing children but does not produce mass lesions.

PBD7 1301-1302

43 (A) Avascular necrosis of bone (osteonecrosis) represents a localized area of bone infarction, most often in a metaphyseal medullary cavity or subchondral epiphyseal location. The femoral head is most often affected. Underlying conditions associated with osteonecrosis include hemoglobinopathies (sickle cell disease in particular), fracture, barotrauma, hypercoagulable states, and hyperlipidemia. Glucocorticoid therapy decreases osteoblastogenesis to promote avascular necrosis, as in this patient with systemic lupus erythematosus and glomerulonephritis. An enchondroma is a benign tumor of hyaline cartilage that arises in the medullary space of young adults. Osteoarthritis may produce some cartilaginous erosion but not collapse or bone infarction. Osteomyelitis typically is not so localized, and there is irregular new bone formation (involucrum). The patient's course is quite short for renal osteodystrophy, which is mediated through chronic renal failure and produces lesions such as osteitis fibrosa cystica.

PBD7 1289-1290   PBD6 1231

44 (A) A ganglion cyst has a thin wall and clear, mucoid content. It arises in the connective tissue of a joint capsule or tendon sheath. The extensor surfaces of the hands and feet are the most common sites, particularly the region of the wrist. Ganglion cysts probably arise following trauma from focal myxoid degeneration of connective tissue to produce a cystic space. They may regress. If not, and they are painful, they can be excised. A lipoma is a mass of adipocytes and is not cystic. Nodular fasciitis is a solid reactive fibroblastic proliferation seen in the upper extremities and trunk of young adults, sometimes occurring after trauma. Rheumatoid nodules are firm, solid masses that typically occur in persons who already have joint involvement with rheumatoid arthritis. A tophus is a solid mass of chalky sodium urate crystals in patients who have a history of gout. Villonodular synovitis is a more diffuse form of giant cell tumor of tendon sheath (a solid mass lesion) and is a proliferation of mononuclear cells resembling synoviocytes.

PBD7 1314-1315   PBD6 1258

45 **(A)** The patient has osteogenesis imperfecta (OI), most likely type I. Type II is the perinatal lethal form, which causes death in utero, at birth, or shortly thereafter. Type III is seen in children and adults and is more severe than type I. Type IV is difficult to distinguish from type III. OI causes osteopenia ("brittle bones") and predisposes to fractures. Patients often have blue sclerae, dental abnormalities, and progressive hearing loss. The perinatal form leads to death in utero, at birth, or shortly thereafter. Absence of HGPRT is an X-linked disorder known as Lesch-Nyhan syndrome and characterized by hyperuricemia. Decreased absorption of vitamin D in the small intestine leads to rickets. Decreased binding of osteoprotegerin to the macrophage RANK receptor is part of the mechanism of osteoporosis. Mutations in the fibroblast growth factor receptor 3 (*FGFR3*) gene can be seen in achondroplasia. Increased interleukin-6 production by osteoblasts occurs in Paget disease of bone and with postmenopausal decrease in estrogen, causing increased bone loss.

BP7 757   BP6 179, 669   PBD7 1279-1281
PBD6 1221-1222

46 **(A)** Achondroplasia is most often the result of a spontaneous new mutation in the fibroblast growth factor receptor 3 (*FGFR3*) gene, leading to abnormal cartilage proliferation at growth plates and affecting mainly endochondral bone growth. The homozygous form is lethal in utero. In Hurler syndrome, mucopolysaccharidosis type I, children are normal at birth but then develop growth retardation, mental retardation, hepatosplenomegaly, and joint stiffness. Juvenile rheumatoid arthritis is not present at birth and leads to a destructive arthritis. Osteogenesis imperfecta may manifest at birth with multiple fractures from severe osteopenia as a result of abnormal type I collagen synthesis. Rickets may occur in childhood from vitamin D deficiency, producing deficient bone mineralization, but dwarfism is not a feature. Vitamin C deficiency causes scurvy and can lead to abnormal bone matrix with mild deformity but not dwarfism. Thanatophoric dysplasia is the most common form of lethal dwarfism and also results from a mutation in *FGFR3*.

BP 756-757   BP6 668-669   PBD7 1279   PBD6 1220-1221

CHAPTER 27

Peripheral Nerve and Skeletal Muscle

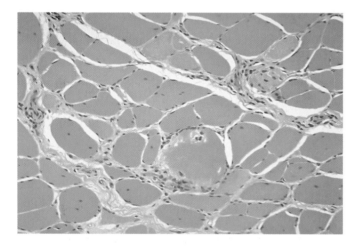

1 A 5-year-old boy develops increasing muscle weakness. He is unable to play with other children because he quickly becomes tired and is unable to keep up with them. On physical examination, he is afebrile. No deformities are noted. He has 4/5 muscle strength in his extremities, with more apparent weakness of the proximal muscles. Laboratory studies show a serum creatine kinase level of 689 U/L. A muscle biopsy is performed. The figure shows the appearance of the biopsy section at low magnification. Which of the following tests would be most appropriate to determine the diagnosis in this boy?

☐ (A) Serum acetylcholinesterase antibody titer
☐ (B) Immunohistochemical staining for dystrophin
☐ (C) Eosinophil count in blood
☐ (D) Presence of oligoclonal bands of immunoglobulin in cerebrospinal fluid
☐ (E) PCR to detect expansion of CGG repeats on Xq27.3

2 A 25-year-old woman has had episodes of numbness and tingling in both hands for several months. The problem typically occurs near the end of the day and makes it difficult for her to use the computer keyboard. The thumb and first two fingers are most affected. There is no pain or swelling, and she does not recall any trauma to the upper extremities. On physical examination, she has decreased sensation to light touch and pinprick over the palmar surface of both hands in the distribution of the first three digits. Thenar muscle atrophy appears to be present. Which of the following conditions is most likely causing her problem?

☐ (A) Repetitive stress injury
☐ (B) Diabetes mellitus
☐ (C) Amyotrophic lateral sclerosis
☐ (D) Acute intermittent porphyria
☐ (E) Varicella-zoster virus infection

3 A 63-year-old man has been receiving hemodialysis for chronic renal failure and has noted increasing loss of sensation in his legs for the past 4 years. On physical examination, there is symmetrically decreased sensation over both lower extremities. He has no decrease in strength or abnormality of gait. Which of the following is most likely to produce these findings?

❏ (A) Guillain-Barré syndrome
❏ (B) Cerebral astrocytoma
❏ (C) Cerebral infarction
❏ (D) Diabetes mellitus
❏ (E) Multiple sclerosis

4 A 17-year-old boy has had generalized muscle pain with fever for 1 week. Over the past 2 days, he has developed increasing muscular weakness and diarrhea. On physical examination, his temperature is 38°C. All of his muscles are tender to palpation, but he has a normal range of motion and no significant decrease in muscle strength. Laboratory findings include hemoglobin of 14.6 g/dL, hematocrit 44.3%, MCV 90 μm³, platelet count 275,000/mm³, and WBC count 16,700/mm³ with differential of 68% segmented neutrophils, 6% bands, 10% lymphocytes, 4% monocytes, and 12% eosinophils. Which of the following is the most likely diagnosis?

❏ (A) Duchenne muscular dystrophy
❏ (B) Polymyositis
❏ (C) Poliomyelitis
❏ (D) Trichinosis
❏ (E) Diabetes mellitus

5 A 35-year-old man has experienced increasing weakness of the pelvic and shoulder girdle muscles for several years. On physical examination, he has 4/5 motor strength in all extremities. There is no pain or deformity, and his range of motion is normal. He has no gait abnormality and no tremors. There are no focal neurologic deficits. He is afebrile. A deltoid biopsy is performed, and Western blot analysis shows reduced amounts of dystrophin with an abnormal molecular weight. Which of the following is the most likely diagnosis?

❏ (A) Amyotrophic lateral sclerosis
❏ (B) Becker muscular dystrophy
❏ (C) Duchenne muscular dystrophy
❏ (D) Lambert-Eaton syndrome
❏ (E) McArdle disease
❏ (F) Myasthenia gravis
❏ (G) Myotonic dystrophy
❏ (H) Polymyositis
❏ (I) Werdnig-Hoffmann disease

6 A 40-year-old man had an influenza-like illness for 1 week. A few days later, he experienced a rapidly progressive, ascending motor weakness that required intubation and mechanical ventilation. On physical examination, he is now afebrile and has 3/5 motor strength in his extremities. A lumbar puncture is performed and yields clear, colorless CSF under normal pressure. The CSF has a slightly elevated protein

concentration but a normal glucose level and a cell count with only a few mononuclear cells. The patient recovers in 3 weeks. If lymphocytic infiltrates were seen in peripheral nerves along with segmental demyelination at the time he initially saw his physician, which of the following would be the most likely diagnosis?

❏ (A) Guillain-Barré syndrome
❏ (B) Multiple sclerosis
❏ (C) Amyotrophic lateral sclerosis
❏ (D) Varicella-zoster virus infection
❏ (E) Vitamin B$_{12}$ (cobalamin) deficiency

7 For the past month, a 56-year-old man has experienced worsening double vision and eyelid drooping, particularly toward the end of the day. He also has had difficulty chewing his food at dinner time. He was diagnosed with Sjögren syndrome more than a decade ago. On physical examination, he has 5/5 motor strength in his extremities that decreases to 4/5 strength with repetitive movement. There is no pain on palpation and no decrease in joint mobility. Which of the following laboratory findings is most likely to be reported for this patient?

❏ (A) Elevated serum creatine kinase level
❏ (B) Acetylcholine receptor antibody positivity
❏ (C) Peripheral blood eosinophilia
❏ (D) Increased serum cortisol level
❏ (E) Anti-histidyl t-RNA synthetase (anti-Jo-1) titer 1:512

8 A 72-year-old man has had a 7-kg weight loss, proximal muscle weakness, and difficulty with urination for the past several months. On physical examination, he has 4/5 muscle strength in his extremities with repetitive motion. He has no muscle pain or loss of mobility. Laboratory studies show that he does not have serum antibodies to acetylcholine receptor. The patient was prescribed anticholinesterase agents but shows no improvement. Which of the following underlying conditions is most likely to be present?

❏ (A) Chronic hepatitis C
❏ (B) Duchenne muscular dystrophy
❏ (C) Small cell lung carcinoma
❏ (D) Lead poisoning
❏ (E) Diabetes mellitus

9 A 56-year-old woman has had increasing generalized muscle weakness for the past 2 months. On physical examination, she has 3/5 motor strength in both upper and lower extremities. She has fat redistribution in the upper trunk and rounded facies. Ecchymoses are scattered over the extremities. She is afebrile, and her blood pressure is 155/90 mm Hg. A biopsy of the gastrocnemius muscle is performed, and histochemical staining of the specimen shows type II muscle fiber atrophy. Which of the following is the most likely diagnosis?

❏ (A) Cushing syndrome
❏ (B) McArdle disease
❏ (C) Duchenne muscular dystrophy
❏ (D) Myasthenia gravis
❏ (E) Polymyositis

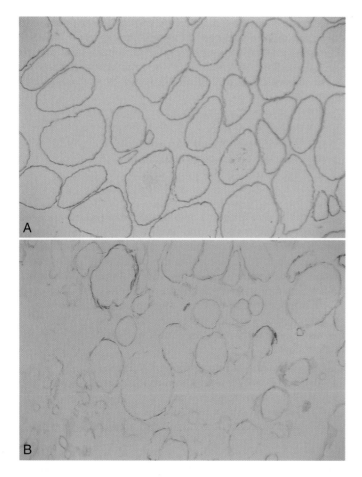

A

B

10 A 44-year-old man has had worsening exercise intolerance for the past year. On physical examination, he has 4/5 motor strength in the extremities but has no muscle pain or loss of joint mobility. He has pitting edema to the knees. A chest radiograph shows cardiomegaly with pulmonary edema and pleural effusions. A deltoid muscle biopsy is performed. The immunohistochemical staining pattern with antibody to dystrophin is shown in the figure (A, normal; B, patient). Which of the following is the most likely diagnosis?

❑ (A) Werdnig-Hoffmann disease
❑ (B) Polymyositis
❑ (C) Becker muscular dystrophy
❑ (D) Amyotrophic lateral sclerosis
❑ (E) Myasthenia gravis
❑ (F) Myotonic dystrophy

11 A 40-year old man sees his physician for a routine checkup. On physical examination, there are no abnormal findings. A chest radiograph shows small focal calcifications in the diaphragmatic leaves. Which of the following is most likely to cause this appearance on the radiograph?

❑ (A) Lambert-Eaton syndrome
❑ (B) McArdle disease
❑ (C) Mitochondrial myopathy
❑ (D) Polymyositis
❑ (E) Trichinosis
❑ (F) Werdnig-Hoffmann disease

12 A 35-year-old woman has been experiencing muscle weakness for several weeks. When she drives her automobile for long distances, she has difficulty keeping her eyes open because her eyelids droop and she experiences double vision. She works as a secretary, and the problems worsen as the day progresses. Which of the following laboratory findings is most likely to be reported for this patient?

❑ (A) Increased serum level of acetylcholine receptor antibody
❑ (B) Loss of staining of muscle for dystrophin
❑ (C) Increased serum CK level
❑ (D) Elevated serum ANA level
❑ (E) Increased CSF protein concentration

13 A 55-year-old man comes to the physician because he has had a foot ulcer for 2 months that has not healed. Physical examination shows a 2-cm shallow, nonhealing ulceration of the left medial malleolus. There is symmetric decreased sensation in the distal regions of the lower extremities. The patient has a history of multiple urinary tract infections resulting from difficulty in completely emptying the bladder. He is impotent. Which of the following pathologic findings is most likely to be present in the peripheral nerves?

❑ (A) Wallerian degeneration
❑ (B) Acute inflammation
❑ (C) Onion bulb formation
❑ (D) Endoneurial lymphocytic infiltration
❑ (E) Axonal neuropathy

14 A 42-year-old man has had increasing progressive muscle weakness in both arms and legs and dysarthria and difficulty in swallowing for the past 2 years. He is now wheelchair-bound. Physical examination shows 3/5 motor strength in all extremities. He has no muscle pain on palpation, no deformities or loss of joint mobility, and no tremor. A biopsy of the quadriceps muscle is performed, and microscopic examination shows a pattern of grouped atrophy of the myofibers. Which of the following is the most likely diagnosis?

❑ (A) Werdnig-Hoffmann disease
❑ (B) Amyotrophic lateral sclerosis
❑ (C) Becker-type muscular dystrophy
❑ (D) Myasthenia gravis
❑ (E) Mitochondrial myopathy

15 A 16-year-old boy has a deep laceration of the upper left anterior thigh. The bleeding is stopped. On physical examination, he has loss of sensation in and movement of the left foot. The wound is surgically repaired, and he receives physical therapy. How long will it take him to regain the use of his left foot?

❑ (A) 1 day
❑ (B) 1 week
❑ (C) 1 month
❑ (D) 1 year

16 A 41-year-old woman has noted marked pain in the right foot for the past 2 months. The pain makes it difficult for her to wear high-heeled shoes and seems to be worse at the end of the day. On physical examination, she has severe pain on palpation of the interdigital space between the second and third toes. There is no swelling or erythema of the foot. Motor strength in the lower extremities appears to be normal. Which of the following has most likely produced these findings?

❑ (A) Diabetes mellitus type 1
❑ (B) Diabetes mellitus type 2
❑ (C) Entrapment neuropathy
❑ (D) Lead poisoning
❑ (E) Thiamine deficiency
❑ (F) Vitamin B$_{12}$ (cobalamin) deficiency
❑ (G) Wallerian degeneration

17 A 16-year-old boy has had two episodes of sudden loss of motor function with residual weakness in his right arm and right leg in the past 2 years. He has had muscle weakness and a seizure disorder since childhood. During the past year, he has had difficulty with memory and performing activities of daily living. On physical examination, he has short stature. He has 4/5 motor strength in all extremities, with no muscle tenderness. Laboratory studies show Na$^+$ of 141 mmol/L, K$^+$ 4.1 mmol/L, Cl$^-$ 95 mmol/L, CO$_2$ 19 mmol/L, glucose 71 mg/dL, creatinine 1.1 mg/dL, and lactic acid 9.2 mmol/L. A gastrocnemius muscle biopsy is performed, and microscopic examination shows ragged red fibers. On electron microscopy, the myofibrils have "parking lot" inclusions. The boy's mother and grandmother had similar findings, but his father and grandfather did not. Which of the following most likely explains the pathogenesis of his disease?

❑ (A) Abnormal voltage-gated calcium channel
❑ (B) Antibodies to acetylcholine receptor
❑ (C) Cytotoxic CD8 lymphocytes
❑ (D) Decreased sarcolemmal dystrophin
❑ (E) Deficient mitochondrial enzyme
❑ (F) Increased CTG repeat sequences at 19q13.2–13.3

18 A 62-year-old woman has a slowly enlarging mass anterior to the right ear. Surgery is performed to remove a pleomorphic adenoma of the parotid gland. The tumor has infiltrated the overlying soft tissue, and the surgeon must remove a portion of the facial nerve to obtain an adequate margin. He places a 2-cm nerve graft in the excised area. Which of the following best describes the most likely outcome during the first week after surgery?

❑ (A) Appearance of acute inflammation around the graft
❑ (B) Formation of a traumatic neuroma
❑ (C) Grouped atrophy of facial muscles
❑ (D) Growth of recurrent tumor along the nerve graft
❑ (E) Wallerian degeneration in the distal facial nerve

19 A 30-year-old woman has had gradually increasing muscle weakness with myalgia for the past year. She now has difficulty getting up from a chair or climbing stairs. However, she does not have weakness of her hand muscles. Physical examination reveals a fine violaceous rash on her face, predominantly palpebral. Dusky flat red patches are present on her elbows, knees, and over her knuckles. Laboratory serum studies show creatine kinase of 620 U/L.

Electromyography shows increased spontaneous activity with fibrillations, complex repetitive discharges, and positive sharp waves. A deltoid biopsy is performed and on microscopic examination shows a mononuclear inflammatory cell infiltrate around small blood vessels and groups of atrophic myofibers at the periphery of fascicles. Which of the following mechanisms is most likely responsible for her disease?

❑ (A) Myofiber injury by CD8+ T-cells directed against muscle antigens
❑ (B) T-cell mediated peripheral nerve injury induced by *Mycoplasma pneumoniae* infection
❑ (C) Antibody and complement mediated injury to the microvasculature
❑ (D) Mutation in agene encoding for voltage-gated clacium channels
❑ (E) Expansion of CTG repeat sequences on chromosome 19q13.2

ANSWERS

1 **(B)** The onset of muscle weakness in childhood suggests an inherited muscular dystrophy. The biopsy specimen shows variation in muscle fiber size and increased connective tissue between the fibers. This morphologic finding in a boy strongly suggests X-linked muscular dystrophy. Immunohistochemical staining for dystrophin would show an absence of dystrophin, confirming the diagnosis of Duchenne muscular dystrophy. Antibodies to the acetylcholine receptor are found in myasthenia gravis, which is characterized by weakness in muscles after repetitive use. Eosinophilia may be present in allergic or parasitic disorders, including trichinosis. Oligoclonal immunoglobulin bands in the cerebrospinal fluid are a feature of multiple sclerosis. Expansion of CGG repeats on Xq27.3 is diagnostic of familial mental retardation.

BP7 780-782   BP6 689-690   PBD7 1336-1338
PBD6 1281-1282

2 **(A)** This patient has carpal tunnel syndrome, a form of compression neuropathy, which results from entrapment of the median nerve beneath the flexor retinaculum at the wrist. Women are more commonly affected than men, and the problem is often bilateral. The most common cause is excessive repetitive use of the wrist. Conditions such as hypothyroidism, amyloidosis, and edema with pregnancy also diminish the space in the carpal tunnel. Diabetes mellitus leads to a symmetric distal sensorimotor neuropathy. Amyotrophic lateral sclerosis results in progressive symmetric weakness from loss of motor neurons. Acute intermittent porphyria can lead to a hereditary form of motor and sensory neuropathy. Infection with varicella-zoster virus produces a painful neuropathy in a dermatomal distribution pattern.

BP7 847   BP6 742-743   PBD7 1335   PBD6 1280

3 **(D)** The most common cause of a predominantly sensory peripheral neuropathy is diabetes mellitus. Long-standing diabetes mellitus also gives rise to renal failure. Guillain-Barré syndrome produces a rapidly ascending paralysis. Sensorimotor disturbances are typically not seen with intracranial mass lesions such as astrocytomas. A cerebral infarction could lead to decreased motor activity and sometimes to sensory loss, although not in a symmetric pattern. The demyelinating lesions of multiple sclerosis can produce many signs and symptoms, but symmetric lesions should suggest another disease process.

BP7 847   BP6 742-743   PBD7 1334   PBD6 1279

4 **(D)** Muscle pain with fever and eosinophilia suggests a parasitic infestation of the skeletal muscles, most likely trichinosis. This results from ingesting poorly cooked infected meat. Duchenne muscular dystrophy is a noninflammatory myopathy that begins in early childhood. Polymyositis is an autoimmune condition characterized by muscle inflammation but no eosinophilia. Poliomyelitis can lead to muscle weakness but is noninflammatory. Diabetes mellitus can lead to peripheral vascular disease and gangrene, but this complication would be rare at age 17.

BP7 312, 780   BP6 689   PBD7 407-408   PBD6 394-395

5 **(B)** This patient has Becker muscular dystrophy. This congenital condition is similar to Duchenne muscular dystrophy in that it has an X-linked pattern of inheritance and there is a mutation in the dystrophin gene. However, in Becker muscular dystrophy, dystrophin is abnormal, not absent, resulting in less severe muscle disease than that of Duchenne muscular dystrophy. The typical patient is a middle-aged man. Amyotrophic lateral sclerosis is a progressive disease with a neurogenic form of muscle atrophy resulting from loss of motor neurons. Lambert-Eaton syndrome is a myasthenia-like paraneoplastic condition. McArdle disease is caused by a deficiency in muscle phosphorylase and does not produce progressive weakness. Myasthenia gravis results from acetylcholine receptor antibody and leads to progressive weakness. Myotonic dystrophy is an X-linked disorder characterized by facial and upper body weakness, cataracts, gonadal atrophy, cardiomyopathy, and dementia. Polymyositis is an autoimmune disorder with myalgia. Werdnig-Hoffman disease is a spinal muscular atrophy resulting from loss of motor neurons in infancy.

BP7 780-782   BP6 689-690   PBD7 1336-1338
PBD6 1281-1282

6 **(A)** The patient's history is typical of Guillain-Barré syndrome. This uncommon disorder most often follows a viral or mycoplasmal infection. It is believed to be caused by generation of myelin-reactive T cells, somehow triggered by viral infection. The paralysis of respiratory muscles may be life threatening, although many patients recover after weeks of ventilatory support. Various presentations are possible in multiple sclerosis, but the plaques of demyelination are generally not large or diffuse enough to cause paralysis of the respiratory muscles. Amyotrophic lateral sclerosis is associated with slowly progressive muscle weakness. Mechanical ventilation may eventually be necessary. Varicella-zoster virus infection most often involves the skin in a dermatomal distribution from a spinal nerve root. Vitamin B$_{12}$ deficiency results in subacute progressive degeneration of the spinal cord plus sensorimotor disturbances in the extremities.

BP7 848   BP6 743   PBD7 1331   PBD6 1275-1276

7 **(B)** This patient has myasthenia gravis, with muscle weakness resulting from loss of motor end-plate function. This disorder is caused by an antibody-mediated loss of acetylcholine receptors at neuromuscular junctions. Myopathic diseases such as muscular dystrophies are accompanied by increased levels of serum creatine kinase. Parasitic infection with *Trichinella spiralis* can lead to eosinophilia. Generalized muscle weakness with type II muscle fiber atrophy occurs in glucocorticoid excess. The anti-Jo-1 antibody is

present in polymyositis. Sjögren syndrome does not cause muscle weakness with use.

BP7 115, 779-780   BP6 88, 689   PBD7 1344   PBD6 1289

8 **(C)** This patient has a paraneoplastic syndrome called Lambert-Eaton myasthenic syndrome. Like many of the paraneoplastic syndromes, it is most often associated with small cell carcinoma of the lung. Persons with chronic viral hepatitis may have generalized malaise and weakness that is not related to specific muscle disease. Duchenne muscular dystrophy is an X-linked disease that manifests early in childhood. Lead poisoning leads to peripheral neuropathy. Diabetes mellitus may also produce peripheral neuropathy.

BP7 780   PBD7 1344-1345   PBD6 1289

9 **(A)** Type II atrophy can occur with glucocorticoid excess and after prolonged immobilization. Routine light microscopy may not allow the physician to distinguish type II atrophy from denervation atrophy. Histochemical staining for ATPase must be performed. There is a deficiency of myophosphorylase enzyme in McArdle disease, leading to muscle pain and cramping with vigorous exercise. Duchenne muscular dystrophy is an X-linked condition and is, therefore, rare in females. Onset is in early childhood. Antibodies to the acetylcholine receptor cause the muscular weakness in myasthenia gravis. Polymyositis is an inflammatory condition affecting all fiber types.

BP7 779   BP6 688   PBD7 1209, 1344   PBD6 1288-1289

10 **(C)** The biopsy specimen shows reduced amounts of dystrophin, suggesting Becker muscular dystrophy. In Duchenne muscular dystrophy, dystrophin is absent because of gene deletion. In keeping with the diagnosis of Becker muscular dystrophy, the patient is older and not severely affected. Both dystrophies are X-linked conditions. Werdnig-Hoffmann disease is a form of spinal muscular atrophy. Onset is at birth, and it results from a genetically determined loss of anterior horn cells. Polymyositis is an autoimmune disease that results from a T-cell–mediated attack on muscle fibers, causing muscle fiber degeneration with inflammation. Amyotrophic lateral sclerosis is a denervation atrophy seen in adults, with loss of anterior horn cells in the spinal cord and cranial nerve nuclei. Myasthenia gravis results from acetylcholine receptor antibody, and there is minimal structural change to the muscle. Myotonic dystrophy is an X-linked disorder characterized by facial and upper body weakness, cataracts, gonadal atrophy, cardiomyopathy, and dementia.

BP7 780-782   BP6 689-690   PBD7 1336-1338
PBD6 1281-1282

11 **(E)** Trichinosis is caused by ingestion of uncooked or poorly cooked meat containing *Trichinella spiralis* organisms. Most cases are asymptomatic because few organisms are ingested. One clue to past infection is the appearance of the calcified encysted organisms in muscle. The most active muscles, such as the diaphragm, tend to be involved preferentially. Lambert-Eaton syndrome is a myasthenia-like paraneoplastic condition. McArdle disease is caused by a deficiency in muscle phosphorylase and does not produce progressive weakness. Mitochondrial myopathies such as Leigh disease can begin in childhood or adulthood, with progressive weakness. Polymyositis is an autoimmune disorder with myalgia.

Werdnig-Hoffman disease is a spinal muscular atrophy resulting from loss of motor neurons in infancy.

BP7 312,780   BP6 689   PBD7 407-408   PBD6 394-395

12 (A) The clinical findings are highly suggestive of myasthenia gravis, a condition caused by antibodies to the acetylcholine receptor. Muscles that undergo repetitive use are most affected. As the course of untreated disease progresses, larger muscle groups and respiratory muscles can be affected. Thymic abnormalities, including thymomas, are associated with myasthenia gravis. Lack of dystrophin on muscle fibers is typical of Duchenne muscular dystrophy. An increased creatine kinase level can be seen in many types of muscle diseases, because myofibers are rich in creatine kinase. A positive ANA test result suggests an underlying autoimmune disease.

BP7 115, 779-780   BP6 688-689   PBD7 1344   PBD6 1289

13 (E) The features described are consistent with a peripheral neuropathy associated with diabetes mellitus. Motor and sensory nerves are involved, and there may also be an autonomic neuropathy. Histologic examination shows an axonal neuropathy with segmental demyelination. Difficulty in emptying the urinary bladder and impotence are results of autonomic neuropathy. Longer nerves are affected first; this explains the lower leg involvement and accounts for many cases of "diabetic foot," with trauma and subsequent ulceration. Wallerian degeneration typically occurs with traumatic transection of a nerve. Acute inflammation is not generally seen in neuropathies. Onion bulb formation is a feature of the hereditary neuropathy known as Refsum disease. Lymphocytic infiltrates may be seen in Guillain-Barré syndrome.

BP7 847   BP6 572   PBD7 1334   PBD6 1279

14 (B) Amyotrophic lateral sclerosis (ALS) is also known as Lou Gehrig disease, named for the famous New York Yankee first baseman afflicted with the disorder. Lower and upper motor neurons can be affected, resulting in a denervation-type pattern of muscular atrophy. This occurs because an individual neuron innervates a group of muscle fibers. Bulbar involvement denotes a more rapid course. Werdnig-Hoffman disease is also a neuropathic disease with grouped atrophy, but onset is in infancy. The other listed options are not associated with denervation.

BP7 778-779   BP6 687-688   PBD7 1335, 1396-1397
PBD6 1273, 1338

15 (D) Laceration of the femoral nerve results in Wallerian degeneration distal to the injury. Realignment of the nerve is accompanied by axonal sprouting. The new axons will find the residual myelin sheaths and grow down at the rate of about 2 mm/day, taking 1 year for the distance of a lower extremity. Thus, there can be reinnervation of the muscle, but there will be type grouping of the muscle fascicles that are reinnervated.

BP7 847   BP6 742   PBD7 1329-1330   PBD6 1274-1275

16 (C) Fashion may have a price. The patient has a Morton neuroma, a form of compressive neuropathy in which a plantar nerve is trapped between metatarsal heads. Chronic injury leads to growth of a tangled mass of axons, fibroblasts, and perineural cells. The toxic disorder (lead poisoning) and metabolic disorders (beriberi with thiamine deficiency or subacute combined degeneration with cobalamin deficiency) are not as focal. Diabetic neuropathy, which occurs in either type 1 or type 2 disease, is bilateral. It is characterized by loss of sensation, which may be a predisposing factor for foot trauma. Wallerian degeneration is a dying-back neuropathy associated with severing of a nerve; a neuroma may form at the site of injury.

BP7 847   BP6 742-743   PBD7 1335   PBD6 1280

17 (E) Oxidative phosphorylation in mitochondria can be affected by mitochondrial genes, which are separate from those on chromosomes in the cell nucleus. These abnormal genes can lead to mitochondrial myopathies, encephalopathies, and deafness. In this case, there is mitochondrial encephalopathy with lactic acidosis and strokelike episodes (MELAS). There is a maternal pattern of inheritance for mitochondrial genes. An abnormal voltage-gated calcium channel is seen in one of the channelopathies; it causes hypokalemic periodic paralysis. Channelopathies are typically inherited in an autosomal dominant fashion. Antibodies to acetylcholine receptor cause myasthenia gravis; its sole manifestation is muscle weakness. Cytotoxic CD8 cells mediate the muscle injury in polymyositis. Decreased sarcolemmal dystrophin is present in Becker muscular dystrophy; dystrophin is absent in Duchenne muscular dystrophy. The dystrophin gene is located on the X chromosome. Increased CTG repeats occur in myotonic dystrophy, which is X-linked.

BP7 15,235-236   BP6 16,199   PBD7 1341-1342
PBD6 1287

18 (E) The axons distal to the point of injury or transection will degenerate. The Schwann cells that remain can guide the regrowing nerves. Macrophages help to remove myelin-derived debris from the area of nerve injury, but acute inflammation is not a typical feature of diseases involving peripheral nerves. Traumatic neuromas may occur following transection. The purpose of the graft is to guide orderly regrowth. A tumor is unlikely to follow a nerve, although a feature of a malignant tumor is a tendency to invade nerves. Grouped atrophy occurs later with progression of disease when denervation is followed by reinnervation.

BP7 847   BP6 742-743   PBD7 1329-1330
PBD6 1274-1275

19 (C) The clinical features and histologic findings are typical of dermatomyositis, an immunologically mediated form of inflammatory myopathy. In these patients antibodies and complement damage small capillaries, resulting in a characteristic perifascicular myofiber atrophy. The CD8+ T cells are believed to be important in the pathogenesis of polymyositis. T-cell mediated myelin injury is seen with the Guillain–Barré syndrome, causing an acute ascending paralysis. Mutations in ion channel genes give rise to various channelopathies, including hypokalemic periodic paralysis and malignant hyperthermia. Expansion of CTG repeats is seen with myotonic dystrophy.

BP7 143-144   PBD7 1342-1343

CHAPTER 28

The Central Nervous System

1 A 46-year-old man who is an intravenous drug user is admitted to the hospital because he has had increasing headache and high fever for the past 24 hours. On physical examination, his temperature is 38.4°C, pulse 85/min, respirations 18/min, and blood pressure 125/85 mm Hg. CT scan of the head shows no mass lesion or midline shift. A lumbar puncture is performed. The CSF shows an increased protein concentration and a decreased glucose level. Which of the following infectious agents is most likely to produce these findings?

❏ (A) JC papovavirus
❏ (B) *Mycobacterium tuberculosis*
❏ (C) *Staphylococcus aureus*
❏ (D) Herpes simplex virus
❏ (E) *Toxoplasma gondii*

2 The family of a 63-year-old woman noticed that she has become more forgetful over a period of 6 weeks. One month later, the woman has difficulty ambulating and is unable to care for herself. On physical examination, she has myoclonus. She is afebrile. CT scan of the head shows minimal cerebral atrophy, which is nearly consistent for age. An EEG shows low-amplitude, slow background activity with periodic complexes and occasional repetitive, sharp waves with intervals of 0.5 to 1 sec. Which of the following histologic abnormalities is most likely to be found in the cerebral cortex?

❏ (A) Numerous neuritic plaques
❏ (B) Plaques of demyelination
❏ (C) Lewy bodies
❏ (D) Microglial nodules
❏ (E) Spongiform encephalopathy

3 A 49-year-old man with an acute psychosis is being examined by a nurse practitioner. The man tells her that he has a lengthy history of chronic alcoholism. He has difficulty performing a finger-to-nose test, and there is paralysis of the lateral rectus muscles. A deficiency of which of the following nutrients is most likely to produce these findings?

❏ (A) Folate
❏ (B) Niacin
❏ (C) Cobalamin
❏ (D) Pyridoxine
❏ (E) Thiamine

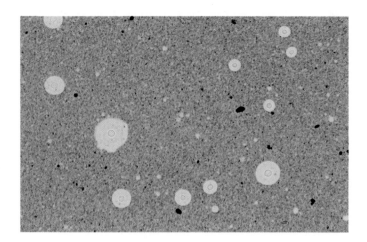

4 A 39-year-old man with a 10-year history of HIV infection sees the physician because he has had a severe headache for 4 days. On physical examination, there is no papilledema. A lumbar puncture is performed, and there is a slightly increased opening pressure. Laboratory analysis of the CSF shows a few mononuclear cells, no neutrophils, no RBCs, normal glucose level, and normal protein concentration. An India ink preparation of the CSF is shown in the preceding figure. Which of the following organisms is most likely to produce these findings?

☐ (A) *Staphylococcus aureus*
☐ (B) *Mycobacterium tuberculosis*
☐ (C) *Listeria monocytogenes*
☐ (D) *Toxoplasma gondii*
☐ (E) *Cryptococcus neoformans*

5 A 40-year-old previously healthy man is brought to the emergency department after sudden onset of a grand mal seizure. Physical examination yields no remarkable findings except for a 1-cm darkly pigmented skin lesion on the upper back. CT scan of the head shows five sharply circumscribed, 1- to 2.5-cm mass lesions located in the cerebral hemispheres at the gray-white junction of the parietal and frontal lobes. Which of the following is the most likely diagnosis?

☐ (A) AIDS
☐ (B) Metastases
☐ (C) Infective endocarditis
☐ (D) Neurofibromatosis type 1
☐ (E) Cysticercosis

6 A 25-year-old previously healthy woman has acute onset of confusion and disorientation followed by a generalized tonic-clonic seizure. On admission to the hospital, she is afebrile and her blood pressure is 110/65 mm Hg. No papilledema is observed. Serum and urine drug screening results are negative. CT scan of the head shows a 3-cm recent hemorrhage in the left temporal lobe. A lumbar puncture is performed, and the CSF shows only a few mononuclear cells and normal glucose and protein levels. Infection with which of the following organisms is the most likely cause of her disease?

☐ (A) Cytomegalovirus
☐ (B) *Neisseria meningitidis*
☐ (C) Herpes simplex virus
☐ (D) Eastern equine encephalitis virus
☐ (E) *Aspergillus niger*

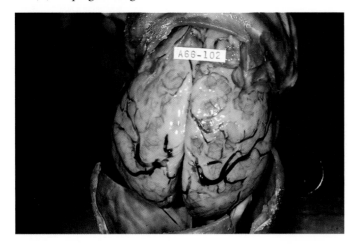

7 A healthy 20-year-old man has a mild pharyngitis, followed a few days later by sudden onset of a severe headache. Physical examination shows nuchal rigidity. His temperature is 38.8°C, pulse 98/min, respirations 26/min, and blood pressure 95/45 mm Hg. The gross appearance of a representative section of the surface of the brain is shown in the preceding figure. Which of the following is most likely to have produced this clinical and histologic picture?

☐ (A) *Cryptococcus neoformans*
☐ (B) *Mycobacterium tuberculosis*
☐ (C) *Toxoplasma gondii*
☐ (D) Poliovirus
☐ (E) *Neisseria meningitidis*

8 A 53-year-old man with a lengthy history of chronic alcoholism has had an increasingly clouded sensorium over the past 2 days. On physical examination, he has a flapping tremor of his outstretched hands. MR imaging of the brain shows no abnormalities. Which of the following laboratory findings is most likely to account for these symptoms?

☐ (A) Hyponatremia
☐ (B) Hypoglycemia
☐ (C) Elevated hemoglobin A_{1c} level
☐ (D) Elevated carboxyhemoglobin level
☐ (E) Hyperammonemia

9 A 68-year-old woman with a 7-year history of progressive dementia dies of bronchopneumonia. At autopsy, there is cerebral atrophy in a predominantly frontal and parietal lobe distribution. Microscopic examination of the brain shows numerous neuritic plaques in the hippocampus, amygdala, and neocortex. Congo red staining demonstrates amyloid in the media of the small peripheral cerebral arteries. Which of the following conditions is likely to be the most important factor in the development of her disease?

☐ (A) HLA-DR3/DR4
☐ (B) Expansion of CAG repeats on chromosome 4p16
☐ (C) Inheritance of the ε4 allele at the ApoE4 gene
☐ (D) Inheritance of a mutant prion gene
☐ (E) Deficiency of thiamine

10 A 72-year-old woman trips on a toy truck left at the top of a flight of stairs by a grandchild and falls down the stairs. She does not lose consciousness. About 36 hours later, she develops a headache and confusion and is taken to the emergency department. On physical examination, she is conscious and has a scalp contusion on the occiput. Which of the following is the most likely location of an intracranial hemorrhage in this patient?

☐ (A) Pontine
☐ (B) Subarachnoid
☐ (C) Basal ganglia
☐ (D) Epidural
☐ (E) Subdural

11 A previously healthy 26-year-old medical student has headaches for several weeks. She has increasing malaise. Physical examination yields no remarkable findings. CT scan of the head shows no abnormalities. A lumbar puncture is performed and yields clear, colorless CSF with a normal opening pressure. Laboratory analysis of the CSF shows a normal glucose concentration and a minimally increased protein level. A few lymphocytes are present, but there are no neutrophils. A Gram stain and India ink preparation of the CSF are negative. Her condition gradually improves over the next several months. Serum serologic tests are most likely to show an elevated titer of antibodies to which of the following infectious agents?

❑ (A) *Toxoplasma gondii*
❑ (B) *Listeria monocytogenes*
❑ (C) *Cryptococcus neoformans*
❑ (D) *Neisseria meningitidis*
❑ (E) Echovirus

12 A 45-year-old previously healthy man has developed headaches over the past month. On physical examination, there are no remarkable findings. A cerebral angiogram shows a 7-mm saccular aneurysm at the trifurcation of the right middle cerebral artery. Which of the following is most likely to result from this lesion?

❑ (A) Epidural hematoma
❑ (B) Subarachnoid hemorrhage
❑ (C) Subdural hematoma
❑ (D) Cerebellar tonsillar herniation
❑ (E) Hydrocephalus

13 A 55-year-old man dies of aspiration pneumonia after a 6-year illness, characterized by progressive, symmetric muscular weakness. At autopsy, the brain and spinal cord appear normal on gross examination. Microscopic sections show gliosis in the motor cortex, pallor of the lateral corticospinal tracts, and neuronal loss in the anterior horns of the spinal cord. Which of the following is the most likely underlying cause of death?

❑ (A) Becker muscular dystrophy
❑ (B) Neurofibromatosis type 2
❑ (C) Guillain-Barré syndrome
❑ (D) Creutzfeldt-Jakob disease
❑ (E) Amyotrophic lateral sclerosis

14 A 19-year-old snowboarder wearing protective equipment consisting of a baseball cap, baggy shorts, and a letterman's jacket flew off a jump and hit a tree. He was initially unconscious and then "came to" and wanted to try another run, but his friends thought it best to call for help. On the way to the emergency department, he became comatose. Physical examination shows left papilledema. Skull radiographs show a linear fracture of the left temporal-parietal region. A serum drug screen is positive for cannabinoids. This clinical picture is most consistent with which of the following lesions?

❑ (A) Contusion of frontal lobes
❑ (B) Epidural hematoma
❑ (C) Ruptured berry aneurysm
❑ (D) Acute leptomeningitis
❑ (E) Acute subdural hematoma

15 An 18-year-old university student has had decreased vision on the left for 6 months. On physical examination, there is papilledema on the right. She has 14 scattered, 2- to 5-cm flat, hyperpigmented skin lesions with irregular borders on the extremities and torso. CT scan of the head shows no intracranial hemorrhage and no edema or midline shift, but there is a mass in the region of the right optic nerve. An optic nerve glioma is excised. Eight months later, she returns for a follow-up examination, and a mass is palpated on the right wrist. Histologic examination of the mass is most likely to show which of the following neoplasms?

❑ (A) Schwannoma
❑ (B) Lipoma
❑ (C) Fibrosarcoma
❑ (D) Meningioma
❑ (E) Hemangioma

16 A 62-year-old man has had increasing difficulty with voluntary movements because of muscular rigidity. On physical examination, he has difficulty initiating movement, but he can keep moving if he follows someone walking ahead of him. He has an expressionless facies. When he is sitting, his hands have a "pill-rolling" tremor. Which of the following pathologic findings in the brain is most likely to be present?

❑ (A) Hippocampal neurofibrillary tangles
❑ (B) Neuronal loss with gliosis in caudate
❑ (C) Hemosiderosis and gliosis of mamillary bodies
❑ (D) Loss of pigmented neurons in substantia nigra
❑ (E) Alzheimer type II gliosis in basal ganglia

17 An 18-year-old boy sustains severe blunt head trauma in a motor vehicle accident. He is comatose on arrival at the emergency department and has no spontaneous movements. There is bilateral papilledema. The boy dies 1 day after the accident. At autopsy, there is a midbrain hemorrhage, arranged in a linear ventral-to-dorsal direction, and bilateral uncal and cerebral herniation. Which of the following mechanisms is most likely to result in this type of hemorrhage?

❑ (A) Tearing of the cerebral (dural) bridging veins
❑ (B) Laceration of the middle meningeal artery
❑ (C) Stretching of perforating basilar artery branches
❑ (D) Rupture of an internal carotid saccular (berry) aneurysm
❑ (E) Sudden decrease in systemic blood pressure

18 A 38-year-old woman who fell to the ground and hit her head is taken to the emergency department. There are no remarkable findings on physical examination. CT scan of the head shows no hemorrhage or fracture, but there is a 5-cm mass beneath dura that compresses the underlying left superolateral parietal lobe. The mass is surgically removed. Histologic analysis shows elongated cells with pale, oblong nuclei and pink cytoplasm with occasional psammoma bodies. Which of the following is the most likely diagnosis?

❑ (A) Meningioma
❑ (B) Tuberculoma
❑ (C) Medulloblastoma
❑ (D) Schwannoma
❑ (E) Ependymoma

19 A 47-year-old woman is brought to the physician by family members, who report that she has become more forgetful in the past few months. She is emotionally labile and often cries. She is disturbed and depressed by these developments because her mother died a few years after experiencing the same symptoms. On physical examination, she has some choreiform movements of her extremities. Which of the following laboratory findings is most likely to be present?

❏ (A) Decreased level of hexosaminidase A enzyme
❏ (B) Mutation in presenilin genes
❏ (C) Extra chromosome 21
❏ (D) Abnormal prion protein
❏ (E) Increased trinucleotide CAG repeats

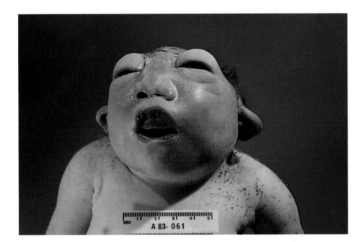

20 A 30-year-old woman, G 3, P 2, is in the third trimester of pregnancy. She has noted minimal fetal movement throughout the pregnancy. An ultrasound study shows normal amniotic fluid volume, normally implanted placenta, and the abnormality represented by the 36-week-gestational-age fetus shown above. Which of the following laboratory findings is most likely to be present?

❏ (A) Fetal hyperbilirubinemia with anemia
❏ (B) High maternal cytomegalovirus IgM titer
❏ (C) Elevated maternal serum α-fetoprotein level
❏ (D) Elevated maternal hemoglobin A_{1c} level
❏ (E) 47,XX,+21 fetal karyotype

21 A 71-year-old woman sustains blunt head trauma in a motor vehicle accident. On admission to the hospital, she is conscious but disoriented. CT scan of the head shows a right temporal bone fracture and mild cerebral edema. One day later, laboratory studies show serum Na^+ 109 mmol/L, K^+ 3.9 mmol/L, Cl^- 82 mmol/L, CO_2 23 mmol/L, glucose 73 mg/dL, and creatinine 1.0 mg/dL. The hyponatremia is corrected over the next 2 hours with intravenous fluid and electrolyte therapy and diuretics. She then becomes obtunded. No papilledema is seen on funduscopic examination. Which of the following complications has most likely occurred?

❏ (A) Cerebellar tonsillar herniation
❏ (B) Intraventricular hemorrhage
❏ (C) Subacute combined degeneration of the cord
❏ (D) Wernicke-Korsakoff syndrome
❏ (E) Central pontine myelinolysis

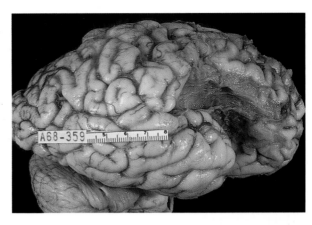

22 A 68-year-old woman suddenly lost consciousness and fell to the ground. When she became arousable, she was unable to move her left arm or leg and had difficulty speaking. On physical examination, her temperature was 37°C, pulse 81/min, respirations 18/min, and blood pressure 135/85 mm Hg. She did not regain function on her left side. Six months later, she died of pneumonia. The gross appearance of the brain at autopsy is shown above. The figure most likely represents which of the following lesions?

❏ (A) Organizing subdural hematoma
❏ (B) Arteriovenous malformation
❏ (C) Recent cerebral infarction
❏ (D) Contusion from blunt trauma
❏ (E) Remote cerebral infarction

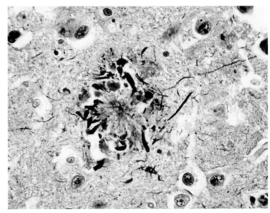

Courtesy of Eileen Bigio, MD, Department of Pathology, University of Texas Southwestern Medical School, Dallas, TX.

23 An autopsy study is conducted of patients who died at ages ranging from 55 to 80 years. A subset of these patients has cerebral atrophy with brain weights that are less than normal for age and body size. On gross examination, these brains show hydrocephalus ex vacuo, but there are no focal lesions. The photomicrograph above shows the microscopic appearance of a representative section of cerebral neocortex when examined under high power with Bielschowsky silver stain. Which of the following symptoms is most likely to be recorded in the medical histories of this subset of patients?

❏ (A) Symmetric muscular weakness
❏ (B) Gait disturbances
❏ (C) Progressive dementia
❏ (D) Grand mal seizures
❏ (E) Choreiform movements

24 A fetus is stillborn at 34 weeks' gestation to a 33-year-old woman, G 3, P 2, whose two previous pregnancies resulted in normal term infants. On examination, the fetus is observed to be hydropic. Autopsy of the fetus shows marked organomegaly, and the brain has extensive necrosis in a periventricular pattern, with focal calcifications. Which of the following congenital infections is most likely to produce these findings?

❑ (A) *Listeria monocytogenes*
❑ (B) HIV
❑ (C) Herpes simplex virus
❑ (D) Cytomegalovirus
❑ (E) Group B streptococcus

25 A 10-year-old boy has had persistent headaches for the past 3 months. On physical examination, he is afebrile. He has an ataxic gait. CT scan of the head shows a 4-cm cystic mass in the right cerebellar hemisphere. Cerebral ventricles are enlarged. A lumbar puncture is performed. The CSF protein concentration is elevated, but the glucose level is normal. Neurosurgery is performed, and the mass is removed and sectioned. On gross examination, the mass is a cyst filled with gelatinous material. The cyst has a thin wall and a 1-cm mural nodule. Microscopically, the mass is composed of cells that stain positive for GFAP and have long, hair-like processes. Which of the following is the most likely diagnosis?

❑ (A) Astrocytoma
❑ (B) Hemangioblastoma
❑ (C) Medulloblastoma
❑ (D) Meningioma
❑ (E) Metastatic carcinoma
❑ (F) Non-Hodgkin lymphoma
❑ (G) Oligodendroglioma
❑ (H) Schwannoma

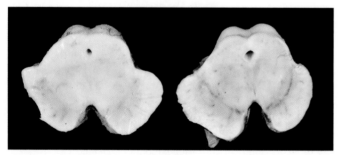

Courtesy of Eileen Bigio, MD, Department of Pathology, University of Texas Southwestern Medical School, Dallas, TX.

26 A 55-year-old man had increasing difficulty with initiation of voluntary movements and increasing inability to perform activities of daily living for 1 year. He became bedridden and died of pulmonary thromboembolism. The gross appearance of the midbrain of this patient is shown on the left; on the right is a section through normal midbrain. Which of the following additional clinical features is most closely associated with this lesion?

❑ (A) Pill-rolling tremor at rest
❑ (B) Symmetric weakness in the extremities
❑ (C) Choreiform movements
❑ (D) Difficulty with short-term memory
❑ (E) Paraplegia

27 A 43-year-old previously healthy woman has had a headache and fever for the past 2 weeks. She recently had a severe respiratory tract infection. On physical examination, her temperature is 38.3°C. There is no papilledema. She has no loss of sensation or motor function, but there is decreased vision in the left half of her visual fields. A CT scan of the head shows a sharply demarcated, 3-cm ring-enhancing lesion in the right occipital region. A lumbar puncture is performed, and laboratory analysis of the CSF shows a cell count of 4 lymphocytes and 8 neutrophils and increased protein and normal glucose levels. Which of the following is the most likely diagnosis?

❑ (A) Glioblastoma multiforme
❑ (B) Multiple sclerosis
❑ (C) Subacute infarction
❑ (D) Cerebral abscess
❑ (E) Metastatic carcinoma

28 In the past 3 months, a 79-year-old man has had several episodes of sudden dysarthria, a feeling of weakness in his hands, and dizziness. These episodes usually last less than 1 hour, and then he feels fine. Today, he suddenly lost consciousness while walking to the bathroom in his house and fell to the floor. On regaining consciousness several minutes later, he was unable to move his right arm or to speak clearly. Which of the following pathologic findings in the brain best explains this patient's symptoms?

❑ (A) Frontal lobe astrocytoma
❑ (B) Subdural hematoma
❑ (C) Cerebral atherosclerosis
❑ (D) Arteriovenous malformation
❑ (E) Meningoencephalitis

29 A 26-year-old man states that 3 years ago he experienced paresthesias of his left arm and had difficulty walking, but these problems diminished. During the past year, he developed difficulty seeing from his left eye. Six months ago, he had difficulty writing with his right hand. On physical examination, there is decreased visual acuity on the left and no papilledema and no retinal lesions. There is decreased motor strength and decreased sensation in the right hand and forearm. MR imaging of the brain shows focal areas of brightness in periventricular white matter and in the left optic nerve. A lumbar puncture is performed. Which of the following findings is most likely to be present on examination of the CSF?

❑ (A) Cryptococcal antigen
❑ (B) Oligoclonal bands of immunoglobulins
❑ (C) Malignant cells
❑ (D) Xanthochromia
❑ (E) Antitreponemal antibodies

30 A 42-year-old man has had increasing difficulty performing activities of daily living for the past year because of worsening choreiform movements. His family reports that his behavior has changed, although his memory remains intact. His older brother is similarly affected. On physical examination, he is afebrile and normotensive. Cranial nerves are intact. He has no motor weakness and no sensory deficits. Which of the following findings in the CNS is most likely to be present?

❏ (A) Loss of pigmented neurons in the substantia nigra
❏ (B) Congophilic angiopathy of the cerebral cortex
❏ (C) Atrophy and gliosis of the caudate nuclei
❏ (D) Loss of motor neurons in the cerebral cortex and brain stem
❏ (E) Multiple lacunar infarcts within the basal ganglia

31 A 12-year-old girl had progressively diminishing neurologic function over a period of 3 years. She had difficulty with movement, decreased mental ability, and loss of control over bladder and bowel functions. While in the hospital, she contracted pneumonia and died. At autopsy, the brain is atrophic, and the centrum semiovale and central white matter are shrunken, gray, and translucent on gross examination. Microscopically, there is widespread myelin loss with sparing of subcortical U fibers. Which of the following degenerative CNS diseases best explains the course of this illness?

❏ (A) Metachromatic leukodystrophy
❏ (B) Progressive multifocal leukoencephalopathy
❏ (C) Acute disseminated encephalomyelitis
❏ (D) Tay-Sachs disease
❏ (E) Multiple sclerosis

32 An 80-year-old resident of a nursing home is admitted to the hospital because of recent onset of fluctuating levels of consciousness. On physical examination, she is arousable but disoriented and irritable. Vital signs include temperature of 36.9°C and blood pressure of 130/85 mm Hg. There is papilledema on the right. CT scan of the head shows a collection of blood in the subdural space on the right. Which of the following most likely produced these findings?

❏ (A) Tear of bridging veins
❏ (B) Rupture of saccular aneurysm
❏ (C) Bleeding from an arteriovenous malformation
❏ (D) Laceration of the middle meningeal artery
❏ (E) Thrombosis of the middle cerebral artery

33 While working at her desk as an accountant, a 50-year-old woman develops sudden, severe headache and is taken to the emergency department. On examination, she has nuchal rigidity. A lumbar puncture is performed. The CSF shows numerous RBCs, no neutrophils, a few mononuclear cells, and a normal glucose level. The Gram stain result is negative. Which of the following events has most likely occurred?

❏ (A) Middle cerebral artery thromboembolism
❏ (B) Tear of subdural bridging veins
❏ (C) Ruptured intracranial berry aneurysm
❏ (D) Bleeding from cerebral amyloid angiopathy
❏ (E) Hypertensive basal ganglia hemorrhage

34 A 20-year old man with HIV infection has had a decreased level of consciousness for the past week. He now experiences a seizure. On physical examination, his temperature is 37.6°C. MR imaging of the brain shows several 1- to 3-cm ring-enhancing lesions in the cerebral gray matter bilaterally. A stereotaxic biopsy is performed. Which of the following pathologic findings is most likely to be present on microscopic examination of the biopsy specimen?

❏ (A) Large atypical lymphocytes
❏ (B) Budding cells with pseudohyphae
❏ (C) Spongiform encephalopathy
❏ (D) *Toxoplasma* pseudocysts
❏ (E) Metastatic squamous cell carcinoma

35 A 5-year-old boy has complained of headaches for the past week. His gait has become ataxic. After sudden onset of vomiting, he is brought to the emergency department, where he becomes comatose. On physical examination, he is afebrile. CT scan of the head shows the presence of a 4-cm mass in the cerebellar vermis and dilation of the cerebral ventricles. A lumbar puncture is performed. Cytologic examination of the CSF shows small cells with dark blue nuclei and scant cytoplasm. Which of the following neoplasms is most likely to explain these findings?

❏ (A) Schwannoma
❏ (B) Ependymoma
❏ (C) Glioblastoma multiforme
❏ (D) Medulloblastoma
❏ (E) Metastatic carcinoma

36 Three months ago, a 27-year-old woman had an episode of weakness, which she attributed to job stress and fatigue. She now sees her physician because she has had decreased vision in her left eye for the past week. The neurologic examination shows mild residual weakness with 4/5 motor strength in the right lower extremity. A lumbar puncture is performed. Laboratory examination of the CSF shows increased IgG levels with prominent oligoclonal bands. MR imaging of the brain shows small, scattered, 0.5-cm areas consistent with demyelination, most of which are located in periventricular white matter. Which of the following is the most appropriate information to give the patient about these findings?

❏ (A) No further neurologic problems will be experienced
❏ (B) Relapses and remissions will occur over many years
❏ (C) This disease can be passed on to your children
❏ (D) Further debilitation and death will occur within 5 years
❏ (E) A test for HIV will be positive

37 A 60-year-old man had sudden loss of consciousness. On physical examination, he had left hemiplegia. He did not regain consciousness and died of pneumonia. At autopsy, there is a large, hemorrhagic infarct in the right parietal region. Microscopically, a thromboembolus is found in a peripheral cerebral artery branch at the gray-white junction near the infarct. Which of the following underlying disease processes was most likely present?

❏ (A) Hypertension with chronic renal failure
❏ (B) Rheumatic heart disease with left atrial mural thrombosis
❏ (C) Chronic alcoholism with micronodular cirrhosis
❏ (D) AIDS with a low CD4+ T lymphocyte count
❏ (E) Papillary thyroid carcinoma with metastases to bone

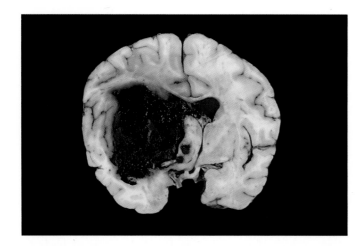

38 A 55-year-old man suddenly loses consciousness while driving his truck, but he is traveling at a slow speed and comes to a stop without a collision. Paramedics arrive but are unable to arouse him. On physical examination, there is bilateral papilledema. He has no spontaneous movements. The gross appearance of the brain at autopsy is shown. Which of the following underlying conditions is most likely to have resulted in this lesion?

- ❑ (A) Thromboembolism
- ❑ (B) Metastatic carcinoma
- ❑ (C) Multiple sclerosis
- ❑ (D) Systemic hypertension
- ❑ (E) Chronic alcoholism

39 A 49-year-old woman has had a severe headache for 2 days. On physical examination, she is afebrile and normotensive. Funduscopic examination shows papilledema on the right. One day later, she has right pupillary dilation and impaired ocular movement. She then becomes obtunded. Which of the following lesions best explains these findings?

- ❑ (A) Hydrocephalus ex vacuo
- ❑ (B) Transtentorial medial temporal herniation
- ❑ (C) Ruptured middle cerebral berry aneurysm
- ❑ (D) Chronic subdural hematoma
- ❑ (E) Occipital lobe infarction
- ❑ (F) Frontal lobe abscess

40 A 56-year-old man sees his physician after a single episode of grand mal seizure. On physical examination, he is afebrile and normotensive. Motor strength is intact, and there is no loss of sensation. Cranial nerves are intact. His mental function is not diminished. Brain MR imaging shows three solid, 1- to 3-cm mass lesions, without ring enhancement or surrounding edema, located at the gray-white junction in the right and left frontal lobes. The cerebral ventricles appear normal in size. Which of the following is the most likely diagnosis?

- ❑ (A) Glioblastoma multiforme
- ❑ (B) Hemangioblastoma
- ❑ (C) Medulloblastoma
- ❑ (D) Meningioma
- ❑ (E) Metastatic carcinoma
- ❑ (F) Non-Hodgkin lymphoma
- ❑ (G) Oligodendroglioma
- ❑ (H) Schwannoma

41 A 25-year-old man has complained of headaches for the past 5 months. During that time, family members noticed that he was not as mentally sharp as he has been in the past and that he has become more emotionally labile. Over a 2-week period, he has a generalized seizure, followed by three more seizures. On physical examination, there is no papilledema or movement disorder. CT scan of the head shows a 2-cm mass in the right frontal lobe. A stereotactic biopsy of this lesion shows only gliosis, as well as evidence of recent and remote hemorrhage. The mass is removed, and histologic examination shows a conglomerate of various-sized tortuous vessels surrounded by gliosis. Which of the following is the most likely diagnosis?

- ❑ (A) Arteriovenous malformation
- ❑ (B) Organizing abscess
- ❑ (C) Angiosarcoma
- ❑ (D) Prior head trauma
- ❑ (E) Ruptured saccular aneurysm
- ❑ (F) Multiple sclerosis plaque

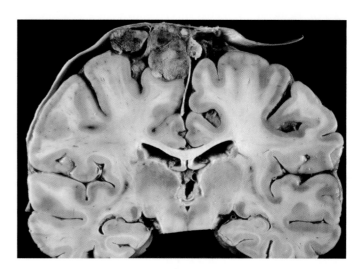

42 A 45-year-old woman sees the physician because she has had unilateral headaches on the right for the past 5 months. Physical examination yields no remarkable findings. The lesion seen on CT scan of the head is shown in this gross photograph of the brain. Which of the following is the most likely diagnosis?

- ❑ (A) Meningioma
- ❑ (B) Astrocytoma
- ❑ (C) Ependymoma
- ❑ (D) Metastasis
- ❑ (E) Tuberculoma

43 A 72-year-old woman had experienced progressive memory problems for several years. During the past year, she often became lost while walking in her own neighborhood and was unable to find her way home. More recently, she was unable to find the bathroom in her own house and could not recognize family members. On physical examination, she is found to have dementia, but there are no other remarkable findings. One year later, she dies of pulmonary thromboembolism. Examination of the brain at autopsy is most likely to show which of the following pathologic findings?

- ❑ (A) Many Lewy bodies in the substantia nigra
- ❑ (B) Atrophy and gliosis of the caudate nuclei
- ❑ (C) Neocortical neuronal Pick bodies
- ❑ (D) Oligodendroglial cytoplasmic inclusions
- ❑ (E) Numerous neocortical senile plaques

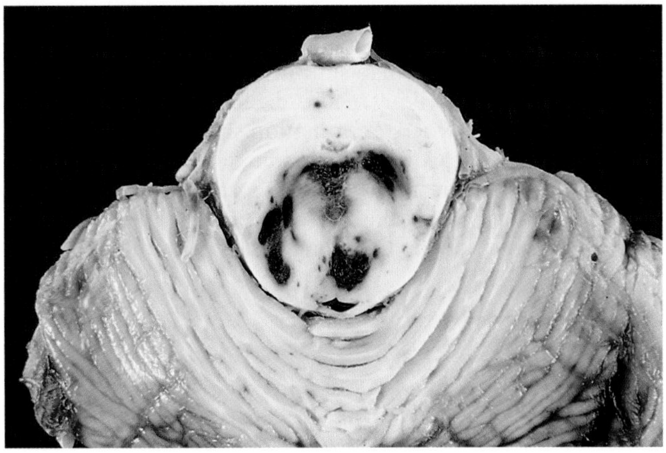

44 A 45-year-old man developed a severe headache and fever over a period of 2 days. On physical examination, he had nuchal rigidity. His temperature was 38.5°C. A lumbar puncture was performed. Analysis of the CSF showed gram-positive cocci in chains, and *Streptococcus pneumoniae* was cultured. Despite antibiotic therapy, he died. The gross appearance of a section of the brain at autopsy is shown. Based on this appearance, which of the following complications most likely resulted from this patient's infection?

- ❑ (A) Uncal herniation
- ❑ (B) Hydrocephalus
- ❑ (C) Abscess formation
- ❑ (D) Subarachnoid hemorrhage
- ❑ (E) Laminar cortical necrosis

45 A 41-year-old woman has had diminished hearing for the last 4 months. On physical examination, she has decreased hearing on the left. Sound lateralizes to the right ear on the Weber tuning fork test. CT scan of the head shows a sharply circumscribed, 4-cm mass adjacent to the left pons that extends toward the left inferior cerebellar hemisphere. Which of the following neoplasms is most likely to be present in this patient?

- ❑ (A) Meningioma
- ❑ (B) Astrocytoma
- ❑ (C) Schwannoma
- ❑ (D) Medulloblastoma
- ❑ (E) Ependymoma

46 A 48-year-old man has noticed speech difficulties for 2 months. On physical examination, he has weakness on the left side. MR imaging of the brain shows a large, irregular 6-cm mass in the centrum semiovale of the right cerebral hemisphere that extends across the corpus callosum. Stereotactic biopsy of the mass shows areas of necrosis surrounded by nuclear pseudopalisading. The neoplastic cells within the mass are hyperchromatic. Which of the following neoplasms is most likely to be present in this patient?

- ❑ (A) Medulloblastoma
- ❑ (B) Glioblastoma multiforme
- ❑ (C) Metastatic lung carcinoma
- ❑ (D) Malignant melanoma
- ❑ (E) Cystic astrocytoma

47 A 37-year-old man who is HIV-1 positive has had increasing memory problems for the past year. He is depressed. During the past 3 months, he has had increasing problems with motor function and is now unable to stand or walk. For the past 3 days, he has had fever, cough, and dyspnea. A bronchoalveolar lavage shows cysts of *Pneumocystis jirovecii*. MR imaging of the brain shows diffuse cerebral atrophy; no focal lesions are identified. On microscopic examination of the brain, which of the following findings is most likely to be present?

- ❑ (A) Plaques of demyelination in periventricular white matter
- ❑ (B) Neocortical senile plaques and neurofibrillary tangles
- ❑ (C) Multiple lacunar infarcts in basal ganglia
- ❑ (D) Spongiform change involving cerebellum and neocortex
- ❑ (E) White matter microglial nodules with multinucleate cells

48 A term infant is born to a 32-year-old woman whose pregnancy was uncomplicated. A newborn physical examination shows a small lower lumbar skin dimple with a protruding tuft of hair. A radiograph shows that the underlying L4 vertebra has lack of closure of the posterior arches. Which of the following is the most likely diagnosis?

- ❑ (A) Dandy-Walker malformation
- ❑ (B) Spina bifida occulta
- ❑ (C) Tuberous sclerosis
- ❑ (D) Arnold-Chiari malformation
- ❑ (E) Meningomyelocele

49 A 5-year-old boy has been irritable for the past 2 days and has complained of an earache for the past 5 days. On physical examination, he has a temperature of 39.1°C. A lumbar puncture is performed, and laboratory examination of the CSF shows numerous neutrophils, slightly increased protein level, and decreased glucose concentration. On Gram staining of the CSF, which of the following is most likely to be seen microscopically?

- ❑ (A) No organisms
- ❑ (B) Gram-positive cocci
- ❑ (C) Gram-negative diplococci
- ❑ (D) Short gram-positive rods
- ❑ (E) Gram-negative bacilli

50 A 55-year-old man who had been healthy all his life now has progressive, symmetric muscular weakness. Two years ago, he noted weakness in the area of the head and neck, which caused difficulty with speech, eye movements, and swallowing. In the past year, the weakness in the upper and lower extremities has increased, and he can no longer stand, walk, or feed himself. His mental function remains intact. Which of the following is the most likely diagnosis?

- ❑ (A) Amyotrophic lateral sclerosis
- ❑ (B) Huntington disease
- ❑ (C) Multiple sclerosis
- ❑ (D) Guillain-Barré syndrome
- ❑ (E) Parkinson disease

51 A neonate is born prematurely at 28 weeks' gestation to a 22-year-old primigravida. The infant is initially stable, and a newborn physical examination shows no abnormalities. The infant becomes severely hypoxemic 24 hours later, and seizure activity is observed. There is poor neurologic development during infancy. CT scan of the head shows symmetrically enlarged cerebral ventricles at 8 months of age. Which of the following perinatal complications most likely produced these findings?

- ❏ (A) Germinal matrix hemorrhage
- ❏ (B) Down syndrome
- ❏ (C) Kernicterus
- ❏ (D) Congenital cytomegalovirus infection
- ❏ (E) Medulloblastoma

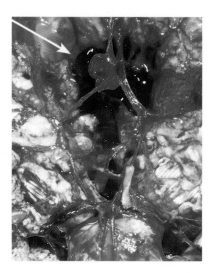

52 A 79-year-old woman was driving her automobile when she had a sudden, severe headache. She drove to a service station, stopped the vehicle, and slumped over the wheel. She was taken to the emergency department, where she remained comatose and died 6 hours later. The gross appearance of the brain at autopsy is shown. Which of the following is the most likely diagnosis?

- ❏ (A) Hemorrhage in a glioblastoma multiforme
- ❏ (B) Thromboembolization with cerebral infarction
- ❏ (C) Tearing of the bridging veins
- ❏ (D) Rupture of a berry aneurysm
- ❏ (E) Hyaline arteriolosclerosis with hemorrhage

53 A study is conducted to identify etiologies of neuronal loss in patients aged 18 to 90 years who died in the hospital from a natural manner of death and who had autopsies performed. Histologic sections are taken from multiple areas of the brain in each patient. The sections are analyzed for the appearance of red, shrunken neurons, decreased numbers of neurons, or absent neurons. A subset of patients is identified in which the hippocampal pyramidal cells, the cerebellar Purkinje cells, and the superior parasagittal neocortical pyramidal cells are affected. The medical records of these patients are reviewed to determine what risk factors for neuronal loss were present before death. Which of the following conditions is most likely to be the major cause of neuronal loss in this subset of patients?

- ❏ (A) Autoimmunity
- ❏ (B) Chemotherapy
- ❏ (C) Diabetes mellitus
- ❏ (D) HIV infection
- ❏ (E) Global hypoxia
- ❏ (F) Lead ingestion
- ❏ (G) Poor nutrition

54 An 83-year-old woman slips in the bathtub in her home and falls backward, striking her head. She is taken to the emergency department, where examination shows a 3-cm reddish, slightly swollen area over the occiput. She is arousable but somnolent. There are no motor or sensory deficits. There is no papilledema. CT scan of the head is performed. Acute hemorrhage in which of the following locations is most likely to be seen?

- ❏ (A) Basis pontis
- ❏ (B) Cerebral ventricle
- ❏ (C) Epidural space
- ❏ (D) Inferior frontal lobe
- ❏ (E) Putamen
- ❏ (F) Sella turcica

55 A 36-year-old woman is involved in a motor vehicle accident. She is not wearing a safety belt and is ejected from the vehicle. When paramedics arrive, her vital signs are stable with pulse of 80/min, respirations 17/min, and blood pressure 125/80 mm Hg. On examination in the emergency department, she has multiple contusions and abrasions over the skin of her head, torso, and extremities. There is no papilledema, no decerebrate posturing, and she has no spontaneous movements. She is not conscious. CT scan of the head shows no intracranial hemorrhage or edema and no skull fractures. She remains in a persistent vegetative state. Which of the following lesions is most likely to be present in this patient?

- ❏ (A) Acute hydrocephalus
- ❏ (B) Cerebellar tonsillar herniation
- ❏ (C) Diffuse axonal injury
- ❏ (D) Hypoxic neuronal damage
- ❏ (E) Multiple cortical contusions
- ❏ (F) Myelinolysis

56 A 77-year-old woman with a 6-year history of small lymphocytic lymphoma was found on physical examination to have no loss of mental, motor, or sensory functions. Her temperature was 37.8°C, pulse 77/min, respirations 18/min, and blood pressure 155/95 mm Hg. She died of *Staphylococcus epidermidis* septicemia while undergoing chemotherapy. At autopsy, there is cardiomegaly with left ventricular hypertrophy. The kidneys are small with irregular granular surfaces. The brain shows a mild amount of cortical atrophy but no ex vacuo ventricular dilation. There is a 0.4-cm cystic area in the left putamen and a similar 0.5-cm lesion in the basis pontis. Which of the following is the most likely pathogenesis of these cystic lesions?

- ❏ (A) Anemia
- ❏ (B) Arteriolosclerosis
- ❏ (C) Chemotherapy
- ❏ (D) *Staphylococcus epidermidis* infection
- ❏ (E) Progressive multifocal leukoencephalopathy
- ❏ (F) Thromboembolism

57 A 63-year-old man had increasing irritability over a period of 3 years. He spent a lot of time wandering about his neighborhood, complaining to the neighbors about everything. He had no memory loss and was always able to find his way home. The neighbors were pleased when he developed aphasia. On physical examination, there were no motor or sensory deficits and no gait disturbances or tremor. MR imaging of the brain showed bilateral marked temporal and frontal lobe gyral atrophy. One year later, he died of pneumonia. At autopsy, the frontal cortex microscopically shows extensive neuronal loss, and some remaining neurons show intracytoplasmic, faintly eosinophilic, rounded inclusions that stain immunohistochemically for tau protein. Which of the following is the most likely diagnosis?

- ❑ (A) Alzheimer disease
- ❑ (B) Huntington disease
- ❑ (C) Leigh disease
- ❑ (D) Multiple system atrophy
- ❑ (E) Parkinson disease
- ❑ (F) Pick disease
- ❑ (G) Vascular dementia

58 A 20-year-old mentally retarded woman saw the physician because she had flank pain for 1 week. Physical examination showed right costovertebral angle tenderness. Patches of skin, some of which appeared leathery (shagreen patches) and some hypopigmented (ash-leaf patches), were scattered over her body. There was a subungual nodule on her right index finger. An abdominal CT scan showed bilateral renal cysts and tumor masses. MR imaging of the brain showed subependymal nodules as well as 1- to 4-cm cortical foci with loss of the gray-white distinction. A chest CT scan showed a 3-cm mass involving the interventricular septum. Two years later, she has sudden, severe headache. MR imaging now shows a nodule obstructing the cerebral aqueduct. Neurosurgery is performed, and a subependymal giant cell astrocytoma is removed. Which of the following is the most likely diagnosis?

- ❑ (A) Down syndrome
- ❑ (B) Krabbe disease
- ❑ (C) Neurofibromatosis type 1
- ❑ (D) Neurofibromatosis type 2
- ❑ (E) Tuberous sclerosis
- ❑ (F) Von Hippel–Lindau disease

59 A 40-year-old man, who rarely had headaches, now has been experiencing headaches for the past 6 months. He comes to the physician because of a seizure that occurred 1 day ago. On physical examination, there are no remarkable findings. MR imaging of the brain shows a solitary, circumscribed 3-cm mass in the right parietal centrum semiovale. The mass has small cysts and areas of calcification and hemorrhage. Neurosurgery is performed, and the mass is removed. Microscopically, the mass consists of sheets of cells with round nuclei that have granular chromatin. The cells have a moderate amount of clear cytoplasm. These cells mark with GFAP

by immunohistochemical staining. The patient receives adjuvant radiation and chemotherapy, and there is no recurrence. Which of the following neoplasms was most likely present in this patient?

- ❑ (A) Astrocytoma
- ❑ (B) Diffuse large B-cell lymphoma
- ❑ (C) Germ cell tumor
- ❑ (D) Glioblastoma multiforme
- ❑ (E) Medulloblastoma
- ❑ (F) Metastatic renal cell carcinoma
- ❑ (G) Oligodendroglioma

60 A 46-year-old woman has had increasing weakness and loss of sensation in the lower extremities for the past 5 months. She comes to the physician because she has been unable to walk without assistance for the past week. On physical examination, there is 4/5 motor strength in the right lower extremity and 3/5 in the left lower extremity. There is bilateral loss of sensation to light touch from the lateral midthigh distally. MR imaging of the spine shows a 1 × 4 cm lesion in the filum terminale. The mass is removed. Microscopically, the mass is composed of cuboidal cells around papillary cores in a myxoid background. Which of the following was most likely present in this patient?

- ❑ (A) Choroid plexus papilloma
- ❑ (B) Ependymoma
- ❑ (C) Meningioma
- ❑ (D) Metastatic transitional cell carcinoma
- ❑ (E) Neurofibroma
- ❑ (F) Pilocytic astrocytoma
- ❑ (G) Schwannoma

61 A 52-year-old woman has had malaise for the past 6 months. On physical examination, there are no remarkable findings. Laboratory studies show hemoglobin of 9.3 g/dL, hematocrit 27.9%, platelet count 549,000/mm³, and WBC count 282,000/mm³ with 64% segmented neutrophils, 10% bands, 3% metamyelocytes, 2% myelocytes, 2% lymphocytes, 1% monocytes, 9% eosinophils, and 9% basophils. She undergoes chemotherapy. Two months later, she develops neurologic deficits with ataxia, motor weakness in the right arm, difficulty swallowing, and sensory changes in the left leg. MR imaging of the brain shows irregular areas of increased attenuation in white matter of the cerebral hemispheres and the cerebellum. A stereotaxic biopsy shows perivascular chronic inflammation, marked gliosis, large reactive astrocytes with bizarre nuclei, and intranuclear inclusions within oligodendroglia. Which of the following infections is most likely to have caused these findings?

- ❑ (A) Cytomegalovirus
- ❑ (B) Herpes simplex virus
- ❑ (C) JC papovavirus
- ❑ (D) Rabies virus
- ❑ (E) Rubeola virus
- ❑ (F) West Nile virus

62 A 39-year-old man who has been infected with HIV for at least 8 years has received no antiretroviral therapy. He has had left-sided weakness for the past month. He sees the physician 1 day after experiencing a generalized seizure. On physical examination, he is afebrile. There is 4/5 motor strength in the left upper extremity. CT scan of the head shows no intracranial hemorrhage, but there is a midline shift. MR imaging of the brain shows a 4-cm mass in the region of the putamen near the right internal capsule, a 3-cm mass in the right centrum semiovale, and a 1-cm mass near the splenium of the corpus callosum. These masses are circumscribed and solid. A lumbar puncture is performed, and analysis of the CSF shows an elevated protein concentration and a normal glucose level. Cytologic examination shows large cells with large nuclei and scant cytoplasm that mark with CD19 but not with GFAP or cytokeratin. Which of the following is the most likely diagnosis?

- (A) Cytomegalovirus encephalitis
- (B) Glioblastoma multiforme
- (C) Kaposi sarcoma
- (D) Large B-cell lymphoma
- (E) Progressive multifocal leukoencephalopathy
- (F) Toxoplasmosis

63 A 60-year-old woman had problems related to movement for 5 years. Physical examination showed cogwheel rigidity of limbs and a festinating gait, which she had difficulty initiating. Her face was expressionless. She was given levodopa, and her condition improved. Two years later, she had difficulty performing activities of daily living and showed marked cognitive decline. She died of aspiration pneumonia. Autopsy findings include mild cerebral atrophy and loss of substantia nigra pigmentation. Microscopically, there is loss of pigmented neurons, and the remaining substantia nigra neurons and cortical neurons show spheroidal, intraneuronal, cytoplasmic, eosinophilic inclusions. Immunohistochemical staining for which of the following proteins is most likely to be positive in these inclusions?

- (A) α-Synuclein
- (B) Amyloid precursor protein
- (C) Apolipoprotein E
- (D) Huntingtin
- (E) Presenilin
- (F) Tau protein

64 A 70-year-old woman comes to the physician because of an episode 2 days earlier during which she lost consciousness for several minutes. Afterward, she had difficulty speaking clearly and had paresthesias in the lower right arm that persisted for several minutes. On physical examination, there is 4/5 motor strength in the right upper extremity and decreased sensation to pinprick on the ulnar aspect of the lower right arm and hand. There are bilateral carotid bruits. A lumbar puncture is performed with normal opening pressure. Laboratory studies on 10 mL of clear, colorless CSF show 2 mononuclear WBCs/mm³, no RBCs, protein concentration of 40 mg/dL, and glucose concentration of 70 mg/dL. The serum glucose concentration is 95 mg/dL. A CT scan of the head shows no intracranial hemorrhage, but there is a slight midline shift; MR imaging of the brain shows an ill-defined area of edema near the left internal capsule. Which of the following laboratory findings is most suggestive of the risk factor for this patient's disease?

- (A) Positive antiphospholipid antibody test result
- (B) Blood culture positive for *Streptococcus pneumoniae*
- (C) Elevated serum concentration of very long chain fatty acids
- (D) Hyperammonemia
- (E) Hypercholesterolemia
- (F) Oligoclonal bands on CSF electrophoresis
- (G) Positive ANA test result
- (H) Positive serologic test result for syphilis

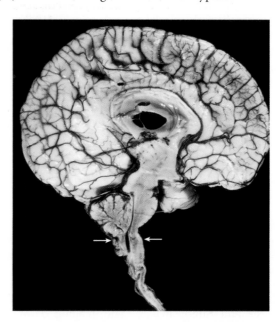

65 A 15-year-old girl is brought to the physician because she has had progressive difficulty speaking during the past 6 months. She becomes dizzy and falls frequently. She complains of headache as well as facial and neck pain. During the past month, she has had decreasing bladder and bowel control. On physical examination, there is loss of pain and temperature sensation over the nape of the neck, shoulders, and upper arms, but vibration and position sensation are preserved. She has muscle wasting in the lower neck and shoulders. MR imaging of the spinal cord shows cervical and thoracic enlargement with a CSF collection dilating the central canal. An MR image of the brain demonstrates gross findings similar to those shown in the figure. Which of the following is the most likely diagnosis?

- (A) Arnold-Chiari II malformation
- (B) Cerebral palsy
- (C) Dandy-Walker malformation
- (D) Holoprosencephaly
- (E) Multiple sclerosis
- (F) Polymicrogyria

66 An infant was born at 36 weeks' gestation to a 22-year-old primigravida. A fetal screening ultrasound study at 18 weeks showed a single large cerebral ventricle and fused thalami. On physical examination at birth, the infant was small for gestational age and had multiple anomalies, including postaxial polydactyly of hands and feet, cyclopia, microcephaly, cleft lip and palate, and rocker bottom feet. The infant died 1 hour after birth. Which of the following CNS abnormalities best explains these findings?

☐ (A) Anencephaly
☐ (B) Arnold-Chiari II malformation
☐ (C) Dandy-Walker malformation
☐ (D) Holoprosencephaly
☐ (E) Periventricular leukomalacia
☐ (F) Subdural hematoma

67 An 86-year-old man has become progressively unable to live independently for the past 10 years, and he now requires assistance with bathing, dressing, toileting, feeding, and transfers in and out of chairs and bed. On physical examination he has no motor or sensory deficits. He cannot give the current date or state where he is. Six months later he suddenly becomes comatose and dies. At autopsy there is a large superficial left parietal lobe hemorrhage. Histologic examination of the brain shows numerous neocortical neuritic plaques and neurofibrillary tangles. The peripheral cerebral arteries and the core of each plaque stain positively with Congo red. Which of the following mechanisms is most likely responsible for his disease?

☐ (A) Aggregation of Aβ peptide
☐ (B) Conformational change in the prion protein (PrP)
☐ (C) Mutations in the *tau* gene
☐ (D) Mutations in the *frataxin* gene
☐ (E) Dopamine deficiency
☐ (F) Expansion of polyglutamine repeats

ANSWERS

1 **(C)** Headache, fever, a high CSF protein level, and a low glucose concentration all point to bacterial meningitis. *Staphylococcus aureus* is a common infection among intravenous drug users. This patient does not have a mass lesion of toxoplasmosis or focal lesions of progressive multifocal leukoencephalopathy (PML) that may be associated with AIDS. PML is associated with the JC papovavirus. A tuberculous meningitis has a more insidious onset. Herpes simplex virus produces encephalitis, not meningitis. Toxoplasmosis, which may occur in immunocompromised patients, produces parenchymal abscesses, not meningitis.

BP7 825-826   BP6 726-727   PBD7 1369-1370
PBD6 1314-1315

2 **(E)** This patient has a rapidly progressive dementia that is most consistent with Creutzfeldt-Jakob disease (CJD). CJD is one of a group of diseases that are called spongiform encephalopathies, because they produce a vacuolated appearance of the cortex. CJD occurs in sporadic or familial forms and is believed to be caused by prions. The normal prion proteins of the brain, designated PrP^c, can undergo conformational change to PrP^sc, which then induces further change in PrP^c to PrP^sc. This patient's age and clinical findings are characteristic of the sporadic type of CJD, which may arise from spontaneous mutation or from exposure to PrP^sc. Variant CJD (vCJD), which may be possibly linked to exposure to bovine spongiform encephalopathy, occurs in much younger patients and does not produce the characteristic EEG findings. Neu-

ritic plaques are seen in Alzheimer disease, which occurs over many years. The demyelinating plaques of multiple sclerosis develop over years, as do the Lewy bodies of Parkinson disease and diffuse Lewy body disease. Microglial nodules may be seen in persons with AIDS.

BP7 830-832   BP6 730-731   PBD7 1380-1382
PBD6 1323-1324

3 **(E)** This patient has Wernicke disease, which results from a deficiency of vitamin B₁ (thiamine). Wernicke disease is uncommon in persons who have a varied diet, but those with a history of chronic alcoholism may not have a well-balanced diet. Capillary proliferation, hemorrhage, necrosis, and hemosiderin deposition are often found in the mamillary bodies and the periaqueductal gray matter, resulting in paralysis of the extraocular muscles. If memory problems with confabulation are observed, the term Wernicke-Korsakoff syndrome is used. Dementia may be present in niacin deficiency. Folate deficiency does not produce CNS signs. A deficiency of pyridoxine may result in a peripheral neuropathy. Subacute combined degeneration of the spinal cord may be seen in vitamin B₁₂ (cobalamin) deficiency.

BP7 839-840   BP6 738   PBD7 423, 457, 1399
PBD6 1341

4 **(E)** This patient's immunocompromised state has resulted in infection with *Cryptococcus neoformans*, which is distributed worldwide. Most *Cryptococcus* infections probably start in the lung, but the CNS is the second most commonly involved area, and meningitis is the most typical manifestation. Cryptococci can be visualized by an India ink test, because the thick, gelatinous capsule of the fungus does not stain black with the dye. Septicemia caused by *Staphylococcus aureus* or disseminated *Mycobacterium tuberculosis* infection is common in AIDS, but it does not commonly produce lesions in the CNS. *Listeria* is infrequently seen in AIDS; it can cause meningitis, but the organisms are not visualized with India ink. *Toxoplasma gondii* is a frequent cause of CNS disease in AIDS, but the organisms are found in parenchymal abscesses, not in the CSF.

BP7 311, 826   BP6 727-728   PBD7 399, 1378
PBD6 1322

5 **(B)** Metastases are typically multiple and are found at the gray-white junction, where peripheral arteries branch and narrow acutely. Metastases from malignant melanomas are often widely disseminated, with multiple mass lesions in organ sites of involvement. AIDS is not associated with metastatic disease to the brain; although primary infections such as toxoplasmosis could produce focal lesions, they would not occur only at the gray-white junction, and they would be ring enhancing. Septic emboli from endocarditis could be found in a similar distribution, but the patient would be septic, and abscesses often show enhancement on CT scan or MR imaging. Cysticerci are irregularly distributed in the parenchyma and are typically 1 cm or smaller. The neurofibromas and schwannomas of neurofibromatosis type 1 are peripheral, not cortical.

BP7 836-837   BP6 735   PBD7 1410   PBD6 1351

6 **(C)** Hemorrhagic lesions of the temporal lobes are characteristic of herpes simplex virus infection; cases are few and usually sporadic, occurring in apparently healthy persons. Cytomegalovirus infection occurs in neonates and in immunocompromised adults, but it does not produce hemorrhagic lesions. Meningococcal infections produce a meningitis. Arboviral infections produce focal lesions that may have an associated vasculitis with hemorrhage, but the CSF protein is usually elevated, and there is a neutrophilic pleocytosis. The lesions of aspergillosis can be hemorrhagic, but they are typically seen in immunocompromised persons.

BP7 828-829   BP6 729   PBD7 1373-1374
PBD6 1318-1319

7   (E) This patient's clinical signs and symptoms are typical of acute meningitis, and there is a purulent exudate on the cerebral convexities, indicative of bacterial infection. At his age, a common etiologic agent is *Neisseria meningitidis*. Cryptococcosis should be considered in immunocompromised patients. Tuberculous meningitis does not manifest so acutely, and the exudate is typically on the base of the brain. Cerebral toxoplasmosis may occur in immunocompromised patients, but the lesions are parenchymal abscesses, not meningitis. Poliomyelitis could occur after pharyngitis, but onset is insidious, with increasing paralysis from loss of motor neurons. It does not cause meningitis.

BP7 825-827   BP6 726-727   PBD7 1369-1370
PBD6 1314-1315

8   (E) This patient has asterixis, a condition resulting from liver failure with hepatic encephalopathy that can occur in severe liver disease from a variety of causes including commonly chronic alcoholism. Hyperammonemia is a feature of liver failure. Hyponatremia from diabetes insipidus may result in obtundation. Severe hypoglycemia can damage neurons in the hippocampus and neocortex. An elevated hemoglobin A_{1c} level suggests a diagnosis of diabetes mellitus, and diabetic patients are most prone to peripheral neuropathies and autonomic neuropathies. Carbon monoxide poisoning can produce obtundation and coma.

BP7 598, 840   PBD7 1400   PBD6 1342

9   (C) The clinical history of dementia, and the presence of numerous neuritic plaques and amyloid deposition in blood vessel walls, is characteristic of Alzheimer disease. The ε4 allele of the ApoE4 gene increases the risk of developing Alzheimer disease by unknown mechanisms. There is no association between HLA genes and this disease. Expansion of CAG repeats on chromosome 4p16 causes Huntington disease. Mutant prion genes give rise to spongiform encephalopathies, such as Creutzfeldt-Jacob disease. Deficiency of thiamine in chronic alcoholism causes Wernicke-Korsakoff syndrome.

BP7 841-843   BP6 739   PBD7 1385-1389
PBD6 1329-1333

10   (E) This patient has a subdural hematoma resulting from tearing of the bridging veins beneath the dura. These veins are at risk of tearing with head trauma, particularly in the elderly, in whom some degree of cerebral atrophy may be present. Pontine hemorrhages are likely to be Duret hemorrhages. Subarachnoid hemorrhage could occur in contusions with trauma. Basal ganglia hemorrhages are most often associated with hypertension. Epidural hemorrhages are most

often preceded by a blow to the head that tears the middle meningeal artery; there is commonly a "lucid" interval between an initial loss of consciousness occurring with trauma and the later accumulation of blood.

BP7 819   BP6 722   PBD7 1359-1360   PBD6 1305

11   (E) This patient had an acute lymphocytic meningitis, which is most typically caused by a virus, such as West Nile virus, an equine encephalitis virus, or an echovirus. It is sometimes referred to as aseptic meningitis, because routine Gram staining and bacterial cultures are negative. Most cases are self-limited, occur in immunocompetent persons, and resolve without significant sequelae. Listerial and meningococcal infections are seen sporadically and have a neutrophilic response. Cryptococcal and toxoplasmal infections can occur in immunocompromised patients, but the India ink test would be positive in the former, and the CT scan would show focal lesions in the latter.

BP7 826   BP6 727   PBD7 1370, 1373   PBD6 1315

12   (B) Intracranial aneurysms are typically saccular and slowly enlarge over time. Those that reach 4 to 7 mm are at greatest risk of rupture. Rupture occurs into the subarachnoid space at the base of the brain, where the cerebral arterial distribution originates around the circle of Willis and where saccular aneurysms are most likely to arise. Epidural hematomas arise from a tear of the middle meningeal artery, typically as a result of head trauma. Trauma can also cause a tear of bridging veins that produces a subdural hematoma. Neither a berry aneurysm nor the bleeding that results is likely to cause a mass effect and herniation. In some cases of survival after rupture of a berry aneurysm, a noncommunicating hydrocephalus results from organization of the subarachnoid hemorrhage.

BP7 816-818   BP6 720   PBD7 1366-1368
PBD6 1311-1312

13   (E) Amyotrophic lateral sclerosis causes loss of upper motor neurons, leading to progressive muscular weakness from grouped atrophy of skeletal muscle fibers (denervation atrophy). Becker muscular dystrophy can produce progressive weakness in middle-aged men as a result of the decreased dystrophin level in muscle, but the CNS is not affected. In neurofibromatosis, mass lesions may be seen, including neurofibromas, schwannomas, meningiomas, and gliomas. Guillain-Barré syndrome is a form of rapidly ascending paralysis that occurs over weeks. Creutzfeldt-Jakob disease is a rapidly progressive form of dementia that results in death in less than 1 year in most cases.

BP7 846   BP6 741   PBD7 1396-1397   PBD6 1338

14   (B) The "lucid" interval is a classic feature of an epidural hematoma. In an acute subdural hematoma or a ruptured aneurysm, there typically is no lucid interval but instead a sudden and progressive worsening of symptoms. Contusions do not progressively worsen. Leptomeningitis is not associated with trauma. Because cannabinoids are stored in adipose tissue and released irregularly for up to 1 month after the last use (or even after secondhand exposure in a smoke-filled room), low levels may be detected for weeks or may appear and disappear.

BP7 818-819   BP6 721-722   PBD7 1358-1359
PBD6 1304-1305

15 (A) The multiple pigmented skin lesions and optic nerve glioma strongly suggest the diagnosis of neurofibromatosis type 1. Patients with this condition, which has an autosomal dominant inheritance, have multiple large café-au-lait spots on the skin, and there is a propensity for development of multiple nerve sheath tumors (schwannomas or neurofibromas). CNS gliomas may also occur. The nerve sheath tumors may become malignant and metastasize, most commonly to the lungs. Of the other neoplasms listed, only meningioma is associated with neurofibromatosis type 1, but it occurs intracranially.

BP7 226-227, 848-849   BP6 725, 743   PBD7 1411-1413
PBD6 1354

16 (D) This patient has Parkinson disease. The most characteristic feature is loss of dopamine-secreting pigmented neurons in the substantia nigra of the midbrain. Some patients with Parkinson disease also have dementia, and Lewy bodies may be found. Neurofibrillary tangles in the neocortex are a feature of Alzheimer disease. Huntington disease affects the caudate. Wernicke-Korsakoff syndrome is caused by vitamin B_1 (thiamine) deficiency and affects the mamillary bodies; hemorrhages in this area eventually give rise to the deposition of hemosiderin. Alzheimer type II gliosis is seen in chronic alcoholism.

BP7 844   BP6 740-741   PBD7 1391-1393
PBD6 1333-1334

17 (C) In herniation of the brain stem, branches of the basilar artery are kinked. This gives rise to hemorrhagic infarcts in the midbrain and pons. Such infarcts, called Duret hemorrhages, have a typical ventral-to-dorsal orientation and occur in the midline or paramedian regions. Tearing of bridging veins gives rise to subdural hematomas. Rupture of the middle meningeal artery gives rise to epidural hematomas. Hemorrhage resulting from berry aneurysms is subarachnoid. Sudden global hypoxia resulting from hypotension gives rise to widespread brain infarction.

BP7 812-813   BP6 716-722   PBD7 1352-1353
PBD6 1298, 1304-1312

18 (A) Meningiomas typically are circumscribed lesions that arise from meningothelial cells of the arachnoid and appear grossly attached to the overlying dura. They are most often seen in adult women. A parasagittal, sphenoid ridge, or subfrontal location is typical. Tuberculomas from disseminated tuberculosis are rare and usually occur at the base of the brain. Medulloblastomas are tumors of the posterior fossa that occur in children. The most typical location for a schwannoma is at the cerebellopontine angle, involving the eighth cranial nerve. Ependymomas arise in ventricles.

BP7 836   BP6 734-735   PBD7 1409-1410
PBD6 1350-1351

19 (E) This patient has Huntington disease, a progressive degenerative disorder that affects the caudate nuclei. This disease is caused by an abnormal expansion of the trinucleotide CAG in the *huntingtin* gene on chromosome 4. The more repeats, the earlier is the onset of the disease. Tay-Sachs disease of infancy and childhood is caused by a deficiency of hexosaminidase A. Mutations in presenilin genes cause familial Alzheimer disease. The risk of Alzheimer disease increases with increased levels of apoprotein E. Trisomy 21 results in mental retardation present at birth. About 10% of Creutzfeldt-Jakob disease cases are genetically determined, with the inheritance of an abnormal prion protein that leads to spongiform encephalopathy in later adult life.

BP7 844-846   BP6 741   PBD7 1393-1394
PBD6 1335-1338

20 (C) The findings indicate anencephaly, a form of severe neural tube defect that results from failure of formation of the fetal cranial vault. This is one of the most common CNS malformations seen at birth. The defect allows fetal α-fetoprotein to enter amniotic fluid and reach the maternal circulation. Neural tube defects are not associated with neonatal jaundice. Cytomegalovirus infection can produce extensive parenchymal necrosis but not loss of the fetal cranial vault. Diabetes mellitus, suggested by an elevated hemoglobin A_{1c} concentration, can increase the risk of malformations (e.g., holoprosencephaly in the CNS) but not neural tube defects. Down syndrome (trisomy 21) may be associated with brachycephaly, but rarely with anencephaly.

BP7 821-823   BP6 723-724   PBD7 1353-1354
PBD6 1299-1300

21 (E) The rapid correction of hyponatremia is one of the common antecedents to demyelination in the basis pontis. Herniation is unlikely, because cerebral edema would cause papilledema. Intracranial hemorrhages would not result from electrolyte and fluid disturbances. A subacute combined degeneration of the spinal cord occurs slowly as a consequence of vitamin B_{12} (cobalamin) deficiency. Wernicke-Korsakoff syndrome is now a rare accompaniment to chronic alcoholism that affects mamillary bodies and periaqueductal gray matter.

BP7 838   BP6 737   PBD7 1385   PBD6 1329

22 (E) The lesion is a remote cerebral infarction. A large cystic area has resulted from resolution of a liquefactive necrosis after vascular injury in the distribution of the middle cerebral artery. A recent infarction may appear softened, but it takes weeks to months for macrophages to clear the debris of liquefactive necrosis and leave a cystic space. A vascular malformation has irregular vascular channels that give a mass effect with a dark red to bluish appearance. A contusion could produce some minimal focal loss of cortex with brown hemosiderin staining. An organizing subdural hematoma would leave a uniform area of compression with flattening of the hemisphere.

BP7 814-815   BP6 718   PBD7 1361-1365
PBD6 1308-1309

23 (C) This lesion is a senile (or neuritic) plaque with a rim of dystrophic neurites surrounding an amyloid core. Alzheimer disease is a progressive dementia marked by plaques and neurofibrillary tangles. This is the most common form of dementia. Symmetric muscular weakness suggests amyotrophic lateral sclerosis. Gait disturbances occur in Parkinson disease. Seizures are associated with many lesions, but often a pathologic finding is not discernible. Choreiform movements suggest Huntington disease.

BP7 841-843   BP6 739-740   PBD7 1386-1388
PBD6 1329-1331

24 (D) Cytomegalovirus (CMV) infection is one of the congenital TORCH infections, and it can become widely disseminated to affect the CNS. Periventricular necrosis is characteristic of CMV infection. Failure of the heart in utero causes hydrops fetalis. Listeriosis can produce focal microabscesses in various organs, but usually there is minimal necrosis. HIV infection produces no significant CNS findings in the perinatal period. Herpes simplex virus infection of neonates typically occurs during passage through the infected birth canal, not in utero. Group B streptococcal infections cause premature rupture of membranes and sepsis without significant CNS findings.

BP7 242, 310, 829   BP6 729   PBD7 366-367, 1374
PBD6 376, 1319

25 (A) Most malignant neoplasms of the brain in children are in the posterior fossa. The two most common neoplasms at this site are cystic cerebellar astrocytoma and medulloblastoma. The type of astrocytoma seen at this location is a pilocytic astrocytoma, and it has a better overall prognosis than do glial neoplasms in adults. Both may enlarge and block CSF flow, causing hydrocephalus. Medulloblastomas often occur in the cerebellar midline and are composed of small, round, blue cells. A hemangioblastoma is a rare cystic mass in adults, typically arising in the cerebellum, and may be associated with polycythemia. Meningiomas occur in adults; they are circumscribed, solid mass lesions adjacent to the dura, and may be multiple in neurofibromatosis. Brain metastases are rare in children, because most are metastatic carcinomas. Cerebral lymphomas are rare, except in persons with HIV infection. Oligodendrogliomas are solitary, circumscribed mass lesions in the cerebral hemisphere of adults. A schwannoma typically arises in the eighth cranial nerve in adults.

BP7 833   BP6 733-734   PBD7 1403-1404
PBD6 1348-1349

26 (A) Loss of pigmented dopaminergic neurons in the substantia nigra of the midbrain is most characteristic of Parkinson disease. Pill-rolling tremors at rest are typical of this disorder. Symmetric weakness suggests a motor neuron disease. Paraplegia suggests a disruption in the motor pathways, such as an infarction. Choreiform movements suggest Huntington disease, which affects the caudate, not the substantia nigra. Short-term memory problems suggest hippocampal lesions.

BP7 844   BP6 740-741   PBD7 1391-1393
PBD6 1333-1334

27 (D) A cerebral abscess is most often a complication of an infection, such as pneumonia, that occurred days to weeks earlier. The bacteria spread hematogenously. As the abscess organizes, it is ringed by fibroblasts that deposit collagen; this feature is characteristic of an abscess in the CNS. A neoplasm may be ring enhancing on occasion, but a glioblastoma multiforme is not well demarcated, and metastases are typically multifocal. A multiple sclerosis plaque is not as large and does not typically have ring enhancement. An infarct would produce sudden signs and symptoms that improve over time, and the CSF protein would not be increased.

BP7 827   BP6 728-729   PBD7 1371   PBD6 1315-1316

28 (C) The brief episodes of neurologic dysfunction represent transient ischemic attacks (TIAs) and are a prodrome to stroke in many cases. Atherosclerotic cerebrovascular disease is a common antecedent to cerebral infarction. A neoplasm is unlikely to produce such sudden symptoms and signs. A subdural hematoma, which most frequently results from head trauma sustained in a fall, is unlikely to develop in a few minutes and would not explain the TIAs. A vascular malformation most often produces symptoms caused by bleeding in young adults. Meningoencephalitis may produce general features such as headache, confusion, and seizures, but not sudden localizing signs.

BP7 813-815   BP6 718   PBD7 1361-1363
PBD6 1308-1310

29 (B) This shifting spectrum of clinical findings over time in a young adult suggests the diagnosis of multiple sclerosis. The plaques of demyelination that give rise to the differing symptoms can be found in various locations, but they most often occur in periventricular white matter. CSF immunoglobulins are increased, and most patients show oligoclonal bands of IgG. Cryptococcal meningitis would manifest more acutely with meningeal signs. Primary or malignant brain tumors are not common at this age and would not have such a long course without serious sequelae. Xanthochromia from hemorrhage would suggest a more acute problem. Neurosyphilis is rare at this age and would not cause localizing signs.

BP7 837-838   BP6 736   PBD7 1382-1385
PBD6 1326-1327

30 (C) The findings point to Huntington disease, which has an autosomal dominant inheritance pattern and an onset in middle age. It results from increased trinucleotide repeat mutations in the *huntingtin* gene on chromosome 4, which normally has 6 to 34 CAG copies. There may be 40 to 55 copies in patients with typical Huntington disease and as many as 70 repeats in persons with earlier onset of the disease. These patients have atrophy, with loss of neurons and gliosis in the caudate, putamen, and globus pallidus. The loss of pigmented neurons is typical of Parkinson disease. Congophilic angiopathy can be seen in Alzheimer disease. Loss of motor neurons is a feature of amyotrophic lateral sclerosis. Multiple lacunar infarcts may be seen in chronic hypertension.

BP7 844-846   BP6 741   PBD7 184, 1393-1394
PBD6 1335-1336

31 (A) In children, an inherited form of CNS disease that accounts for a progressively worsening course should be suspected. The leukodystrophies affect white matter extensively and cause myelin loss and abnormal accumulations of myelin. A variety of lysosomal enzyme defects lead to these disorders, which are characterized by failure of generation or maintenance of myelin. However, there are no discrete plaques of demyelination, in contrast to multiple sclerosis. Sparing of subcortical myelin (U fiber) is often seen in leukodystrophies. Progressive multifocal leukoencephalopathy is an infectious lesion that occurs in immunocompromised adults. Tay-Sachs disease affects infants. Acute disseminated encephalomyelitis is a postinfectious process with abrupt onset.

BP7 838-839   BP6 737   PBD7 1397-1398   PBD6 1340

32 (A) Tearing of bridging veins gives rise to an acute subdural hematoma. This almost always results from head trauma in which there has been a fall. The risk of hemorrhage is greater in elderly persons because of cerebral atrophy, which leaves the bridging veins beneath the dura at the vertex more vulnerable to traumatic tearing. When saccular (berry) aneurysms rupture, the bleeding is typically subarachnoid and at the base of the brain. Arteriovenous (vascular) malformations are often located within the parenchyma of a hemisphere, and bleeding from them occurs more often in young adults. A tear of the middle meningeal artery can occur in head trauma (e.g., a blow to the head), but it results in an acute epidural hematoma. Thrombosis of an intracranial artery may result in an infarction, which can be hemorrhagic, but the hemorrhage typically does not extend into subarachnoid or subdural locations.

BP7 819   BP6 722   PBD7 1359-1360   PBD6 1305

33 **(C)** About 1 in 100 persons has a saccular (berry) aneurysm. Although this lesion is present at birth as a congenital defect in the arterial media at intracerebral artery branch points, it can manifest later in life with aneurysmal dilation and possible rupture. These aneurysms are the most common cause of spontaneous subarachnoid hemorrhage in adults. Thromboemboli can cause infarctions, most often in the distribution of the middle cerebral artery in cortex, and embolic infarcts can be hemorrhagic, but the blood typically does not reach the CSF. A subdural hematoma results from a tear of bridging veins. The bleeding from amyloid angiopathy is in peripheral cortex. A hypertensive hemorrhage tends to remain in the brain parenchyma.

BP7 816-817   BP6 720   PBD7 1366-1368
PBD6 1311-1312

34 **(D)** Toxoplasmosis is one of the more common opportunistic infections that affect the CNS in patients with AIDS. Toxoplasmosis produces abscesses that organize on the periphery to produce a bright ring on CT and MR imaging scans. Lymphomas can also produce this picture, but they generally occur as fewer, larger masses or as a solitary mass. *Candida* infections of the CNS are rare, and disseminated candidiasis in AIDS is uncommon. A spongiform encephalopathy, such as Creutzfeldt-Jakob disease, typically has no grossly visible or radiographic findings. Metastatic carcinoma is uncommon at this age.

BP7 827-828   BP6 729   PBD7 1378-1379   PBD6 1323

35 **(D)** The clinical features, location, and cytologic findings all point to the diagnosis of medulloblastoma. Most intracranial neoplasms in children are located in the posterior fossa. The medulloblastoma, one of the "blue cell tumors" of childhood, arises in the midline, and the cells can seed into the CSF. Schwannomas are benign neoplasms that do not seed the CSF. Ependymomas can occur in children, but they typically arise in the ventricles. A glioblastoma multiforme could also seed the CSF, but this neoplasm occurs in adults. Metastatic disease is uncommon in children.

BP7 834-835   BP6 734   PBD7 1407-1408
PBD6 1346-1348

36 **(B)** This patient has multiple sclerosis with plaques of demyelination. The course of multiple sclerosis is variable, with many relapses and remissions, and some patients are affected more than others. Some patients have minimal problems, but most can be expected to have further neurologic

problems. Severe neurologic impairment and death are unlikely, and most patients live for decades. There is no defined inheritance pattern. Multiple sclerosis is not associated with HIV infection. The neurologic problems observed in HIV-infected persons are related mainly to dementia.

BP7 837-838   BP6 736   PBD7 1382-1385
PBD6 1326-1327

37 **(B)** Thromboembolic disease leading to cerebral infarcts most often results from a cardiac disease (e.g., endocarditis, mural thrombosis, prosthetic valvular thrombosis). Hypertension is associated with basal ganglia, pontine, and cerebellar hemorrhages and with small lacunar infarcts in basal ganglia. Head trauma with hemorrhage is more common in persons with chronic alcoholism. AIDS is not associated with significant cardiovascular or cerebrovascular diseases. Metastatic carcinomas may be found at the gray-white junction, but they do not typically produce infarction.

BP7 814-815   BP6 718-719   PBD7 1363-1365
PBD6 1308-1310

38 **(D)** Hypertensive hemorrhages are most likely to arise in the basal ganglia, thalamus, cerebral white matter, pons, or cerebellum. Multiple hemorrhages are uncommon. The small vessels weakened by hyaline arteriolosclerosis are prone to rupture. Thromboemboli can produce cerebral infarctions, sometimes with hemorrhage, and usually involve the cerebral cortex. Metastases are typically multiple and peripheral at the gray-white junction. The plaques of multiple sclerosis occur in white matter and do not bleed. Chronic alcoholism predisposes to falls with subdural hematomas or contusions.

BP7 816   BP6 719   PBD7 1366   PBD6 1310

39 **(B)** The papilledema and the herniation are a consequence of brain swelling. The herniation of the uncus results in a third cranial nerve palsy as the nerve is compressed. Rupture of a berry aneurysm produces subarachnoid hemorrhage at the base of the brain, which is less likely to result in a mass effect. There is no pressure effect with hydrocephalus ex vacuo, which is a consequence of atrophy. A chronic subdural hemorrhage accumulates slowly enough that herniation may not occur. An infarct is not likely to produce significant associated brain swelling. An abscess may cause some associated brain swelling, but this patient is afebrile.

BP7 811-812   BP6 716   PBD7 1352-1353   PBD6 1298

40 **(E)** Multiple discrete neoplasms in the CNS are more likely to be metastases than a primary brain tumor. Tumor cells may reach the brain in the form of emboli through the cerebral arterial circulation. Most embolic events occur at the gray-white junction, where narrowing and acute branching of the vessels tend to trap emboli. The distribution of the middle cerebral artery, which receives the most blood, is the most likely location. Glioblastomas are large, malignant primary glial neoplasms; they are invasive but do not appear as multiple small lesions. A hemangioblastoma is a rare cystic mass in adults, typically arising in the cerebellum, and may be associated with polycythemia. Medulloblastomas are cerebellar neoplasms that occur in children. Meningiomas are circumscribed, solid mass lesions adjacent to the dura; they may be multiple in persons with neurofibromatosis. Cerebral lymphomas are rare, except in patients with HIV infection.

Oligodendrogliomas are solitary, circumscribed mass lesions that occur in the cerebral hemispheres of adults. A schwannoma typically arises in the eighth cranial nerve.

BP7 836-837   BP6 735   PBD7 1410   PBD6 1351

41 (A) Arteriovenous malformations most often occur in the cerebral hemisphere of a young adult and can be removed by a neurosurgeon. There may be slow leakage of blood from the lesion over time, resulting in the clinical symptoms and the gliosis seen on biopsy in this case. An abscess would have an organizing wall with collagen and gliosis but no prominent larger vessels. An angiosarcoma is not a primary lesion in the brain parenchyma. Head trauma generally produces contusions and hematomas on the surface but not hemorrhages in the brain parenchyma. A ruptured aneurysm can, in some cases, extend upward into parenchyma; with this complication, the outcome is always fatal. A plaque of demyelination in multiple sclerosis can appear as a mass, but its features include loss of myelin with gliosis and macrophages, not vascular abnormalities.

BP7 818   BP6 721   PBD7 1367-1368   PBD6 1313

42 (A) This tan-yellow mass is a meningioma, a benign tumor that arises in meningothelial cells beneath the dura. Gliomas are most often found within a cerebral hemisphere in an adult. Ependymomas are seen within ventricles or on the distal spinal cord. The parasagittal location is unusual for a metastatic lesion, although some malignancies, such as breast carcinomas, may involve the dura in a diffuse fashion. Tuberculomas are rare complications of disseminated tuberculosis and often appear at the base of the brain.

BP7 836   BP6 734-735   PBD7 1409-1410
PBD6 1350-1351

43 (E) This patient has Alzheimer disease, a progressive dementia marked by plaques and neurofibrillary tangles. This is the most common form of dementia. Other forms of dementia include diffuse Lewy body disease, Huntington disease with caudate atrophy, Pick disease, and various forms of multisystem atrophy. The number of senile plaques normally increases with age, but persons with Alzheimer disease have many more plaques, and this finding is diagnostic of the disease. Oligodendroglial inclusions are seen in progressive multifocal leukoencephalopathy.

BP7 841-843   BP6 739-740   PBD7 1386-1389
PBD6 1329-1333

44 (A) The brain stem shows linear midline hemorrhages, called Duret hemorrhages. The acute bacterial meningitis led to brain swelling with edema and subsequent herniation with Duret hemorrhages in the pons. Although not seen in this figure, an infection could organize with scarring of foramina to produce a noncommunicating hydrocephalus, or it could scar the vertex and impair reabsorption of CSF at the arachnoid granulations to produce a communicating hydrocephalus. An abscess infrequently complicates meningitis; conversely, an abscess in a paranasal sinus or mastoid air cell may extend into the cranial cavity to cause meningitis. The small meningeal vessels do not bleed due to inflammation caused by a meningitis. Laminar necrosis could occur after brain death, but this finding is not specific for meningitis.

BP7 812-813   BP6 716   PBD7 1352-1353   PBD6 1298

45 (C) A schwannoma in this location is also known as a cerebellopontine angle tumor. Schwannomas in this location arise from the eighth cranial nerve; they are also called acoustic neuromas. Most schwannomas are benign, slow-growing tumors that can be resected. Meningiomas are rare at this location. Astrocytomas most often involve the hemispheres of adults and the cerebellum of children. Medulloblastomas likewise typically arise in the cerebellum in children. Ependymomas arise in the ventricular system, often in the fourth ventricle.

BP7 848-849   BP6 743   PBD7 1411-1412   PBD6 1352

46 (B) The location in the cerebral hemispheres and the presence of necrosis with pseudopalisading are characteristic of an aggressive brain tumor called glioblastoma multiforme. This is the most malignant form of glioma. These neoplasms can infiltrate widely within the CNS, particularly along white matter tracts. The prognosis is poor. Metastases usually are found at the gray-white junction and are multiple. Medulloblastomas and cystic astrocytomas are neoplasms located in the posterior fossa in children. Primary CNS melanomas are rare.

BP7 832-833   BP6 732   PBD7 1401-1403
PBD6 1343-1345

47 (E) This patient has AIDS dementia complex late in the course of his HIV infection. HIV-1 produces an encephalitis that is characterized by a collection of reactive microglial cells (microglial nodules). HIV-1–infected mononuclear cells, particularly macrophages, can fuse to form multinucleate cells, which are seen in association with microglial nodules. Plaques of demyelination are typical of multiple sclerosis. Senile plaques and tangles are typical of Alzheimer disease and are unlikely to manifest at this patient's age. Lacunar infarcts are small, cavitary infarcts that result from arteriolosclerosis of the deep penetrating arteries and arterioles. Such arteriolar lesions occur in persons with long-standing hypertension and are unlikely to be found in a 37-year-old man. Spongiform change suggests Creutzfeldt-Jakob disease, a rapidly progressive dementia unrelated to HIV infection.

BP7 829-830   BP6 730   PBD7 1375-1376
PBD6 1320-1321

48 (B) Spina bifida occulta is the mildest form of neural tube defect. It is characterized by defective closure of the vertebral arches with intact meninges and spinal cord. A radiograph may demonstrate its presence in up to 20% of the population. A Dandy-Walker malformation is detected by ultrasonographic evidence of a cyst in the fourth ventricle and agenesis of the cerebellar vermis. Tuberous sclerosis is a rare disease that causes firm hamartomatous "tubers" in the cortex. In an Arnold-Chiari malformation, there is a small posterior fossa and extension of the cerebellum into the foramen magnum, as well as a lumbar meningomyelocele. Meningomyeloceles are open neural tube defects.

BP7 821-822   BP6 724   PBD7 1354   PBD6 1300-1302

49 (E) This patient has acute bacterial meningitis. In his age group, the most common etiologic organism is now *Streptococcus pneumoniae*, a gram-positive coccus. The number of CNS infections with *Haemophilus influenzae*, a gram-negative bacillus, in this age group has decreased due to widespread immunization. Pneumococci are also likely to be seen in an adult. The gram-negative diplococci of *Neisseria meningitidis* are seen in young adults. The short, gram-positive rods of *Listeria monocytogenes* appear sporadically or in epidemics caused by food contamination. The gram-negative bacilli of *Escherichia coli* are most often seen in neonates. With these clinical and CSF features, it would be unusual if bacteria were not present in the CSF.

BP7 825-827   BP6 725-726   PBD7 1369-1370
PBD6 1315

50 **(A)** The progressive and symmetric nature of this patient's disease is a classic feature of amyotrophic lateral sclerosis (ALS). The muscles show a denervation type of grouped atrophy from loss of upper motor neurons. The "bulbar" form of ALS affects mainly cranial nerve nuclei and has a more aggressive course. Huntington disease causes abnormal movements, not weakness, and there can be associated dementia over time. Mental function is preserved in ALS. The demyelinating plaques of multiple sclerosis can produce a variety of motor signs and symptoms over time, but symmetry is not a feature of this disease. Guillain-Barré syndrome usually occurs after a viral infection and manifests as a rapidly progressive ascending motor weakness. Parkinson disease is characterized by rigidity and involuntary movements, not by muscular weakness.

BP7 846   BP6 741-742   PBD7 1396-1397
PBD6 1338-1339

51 **(A)** Germinal matrix hemorrhage is the most common cause of intraventricular hemorrhage in premature infants. The germinal matrix, composed of highly vascularized tissue with primitive cells, is most prominent between 22 and 30 weeks' gestation. Hemorrhages within this area readily occur in common neonatal problems such as hypoxemia, hypercarbia, acidosis, and changes in blood pressure. Hemorrhages in the germinal matrix can extend into the cerebral ventricles and from there into the subarachnoid space. Smaller hemorrhages can resolve without sequelae. With larger hemorrhages, organization of the blood in the aqueduct of Sylvius or the fourth ventricle or foramina of Luschka may obstruct the flow of CSF, producing hydrocephalus. Infants with Down syndrome may have vascular malformations that can bleed into the parenchyma. The bilirubin staining of kernicterus does not result in scarring. Cytomegalovirus infection can cause considerable necrosis of the brain parenchyma, but not hemorrhage. Medulloblastomas are tumors that occur in children (not typically in infants) that could cause obstruction of CSF flow.

BP7 824   BP6 725-726   PBD7 1356   PBD6 1302

52 **(D)** The figure shows an aneurysm in the circle of Willis and extensive subarachnoid hemorrhage. The hemorrhage occurs at the base of the brain, because berry aneurysms involve the circle of Willis and its branches. The vasospasm caused by the leakage of blood can lead to ischemia that further complicates the course. A glioblastoma often has extensive necrosis and some hemorrhage, but the blood remains intraparenchymal. Thromboembolic infarctions can be hemorrhagic, because the embolus does not completely occlude the vessel, but the hemorrhage is localized. Rupture of bridging veins occurs at the vertex beneath the dura, producing a subdural hematoma. Hypertensive hemorrhages most often occur in the basal ganglia, the pons, or the cere-

bellum from rupture of small arteries in hyaline arteriolosclerosis, and the blood typically remains intraparenchymal.

BP7 816-818   BP6 720   PBD7 1366-1368
PBD6 1311-1312

53 **(E)** The neurons that are most sensitive to anoxia reside in the hippocampus, along with the Purkinje cells and the larger neocortical neurons. In addition, the first areas in the neocortex to be affected are the "watershed" areas between the three major cerebral circulations, including the watershed located superiorly between the anterior cerebral and middle cerebral circulations, as in this study. "Red" shrunken neurons, especially in the areas mentioned, are typically seen in the early stages of global hypoxia, as may occur in a severe hypotensive episode. Focal hypoxia leads to infarcts. Autoimmunity can lead to vasculitis and subsequent hypoxemia. Chemotherapy tends to damage actively dividing cells more severely. Diabetes mellitus causes atherosclerosis, which can lead to hypoxemia. HIV infection can produce an encephalitis, and there can be opportunistic infections of the CNS. Lead poisoning leads to encephalopathy, not ischemia. Poor nutrition with a deficiency of thiamine (vitamin B_1) can lead to Wernicke disease, which affects the mamillary bodies and periaqueductal gray matter most severely.

BP7 813-814   BP6 717   PBD7 1350-1351
PBD6 1307-1308

54 **(D)** This patient has the classic "contrecoup" type of injury, in which the moving head strikes an object and the force is transmitted to the opposite side of the head. A fall backward is most likely to produce contusions to the inferior frontal lobes, temporal tips, and inferior temporal lobes. A blow to a stationary head is more likely to produce a "coup" injury directly adjacent to the site of the blow. Hemorrhage into the pons is typical of a Duret hemorrhage, seen in medial temporal lobe herniation. Hemorrhage into the cerebral ventricles may occur in premature infants from germinal matrix hemorrhage; in adults, it is not common but may occur with dissection of blood from an intraparenchymal lesion. A blow to the side of the head is more likely to lacerate the middle meningeal artery and produce an epidural hematoma. Putaminal hemorrhage is most likely to occur in hypertension. Subarachnoid hemorrhage at the base of the brain may dissect into the sella.

BP7 819-821   BP6 722-723   PBD7 1357-1358
PBD6 1303-1304

55 **(C)** Angular acceleration with torsional forces applied to white matter tracts can cause stretching and tearing of axons, followed by axonal swelling or "retraction balls" within hours. Acute hydrocephalus requires a blockage of CSF flow, and there is no mass lesion, hemorrhage, or brain swelling in this case. Herniation requires brain swelling or a large hemorrhage or a mass that enlarges rapidly. Hypoxic injury is most likely to affect neurons of the hippocampus, Purkinje cells, and cortical neurons in watershed areas first; this patient's vital signs suggest that this did not occur. Contusions represent areas of superficial cortical hemorrhage. Central pontine myelinolysis can occur from rapid correction of hyponatremia.

BP7 819-821   BP6 722-723   PBD7 1358-1359
PBD6 1304

56 (B) These small cavitary lesions are lacunar infarcts. They are relatively common findings at autopsy, because arteriosclerosis (linked to hypertension) is common. These lesions are considered incidental findings when there are few and they are small and scattered. This patient's cardiac and renal findings suggest hypertension. Anemia may lead to hypoxemia with neuronal loss, but not to focal infarction. Chemotherapy typically damages more actively dividing cells first. Sepsis can lead to abscesses and meningitis, and septic emboli can cause mycotic aneurysms and hemorrhage. Progressive multifocal leukoencephalopathy is a disease of the white matter that produces soft granular lesions; it is caused by JC papovavirus infection in immunocompromised persons. Thromboembolism can produce infarctions, but they typically occur in the distribution of the major cerebral arteries.

PBD7 1368-1369   PBD6 1313-1314

57 (F) Pick disease has clinical features similar to those of Alzheimer disease, but initially it causes less memory loss and more behavioral changes. The "knifelike" gyral atrophy of frontal and temporal lobes and relative sparing of parietal and occipital lobes are characteristic of Pick disease. Pick bodies are seen in remaining neurons, but the neuritic plaques and neurofibrillary tangles seen in Alzheimer disease are not increased. Huntington disease affects mainly the caudate nuclei and basal ganglia; onset occurs in middle age, and choreiform movements are common. Leigh disease is one of the mitochon-drial encephalomyopathies that can cause muscular weakness and neurologic deterioration beginning at a young age. Multiple system atrophy (MSA) has features that overlap those of striatonigral degeneration, olivopontocerebellar atrophy, and Shy-Drager syndrome; most patients with MSA exhibit symptoms similar to those of Parkinson disease. MSA is characterized microscopically by the appearance of glial cytoplasmic inclusions. In Parkinson disease, loss of pigmented neurons in the substantia nigra leads to movement problems. Vascular dementia, or multiinfarct dementia, can have clinical features that mimic those of Alzheimer disease, but there are multiple small infarcts that collectively produce dementia, and the neurologic decline happens in a stepwise fashion.

BP7 843-844   PBD7 1390   PBD6 1333

58 (E) Tuberous sclerosis is one of the phakomatoses—rare inherited disorders in which hamartomas and neoplasms develop throughout the body, as well as cutaneous abnormalities. Persons with tuberous sclerosis have cortical tubers, which are hamartomas of neuronal and glial tissue; other characteristic findings include renal angiomyolipomas, renal cysts, subungual fibromas, and cardiac rhabdomyomas. In Down syndrome (trisomy 21), patients may develop acute leukemia, but not brain neoplasms, and those who survive to middle age develop Alzheimer disease. Krabbe disease is a leukodystrophy that results in deficiency of galactocerebroside β-galactosidase and an onset of neurologic deterioration in infancy. Neurofibromatosis type 1 (NF-1) is characterized by deforming cutaneous and visceral neurofibromas, cutaneous café-au-lait spots, and neurofibrosarcomas. In NF-2, acoustic schwannomas, meningiomas, gliomas, and ependymomas are present. Von Hippel–Lindau disease is characterized by

hemangioblastomas in the cerebellum, retina, and spinal cord, as well as by pheochromocytomas.

BP7 215, 821   BP6 179, 725   PBD7 1413
PBD6 1354-1355

59 (G) Oligodendrogliomas tend to have a better prognosis than most other glial neoplasms. Astrocytomas tend to be less circumscribed. Diffuse large B-cell lymphomas can occur in association with AIDS; they are negative for GFAP but positive for CD19 and CD20. Intracranial germ cell tumors are most likely to arise in the pineal body. Glioblastomas are highly aggressive, infiltrative gliomas. Medulloblastomas are posterior fossa tumors that occur in children. Renal cell carcinoma has cells with clear cytoplasm, but it is not positive for GFAP and often produces multiple metastases. In rare cases, removal of a solitary metastasis of renal cell carcinoma can be beneficial.

BP7 833-834   BP6 733   PBD7 1404   PBD6 1346

60 (B) This patient had the myxopapillary variant of ependymoma, which is more common in adults than in children. The tumors that arise in the ventricles (usually the fourth ventricle) are more common in the first two decades of life. Choroid plexus papillomas are rare tumors that arise in the cerebral ventricles. Meningiomas most often arise in the cranial cavity and have plump, pink, round to spindle-shaped cells, often with psammoma bodies. Metastases to the spinal cord are uncommon. Neurofibromas are more likely to arise in peripheral nerves, although in neurofibromatosis type 1, they can arise in many sites. A pilocytic astrocytoma is one of the common pediatric primary intracranial neoplasms; it arises in the posterior fossa. A schwannoma most often occurs in the eighth cranial nerve, although neurofibromatosis may be associated with multiple schwannomas.

BP7 834   BP6 733   PBD7 1405   PBD6 1346-1347

61 (C) This patient has progressive multifocal leukoencephalopathy, which is caused by the JC papovavirus and occurs in immunocompromised persons, including those with AIDS. The patient was treated for chronic myelogenous leukemia. Cytomegalovirus infection also complicates the course of immunocompromised patients, but it causes large intranuclear inclusions, most often in endothelial cells. Herpes simplex virus is not common, even in immunocompromised patients, and it most often produces a hemorrhagic encephalitis in temporal lobes. Rabies virus produces CNS excitability with convulsions, meningismus, and hydrophobia. Subacute sclerosing panencephalitis is a rare complication of measles (rubeola) virus infection and leads to progressive mental decline, spasticity, and seizures. West Nile virus, like many arboviruses, can cause a meningoencephalitis.

BP7 830   BP6 730   PBD7 1376-1377   PBD6 1321

62 (D) Non-Hodgkin lymphomas, including large B-cell lymphomas, are not common in the brain, but they may be seen in immunocompromised persons, particularly those with AIDS. They tend to be multifocal. Cytomegalovirus infection is common in AIDS, but it is unlikely to produce mass lesions. A glioblastoma multiforme can be a large infiltrative and destructive mass, but the cells are typically GFAP positive and CD19 negative. Kaposi sarcoma can occur in association with HIV infection, but CNS involvement is rare, and the cells are

CD34 positive. Progressive multifocal leukoencephalopathy produces granular white matter lesions with large, bizarre oligodendrocytes infected with JC papovavirus. Toxoplasmosis can produce multiple mass lesions, but they are chronic abscesses that are filled with necrotic material and surrounded by gliosis; toxoplasma pseudocysts may be found in the abscesses.

BP7 835   BP6 734   PBD7 1408   PBD6 1349-1350

63 **(A)** This patient has findings of dementia with Lewy bodies (DLB), a form of dementia with clinical features similar to those of Alzheimer disease and idiopathic Parkinson disease (IPD). Mutations in the gene for α-synuclein have been linked to IPD, and Lewy bodies can be found in the substantia nigra neurons, but the clinical dementia as well as cortical Lewy bodies point to DLB. Amyloid precursor protein (APP) is encoded by a gene on chromosome 21 (perhaps explaining early Alzheimer disease in trisomy 21) and is processed to form the Aβ amyloid of neuritic plaques in Alzheimer disease. The ε4 allele of apolipoprotein E can bind Aβ and increase the risk of Alzheimer disease. Huntingtin is the protein product of the *HD* gene in Huntington disease. Presenilin 1 and 2 mutations can increase production of Aβ and increase the risk of early-onset Alzheimer disease. Tau protein is found in neurofibrillary tangles of Alzheimer disease and in Pick bodies of Pick disease.

BP7 844   PBD7 1386, 1392   PBD6 1333-1334

64 **(E)** This patient has findings consistent with an acute cerebral infarction from obstruction of blood flow causing focal cerebral ischemia. After 2 days, there will be some cerebral softening and edema with ischemia of neurons, but little else. Hypercholesterolemia is a risk factor for atherosclerosis, which is the major cause of thrombotic cerebral arterial occlusions. The antiphospholipid syndrome can produce thrombotic and embolic disease, but an embolic "stroke" is typically hemorrhagic, and antiphospholipid syndrome is uncommon at this age. A positive blood culture suggests sepsis with the possibility of meningitis or cerebral abscess formation, but abscesses typically have ring enhancement on CT imaging studies. Elevated serum levels of very long chain fatty acids are present in patients with adrenoleukodystrophy, a rare disorder that leads to myelin loss at an early age. Hyperammonemia occurs in hepatic encephalopathy with liver failure; it produces Alzheimer type II gliosis but no focal or gross lesions. Oligoclonal bands are characteristic of multiple sclerosis, which typically has an onset in youth or middle age, with formation of plaques of demyelination in white matter. The ANA test result is positive in many autoimmune diseases and may be accompanied by vasculitis, which can produce scattered areas of ischemic injury, resulting in a clinical picture of encephalopathy. Neurosyphilis is now rare; it does not produce focal ischemic lesions.

BP7 814-815   BP6 717-719   PBD7 1361-1365
PBD6 1308-1310

65 **(A)** This patient has an Arnold-Chiari II malformation, which results in a small posterior fossa, misshapen midline cerebellum with downward displacement of the vermis, and tenting of the tectal plate. The MR image in this case is characteristic of hydromyelia. Cerebral palsy is a general term describing nonprogressive motor deficits that are present from birth. A Dandy-Walker malformation includes hypoplasia or absence of the cerebellar vermis, as well as cystic enlargement of the posterior fossa. Holoprosencephaly is a severe malformation with total (alobar) or incomplete (semilobar) separation of the cerebral hemispheres in brain development. Multiple sclerosis results in white matter plaques of demyelination, not malformation. Polymicrogyria is characterized by numerous, small, irregularly formed gyral contours.

BP7 823   BP6 724   PBD7 1355-1356   PBD6 1301

66 **(D)** Holoprosencephaly is a midline defect in which there is absent (alobar) or partial (semilobar) cerebral hemispheric development. It can occur in trisomy 13, as in this case, with other midline defects. It may also be seen in cases of maternal diabetes mellitus. Anencephaly is the absence of a fetal cranial vault, which leads to absence of most of the brain. An Arnold-Chiari II malformation results in a small posterior fossa, a misshapen midline cerebellum with downward displacement of the vermis, and tenting of the tectal plate. A Dandy-Walker malformation is characterized by aplasia or hypoplasia of the cerebellar vermis, cystic enlargement of the fourth ventricle, and hydrocephalus. Periventricular leukomalacia is a form of perinatal injury that is caused by hypoxic-ischemic events or infections. A subdural hematoma results from trauma.

BP7 823   BP6 725   PBD7 1355   PBD6 1300-1301

67 **(A)** This patient had Alzheimer disease (AD) complicated by cerebral amyloid angiopathy and terminal hemorrhagic stroke. Formation and aggregation of the Aβ peptide is now considered central to the pathogenesis of AD. Aβ peptide is derived from abnormal processing of amyloid precursor protein (APP) by β- and γ-secretases. When APP, a transmembrane protein, is cleaved by α-secretases, followed by γ-secretases, a soluble non-toxic fragment is formed. However, cleavage by β-secretase and then γ-secretase gives rise to Aβ peptides that aggregate and form the amyloid cores of neuritic plaques. Conformational change in prion protein leads to Creutzfeldt-Jakob disease, a rapidly progressive dementia with spongiform encephalopathy but not neuritic plaques or amyloid deposition. Although abnormally phosphorylated forms of tau protein are found in neurofibrillary tangles seen in AD, there is no mutation of the *tau* gene, nor are the tangles considered primary in the pathogenesis of AD. Mutation of the *tau* gene gives rise to frontotemporal dementia with Parkinsonism. Mutations in the *frataxin* gene lead to Friedreich ataxia, an autosomal-recessive progressive illness, generally beginning in the first decade of life. Loss of dopaminergic neurons with deficiency of dopamine is central to the pathogenesis of Parkinson disease. Expansion of polyglutamine repeats due to CAG trinucleotide repeat-expansion underlies Huntington disease.

BP7 841-843   PBD7 1386-1389

CHAPTER 29

The Eye

PBD7 Chapter 29: The Eye

PBD6 Chapter 31: Diseases of the Eye

1 A 29-year-old woman seeks medical attention because she has had pain in the right eye for the past 2 days. On physical examination, there is no conjunctival erythema or vascular injection. Funduscopic examination shows no retinal lesions. A slit-lamp examination with fluorescein dye shows a dendritic ulcer on the right cornea. Which of the following most likely produced these findings?

- ❏ (A) Trachoma
- ❏ (B) Herpes simplex virus infection
- ❏ (C) Excessive sunlight exposure
- ❏ (D) Cytomegalovirus infection
- ❏ (E) Vitamin A deficiency

2 A 31-year-old man has increasing difficulty seeing at night but has no problems with his vision during the day. Three years later, his daytime visual acuity is also decreasing. Funduscopic examination shows a branching reticulated pattern to the retina. The optic disc appears pale and waxy, and there is attenuation of retinal blood vessels. These findings are most characteristic of which of the following conditions?

- ❏ (A) Macular degeneration
- ❏ (B) Hypertensive retinopathy
- ❏ (C) Retinitis pigmentosa
- ❏ (D) Proliferative retinopathy
- ❏ (E) Arteriosclerotic retinopathy

3 After an uncomplicated pregnancy, a 20-year-old woman gives birth at term to a male infant. No abnormalities are noted on a newborn physical examination. During infancy, a well-infant checkup shows leukokoria in the right eye. The eye is enucleated. Molecular analysis of the enucleated tumor cells indicates loss of both normal alleles of the *RB* gene. In comparison, skin fibroblasts of the infant do not show any abnormality at the *RB* locus. Which of the following statements regarding the clinical appearance of this infant is most accurate?

- ❏ (A) A predisposition to develop this tumor was inherited
- ❏ (B) His siblings have an increased risk of developing retinoblastoma
- ❏ (C) He is at increased risk of developing osteosarcoma in later life
- ❏ (D) Both copies of the *RB* gene were lost because of mutations in retinoblasts
- ❏ (E) He is at a high risk of developing retinoblastoma in the left eye

4 A 63-year-old woman was diagnosed with type 2 diabetes mellitus at the age of 18 years. She has had increasing difficulty with her vision for the past 10 years. Her most recent hemoglobin A_{1c} level is 9%. Which of the following pathologic findings is most likely to be found on funduscopy?

- ❏ (A) Corneal stromal dystrophy
- ❏ (B) Retrolental fibroplasia
- ❏ (C) Granulomatous uveitis
- ❏ (D) Capillary microaneurysms
- ❏ (E) Papilledema

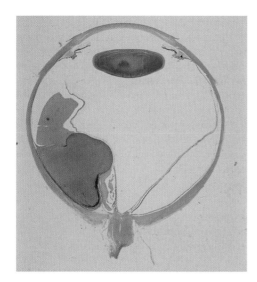

5 A 61-year-old woman experienced sudden loss of part of the vision in the left eye, which occurred "as though a shade had been pulled across" her field of view. On funduscopic examination, there is a uveal mass. The enucleated eye is shown in transverse section above. Which of the following is the most likely diagnosis?

❑ (A) Granulomatous uveitis
❑ (B) Melanoma
❑ (C) Toxoplasmosis
❑ (D) Malignant hypertension
❑ (E) Ocular trauma with hematoma
❑ (F) Retinoblastoma
❑ (G) Proliferative retinopathy

6 A 50-year-old man was not using protective goggles while ripping plywood on his table saw and suffered a penetrating injury to the left eye. A wood splinter is removed. On funduscopic examination, there appears to be a partial uveal prolapse, but he has vision in the left eye. Three weeks later, he has loss of accommodation, photophobia, and blurred vision in the right eye. Choroidal infiltrates are now seen on funduscopic examination. Which of the following is the most likely diagnosis?

❑ (A) Undiagnosed trauma
❑ (B) Aspergillosis
❑ (C) Sarcoidosis
❑ (D) Fuchs dystrophy
❑ (E) Sympathetic ophthalmia

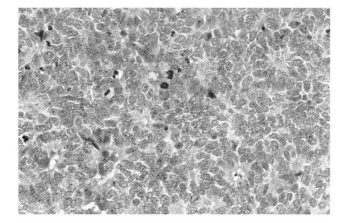

7 A 3-year-old boy has been observed by his parents to be increasingly clumsy for the past 6 months. He is brought to the physician, who notes leukocoria with absence of the red reflex in the left eye. The eye is enucleated, and the microscopic appearance of an intraocular mass is shown in the preceding figure. Which of the following is the most likely diagnosis?

❑ (A) Metastatic adenocarcinoma
❑ (B) Retinoblastoma
❑ (C) Squamous cell carcinoma
❑ (D) Glioma
❑ (E) Melanoma
❑ (F) Medulloblastoma
❑ (G) Neuroblastoma

8 A 62-year-old woman has had decreasing vision for the past year. She now has increasing headaches. She has worn glasses since childhood because of myopia. Funduscopic examination shows deepening of the optic cup with excavation. The retina appears normal. Screening of which of the following would have detected the disease that led to these findings?

❑ (A) Serum glucose
❑ (B) Serum cholesterol
❑ (C) Homocystine in urine
❑ (D) Blood pressure
❑ (E) Intraocular pressure

9 A pharmaceutical company is developing a product that will be useful to prevent age-related visual loss. A cohort of individuals between 60 and 80 years of age is followed for 5 years with periodic examinations of visual acuity, funduscopy, and fluorescein angiography. Some of these individuals develop progressive loss of vision characterized initially by diffuse deposits in Bruch's membrane and by atrophy of retinal pigment epithelium. Later, a subset of these patients has a further decline in vision due to development of choroidal neovascularization. An antagonist to which of the following molecules is most likely to be useful in reducing vision loss in this subset of patients?

❑ (A) Platelet-derived growth factor (PDGF)
❑ (B) Vascular endothelial growth factor (VEGF)
❑ (C) Transforming growth factor-β (TGF-β)
❑ (D) Insulin-like growth factor (IGF)
❑ (E) Epidermal growth factor (EGF)

10 The parents of a 6-year-old child notice that she has decreased vision. Examination of the eye shows diffuse punctate inflammation of the cornea as well as pannus extending as a growth of fibrovascular tissue from conjunctiva onto the cornea. Microscopic examination of a corneal scraping shows lymphocytes, plasma cells, neutrophils, and scattered corneal epithelial cells that have cytoplasmic inclusion bodies. Which of the following infectious agents is most likely to produce these findings?

❑ (A) Herpes simplex virus
❑ (B) *Treponema pallidum*
❑ (C) Cytomegalovirus
❑ (D) Rubella virus
❑ (E) *Chlamydia trachomatis*

11 A 68-year-old woman has had decreased visual acuity for the past 5 years. She has no ocular pain. Her intraocular pressure is normal. Findings on funduscopic examination include arteriolar narrowing, flame-shaped hemorrhages, cotton-wool spots, and hard, waxy exudates. Which of the following is the most likely diagnosis?

- ❏ (A) Chronic hypertension
- ❏ (B) Retinitis pigmentosa
- ❏ (C) Advanced atherosclerosis
- ❏ (D) Diabetes mellitus
- ❏ (E) Cerebral edema

12 A 30-year-old man has had decreasing vision for the past 3 years and now has severely impaired vision in both eyes. His brother is similarly affected. Both parents have normal vision. Examination shows diffuse cloudiness of the anterior stroma with aggregates of gray-white opacities in the axial region of the corneal stroma. He undergoes corneal transplantation. The diseased corneas show basophilic deposits in the stroma that stain positively for keratan sulfate. Which of the following is the most likely diagnosis?

- ❏ (A) Cataracts
- ❏ (B) Keratomalacia
- ❏ (C) Macular dystrophy
- ❏ (D) Pterygium
- ❏ (E) Trachoma

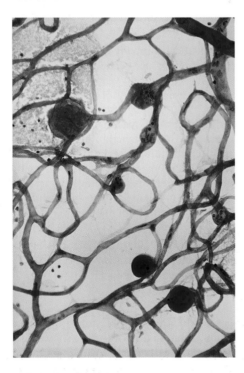

13 A 68-year-old woman who had chronic renal failure for 10 years died of an ischemic cardiomyopathy. This figure shows a preparation of human retina removed at autopsy. The changes seen in the retina are most characteristic of which of the following diseases?

- ❏ (A) Systemic lupus erythematosus
- ❏ (B) Malignant hypertension
- ❏ (C) Diabetes mellitus
- ❏ (D) Amyloidosis
- ❏ (E) Polycystic kidney disease

14 A 15-year-old African-American boy has experienced fatigue for the past 10 years. Physical examination is not remarkable. Laboratory investigations show hemoglobin 8.0 g/dL, hematocrit 24.7%, MCV 95 μm^3, and total serum bilirubin 2.1 mg/dL. The serum AST, ALT, albumin, and total protein are normal. His prothrombin time and partial thromboplastin time are normal. Examination of his peripheral blood smear shows reticulocytosis and polychromasia with occasional deformed RBCs shaped like crescents. This patient is at increased risk for developing which of the following ocular complications?

- ❏ (A) Cataract
- ❏ (B) Uveitis
- ❏ (C) Keratoconus
- ❏ (D) Intraretinal hemorrhage
- ❏ (E) Secondary angle closure glaucoma

15 A 25-year-old woman with preeclampsia gives birth prematurely at 32 weeks' gestation. The infant's Apgar scores are 4 and 6 at 1 and 5 minutes. The infant has hyaline membrane disease and is intubated and administered positive pressure ventilation with 100% inspired oxygen. The infant survives and is discharged on the 23rd day of life. Two months later, the mother notices that the infant does not respond visually to her presence. The infant is examined and is found to be blind. Which of the following is the most likely diagnosis?

- ❏ (A) Keratomalacia
- ❏ (B) Retrolental fibroplasia
- ❏ (C) Macular degeneration
- ❏ (D) Cataracts
- ❏ (E) Retinitis pigmentosa

16 A 70-year-old man suddenly lost the upper half of the visual field in the right eye. Before this event, he has had decreasing visual acuity in both eyes for the past 6 years. On physical examination, his height is 170 cm (5 ft 8 in) and weight is 92.5 kg (BMI 32). Laboratory studies show a fasting serum glucose level of 165 mg/dL. Which of the following underlying pathologic processes is most likely to account for the sudden loss of vision in the right eye?

- ❏ (A) Retinitis pigmentosa
- ❏ (B) Macular degeneration
- ❏ (C) Dendritic corneal ulcer
- ❏ (D) Uveal melanoma
- ❏ (E) Traction retinal detachment

17 A 76-year-old woman has had decreasing vision, mainly in a central pattern, for the past 3 years. She has no ocular pain. Intraocular pressures are normal. There are no abnormalities of the cornea or crystalline lens. On funduscopic examination, the retinal pigment epithelium appears atrophic and deposits are seen in Bruch's membrane. Which of the following is the most likely diagnosis?

- ❏ (A) Retinitis pigmentosa
- ❏ (B) Proliferative retinopathy
- ❏ (C) Retinal detachment
- ❏ (D) Macular degeneration
- ❏ (E) Retrolental fibroplasia

18 A 29-year-old woman has developed malaise with nausea over the past month. On physical examination, she has an erythematous rash on the cheeks of her face. Laboratory studies show a serum creatinine level of 3.3 mg/dL, urea nitrogen of 33 mg/dL, positive ANA 1:2048, and positive anti–double-stranded DNA 1:512. A renal biopsy specimen shows a proliferative glomerulonephritis. She receives long-term high-dose glucocorticoid therapy. Which of the following ocular complications is this patient most likely to develop?

❑ (A) Background retinopathy
❑ (B) Macular degeneration
❑ (C) Granulomatous uveitis
❑ (D) Cataracts
❑ (E) Corneal stromal dystrophy

19 A 70-year-old man who was diagnosed with diabetes mellitus 30 years ago is recovering from right hip replacement surgery after sustaining a femoral neck fracture in a fall 3 weeks ago. He has had a worsening headache for the past 3 days. On physical examination, he is afebrile and normotensive. On funduscopic examination, there is papilledema of the left eye. Which of the following is the most likely cause of the papilledema?

❑ (A) Diabetes mellitus
❑ (B) Glaucoma
❑ (C) Macular degeneration
❑ (D) Optic neuritis
❑ (E) Subdural hematoma

20 Over the past 2 years, a 78-year-old woman has had increasing visual problems that are worse in the right eye. She is unable to see clearly when looking straight ahead because of cloudiness and opacification and has great difficulty reading printed material. Her peripheral vision is better. Which of the following pathologic processes is most likely to have occurred?

❑ (A) Retinal macular degeneration
❑ (B) Keratomalacia
❑ (C) Sympathetic ophthalmia
❑ (D) Glaucoma
❑ (E) Nuclear sclerosis of the lens

21 A 54-year-old man has had decreasing visual acuity in the right eye. The ophthalmologist notices a 15-mm choroidal mass on funduscopic examination. One week later, the patient experiences a sudden loss of vision in the right eye "as though someone pulled a window shade down halfway." Which of the following is the most likely diagnosis?

❑ (A) Uveal melanoma
❑ (B) Diabetic retinopathy
❑ (C) Sarcoidosis
❑ (D) Glaucoma
❑ (E) Cytomegalovirus infection

22 For the past 36 hours, a 76-year-old man has experienced increasing pain accompanied by clouded vision in the right eye. He has worn corrective lenses for hyperopia for the past 70 years. On physical examination, there are no lesions of the cornea or crystalline lens. On funduscopic examination, there is excavation of the optic cup on the right. Which of the following is most likely to produce these findings?

❑ (A) Deposition of amyloid within the vitreous of the posterior chamber
❑ (B) Dislocation of the crystalline lens into the anterior chamber
❑ (C) Increased production of aqueous humor by the ciliary body
❑ (D) Increased resistance to outflow of aqueous into Schlemm's canal
❑ (E) Narrowed anterior chamber angle obstructing outflow of aqueous humor
❑ (F) Thromboembolism to the central retinal artery

ANSWERS

1 **(B)** The most common cause of corneal ulcers is infection with herpes simplex virus. Such ulcers can perforate through to the globe, which is a medical emergency. Some chronic herpetic corneal infections cause localized opacity. Lymphocytes and plasma cells are present as well as viral inclusions in the corneal epithelial cells. Trachoma, an infection seen most often in children, produces inflammation leading to extensive corneal and conjunctival scarring. Some chronic herpetic corneal infections cause localized opacity. Lymphocytes and plasma cells are present as well as viral inclusions in the corneal epithelial cells. Excessive exposure to sunlight can predispose to malignancy; for example, a carcinoma in situ that produces a white, shiny lesion (leukoplakia). Cytomegalovirus infection rarely causes corneal lesions. It can cause retinitis in congenital infections and in immunocompromised adults. Vitamin A deficiency causes keratomalacia and scarring.

PBD7 1428   PBD6 1362-1363

2 **(C)** Retinitis pigmentosa can be inherited in a variety of patterns, and progression of disease is variable. Night blindness caused by loss of rod photoreceptors is an early symptom. Later, the cones also begin to degenerate, producing blindness. Macular degeneration is seen in elderly persons. Vascular changes are seen with hypertensive and arteriosclerotic retinopathies. Neovascularization is a feature of diabetic proliferative retinopathy.

PBD7 1442   PBD6 1370-1371

3 **(D)** This infant has a sporadic form of retinoblastoma, because the somatic cells have normal *RB* genes. Both mutations probably arose in the retinoblasts. The infant did not inherit susceptibility to develop retinoblastoma, because both copies of the *RB* gene are normal in unaffected somatic cells (fibroblasts). If he had inherited one copy of the mutant (or deleted) *RB* gene, all the cells in the body would have only one normal copy of the *RB* gene. His siblings are at no increased risk of developing retinoblastoma, and he is at no increased risk of developing osteosarcoma. For similar reasons, risk of developing a retinoblastoma in the left eye is also no greater than that of the general population.

BP7 255   PBD7 1442-1443   PBD6 1372

4 **(D)** Formation of capillary microaneurysms is a common presenting clinical sign in background diabetic retinopathy. Generally, the retinopathy begins to develop at least 15 to 20 years after the initial diagnosis of diabetes mellitus type 1 or type 2. Corneal stromal dystrophies are typically inherited conditions. Retrolental fibroplasia is a complication of high-dose oxygen therapy for neonates. Granulomatous uveitis can be produced by a variety of conditions such as sarcoidosis and sympathetic ophthalmia. Papilledema results from increased intracranial pressure.

BP7 651   BP6 571   PBD7 1197, 1437-1439
PBD6 1369-1370

5 **(B)** The patient has a pigmented uveal mass with retinal detachment. After skin, the eye is the most common site of melanoma. This is the most common intraocular malignancy in adults. Granulomatous uveitis can occur from sarcoidosis, but the inflammation does not produce a large mass lesion. Toxoplasmosis can produce small foci of inflammation but not a mass. Hypertensive retinopathy can produce small hemorrhages. Ocular trauma may lead to sympathetic ophthalmia with inflammation but has no mass effect. Retinoblastoma most often occurs in children, and the tumor is not pigmented. Diabetic proliferative retinopathy can also cause a sudden retinal detachment, but there is no mass lesion.

PBD7 1434-1436   PBD6 1365-1367

6 **(E)** Sympathetic ophthalmia is an unusual, but devastating, complication of penetrating ocular trauma that results from the release of an antigen from one eye and causes an inflammatory reaction in the opposite eye. To avoid this complication, the traumatized eye must be removed before inflammation begins in the opposite eye. Trauma alone cannot produce this spectrum of findings. Infection with *Aspergillus* is unlikely to become disseminated in a nonimmunocompromised person and is not typically associated with traumatic lesions. Sarcoidosis can affect the eye, but lesions in the choroid are uncommon. Fuchs dystrophy is an inherited condition that affects the corneal endothelium.

PBD7 1433   PBD6 1364-1365

7 **(B)** Retinoblastoma is the most common malignant ocular neoplasm in children. Histologically, there is clustering of cuboidal or short columnar cells around a central lumen. These clusters are sometimes called Flexner-Wintersteiner rosettes. This tumor can spread to the orbit or along the optic nerve. Adenocarcinomas and squamous cell carcinomas are uncommon neoplasms in children. Gliomas may affect the optic nerve in a child, but the microscopic pattern does not include the rosettes shown. Melanomas of the eye are seen in adults and have spindle or polygonal cell patterns. Medulloblastomas are cerebellar malignancies in children. Neuroblastomas are pediatric neoplasms arising in adrenal or extra-adrenal paraganglia. Retinoblastomas, medulloblastomas, and neuroblastomas are all forms of "small, round, blue cell tumors" seen in children.

BP7 254-255   BP6 212-213   PBD7 1442-1443
PBD6 1372-1373

8 **(E)** The patient has glaucoma. Increased intraocular pressure is believed to cause the loss of nerve fibers, resulting in a characteristic cupped excavation of the optic disc. Because there are no obvious early signs or symptoms, screening is important for detection. Glaucoma has several causes; a variety of medications are used to treat the disease. Hyperglycemia suggests a diagnosis of diabetes mellitus, which can increase the risk of glaucoma. An increased cholesterol level suggests an increased risk of arteriosclerotic diseases. Homocystinuria is a rare condition that also increases the risk of atherosclerosis. Hypertension can produce a retinopathy.

PBD7 1430-1432, 1444-1445   PBD6 1374-1375

9 **(B)** Age-related macular degeneration (ARMD) is the leading cause of visual loss in the Western world. Its advanced stages (exudative ARMD) are characterized by extensive choroidal neovascularization that is driven by the local production of VEGF. Clinical trials now in progress indicate that anti-VEGF agents reduce neovascularization and visual loss. None of the other listed factors affects angiogenesis.

PBD7 1441-1442

10 **(E)** Trachoma is one of the major causes of blindness worldwide. The initial inflammation is followed by progressive scarring of the conjunctiva and cornea. Herpetic keratitis can result in ulceration and scarring; herpesviruses have intranuclear inclusions. Congenital infections with *Treponema pallidum* result in an interstitial keratitis. In children, cytomegalovirus, one of the herpesviruses, is a rare cause of ocular infection. It produces prominent intranuclear inclusions. Congenital rubella, which is now a rare disease because of immunization, produces a retinopathy.

PBD7 394-395, 1425   PBD6 1361-1362

11 **(A)** Hypertensive retinopathy results from longstanding hypertension, with progressive changes that begin with generalized narrowing of the arterioles and proceed to the changes seen in this case. Retinitis pigmentosa is an inherited condition that may begin later in life (but usually earlier) and produces a waxy pallor of the optic disc. Arteriosclerotic retinopathy causes vascular changes, including arteriovenous nicking and hyaline arteriolosclerosis with "copper-wire" and "silver-wire" arterioles. A variety of findings are associated with diabetic retinopathy, including capillary microaneurysms, cotton-wool spots, arteriolar hyalinization, and more severe changes of proliferative retinopathy with neovascularization. Cerebral edema may result in papilledema.

PBD7 1436-1438   PBD6 1370

12 **(C)** There are several forms of inherited corneal stromal dystrophy, and most are autosomal dominant. However, the most severe form is macular dystrophy, which has an autosomal recessive form of inheritance. It is essentially a form of mucopolysaccharidosis confined to the cornea in which keratan sulfate is deposited. Cataracts are seen most often in the elderly and result from opacifications of the crystalline lens. Keratomalacia can be a consequence of vitamin A deficiency. A pterygium is a localized area of basophilic degeneration of conjunctival epithelium that extends onto the cornea. Trachoma is caused by infection with *Chlamydia trachomatis*.

PBD7 1428-1429   PBD6 1363

13 (C) Microaneurysms in the retinal vessels are seen in persons with diabetes mellitus. Several other changes can also occur in diabetes, including hemorrhages, arteriolar hyalinization, cotton-wool spots, neovascularization, and fibroplasia. All other conditions listed can also cause renal failure, but retinal microaneurysms are not seen.

BP7 651   PBD7 1437-1439   PBD6 1369-1370

14 (D) This patient has sickle cell anemia in which the sickled RBCs can occlude the retinal microvasculature as oxygen tension falls and the RBCs assume a sickle shape. These vascular occlusions can cause pre-retinal, intraretinal, and subretinal hemorrhages. Organization of pre-retinal hemorrhages can cause retinal traction and detachment. Cataracts are most commonly age-related but may be secondary to systemic diseases such as galactosemia, diabetes mellitus, and Wilson disease. Uveitis may occur locally or be part of systemic diseases such as sarcoidosis. Keratoconus is characterized by progressive thinning of the cornea without any inflammation that leads to an abnormal shape that is more conical than spherical, giving rise to severe astigmatism. This form of corneal degeneration can occur sporadically or in association with a systemic disease such as Marfan syndrome. Secondary angle closure glaucoma is caused by inflammation of the uvea and consequent formation of a neovascular membrane that blocks the trabecular meshwork.

PBD7 1439

15 (B) Retrolental fibroplasia results from oxygen toxicity to the immature retinal vasculature, leading to neovascularization of the retina with ingrowth into the vitreous. In some cases, scarring continues and causes retinal detachment. Keratomalacia is a feature of vitamin A deficiency that develops over a longer period. Macular degeneration is a disease of the elderly. Cataracts are also seen in older persons. Retinitis pigmentosa can be inherited in a variety of patterns and has a variable onset from childhood through older age.

PBD7 1439   PBD6 1368-1369

16 (E) The clinical features described suggest retinal detachment, which occurs in a late stage of proliferative retinopathy associated with diabetes mellitus. The neovascularization results in a membrane with fibrosis that increases traction on the retina, leading to sudden detachment. Retinitis pigmentosa is an inherited, degenerative condition that is not related to diabetes mellitus. Macular degeneration is a common cause of decreased vision in the elderly but not of retinal detachment. Dendritic corneal ulceration suggests infection with herpes simplex virus. Uveal melanomas may cause retinal detachment, but they are not a feature of diabetes mellitus.

BP7 651   BP6 571   PBD7 1436   PBD6 1370

17 (D) Macular degeneration is most often an age-related condition and is the most common cause of decreased vision in the elderly. An absence of retinal vessels in the center of the macula may contribute to this disease, because the retina has high metabolic demands. The disease may result in fibrous metaplasia and scarring of the macular region, causing permanent loss of central vision. Retinitis pigmentosa is an inher-

ited disorder that produces a characteristic waxy pallor of the optic disc. Proliferative retinopathy is characterized by neovascularization of the retina. Retrolental fibroplasia is a complication of high-dose oxygen therapy for neonates (often premature).

PBD7 1441-1442   PBD6 1371

18 (D) Cataracts of the crystalline lens are an important complication of systemic therapy with glucocorticoids. This patient has systemic lupus erythematosus with lupus nephritis. Cataracts can be caused by aging, diabetes mellitus, glaucoma, ultraviolet light, or irradiation. Retinopathy is most often a feature of diabetes mellitus or hypertension. Macular degeneration is a disease of aging. Granulomatous uveitis occurs with sarcoidosis. Stromal dystrophies are inherited conditions that affect the cornea.

PBD7 1431   PBD6 1367-1368

19 (E) Papilledema results from increased intracranial pressure produced by cerebral edema, intracranial hemorrhage, or rapidly expanding masses. This patient has a slowly forming subdural hematoma as a result of his prior fall. The blood collecting in the subdural space leads to increased intracranial pressure. Diabetes mellitus can cause retinopathy, cataracts, and glaucoma. Glaucoma, with increased intraocular pressure, produces optic cup excavation (the opposite of papilledema). Macular degeneration affects the fovea more severely. Optic neuritis leads to decreased visual acuity and is most often a complication of multiple sclerosis.

PBD7 1443-1444   PBD6 1373-1374

20 (E) Nuclear sclerosis of the lens gives rise to cataracts in aging persons. This change causes opacification due to compression of the lens fibers in the central (nuclear) portion of the lens. Macular degeneration also occurs in the elderly and results in loss of central vision, but it does not cause cloudiness. Keratomalacia can produce corneal scarring with opacification, but not in a central distribution pattern. Sympathetic ophthalmia in one eye occurs after trauma to the other eye. Glaucoma results from increased intraocular pressure and damages the optic nerve, but it is not characterized by loss of central vision.

PBD7 1431   PBD6 1367-1368

21 (A) Uveal melanomas can involve the choroid, the iris, or the ciliary body. They are often pigmented. In addition to causing retinal detachment, as in this case, they may cause choroidal hemorrhage or macular edema. Retinal detachment can occur with diabetic retinopathy, but there is no mass effect. Choroidal and corneal granulomatous inflammation can occur with sarcoidosis, but retinal detachment does not occur. Glaucoma is characterized by increased intraocular pressure. Cytomegalovirus infection can produce focal lesions from inflammation, but retinal detachment is uncommon.

BP7 806   PBD7 1434-1435   PBD6 1365-1367

22 (E) In some older persons with hyperopia, the iris is displaced forward to narrow the angle at the anterior chamber, obstructing flow of aqueous humor, so-called primary "angle-closure" glaucoma, which presents with acute pain. Increased pressure on the optic nerve causes excavation and produces progressive visual loss. Amyloid deposition is quite rare and does not increase intraocular pressure. Crystalline lens dislocation can occur with trauma and with Marfan syndrome. Increased production of aqueous humor is a rare cause of glaucoma. Increased resistance to outflow of aqueous into Schlemm's canal is typical of primary "open-angle" glaucoma, which occurs in persons with myopia. Thrombosis or embolism to the central retinal artery can lead to occlusion with edema, pallor, and a "cherry red" spot in the fovea; unless the ischemia is of short duration, blindness will result.

PBD7 1430-1432   PBD6 1374-1375

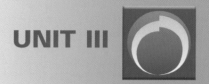

Final Examination

CHAPTER 30

Final Review and Assessment

1 A 47-year-old white man has had increasing orthopnea and worsening pedal edema for the past 3 years. He complains of worsening arthritis involving his hands, knees, hips, and elbows. On physical examination, he has decreased range of motion of the lower legs but no apparent joint deformities, warmth, or swelling. There is a brownish hue to his skin, although it is winter and he rarely goes outdoors. Laboratory findings show hemoglobin of 13.7 g/dL, hematocrit 40.8%, MCV 90 μm^3, platelet count 213,500/mm^3, WBC count 6690/mm^3, Na^+ 141 mmol/L, K^+ 4.2 mmol/L, Cl^- 101 mmol/L, CO_2 24 mmol/L, glucose 201 mg/dL, creatinine 1.2 mg/dL, and calcium 8.2 mg/dL. Which of the following underlying diseases is most likely to explain these findings?

- ❑ (A) β-Thalassemia minor
- ❑ (B) Diabetes mellitus type 1
- ❑ (C) Familial hypercholesterolemia
- ❑ (D) Hereditary hemochromatosis
- ❑ (E) Rheumatoid arthritis

2 A 34-year-old woman has had increasing lethargy for the past 8 months. During this time, she has experienced increased sensitivity to sunlight and now rarely goes outdoors during the day. She has pain in her hands, elbows, knees, and feet and muscle aches in her arms and legs. She has had increasing dyspnea for the past week. Physical examination shows no joint deformities, swelling, or redness. On auscultation of the chest, a friction rub is audible. A chest radiograph shows bilateral pleural effusions. Laboratory findings show hemoglobin of 11.6 mg/dL, hematocrit 34.3%, MCV 84 $\mu m3$, platelet count 133,400/mm^3, WBC count 4610/mm^3, Na^+ 140 mmol/L, K^+ 4.0 mmol/L, Cl^- 99 mmol/L, CO_2 25 mmol/L, glucose 80 mg/dL, creatinine 2.4 mg/dL, and calcium 7.9 mg/dL. Which of the following additional laboratory tests is most helpful to diagnose her underlying condition?

- ❑ (A) Acetylcholine receptor antibody
- ❑ (B) Anti-DNA topoisomerase antibody
- ❑ (C) Anti–glomerular basement membrane antibody
- ❑ (D) Antimicrosomal antibody
- ❑ (E) Antimitochondrial antibody
- ❑ (F) Antinuclear antibody

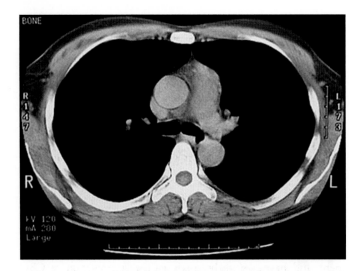

3 A 40-year-old woman has had increasing muscle weakness for the past 5 months. This difficulty is exacerbated by repetitive activities, such as word processing at her computer keyboard. She has trouble keeping her eyes open toward the end of the day and has double vision. She has no muscle aches or pains. On physical examination, she has no apparent muscle atrophy, although muscle strength is slightly decreased in all extremities. There is no joint deformity, pain, or redness. Her lungs are clear to auscultation, and her heart rate is regular. A chest CT scan is shown. Which of the following serologic laboratory tests will be most helpful in diagnosing her underlying condition?

- ❑ (A) Acetylcholine receptor antibody
- ❑ (B) Anti-DNA topoisomerase
- ❑ (C) Anti–glomerular basement membrane antibody
- ❑ (D) Antimitochondrial antibody
- ❑ (E) Antinuclear antibody

4 A 24-year-old previously healthy man who smokes one pack of cigarettes per day and who works as a histotechnologist has developed a cough with bloody sputum over the past 2 days. He has increasing lethargy and nausea. A chest radiograph shows diffuse infiltrates most pronounced in the lower lobes. Laboratory findings show hemoglobin of 13.7 g/dL, hematocrit 40.6%, MCV 91 μm³, platelet count 361,000/mm³, WBC count 7385/mm³, Na⁺ 144 mmol/L, K⁺ 4.3 mmol/L, Cl⁻ 103 mmol/L, CO₂ 26 mmol/L, creatinine 3.8 mg/dL, urea nitrogen 36 mg/dL, and glucose 75 mg/dL. An abdominal ultrasound scan shows normal-sized kidneys. A renal biopsy specimen shows a crescentic glomerulonephritis. Which of the following mechanisms most likely produced this patient's pulmonary disease?

- ❑ (A) Antibody directed against basement membrane collagen
- ❑ (B) Complement activation by circulating antigen-antibody complexes
- ❑ (C) Activation of macrophages by CD4 lymphocytes
- ❑ (D) Increased pulmonary venous pressure
- ❑ (E) Release of inflammatory mediators from mast cells

5 A 56-year-old man has noticed increasing abdominal girth and decreased libido for the past 7 months. Physical examination shows an enlarged abdomen with a fluid wave but no tenderness or masses; the spleen tip is palpable. Bibasi-lar crackles are audible on auscultation of the chest. There is 1 + pitting edema to the knees. The testes are smaller than normal but without masses. Laboratory findings show hemoglobin of 12.2 g/dL, hematocrit 36.9%, MCV 103 μm³, platelet count 189,400/mm³, WBC count 5762/mm³, Na⁺ 138 mmol/L, K⁺ 3.9 mmol/L, Cl⁻ 98 mmol/L, CO₂ 24 mmol/L, creatinine 1.1 mg/dL, glucose 88 mg/dL, total protein 5.7 g/dL, albumin 2.7 g/dL, AST 167 U/L, ALT 69 U/L, alkaline phosphatase 48 U/L, total bilirubin 1.5 mg/dL, and prothrombin time 23 sec. Which of the following is the most likely diagnosis?

- ❑ (A) Adrenal atrophy
- ❑ (B) Aortic valvular stenosis
- ❑ (C) Autoimmune gastritis
- ❑ (D) Chronic glomerulonephritis
- ❑ (E) Hypertrophic cardiomyopathy
- ❑ (F) Micronodular cirrhosis

6 A 33-year-old woman, G 3, P 0, who has had two spontaneous abortions, is in the second trimester of her third pregnancy. An ultrasound at 18 weeks' gestation revealed symmetric growth retardation. At 25 weeks' gestation, she gives birth to a stillborn fetus and experiences sudden onset of dyspnea. A pulmonary ventilation/perfusion scan indicates a high probability of thromboembolism. Four months later, she experiences an altered state of consciousness and sudden loss of movement in the right arm. A cerebral angiogram shows occlusion of a branch of the left middle cerebral artery. Laboratory findings show hemoglobin of 13.4 g/dL, hematocrit 40.3%, MCV 91 μm³, platelet count 124,000/mm³, WBC count 5530/mm³, prothrombin time 13 sec, partial thromboplastin time 46 sec, positive anticardiolipin antibody, positive serologic test result for syphilis, and negative ANA. Which of the following best explains these findings?

- ❑ (A) Antiphospholipid syndrome
- ❑ (B) Myeloproliferative disorder
- ❑ (C) Thrombophlebitis
- ❑ (D) *Treponema pallidum* infection
- ❑ (E) Trousseau syndrome
- ❑ (F) Von Willebrand disease

7 A 20-year-old man has sudden onset of severe abdominal and back pain and dyspnea. His medical history indicates similar episodes over a 12-year period. One year ago, he had osteomyelitis of the left hip; the bone culture was positive for *Salmonella enteritidis*. On physical examination, his lungs are clear to auscultation, but he has tachycardia. Palpation of the abdomen reveals diffuse tenderness with rigidity of abdominal musculature but no apparent masses. A CT scan of the chest shows prominent pulmonary veins but no infiltrates. An abdominal CT scan shows the presence of multiple 0.5- to 1-cm stones in the gallbladder, a very small spleen, and prominent hepatic veins. An abdominal radiograph shows no free air. CBC shows hemoglobin of 10.2 g/dL, hematocrit 30.9%, MCV 99 μm³, RDW 22, platelet count 189,300/mm³, and WBC count 6320/mm³. Which of the following additional laboratory test findings is most likely to be reported?

- ❑ (A) Amylase 694 U/L
- ❑ (B) Positive anticardiolipin antibody
- ❑ (C) Calcium 12.3 mg/dL
- ❑ (D) Ferritin 710 ng/mL
- ❑ (E) Haptoglobin 1 mg/dL
- ❑ (F) Triglyceride 1140 mg/dL

8 A 24-year-old woman has developed right-sided facial pain over the past 24 hours. During that time, she has become lethargic and obtunded. Her medical history shows a 5-kg weight loss over the past 6 months, despite increasing caloric intake. On physical examination, there is swelling with marked tenderness over the right maxilla, exophthalmos on the right side, diffuse abdominal pain, poor skin turgor, and dry mucous membranes. Her temperature is 37.7°C. She has tachycardia, but no murmurs, and tachypnea; the lung fields are clear. Laboratory findings show hemoglobin of 13.1 g/dL, hematocrit 39.4%, Na^+ 131 mmol/L, K^+ 4.6 mmol/L, Cl^- 92 mmol/L, CO_2 9 mmol/L, glucose 481 mg/dL, and creatinine 1.0 mg/dL. An arterial blood gas measurement shows pH of 7.2, PO_2 98 mm Hg, PCO_2 28 mm Hg, and bicarbonate 10 mmol/L. Fine-needle aspiration of the right maxillary region is performed. Which of the following organisms is most likely to be present in this aspirate?

- [ ] (A) *Actinomyces israelii*
- [ ] (B) *Bacillus anthracis*
- [ ] (C) Cytomegalovirus
- [ ] (D) *Clostridium perfringens*
- [ ] (E) *Cryptococcus neoformans*
- [ ] (F) *Mucor circinelloides*
- [ ] (G) *Pseudomonas aeruginosa*

9 A 30-year-old man is infertile and has a low sperm count. He also has a chronic diarrhea with elevated quantitative stool fat. He has had recurrent, severe respiratory tract infections since early childhood. As a neonate, he had bowel obstruction from meconium ileus. He is most likely to have an abnormality involving which of the following genes?

- [ ] (A) *CFTR*
- [ ] (B) *FGFR*
- [ ] (C) *G6PD*
- [ ] (D) *HFE*
- [ ] (E) *NF1*
- [ ] (F) *p53*

10 A 54-year-old man has had nausea for the past 6 months, but he does not report hematemesis. He has increasing malaise. On physical examination, he has decreased sensation to pinprick and light touch over the lower extremities bilaterally. He exhibits mild ataxia when walking. An upper gastrointestinal endoscopy study shows the absence of gastric rugal folds but no ulceration or mass. Which of the following laboratory findings is most likely to be reported?

- [ ] (A) Positive anti-Smith antibody
- [ ] (B) Deficiency of factor V
- [ ] (C) Positive *Helicobacter pylori* antibody
- [ ] (D) MCV 125 μm³
- [ ] (E) Urine glucose 4+

11 A 33-year-old man has experienced onset of chest pain, diaphoresis, and dyspnea over the past 6 hours. In the emergency department, he has a serum troponin I level of 6 ng/mL. Additional laboratory findings include hematocrit of 41%, hemoglobin A_{1c} 4.2%, total serum cholesterol 482 mg/dL, and serum triglyceride 160 mg/dL. Emergent coronary angiography shows 65% stenosis of the left circumflex artery and 70% stenosis of the left anterior descending artery. Angioplasty is performed. One year later, he experiences a series of transient ischemic attacks. He also has pain in the lower extremities when walking more than 300 meters. He is given a drug that inhibits hepatic HMG CoA reductase. The pathogenesis of his underlying disease is most likely related to a reduction in which of the following?

- [ ] (A) β Cells
- [ ] (B) Glucose transport proteins
- [ ] (C) Hepatocytes
- [ ] (D) Intimal smooth muscle cells
- [ ] (E) LDL receptors

12 Several children between the ages of 6 and 10 in the same community have been reported by the local physician to have similar symptoms. They are all doing poorly in school, which has been attributed to behavioral problems. Their parents state that these children have poor appetites, complain of nausea, and have frequent headaches. On physical examination, they have decreased sensation to touch over the lower extremities. They exhibit loss of fine motor control of movement and have a slightly ataxic gait. A representative CBC shows hemoglobin of 11.8 g/dL, hematocrit 35.2%, MCV 82 μm³, platelet count 282,300/mm³, and WBC count 4745/mm³. Examination of the peripheral blood smear shows basophilic stippling of the RBCs. Serum chemistries show Na^+ 144 mmol/L, K^+ 4.4 mmol/L, Cl^- 105 mmol/L, CO_2 26 mmol/L, glucose 69 mmol/L, creatinine 1.4 mg/dL, calcium 7.7 mg/dL, total protein 6.6 g/dL, albumin 4.3 g/dL, AST 43 U/L, ALT 28 U/L, alkaline phosphatase 189 U/L, and total bilirubin 1.1 mg/dL. Excessive chronic ingestion of which of the following substances is most likely to explain these findings?

- [ ] (A) Fluoride
- [ ] (B) Lead
- [ ] (C) Methanol
- [ ] (D) Monosodium glutamate
- [ ] (E) Vitamin A
- [ ] (F) Zinc

13 A 45-year-old previously healthy woman has had a chronic nonproductive cough for the past 2 months. During the past 3 weeks, she has had increasing dyspnea as well as arthralgias. One week ago, her cough was productive of blood-streaked sputum. She does not smoke. Physical examination shows temperature of 37.5°C, pulse 77/min, respirations 17/min, and blood pressure 140/90 mm Hg. On auscultation, bilateral crackles are audible in the lungs. A chest radiograph shows bilateral nodular and cavitary infiltrates, but there are no masses. Laboratory findings show hemoglobin of 11.7 g/dL, hematocrit 35.2%, platelet count 217,000/mm³, WBC count 6330/mm³, serum glucose 72 mg/dL, creatinine 2.6 mg/dL, and urea nitrogen 25 mg/dL. Urinalysis shows specific gravity of 1.017, pH 6.5, 1+ proteinuria, 2+ hematuria, and no glucose or ketones. A transbronchial biopsy specimen shows necrotizing granulomatous vasculitis of the alveolar capillaries and small peripheral pulmonary arteries. A renal biopsy specimen shows a crescentic glomerulonephritis. Which of the following serologic test results is most likely to be positive?

- [ ] (A) Anti-DNA topoisomerase I
- [ ] (B) Anti–glomerular basement membrane antibody
- [ ] (C) Anti–Jo-1 antibody
- [ ] (D) Antimitochondrial antibody
- [ ] (E) C-ANCA
- [ ] (F) ANA
- [ ] (G) Antiribonucleoprotein antibody

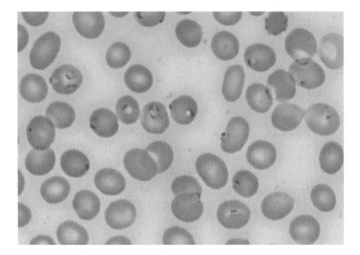

15 A 40-year-old man has been bothered by oral candidiasis for the past year. On physical examination, he has muscle wasting. His weight is 70% of normal for his height and age. He has generalized nontender lymphadenopathy but no hepatosplenomegaly. A skin lesion on his forearm is shown in the preceding figure. Laboratory findings show hemoglobin of 12.2 g/dL, hematocrit 36.5%, MCV 85 μm³, platelet count 188,000/mm³, and WBC count 3460/mm³ with 78% segmented neutrophils, 4% bands, 10% lymphocytes, 6% monocytes, and 2% eosinophils. Infection with which of the following organisms is most likely to produce these findings?

- ❏ (A) Hepatitis C virus
- ❏ (B) Herpes simplex virus
- ❏ (C) HIV
- ❏ (D) *Mycobacterium leprae*
- ❏ (E) *Plasmodium vivax*
- ❏ (F) *Staphylococcus aureus*
- ❏ (G) *Streptococcus pyogenes*

14 A 7-year-old child has had worsening headaches and obtundation for the past 2 days. Physical examination shows temperature of 39.5°C, pulse 103/min, respirations 18/min, and blood pressure 90/55 mm Hg. There is bilateral papilledema on funduscopic examination. No focal neurologic deficits are noted. Palpation of the abdomen reveals hepatosplenomegaly. Laboratory findings show hemoglobin of 9.5 g/dL, hematocrit 28.8%, MCV 101 μm³, platelet count 145,000/mm³, WBC count 6920/mm³, Na⁺ 146 mmol/L, K⁺ 5.5 mmol/L, Cl⁻ 106 mmol/L, CO₂ 26 mmol/L, creatinine 2.3 mg/dL, urea nitrogen 22 mg/dL, LDH 1095 U/L, and amylase 45 U/L. The peripheral blood smear is shown. Which of the following infectious agents is most likely to produce these findings?

- ❏ (A) *Babesia microti*
- ❏ (B) *Borrelia burgdorferi*
- ❏ (C) *Leishmania donovani*
- ❏ (D) *Plasmodium falciparum*
- ❏ (E) *Trypanosoma gambiense*
- ❏ (F) *Wuchereria bancrofti*

16 A 30-year-old man comes to the physician because he has had joint pain in the right hip and left elbow and a headache for the past week. One month ago, he had similar pain in the left hip and knee, which slowly resolved. He remembers having a ringlike skin rash on his left thigh several months ago after a tick bite. On physical examination, there is joint tenderness but no swelling or deformity of the right hip and left elbow. His heart rate is slightly irregular. Which of the following infectious agents is most likely to produce these findings?

- ❏ (A) *Streptococcus pyogenes*
- ❏ (B) *Staphylococcus aureus*
- ❏ (C) *Borrelia burgdorferi*
- ❏ (D) *Mycobacterium tuberculosis*
- ❏ (E) Parvovirus B19
- ❏ (F) *Yersinia enterocolitica*

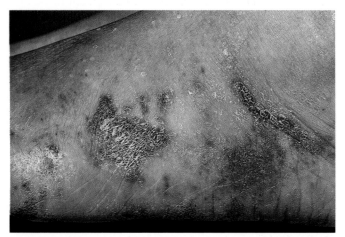

Courtesy of Christopher D.M. Fletcher, MD, Brigham and Women's Hospital, Boston, MA.

17 A 9-year-old girl has become increasingly listless over the past year. On physical examination, she has pitting edema to the thighs, muscle wasting, a protuberant abdomen with a fluid wave, areas of scaling skin with decreased pigmentation, and patches of hair that are irregularly pigmented. No ecchymoses are noted. She is 75% of ideal body weight, but her height is normal. Which of the following laboratory findings is most likely to be present?

- ❏ (A) Hyperhomocysteinemia
- ❏ (B) Hyperuricemia
- ❏ (C) Hypercalcemia
- ❏ (D) Hypoprothrombinemia
- ❏ (E) Hypoalbuminemia
- ❏ (F) Hypoinsulinemia

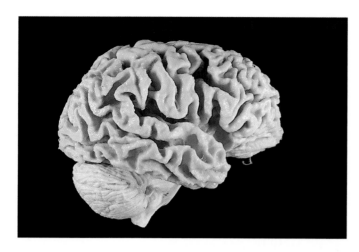

- ❑ (A) Calcium pyrophosphate dihydrate
- ❑ (B) Cholesterol
- ❑ (C) Cystine
- ❑ (D) Hydroxyapatite
- ❑ (E) Sodium urate

20 A 38-year-old woman has had malaise and arthralgias for the past 14 months. Over the past month, she has developed areas of purpura on the distal extremities. On physical examination, her temperature is 37°C, pulse 81/min, respirations 14/min, and blood pressure 140/90 mm Hg. She has scleral icterus and 1- to 3-cm areas of reddish-purple discoloration on her skin. Several of these areas show focal ulceration. Laboratory findings show total protein of 7.1 g/dL, albumin 3.3 g/dL, AST 87 U/L, ALT 95 U/L, alkaline phosphatase 80 U/L, total bilirubin 4.0 mg/dL, and direct bilirubin 3.1 mg/dL. Serologic test results are positive for anti-HCV and negative for anti-HBs and IgM anti-HAV. Urinalysis shows 4+ proteinuria and 1+ hematuria. CT scan of the abdomen shows a small amount of ascites, mild hepatomegaly, and no splenomegaly or lymphadenopathy. A biopsy specimen of an ulcerated skin lesion shows leukocytoclastic vasculitis involving the upper dermis. Which of the following is the most likely diagnosis?

- ❑ (A) Autoimmune hemolytic anemia
- ❑ (B) Hepatocellular carcinoma
- ❑ (C) Hereditary hemochromatosis
- ❑ (D) Mixed cryoglobulinemia
- ❑ (E) Multiple myeloma

18 A 61-year-old man has become more withdrawn and less active over the past 2 years. He spends most of his day in bed, although he appears to have minimal difficulty with movement. He has become less talkative. On physical examination, he has 5/5 motor strength in all extremities; there is no apparent tremor or ataxia. There are no focal neurologic deficits. He can remember only one of three objects after 3 minutes. His mood is depressed. His condition improves somewhat with use of ginkgo biloba extract, but 1 year later he has an episode of aspiration while eating and dies 1 week later of pneumonia. At autopsy, the brain weighs 1000 g. The gross appearance is shown. Which of the following microscopic findings is most likely to be seen in the frontal cortex?

- ❑ (A) Spongiform change
- ❑ (B) Intranuclear inclusions
- ❑ (C) Alzheimer type II cells
- ❑ (D) Aβ amyloid deposits
- ❑ (E) Arteriolosclerosis
- ❑ (F) Loss of pigmented neurons
- ❑ (G) Absence of Betz cells

19 A 51-year-old man has had increasing lethargy over the past year. On physical examination, his temperature is 37°C, pulse 80/min, respirations 15/min, and blood pressure 145/90 mm Hg. He has deformity with increased size, and there is decreased range of motion of the first three metacarpophalangeal (MCP) joints on the right and the second two MCP joints on the left. There is a 2-cm firm, painless nodule over the left olecranon bursa. A similar 1-cm nodule is palpated in the helix of the right ear, and another 1.5-cm nodule is palpable over the right Achilles tendon. Urinalysis shows specific gravity of 1.012, pH 5.5, 1 + hematuria, 1 + proteinuria, and no glucose. The serum urea nitrogen level is 31 mg/dL, and the creatinine is 3.2 mg/dL. The total serum cholesterol is 222 mg/dL. Aspiration of material from the nodule at the left elbow is performed. Which of the following types of crystals is most likely to be seen microscopically in this aspirate?

21 A 41-year-old woman has had increasing lethargy and weakness over the past 3 years. She complains of being cold most of the time and wears a sweater in the summer. One year ago, she had menorrhagia but now has oligomenorrhea. She has difficulty concentrating, and her memory is poor. She has chronic constipation. On physical examination, her temperature is 35.5°C, pulse 54/min, respirations 13/min, and blood pressure 110/70 mm Hg. She has alopecia, and her skin appears coarse and dry. Her face, hands, and feet appear puffy, with a doughlike consistency to the skin. Laboratory findings show hemoglobin of 13.8 g/dL, hematocrit 41.5%, AST 26 U/L, ALT 21 U/L, total bilirubin 1.0 mg/dL, Na⁺ 140 mmol/L, K⁺ 4.1 mmol/L, Cl⁻ 99 mmol/L, CO₂ 25 mmol/L, glucose 73 mg/dL, and creatinine 1.1 mg/dL. Which of the following serologic test findings is most likely to be positive?

- ❑ (A) Anticentromere antibody
- ❑ (B) Anti–DNA topoisomerase antibody
- ❑ (C) Antimitochondrial antibody
- ❑ (D) Antinuclear antibody
- ❑ (E) Antiribonucleoprotein antibody
- ❑ (F) Anti–thyroid peroxidase antibody

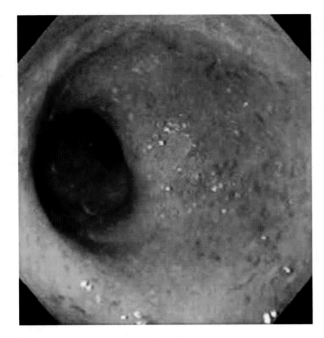

22 A 64-year-old man develops a low-volume mucoid diarrhea. He has had about five bowel movements per day, accompanied by cramping abdominal pain for the past 2 months. The stool is occasionally blood-streaked. On physical examination, he appears pale. Vital signs include temperature of 37.2°C, pulse 84/min, respirations 15/min, and blood pressure 115/75 mm Hg. A colonoscopy is performed, and a representative image of the mucosa from the rectum to the lower portion of the sigmoid is shown above. The remaining colonic mucosa appears normal. Biopsy specimens of the affected colon show mucosal crypt distortion, focal crypt abscesses, and mixed inflammatory infiltrates extending to the lamina propria. Over the next 2 years, the patient develops polyarthritis with no joint deformity, as well as uveitis and chronic active hepatitis. Which of the following inflammatory diseases is he most likely to develop?

❑ (A) Dermatitis herpetiformis
❑ (B) Rheumatoid arthritis
❑ (C) Orchitis
❑ (D) Thyroiditis
❑ (E) Primary sclerosing cholangitis
❑ (F) Atrophic gastritis

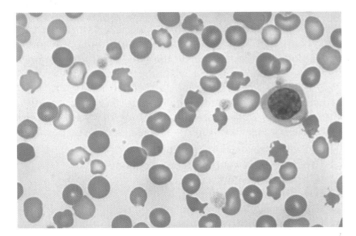

23 A 16-year-old girl has had a history of fatigue and weakness for her entire life. She has not undergone puberty. On physical examination, secondary sex characteristics are not well developed. She has hepatosplenomegaly. CBC shows hemoglobin of 9.1 g/dL, hematocrit 26.7%, MCV 66 μm³, platelet count 89,000/mm³, and WBC count 3670/mm³. The peripheral blood smear is shown in the preceding figure. Additional laboratory findings include serum glucose of 144 mg/dL, TSH 6.2 mU/mL, and ferritin 679 ng/mL. A mutation involving which of the following genes is most likely to be present?

❑ (A) AAT
❑ (B) β-Globin
❑ (C) CFTR
❑ (D) G6PD
❑ (E) HFE
❑ (F) NADPH oxidase
❑ (G) Ankyrin

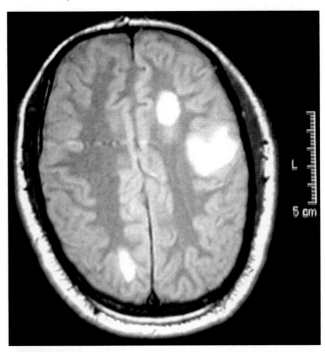

24 Over the past 2 years, a 44-year-old man has noticed a decline in dexterity of his right hand in his work as an auto mechanic. His right hand strength is weaker than the left. One year ago, he experienced painful burning sensations in the left upper extremity. He has been bothered by decreased visual acuity in the left eye for the past month. He is insensitive to heat, and upon taking a hot shower, his vision worsens. On physical examination, he is afebrile and his blood pressure is normal. Motor strength in the right extremity is 4/5 but 5/5 elsewhere. Vision in the left eye is 20/100 and 20/40 in the right eye. One year later, he reports chronic constipation and urinary urgency, hesitancy, and incontinence. An MR image of the brain is shown above. Which of the following is the most likely diagnosis?

❑ (A) Diabetes mellitus
❑ (B) Graves disease
❑ (C) HIV infection
❑ (D) Multiple sclerosis
❑ (E) Myasthenia gravis
❑ (F) Systemic lupus erythematosus

25 A 22-year-old woman has experienced bizarre changes in her behavior over the past year, culminating in her withdrawal from college. She is diagnosed with bipolar disorder. Over the next year, she develops neurologic manifestations that include resting and intention tremors, rigidity, chorea, dysphagia, and dysarthria. On physical examination, she has bilateral Babinski responses. There are ringlike deposits of gold-colored material involving the cornea bilaterally, but her vision is not decreased. One year later, she has an illness that lasts several weeks, with nausea, vomiting, and malaise as well as scleral icterus. Laboratory findings include serum AST of 100 U/L, ALT 122 U/L, alkaline phosphatase 105 U/L, total bilirubin 4.5 mg/dL, glucose 77 mg/dL, and creatinine 0.9 mg/dL. Serologic test results for hepatitis A, B, and C are negative. This episode subsides without treatment, but she eventually develops cirrhosis. A mutation in a gene encoding for which of the following substances is most likely to be present?

❏ (A) α-1-Antitrypsin
❏ (B) CFTR
❏ (C) Galactose-1-phosphate uridyl transferase
❏ (D) Glucocerebrosidase
❏ (E) Glucose-6-phosphatase
❏ (F) Copper-transporting ATPase

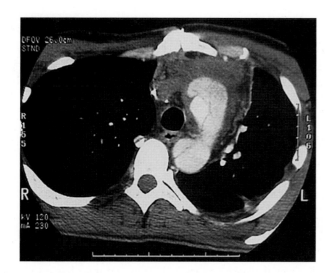

26 A 57-year-woman with a history of untreated hypertension who has smoked one pack of cigarettes per day for the past 40 years experiences a sudden loss of consciousness. On physical examination, her temperature is 37.1°C, pulse 70/min and irregular, respirations 18/min, and blood pressure 90/40 mm Hg. Carotid and radial pulses are diminished compared with femoral and posterior tibial pulses. Auscultation of the chest reveals faint heart sounds; lung fields are clear. A chest radiograph shows a widened mediastinum. The chest CT scan is shown. Pericardiocentesis is performed, and there is blood in the aspirate. Which of the following conditions is most likely to produce these findings?

❏ (A) Aortic dissection
❏ (B) Bicuspid aortic valve
❏ (C) Small cell anaplastic carcinoma
❏ (D) Takayasu arteritis
❏ (E) Tertiary syphilis
❏ (F) Thromboangiitis obliterans

27 A 62-year-old woman who has had a chronic cough for years becomes short of breath after climbing a single flight of stairs. A chest radiograph performed 1 year ago showed increased lucency of upper lung fields and bilateral flattening of the diaphragmatic leaves. She has had nausea and vague abdominal discomfort for 6 months. Biopsy specimens from an upper gastrointestinal endoscopic study show a chronic nonspecific gastritis with no detectable *Helicobacter pylori* organisms. During the past month, she has passed red-colored urine on several occasions. Cystoscopic examination shows a 3-cm exophytic mass in the dome of the bladder, and biopsy specimens show a transitional cell carcinoma. Which of the following is the most likely risk factor for this spectrum of findings?

❏ (A) α₁-Antitrypsin deficiency
❏ (B) Chronic alcoholism
❏ (C) Cigarette smoking
❏ (D) Exposure to aniline dye
❏ (E) Vitamin C deficiency

28 A 59-year-old man comes to the physician seeking a prescription for sildenafil after seeing television advertisements regarding erectile dysfunction. He is 168 cm (5 ft 6 in) tall and weighs 93 kg (BMI 33). On physical examination, there are bilateral carotid bruits and a midline palpable abdominal pulsatile mass. Decreased hair is noted over the lower extremities, and a 1-cm shallow ulceration is present in the skin over the right first metatarsal head. He has decreased sensation to light touch and pinprick in the lower extremities. Laboratory findings include hemoglobin of 12.9 g/dL, hematocrit 42%, WBC count 8950/mm³, Na⁺ 140 mmol/L, K⁺ 4.2 mmol/L, Cl⁻ 105 mmol/L, CO₂ 26 mmol/L, glucose 144 mg/dL, and creatinine 1.7 mg/dL. Which of the following laboratory findings is most likely to be present?

❏ (A) Plasma ACTH of 119 pg/mL
❏ (B) Hemoglobin A1C of 8.8%
❏ (C) Plasma homocysteine of 23 μmol/L
❏ (D) Cerebrospinal fluid oligoclonal IgG bands
❏ (E) Serum antiparietal cell antibodies

29 A 42-year-old woman has had increasing weakness, nausea, vomiting, watery diarrhea, and a 5-kg weight loss over the past 7 months. On physical examination, she has generalized muscle weakness, muscle wasting, and increased skin pigmentation. After an upper respiratory tract infection lasting 1 week, she develops abdominal pain and faintness and lapses into a coma. On admission to the hospital, her temperature is 36.9°C, pulse 83/min, respirations 17/min and shallow, and blood pressure 80/40 mm Hg. Laboratory findings show hemoglobin of 13.6 g/dL, hematocrit 43.8%, WBC count 5420/mm³, Na⁺ 129 mmol/L, K⁺ 3.5 mmol/L, Cl⁻ 95 mmol/L, CO₂ 23 mmol/L, glucose 48 mg/dL, and creatinine 0.6 mg/dL. Atrophy of which of the following tissues is most likely to be present?

❏ (A) Adrenal cortex
❏ (B) Islets of Langerhans
❏ (C) Hypothalamus
❏ (D) Parafollicular cells
❏ (E) Pineal gland
❏ (F) Thyroid epithelium

30 A 39-year-old man goes to the physician because he has experienced diminished libido for the past 4 months. Review of systems indicates that he has had frequent headaches over the past 2 months. On physical examination, he has gynecomastia bilaterally, normal-sized testes in the scrotum, and difficulty with peripheral vision. His visual acuity is 20/20 bilaterally. Laboratory findings show Na^+ of 141 mmol/L, K^+ 4.1 mmol/L, Cl^- 102 mmol/L, CO_2 25 mmol/L, glucose 75 mg/dL, and creatinine 1.2 mg/dL. Which of the following neoplasms is most likely to be diagnosed?

- ❏ (A) Adenohypophyseal adenoma
- ❏ (B) Carcinoid tumor
- ❏ (C) Medullary carcinoma
- ❏ (D) Pheochromocytoma
- ❏ (E) Renal cell carcinoma
- ❏ (F) Small cell anaplastic carcinoma

31 A male infant born to a 40-year-old woman, who had an uncomplicated pregnancy, is noted at birth to be at the 70th percentile for height and weight. On physical examination, the infant has bilateral palmar transverse creases and absent distal flexion creases on the fifth digits. The palpebral fissures are oblique. He has brachycephaly. On auscultation of the chest, a holosystolic murmur is audible. During childhood, mental retardation is exhibited, but the child is able to perform activities of daily living. At age 17, the boy has a series of severe upper respiratory tract infections. CBC shows hemoglobin of 10.2 g/dL, hematocrit 30.5%, MCV 89 μm^3, platelet count 103,000/mm^3, and WBC count 19,200/mm^3 with 14% segmented neutrophils, 6% bands, 22% lymphocytes, 13% monocytes, and 45% blasts. Which of the following karyotypes is most likely to be present in this boy?

- ❏ (A) 45,X
- ❏ (B) 46,XY
- ❏ (C) 47,XY, + 13
- ❏ (D) 47,XY, + 18
- ❏ (E) 47,XY, + 21
- ❏ (F) 47,XXY
- ❏ (G) 69,XYY

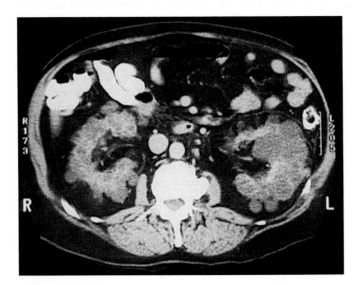

32 A 52-year-old woman has noticed increasing thirst and urine output for the past 6 months. She has become more lethargic and has had decreased mental agility during that time. She has had flank pain on the right during the past month. On physical examination, her temperature is 37°C, pulse 77/min, respirations 14/min, and blood pressure 150/95 mm Hg. There are bilateral palpable masses in the abdomen. An abdominal CT scan is shown in the preceding figure. Urinalysis shows specific gravity of 1.010, pH 6.5, 2+ proteinuria, 2+ hematuria, and no glucose or ketones. Laboratory findings show hemoglobin of 10.4 g/dL, hematocrit 31.3%, glucose 102 mg/dL, AST 30 U/L, ALT 21 U/L, creatinine 5.5 mg/dL, and urea nitrogen 53 mg/dL. One year later, she develops a sudden, severe headache. A CT scan of the head shows a subarachnoid hemorrhage at the base of the brain. Which of the following is the most likely diagnosis?

- ❏ (A) Adult-onset medullary cystic disease
- ❏ (B) Cystinosis
- ❏ (C) Diabetes mellitus type 2
- ❏ (D) Dominant polycystic kidney disease
- ❏ (E) Polyarteritis nodosa
- ❏ (F) Wegener granulomatosis
- ❏ (G) Wilson disease

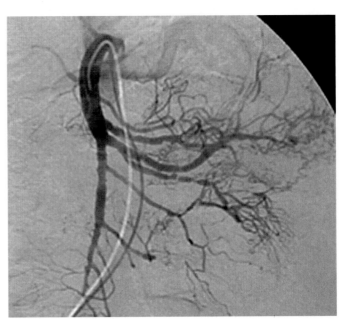

33 A 35-year-old man has had bouts of severe, diffuse abdominal pain over the past 4 months. These bouts have been accompanied by fever, malaise, and myalgias. During one bout, he sees the physician. On physical examination, his temperature is 37.7°C, pulse 81/min, respirations 16/min, and blood pressure 145/90 mm Hg. There is diffuse abdominal tenderness but no masses, and bowel sounds are present. A stool sample is positive for occult blood. Laboratory findings show serum glucose of 73 mg/dL, amylase 44 U/L, AST 54 U/L, ALT 23 U/L, creatinine 2.4 mg/dL, and urea nitrogen 22 mg/dL. A renal biopsy specimen shows acute transmural vasculitis of medium-sized arteries; the glomeruli and tubules are unremarkable. Mesenteric artery angiography is performed and is shown above. Which of the following serologic tests is most likely to be positive in this patient?

☐ (A) Antimitochondrial antibody
☐ (B) C-ANCA
☐ (C) ANA
☐ (D) *Cryptococcus neoformans* antigen
☐ (E) HBsAg
☐ (F) *Histoplasma capsulatum* antibody
☐ (G) p24 antigen

34 A 14-year-old girl who has been in foster care for the past 11 years has not been with one caregiver for more than 1 year at a time. She is brought to the physician by the most recent caregiver, who obtained custody of the child 1 week ago. On physical examination, there are ecchymoses of the trunk, extremities, and gingiva. A hyperkeratotic, papular rash, with 0.4-cm lesions ringed by hemorrhage, is present in a similar distribution. The child has pain on movement of the arms and legs. There is abnormal depression of the sternum with prominence of the ribs and the costochondral junctions. Radiographs of the arms and legs show bowing of the long bones and widening of the metaphyses, with normal calcification. There is a right femoral subperiosteal hematoma. No fractures are noted. CBC shows hemoglobin of 10.8 g/dL, hematocrit 32.4%, MCV 77 μm³, platelet count 201,300/mm³, and WBC count 5730/mm³. Which of the following is most likely to explain these findings?

☐ (A) CFTR gene mutation
☐ (B) Inhibitor of procoagulant factor VIII
☐ (C) Collagen gene mutation
☐ (D) Vitamin C deficiency
☐ (E) Multiple blunt trauma

35 A 10-year-old girl has a respiratory tract infection and is treated with trimethoprim-sulfamethoxazole. Three days later, she develops a sore throat, malaise, fever, and a macular skin rash on the trunk and extremities. Some of the skin lesions have a central raised area of more pronounced erythema. Within a few days, there are erosions of the oral mucosa and small blisters developing on purpuric skin macules. The blisters enlarge slightly and then show epidermal detachment. The total body surface area involved with blistering and detachment is less than 10%. This disease process is most likely mediated by which of the following inflammatory cell types?

☐ (A) CD8 lymphocytes
☐ (B) Eosinophils
☐ (C) Langerhans cells
☐ (D) Macrophages
☐ (E) Neutrophils
☐ (F) Natural killer cells

36 Within the past 24 hours, a 26-year-old previously healthy woman has developed a high fever and generalized diffuse erythematous macular rash resembling a sunburn. She is menstruating, and her menstrual cycles are regular. She has nausea, vomiting, abdominal pain, diarrhea, myalgias, sore throat, headache, and dizziness. On physical examination, her temperature is 39.4°C, pulse 101/min, respirations 18/min, and blood pressure 90/40 mm Hg. She has oropharyngeal and conjunctival hyperemia. The vaginal mucosa is erythematous. A tampon is present in the vagina vault. She is disoriented, but there are no neurologic deficits. Laboratory findings show hemoglobin of 13.5 g/dL, hematocrit 41.4%, platelet count 100,000/mm³, WBC count 11,200/mm³, glucose 70 mg/dL, creatinine 2.5 mg/dL, total bilirubin 2.4 mg/dL, AST 82 U/L, and ALT 29 U/L. A chest radiograph shows no abnormal findings. She receives supportive therapy of nafcillin with clindamycin and improves, but skin and mucous membrane desquamation is noted 10 days later. These findings are most likely produced by an exotoxin elaborated by which of the following organisms?

☐ (A) *Bacillus anthracis*
☐ (B) *Clostridium perfringens*
☐ (C) Enterococcus
☐ (D) *Listeria monocytogenes*
☐ (E) *Staphylococcus aureus*
☐ (F) *Vibrio cholerae*

37 A 21-month-old child has had recurrent otitis media complicated by mastoiditis for the past 3 months. On physical examination, there is a seborrheic eruption on the skin of the trunk and scalp. Hepatosplenomegaly and generalized nontender lymphadenopathy are present. A chest radiograph shows bilateral 0.5- to 2-cm pulmonary nodules, and there is a 1-cm lesion on the right clavicle and a 1.5-cm lesion on the left seventh rib, both osteolytic. Laboratory findings show hemoglobin of 10.4 g/dL, hematocrit 31.2%, platelet count 93,400/mm³, WBC count 5780/mm³, glucose 72 mg/dL, and creatinine 0.5 mg/dL. A bone marrow biopsy specimen shows reduced hematopoiesis with increased numbers of large cells having oval vesicular nuclei and vacuolated cytoplasm that mark immunocytologically for CD1a. Which of the following is the most likely diagnosis?

☐ (A) Acute lymphoblastic leukemia
☐ (B) Gaucher disease
☐ (C) Langerhans cell histiocytosis
☐ (D) Leishmaniasis
☐ (E) Multiple myeloma
☐ (F) Myelodysplastic syndrome

38 A 4-year-old girl has become increasingly listless over the past year. The child is at the 25th percentile for height and weight. On physical examination, there is pubic hair and clitoral and breast enlargement. There is no hepatomegaly, splenomegaly, or lymphadenopathy. The neurologic examination is unremarkable. Laboratory findings show hemoglobin of 13.7 g/dL, hematocrit 41.8%, WBC count 7120/mm³, Na⁺ 128 mmol/L, K⁺ 4.8 mmol/L, Cl⁻ 99 mmol/L, CO₂ 21 mmol/L, glucose 69 mg/dL, and creatinine 0.5 mg/dL and ACTH 95 pg/mL with loss of diurnal rhythm of secretion. Which of the following disease processes is most likely to be associated with these findings?

☐ (A) Anaplastic carcinoma of the thyroid
☐ (B) Bilateral adrenal hyperplasia
☐ (C) Islet cell adenoma
☐ (D) Medullary carcinoma of the thyroid
☐ (E) Neuroblastoma of the adrenal
☐ (F) Pituitary microadenoma
☐ (G) Suprasellar craniopharyngioma

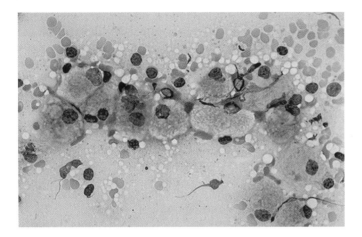

39 A 10-month-old infant is not meeting developmental milestones and is below ideal weight and height. One week ago, the parents noted an episode of convulsions. On physical examination, the infant has hepatosplenomegaly and generalized nontender lymphadenopathy. There is tenderness on palpation of the right upper extremity. No focal neurologic deficits are present, but the infant's attention and movement are diminished. A radiograph of the right arm shows a healing fracture. Laboratory findings show hemoglobin of 9.7 g/dL, hematocrit 28.4%, platelet count 76,700/mm³, WBC count 4200/mm³, glucose 78 mg/dL, and creatinine 0.4 mg/dL. A bone marrow biopsy is performed, and the microscopic appearance of the biopsy specimen is shown. The infant is most likely to have the near absence of which of the following enzymes?

- ❑ (A) α-L-Iduronidase
- ❑ (B) α-1,4-Glucosidase
- ❑ (C) Arylsulfatase A
- ❑ (D) Glucocerebrosidase
- ❑ (E) Glucose-6-phosphatase
- ❑ (F) Hexosaminidase A
- ❑ (G) Hexosaminidase B
- ❑ (H) Sphingomyelinase

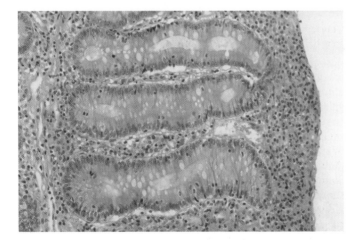

40 A 39-year-old man states that he has had watery diarrhea and flatulence for the past 8 months. He also reports increasing fatigue and a 4-kg weight loss. He has had urticarial plaques on extensor surfaces of the elbows and knees and on the upper back for the past month. Some of the plaques have small, grouped vesicles. A biopsy specimen of one of the skin lesions shows neutrophils at the tips of dermal papillae with overlying basal cell vacuolization. Under immunofluorescence microscopy, granular IgA deposits appear at the tips of dermal papillae. The microscopic appearance of a jejunal biopsy is shown. More than 20 years later, the patient has a T-cell lymphoma of the jejunum. Antibody to which of the following is most likely to produce this disease?

- ❑ (A) Desmoglein 3
- ❑ (B) Double-stranded DNA
- ❑ (C) Gliadin
- ❑ (D) Histone
- ❑ (E) Ribonucleoprotein
- ❑ (F) Type IV collagen

41 For the past month, a 33-year-old woman has had burning epigastric pain and nausea and vomiting. An upper gastrointestinal endoscopic study shows multiple 1-cm shallow gastric antral and proximal duodenal ulcerations. She is treated with omeprazole and improves. One year later, she has an episode of severe, colicky lower abdominal pain and hematuria and passes a calcium oxalate calculus. One month later, she notes galactorrhea, and over the next 2 months ceases to menstruate. She is given a dopamine agonist and improves. Laboratory findings show Na⁺ 140 mmol/L, K⁺ 4.0 mmol/L, Cl⁻ 101 mmol/L, CO₂ 25 mmol/L, calcium 11.1 mg/dL, phosphorus 2.4 mg/dL, and creatinine 1.1 mg/dL. Which of the following gene mutations with associated neoplasms is most likely to develop in this patient?

- ❑ (A) Islet cell adenoma—*MEN1*
- ❑ (B) Medullary carcinoma—*RET*
- ❑ (C) Non-Hodgkin lymphoma—*BCL6*
- ❑ (D) Osteoma—*APC*
- ❑ (E) Pheochromocytoma—*RET*
- ❑ (F) Renal cell carcinoma—*VHL*

42 A 60-year-old man has pain in his hands and feet on arising in the morning. The pain persists for almost 2 hours and is aggravated by movement. He would rather stay in bed. He has weakness, easy fatigability, and anorexia and reports a 6-kg weight loss over the past 2 years. On physical examination, his temperature is 37.4°C, pulse 74/min, respirations 20/min, and blood pressure 110/70 mm Hg. There is warmth, tenderness, and limitation of motion of the joints of his hands. Over the next 5 years, he develops joint deformities. A chest radiograph shows extensive interstitial lung disease and a prominent right-sided heart border. Spirometry reveals decreased FEV₁ and FVC. Additional findings include 1-cm firm, subcutaneous nodules over the olecranon bursae and Achilles tendons. Which of the following is the most likely diagnosis?

- ❑ (A) Caplan syndrome
- ❑ (B) Carney syndrome
- ❑ (C) Churg-Strauss syndrome
- ❑ (D) Felty syndrome
- ❑ (E) Hamman-Rich syndrome
- ❑ (F) Kartagener syndrome
- ❑ (G) Trousseau syndrome

43 A 40-year-old man has noticed worsening myalgias and increasing difficulty swallowing over the past 2 years. When exposed to cold, the skin of his hands turns white. On physical examination, he has an erythematous rash extending across the bridge of his nose. There is swelling and warmth in the joints of his hands. Laboratory findings show hemoglobin of 12.2 g/dL, hematocrit 36.5%, platelet count 180,000/mm³, WBC count 4510/mm³, serum glucose 72 mg/dL, total bilirubin 1.0 mg/dL, AST 41 U/L, ALT 19 U/L, alkaline phosphatase 69 U/L, creatine kinase 483 U/L, and creatinine 1.3 mg/dL. The presence of antibodies to which of the following is most characteristic of his condition?

- ❏ (A) ANCA
- ❏ (B) Cyclic citrullinated peptide
- ❏ (C) Histone
- ❏ (D) Smith
- ❏ (E) Thyroid peroxidase
- ❏ (F) U1-RNP

44 A 19-year-old man is found unconscious by his roommate. He is taken to the emergency department, where physical examination shows temperature of 41.2°C, pulse 103/min, respirations 18/min and shallow, and blood pressure 145/100 mm Hg. He develops an intractable cardiac dysrhythmia and dies. At autopsy, the heart is slightly enlarged; microscopically, the distal coronary arteries are thickened. Sections of the brain show a 2-cm area of hemorrhage in the right superior parietal lobe and a 0.5-cm hemorrhage in the medulla. There is a partially cystic 1-cm area with brown discoloration in the left anterior frontal lobe. Which of the following drugs was this patient most likely to have used regularly?

- ❏ (A) Amphetamine
- ❏ (B) Barbiturate
- ❏ (C) Cocaine
- ❏ (D) Ethanol
- ❏ (E) Heroin
- ❏ (F) Marijuana
- ❏ (G) Methamphetamine
- ❏ (H) Phencyclidine

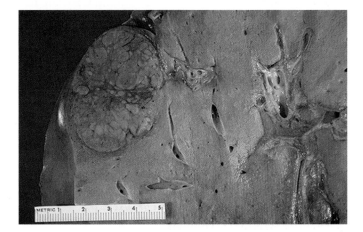

45 A 44-year-old woman has noted dull right upper quadrant pain for the past year. On physical examination there is right upper quadrant tenderness on palpation. An abdominal CT scan shows a 5-cm circumscribed mass in the superior right lobe of the liver. The representative gross appearance of a similar mass is shown. One month later, she experiences sudden onset of dyspnea with diaphoresis. Multiple peripheral perfusion defects are seen on a pulmonary ventilation/perfusion scan. Which of the following combinations of pharmacologic agents taken by this patient regularly is most likely to be associated with these findings?

- ❏ (A) Allopurinol and sulfamethoxazole
- ❏ (B) Ethynyl estradiol and norethindrone
- ❏ (C) Ibuprofen and acetylsalicylic acid
- ❏ (D) Isoniazid and rifampicin
- ❏ (E) Phenacetin and acetaminophen
- ❏ (F) Prednisone and cyclophosphamide

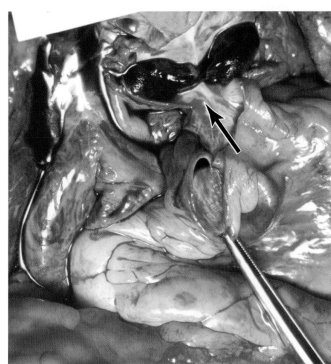

Courtesy of Dr. Linda Margraf, Department of Pathology, University of Texas Southwestern Medical School, Dallas, TX.

46 A 90-year-old woman died suddenly. Autopsy shows a 5-cm skin ulceration extending to the sacrum. She has diffuse muscle wasting; a microscopic section shows decreased size of muscle fibers without inflammation or fibrosis. Her bones demonstrate marked osteoporosis, and there is vertebral column kyphosis. A finding on examination of the lungs is shown. There a right lower lobe pneumonia. Which of the following conditions is most likely to predispose this patient to the pathologic findings seen at autopsy?

- ❏ (A) Antiphospholipid syndrome
- ❏ (B) Aplastic anemia
- ❏ (C) Chronic alcoholism
- ❏ (D) Elder abuse with blunt trauma
- ❏ (E) Immobilization
- ❏ (F) Malnutrition

47 A 29-year-old man has had a low-grade fever for the past 2 weeks. He has had increasing fatigue and a 2-kg weight loss during this time. On physical examination, his temperature is 37.5°C, pulse 80/min, respirations 17/min, and blood pressure 150/70 mm Hg. His spleen tip is palpable, and there is left upper quadrant tenderness. There is bilateral costovertebral angle tenderness. A diastolic murmur is heard at the left sternal border. Subungual hemorrhages are noted on the digits of his hands. A needle track is present in the left antecubital fossa. Laboratory findings show hemoglobin of 13.6 g/dL, hematocrit 41.8%, platelet count 228,000/mm³, WBC count 11,200/mm³, glucose 66 mg/dL, AST 101 U/L, ALT 28 U/L, alkaline phosphatase 89 U/L, amylase 45 U/L, and total bilirubin 0.9 mg/dL. Urinalysis shows 1 + hematuria and both WBCs and WBC casts. A chest radiograph shows a 3-cm nodule with an air-fluid level in the right upper lobe. Which of the following organisms is most likely to be cultured from his blood?

- (A) *Candida albicans*
- (B) *Cryptococcus neoformans*
- (C) *Escherichia coli*
- (D) *Listeria monocytogenes*
- (E) *Staphylococcus aureus*
- (F) *Streptococcus pyogenes*
- (G) *Yersinia enterocolitica*

48 A 41-year-old woman has had headaches with blurred vision for the past 3 days. Over the past day, she has developed increasing mental confusion. On admission to the hospital, her temperature is 37.9°C, pulse 104/min, respirations 25/min, and blood pressure 70/40 mmHg. On physical examination, she has petechial hemorrhages over her arms and trunk. A stool sample is positive for occult blood. Laboratory findings show hemoglobin of 9.1 g/dL, hematocrit 27.2%, MCV 92 μm³, RDW 19%, platelet count 8900/mm³, and WBC count 8950/mm³. The peripheral blood smear shows schistocytes. A serum electrolyte panel shows Na⁺ 147 mmol/L, K⁺ 5.0 mmol/L, Cl⁻ 105 mmol/L, CO₂ 26 mmol/L, creatinine 3.3 mg/ dL, urea nitrogen 32 mg/dL, and glucose 80 mg/dL Ultra-large multimers of von Willebrand factor are present in plasma. Which of the following therapies should she receive emergently?

- (A) Two units of packed RBCs
- (B) Six-pack of platelets
- (C) Dobutamine
- (D) Exploratory laparotomy
- (E) Plasmapheresis
- (F) Prednisone

49 A 30-year-old woman has noted a 5-kg weight gain over the past 3 months and has not had a menstrual period during that time. She has experienced upper abdominal pain for the past month. Physical examination shows abdominal enlargement with apparent ascites. There is no peripheral edema. She has a positive pregnancy test. Additional laboratory findings show hemoglobin of 13.2 g/dL, hematocrit 39.7%, WBC count 12,300/mm³, glucose 80 mg/dL, AST 581 U/L, ALT 611 U/L, total bilirubin 1.3 mg/dL, total protein 6.2 g/dL, and albumin 3.5 g/dL. An abdominal ultrasound scan shows hepatomegaly with heterogenous echogenicity, and there is an intrauterine gestation with a fetus estimated at 12 weeks' size. Which of the following pathologic findings is most likely to be present?

- (A) Choledocholithiasis
- (B) Chronic passive congestion
- (C) Hepatic venous thrombosis
- (D) Hepatocellular adenoma
- (E) Metastatic choriocarcinoma
- (F) Microvesicular steatosis

50 A 25-year-old woman has had increasingly frequent infections over the past 5 years. His most recent respiratory infection was due to *Streptococcus pneumoniae*. He now has a watery diarrhea. On physical examination, he is below ideal weight. There is a vesicular rash in the T10 dermatomal distribution on the left. Laboratory findings include hemoglobin of 14.3 g/dL, hematocrit 43.2%, platelet count 290,600/mm³, and WBC count 7200/mm³ with 55% segmented neutrophils, 2% bands, 35% lymphocytes, 6% monocytes, and 2% eosinophils. Quantitative immunoglobulins include IgA of 22 mg/dL, IgG 175 mg/dL, and IgM 40 mg/dL. Lymphocyte subsets by flow cytometry show CD4 cells (absolute) of 630/μL, CD8 cells (absolute) 785/μL, B cells 280/μL, and T cells 2010/μL. A stool culture is negative for bacterial pathogens, but a stool culture for ova and parasites shows *Giardia lamblia* cysts. Which of the following is the most likely diagnosis?

- (A) Chronic granulomatous disease
- (B) Common variable immunodeficiency
- (C) Hyper-IgM syndrome
- (D) Leukocyte adhesion deficiency
- (E) Severe combined immunodeficiency

51 A 44-year-old man has had worsening exercise tolerance as well as peripheral edema during the past 5 years. He has noted increasing central opacifications that interfere with vision. He has frontal baldness. During the past 2 years, he has had progressive memory loss with decreasing ability to perform activities of daily living. On physical examination, there is significant atrophy of masseter, temporalis, scalene, deltoid, trapezius, and sternocleidomastoid muscles. There is bilateral testicular atrophy. A glucose tolerance test at 2 hours shows serum glucose of 156 mg/dL. Serum quantitative immunoglobulins show IgG of 450 mg/dL, IgA 303 mg/dL, and IgM 197 mg/dL. His condition worsens over the next 3 years, with increasing muscular weakness, and he succumbs to bronchopneumonia. An abnormality in which of the following gene products is most likely to be present?

- (A) α-1,4-Glucosidase
- (B) Dystrophin
- (C) Fibroblast growth factor receptor 3
- (D) Mitochondrial oxidative phosphorylase
- (E) Myophosphorylase
- (F) Myotonin protein kinase
- (G) Neurofibromin

52 A 4-year-old girl has abrupt onset of vomiting, which remains protracted for 24 hours. On arrival at the emergency department, the child is lethargic and febrile to 37.7°C. The parents state that she had a mild upper respiratory tract illness 3 days ago but was improving, and the only medication she received was acetylsalicylic acid (aspirin). On physical examination, there is poor skin turgor, the lungs are clear, the abdomen is nontender, and the heart rate is regular. Laboratory findings show Na⁺ of 150 mmol/L, K⁺ 4.5 mmol/L, Cl⁻

93 mmol/L, CO$_2$ 30 mmol/L, glucose 60 mg/dL, creatinine 1.1 mg/dL, amylase 25 U/L, AST 386 U/L, ALT 409 U/L, alkaline phosphatase 120 U/L, total bilirubin 1.1 mg/dL, ammonia 80 μmol/L, and prothrombin time 26 sec. The child becomes comatose. Which of the following pathologic findings is most likely to be present in this patient?

- ❑ (A) Common bile duct atresia
- ❑ (B) Hepatic vein thrombosis
- ❑ (C) Hepatoblastoma
- ❑ (D) Intrahepatic duct lithiasis
- ❑ (E) Microvesicular steatosis
- ❑ (F) Multinucleated giant cells

53 A 22-year-old woman has sudden onset of severe lower abdominal pain. Her medical history is remarkable for *Chlamydia trachomatis* cervicitis. On physical examination, her temperature is 36.9°C, pulse 90/min, respirations 17/min, and blood pressure 90/50 mm Hg. There is lower abdominal tenderness but no palpable masses. No vaginal bleeding is present. The rectal examination is unremarkable, and a stool sample is negative for occult blood. Bowel sounds are reduced. An abdominal ultrasound scan is performed, and the uterus appears normal in size with no masses visualized, but there is a right adnexal mass. Culdocentesis is performed, and there is blood in the aspirate. Laboratory findings show hemoglobin of 9.5 g/dL, hematocrit 28.6%, platelet count 269,300/mm^3, and WBC count 9110/mm^3. Which of the following laboratory findings is most likely to be present?

- ❑ (A) Carcinoembryonic antigen increase
- ❑ (B) *Entamoeba histolytica* cysts in stool
- ❑ (C) Factor XIII deficiency
- ❑ (D) Follicle-stimulating hormone decrease
- ❑ (E) Human chorionic gonadotropin elevation
- ❑ (F) Partial thromboplastin time prolonged
- ❑ (G) *Schistosoma haematobium* eggs in urine

54 A 71-year-old woman has had a history of back pain for several months. She recently developed a cough productive of yellowish sputum, and a sputum culture grew *Streptococcus pneumoniae*. On physical examination, she has no lymphadenopathy or hepatosplenomegaly. Laboratory findings show Na$^+$ of 141 mmol/L, K$^+$ 4.2 mmol/L, Cl$^-$ 104 mmol/L, CO$_2$ 26 mmol/L, glucose 79 mg/dL, calcium 9.8 mg/dL, phosphorus 3.1 mg/dL, AST 31 U/L, ALT 24 U/L, alkaline phosphatase 291 U/L, total protein 9.3 g/dL, albumin 4.4 g/dL, urea nitrogen 31 mg/dL, and creatinine 3.8 mg/dL. A skull radiograph shows multiple 1- to 4-cm lytic lesions. Which of the following laboratory findings is most likely to be reported?

- ❑ (A) Bence-Jones proteinuria
- ❑ (B) Increased hemoglobin F
- ❑ (C) Hemoglobin 21.2 g/dL
- ❑ (D) Positive ANA
- ❑ (E) WBC count 450,000/mm^3

55 A 49-year-old man has had increasing knee and hip pain for the past 10 years. The pain is worse at the end of the day. During the past year, he has become increasingly drowsy at work. His wife complains that he is a "world class" snorer. During the past month, he has experienced bouts of sharp, colicky, right upper abdominal pain. On physical examination, his temperature is 37°C, pulse 82/min, respirations

10/min, and blood pressure 140/85 mm Hg. He is 175 cm (5 ft 8 in) tall and weighs 156 kg (BMI 51). Laboratory findings show glucose of 139 mg/dL, total cholesterol 229 mg/dL, and HDL cholesterol 33 mg/dL. An arterial blood gas measurement shows pH of 7.3, PCO_2 50 mm Hg, and PO_2 70 mm Hg. Which of the following conditions is most likely to be present?

- ❑ (A) Hashimoto thyroiditis
- ❑ (B) Hypertrophic cardiomyopathy
- ❑ (C) Laryngeal papillomatosis
- ❑ (D) Nonalcoholic steatohepatitis
- ❑ (E) Panlobular emphysema
- ❑ (F) Rheumatoid arthritis

56 A 51-year-old man living on the island of St. Helena has had a downturn in his political fortunes. Over the past 3 years, and particularly over the past year, he has had increasing bouts of abdominal pain, anorexia, nausea, vomiting, dysuria, lethargy, spiking fevers, diarrhea, constipation, excessive weakness, heavy perspiration, and weight loss. He is given a large dose of calomel (a mercury-containing compound) a few days before his death May 5, 1821, a treatment that has since vanished for good reason. An autopsy shows hepatomegaly (with steatosis?) and ulceration with thickening of the stomach. The autopsy report does not record skin and nail changes, such as hyperkeratosis and hyperpigmentation. If those changes had been present, as well as squamous cell carcinoma of the skin, the findings would have been most suggestive of chronic poisoning with which of the following metals?

- ❑ (A) Arsenic
- ❑ (B) Beryllium
- ❑ (C) Chromium
- ❑ (D) Cobalt
- ❑ (E) Lead
- ❑ (F) Nickel

57 A 37-year-old woman, G 1, P 0, at 30 weeks' gestation has noted increasing pedal edema for the past 2 weeks. During the past week, she has developed headaches and confusion, and she has decreased urine output. She exhibited seizure activity and then lapsed into a coma. On physical examination, her temperature is 36.8°C, pulse 82/min, respirations 18/min, and blood pressure 145/95 mm Hg. Her heart rate is regular, and lung fields are clear. The abdomen is soft, and bowel sounds are present. There is pitting edema to the thighs. No vaginal bleeding is noted, and the cervix is not effaced. Laboratory findings show hemoglobin of 11.9 g/dL, hematocrit 35.8%, platelet count 73,000/mm^3, WBC count 8180/mm^3, glucose 151 mg/dL, total protein 6.6 g/dL, albumin 3.2 g/dL, total bilirubin 2.3 mg/dL, AST 78 U/L, ALT 93 U/L, alkaline phosphatase 253 U/L, and prothrombin time 32 sec. Urinalysis shows specific gravity of 1.024, pH 6, 4 + proteinuria, 1 + glucosuria, and no blood. An ultrasound examination shows a viable 30-week fetus. Which of the following conditions is most likely to be present in this patient?

- ❑ (A) Abruptio placentae
- ❑ (B) Budd-Chiari syndrome
- ❑ (C) Dilated cardiomyopathy
- ❑ (D) HELLP syndrome
- ❑ (E) Hydatidiform mole
- ❑ (F) Reye syndrome
- ❑ (G) Sheehan syndrome

58 A 29-year-old man sees his physician because of burning pain on urination that has persisted for 3 days. There is a urethral discharge. A sample of the exudate is positive by ELISA for *Chlamydia trachomatis*. Three weeks later, the man has increasing stiffness of the knees and ankles and lower back pain. A radiograph of the lumbar spine shows narrowing with sclerosis of the sacroiliac joints. One month later, he develops painful erythema of the penile glans, and the conjunctivae are red. A follow-up examination shows a slightly irregular heart rate and a murmur suggestive of aortic regurgitation. The back pain continues off and on for 5 more months. Which of the following test results is most likely to be positive?

❑ (A) ANCA
❑ (B) ANA
❑ (C) HLA-B27 antigen
❑ (D) Lyme disease
❑ (E) Purified protein derivative
❑ (F) Rapid plasma reagin
❑ (G) Rheumatoid factor
❑ (H) U1-RNP

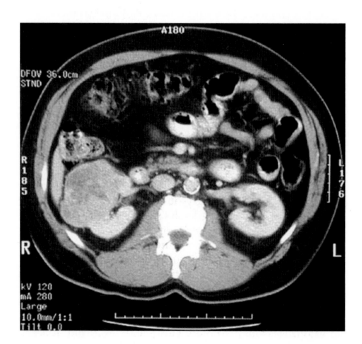

59 A 19-year-old man has been having headaches for the past month. On physical examination, his temperature is 37°C, pulse 77/min, respirations 14/min, and blood pressure 160/95 mm Hg. On funduscopic examination, there are bilateral retinal angiomas. An abdominal CT scan shows a 3-cm mass involving the right adrenal gland. Laboratory testing shows increased urinary catecholamines. The mass is removed surgically. Five years later, he develops a movement disorder with incoordination and ataxia. MR imaging of the brain shows a 2-cm mass in the left cerebellar hemisphere and a 1-cm mass in the vermis. These are removed surgically. Six years later, he has right flank pain with hematuria; his abdominal CT scan is shown. His hemoglobin concentration is 20.3 g/dL,

and hematocrit is 60.9%. Which of the following gene mutations and associated neoplasms does he most likely have?

❑ (A) Beckwith-Wiedemann syndrome—*WT-1*
❑ (B) Denys-Drash syndrome—*MET*
❑ (C) Gardner syndrome—*APC*
❑ (D) Neurofibromatosis type 2—*NF-2*
❑ (E) Tuberous sclerosis—*TSC-1*
❑ (F) Von Hippel-Lindau disease—*VHL*

60 A 43-year-old woman has had increasing difficulty swallowing over the past year. She notices that her hands turn white and are painful on exposure to cold. She remarks, "I may be getting older, but at least I don't have any wrinkles on my face or hands yet." On physical examination, her temperature is 37°C, pulse 68/min, respirations 14/min, and blood pressure 115/75 mm Hg. The skin of her face and hands appears taut and shiny. A punch biopsy of the skin of the hand shows dermal collagenous fibrosis and focal calcification. She receives yearly esophageal dilation for the next 20 years, during which time she develops no serious illnesses. Which of the following serologic test results is most likely to be positive?

❑ (A) Anticentromere antibody
❑ (B) Anti-DNA topoisomerase antibody
❑ (C) Antigliadin antibody
❑ (D) Antimicrosomal antibody
❑ (E) Antimitochondrial antibody
❑ (F) ANCA

61 A 56-year-old man has had increasing lower leg swelling during the past 6 months. He also has had so much difficulty breathing at night that he sleeps propped up on two pillows. On physical examination, his temperature is 37.1°C, pulse 80/min, respirations 17/min, and blood pressure 110/70 mm Hg. On auscultation of the chest, bilateral crackles are audible at the lung bases. The liver span is increased. There is 2+ pitting edema to the thighs. Laboratory findings show hemoglobin of 13.4 g/dL, hematocrit 40.2%, MCV 88 μm³, platelet count 229,300/mm³, and WBC count 6715/mm³. One year later, he develops an acute psychosis. He dies of aspiration pneumonia. At autopsy, there is anterior vermian atrophy and petechial hemorrhages with brown discoloration in the periaqueductal gray matter, as well as shrunken mamillary bodies. A chronic deficiency of which of the following vitamins is most likely to explain these findings?

❑ (A) Vitamin A (retinoic acid)
❑ (B) Vitamin B₁ (thiamine)
❑ (C) Vitamin B₂ (riboflavin)
❑ (D) Vitamin B₃ (niacin)
❑ (E) Vitamin B₁₂ (cobalamin)
❑ (F) Vitamin C (ascorbic acid)
❑ (G) Vitamin D (cholecalciferol)
❑ (H) Vitamin E (α-tocopherol)

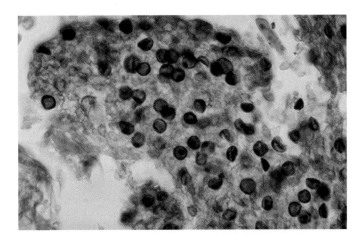

- ❏ (A) Acetylsalicylic acid
- ❏ (B) Acetaminophen
- ❏ (C) Adalimumab
- ❏ (D) Methotrexate
- ❏ (E) Oxycodone
- ❏ (F) Propoxyphene

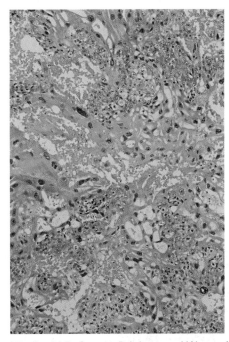

Courtesy of Dr. David R. Genest, Brigham and Women's Hospital, Boston, MA.

62 A 32-year-old woman has had increasing malaise and a 10-kg weight loss over the past 6 months. Physical examination shows muscle wasting, and there is a tan-yellow, plaque-like coating on her tongue. Laboratory testing shows hemoglobin of 12.6 g/dL, hematocrit 37.8%, MCV 85 μm^3, platelet count 188,300/mm³, and WBC count 4320/mm³ with 73% segmented neutrophils, 3% bands, 9% lymphocytes, 14% monocytes, and 1% eosinophils. A scraping of the material from her tongue microscopically shows budding cells with pseudohyphae. Six months later, she develops a watery diarrhea; a stool specimen contains cysts of *Cryptosporidium parvum*. She then develops a fever, cough, and severe dyspnea. Bronchoalveolar lavage is performed, and the microscopic findings are shown. Which of the following laboratory findings is most likely to be present?

- ❏ (A) ANA titer 1:1024
- ❏ (B) CD4 lymphocyte count 111/μL
- ❏ (C) Complement C2 undetectable
- ❏ (D) IgG 88 mg/dL
- ❏ (E) Neutrophil oxidative burst assay <5%
- ❏ (F) Positive RPR

63 A 73-year-old man has had bilateral knee and hip pain for the past 25 years and has taken a medication for this pain for the past 5 years. During the past year, he has noticed increasing frequency of headaches, dizziness, tinnitus, confusion, and nausea. He states that bruises form on his skin with minimal trauma. One week ago, he experienced an episode of hematemesis. On physical examination, his temperature is 37.1°C, pulse 73/min, respirations 18/min, and blood pressure 130/80 mm Hg. There are scattered petechiae on his arms and legs and an area of purpura on his right thigh. His heart rate is regular, and the lungs are clear. No neurologic deficits are noted. Laboratory findings show hemoglobin of 11.1 g/dL, hematocrit 33.1%, MCV 72 μm³, platelet count 317,200/mm³, WBC count 5915/mm³, Na⁺ 139 mmol/L, K⁺ 3.9 mmol/L, Cl⁻ 98 mmol/L, CO_2 19 mmol/L, glucose 76 mg/dL, and creatinine 1.1 mg/dL. The partial thromboplastin time is 27 sec, and the prothrombin time is 13 sec. Platelet function analysis shows decreased aggregation in response to ADP and collagen stimulation. An upper gastrointestinal endoscopic study shows gastric mucosal erythema and a 1.8-cm sharply demarcated, shallow, antral ulceration. Chronic use of which of the following pharmacologic agents is most likely to produce these findings?

64 For the past month, a 16-year-old girl has had increasing heat intolerance, with nervousness and a fine tremor. She has had irregular menstrual cycles since menarche 2 years ago and has not menstruated for 3 months. She has not used contraceptives. One week ago, she noticed a small amount of vaginal bleeding and now has sudden onset of severe abdominal pain. On physical examination, her temperature is 36.9°, pulse 105/min, respirations 17/min, and blood pressure 80/40 mm Hg. There is marked right upper quadrant abdominal tenderness, and bowel sounds are reduced. A stool sample is negative for occult blood. Brownish-colored fluid is noted in the vaginal vault, emanating from a reddish-brown 2-cm mass in the vault. An abdominal ultrasound examination shows several 3- to 6-cm masses in the liver, and the uterus appears enlarged, with a 5-cm mass. An anteroposterior chest radiograph shows several 1- to 3-cm nodules in the lungs. Paracentesis is performed, and there is blood in the aspirate. The microscopic appearance of a biopsy specimen of the vaginal mass is shown. She receives therapy with methotrexate and actinomycin-D and improves. Which of the following neoplasms is most likely to produce these findings?

- ❏ (A) Adenocarcinoma
- ❏ (B) Choriocarcinoma
- ❏ (C) Clear cell carcinoma
- ❏ (D) Leiomyosarcoma
- ❏ (E) Malignant mixed müllerian tumor
- ❏ (F) Sarcoma botryoides

65 A 31-year-old woman, G 1, P 0, is in the second trimester and has not felt any fetal movement. The maternal serum α-fetoprotein level is elevated. An ultrasound examination shows a fetus that is equivalent in size to 18 weeks' gestation. However, several anomalies are noted. The umbilical cord is short, the digits of the left hand are missing, and there is a band extending from the distal left extremity to the edge of an abdominal wall defect. This defect has no covering and is located to the right of the umbilicus, with bowel and liver herniating out through it. There appears to be marked scoliosis. Which of the following is the most likely cause of these findings?

- ❑ (A) Autosomal dominant trait
- ❑ (B) Early amnion disruption
- ❑ (C) Germ-line mosaicism
- ❑ (D) Meiotic nondisjunction
- ❑ (E) Prolonged rupture of fetal membranes
- ❑ (F) Spontaneous new mutation
- ❑ (G) Teratogen exposure
- ❑ (H) Trinucleotide repeat sequence increase

66 A 70-year-old man has had increasing exercise intolerance and difficulty breathing for the past year. His family has noted memory loss and decreased ability to perform activities of daily living for the past 2 years. On physical examination, his temperature is 37.1°C, pulse 70/min, respirations 18/min, and blood pressure 140/80 mm Hg. On auscultation of the chest, rales are audible in the lung bases, and there is a diastolic murmur. He has a marked decrease in sensation to light touch and pinprick over the lower extremities. His gait is ataxic, with the feet widely spaced. He cannot name any of three objects after 3 minutes. He thinks he is an astronaut returned from Mars. An echocardiogram shows aortic regurgitation with a widened aortic root and arch. MR imaging of the brain shows mild diffuse cortical atrophy and meningeal thickening. Infection with which of the following organisms is most likely to produce these findings?

- ❑ (A) *Borrelia burgdorferi*
- ❑ (B) Coxsackievirus B
- ❑ (C) HIV
- ❑ (D) *Mycobacterium leprae*
- ❑ (E) *Mycobacterium tuberculosis*
- ❑ (F) *Treponema pallidum*
- ❑ (G) West Nile virus

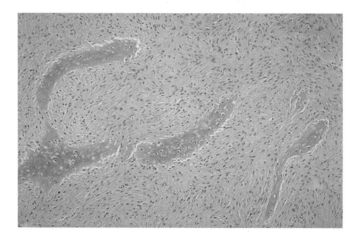

67 A 9-year-old girl has been bothered by right lower leg pain for the past 3 months. On physical examination, she is at the 150th percentile for height. She has a 4 × 5 cm dark café-au-lait spot with a serpiginous border on her right hip and a similar 3 × 6 cm spot on the posterior aspect of her right shoulder. She has significant breast and pubic hair development. A radiograph of the lower leg shows a 3-cm circumscribed, lucent lesion involving the intramedullary right tibial diaphysis, with expansion of surrounding bone. A biopsy of the lesion has the microscopic appearance shown in the preceding figure. An abdominal CT scan shows bilateral adrenal enlargement. MR imaging of the brain shows a gadolinium-enhancing 1.5-cm mass in the sella turcica. Which of the following is the most likely diagnosis?

- ❑ (A) Albers-Schönberg disease
- ❑ (B) Congenital adrenal hyperplasia
- ❑ (C) Maffucci syndrome
- ❑ (D) McCune-Albright syndrome
- ❑ (E) Ollier disease
- ❑ (F) Osteitis deformans

68 A 4-month-old male infant was born at term to an 18-year-old woman, G 1, P 0, who had a normal pregnancy. The woman returned home from work one evening and was told by her boyfriend, who is staying at her home, that the infant died suddenly and unexpectedly. An autopsy shows no external anomalies. The infant's height and weight are at the 40th percentile. Internal examination reveals subarachnoid hemorrhage at the vertex and subdural hemorrhage over the right parietal lobe. The right eye shows petechial hemorrhages at the ora serrata. There is a soft tissue hemorrhage in the right upper arm. There is a recent fracture of the occipital bone. A section of the frontal cortex shows axonal retraction balls in white matter tracts. Which of the following is the most likely diagnosis?

- ❑ (A) α-Thalassemia
- ❑ (B) Congenital syphilis
- ❑ (C) Edwards syndrome
- ❑ (D) Hemophilia A
- ❑ (E) Osteogenesis imperfecta
- ❑ (F) Shaken baby syndrome
- ❑ (G) Sudden infant death syndrome
- ❑ (H) Thanatophoric dysplasia

69 At autopsy, the following spectrum of microscopic findings is noted: hypogastric arterial medial calcific sclerosis, scattered glomerulosclerosis, increased lipofuscin in myocardium and hepatocytes, calcifications in the pineal gland, lack of hematopoiesis in the long bones, and decreased cerebral cortical thickness. Which of the following conditions is most likely to explain these findings?

- ❑ (A) Aging
- ❑ (B) Chronic alcoholism
- ❑ (C) Cystic fibrosis
- ❑ (D) Diabetes mellitus
- ❑ (E) HIV infection
- ❑ (F) Vitamin C deficiency

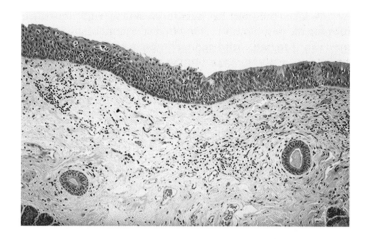

70 A 5-year-old child who has received no medical care since birth has had gradual onset of markedly decreased vision bilaterally. The child also has a history of increased respiratory tract infections due to *Haemophilus influenzae*, *Streptococcus pneumoniae*, *Klebsiella pneumoniae*, and rubeola. The representative microscopic appearance of the bronchial mucosa is shown. The child has also passed several urinary tract calculi. On physical examination, generalized papular dermatosis is noted. The child has xerophthalmia, and there is marked keratomalacia with corneal clouding. Bilateral crackles are audible in the lungs on auscultation. Which of the following disease processes is most likely to lead to these findings?

❏ (A) Cystic fibrosis
❏ (B) Congenital syphilis
❏ (C) HIV infection
❏ (D) Kartagener syndrome
❏ (E) Vitamin A deficiency

71 A 47-year-old woman has had increasing abdominal enlargement, with no significant pain, and diarrhea for the past 3 months. She goes to the physician, who performs a cursory physical examination and obtains a stool culture that is negative. The diagnosis is irritable bowel syndrome. She continues to have increasing abdominal enlargement over the next month, reaching the size of a 5-month pregnancy. She sees another physician, who finds a fluid wave on examination of the abdomen. An abdominal CT scan shows massive ascites and scattered 0.5- to 1.5-cm cystic to solid nodules on the surfaces of the bowel and abdominal wall. Paracentesis yields a yellow, slightly cloudy fluid with a high protein content. Cytologic examination of the fluid shows clusters of malignant cells. Laboratory studies show a positive CA-125 and a negative carcinoembryonic antigen test result. Which of the following is the most likely neoplasm?

❏ (A) Adenocarcinoma of the ileum
❏ (B) Carcinoid tumor
❏ (C) Endometrioid carcinoma
❏ (D) Malignant mesothelioma
❏ (E) Serous cystadenocarcinoma
❏ (F) Mucinous cystadenoma

72 A 12-year-old boy develops fever, accompanied by occasional headaches, malaise, fatigue, and nausea after being bitten by a dog. One day later, he experiences episodes of rigidity, hallucinations, breath holding, and difficulty swallowing due to uncontrollable oral secretions. Dr. Louis Pasteur is called upon. "The death of this child appearing to be inevitable, I decided, not without lively and sore anxiety, as may well be believed, to try . . . the method which I had found constantly successful with dogs. Consequently, 60 hours after the bites [the child] was inoculated under a fold of skin with half a syringeful of the spinal cord of a rabbit. In the following days, fresh inoculations were made. I thus made thirteen inoculations." The boy survived. Which of the following pathologic findings is most characteristic of the boy's disease?

❏ (A) Anterior horn cell loss
❏ (B) Gummatous necrosis
❏ (C) Multinucleated giant cells
❏ (D) Necrotizing vasculitis
❏ (E) Negri bodies
❏ (F) Pseudocysts with bradyzoites
❏ (G) Spongiform encephalopathy

73 An 18-year-old woman has had recurrent acute attacks of dyspnea for the past 10 years. Between these attacks she has no medical problems. She is brought to the emergency department within an hour of onset of the latest episode. On physical examination her temperature is 37.4 C, pulse 110/min, respiratory rate 18/min, and blood pressure 110/70 mm Hg. Expiratory wheezes are auscultated over the chest bilaterally. A chest x-ray shows bilateral radiolucency with no masses or infiltrates. Pulmonary function studies show severe limitation of airflow that is relieved upon injection of epinephrine. Sputum cytologic examination shows abundant mucus with an inflammatory infiltrate dominated by eosinophils, but mixed with neutrophils and macrophages. Which of the following immunologic mechanisms is of primary importance in the pathogenesis of her disease?

❏ (A) Differentiation and activation of the T_H2 subset of CD4+ T cells
❏ (B) Recruitment and activation of neutrophils and macrophages by IL-8
❏ (C) Recruitment and activation of monocytes by interferon-γ
❏ (D) Stimulation and proliferation of bronchial smooth muscle cells by ADAM-33
❏ (E) Recruitment and activation of eosinophils by exotoxin

74 As a student in the health sciences, you have just finished this review book, learning to apply your knowledge base in pathology to clinical and experimental scenarios of human disease states. Which of the following represents your best application of this knowledge?

❏ (A) Collegial consultation
❏ (B) Compassionate care
❏ (C) Differential diagnosis
❏ (D) Lifelong learning
❏ (E) Patient education
❏ (F) Research projects

ANSWERS

1 (D) The C282Y mutation in the *HFE* gene can be found in one of nine persons of Celtic heritage and causes increased absorption of dietary iron. In male patients about 40 years of age, the increased iron stores lead to organ dysfunction, typically involving the heart (cardiomyopathy with congestive heart failure), pancreas (diabetes mellitus), skin (increased pigmentation), and joints (arthritis). In women, increased iron loss through menses delays the onset of this disease for 20 more years. A patient with β-thalassemia would have anemia, although the ineffective erythropoiesis leads to excessive iron absorption. Although this patient has diabetes mellitus and an increased glucose level, diabetes mellitus type 1 does not explain all the findings, such as the arthritis. Familial hypercholesterolemia could lead to coronary artery disease and heart failure, but it does not explain the patient's diabetes or arthritis. Rheumatoid arthritis typically leads to joint deformities and mostly involves small joints.

BP7 615-617   BP6 538-540   PBD7 908-910
PBD6 586-587, 873-875

2 (F) The patient has findings consistent with systemic lupus erythematosus: photosensitivity, renal failure, body cavity effusions, pericarditis, arthralgias, myalgias, and cytopenias. The antinuclear antibody test is the most sensitive screening test for SLE, and if positive can be followed by the more specific anti-double stranded DNA antibody test. Acetylcholine receptor antibody may be seen in myasthenia gravis, which would explain muscle weakness but not pain. Anti-DNA topoisomerase is seen in scleroderma, in which there is renal failure and skin thickening but not photosensitivity. Anti–glomerular basement membrane antibody can be seen in Goodpasture syndrome and renal failure but not arthralgias, myalgias, or cytopenias. Antimicrosomal (anti–thyroid peroxidase) antibody is associated with autoimmune thyroid diseases, mainly Hashimoto thyroiditis but also Graves disease. Antimitochondrial antibody may be seen in primary biliary cirrhosis, which leads to malaise but not to renal failure or photosensitivity.

BP7 130-136   BP6 102-109   PBD7 227-236
PBD6 216-225

3 (A) The findings listed describe myasthenia gravis. The chest CT scan shows a mass posterior to the sternum just below the clavicles. Thymic disorders are common in myasthenia gravis, either thymic hyperplasia or thymoma (as in this case). Antibodies against the acetylcholine receptor disrupt myoneural junction function. Anti-DNA topoisomerase is seen in scleroderma, in which there is renal failure and skin thickening but not muscle weakness after use. Anti–glomerular basement membrane antibody can be seen in Goodpasture syndrome, a form of rapidly progressive glomerulonephritis, often with pulmonary hemorrhage. Antimitochondrial antibody may be seen in primary biliary cirrhosis. ANA is characteristic of many systemic autoimmune diseases, most often systemic lupus erythematosus, which can be accompanied by myalgias but not by muscle weakness with repetitive movement.

BP7 115, 779-780   BP6 390-391, 688-689
PBD7 211, 706-708, 1344   PBD6 1289

4 (A) This patient has findings associated with Goodpasture syndrome, in which there is antibody directed against the glomerular basement membrane, which also acts on basement membrane in the lung to produce pulmonary hemorrhage and hemoptysis. Circulating immune complexes are more likely to be seen in autoimmune diseases such as systemic lupus erythematosus. Macrophage activation is more typical of chronic inflammation and granulomatous inflammation with type IV hypersensitivity. Pulmonary hemorrhage with right-sided congestive heart failure is not part of the acute onset of Goodpasture syndrome. Release of mediators such as histamine from mast cells is typical of anaphylaxis with type I hypersensitivity.

BP7 473-474, 514, 523, 524   BP6 444, 452-453
PBD7 745-746, 968, 977   PBD6 945, 951

5 (F) This patient's findings of ascites, edema, and splenomegaly together with laboratory evidence of hepatic dysfunction suggest a hepatic disorder with portal hypertension, and the most common cause is hepatic cirrhosis from chronic alcohol abuse. Decreased estrogen metabolism results in testicular atrophy. The findings of right- and left-sided congestive heart failure are associated with alcoholic dilated cardiomyopathy. Macrocytic anemia is common, and the AST level is slightly higher than the ALT, features typical of chronic alcoholism. Addison's disease due to adrenal atrophy would not produce hypoalbuminemia or liver enzyme elevations, and the glucose level is often lower. Aortic stenosis may explain the pulmonary edema. Autoimmune gastritis may lead to gastric mucosal atrophy, loss of parietal cells, and megaloblastic anemia but not to hepatic abnormalities. In chronic glomerulonephritis severe enough to produce a hepatorenal syndrome, the renal failure would be much worse and would be indicated by a high serum creatinine. Dilated cardiomyopathy is a type of cardiomyopathy typical of chronic alcoholism.

BP7 612-613   BP6 523-524   PBD7 904-907
PBD6 853-855

6 (A) Some patients with antiphospholipid syndrome (APS) have systemic lupus erythematosus, but others (like this patient) do not. Both arterial and deep venous thrombosis can occur in APS, with increased risk particularly of cerebral arterial thrombosis. Anticardiolipin antibody often leads to a false-positive serologic test result for syphilis (*Treponema pallidum* infection). Thrombocytopenia often is present. APS should be considered in women who have recurrent miscarriages. Polycythemia vera is a myeloproliferative disorder that predisposes to thrombosis, but the patient's WBC count and hemoglobin do not support this diagnosis. Thrombophlebitis occurs more frequently in pregnancy, but this explains only venous thrombosis and not the anticardiolipin antibodies. Trousseau syndrome, a hypercoagulable state associated with an underlying malignancy, can explain both venous and arterial thromboses but not the anticardiolipin antibodies. The patient's age militates against cancer. Von Willebrand disease is a bleeding disorder without thrombotic complications.

BP7 91, 131   BP6 70, 103   PBD7 132-135
PBD6 126, 218, 986

7 (E) The patient has findings that are consistent with sickle cell anemia (hemoglobin SS) with abdominal crisis and vertebral bone marrow infarction. The haptoglobin is low as a result of sickle cell crisis with hemolysis. The continued hemolysis leads to formation of pigmented gallstones. "Autosplenectomy" is a consistent finding. There is a predisposition to aseptic necrosis and osteomyelitis, particularly with *Salmonella*. The MCV is high because of reticulocytosis, and the RDW is quite high because of sickling and hemolysis. An elevated amylase level could be seen in acute pancreatitis, which could occur with gallstones, but this would not explain the anemia or the undetectable spleen. Antiphospholipid syndrome (APS) with anticardiolipin antibodies leads to thrombosis, but the abdomen is not the typical location, and the anemia is not explained by APS. Pancreatitis can complicate hypercalcemia and hypertriglyceridemia, but this does not explain the anemia or undetectable spleen. An increased serum ferritin level indicates increased iron stores, which is most typical of hemochromatosis. This condition could complicate β-thalassemias but not sickle cell disease, unless the patient has received many blood transfusions.

BP7 400-403   BP6 345-347   PBD7 628-632
PBD6 611-615

8 (F) This patient has type 1 diabetes mellitus with ketoacidosis, which is the setting for infection by *Mucor* in the paranasal sinuses, an otherwise unusual infection. T- and B-cell function is generally maintained in diabetes mellitus, although neutrophilic function may be depressed, so bacterial infections (staphylococcal, streptococcal, and coliform organisms) most often complicate diabetes mellitus. Actinomycosis can produce chronic subcutaneous abscesses, usually in the neck, lung, or abdomen and usually following trauma or tissue devitalization. Cutaneous anthrax is rare and produces a localized eschar or ulcerated region. Cytomegalovirus and cryptococcal infections are typically seen in immunocompromised persons with diminished cell-mediated immunity. *Clostridium perfringens* appears in the setting of soft tissue infections with gas gangrene. *Pseudomonas* infections are frequent nosocomial infections of the urinary and respiratory tracts.

BP7 494, 652   BP6 564-566, 572   PBD7 1190-1203
PBD6 913, 924-926

9 (A) The patient has findings consistent with cystic fibrosis; agenesis of the vas deferens is a common finding and leads to infertility. With good medical care, persons with cystic fibrosis are living longer, and childbearing becomes an issue. Disorders of fibroblast growth factor receptor (*FGFR*) can include dwarfism. Glucose-6-phosphatase deficiency results in hemolysis on exposure to oxidants such as antimalarial drugs (e.g., primaquine). The *HFE* gene is abnormal in hereditary hemochromatosis; however, the patient is young for the onset of this disease. *NF1* (neurofibromatosis) is associated with the appearance of a variety of neoplasms, including neurofibromas, pheochromocytomas, and gliomas. *p53* is a tumor

suppressor gene, and loss of both alleles can promote the appearance of a variety of malignancies, mainly carcinomas.

BP7 248-251   BP6 207-209   PBD7 489-495
PBD6 477-481

10 (D) The patient has pernicious anemia due to atrophic gastritis, with lack of intrinsic factor to bind dietary vitamin B_{12} for absorption. This condition has led to megaloblastic anemia and subacute combined spinal cord degeneration of dorsal and lateral tracts. The anti-Smith antibody is a feature of systemic lupus erythematosus, which has many manifestations but not typically gastritis or spinal cord degeneration. Factor V (Leiden) deficiency is a risk factor for recurrent thrombosis. *Helicobacter pylori* infection leads to gastritis (not typically atrophic) but not to neurologic problems. An elevated urine glucose level suggests diabetes mellitus, which may lead to peripheral neuropathy but not to gastritis.

BP7 413-414   BP6 356-357   PBD7 638-642
PBD6 623-626

11 (E) This patient with acute myocardial infarction, cerebrovascular disease, and peripheral vascular disease has features suggestive of heterozygous familial hypercholesterolemia, in which a mutation in the gene encoding for the LDL receptor is present. Such persons have early, accelerated atherosclerosis. The "statin" drugs are HMG CoA reductase inhibitors that suppress endogenous cholesterol synthesis and increase LDL receptor synthesis. The patient does not have findings consistent with diabetes mellitus, another disease that promotes atherosclerosis, because his hemoglobin A_{1c} level is normal, indicating that hyperglycemia has not been present. In type 1 diabetes mellitus, there is reduced β cell mass; in type 2 diabetes mellitus, there can be a reduction in glucose transport proteins. Although glucose metabolism and lipoprotein metabolism are important liver functions, liver disease does not tend to produce atherosclerosis, and the liver can regenerate hepatocytes. Proliferation of intimal smooth muscle cells is part of the formation of arterial atheromas.

BP7 218-220   BP6 182-184   PBD7 156-159
PBD6 152-153, 505

12 (B) These findings are characteristic of lead poisoning, which is mainly manifested by neurologic disorders, particularly in children. Lead absorption is enhanced by zinc deficiency; zinc is a trace metal. Lead inhibits heme incorporation into hemoglobin, leading to increased amounts of zinc protoporphyrin with anemia. Fluoride is added in small quantities to drinking water to reduce the prevalence of dental caries, and increased amounts produce fluorosis, which discolors the teeth. Methanol poisoning is acute and can lead to acidosis, respiratory depression, CNS depression, and blindness. Monosodium glutamate (MSG) is an additive in many foods, and in some persons, it causes an acute reaction characterized by nausea, dizziness, and flushing. Vitamin A toxicity leads to CNS findings resembling a brain tumor.

BP7 278-280   BP6 232-234   PBD7 432-433
PBD6 420-421

13 (E) This patient has Wegener granulomatosis, a multisystem vasculitis that most often involves the lungs and kidneys. C-ANCA is positive in 95% of patients with Wegener granulomatosis. Anti-DNA topoisomerase I antibody can be seen in diffuse scleroderma, which produces pulmonary interstitial fibrosis and renal hyperplastic arteriolosclerosis. Anti–glomerular basement membrane antibody is seen in Goodpasture syndrome, which does produce crescentic glomerulonephritis and pulmonary hemorrhage but not necrotizing vasculitis. Anti–Jo-1 antibody accompanies polymyositis/dermatomyositis. Antimitochondrial antibody accompanies primary biliary cirrhosis. ANA is positive in many autoimmune diseases, principally systemic lupus erythematosus (SLE), which can produce a vasculitis but not a necrotizing granulomatous vasculitis. Anti-RNP antibody is positive in cases of mixed connective tissue disease, which overlaps SLE, scleroderma, rheumatoid arthritis, and polymyositis, but it usually does not entail significant renal or pulmonary involvement.

BP7 351-352   BP6 295-296   PBD7 535-537, 541-542, 746, 977   PBD6 522-523

14 (D) This child has cerebral malaria, and the smear shows numerous ring forms of the parasites in RBCs. The parasites adhere to the vascular endothelium and lead to ischemia in various organs, including the brain with consequent acute cerebral edema. There is hemolytic anemia. The liver and spleen become progressively enlarged. Babesiosis is a rare, tick-borne disease found in the northeastern US, which can produce a hemolytic anemia, but the organisms produce a classic "tetrad" in RBCs. Lyme disease, caused by *Borrelia burgdorferi*, is best known for producing chronic arthritis, but meningoencephalitis, neuritis, and neuropathy may complicate this illness. Leishmaniasis, caused by *Leishmania donovani*, produces mainly visceral disease without cerebral findings. Sleeping sickness, caused by *Trypanosoma gambiense*, tends to be a chronic disease, whereas *T. rhodesiense* is more acute, causing brain dysfunction (sleeping sickness). *Wuchereria bancrofti* produces lymphatic filariasis with elephantiasis.

BP7 408-409   BP6 352-353   PBD7 401-403
PBD6 389-391

15 (C) The reddish-purple nodular lesion is typical of Kaposi sarcoma in a patient with wasting syndrome, oral thrush, and lymphopenia characteristic of HIV infection with AIDS. Hepatitis C virus is unlikely to produce skin lesions or lymphopenia of this degree. Herpes simplex virus infections may be seen more frequently in HIV infection, but the lesions are typically vesicular and are located in the perioral or perianal regions. Hansen disease, caused by *Mycobacterium leprae* infection, may produce a faint reddish rash that fades, followed by hypopigmentation or anesthesia of affected skin and sometimes nodular deforming lesions developing over years. Malaria due to *Plasmodium vivax* can produce anemia with a pale appearance to the skin. Staphylococcal skin infections tend to produce localized abscesses, such as furuncles and boils. Streptococcal skin infections may manifest as abscesses or as cellulitis.

BP7 156-157, 358-359   BP6 125, 305-307   PBD7 256-257, 548-550   PBD6 248-249, 535-537

16 (C) This patient has Lyme arthritis, meningitis, and carditis, as well as a past history of erythema chronicum migrans. The arthritis may appear from weeks to a couple of years after a bite from the vector, the deer tick (*Ixodes*), and can be migratory and involve the large joints. Streptococci

may cause an acute arthritis, although a polyarthritis with rheumatic fever due to group A streptococcal infection can occur along with carditis. *Staphylococcus aureus* causes an acute suppurative arthritis. Tuberculosis tends to produce a chronic arthritis associated with osteomyelitis of the large joints, leading to ankylosis and deformity. Viral arthritis can be acute to subacute but generally is mild. *Yersinia enterocolitica* can cause an enteropathic arthritis with an abrupt onset but a year-long course in HLA-B27–positive persons.

BP7 777   BP6 686-687   PBD7 392-393, 1310
PBD6 388, 389, 1253

17 (E) The child has features of protein-energy malnutrition characteristic of kwashiorkor; the decreased protein intake translates to diminished albumin synthesis by the liver. The decreased plasma oncotic pressure from hypoalbuminemia leads to peripheral edema and ascites. The hair and skin changes and the muscle wasting also reflect decreased protein synthesis. An increased plasma homocysteine level is a risk factor for accelerated atherosclerosis, which could lead to heart disease and congestive failure, but this takes decades to occur and does not explain the skin and hair findings. Hyperuricemia is seen in gout, which mainly leads to arthritis. Hypercalcemia can lead to ulcer disease, pancreatitis, stone formation, cardiac arrhythmias, and mental status changes. In the absence of signs of bleeding, including skin ecchymoses, a decreased prothrombin time is unlikely. An absolute decrease in insulin is indicative of type 1 diabetes mellitus, which could also lead to eventual heart disease and congestive heart failure, but decades later.

BP7 292   BP6 244-246   PBD7 447-449   PBD6 436-438

18 (D) The findings are most characteristic of Alzheimer disease, which is progressive over several years. The brain is slightly decreased in size, with narrower gyri and widened sulci in all lobes except the occipital lobes. There is ex vacuo ventricular dilation. Microscopically, there are neuritic plaques with Aβ amyloid cores. Spongiform change is most likely to occur in a rapidly progressive dementia (over weeks to months) such as Creutzfeldt-Jakob disease. Intranuclear inclusions may be seen in viral infections such as cytomegalovirus or herpes simplex virus, and these are more acute illnesses in which focal neurologic findings are more likely to be seen. Alzheimer type II cells, despite the eponym, are not part of Alzheimer disease, but are seen with increased blood ammonia levels as a consequence of hepatic failure—hepatic encephalopathy. Arteriolosclerosis can occur in association with hypertension. Loss of pigmented neurons occurs in Parkinson disease, and the loss is in the substantia nigra of the midbrain, not the neocortex. Absence of Betz cells may be seen in amyotrophic lateral sclerosis, in which there is progressive muscular weakness.

BP7 841-843   BP6 739-740   PBD7 1385-1389
PBD6 1329-1333

19 (E) The findings are most typical of gouty arthritis. Gout can lead to renal failure and to tophaceous deposits in soft tissues as well as joints, and it is often accompanied by hyperlipidemia. Calcium pyrophosphate dihydrate deposition disease is more common in the elderly and usually is asymptomatic; the knees are most often affected, and soft tissue deposition of the crystals away from joints is unlikely.

Cholesterol crystals form in joint cavities following trauma with hemorrhage. Cystine crystals can be seen in the urine in cystinosis, a rare inborn error of metabolism. Hydroxyapatite crystals may be found in joints affected by osteoarthritis, with either acute or chronic presentation.

BP7 774-777 BP6 682-686 PBD7 1311-1314
PBD6 1253-1257

20 **(D)** Persons with hepatitis C infection can develop chronic hepatitis with persistently elevated liver enzymes. Some persons with hepatitis C develop a mixed cryoglobulinemia with a polyclonal increase in IgG. Renal involvement is common, with either nephrotic or nephritic features. Cryoglobulinemic vasculitis leads to skin hemorrhages and ulceration. Autoimmune hemolytic anemia can lead to a predominantly indirect hyperbilirubinemia. Although hepatocellular carcinoma may complicate hepatitis C infection, a mass lesion would be seen on a CT scan, and the alkaline phosphatase level usually is elevated when an intrahepatic mass is present. Chronic liver disease may complicate hereditary hemochromatosis, but these patients usually do not have hepatitis C, and the skin has a slate color, not purpura. Multiple myeloma can increase the serum globulin and produce renal disease, but hepatitis is usually not part of myeloma, nor is vasculitis.

BP7 603-604 BP6 528 PBD7 891, 894-895
PBD6 860-861

21 **(F)** The patient has hypothyroidism, and one of the most common causes is Hashimoto thyroiditis, an autoimmune thyroiditis that eventually leads to thyroid atrophy. Both antimicrosomal (anti–thyroid peroxidase) and antithyroglobulin antibodies may be seen in Hashimoto thyroiditis. Anticentromere antibody is most often associated with limited scleroderma, or CREST syndrome, with sclerodactyly and esophageal dysmotility the most frequent complications. Anti-DNA topoisomerase antibody is most often associated with diffuse scleroderma, with extensive sclerodactyly and renal disease. Antimitochondrial antibody may appear in association with primary biliary cirrhosis producing chronic liver disease. ANA appears in a wide variety of autoimmune diseases, such as systemic lupus erythematosus (SLE), but it is not typical of Hashimoto thyroiditis. Anti-RNP antibody can be seen in mixed connective tissue disease, with overlapping features of SLE, scleroderma, polymyositis, and rheumatoid arthritis.

BP7 731-732 BP6 648-649 PBD7 1169-1170
PBD6 1134-1135

22 **(E)** Ulcerative colitis has a peak age of onset between 15 and 30 years. A second peak occurs between 60 and 80 years of age. The colonoscopic appearance is of a mucosal erythematous and finely granular surface that looks like sandpaper. Extra-intestinal manifestations of ulcerative colitis can occur, including primary sclerosing cholangitis (PSC), uveitis, migratory polyarthritis, and erythema nodosum. Indeed, 60 to 70% of cases of PSC have concurrent inflammatory bowel disease. Dermatitis herpetiformis occurs in patients with celiac disease, both caused by gluten sensitivity. Rheumatoid arthritis is typically associated with Sjögren syndrome. Orchitis is most often a complication of mumps virus infection, particularly in adults. Thyroiditis may occur in association with

other autoimmune endocrinopathies, such as Addison disease. Atrophic gastritis causes pernicious anemia and may also coexist with other autoimmune disorders such as Hashimoto thyroiditis.

BP7 574-577 BP6 500-503 PBD7 846-851
PBD6 818-820

23 **(B)** This patient has β-thalassemia, probably of at least intermediate severity. There is decreased β-globin chain formation, with increased hemoglobin A_2 and F to compensate. There is ineffective erythropoiesis and increased erythropoietin to drive increased iron absorption, leading to iron overload. Chronic anemia requiring transfusion therapy exacerbates hemochromatosis. Iron deposited in endocrine tissues can lead to gonadal, pituitary, thyroid, islet cell, and adrenal failure. Secondary hypersplenism can result from the splenomegaly, with sequestration of platelets and leukocytes. Deficiency of α_1-antitrypsin can lead to pulmonary emphysema or chronic liver disease, or both. The *CFTR* gene is associated with cystic fibrosis. In glucose-6-phosphate deficiency, sensitivity to oxidizing agents causes a hemolytic anemia, but this usually is not ongoing. The *HFE* gene is abnormal in hereditary hemochromatosis, leading to iron overload, but onset of the disease occurs in middle age. Mutations involving NADPH oxidase lead to immunodeficiency in chronic granulomatous disease. The abnormal *ankyrin* gene leads to hereditary spherocytosis and a mild hemolytic anemia with splenomegaly but not to iron overload.

BP7 403-406 BP6 347-350 PBD7 632-635
PBD6 615-618

24 **(D)** The MR image shows white matter plaques of demyelination typical of multiple sclerosis, a disease that has varied neurologic manifestations. The mean age at onset is 30 years, and it rarely occurs after age 60. Optic neuritis, weakness, and sensory changes are frequent manifestations. Diabetes mellitus can produce peripheral neuropathy and retinopathy, but typically in a more symmetric fashion, and white matter plaques are not present. Graves disease can lead to hyperthyroidism with heat intolerance, but neurologic manifestations are not frequent, and diarrhea is typically present. HIV infection can lead to HIV encephalitis, which can involve white matter, although defined plaques are unlikely, and peripheral neuropathy is not frequent. Myasthenia gravis can produce generalized weakness, which becomes worse with repetitive movement and is not focal; there are no white matter changes. Systemic lupus erythematosus can cause cerebritis but without plaques of demyelination, and focal neurologic deficits are not a frequent finding.

BP7 837-838 BP6 736-737 PBD7 1382-1385
PBD6 1326-1327

25 **(F)** The patient has Wilson disease (hepatolenticular degeneration), with Kayser-Fleischer corneal rings due to a mutation in the gene encoding for a copper-transporting ATPase. Excessive copper deposition occurs, particularly in the liver, putamen, and cornea. Psychiatric and neurologic disturbances are common in Wilson disease, and patients often develop chronic liver disease ranging from acute hepatitis to chronic hepatitis to cirrhosis. In α_1-antitypsin deficiency, there can be chronic hepatitis and pulmonary emphysema, but there are no neurologic changes. Cystic fibrosis can lead to pulmonary disease and pancreatic insufficiency. Galactosemia can lead to liver disease and cirrhosis in early childhood. In its most severe form, Gaucher disease can lead to neurologic deterioration but does not lead to chronic liver disease. Von Gierke disease is a form of glycogen storage disease that does not commonly progress to cirrhosis.

BP7 617-618   BP6 540-541   PBD7 910-911   PBD6 875

26 (A) The patient has an aortic dissection that is extending proximally to envelop and partially occlude the great vessels. Proximal dissections may result in minimal or no chest pain. Blood has moved into the mediastinum, causing widening, and into the pericardial cavity, causing tamponade. Risk factors include hypertension and atherosclerosis. In addition, cystic medial necrosis makes aortic dissection a serious risk in persons with Marfan syndrome. A bicuspid aortic valve leads to aortic valvular stenosis but not to aortic rupture. Neoplasms involving the mediastinum, typically hematologic malignancies such as lymphomas, may produce a superior vena cava syndrome, but neoplasms virtually never invade the arterial media, and bleeding from neoplasms is produced from much smaller vessels. Takayasu arteritis can involve the aortic arch and lead to dissection, but this condition is rare and is most likely seen in women younger than 30 years of age. Syphilitic aortitis may produce aortic root dilation and possible rupture, but this is much less common than aortic dissection due to hypertension and atherosclerosis. Thromboangiitis obliterans (Buerger disease) is an uncommon disorder that affects small- to medium-sized arteries in the arms and legs of middle-aged men who smoke.

BP7 343-345   BP6 300-302   PBD7 532-534
PBD6 526-528

27 (C) The patient has findings that are consistent with emphysema. Smoking promotes gastritis. Several malignancies are related to smoking, including urinary tract transitional cell carcinoma and renal cell carcinoma. α_1-Antitrypsin (AAT) deficiency can explain emphysema, but it would be panlobular, and AAT deficiency is not associated with urinary tract neoplasia. Chronic alcoholism can explain gastritis but not emphysema or carcinoma. Aniline dyes increase the risk of transitional cell carcinoma but not of emphysema or gastritis. Vitamin C deficiency can lead to soft tissue hemorrhages and bone pain but not to carcinoma or emphysema.

BP7 459-460   BP6 398-402   PBD7 717-721
PBD6 707-709

28 (B) Hemoglobin A1C elevation occurs in diabetes mellitus. The patient has complications of diabetes mellitus type 2 that are typical of obesity: a "diabetic foot" as a consequence of peripheral neuropathy and decreased sensation, advanced atherosclerosis with carotid arterial occlusion, and an atherosclerotic aortic aneurysm. Autonomic dysfunction with neuropathy can lead to erectile dysfunction. Cushing disease due to an ACTH-secreting pituitary adenoma leads to truncal obesity and easy bruisability of the skin and possibly to secondary diabetes mellitus but not to advanced atherosclerosis. Hyperchomocysteinemia is a risk factor for atherosclerosis but not for neuropathy. The oligoclonal bands of IgG are characteristic for multiple sclerosis, which usually has more focal CNS involvement. Antiparietal cell antibodies occur in pernicious anemia with vitamin B12 deficiency that can lead to

decreased sensation in the lower extremities, but not to atherosclerotic complications.

BP7 646, 649-650   BP6 566-567, 572   PBD7 1197-1205, 1334   PBD6 913, 919-920

29 (A) The patient has Addison disease with bilateral atrophy of the adrenal cortex, which is most often idiopathic and leads to electrolyte changes due to loss of mineralocorticoid secretion, mainly aldosterone; when atrophy is marked, glucocorticoid secretion is diminished. Increased ACTH precursor hormones, resulting from loss of feedback from cortisol production, stimulate skin melanocytes. Stress, including infections, may precipitate an addisonian crisis. Loss of islets of Langerhans is a feature of type 1 diabetes mellitus, with hyperglycemia and possible ketoacidosis as complications. Loss of releasing or inhibiting hormones from the hypothalamus affects the pituitary and leads to multiple endocrinopathies but not specifically to loss of ACTH. Parafollicular cells of the thyroid produce calcitonin, which plays a minor role in calcium homeostasis. The pineal gland produces melatonin, which is involved in circadian rhythms but not in significant disease states. Loss of thyroid hormone from follicular epithelium leads to hypothyroidism typified by modest weight gain, coarse and dry skin, and constipation, but without significant electrolyte disturbances.

BP7 748-749   BP6 661-662   PBD7 1214-1217
PBD6 1160-1161

30 (A) The patient has hyperprolactinemia caused by a prolactinoma, which is the most common tumor of the anterior pituitary. Macroadenomas produce homonymous hemianopsia and can secrete prolactin to cause gynecomastia. A carcinoid tumor can produce a variety of hormones but not prolactin. Medullary thyroid carcinomas can produce calcitonin, which has a minimal effect on calcium homeostasis. Pheochromocytomas can produce excess catecholamines, most often manifested by hypertension. Renal cell carcinomas can be accompanied by a variety of paraneoplastic syndromes, most often polycythemia, hypercalcemia, and Cushing syndrome, but not hyperprolactinemia. Likewise, small cell anaplastic ("oat cell") lung cancers can produce paraneoplastic syndromes, most often Cushing syndrome and the syndrome of inappropriate antidiuretic hormone secretion.

BP7 723-724   BP6 640-641   PBD7 1160-1161
PBD6 1125-1126

31 (E) The child has Down syndrome and has developed leukemia as a complication. The 45,X karyotype is seen in Turner syndrome only in females. The normal 46,XY karyotype is unlikely with the constellation of anomalies present in this case. Trisomies 13 and 18 are far less likely than trisomy 21 to be associated with long-term survival; affected children are more likely to have severe anomalies. The 47,XXY karyotype of Klinefelter syndrome is associated with nearly normal-appearing males of normal intelligence. Triploidy with 69 chromosomes is associated with partial hydatidiform mole and with stillbirth.

BP7 230-232   BP6 193-195   PBD7 175-177, 667
PBD6 170-172

32 (D) About 10% of persons with autosomal-dominant polycystic kidney disease (ADPKD) have a berry aneurysm of the circle of Willis, which may be complicated by rupture and hemorrhage into the subarachnoid space. The cysts of ADPKD may appear in the liver, and rarely in the pancreas. The cysts in adult-onset medullary cystic disease are centrally located in the kidney. Although renal failure does occur in middle age, similar to DPKD, the kidneys are small and shrunken, and there are no cysts in other organs. Abnormal renal resorption of amino acids, including cystine, may lead to formation of cystine crystals and stones in the urine; maple syrup urine disease and severe liver disease may cause such a finding. Diabetic nephropathy includes nephrosclerosis, glomerulosclerosis, pyelonephritis, and papillary necrosis but not cystic disease. Polyarteritis nodosa may produce small microaneurysms of arteries, typically in the kidneys, and may affect multiple organs, but cystic disease is not seen. Wegener granulomatosis is a form of vasculitis that can affect multiple organs, principally the kidneys and lungs, but it does not produce cystic disease. Wilson disease, or hepatolenticular degeneration, leads to chronic liver disease and putaminal degeneration, not cystic disease.

BP7 535-536, 817   BP6 463-464, 720   PBD7 962-965, 1366-1368   PBD6 937-940, 1311

33 **(E)** This patient has findings of "classic" polyarteritis nodosa, and in about one third of cases, the HBsAg is positive. The mesenteric artery angiogram reveals focal distal occlusions and microaneurysms of branches of the superior mesenteric artery. Antimitochondrial antibody is seen in primary biliary cirrhosis. P-ANCA is associated with "microscopic" polyarteritis but not with classic polyarteritis. The ANA test result is positive in a wide variety of autoimmune diseases, principally systemic lupus erythematosus, which can affect the kidney with glomerulonephritis, not typically vasculitis. Cryptococcal antigen can be detected in CSF of patients with meningitis, usually immunocompromised persons. *Histoplasma capsulatum* antibody may be detected in persons with prior exposure to this agent, which mainly causes pulmonary disease. The p24 antigen of HIV is used in testing for congenital infection; HIV does not produce a florid acute vasculitis.

BP7 349-350   BP6 293-295   PBD7 535, 537, 539-540
PBD6 520-521

34 **(D)** Vitamin C deficiency is manifested by a decrease in synthesis of collagen peptides from inadequate hydroxylation of procollagen. Diminished collagen synthesis affects bone matrix formation, vascular integrity, and epithelial function. There is bleeding into joints and soft tissues with minimal trauma. Mutation of the *CFTR* gene gives rise to cystic fibrosis, and malabsorption in cystic fibrosis primarily affects the fat-soluble vitamins A, D, E, and K, with bone changes marked by inadequate mineralization. Hemophilia A, which in some cases can be due to an acquired inhibitor of factor VIII, leads to hemorrhage into soft tissues with hemarthroses and joint deformities, but this condition is typically X-linked and unlikely to affect girls, and skin and bone are not primarily involved. Mutations in a collagen gene can give rise to osteogenesis imperfecta results in multiple fractures with deformity. The lack of fractures in this case makes a diagnosis of trauma less likely, and the skin and epiphyseal changes are not seen with trauma.

BP7 298-301   BP6 257   PBD7 458-460   PBD6 449-450

35 **(A)** This girl has Stevens-Johnson syndrome (SJS), a severe form of erythema multiforme that can complicate infections and drug therapy. Sulfonamides, allopurinol, phenytoin, and carbamazepine are the most likely drugs to be associated with SJS. Cytotoxic (CD8-positive) lymphocytes mediate SJS through epidermal cell necrosis. Eosinophils are common in allergic reactions, including drug allergies, but most of these reactions are accompanied by urticaria and erythema of short duration, without blistering or desquamation. Langerhans cells and macrophages are antigen-presenting cells in the epidermis and dermis that do not directly cause toxic damage to surrounding cells. Neutrophilic exudates are not a feature of SJS, although a leukocytoclastic vasculitis with purpura is a form of drug reaction. Natural killer cells are part of innate immunity and do not participate directly in drug reactions.

BP7 793   BP6 700   PBD7 1255-1256   PBD6 1197-1198

36 **(E)** The patient has toxic shock syndrome. Some strains of *Staphylococcus aureus* produce exotoxins, acting as "superantigens," such as TSST-1, which are T-cell mitogens able to stimulate more than 10% of the body's T cells, provoking an exuberant and dysregulated immune response characterized by release of the cytokines that mediate cell injury. *Bacillus anthracis* can cause anthrax, a serious illness with pneumonia and meningitis as the predominant findings. *Clostridium perfringens* is known to cause wound infections with gas gangrene. Enterococcus generally does not cause such a rapidly progressing illness. Listeriosis is associated with food poisoning and can cause life-threatening disease, but typically without desquamation. *Vibrio cholerae* organisms elaborate a toxin that causes a severe watery diarrhea and little else.

BP7 111   PBD7 345, 359, 371-373   PBD6 136, 366

37 **(C)** The child has Letterer-Siwe disease, an acute disseminated form of Langerhans cell histiocytosis. Acute lymphoblastic leukemia generally produces an elevated WBC count, and cutaneous and skeletal manifestations are rare. Gaucher disease, an autosomal recessive condition resulting from diminished glucocerebrosidase activity, has cells with cytoplasm that resembles crinkled tissue paper, and the course is not as aggressive. *Leishmania donovani* can cause visceral leishmaniasis, but the amastigotes infiltrating the marrow are not positive for CD1a, and the course is usually not as aggressive. Multiple myeloma is seen in older adults and, although lytic bone lesions are common, they are caused by infiltrates of plasma cells. Forms of myelodysplastic syndrome are seen in older adults, with myeloid cells that do not mark for CD1a and numerous ringed sideroblasts in the marrow; some cases progress to acute myelocytic leukemia.

BP7 441   BP6 382-383   PBD7 701-702   PBD6 685-686

38 **(B)** The findings are consistent with an adrenogenital syndrome, characterized by 21-hydroxylase deficiency and salt wasting due to a block in cortisol synthesis and an increase in ACTH secretion stimulating increased androgen production. The rare anaplastic thyroid carcinoma is a neoplasm seen in adults with no hormonal effect. Islet cell adenomas may secrete a variety of hormones, often insulin, glucagon, or somatostatin, which do not produce virilizing signs. Medullary carcinoma of the thyroid is a tumor in adults that can produce calcitonin. Neuroblastomas can be seen in young children, but their hormonal output may produce only hypertension. Pituitary adenomas may destroy remaining pituitary function and lead to hypopituitarism, but a microadenoma is unlikely to do this, and the features in this case suggest increased ACTH secretion. Craniopharyngiomas are typically seen in adolescence to young adulthood and are destructive lesions without hormonal output.

BP7 746-748   BP6 659   PBD7 1211-1214
PBD6 1157-1159

39 (D) This infant has the acute neuronopathic form of Gaucher disease (type II), which is uniformly fatal in children and is much less common than the milder type I, which has prolonged survival into adulthood. The marrow is infiltrated by large cells with abundant pale cytoplasm with the appearance of crumpled tissue paper. α-L-Iduronidase deficiency is seen in Hurler syndrome, characterized by progressive features of corneal clouding, coarse facial features, and mental retardation. α-1,4-Glucosidase deficiency is present in Pompe disease, a glycogen storage disease that causes marked cardiomegaly. Arylsulfatase A deficiency is present in metachromatic leukodystrophy and causes CNS degeneration without visceral organ involvement. Glucose-6-phosphatase deficiency characterizes von Gierke disease; affected persons have hepatomegaly and hypoglycemia. Tay-Sachs disease with cherry red maculae and progressive neurologic deterioration occurs as a result of diminished hexosaminidase A; hexosaminidase B deficiency leads to Sandhoff disease. Sphingomyelinase deficiency leads to Niemann-Pick disease, with foamy appearing macrophages filling tissues of the mononuclear phagocyte system.

BP7 223-224   BP6 186-187   PBD7 163-165
PBD6 158-159

40 (C) This man has celiac sprue complicated by dermatitis herpetiformis. The jejunal biopsy specimen shows mucosal flattening and increased intraepithelial lymphocytes. Persons who have HLA-B8 or HLA-Drw3 are more likely to develop these findings. With a gluten-free diet, the skin lesions resolve in some patients. Antibodies to desmoglein 3, a desmosome protein, are present in pemphigus vulgaris, a vesicular disease of older adults without gastrointestinal tract involvement. Antibodies to double-stranded DNA are highly specific for systemic lupus erythematosus (SLE), which produces erythematous rashes without vesicles. Antihistone antibodies are most characteristic of drug-induced SLE. Anti-RNP antibodies are seen in mixed connective tissue disease, which has elements of SLE, scleroderma, rheumatoid arthritis, and polymyositis. Antibodies to type IV collagen are seen in Goodpasture syndrome, which does not involve skin rashes.

BP7 525, 571   BP6 498, 704   PBD7 843-844, 1262-1263
PBD6 813, 1204-1205

41 (A) The patient has multiple endocrine neoplasia type I (MEN I) with a gastrinoma (arising either in the islets or in the small intestine), a parathyroid lesion (adenoma or hyperplasia), and a prolactinoma. Medullary carcinoma and pheochromocytoma are more typical of MEN II with *RET* gene mutation. Non-Hodgkin lymphomas are more typical of syndromes in which an immunodeficiency state is present, such as AIDS and large cell lymphoma with *BCL-6* mutation. Osteomas may be seen in Gardner syndrome with the adenomatous polyposis coli (*APC*) gene. Renal cell carcinoma may be seen in von Hippel–Lindau disease due to mutation in the *VHL* gene.

BP7 752-753   BP6 664-665   PBD7 1221-1223
PBD6 1166-1167

42 (A) Caplan syndrome includes pneumoconiosis (with progressive massive fibrosis producing restrictive lung disease) coupled with rheumatoid arthritis (RA). Carney syndrome includes atrial and extracardiac myxomas, irregular pigmentation, and endocrinopathies. Churg-Strauss syndrome is a form of pulmonary vasculitis with allergic manifestations. Felty syndrome includes RA with splenomegaly and secondary hypersplenism (anemia, leukopenia, thrombocytopenia). Hamman-Rich syndrome is idiopathic pulmonary interstitial fibrosis. Kartagener syndrome includes absence of ciliary dynein arms leading to bronchiectasis, and situs inversus is present. In Trousseau syndrome, hypercoagulability results from a paraneoplastic effect, and pulmonary thromboembolism is often present.

BP7 270, 273   BP6 228   PBD7 732-733   PBD6 730, 733

43 (F) The patient has mixed connective tissue disease (MCTD), which has overlapping features of systemic lupus erythematosus (SLE), scleroderma, polymyositis, and rheumatoid arthritis. ANCA is most likely to be seen in vasculitides such as Wegener granulomatosis or microscopic polyarteritis. Antibodies to cyclic citrullinated peptide (anti-CCP) have greater than 99% specificity for rheumatoid arthritis, and these patients are more likely to have severe disease. Antihistone antibodies are most characteristic of drug-induced SLE. Anti-Smith antibodies are very specific for SLE. Thyroid peroxidase antibodies are seen in autoimmune thyroid disorders such as Hashimoto thyroiditis and Graves disease.

BP7 143   BP6 115   PBD7 239   PBD6 231

44 (C) This man has features of acute cocaine toxicity with hyperthermia, as well as chronic cocaine use with coronary arteriopathy and cerebral hemorrhagic strokes. The brown discoloration from hemosiderin deposition in the left anterior frontal lobe suggests a subacute to remote hemorrhage. Cocaine is a powerful vasoconstrictor. Like cocaine, amphetamine and methamphetamine are "uppers," or stimulants; however, they do not typically produce arterial changes. Barbiturates are "downers," or depressants. Ethanol is a depressant that can produce liver disease, but the cardiac effect is obscure and results in dilated cardiomyopathy. Heroin is an opiate narcotic that has minimal effects itself, but the typical route of administration is intravenous, and this can lead to numerous infectious complications, such as hepatitis, endocarditis, meningitis, and AIDS. Marijuana is a mild tranquilizer. Phencyclidine is a schizophrenomimetic that causes erratic behavior but not obvious tissue effects.

BP7 282-283   BP6 236-237   PBD7 424-425
PBD6 412-414

45 (B) Thromboembolic events and hepatic adenoma are rare complications of oral contraceptive use. Allopurinol and sulfonamides are associated with hepatic granuloma formation. Aspirin use in children has been associated with Reye syndrome with microvesicular steatosis. Isoniazid has been associated with acute or chronic hepatitis. Phenacetin and acetaminophen use have been associated with analgesic nephropathy, and excessive acetaminophen use may produce acute massive hepatic necrosis. The combination of prednisone and cyclophosphamide is used in aggressive immunosuppressive therapy and results in an immunocompromised state with increased risk of infection.

BP7 277   BP6 70, 231   PBD7 131-132, 922-923 PBD6 414-416

46 (E) This woman has features seen in chronically bedridden persons. There is a large saddle thromboembolus in the pulmonary arterial trunk. The antiphospholipid syndrome can include thromboembolic events, but osteoporosis, decubital ulcers, and muscle wasting are not features. Aplastic anemia leads to high-output congestive heart failure, bleeding diathesis from thrombocytopenia, and risk of infections. Chronic alcoholism produces chronic liver disease that predisposes to bleeding problems, not thrombosis. Blunt trauma is marked by contusions and fractures. Malnutrition could account for decreased bone density from osteomalacia, poor wound healing with skin ulceration, and muscle wasting, but coagulopathy with bleeding is more likely to occur than thromboembolism.

BP7 475-477   BP6 411-413   PBD7 130-135, 742-743 PBD6 703-704

47 (E) The findings are those of subacute bacterial endocarditis, and the needle track in the left arm suggests intravenous drug use as the risk factor. These persons can have both right- and left-sided valvular lesions. The vegetations are likely to embolize, and the septic emboli can lead to infection or infarction of multiple organs from left-sided lesions and of the lungs from right-sided lesions. The pulmonary nodule is likely a lung abscess. The patient probably has acute pyelonephritis from hematogenous infection. *Candida albicans* is a cause of endocarditis in immunocompromised persons. *Cryptococcus neoformans* is a rare cause of endocarditis in immunocompromised persons. *Escherichia coli* is a likely cause of ascending urinary tract infections with pyelonephritis, but it is an uncommon cause of endocarditis. Listeriosis most often results from food or water contamination and can lead to sepsis with meningitis but rarely endocarditis. Streptococcal infections are more likely to cause endocarditis in persons with preexisting valvular heart disease, and the *Streptococcus viridans* group is most often implicated. *Yersinia enterocolitica* can produce enterocolitis, not endocarditis (this organism can persist in stored blood and cause transfusion-related sepsis).

BP7 381-383   BP6 326-328   PBD7 595-598 PBD6 572-576

48 (E) The patient has thrombotic thrombocytopenic purpura (TTP) with the classic pentad of neurologic changes, fever, thrombocytopenia, microangiopathic hemolytic anemia, and decreased renal function. The pathogenesis of TTP is related to release of von Willebrand factor (vWF). Monomers of vWF are linked by disulfide bonds to form multimers with various molecular masses that range to millions of daltons. A vWF-cleaving metalloproteinase in plasma normally prevents the entrance into the circulation (or persistence) of unusually large multimers of vWF. The metalloproteinase is referred to as ADAMTS 13 (a disintegrin

and metalloproteinase, with thrombospondin-1–like domains). In most patients with TTP, plasma ADAMTS 13 activity is less than 5% of normal. The patient's hemoglobin concentration is not low enough to justify transfusion of RBCs. Giving platelets to a patient with TTP will "add fuel to the fire," because the platelets will cause more thrombi to form, resulting in further organ damage. Simple pressor agents such as dobutamine are not primary therapy. Surgery is not indicated, because the injury is occurring in the small vasculature of many organs. Prednisone may be given to a subset of patients who do not respond to plasmapheresis.

BP7 448   BP6 387   PBD7 652-653, 1009-1011   PBD6 986

49 (C) The patient has Budd-Chiari syndrome, a rare condition that can complicate pregnancy or the postpartum state. Hepatic venous occlusion leads to hepatomegaly with severe centrilobular congestion and necrosis, much more pronounced than the typical "nutmeg" liver of chronic passive congestion with right-sided heart failure. Biliary tract obstruction with choledocholithiasis would increase the serum bilirubin to a greater degree than in this patient, and hepatomegaly is not likely. Hepatic adenomas, which can be associated with use of oral contraceptives, are mass lesions, usually several centimeters in size. At 12 weeks' gestation, with a fetus present, choriocarcinoma is very unlikely, and a marked increase in liver enzymes is not likely. Acute fatty liver of pregnancy with microvesicular steatosis produces a more uniform density with hepatomegaly, a condition that is seen in the third trimester of pregnancy.

BP7 624-625   BP6 547   PBD7 917-918   PBD6 883-884

50 (B) In common variable immunodeficiency (CVID), there are normal numbers of T cells with normal to low numbers of B cells, and there is hypogammaglobulinemia with decreased IgG and possibly other immunoglobulin types. CVID occurs in young adults of both sexes, causing increased bacterial infections as well as giardiasis and recurrent herpes simplex (and herpes zoster) infections. The mechanisms are diverse and include failure of B-cell maturation to plasma cells, excessive T-cell suppression, and defective T-helper cell function. A selective abnormality of T-cell activation, as demonstrated by decreased synthesis of interleukins (IL-2, -4, and -5), has been identified in some cases. Other patients have T- and B-cell autoantibodies or a decreased CD4/CD8 ratio. Mutations in genes encoding NADPH oxidase proteins produce chronic granulomatous disease and recurrent infections with *Aspergillus*, *Staphylococcus*, *Serratia*, *Nocardia*, and *Pseudomonas*. In the hyper-IgM syndrome, mutations in the CD40 ligand induce failure in B cells, with low IgG, IgA, and IgE levels but increased IgM; in infancy and childhood, there is increased risk of severe infections with bacterial and viral agents and opportunistic agents such as *Pneumocystis carinii*. Mutations in CD18, the common β chain of integrins, which aid in binding of leukocytes, lead to leukocyte adhesion deficiency with leukocytosis but with absence of suppurative inflammation in areas of tissue necrosis and ulceration caused by *Staphylococcus aureus* and gram-negative enteric bacteria. In severe combined immunodeficiency (SCID), half of cases result from an X-linked mutation for the common γ chain of IL-2, a receptor for many cytokines needed for T-cell development, and the other half of cases result from autosomal recessive mutation in adenosine deaminase with accumulation of purine metabolites toxic to T cells. In SCID, although T cells are primarily involved, there is secondary impairment of B-cell function, so that affected persons have diminished IgG levels and no IgA or IgM, as well as decreased T-cell function, resulting in increased susceptibility to virtually all infectious organisms.

BP7 145, 146   BP6 116   PBD7 242   PBD6 233-234

51 (F) The patient has myotonic dystrophy, a form of muscular dystrophy in which there are increased CTG repeat sequences in the gene. Weakness in skeletal, cardiac, and smooth muscle develops, as well as cataracts, dementia, gonadal atrophy, and hypogammaglobulinemia. Deficiency of α-1,4-glucosidase leads to Pompe disease in infancy. Absence of dystrophin characterizes Duchenne muscular dystrophy, which affects young boys. The *FGFR3* mutation is seen in achondroplasia, a form of short-limbed dwarfism. Mutations in the mitochondrial oxidative phosphorylase genes (mitochondrial myopathies) can produce neurodegenerative disorders and hearing loss, in addition to myopathy. Myophosphorylase is diminished in McArdle disease, which causes muscle pain on strenuous exercise. The neurofibromin gene is mutated in neurofibromatosis type 1, which does not have myopathy as a feature.

BP7 235, 236   BP6 197   PBD7 1338-1339
PBD6 1283, 1285

52 (E) This patient has microvesicular steatosis characteristic of Reye syndrome, which rarely occurs now because the link between aspirin use in children following a fever and hepatic injury has been recognized; it is caused by severe mitochondrial dysfunction in the brain and liver. Biliary atresia with marked hyperbilirubinemia becomes apparent in the neonatal period. Hepatic venous thrombosis leads to Budd-Chiari syndrome, which is typically a disease of adults that complicates such conditions as polycythemia or pregnancy. Hepatoblastomas may be congenital, but they are mass lesions unlikely to be associated with such marked increases in liver enzymes. Intrahepatic lithiasis is unlikely to occur in children and is unlikely to produce marked increases in liver enzymes. Neonatal giant cell hepatitis can produce findings of acute hepatitis in neonates, not in children.

BP7 619   BP6 542   PBD7 881-882, 904   PBD6 869

53 (E) This patient has findings that strongly suggest a ruptured ectopic pregnancy, hence, HCG levels will be increased. Gonococcal and chlamydial infections are risk factors for pelvic inflammatory disease, which increases the risk of ectopic pregnancy. An increase in carcinoembryonic antigen is seen in some gastrointestinal tract neoplasms, but this patient is young to have such malignancies. Amebiasis would produce a bloody diarrhea, and perforation of the colon is uncommon. Factor XIII, which stabilizes fibrin clots, can be deficient, but this is extremely rare. Bleeding is first observed in the neonatal period; older patients may have poor wound healing, intracerebral hemorrhage, infertility (males), and abortion (females). Decreased follicle-stimulating hormone is typical of pituitary failure, which does not explain the bleeding. A ruptured ectopic pregnancy may lead to disseminated intravascular coagulopathy with increased partial thromboplastin time and prothrombin time, but the normal platelet count in this patient suggests that this has not yet occurred.

Schistosomiasis due to *Schistosoma haematobium* can produce hematuria, but the bladder is not perforated.

BP7 701   BP6 620   PBD7 1105-1106   PBD6 1079-1080

54 (A) The findings are those of multiple myeloma with increased M protein and lytic bone lesions producing bone pain; there is increased risk of infection from encapsulated bacteria. Elevated hemoglobin F occurs in some hemoglobinopathies such as β-thalassemias, which do not have hypergammaglobulinemia. Polycythemia can be a feature of myeloproliferative disorders but not myeloma. The ANA test result is positive in autoimmune conditions but not in lymphoproliferative disorders. A markedly elevated WBC count suggests leukemia, typically chronic myelogenous leukemia.

BP7 429-431   BP6 380-382   PBD7 678-681, 1005-1006,
1292   PBD6 664-666

55 (D) This patient is morbidly obese with complications, including obesity hypoventilation syndrome, glucose intolerance, probable sleep apnea, cholelithiasis, and osteoarthritis. Macrovesicular steatosis with hepatomegaly is seen in obesity and may even progress to cirrhosis. Weight gain due to hypothyroidism, which could occur in Hashimoto thyroiditis, is modest and does not lead to morbid obesity. An "obesity cardiomyopathy" resembles dilated cardiomyopathy. Laryngeal papillomatosis, which produces airway obstruction (without snoring), occurs more often in children and is not associated with obesity. The blood gas findings in this case could be seen in emphysema, which is not a complication of obesity; panlobular emphysema is much less common than the centrilobular emphysema associated with smoking. Rheumatoid arthritis tends to involve small joints first, and there is no relationship to obesity.

BP7 303-305   BP6 259-262   PBD7 461-466, 716
PBD6 452-455

56 (A) One hypothesis regarding the death of Napoleon Bonaparte is that he was the victim of arsenic poisoning perpetrated by former enemies. The FBI analyzed a hair sample in 1995 and found increased arsenic levels, but the amount is equivocal. Another hypothesis is that the wallpaper at Longwood House, where he lived, contained copper arsenate and became moldy, releasing arsine vapor. A third hypothesis suggests that he died of the effects of gastric cancer, not related to arsenic ingestion, substantiated by an observation at autopsy, of lymphadenopathy adjacent to the stomach. Chronic arsenic exposure has been associated with a greatly elevated risk of skin cancer and possibly of cancers of the lung, liver (angiosarcoma), bladder, kidney, and colon. Beryllium acutely produces a pneumonitis, and long-term exposure leads to nonnecrotizing granulomas, similar to sarcoidosis. Chromium or nickel exposure may lead to respiratory tract cancers. Cobalt poisoning can produce pulmonary interstitial fibrosis. Lead poisoning can produce abdominal pain, anemia, neuropathy, and decreased mental sharpness, but it is not associated with malignancies.

PBD7 431-432, 1240, 1242   PBD6 274, 309

57 (D) Risk factors for HELLP (hemolysis with elevated liver enzymes and low platelets) syndrome, a variant of severe preeclampsia, include nulliparity, advanced maternal age, diabetes mellitus, preexisting hypertension, a prior history of preeclampsia, and renal disease. Patients with HELLP syndrome may progress to disseminated intravascular coagulation. Emergent delivery is indicated. Abruptio placentae is an acute event marked by severe abdominal pain and vaginal bleeding. Hepatic vein thrombosis in Budd-Chiari syndrome can produce liver necrosis with elevated enzymes; pregnancy is a risk factor, but this does not explain the neurologic and renal findings. Likewise, a dilated cardiomyopathy that can occur in pregnancy does not explain these findings. In hydatidiform mole, preeclampsia is more likely, but 30 weeks is a long time to have it, and a fetus would not be present. Acute fatty liver of pregnancy may resemble Reye syndrome (a disease that occurs in children) and may be preceded by preeclampsia. Sheehan syndrome is postpartum pituitary necrosis leading to hypopituitarism.

BP7 704-705   BP6 622-623   PBD7 1106-1110
PBD6 884, 1082-1084

58 **(C)** The combination of nongonococcal urethritis, arthritis, and conjunctivitis suggests Reiter syndrome, one of the spondyloarthropathies; the changes in the spine can resemble ankylosing spondylitis and can be equally debilitating. ANCA is indicative of forms of vasculitis such as Wegener granulomatosis. The ANA test result is positive in many autoimmune diseases, such as systemic lupus erythematosus (SLE), but it is not a feature of spondyloarthropathies. Lyme disease can include large joint arthritis, but not urethritis or conjunctivitis. The PPD is positive in prior tuberculosis infection, which may include a large joint arthritis. The RPR is a screening test for syphilis, which can include arthritis of large joints (Charcot joint) in the tertiary form, but it takes decades to develop. Rheumatoid factor is a feature of rheumatoid arthritis (RA), which initially manifests more commonly in small joints of the hands and feet. U1-RNP is a marker for mixed connective tissue disease, which has features of RA, scleroderma, polymyositis, and SLE; arthralgias are not accompanied by joint destruction or deformity.

BP7 126, 139, 140   BP6 111   PBD7 223, 1309
PBD6 361, 1252

59 **(F)** Von Hippel–Lindau disease is rare and results from acquired or inherited mutation in a tumor suppressor gene. Beckwith-Wiedemann syndrome includes Wilms tumor, hemihypertrophy, and adrenal cytomegaly. The *MET* oncogene is mutated in papillary renal carcinomas (not associated with other tumors elsewhere) and in Denys-Drash syndrome that also includes Wilms tumor plus gonadal dysgenesis and nephropathy. Gardner syndrome has the same mutation in the adenomatous polyposis coli (*APC*) gene as familial polyposis, but also has osteomas, epidermal cysts, and fibromatoses. Neurofibromatosis type 2 includes schwannomas, meningiomas, gliomas, and ependymomas. Tuberous sclerosis is one of the phakomatoses with cortical hamartomas called tubers, renal angiomyolipomas, cardiac rhabdomyomas, and subungual fibromas.

BP7 356, 539, 751, 821   BP6 466, 663, 725, 734
PBD7 1414   PBD6 533, 909, 1164, 1355

60 **(A)** The patient has features of CREST syndrome, or limited scleroderma. Because her disease has not progressed to include serious pulmonary fibrosis or renal disease, she is less likely to have diffuse scleroderma, which is associated with

the anti-DNA topoisomerase antibody. Gliadin antibodies are seen in celiac disease, which is marked by malabsorption, not esophageal dysmotility. Antimicrosomal (anti–thyroid peroxidase) antibodies are seen in autoimmune thyroid diseases such as Hashimoto thyroiditis and Graves disease. Antimitochondrial antibody appears most frequently in primary biliary cirrhosis. ANCA can be a marker for various forms of vasculitis.

BP7 141-143   BP6 112-114   PBD7 229, 237-239, 800
PBD6 226-229

61 **(B)** The patient has features of Wernicke disease and beriberi, both resulting from thiamine deficiency, which can accompany chronic alcoholism. Vitamin A deficiency leads to night blindness, keratomalacia, and respiratory tract difficulties due to epithelial disorders. Pure vitamin B_2 deficiency is rare and is marked by findings such as neuropathy and cheilosis. Niacin deficiency leads to pellagra with dementia, diarrhea, and photodermatitis. Vitamin B_{12} deficiency leads to subacute combined degeneration of the spinal cord; the MCV in this case is not in the range to cause macrocytosis. Vitamin C deficiency leads to scurvy with anemia, loose teeth, hematomas, and poor wound healing. Vitamin D deficiency in an adult leads to osteomalacia with risk of fractures. Vitamin E deficiency is rare and produces spinal cord changes similar to those of vitamin B_{12} deficiency.

BP7 839-840   BP6 254, 738   PBD7 422-423, 450, 457,
1399   PBD6 412, 447, 1341

62 **(B)** The patient has *Pneumocystis carinii* pneumonia. The spectrum of opportunistic infections, as well as wasting syndrome and lymphopenia, suggests AIDS complicating HIV infection. This spectrum of findings is not typical of autoimmune diseases, which usually are accompanied by opportunistic infections in patients receiving immunosuppressive therapy (e.g., patients with systemic lupus erythematosus who have a positive ANA test result). An SLE-like disease is seen in C2 deficiency. B-cell function tends to be preserved in HIV infection, so marked hypogammaglobulinemia is unlikely to be present. The neutrophil oxidative burst assay is used to test for chronic granulomatous disease, an immunodeficiency condition in which bacterial infections are more likely to appear in children. RPR is a screening test for syphilis, which is a sexually transmitted disease that is not accompanied by immunodeficiency.

BP7 497-498   BP6 430-431   PBD7 240, 345, 361, 715,
747, 756   PBD6 381-382

63 **(A)** Metabolic acidosis, tinnitus, platelet function abnormalities, and gastritis with ulceration are typical effects of excessive aspirin ingestion. Acetaminophen in large quantities may produce hepatotoxicity. Adalimumab, a monoclonal antibody directed against tumor necrosis factor, and methotrexate are drugs used to treat rheumatoid arthritis and do not have antiplatelet effects. Oxycodone is an opiate, and propoxyphene is a nonnarcotic analgesic; these drugs do not have significant effects on the gastrointestinal tract or on platelets.

BP7 278   BP6 231-232   PBD7 428   PBD6 416

64 **(B)** Choriocarcinoma is the most aggressive, and the least common, form of molar pregnancy. It can metastasize widely, particularly to the lungs and vagina and also to the brain, liver, and kidney. The neoplasm is composed of a malignant-appearing syncytiotrophoblast and forms a soft, hemorrhagic mass that can rupture and bleed. In addition, the amount of human chorionic gonadotropin (hCG) produced by a choriocarcinoma is marked; hCG shares the same α-subunit as other glycoprotein hormones, such as thyroid-stimulating hormone (TSH), and thus may enhance the effect of TSH. Fortunately, many choriocarcinomas respond to chemotherapy. Endometrial adenocarcinoma is most often seen in postmenopausal women. Clear cell carcinomas of the vagina most often appear in young women whose mothers were given diethylstilbestrol (DES) during pregnancy. A leiomyosarcoma is an uncommon lesion in adult women and usually produces a large uterine mass. Likewise, a malignant mixed müllerian tumor is a rare neoplasm seen in adult women. Sarcoma botryoides is a neoplasm found in girls younger than 5 years of age.

BP7 703-704   BP6 622   PBD7 1110-1114
PBD6 1087-1089

65 **(B)** The fetus has features of the limb-body wall complex (also known as amniotic band syndrome), which is thought to result from an abnormal event occurring early in embryogenesis that is unrelated to a chromosome or gene defect. Although autosomal dominant genetic defects often involve structural genes, the spectrum of findings in this case does not suggest such a mutation. Germ-line mosaicism explains the appearance of an autosomal dominant trait, such as neurofibromatosis type 1, if multiple children are affected by a disorder and the parents and relatives are not affected. Meiotic nondisjunction underlies many trisomies, principally trisomy 21. Prolonged rupture of fetal membranes leads to the oligohydramnios sequence (Potter sequence) with deformations, but not to absent parts of limbs or abdominal wall defects. Spontaneous new mutations explain some structural gene abnormalities, such as achondroplasia, but not the spectrum of findings reported in this case. Teratogens have varied effects; thalidomide is best known for producing limb defects, but the findings in this case are most characteristic of limb-body wall complex. Trinucleotide repeats are increased in disorders such as fragile X syndrome, Huntington disease, and myotonic dystrophy; these diseases typically manifest after the first year of life.

BP7 238   BP6 200   PBD7 470-471   PBD6 465

66 **(F)** The findings are consistent with tertiary syphilis; specifically, syphilitic aortitis from endarteritis obliterans of the vasa vasorum, which is most marked in the proximal aorta. In addition, the patient has findings of neurosyphilis, with tabes dorsalis and general paresis. A positive VDRL test result on CSF aids in diagnosis. None of the remaining organisms listed produces aortic disease. Neuroborreliosis from Lyme disease can produce aseptic meningitis, encephalopathy, and polyneuropathy. Coxsackievirus B can produce meningoencephalitis and myocarditis. HIV can produce encephalitis characterized by dementia and motor and sensory deficits. Hansen disease, caused by *Mycobacterium leprae* infection, mainly affects the peripheral nerves. Tuberculosis can produce meningoencephalitis or a mass known as a tuberculoma; obstructive hydrocephalus may occur in chronic meningitis.

West Nile virus is most likely to produce severe meningoencephalitis in elderly persons.

BP7 343, 670-673, 826-827   BP6 299-300, 589-592, 728
PBD7 388-391, 532, 1292, 1372   PBD6 362-364, 526, 1317

67 **(D)** This girl has McCune-Albright syndrome, an acquired somatic gene defect that occurs during embryogenesis and leads to excessive cyclic AMP production that fuels endocrine gland activity. As a result, growth hormone–secreting pituitary adenomas, hyperthyroidism, adrenal hyperplasia, and sexual precocity can occur. There are café-au-lait spots. The bone lesions are polyostotic fibrous dysplasia. Most cases of fibrous dysplasia are solitary (monostotic) and unaccompanied by syndromic features. Albers-Schönberg disease is rare and leads to a form of osteopetrosis known as marble bone disease (the manatee normally has similar bone). Congenital adrenal hyperplasia, most often due to an inherited defect in 21-hydroxylase, can lead to sexual precocity but not to bone lesions. Ollier disease is enchondromatosis (cartilaginous tumors in metaphyseal regions of long bones); if soft tissue hemangiomas are also present, it is called Maffucci syndrome. Paget disease of bone (osteitis deformans) affects older persons with monostotic or polyostotic lesions, which initially may be lytic but then become sclerotic; there are no endocrinopathies.

BP7 771   BP6 680   PBD7 1300-1301   PBD6 1243

68 **(F)** The sudden and unexpected nature of the death requires investigation by the medical examiner (coroner), who will notify the local law enforcement agency upon discovery of the findings in this case. The pattern of injuries is consistent with vigorous shaking of the infant. Because the infant's head is larger in proportion to its body than that of an adult, it cannot counter the shaking with neck musculature. Grasping the arms of the infant strongly and pressing or hitting the head against a hard surface increases the risk of internal injuries, including fractures. Axonal retraction balls are a feature of marked stretching and tearing with acceleration-deceleration forces. α-Thalassemia major leads to severe anemia with hydrops noted at birth; α-thalassemia minor leads to mild anemia. Congenital syphilis produces osteochondritis with skeletal deformities, not fractures, and without a bleeding tendency. Edwards syndrome is trisomy 18, which is characterized by multiple external anomalies such as overlapping fingers, cleft lip, and omphalocele. Hemophilia A could account for hemorrhages in a child or adult but not fractures. Osteogenesis imperfecta can account for fractures but not hemorrhages. In sudden infant death syndrome, there would be no signs of trauma. Thanatophoric dysplasia is a lethal form of short-limbed dwarfism.

BP7 819-820, 824   BP6 722-723, 726   PBD7 1358-1359
PBD6 1303-1305

69 **(A)** The findings listed are all seen with increased frequency in elderly persons and are incidental findings with no significant pathologic effect. Chronic alcoholism can produce chronic liver disease progressing to cirrhosis, dilated cardiomyopathy, and Wernicke disease. Cystic fibrosis would be accompanied by bronchiectasis and pancreatic atrophy. Diabetes mellitus causes significant disease through atherosclerosis and arteriolosclerosis, whereas calcific medial sclerosis usually does not cause significant disease. HIV infection leads